W9-AAU-674

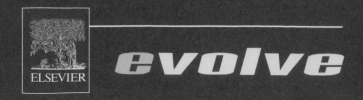

SAUNDERS
Fundamentals
of Medical
Assisting

Fundamentals *of* Medical Assisting

Sue A. Hunt, MA, RN, CMA
Professor and Coordinator
Medical Assisting Program
Middlesex Community College
Lowell, Massachusetts

Jon H. Zonderman, BA, MSJ
Contributing Writer
Orange, Connecticut

SAUNDERS
An Imprint of Elsevier

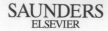

11830 Westline Industrial Drive
St. Louis, Missouri 63146

Notice

ISBN-13: 978-1-4160-4223-5
ISBN-10: 1-4160-4223-7

Executive Editor: Susan Cole
Developmental Editor: Celeste Clingan
Publishing Services Manager: Linda McKinley
Senior Project Manager: Kelly E.M. Steinmann

Printed in Canada

Last digit is the print number: 9 8 7 6 5 4 3 2

This book is dedicated to medical assisting students. Those I have taught over the years were teachers themselves in addition to learners, for each other, for me, and through this book, for students yet to come.

Sue A. Hunt

Contributors

Eugenia M. Fulcher, RN, BSN, MEd, EdD, CMA
Program Director
Swainsboro Technical College
Waynesboro, Georgia
  Unit 6: Special Populations

Ava Gilman, MT (ASCP), BS
Medical Technologist
Veterans Administration Hospital
Nashville, TN
  Unit 5: The Laboratory and Laboratory Tests

Deborah Montone
Dean of Medical Sciences
The Ho Ho Kus School
Ramsey, NJ
  Unit 7: Patient Teaching and Follow-Up
  Unit 8: Financial Management and Health
  Insurance

Lisa Nagle, MS Ed, CMA
Augusta Technical Institute
Augusta, Georgia
  Procedures for Clinical Chapters

Reviewers

Acknowledgments

So many people have helped to transform this project from an idea to a reality, and I cannot thank them all enough. First and foremost I want to express my heartfelt gratitude to Jon Zonderman for assistance with writing and organizing this book and its supplementary materials. The photographs were taken by Jack Foley of Jack Foley Photography, Boston, MA. Jane Snellman, Nick Kaufman Productions, spent hours finding models, supplies and equipment. I am also grateful to Harvard Vanguard for allowing us to its Boston facility for photographs.

I am grateful to the contributors and reviewers who helped with both the textbook and the ancillary materials. Their names are listed in the preceding pages, and the book truly would not have been possible without their assistance.

The project has continued for so long that there have been several editors: Scott Weaver and Rae Robertson, developmental editors at W.B. Saunders, as well as Marie Pelcin. I owe them special thanks for their encouragement and assistance. I am also grateful to the production staff who have kept the project on track.

Finally I must thank Adrianne Williams, senior editor, who has guided this project from inception to completion and provided a tremendous amount of creative energy throughout the entire process. Her vision of educational materials for the twenty-first century inspires all who work with her.

The publisher wishes to acknowledge the permission of the AAMA to use the language of the AAMA Entry-Level Competencies. The publisher also thanks the AMT for permission to use the Registered Medical Assistant Certification Examination Content Summary.

Contents

Chapter 26

Microbiology, Immunology, Chemistry 638

UNIT 6

SPECIAL POPULATIONS 669

Chapter 27

Pediatrics 670

Chapter 28

Geriatrics 698

Chapter 29

Obstetrics 714

Chapter 30

Patients with Chronic and Terminal Diseases 742

Chapter 31

Emergency Care 762

UNIT 7

PATIENT TEACHING AND FOLLOW-UP 797

Chapter 32

Teaching Patients in the Medical Office 798

Chapter 33

Maintaining Health: Nutrition, Exercise, and Self-Examination 824

Chapter 34

Oral Follow-up 846

List of Procedures

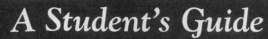

A Student's Guide

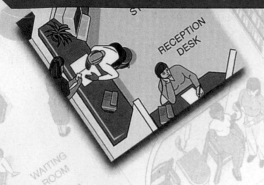

The following pages walk you through some of the main features of this text and its integrated media components. Each feature has been carefully designed to help you achieve one of the three important learning goals of any Medical Assisting education: *content mastery, content application* and *visualization*. We hope you enjoy your study of the exciting and dynamic field of Medical Assisting.

Content Mastery

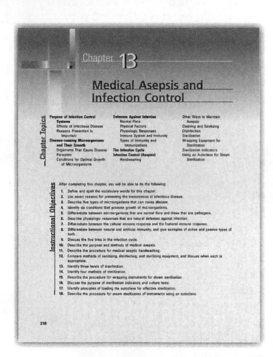

Chapter Openers

Content Outlines
are provided to help you prepare for studying each chapter, and should be reviewed prior to reading the chapter.

Instructional Objectives
help you focus on the theoretical concepts you will be expected to learn throughout the chapter. You can use these when reviewing for quizzes.

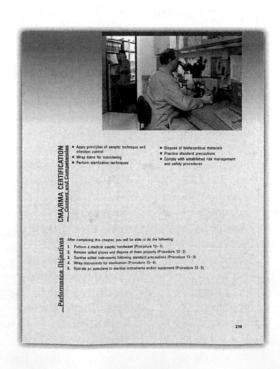

Curriculum Components and Competencies
are identified for each chapter, listing the key information and skills you must learn to satisfy the AAMA and RMA certification exam qualifications.

Performance Objectives
highlight the skills within each chapter that you will be expected to master. You can use these as a checklist to ensure that you've learned all the appropriate Medical Assisting skills.

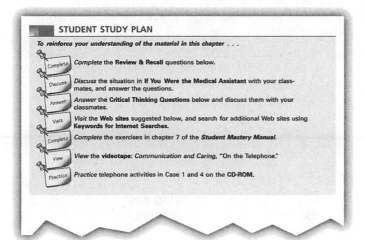

VOCABULARY

calculi (p. 424)
catheter (p. 422)
catheterization (p. 424)
clonus (p. 431)
cryosurgery (p. 426)
cystoscopy (p. 428)
endocervical
    curettage (p. 428)

expiratory reserve volume
    (p. 417)
forced expiratory volume at
    1 second (p. 417)
forced vital capacity
    (p. 417)
inspiratory reserve volume
    (p. 417)

intracervical insemination
    (p. 429)
intrauterine insemination (p. 429)
malignant (p. 415)
motility (p. 426)
precancerous (p. 415)
prostate-specific antigen (p. 429)
residual volume (p. 417)

spirometry (p. 414)
sputum (p. 417)
subclinical (p. 425)
tidal volume (p. 417)
vital capacity (p. 417)

ABBREVIATIONS

AFB (p. 420)
BPH (p. 428)

CSF (p. 431)
FEV₁ (p. 417)

FVC (p. 417)
LEEP (p. 428)

LP (p. 431)
PSA (p. 428)

STD (p. 424)

Vocabulary Terms and Abbreviations Listing

Each chapter begins with a listing of the relevant medical terms and abbreviations that will be introduced in that chapter, along with a page number of where that word first appears and is defined in the chapter. Turn to the glossary for a definition of all terms.

Student Study Plan

STUDENT STUDY PLAN

To reinforce your understanding of the material in this chapter . . .

Complete — Complete the **Review & Recall** questions below.

Discuss — Discuss the situation in **If You Were the Medical Assistant** with your classmates, and answer the questions.

Answer — Answer the **Critical Thinking Questions** below and discuss them with your classmates.

Visit — Visit the **Web** sites suggested below, and search for additional Web sites using **Keywords for Internet Searches.**

Complete — Complete the exercises in chapter 7 of the **Student Mastery Manual.**

View — View the **videotape:** Communication and Caring, "On the Telephone."

Practice — Practice telephone activities in Case 1 and 4 on the **CD-ROM.**

At the end of each chapter is a listing of activities you can do to help you increase your understanding and mastery of the information in that chapter. This plan integrates all the various learning tools available to you in the textbook, workbook, the CD-ROM that accompanies this textbook, plus the companion SIMON web site and *Critical Thinking Skills for Medical Assistants Video Series*. By following the study plan for each chapter, you will ensure your learning success.

Review and Recall

This listing of questions and exercises tests your knowledge of the key content you need to master in each chapter. This challenge session ties into the *Instructional Objectives* listing found at the beginning of each chapter.

 REVIEW & RECALL

1. List three reasons why the telephone is of vital importance to the functioning of the medical office.

2. How are the following used in the medical office: multi-line telephone, facsimile (fax) machine, pager, voice mail?

3. List four types of telephone calls that the medical assistant can handle.

4. List five types of telephone calls where the medical assistant may need to take a message.

5. What information must be included in a telephone message?

6. Identify three types of problem calls.

7. Describe how to place an outgoing call.

SIMON Chapter Quizzes

You can access individual chapter quizzes for each chapter of this textbook on the companion SIMON site by going to www.wbsaunders.com/SIMON/Hunt/ and clicking on **Student Station**. Each quiz contains multiple choice questions, formatted in the style of the AAMA and RMA certification exams, with answers and rationales.

Content Application

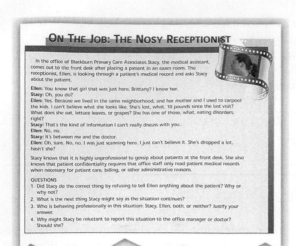

On the Job

Throughout the book, scenarios are introduced to help you apply what you're learning to realistic situations to think about how you would respond. Some are variations of scenarios that appear on the *Critical Thinking Skills for Medical Assistants Video Series*, and these are identified by a video icon. All include prompting questions designed to help you develop good critical thinking and decision making skills.

Focus On

These boxes contain information that will help you focus on and apply one of five important themes that transcend the chapter information. These themes are: professionalism, communication, safety, legal, and patient education.

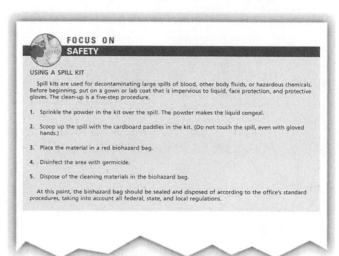

Enrichment Topics

These mini-articles apply chapter content to current medical issues, disease conditions, and diagnostic and treatment developments that are relevant to the information being discussed. These articles add a real-world perspective to what you are learning.

If You Were the Medical Assistant

These scenarios, with thought-provoking questions at the end of each chapter, challenge you to decide how you would handle a variety of realistic situations.

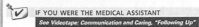

Critical Thinking Questions

These questions at the end of chapters provide additional opportunity for you to apply the information you learn in each chapter to realistic situations you may encounter on the job.

The Virtual Office CD-ROM

The free CD-ROM that comes with your textbook includes three programs designed to have you apply all the content and skills you've learned: *The Virtual Medical Office Challenge* provides four realistic scenarios with you making the decisions and getting feedback on all actions taken, plus a skill-building section that lets you practice both administrative and clinical skills; *The Body Spectrum*, an interactive Anatomy and Physiology workbook that will help you strengthen your knowledge of the body; and *Lytec Medical 2001*, a real medical office computer program that lets you practice all administrative workbook skills electronically.

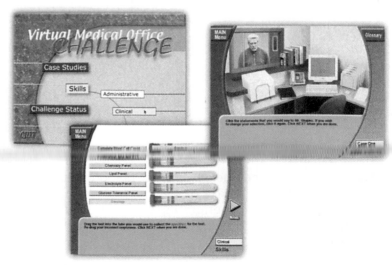

Visualization

An Integrated Organizational Approach

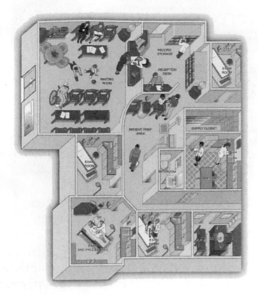

The flow of units in this book has been organized to follow the flow of a patient through the doctor's office. An architectural rendering of a realistic medical office has been created as a type of map to help you visualize where you are within the medical office for each unit.

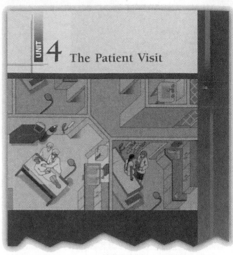

A Virtual Practice

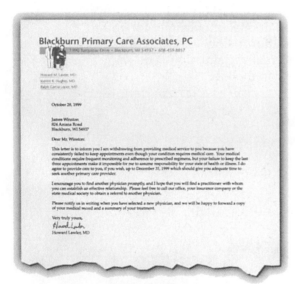

As a way to integrate the material throughout the book, CD-ROM, and videos, a virtual group medical practice has been created, within which case studies and other references have been developed. The group, called Blackburn Primary Care Associates, is a family practice with three doctors and several medical assistants who are based on actual medical assistants who appear in many of the photographs in this text, on the CD-ROM, and on the videos.

Procedure Aseptic Checklists

Procedures requiring one or more aseptic Standard Precaution show a checklist of the precautions you will need to take when performing that skill. By following these lists, you will be protecting both yourself and your patients.

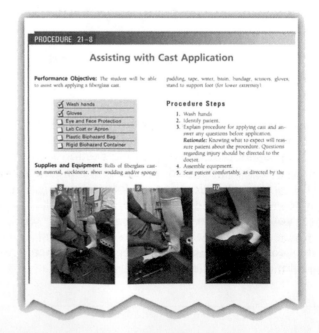

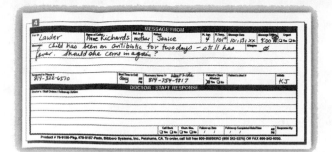

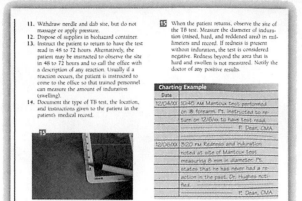

Charting Examples

Wherever necessary, examples have been provided to show how to document and chart patient interactions such as telephone calls. Results and observations from performing certain skills are shown in charting examples that appear at the end of every skill where recording patient information in the medical record is important.

Many important concepts and procedures throughout the book are condensed into at-a-glance tables and figures to help improve your understanding and mastery of information. Many illustrations and photos help you better visualize key tasks, equipment, skill steps, and complex concepts.

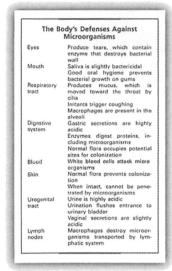

Content At-A-Glance

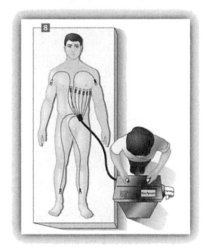

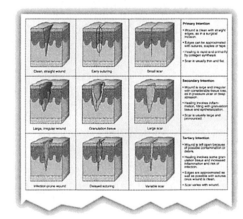

Explore the Web/Companion Web Site

Your book comes with a free unique passcode that can be used to access the companion SIMON web site. This site contains instant access to all internet web sites listed throughout your textbook, plus internet research exercises, study tips, resume-building, job seeking recommendations, and much more! Access this web site at www.wbsaunders.com/SIMON/Hunt/ and get ready to access a virtual world of resources. Lists of key words for internet searches, and internet web sites are provided at the end of each chapter.

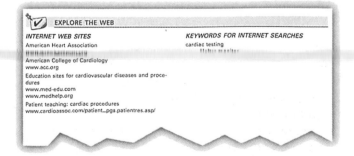

Chapter 1

Welcome!

Welcome to the *Fundamentals of Medical Assisting.*

Medical assisting is a field full of opportunity for people willing and able to work with other professionals in the care and treatment of patients. It is a dynamic field, always changing and always growing.

This book is designed to introduce students to the full range of activities and tasks that medical assistants may undertake. As we begin the 21st century, medical assistants are being asked to undertake increasingly complex tasks, both administrative and clinical. This is happening because of a host of changes in the practice of medicine.

A number of forces have lead to these changes, and it is impossible to study medical assisting without an understanding of the history of health care and the current changes in health care practice. This book places the current scope of the medical assistant's job in the context of these changes and trends.

BECOMING A MEDICAL ASSISTANT

You may have chosen to study medical assisting for many reasons. You may want to work in a field where you feel you are helping people. Medical assistants work in office-based medical practices, in contrast to other medical personnel who work in hospitals that treat critically ill or injured people or in long-term care facilities. In an office-based medical practice, you will have an opportunity to develop long-lasting relationships with patients, working with them in times of good health and routine medical care, as well as in times of illness.

Good medical assistants certainly help patients who come to the medical practice seeking care. You may be most interested in the clinical aspects of medical assisting—helping doctors perform diagnostic procedures, physical examinations, and even surgical procedures. You may be most interested in the opportunities for helping with patient education.

Or you may be most interested in the business aspects of office-based medical practice: administration and management.

Whichever aspect of medical assisting you are most interested in, good medical assistants need to be generalists. They need to learn about and appreciate all aspects of the office's clinical, administrative, and patient-education activities.

Regardless of why you have entered this field, you still may be surprised by all the different things medical assistants do. Especially if you work in a smaller office, you will have to assist the doctor or doctors with checking patients in, taking medical histories, performing examinations and treatments, filing insurance claims, purchasing equipment and medications, and a host of other activities (Figure 1–1).

HOW THIS BOOK IS ORGANIZED

Traditionally, medical assisting has been seen as a two-part field of study. In a medical office, both administrative tasks and clinical tasks need to be done. Therefore, medical assistant students must acquire both administrative skills and competencies, and clinical skills and competencies.

Administrative tasks include assisting new patients to fill out their information forms; preparing doctors' schedules, patient files, and the day's schedule; assisting patients with payments for services and filling out insurance forms; filing insurance claims for the office; transcribing doctors' dictation about patient visits; purchasing equipment, medications, and supplies; and processing incoming mail and telephone calls.

Clinical tasks include taking patient vital signs; performing simple diagnostic tests; assisting young, old, or frail patients; performing laboratory tests in the office's lab; sterilizing equipment and examination rooms be-

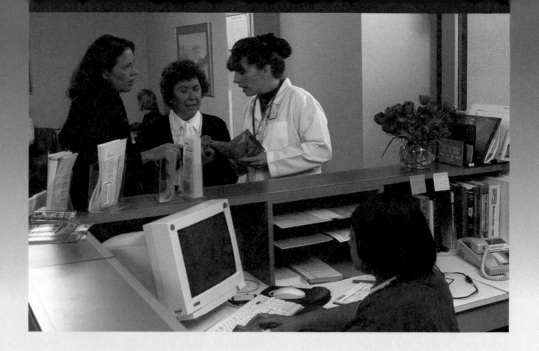

tween patients; checking equipment at the beginning and end of the day; and assisting the doctor with examinations, diagnostic procedures, treatments, and surgeries.

Many students have more interest in one of these two aspects of medical assisting than the other. But to become certified, students must learn both sets of skills and competencies. This is becoming increasingly im-

portant as patient care and business management become more tightly linked because of managed care, which forces independent doctors' offices to more closely coordinate care with other doctors, providers of other medical services such as rehabilitation and home health care, and insurance providers.

Traditionally, comprehensive medical assisting textbooks have been organized along this two-part scheme.

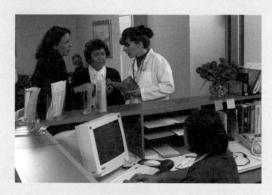

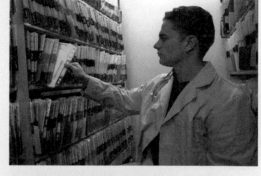

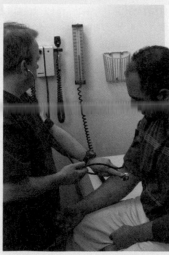

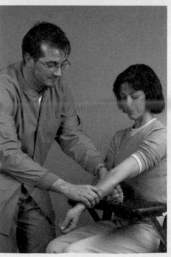

➢ Figure 1–1 Working in a medical office involves a variety of clinical and administrative tasks.

Most begin with administrative skills and competencies, followed by the clinical side of things.

In this book, the flow of the units has been organized in such as way as to follow the flow of a patient through the doctor's office. After a few chapters that set the stage, discussing the basic activities of a medical office and the necessity for medical assistants to act and communicate in a professional manner, the book moves into daily tasks, from opening the office door, switching on the equipment and checking for voice messages, faxes, and e-mails, to making the final evening follow-up telephone calls and closing the office. In the ever-more tightly integrated field of office-based medical practice, it is important for the medical assistant to think in terms of the flow of tasks from one to the next rather than separating tasks into administrative or clinical.

In between opening and closing the office is a day full of encounters with patients and insurance providers, as well as others who are integral to maintenance of the doctor's office as a business that provides professional services—from the pharmaceutical company representative to the technician who fixes the photocopier, possibly to a medical school faculty member with whom the doctor is working on a lecture he or she will present to medical students about office-based medicine.

Each patient encounter has both administrative and clinical tasks associated with it. The encounter begins with checking the patient off against the schedule and assisting the patient to fill out any necessary paperwork, moves to taking vital signs (height, weight, temperature, blood pressure), to the examination or treatment, any necessary laboratory work, and then to patient education, follow-up referrals, and dealing with payment and insurance matters.

Throughout the book, a clear message will come through that medical assistants must focus on four things:

1. Professionalism
2. Communication
3. Safety
4. Patient and family instruction

Professionalism means showing patients and others that the medical assistant has a firm command not only of technical knowledge and skills, but also of legal and ethical requirements for both those who provide medical care and those who run a business.

Communication means knowing how to speak clearly and listen closely, to pass information and knowledge to others, and to gather information from them. A medical assistant will often spend more time with a patient than a doctor will, and many patients feel less anxious talking to a medical assistant than to a doctor. Being a good listener is part of being a good communicator.

Safety—for patients, staff, and visitors—is key in a medical practice. Many safety precautions—especially those that involve staff safety when dealing with patients who may have infectious diseases—are mandated by federal and/or state laws and regulations. But many other safety precautions involve more common sense and good housekeeping practices. Regardless, they are all important.

Finally, medical assistants are increasingly being asked to instruct patients and their families about acute conditions such as wound healing and chronic illnesses such as asthma. Education is more than simple communication; it is establishing a relationship with the patient and his or her family such that the medical assistant is trusted as both an expert and a friendly face and voice with whom to talk and ask questions.

YOUR ROLE AS A MEDICAL ASSISTANT

As a medical assistant, you really are an *assistant*. Your function is to assist—or help—the doctor in a process where the doctor leads and you follow. The tricky part is balance.

You have to know what the doctor is going to do, or need, next. This means that you have to know a little bit about what the doctor is thinking. This is the medical part, and this is why you have to learn about anatomy and physiology, about diseases, and about laboratory and diagnostic tests.

You also have to learn how the doctor and other members of the health care team talk about what they are doing, and how they conceptualize what they are doing (Figure 1–2). The doctor in our health care system operates based on principles of science, tempered with real concern for others and an ability to make a one-to-one human connection with them.

As a patient describes problems, the doctor tries to fit them into known and tested categories, using a rigorous process that involves gathering information in a systematic way and testing that information against various known disease categories to see what can be excluded and what must continue to be included as possible causes of the patient's problem.

Most medical problems get better over time. One important task for doctors is to look at hundreds of people and try to zero in on those sets of symptoms that meet two criteria: those that indicate that a severe problem exists or could develop if not treated, and those for which an effective treatment exists.

In addition to assisting the doctor to perform this information gathering, the medical assistant also assists the patient to understand what will go on, is going on, or has been going on during the encounter with the doctor, and what will happen in future visits, procedures, or visits to other medical professionals to whom the patient is being referred.

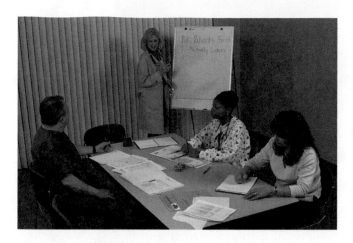

> **Figure 1–2** The medical assistant is an important member of the health care team.

So, you see, the role of "assisting" means more than simply helping to undertake individual activities. The medical assistant helps the doctor(s) in a medical practice to manage all of the pieces that go into maintaining relationships with hundreds of other human beings—in this case the patients who utilize the practice's services.

CHAPTER ORGANIZATION

Chapters are organized so the student can follow easily and integrate chapter materials as he or she moves through it. Each chapter opens with a topic outline, learning objectives, and a list of vocabulary words and abbreviations. The vocabulary word is not defined at the chapter opening; rather, the first time the word is encountered it is printed in boldface and defined in the proper context.

Each chapter opening also identifies a list of curriculum components and competencies designed to help the student prepare for the certification examination for Certified Medical Assistant (CMA) or Registered Medical Assistant (RMA). Medical assisting programs are accredited either by the Commission on Accreditation of Allied Health Education Programs (CAAHEP), the Accrediting Bureau of Health Education Schools/Programs (ABHES), or other agencies. A graduate of an accredited medical assisting program is eligible to take one of the certification examinations.

At the end of each chapter is a student study plan, which includes a set of **Review & Recall** questions about the chapter, a case study called **If You Were the Medical Assistant,** and **Critical Thinking Questions** based on information provided in the chapter. It also includes a section called **Explore the Web** where we provide useful Web sites containing more information about the topics covered in the chapter, as well as suggest some keywords to use to search for other Internet sites.

THE PRACTICE

As a way to integrate the material through the book even more tightly, a group medical practice has been created, within which case studies and other references have been developed.

The group, called Blackburn Primary Care Associates, is a family practice with three doctors and several medical assistants. These medical assistants are based on the actual medical assistants who appear in many of the photographs in this textbook and who helped prepare the videos designed to be used with it. Some of the medical assistants are young and have only a little experience; others have worked in the field for several years.

Students will learn about real-life situations by discussing case studies in each chapter, by completing activities on the companion CD-ROM, and by discussing scenes from the videos that are available for classroom use. Many of the book's case studies have been excerpted from the CD-ROM or the videos.

EXPAND YOUR KNOWLEDGE

Becoming an effective medical assistant means far more than learning and memorizing facts. Employers in the health care field need employees who can think on their feet. A good medical assistant needs to be able to analyze a situation and respond appropriately, even if he or she has never come across that exact situation before. To do this, a medical assisting student must learn how to take a piece of knowledge and use it in many different situations.

An effective medical assistant must also be a lifelong learner, a person who is constantly seeking to expand his or her knowledge, skills, and experiences. To do this, he or she must:

1. Master a knowledge base related to the profession of medical assisting.
2. Learn a set of skills and procedures that are critical to performing the tasks necessary to maintain a smoothly running medical practice.
3. Use disciplined, critical thinking as a tool for reflecting before and after implementing any particular action.
4. Keep up to date with changes in the field, and know how to research information in order to do so.

Knowledge Base

The knowledge base for medical assistants includes scientific topics such as anatomy, physiology, medicine, and pharmacology; psychology, human relations, and communications; medical law and ethics; medical ter-minology; and background knowledge related to the administrative and clinical procedures performed in the medical offices. This textbook assumes that students have a background in anatomy and physiology, medical terminology, and psychology.

Administrative and Clinical Procedures

A graduate of a medical assisting program needs more than just knowledge. He or she must be prepared to work as an employee, performing any of the tasks of a medical assistant.

Competency in a particular task requires an understanding of the steps needed to complete the task, the correct order in which to complete the steps, and the ability to perform each step correctly. Students will learn the steps involved in each task by studying the procedures in this textbook. The Student Mastery Manual also contains checklists to validate that students have practiced and/or mastered the procedures. The CD-ROM also contains many opportunities to practice skills.

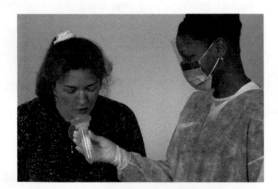
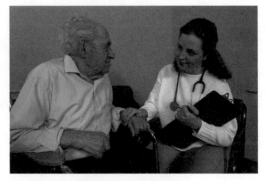
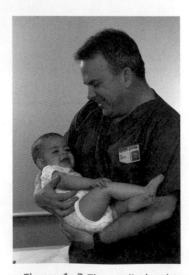
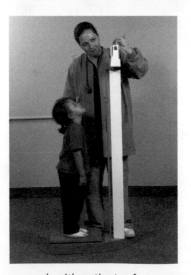

➤ **Figure 1–3** The medical assistant may work with patients of any age.

Critical Thinking

The term *critical thinking* is often used to refer to the mental activity involved in putting knowledge into practice. Working as a professional medical assistant requires making decisions about what to do and when to do it, predicting the consequences of your actions, evaluating how effective your activities have been, and planning for the future.

Critical thinking might be thought of as "the art of thinking about your thinking while you are thinking." The critical thinker constantly asks why he or she thinks about things in a particular way. By constantly questioning one's own thinking, a person is able to be more receptive to new ideas, to other points of view, and to alternative techniques for performing tasks.

A critical thinker does not fall into the trap of saying "we do this because this is the way we have always done it." A critical thinker is open to new ideas and insights. And a critical thinker is sensitive to differences in the way people of different cultures, generations, gender, or sexual orientation view the world (Figure 1–3). Critical thinking in a medical assistant can make that person a better listener and a better patient teacher.

Various intellectual skills can be used to reflect on and process information, based on values that include clarity, accuracy, precision, sound evidence, consistency, and fairness. Table 1–1 lists some of these skills, with examples.

The student who puts significant effort into improving critical thinking skills will receive lifelong personal and professional rewards.

Using the Internet to Find Information

The Internet is an incredible resource. Using the Internet, a student can tap into literally thousands of subjects, ranging from the federal government's safety and health regulations regarding medical offices and laboratories to Web sites about particular diseases he or she may encounter while working in an externship or later on the job.

This book gives Web site addresses at the end of each chapter as well as keywords to use for conducting Internet searches. But simply "surfing" the Web creatively—like wandering the stacks in a gigantic library—can lead to informative, interesting, and fun Web sites.

Conducting Internet research is easy. If you know the Web site address, you can type it in, and the browser software will go to that site's server and bring the site up on your computer. Every Web site address begins with **http://** (*http* means hypertext transmission protocol and gives the computer instructions to find the proper site.) In reality, typing in **www.** and then the name of the Web site, will get you there.

Table 1–1	Critical Thinking Skills

Critical thinking uses clarity, accuracy, precision, relevance, depth, and logic to reflect on the past (including one's thinking about the past) and plan for the future. Below is a partial list of critical thinking skills with brief discussions and/or examples of their use.

Making Comparisons
Identifying similarities and differences helps us categorize information. This can increase efficiency and understanding. If we discover a new animal, part of learning to understand it will involve questions about how it is like or not like other animals we already know a lot about.

Expressing Problems Clearly
Suppose a medical assistant works for a doctor who often seems to be irritated with the medical assistant, who then feels like things are not going well. By clarifying what the problem is, solutions can be proposed.

Determining Relevance
Deciding whether something has a bearing on the matter at hand is important when assessing an emergency, for example. Which is more relevant, a large red stain on the shirt of an accident victim or a missing shoe?

Demonstrating Reasoned Judgment
Using logic and reason to back up ideas is the opposite of defending ideas based on feelings and emotions. The medical assistant may not want to make an infant cry by giving it an immunization, but he or she knows that scientific studies show that the prevention of communicable diseases will benefit both the baby and society.

Identifying Alternatives
Often we want to try out the first solution we think of rather than thinking the problem through. Continuing to think of solutions may lead to a better idea, often one containing elements of several ideas.

Predicting Consequences
Thinking about the possible results of an action is faster and more efficient than actually trying out every possibility.

Identifying Assumptions
If a child asks for a glass of milk, I assume that the child is thirsty. I assume that a cup of milk would be satisfactory. I assume that the child knows how to drink from a glass. If the child wants to feed a stray kitten, my assumptions may prevent me from helping the child effectively.

Recognizing Bias or Prejudice
The tendency to think or feel a certain way can influence how we interpret situations or how we act. What might happen if a medical assistant assumes that elderly people are always hard of hearing?

Distinguishing False from Accurate Information
All kinds of information are available, but it is often difficult to know how reliable any piece of information is. In addition we do not always know whether our own memories are accurate. It is important to check information using reliable sources, especially when accuracy is important, as for example when preparing a patient for a diagnostic test.

If you don't know the site's address, you can search using keywords. Any Web browser has within it a search engine, a software program that searches all of the registered Web sites for the keyword and brings up a list of the most logical sites.

The more specific you can be with your keywords, the better. For instance, the keyword *angel* brings up references to religious Web pages, Web pages with inspirational stories about people who do good deeds, and Web pages for dating services. The keyword *investor* brings up thousands of references about stocks, bonds, real estate, and other kinds of financial investments. Combining the keywords into *angel investor* brings up a listing of fewer than a dozen sites that specialize in individuals who make private investments in new companies, who are known in the investment world as angels.

In a similar way, a search on the word *medical* would bring up thousands of potential sites, known as "hits." A search of the word *assistant* would also bring up thousands of hits. By combining these two keywords into *medical assistant*, you can narrow your search to only those sites that focus on medical assisting.

Once you find a site that is useful to you, you can get back to that site without having to type in the Web site address each time. To do this, simply add the site to your list of "bookmarks" or "favorites." On future visits to the Internet, you can simply click on bookmarks or favorites (depending on the program you use), bring up the list of sites you are holding in your easy-to-reach group, and click on the site you wish to visit.

COMPANION RESOURCES TO THE TEXTBOOK

Each chapter in the textbook also has a companion chapter in both the **Student Mastery Manual** and the accompanying pocket guide. Mastery manual exercises should be done after completing each chapter to reinforce the lesson. The pocket guide is a quick reference that can be used at work or externship so you don't have to have the textbook available at all times.

In addition, there are many case-study exercises and skills practice exercises you can perform on the accompanying CD-ROM. The CD-ROM is designed to provide practice for selected skills and also allows students to manage simulated patient situations.

Finally, the set of six videos also serves as a companion to this text. These videos not only reinforce the messages about professionalism, clear communication, safe working, and proper technique in performing vital signs, medical history taking, medication administra-

tion, and blood drawing, but they also help the student to develop critical thinking skills and encourage students to analyze and discuss situations that could take place in a medical office.

In the videos, real medical assistants work with actors playing the patients. Scenes are designed that create problems for the medical assistant to respond to. Following each scene, there is an opportunity for students to discuss how the medical assistant responded to the "patient." Then, the actual medical assistant discusses the interaction.

GOOD STUDY HABITS

We have provided you with source material in a variety of forms, but it is up to you to use those materials well. Good study habits are the key to absorbing the enormous amount of material presented in a medical assisting curriculum.

How, where, and when to study are matters of personal style; for many they are also dictated by other influences, such as family obligations and jobs.

The best studying is done in quiet, familiar surroundings. This might be in the school library, your bedroom, or even at the kitchen table. The best studying is also done at the same time each day, rather than in bits and pieces when possible. For some, this is the afternoon after classes; for others, the evening after children have gone to bed; for still others it is in the early morning before everyone else is awake.

The key is to find your best place and time, and try to stick to it.

How to absorb information is also a matter of personal style.

Some people find that rereading information after it has been presented by a teacher is helpful. Others find that taking brief notes during lectures, then forcing themselves to remember the content and expand their notes into more depth after class is the best reinforcement tool.

Still others find that studying with a friend or in a small study group is the most helpful. Some study groups quiz each other on material. Others assign a particular aspect of each week's material to each member; after the members explore their assigned aspect in depth, the members each present their work to each other and they all learn from one another.

A JOURNEY, NOT A DESTINATION

Because medical assisting is a rapidly changing field, being a medical assistant is not really a destination, but a continuous journey during which an individual constantly learns new information, adds new skills, refines techniques of patient interaction, and adapts to changes in health care.

This book is not the final word. It cannot be. You will enter the world of work with a defined set of skills. But the experiences of those you work with—other medical assistants, doctors and other licensed medical service providers, business and finance managers, and patients—will assist you as you pursue professional growth and lifelong learning.

So welcome to the field of medical assisting and good luck.

UNIT 1 The Medical Office

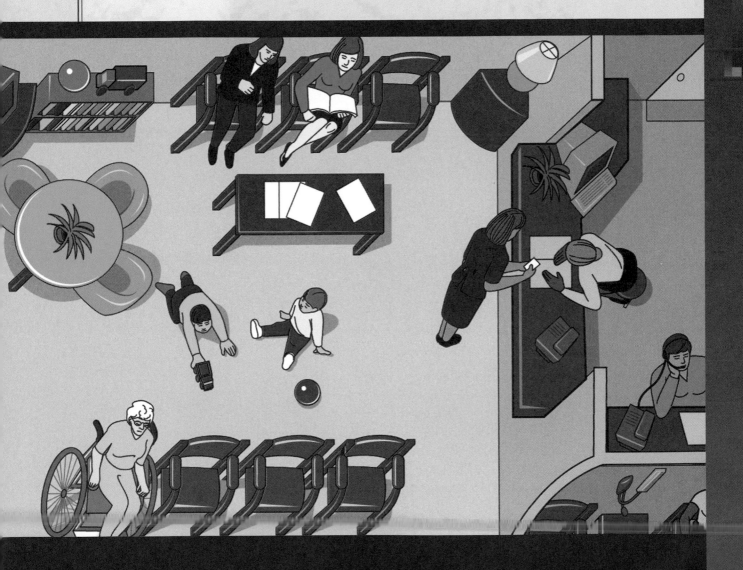

Chapter 2

In the Typical Medical Office

Instructional Objectives

After completing this chapter, you will be able to do the following:

1. Define and spell the vocabulary words for this chapter.
2. Describe the development of the medical assisting profession.
3. List the tasks in the medical office that may be completed by the medical team.
4. Identify administrative activities, clinical activities, interpersonal activities, and office management activities that may be part of the medical assistant's role.
5. List the flow of activities for a patient who makes an office visit.
6. Describe the function and activities performed in each of the four basic areas of the medical office.
7. List several additional areas that are found in many medical offices.
8. Identify the three types of physician office laboratories.
9. List government agencies and/or laws that regulate activities in the medical office.
10. Identify members of the health care team who may work in the medical office or with the medical office staff.
11. Describe the scope of decision-making authority of a medical assistant when working as a health care team member.
12. Describe briefly how Western medicine has evolved to the modern medical model.
13. Explain the general trends influencing the practice of medicine today.
14. Compare and contrast fee-for-service insurance plans with managed care as they affect both patients and doctors.

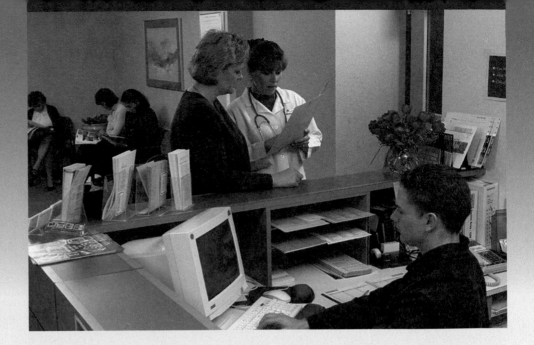

- Understand legal guidelines and requirements for health care
- Understand workplace dynamics
- Understand allied health professions and credentialing
- Perform within legal and ethical boundaries

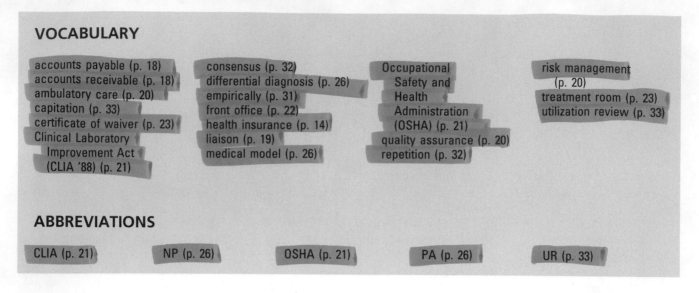

VOCABULARY

accounts payable (p. 18)
accounts receivable (p. 18)
ambulatory care (p. 20)
capitation (p. 33)
certificate of waiver (p. 23)
Clinical Laboratory
    Improvement Act
    (CLIA '88) (p. 21)

consensus (p. 32)
differential diagnosis (p. 26)
empirically (p. 31)
front office (p. 22)
health insurance (p. 14)
liaison (p. 19)
medical model (p. 26)

Occupational
Safety and
Health
Administration
(OSHA) (p. 21)
quality assurance (p. 20)
repetition (p. 32)

risk management
    (p. 20)
treatment room (p. 23)
utilization review (p. 33)

ABBREVIATIONS

CLIA (p. 21)   NP (p. 26)   OSHA (p. 21)   PA (p. 26)   UR (p. 33)

Medical assistants work in a variety of medical office situations: in private doctor's offices, public or community health centers (often called health clinics), and outpatient departments of hospitals. Medical assistants perform various clinical and administrative tasks. Each doctor or group of doctors works in a slightly different way and expects different things of the medical assistants employed in their practice. But although each medical practice is unique, every medical office has a number of things in common.

This chapter will discuss the various physical settings in a medical office, the kinds of activities that take place in the medical office, and who on the medical office team is responsible for these activities.

The chapter is broken into six major parts:

1. Historical development of the role of the medical assistant
2. Role of the medical assistant
3. What takes place in a medical office
4. Parts of the medical office
5. The health care team
6. How medical office care fits into the medical care system.

Before discussing the specifics of medical office work, it is important to understand a little about how medical care, and the role of the medical assistant, got to where it is today.

HISTORICAL DEVELOPMENT OF THE ROLE OF THE MEDICAL ASSISTANT

As recently as 1950, most doctors established their own practice when they finished their medical education and hospital training. A doctor usually saw patients with no assistance, except possibly his wife (almost all doctors were men), who answered the telephone and often did the billing.

The doctor spent a good part of each day making house calls, where he examined patients with only the equipment he could carry in his doctor's bag. Patients who went to the doctor's office (often a room in his house, or the first floor of a building, with the doctor living in an apartment above) may or may not have had an appointment. They expected to wait to be seen.

Health insurance, if the patient had any, paid only for hospitalization, and usually the patient completed most of the paperwork. Health insurance is a system by which a person or the person's employer pays an insurance company a yearly amount of money, and the insurance company pays some or most of the person's medical expenses for that year. The theory behind insurance is that, although a few people will have large medical bills over the course of the year, most people will have small bills. By setting the fee for everyone at a level above the actual cost of care for most people, the insurance company can pay for the care of the well, the occasionally ill, and the often ill, and still make a profit.

In the first 20 years after World War II, before the increasing use of technology caused medical costs to skyrocket, a doctor probably charged $2 to $5, possibly $10, for an office visit, a sum that seems small today. For some patients, however, even this small charge was more than a day's pay. For doctors, the low fee was enough, because the expenses of his practice were also low. In fact, doctors rarely pressed poor patients for full payment. They always had many patients who owed them money; it was not uncommon for patients to pay tiny amounts weekly for many months or even years, especially parents of young children. Doctors would even barter—exchange goods or services—for medical care.

In the past 40 years, the practice of medicine has changed dramatically. Today, a medical practice is a business that, depending on the number of doctors who work there and the type of medical specialty, can have an annual income of millions of dollars. The reasons for these changes are complex.

Government health insurance programs—first for the medically needy, and later for the elderly and disabled, and for dependents of military personnel—began to pay for doctor's office visits. From 1950 to 1965, the Medicaid program was funded by individual states to provide health insurance for the medically needy. As part of the Social Security Act of 1965, the U.S. Congress created the Medicare program (Title 18) to provide health insurance for the elderly and disabled, and introduced Title 19, which made the Medicaid program a joint federal/state program and set requirements for coverage. A year later, Congress authorized and the Department of Defense established the Civilian Health and Medical Program of the Uniformed Services (CHAMPUS) to provide health insurance for dependent spouses and children of active-duty military personnel.

By the 1970s, private health insurance also began to pay for office visits in addition to hospital expenses. This shift to so-called "third-party payers" required more detailed medical records and a medical office staff that could help patients understand insurance claims forms and later fill out those claim forms. Today, most insurers pay doctors directly rather than reimbursing individuals after they have personally paid.

Advances in medical science made many more diagnostic tests and treatment available and even necessary for good medical care. For example, any doctor who practices family medicine or adult internal medicine will have an electrocardiogram (EKG) machine in his or her office today, and EKGs are routinely performed at physical exams of people over 40. There is no reason for the doctor to spend the time performing this test, so it is left to the medical assistant.

Even as diagnostic and treatment equipment has increased in amount and in complexity, so too has the clerical equipment used in a doctor's office. Today there are fax machines, intercoms and answering systems, photocopiers, and computers.

Doctors send claims to a number of different insurance companies. Many insurance plans require prior approval for certain procedures, referrals to specialists, or surgical care. Some insurance companies and even government programs use electronic claims filing via e-mail and electronic payments directly into doctor's office accounts at banks. This creates a need not only for more staff, but also for more highly trained staff.

Doctors have also stopped or at least greatly reduced the number of house calls they make. Because of this, they need more office space. In addition, patients with more complex needs are seen in doctor's offices, rather than the hospital emergency room or outpatient department. Sometimes patients must occupy an exam or treatment room for a long time, such as when an individual with asthma is receiving an inhalation treatment.

Finally, since the 1970s doctors have practiced what has come to be called "defensive medicine." Because of the fear of a malpractice lawsuit, and the high cost of malpractice insurance, doctors perform every test necessary to rule out even the most unlikely cause of an illness.

All of these factors—increased medical equipment, increased clerical equipment, and increased space—push up the overhead costs of running a medical office. This forces doctors to see more patients, which in turn encourages the doctor to transfer many procedures to the rest of the medical staff. Increasing costs also have encouraged doctors to band together into group practices, to share the burdens of equipment, staff, and space.

Today, the solo-practice doctor is a rarity. More common are groups of three to six doctors who practice the same specialty of medicine—pediatrics, adult medicine, obstetrics and gynecology, or surgery—or one of the dozens of subspecialties such as cardiology (care of the heart), pulmonary medicine (care of the lungs), or gastroenterology (care of the intestinal tract). By rotating who makes hospital rounds, who takes after-hours and weekend calls from patients, and sometimes even who sees patients in which of the group's different physical locations, doctors are able to maximize their efficiency as well as their effectiveness and still have time for their own families.

Multi-specialty clinics, which vary in size from about 10 to more than 30 doctors, usually also have a laboratory and vision care personnel, and sometimes have a pharmacy and on-site x-ray facilities.

Patients today are charged between $50 and $100 for the typical doctor's office visit and additional charges for diagnostic tests or treatments. Most patients have some kind of insurance, which pays for some or all of the office visit. Doctors usually fill out and submit the claim forms, and most insurance companies pay a discount from the actual price charged for the service. Doctors may also participate in health maintenance organization (HMO) networks. Patients enrolled in HMOs pay the doctor a small co-payment, with the rest of the charges paid by the HMO. HMOs have changed the face of American medical care since the mid-1980s, and will be examined in greater detail in chapter 38, in the discussion of how to file various forms of health insurance claims.

As services expanded, doctors hired nurses to help them in their offices. This helped ease their burden of performing procedures and caring for patients; but nurses were often unable and unwilling to assist with

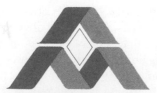

> **Figure 2–1** Logo of the American Association of Medical Assistants (Courtesy of the AAMA)

the administrative aspects of the practice. As a result, many doctors found a willing candidate and trained that person to assist with both patient care and administrative duties. This position evolved over time into what today is called a medical assistant.

Medical assistants from 15 states organized to form the American Association of Medical Assistants (AAMA) in 1956, and the profession was recognized by the U.S. Department of Education in 1978. The AAMA and other organizations, especially the American Medical Technologists (AMT), have worked for the professionalization of medical assisting, including defining the scope of training necessary. Recognizing that uniform training is necessary, various organizations developed curricula, as well as accrediting medical assisting programs and validating credentials of medical assistants through examinations. Issues of licensing and accreditation are described in more detail in chapter 4.

The current definition of a medical assistant, as expressed by the AAMA in 1999, is as follows:

Medical assisting is an allied health profession whose practitioners function as members of the health care delivery team and perform administrative and clinical procedures.

Figure 2–1 shows the logo of the American Association of Medical Assistants.

ROLE OF THE MEDICAL ASSISTANT

To run a larger medical office, a group of doctors often employs a team of allied health professionals and office professionals. These usually include:

■ A front-office medical assistant or receptionist, who answers telephones, makes appointments by phone or in person, operates a computer, checks patients in, and collects co-payments (Figure 2–2).
■ A clinical staff of medical assistants and/or nurses who prepare patients for examinations, take vital signs, perform diagnostic tests, assist with exams and procedures, and maintain the examination area supplies and equipment (Figure 2–3).

■ A financial staff, who fill out insurance forms, post charges and payments, and collect overdue accounts (Figure 2–4). Medical assistants also perform these tasks.
■ Consultants for both clinical and administrative areas, such as laboratory technologists, or accountants.

In addition, some offices have a laboratory staff as well, who perform lab tests on samples taken from patients. These tests range from a simple rapid strep test for strep throat to complex tests, such as a Chem 20, in which a machine does 20 chemical tests on a single sample of blood, with the results printed on a single page within minutes. Offices that send their lab work out to commercial labs for complex tests often don't employ laboratory technicians but have medical assistants obtain specimens and perform simple lab tests.

In a smaller medical office, most or all of these tasks fall to the medical assistant. Therefore, every medical assisting student needs to know and understand all of the various tasks a medical assistant may be asked to undertake. These fall into four categories:

One category is made up of administrative activities, such as setting up appointments, maintaining medical and financial records, and handling billing procedures. The second is made up of clinical activities, such as collecting and processing specimens, preparing patients for examinations and treatments, and assisting the doctor with examinations and treatments. The third area is interpersonal activities, such as performing patient education, obtaining referrals, and coordinating community resources for patients. The fourth area is managing the office, which includes tasks such as maintaining supply inventory, maintaining personnel policies and procedures, and promoting safety of patients and staff.

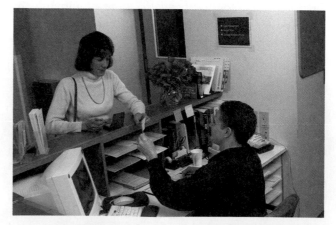

> **Figure 2–2** Medical assistant at reception desk

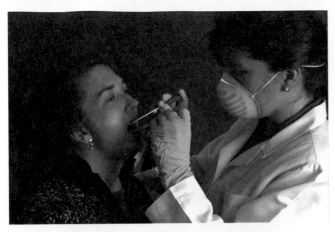

➤ **Figure 2-3** Medical assistant obtaining throat culture

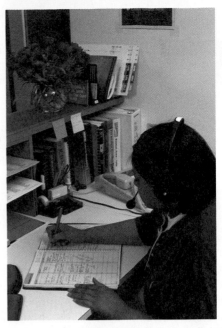

➤ **Figure 2-5** Medical assistant making an appointment

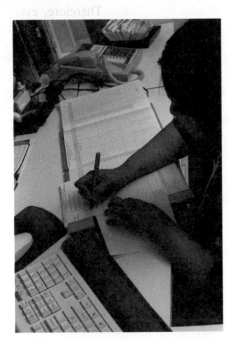

➤ **Figure 2-4** Medical assistant posting financial charges

The Medical Assistant's Administrative Activities

A host of administrative activities must be performed on a daily basis in a medical office. We like to think of a doctor's office as a place where patients receive medical treatment, but in reality much of the activity in a doctor's office involves moving paperwork through specified processes. The medical assistant is responsible for a number of these activities; some di-

rectly involve the patient and the patient's records, and others involve financial matters:

1. Scheduling appointments, both over the telephone and in person for follow-up appointments, is a primary responsibility. Many patients also need appointments made with other medical facilities, either for referral to a specialist, a diagnostic procedure, outpatient surgery, continuing therapy or rehabilitation, or hospital admission. Some patients may need to schedule multiple appointments with other facilities as the result of a single office visit. The medical assistant must learn the procedure for making and documenting such an appointment (Figure 2-5).

2. Every patient visit generates a paper trail that is necessary for the doctor to be paid for the services provided. The medical assistant must know how to enter the correct charges, depending on the type of visit (brief, standard, extended, or new patient), and the procedures and/or diagnostic tests performed.

These charges are entered either into the office computer or into various records, such as the day sheet and patient ledger, to generate a bill to the patient or the patient's insurance company. Sometimes, the patient makes a co-payment at the time of the visit, and the remainder of the charges are billed to the insurance company (Figure 2–6). In turn, these charges create the **accounts receivable,** money that is owed to the doctor for services performed. In larger offices and clinics, a separate business office usually handles financial matters.

3. Each patient encounter with a clinician—doctor, advanced-practice nurse (also called a nurse practitioner [NP]), or physician's assistant (PA)—is followed by charting of the patient's visit. Many clinicians prefer to dictate their patient notes rather than write them or type them into the chart. A medical assistant may be asked to perform medical transcription on these dictations, typing up the notes and placing them into the chart. Some larger offices employ a full-time medical transcriptionist; some offices use an outside medical transcription service (Figure 2–7). Some offices have computer equipment in each examination room to perform automated, computerized medical-record charting.

4. On a regular basis, checks and cash need to be deposited in the office's bank account. Preparing bank deposits and recording the deposits into the office's checkbook is an activity that medical assistants often perform.

5. Every business has bills to pay. These include rent (or mortgage, if the office is owned), electricity, lease payments on equipment, staff salaries, and a number of other regular payments such as liability and malpractice insurance. Medical assistants, or business office personnel, usually write these checks and maintain records of

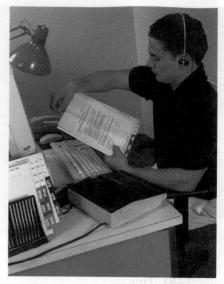

> **Figure 2–7** Medical assistant performing transcription

these and other **accounts payable**—bills owed by the office. (Some offices have an outside bookkeeping service perform these tasks, and even in many offices that pay their own regular bills, salary is handled by an outside payroll service.)

The Medical Assistant's Clinical Activities

The clinical part of what goes on in a doctor's office also creates a number of activities for the medical assistant. These fall into two general areas: carrying out diagnostic procedures and assisting with patient care.

In the diagnostics area, medical assistants are often asked to collect and process specimens such as urine, perform diagnostic tests such as EKGs, and screen and follow up patient test results, such as from a strep test, pregnancy test, or blood sample.

In the area of assisting with patient care, medical assistants perform seven primary activities:

1. They screen patient phone calls and visits, determining which patients need to be seen most urgently, which can be seen in a less urgent fashion, and which can be dealt with via a telephone consultation with a doctor.

2. They take medical histories and check vital signs. This is a big timesaver for the doctor. Weighing the patient; measuring temperature, pulse, respiration, and blood pressure; and noting the chief complaint for the visit takes up to 5 or 10 minutes for each patient. Having this done by a medical assistant allows the doctor to see at least one extra patient per hour.

3. Between each patient visit, the medical assistant prepares the examination and/or treatment room

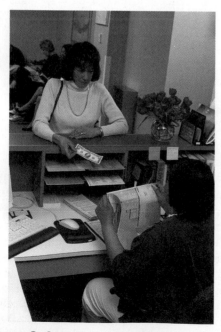

> **Figure 2–6** Medical assistant taking a co-payment

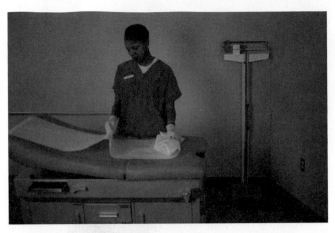

➤ Figure 2–8 Medical assistant preparing an exam room

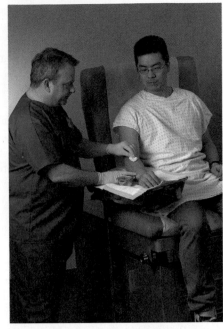

➤ Figure 2–9 Medical assistant preparing a patient for minor surgery

(Figure 2–8). This involves making sure there is fresh paper on the table, that the proper instruments are available for the next examination or procedure, and that the necessary equipment is available and in working order.

4. Medical assistants prepare patients for exams or procedures, and assist the doctor with those exams or procedures. These activities involve everything from helping to settle a patient into an exam room to helping shift a patient into different positions for portions of the exam; to passing instruments and supplies to the doctor while he or she performs a procedure; to removing sutures, bandaging, and changing dressings (Figure 2–9).
5. Medical assistants perform routine diagnostic tests such as EKGs, collect specimens, and perform routine laboratory tests, such as urinalysis.
6. Medical assistants prepare and administer medications and immunizations. This sounds like a straightforward activity, but in reality it calls for concentration and precision.
7. Sometimes a medical assistant also has to perform emergency care and administer first aid. This does not happen often, but every medical assistant must be prepared.

The Medical Assistant as a Liaison (Interpersonal Activities)

To act as a liaison has a specific meaning. A **liaison** serves the purpose of communicating between individuals, groups, or units. The medical assistant, in her or his liaison role, serves as a means of communicating between the doctor and the patient and between the doctor's office (on behalf of the patient) and specialists to whom the patient is being referred.

The medical assistant also serves as a liaison between the patient and outside agencies, for example, when he or she sets up diagnostic tests; and between

the patient or the doctor and community agencies, such as the Visiting Nurse Association or hospice, when the medical assistant helps to locate community resources that can provide needed services for a patient.

Instructing patients can also be seen as part of the liaison role, as the medical assistant actually conveys the information to the patient that the doctor wants the patient to have. Once on the job, the medical assistant may serve as a resource for other medical assistants in the office by locating speakers to give continuing education talks, or by preparing educational materials and presenting community education programs herself or himself.

The Medical Assistant and Office Management Activities

Especially in smaller offices, medical assistants serve as office managers. This entails four groups of activities:

1. Operational activities involve maintaining the inventory of supplies, everything from purchasing tongue blades and gauze to contracting with a uniform service to launder the staff's white coats. It also involves evaluating and recommending changes in the supplies purchased and evaluating new equipment for potential purchase or lease.
2. The second group of activities involves personnel policy and procedures. Businesses are always reviewing their policies and procedures, and updating and revising them as necessary. As offices

move from one or two doctors and a small staff working "as a family" to a larger organization, policies and procedures become more important to standardize the way all employees are dealt with.

3. **Risk management** is the development of policies and procedures that minimize the chances of the practice being sued by a patient or disciplined by a regulatory agency. Every doctor's office needs to have one person responsible for risk management, which involves, among other areas, the promotion of health and safety for office personnel and patients, maintenance of proper infection control measures, fire prevention, and the proper disposal of hazardous waste and controlled substances.

4. Record keeping is an important activity for the individual who manages a medical office. In addition to patient records, many other kinds of records must be kept. For example, the office must maintain records for controlled substances (drugs that have the potential for abuse or addiction).

Every doctor has what amounts to a license to dispense controlled substances, and a federal controlled substance identification number, issued by the Drug Enforcement Administration (DEA). Doctors must keep inventory records each time they purchase a controlled substance for office use and each time they dispense a controlled substance from the office. Doctors can be audited by the DEA and can have their licenses suspended for writing unnecessary prescriptions for controlled substances or prescriptions that are not justified by the medical records.

Records must also be kept for **quality assurance**, the process of auditing records to make sure that proper procedures have been followed and proper care has been given. Doctor's offices with laboratories must have a quality-control plan and keep quality-control records. Offices must also maintain information about all potentially hazardous materials used in the office (called Material Safety Data Sheets).

Every doctor's office maintains contractual relationships with a host of other businesses. The office is usually rented, although some practices own an office condominium or a building for their space. Diagnostic equipment (such as ultrasound machines) and office equipment (such as computers) are often leased and may have a maintenance contract. Doctors may have a contract with an answering service, as well as with a company that sells and services pagers, and maybe even with a company that supplies cell phones and monthly service.

Medical records, personnel records, and financial records necessary for tax purposes and liability insurance policies all need some dedicated attention as well.

WHAT TAKES PLACE IN A MEDICAL OFFICE?

There is no such thing as a "typical" medical office. The style of any particular medical office depends on the personality of the doctor or doctors who practice there, as well as the general population of patients who come there. Regardless of the doctor's personality and the patients' personal background, the same kinds of activities occur in any doctor's office setting.

Today, the trend in medical care is toward an increasing amount of **ambulatory care**—defined as the patient coming to the care rather than the patient receiving care in a home or hospital setting. To take advantage of ambulatory care, the patient must be able to walk into the doctor's office, or at the very least be brought to the office in a wheelchair. In addition to private doctor's offices, offices of doctors who make up a staff HMO, community health centers, and hospitals are increasingly making more space available for outpatient clinics.

Whatever the organizational setup of the doctor's office where you work—private practice, public or community health center, or hospital-based outpatient clinic—the flow of activities for each patient will be the same. The patient will:

1. Enter the office
2. Give the office staff personal and payment information
3. Be seen by a doctor (or by a nurse practitioner or physician assistant if the practice uses such personnel)
4. Receive a diagnosis, treatment, or a referral to another health care provider
5. Possibly undergo diagnostic or laboratory tests, in which various specimens may be taken in the office and either processed through the office laboratory or sent out to an outside laboratory for evaluation
6. Be sent home or be admitted to the hospital.

Figure 2–10 is a flowchart of how a patient would move through the office.

After a visit, the doctor's office begins the process of receiving payment for its services, either from a private insurance plan, a government-funded insurance program, and/or from the patient, who may be responsible for a co-payment, a percentage of the charges, or the entire bill if he or she does not have insurance.

After the examination and before going home, the patient may make an appointment for follow-up care and receive instructions, either about steps to take before undergoing a particular test or procedure in the future or about medication that is being prescribed. Patients who are seen regularly because of a chronic illness may spend time with a doctor, nurse, or medi-

```
                                                          ┌──────────────┐
                                                          │  send out    │
                                                          │  specimens   │
                                                          └──────────────┘
                                                                 ▲
   Reception      Patient                                        │
    area          preparation    Exam room      Laboratory       Home          Follow-up
┌───────────┐  ┌───────────┐  ┌───────────┐  ┌───────────┐  ┌───────────┐  ┌─────────────────┐
│Appointment│  │Vital signs│  │Chief      │  │Specimen   │  │           │  │Return appointment,│
│and Insurance│ │height,    │  │complaint  │  │collection │  │instructions,│ │Telephone call,  │
│info (copay if│ │weight    │  │history    │  │testing    │  │prescriptions│ │Referrals        │
│necessary) │  │           │  │examination│  │           │  │           │  │                 │
└───────────┘  └───────────┘  └───────────┘  └───────────┘  └───────────┘  └─────────────────┘
```

Treatment room

Diagnostic tests Treatments

Outpatient testing

Submit and collect insurance

➤ **Figure 2–10** Patient progress through a medical office

cal assistant reviewing the patient's individual treatment plan.

Increasingly, doctors are providing all of their patients with health education materials in the waiting room, either in the form of pamphlets or article reprints or as health education videos or health news reports specially prepared for viewing in doctor's offices.

PARTS OF THE MEDICAL OFFICE

A doctor's office has a number of different physical spaces in it. Each space has a particular purpose. Every doctor's office has four basic areas:

reception area and waiting room
front office
examination and treatment rooms
medical records storage, which may be in the front
   office or, more commonly, in a separate room.

In most offices, doctors also have their own office (sometimes called a consultation room), separate from

exam rooms. But some doctors have exam tables in their offices, combining the two spaces in one room.

Larger offices may have several additional areas:

office laboratory
treatment rooms, in addition to examination rooms
   (Not all doctors perform treatments as such, or if
   treatments are needed they may be given in an
   exam room. Some offices that perform a lot of
   treatments also have a treatment setup room.)
business office, which is separate from the front
   office (reception, telephones, appointments) and
   is sometimes known as the "back office"
lunch/break room for staff.

All doctor's offices must meet a number of specifications laid out by regulatory agencies. These include the federal **Occupational Safety and Health Administration (OSHA)**, which regulates workplace health and safety. They also must meet the specifications of the Americans with Disabilities Act, which requires that doorways be at least 3 feet wide and hallways at least 5 feet wide. Restroom facilities must be available for both patients and staff. Office laboratories are regulated by the **Clinical Laboratory Improvement Act (CLIA '88)**. Local boards of health also inspect and regulate hospitals and clinics.

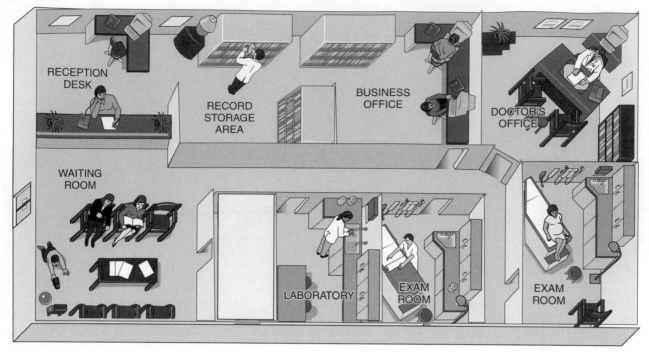

> Figure 2–11 Layout of a small medical office

Figures 2–11 and 2–12 show typical doctor's office layouts.

Four Basic Areas

Let's look at the basic medical office areas in a little more detail. First I'll discuss the various locations, then go back and talk about the equipment that will be found in each area.

The reception area and waiting room are the first place any new or prospective patient will see. First impressions are important. The waiting room should be clean and well lit. Furniture should be arranged and not haphazardly placed. Up-to-date general-interest reading material should be available; many doctors also have patient education materials available in the waiting room. Waiting rooms in pediatric and family-practice offices also have toys available for children. Large pediatric practices may have a separate waiting room for sick children or for adolescents.

There should be enough chairs for two people per patient visit, multiplied by the number of patients seen in 2 hours. The waiting room needs to present a calm atmosphere and look professional. Usually, the waiting area is carpeted. It should have comfortable chairs, grouped in blocks rather than just lined up around the walls. Colors should be muted, and music should be soft. Red, yellow, and orange are typically avoided;

today, doctor's office decor often uses shades of green, dusty pink, or salmon. Music is usually a tape or radio station of the "easy listening" variety.

The reception area connects the front office to the waiting room. The receptionist should greet each patient as he or she enters the waiting room. Most reception areas have a counter so the patient can fill out or sign forms, and many have a sliding window so patients cannot hear the conversations that are occurring behind the receptionist.

The **front office** is usually where the business transactions between patient and office staff occur. Patients check in here when they enter the office. New patient forms are received here and health insurance cards are copied. Co-payments are taken from patients whose insurance is provided through HMOs. In smaller offices, posting of patient charges, billing, and insurance forms are processed here; larger offices have a separate office for billing and processing insurance claims.

The receptionist makes follow-up appointments and answers the telephones. In smaller offices, the receptionist also makes telephone appointments; larger offices have one or two people who work as dedicated appointment schedulers; they are usually located in the business office.

Many offices have a small open area to take vital signs such as blood pressure, as well as height and weight, and to process simple lab tests, especially if there is no larger lab in the office (Figure 2–13). This allows the medical assistant to obtain preliminary data while the exam rooms are occupied. There is usually a telephone in this area so that clinical personnel can talk to patients about medical problems, take lab results, and make calls related to clinical care.

Examination rooms are designed for the convenience of the doctor and assisting personnel who will work there. However, they need to also be as comfortable and calming to the patient as possible. Reading material should be available in each exam room. Although good scheduling will ensure that patients will not wait too long in exam rooms for a doctor, emergency phone calls, "corridor consults" with colleagues, and other short delays may occur.

Many doctors also perform treatments or diagnostic procedures in exam rooms; complex procedures (such as suturing a laceration) may be performed in larger rooms with extra equipment and/or supplies. These are called **treatment rooms.**

The medical records storage may be located near the reception area, in the business areas, adjacent to the patient preparation area, or in a separate room. Charts of current patients—those who have been seen within the past 2 to 3 years—are kept in the records storage area in the office. Inactive charts are removed regularly and stored in a less accessible location, such as the basement of the building, or off-site in a facility that maintains records in storage. Charts needed for patients who will be coming in during a specified period—morning, afternoon, or an entire day—are removed from the storage area and prepared for use.

Some practices are moving away from paper records to computerized medical records. In this case, patient records are stored on a computer's hard disk and are simply pulled up from the database as necessary.

Additional Areas Found in Many Offices

The 1988 amendments to CLIA (CLIA '88) allow doctor's offices to establish one of three different categories of laboratory:

■ A **certificate of waiver** is a process by which a doctor's office can be granted permission under CLIA for staff to perform low-complexity tests that require no special certification to perform, and no experimental equipment.

■ A laboratory certified for moderate-complexity tests can perform such tests as cultures, electrophoresis, and blood tests using machine analysis. Although not required, it is recommended that such a lab be run by a licensed or certified individual, such as a certified medical assistant or a medical technologist.

■ A laboratory certified for high-complexity tests can perform tests that result in a final diagnosis. It can also engage in research studies and experimental testing. Such a laboratory must be run by a doctor

trained as a pathologist, and all testing must be performed by medical laboratory technologists.

CLIA '88 specifies who can supervise labs and lays out the process for inspection and accreditation. It sets strict guidelines for quality control, quality assurance, handling of hazardous materials, documentation, and proficiency training. Offices that perform only certificate of waiver tests may perform lab testing in the patient preparation area. Ideally, the bathroom is adjacent to this area, with an opening in the wall so that urine samples can be passed directly into the lab area.

Chapters 23 to 26 of this book are devoted to a detailed discussion of the doctor's office laboratory.

Other areas may be present in some, if not most, doctors' offices.

Doctor's private offices are often a reflection of the doctor's personal taste. This room is where a doctor meets privately with patients, patients' families, and other visitors. He or she usually displays degrees and certificates of membership in professional organizations on the walls of the office. Even if the practice has a small library for the use of all staff, doctors will usually have at least a few important references in this office. Art and memorabilia that shows the doctor's personal taste also helps to make the private office a pleasant place for the doctor to do quiet work and hold meetings.

Some medical practices will separate their business office from the rest of the office. If the practice has one or more satellite locations, the billing and insurance is usually done in the practice's main office for all locations. Some offices contract billing and insurance claim processing to an outside company, which may even be located in another state.

Depending on the type of medical practice, particular rooms may be set aside for specific treatments or diagnostic procedures. Having a separate room makes it easier because:

All necessary supplies and instruments are in one room.
Necessary equipment may not be portable.
Patients who do not need the particular treatment may be uncomfortable seeing the equipment or instruments.

Types of special rooms might include

1. A pediatrics exam/treatment room in a family practice group's office
2. Surgical procedure room in a general surgery group's office
3. A room for more complex testing, such as colposcopy, nonstress testing, and pelvic ultrasounds, in a group practice specializing in obstetrics/gynecology
4. A trauma room in a large clinic or community health semi-rural internal medicine group's office

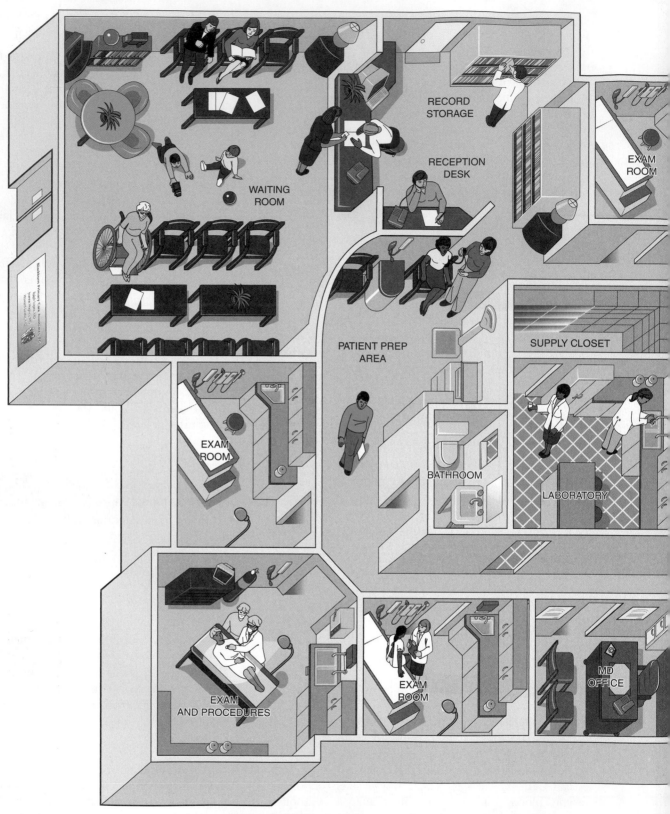

➢ Figure 2–12 Layout of a large medical office

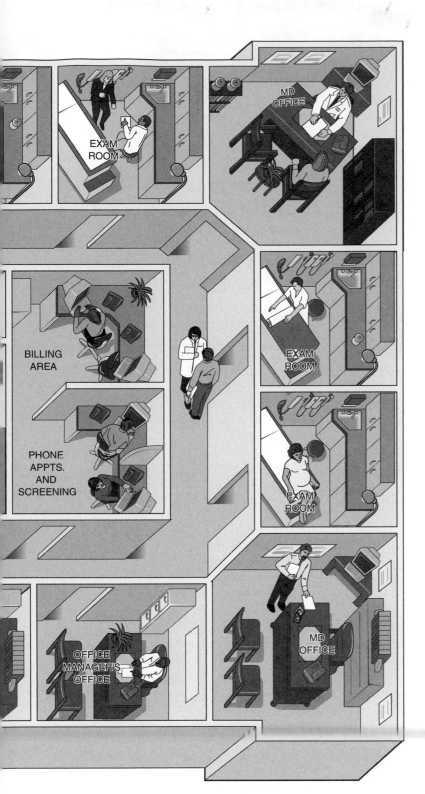

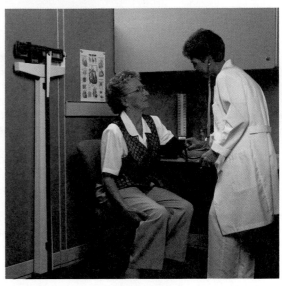

➤ **Figure 2–13** Patient preparation area with medical assistant measuring blood pressure

Recognizing the needs of staff for a quiet place to take their breaks and eat their lunch, newer offices often include a staff break/lunchroom. This room may have a refrigerator and microwave for staff to prepare lunches they bring from home. There should be at least one table and chairs. The break/lunchroom should not double as a storage area, and staff should avoid using the room for meetings that deprive others use of the room.

Although the break/lunchroom is to be used for "down time," a telephone and office intercom should be located in the room, so staff can be paged in an emergency or can take important phone calls.

THE HEALTH CARE TEAM

A medical assistant works as a member of a dedicated team. Each doctor or group of doctors expects medical assistants to fill a slightly different role within the office team. This role will depend on the style of the practice, the region of the country where the practice is located, and what other types of medical professionals staff the team.

As the operations of a medical practice become more complex, doctors are hiring people with more specialized medical business and medical management experience to run the business side of the office. In these offices medical assistants play more of a clinical role. In smaller offices, and often in rural areas where it is harder to find office management professionals, medical assistants continue to perform many administrative activities, and may perform both clinical and

---

The Medical Model

The medical model is a term often used to describe how doctors and others trained in Western medicine view health, disease, wellness, and treatment. Understanding this concept, and how a doctor assesses a patient, helps a medical assistant to function as a more effective health care team member.

Doctors in the United States are trained to observe a condition and ask what examinations, laboratory tests, and diagnostic procedures are necessary to determine the cause of the condition. This methodology is based on ruling out conditions, working from the most simple to the most complex. This is called making a differential diagnosis. At each step, as one possible cause is ruled out, the doctor asks, "What do I need to know to determine for certain what the cause of this condition is or to determine for certain that this condition could not have been caused by something else?"

Various members of the health care team may carry out the tests or treatments, assess the patient, and provide information. The doctor or other primary care provider heads the team and makes decisions about patient care based on the patient's diagnosis.

---

administrative activities. See the box above, which describes what is called "The Medical Model," and "Focus On: History of the Medical Model."

This section of the chapter will first describe the members of the medical team and their roles. Then it will discuss the concept of working as a team and what that means for the medical assistant as a team member.

Members of the Health Care Team

The members of the medical team who typically work in an outpatient office—be it a private practice, a community or public health clinic, or a hospital clinic—are:

doctors
medical assistants
one or more nurses
a business manager
secretary/receptionist(s)
insurance specialist(s)
medical transcriptionist(s)
file clerk(s).

Some doctors, especially those in primary-care adult medicine and pediatrics, have come to rely increasingly

on nurse practitioners (NPs) or physician assistants (PAs) to see patients on routine visits. Public health clinics and community health centers also usually depend on these nondoctor clinicians for much routine patient care.

If the office performs moderate- or high-complexity laboratory tests, a certified medical technologist may also be on the staff.

Hospital or community-based clinics will possibly also have a staff of social workers, outreach workers, and case managers to provide social services to patients.

Obstetrics/gynecology practices may also have certified nurse midwives.

Table 2–1 lists the various allied health professions and the educational requirements necessary for certification or licensure.

Doctors and Other Primary Care Providers

Doctors either have an MD (medical doctor) or DO (doctor of osteopathy) degree, either of which is received after 4 years of college, then 4 years of medical school. In addition, doctors complete a hospital-based, intensive training period called residency, which lasts from 2 to 7 years, depending on the specialty. To receive a medical license from the state where he or she will practice, the doctor must pass Parts I, II, and III of the United States Medical Licensing Examination (USMLE). The first two parts of the exam are taken during medical school, but Part III cannot be taken until the doctor has completed at least one year of residency (sometimes called an internship).

If a doctor wants to be "board certified" in a specialty, he or she must pass another exam, administered by the certification board of the particular specialty. The doctor does not need to be board certified to obtain a license.

A physician assistant must have at least 2 years of college, plus 2 years of physician assistant school. A physician assistant usually specializes—for instance, in pediatrics or adult medicine—and manages a group of patients receiving routine care. He or she must practice with a doctor. All states except Mississippi have laws regulating physician assistants; most states require a license for a physician assistant to practice.

An nurse practitioner is a registered nurse (RN) who studies in a program in advanced practice nursing, a program that usually grants a Master of Science in Nursing (MSN) degree. Nurse practitioners can specialize in pediatrics (PNP) or family practice (FNP).

The scope of a nurse practitioner's ability to practice independently is determined by each state. In all states, nurse practitioners are allowed to carry a caseload and manage routine patient care. Some states allow nurse practitioners to write prescriptions; in other states a doctor must cosign the order. In some states, nurse practitioners are allowed to practice independently, but

Table 2-1	Allied Health Professionals	
Occupation	Credentials	Responsibilities
Certified Coding Specialist	CCS (certified coding specialist) (certificate or associate degree)	Assigns codes to diagnoses and procedures
Certified Coding Specialist—Physician-based	CCS-P (certificate or associate degree)	Has expertise in physician-based settings
Certified Medical Assistant, Registered Medical Assistant	CMA or RMA (certificate or associate degree)	Performs administrative and clinical tasks in ambulatory care
Licensed Practical (Vocational) Nurse	LPN or LVN (certificate)	Performs direct patient care and clinical procedures
Medical Laboratory Technician	MLT (associate degree)	Performs lab tests in the clinical laboratory
Medical Secretary	CMS (associate degree)	Specializes in administrative procedures in a health care setting
Medical Technologist	MT (bachelor degree)	Performs lab tests and supervises the MLT
Nurse Practitioner	NP (additional training beyond bachelor's degree, usually a master's degree)	Specializes in a specific area and often manages routine patient care
Occupational Therapist	OT (bachelor's degree)	Plans therapeutic activities for rehabilitation, especially for activities of daily living
Occupational Therapist Assistant	OTA (associate degree)	Carries out treatment to assist in rehabilitation as planned and supervised by the occupational therapist
Physical Therapist	PT (additional training beyond bachelor's degree, usually a master's degree)	Plans exercises for large muscle groups for rehabilitation and performs exercises
Physical Therapist Assistant	PTA (associate degree)	Performs exercise program as planned by and supervised by the physical therapist
Physician's Assistant	PA (bachelor's degree)	Manages routine patient care under the supervision of a physician
Radiological Technologist	RT (associate degree or bachelor's degree)	Takes X-rays and assists with special radiographic examinations
Registered Health Information Administrator	RHIA (bachelor's degree) (formerly (RRA [Registered Record Administrator])	Administers the record department of a health care setting
Registered Health Information Technician	RHIT (associate degree) (formerly ART [Accredited Record Technician])	Works with patient information and records
Registered Nurse	RN (associate degree or bachelor's degree)	Performs nursing duties and also often supervises nursing assistants and LPNs
Registered Respiratory Therapist	RRT (associate degree)	Provides respiratory treatments and manages patients on ventilators

in most they must practice in an office with MDs or DOs present for consultation. In a few states, nurse practitioners are allowed to admit patients to hospitals.

Effective Teamwork

Working as a effective health care team does not just happen. To be effective, team members work together to provide appropriate care for each patient. The more people are involved, the more crucial this teamwork is. Each member of the team must be committed to:

problem solving
focusing
communicating
meeting.

Teamwork is reinforced at regular staff meetings, which can be directed by either the medical or business director of the office, depending on the particular topics of the meeting. But the true test of teamwork occurs in providing patient care among the entire group of health care professionals.

Each health care team member has a certain responsibility and restrictions on activities and areas about which he or she is allowed to make decisions. Sometimes this scope is defined by federal or state law. For example, medical assistants are allowed to administer injections in some states, but in others they cannot.

The Medical Assistant as a Team Member

The medical assistant must learn what areas fall within the proper scope of decision-making responsibility. This may vary. Generally, on the clinical side, these areas will be limited to patient safety and comfort needs, as well as possibly to anticipating diagnostic tests that will be needed. In the area of supplies, the medical assistant may have more freedom to make decisions.

Remember, a medical assistant can anticipate a diagnostic test by, for example, collecting a sample or wheeling in the EKG machine, but he or she should not perform a diagnostic test without direction from a doctor or other primary care provider.

A medical assistant can also anticipate teaching needs, prepare materials, and instruct patients about diagnostic tests or routine health practices. But the medical assistant cannot give advice to the patient. Again, that is the job of the doctor or other licensed professionals who have been authorized to do so.

Finally, a medical assistant can observe a patient and inform the clinician who will examine that patient about what has been observed. If office policy allows, the observation can be written in the patient's record, but using descriptive language only, not any words that can be interpreted to diagnose the patient's condition.

HOW MEDICAL OFFICE CARE FITS INTO THE HEALTH CARE SYSTEM

Three trends running in parallel through modern medicine are leading to an increasingly important role for office-based, or ambulatory, health care.

One trend is the desire by those who pay the bills—employers, the federal and state governments, and insurance companies—to reduce the costs of health care whenever and wherever possible.

A second trend is the ability for doctor's practices and other outpatient clinics to provide a broad range of diagnostic and treatment services without having to put patients in the hospital. This has occurred because of the high cost of hospitalization, the decreased cost of diagnostic equipment, and the development in some cases of less invasive surgical procedures.

The third trend is an increased understanding, through empirical evidence and research on outcomes, that people *feel better* the less they must be confined to a hospital or go to a hospital for treatment.

Shift from Hospital to Community-Based Health Care

Many people today liken a hospital to a factory, a place where processes are rigid and routinized. This may be good for reducing costs and for measuring outcomes. But it is not good for the emotional well-being of those treated there.

Being able to be diagnosed and treated in an outpatient setting allows people to feel more in control of their lives as medical patients. This is especially important for people who have frequent contact with the medical system—infants and children, the elderly, and those with chronic illnesses.

The outpatient office—be it private practice, public clinic, or hospital-based clinic—is part of an integrated web of community-based health care providers that includes:

primary care doctors
medical specialists
dentists, orthodontists, and oral surgeons
psychologists, social workers, and case managers
substance-abuse treatment providers
nutritionists and dietitians
audiologists
optometrists and opticians
podiatrists
home health care providers
home infusion providers
satellite dialysis centers
mobile examination facilities.

Working together, these health care providers can keep many people who would have been hospitalized for long periods or possibly even institutionalized 50, 25, or even 10 years ago living independently or semi-independently in the community.

Today the hospital's role is to provide acute care only. The patient's condition must be unstable or require constant regulation of therapy. If the patient does not meet these strict criteria, he or she either goes home to be followed as an outpatient or is transferred to a rehabilitation facility for intense regular rehabilitative treatment or to a nursing home for long-term maintenance care.

Managed Care Versus Patient Care: Competing Forces Facing the Medical Office in the 21st Century

Traditionally, medical care in the United States was paid for on a fee-for-service basis. Each service was billed and paid for as a separate charge: so much for the office visit, so much for the EKG, so much for the urinalysis, and so on. Fee-for-service payments can be

FOCUS ON
PROFESSIONALISM

THE MEDICAL ASSISTANT'S SCOPE OF DECISION-MAKING AUTHORITY

As you read the following scenarios, ask yourself if you think it is within a medical assistant's scope of decision-making authority to take action, and what action you might take.

1. You bring Ms. Richards into an examination room, and while getting her a gown you notice it is the last in the drawer. Do you think you should get a handful from the supply closet and bring them in the next time you come into the room? The answer is, of course you should.

2. While you are weighing Mr. Jackson, he tells you he needs to use the toilet. You know from the chart that at this visit the patient will need to give a urine specimen. Should you provide him with a specimen container and ask that he give the specimen now, even though you usually do it later in the exam? Again, the answer is yes. This is a good example of anticipating a diagnostic need. Even if you are not sure if the specimen will be needed, it cannot hurt to obtain it and avoid the possibility that the patient will not be able to produce a specimen 15 or 30 minutes later.

3. Dr. Lopez was delayed at the hospital and has been running late all day. You usually weigh each patient and take blood pressure before the exam, but Dr. Lopez is coming into the exam room just as you bring Mrs. Costello in. Should you delay the exam by doing weight and blood pressure? Or should you get Ms. Fredericks into another exam room, do the weight and blood pressure on her, then come in and do weight and blood pressure on Mrs. Costello while Dr. Lopez sees Ms. Fredericks?

   This is one where the first time it happens you're going to have to ask Dr. Lopez what his or her preference is in this situation. Dr. Lopez may find it easier to mentally "get into" the exam by seeing those weight and blood pressure numbers. On the other hand, Dr. Lopez's colleague, Dr. Hughes, may find it just as easy to have two exams happening essentially simultaneously, getting data such as weight and blood pressure from both in a more random fashion.

   How you ask Dr. Lopez or Dr. Hughes about their preference on issues like patient flow says a lot about how you work as a team member. Even if you have been given some preparation about an issue from the head medical assistant in the office, you might want to double-check with the doctor the first time it comes up.

   Remember also that you may use your powers of observation, but you are not the person who acts on those observations. You should note your observation, either in the chart, verbally to the doctor, or on a note attached to the chart by a paper clip or a self-sticking note, depending on the policy in your office. You may not use any term that could be interpreted as a diagnosis.

   You can say, "The patient complains of a rash and the skin on his arms is red, raised, flaky, and contains a few open sores." You *cannot* say, "The patient has dermatitis on his arms" because dermatitis—inflammation of the skin—is a diagnosis. An important thing to focus on during your training is how to identify diagnostic terms.

4. You notice, while weighing Mr. Jeffreys, that he is visibly short of breath and sweating. Should you tell this to the doctor? You need to communicate this information. After sitting in an exam room for 3 or 4 minutes waiting for the doctor, the patient's breathing may become regular and he may stop sweating. But the doctor should be aware that he was in that condition 3 minutes ago.

thought of as ordering food at a restaurant a la carte: so much for the main course, so much for a salad, so much for coffee.

Health care providers got into the habit of providing Cadillac level care for everyone with health insurance, because the insurance paid for every test and every procedure. Doctors' incomes soared between the end of World War II and the early 1980s. With the increasing costs of diagnostic testing, hospital services, and office visits, the cost of medical care increased far more rap-

idly than the cost of other goods and services in the U.S. economy. (In technical economic terms, health care inflation increased much more rapidly than the general rate of inflation.)

During this time, ever better health insurance, untaxed, became a standard employee benefit at many companies. The first kind of health insurance offered, in the 1950s and 1960s, was coverage for hospital care. Coverage for office visits became standard in the 1970s.

FOCUS ON
HISTORY OF THE MEDICAL MODEL

Within the medical model every condition is described scientifically and clinically, and objective criteria are given by which a doctor can make a diagnosis. With this system, the tendency is that body systems and groups of diseases get compartmentalized. More and more doctors develop special interests.

The advantage of this is that patients with rare diseases or severe conditions can usually find at any major medical center a doctor who makes a practice of dealing with that specific condition. The disadvantage has been that in the U.S. medical system in the second half of the 20th century too many doctors specialized and not enough trained broadly to provide primary care to all communities. Another disadvantage of specializing is that the doctor may tend to focus more on the disease than the patient as a person.

Historians argue about where exactly to place the beginning of the modern medical model. A good place to start might be with the English scientist William Harvey (1578–1657), who rejected the traditional belief that blood was made up of "spirits" and that body fluids were "humors." Harvey was responsible for the theory—later proved true—that blood flows from the heart to the lungs, throughout the body via arteries and back to the heart via veins.

The first microscopic lens was invented in 1677 by Antonie van Leeuwenhoek (1632–1723). van Leeuwenhoek saw through his microscope yeasts, molds, and algae. He also identified red blood cells, adding evidence to the theory that diseases could be caused by particles too small to be seen with the eyes.

Throughout the 19th century, a host of scientists and doctors advanced the understanding of the cause of disease. Some found ways to combat disease without understanding the mechanism by which the disease acted; others determined the actual cause of a particular disease.

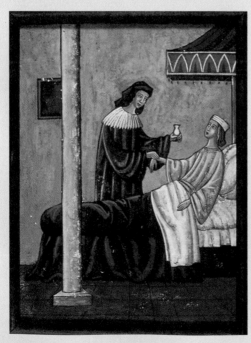

➤ **Figure 2–A** Doctor in the Middle Ages taking patient's pulse and holding a flask of urine (From the Blocker History of Medicine Collection)

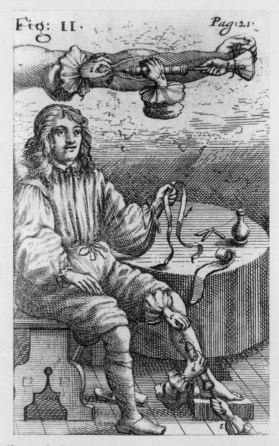

➤ **Figure 2–B** Extracting blood for a transfusion, 18th century (Courtesy of the National Library of Medicine)

In the 1840s, the Viennese obstetric assistant Ignaz Semmelweis, determined to solve the problem of puerperal fever, or so-called childbed fever, a fatal illness of women who had just given birth. He believed that doctors were infecting women by transferring bacteria from one woman to another.

Semmelweis conducted what today would be called an epidemiologic study. He studied the records of women who had died and determined which doctors and medical students had attended which birth. His study of the records led him to conclude that most of the women who died had been attended to by doctors and medical students who had come into the birthing room directly from the anatomy lab, where they had worked with cadavers, without first washing their hands. Most of Semmelweis's colleagues dismissed his notion that simple handwashing could reduce childbirth deaths as nonsense, and during his lifetime, Semmelweis was ridiculed. It was not until decades later that doctors regularly began washing their hands.

The Scottish surgeon Joseph Lister (1827–1912) worked on similar ideas to develop the first practice of antisepsis (cleaning areas where germs may be) and later asepsis (creating a germ-free environment.) Lister started by pouring carbolic acid on the wounds of those who had just had surgery. Over time, he found milder substances. Lister found that far fewer patients who were treated with these substances died from gangrene that developed in their open wounds.

Semmelweis, Lister, and others worked **empirically,** which means they determined a result through experimentation that proved the event could be **replicated,** or performed repeatedly with the same results. They never completely understood what caused infectious diseases. Other scientists sought to determine that bacteria caused specific diseases.

The German doctor Robert Koch (1843–1910) is called the Father of Microbiology because of his work with specific bacteria such as *Mycobacterium tuberculosis,* the bacterial agent that causes tuberculosis. Koch also isolated the bacterial agent that causes anthrax. Koch grew the anthrax bacterium in a number of different liquid media in his laboratory; all of them carried the same virulence, the potential for infection. Koch established that bacteria do not die out naturally. Today we know that it is possible to break the chain of illness by keeping those who are contagious away from those who are vulnerable to disease.

Koch's methods are today known as Koch's Postulates, which are used to prove that a particular infectious agent is causing a disease in more than one individual:

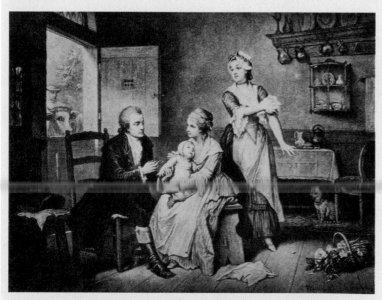

➢ **Figure 2–C** Edward Jenner vaccinating an infant (Courtesy of the National Library of Medicine)

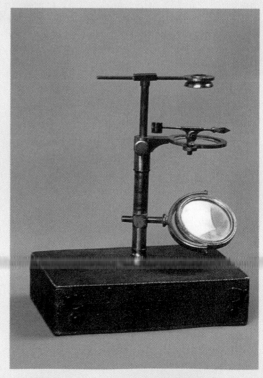

➢ **Figure 2–D** Early microscope, about 1765 (From the Blocker History of Medicine Collection)

Focus On continued on next page

1. Isolate an organism.

2. Inject the organism into a healthy animal.

3. The animal becomes sick.

4. Recover the same organism from the sick animal.

The work of Louis Pasteur and Koch, among others, helped set the stage for the understanding of infectious disease and for worldwide vaccination programs to eradicate smallpox and to try to eradicate the "childhood illnesses" of mumps, measles, and rubella (German measles).

The first vaccination actually had occurred a century earlier. Edward Jenner (1749–1823), an English doctor in the farming country of Gloucestershire, used the pus from one person's cowpox lesion to vaccinate another individual against smallpox in 1796.

Cowpox is a variant of smallpox. It is lethal to animals but relatively harmless to humans. For centuries, people had realized that people who had been infected with cowpox did not develop small-pox. Today, we understand that what had happened was that their immune systems had developed antibodies that prevented smallpox infection by attacking the smallpox virus.

Before Jenner, doctors had tried to immunize people against smallpox through a method known as "variolation," deliberately infecting a person with a mild smallpox infection by taking the pus from a smallpox lesion. Variolation usually led to only mild cases of smallpox in those deliberately infected, but they remained contagious and unfortunately were able to pass on lethal cases to others.

Jenner used "humanized cowpox," taking pus from a lesion on a human and rubbing it into an open wound on another human. A couple of weeks later, he inoculated the second person with smallpox. Not only did the individual not become ill, but he also was not contagious. A century later Pasteur would discover fully the mechanism by which vaccination works.

See Table 2–2, Milestones in the History of Medicine.

The basic work of these scientists has led to the scientific method used today, in the basic sciences as well as in medicine. The goal of scientific study is error-free understanding of the world and all its parts. Two means of checking for correctness are repetition and consensus. Scientific investigation usually limits itself to those phenomena that can be induced to repeat themselves, preferably whenever desired. To become scientifically valid, a phenomenon must be checked and rechecked through repeated experimen-tation, and different observers must reach consensus, agreeing about what has been seen.

Although consensus increases the likelihood that an observation is not in error, it is still possible for a large group of people to be influenced by the same bias so that the entire group is mistaken or has an incomplete understanding.

The increase in the quantity of health care services and the increase in the costs of that care did not happen all at once.

In the 1960s, the federal government became the largest provider of health insurance. Through Medicaid, which provides health insurance for the poor; Medi-care, which provides health insurance for the elderly, disabled, and those with end-stage kidney disease; and CHAMPUS (now called TRICARE), which provides health insurance for dependents of active-duty military personnel, the federal government is today the primary insurer for more than 50 million Americans.

These plans, which paid for office visits, greatly in-creased the number of Americans who had medical insurance. There was little incentive for the consumer (the patient) to control costs, because insurance was covering those costs and in most cases was "free" to the consumer.

Although most Americans who were insured did not feel that they were "paying" for their medical care, they were, indirectly. The huge increases in health care costs were one of the major sources of the generally high rates of inflation in the 1970s. Employers, who paid for the insurance, had to pay ever-rising premiums and offset these large premium increases with small in-creases in cash wages, which did not keep up with inflation. So American workers did, in fact, pay for health insurance and health care costs in lower pur-chasing power for the cash they received as salary.

The expansion of health care to cover office visits originally only covered visits for illness or injury and did not cover so-called routine care (well-child visits, immunizations, regular check-ups, or physical exams).

Health Maintenance Organizations (HMOs) were originally formed to cover the costs of routine care. The HMO concept was based on the belief that con-sistent, routine care would help prevent later expensive care by increasing prevention and promoting early de-tection and diagnosis of chronic and life-threatening medical conditions. The HMO movement, which

Table 2–2	**Milestones in the History of Medicine**

3000 B.C.	Writings about the circulation of blood in China
460 B.C.	Birth of **Hippocrates** (called Father of Medicine) in Greece—based medical care on observation and believed that illness was a natural biological event
1514–1564	**Andreas Vesalius**—wrote the first relatively correct anatomy textbook
1578–1657	**William Harvey**—discovered circulation of blood (England)
1632–1723	**Antonie van Leeuwenhoek**—discovered the microscope (Holland) **Medical schools in the great cities of Europe (London, Paris, Leyden)**
1728–1793	**John Hunter**—developed surgical techniques used in surgery
1749–1823	**Edward Jenner**—first vaccine for smallpox (England)
1818–1865	**Ignaz Semmelweis**—theorized that handwashing prevents childbirth fever (Austria); his theories were rejected during his lifetime and not accepted until the work of Pasteur and Lister
1822–1895	**Louis Pasteur**—pasteurization of wine, beer, and milk to prevent growth of microorganisms; microbiology (France).
1820–1910	**Florence Nightingale**—began training for nurses; established first nursing school; before this time nurses received no training and the profession had very little status (England).
1821–1912	**Clara Barton**—founded the American Red Cross (U.S.)
1821–1910	**Elizabeth Blackwell**—first woman to complete medical school in the U.S.; established a medical school in Europe for women only
1827–1912	**Joseph Lister**—demonstrated that microorganisms cause illness; his experiments with phenol, carbolic acid, and other antiseptics laid the groundwork for modern surgery (England).
mid-1800s	**First large hospitals established in U.S. cities, such as Bellevue, Johns Hopkins, and Massachusetts General** Discovery of **anesthesia** in U.S. is credited to a Southern doctor named **Crawford Williamson Long.**
1843–1910	**Robert Koch**—isolated the bacteria which cause anthrax and cholera; established principles to determine that a specific bacteria causes a specific disease (German).
1845–1923	**Wilhelm Roentgen**—discovered X-rays (Germany) based on the discovery of radium and radioactivity by **Marie (1867–1934) and Pierre Curie (1859–1906)**
1881–1955	**Alexander Fleming**—discovered penicillin (England); identified it in 1929, but an efficient method of producing large amounts was not developed until needed in World War II. Other antibiotic medications, such as sulfa, were soon discovered.
1891–1941	**Frederick Banting**—co-discoverer of insulin with Charles Best and John Macleod in 1922
1906–1993	**Albert Sabin**—developed oral polio vaccine
1914–1995	**Jonas Salk**—developed parenteral polio vaccine

gained acceptance in the 1970s, pushed traditional health insurance companies to provide coverage for routine care.

In the late 1970s, insurance companies began to respond to escalating health care costs by reviewing care to find out if it was medically necessary. This process, called utilization review (UR), identified patients who, according to the insurance companies, no longer needed to be hospitalized. Originally, UR was used by Medicare and Medicaid, but other insurance companies soon realized that shortening hospital stays was an important way of reducing overall health care costs. The combination of HMO insurance plans and strict utilization review for hospitalized patients is the basis of what we call managed care.

The original HMO model had two components: insurance and the provision of services, which included diagnostic tests and pharmacy. Doctors were employees. The HMO established a contractual relationship with a hospital for inpatient services, and patients had to go to the specific hospital with which the HMO had a contract.

In the later 1980s, a second type of HMO model came into being, based on networks of doctors who agreed to provide care for HMO patients. Some of these networks operated under the old fee-for-service plans, but agreed to discounted fees from the HMOs in exchange for access to the rapidly growing patient populations enrolled in HMOs. Increasingly, such "open-panel" HMOs pressed primary care doctors to provide all office care for patients for an annual rate; this type of payment is called capitation.

Under the capitation system, the doctor receives a certain amount of money monthly for each member of the HMO plan for whom he or she provides primary care services. Specialists also have contracts with HMOs to provide their services for a set fee per visit. In most capitation plans, the fees to specialists must be paid by the primary care doctor who refers the patient; this puts the burden on doctors to provide most care to each patient in a primary care setting to maximize the amount of the capitation fee he or she gets to keep.

The HMO movement in general, and the capitation system in particular, put the burden on doctors to compete with each other to provide the most care for the least money. As a result, doctors feel pressure to reduce hospitalizations and the number of days patients stay in the hospital and to use generic instead of brand-name drugs. (Generics are identical in chemical formulation to brand-name drugs and can only be manufactured after the brand-name drug's patent protection has expired.)

Capitation also puts pressure on doctors to see more patients, spend less time with each patient, and justify all services, including diagnostic tests and referrals. The expense of handling sicker patients is expected to be balanced by those patients who use less than the average amount of medical services.

In addition, HMOs have tried to reduce their costs for prescription medications by restricting what drugs doctors can prescribe by devising lists of approved drugs. These so-called formularies usually limit doctors to one or two of the less expensive drugs for each possible medical condition, unless the doctor can show that those drugs have been ineffective for his or her patient and that a more expensive drug is needed.

Some HMOs provide for treatment of chronically ill patients, who must see specialists frequently, through excess payments to either the primary care doctor holding the capitation contract or directly to the specialist through some kind of capitation override system.

Despite these measures, however, in the late 1990s, insurance premiums began to increase at more than double and even triple the underlying rate of inflation. HMOs, even those that had instituted capitation in the early 1990s, saw their ability to limit costs severely hampered. In addition, prescription drug costs increased more than 15 percent a year in the late 1990s.

Consumers and doctors both became increasingly upset about the control of medical practice exacted by insurance companies. And doctors began banding together in larger groups—either large practices or individual practice associations (IPAs), which are groups of solo or small group practices—to negotiate more rigorously with HMOs. It remains to be seen how managed care will evolve and respond to consumer and doctor dissatisfaction.

Each form of providing health care services has advantages and disadvantages. A comparison of managed care and fee-for-service care is shown in Table 2–3.

CONCLUSION

Whether you work in a general medical, pediatric, or obstetric practice, or in a specialty practice; whether in a private practice, a community health center, or a hospital clinic; whether in a practice that focuses on treatments or on preventive health care, your work as a medical assistant will be rewarding. You will be an important member of a team dedicated to the well-being of others, to the compassionate care of people at their most vulnerable.

Table 2–3	Comparison of Managed Care and Traditional Fee-for-Service Plans	
	Managed Care	Traditional Fee-for-Service
	Doctor Choice Patient must see a member doctor. Primary provider refers to specialists. Patient may be seen by a provider other than own primary provider.	*Doctor Choice* Patient can see any doctor. Patient can choose to see a specialist. Patient always sees doctor of choice.
	Services Plan pays for routine and preventive care as well as illness and injury. Each plan has own guidelines and schedules about how often routine procedures can be done. Each plan has guidelines about what type of tests and treatments can be ordered for a specific diagnosis. Plan pays part or all of medication, although the patient may be responsible for a greater portion if the medication is not on the list approved by the plan. Plan pays part or all of other services such as eye exams and glasses.	*Services* Plan covers illness or injury only. Doctor can order any tests or treatments. Medications are not covered. Nonmedical services are not covered.
	Patient Payments Patient pays a set fee (co-payment) for each visit or service.	*Patient Payments* Patient pays an annual fee (deductible) and set percent of each service (coinsurance).
	Insurance Payments Doctor may receive an annual payment for each patient (capitation) or may be paid by service at a significant discount from usual charge for the service.	*Insurance Payments* Doctor is paid by service; actual amount varies according to insurance; government plans may pay much less than the usual charge for the service.

STUDENT STUDY PLAN

To reinforce your understanding of the material in this chapter . . .

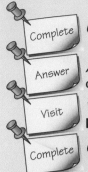

Complete the **Review & Recall** questions below.

Answer the **Critical Thinking Questions** below, and discuss them with your classmates.

Visit the **Web sites** suggested below and search for additional Web sites using **Keywords for Internet Searches**.

Complete the exercises in chapter 2 of the **Student Mastery Manual**.

REVIEW & RECALL

1. In what year was the American Association of Medical Assistants founded? In what year was the profession recognized by the U.S. Department of Education?

2. List four areas of responsibility of the medical assistant, and give specific duties in each area.

3. Describe activities that take place in the four basic areas of the medical office.

4. Identify several members of the health team, including primary care providers and allied health care personnel.

5. List the three types of medical office laboratories and identify two government agencies that are responsible for their regulation.

6. Identify three trends that have a significant impact on modern medical care in the doctor's office.

CRITICAL THINKING QUESTIONS

1. Compare and contrast the education and responsibilities of a doctor with those of a medical assistant.

2. Choose a medical discovery such as the circulation of blood, the microscope, immunization, or hand washing, and imagine what health care might be like if this discovery had never been made.

3. Imagine that you must choose between two health care plans offered by your employer—one a traditional fee-for-service plan and the other a managed care plan. Discuss the factors that influence your choice. What kind of research will you need to do before making a choice between the two plans?

4. What responsibilities do medical assistants usually have in the area where you live? Discuss how you can get information to answer this question, and then research the topic.

5. What are the advantages and disadvantages of a team approach to patient care, based on your own experience of teamwork? Describe your own strengths and weaknesses as a team member or team player. How can you use your educational experience to improve your teamwork?

EXPLORE THE WEB

INTERNET WEB SITES

AAMA—American Association of Medical Assistants
www.aama-ntl.org

Education of doctors
www.medicalstudent.com

Health statistics
www.cdc.gov/nchswww
www.naphsis.org

Insurance

    Medicare
    www.medicare.gov

    Medicaid
    www.medicaidfaq.com

managed care
www.mceconnection.com

laboratory regulation
www.phppo.cdc.gov/clia/default.asp

KEYWORDS FOR INTERNET SEARCHES

CLIA-Clinical Laboratory Improvement Amendments
    managed care
    medical assisting
    medical history
    medical licensure

Chapter 3

What Kinds of Health Care Do Patients Look for and Why?

Instructional Objectives

After completing this chapter, you will be able to do the following:

1. Define and spell vocabulary words for this chapter.
2. Describe the levels of Maslow's hierarchy of needs.
3. List factors that affect patient expectations of health care.
4. Identify different ways that medical care is provided.
5. Describe medical specialties and subspecialties.
6. Describe three basic types of medical practice.
7. Differentiate among complementary, alternative, and non-Western medical care.
8. Compare and contrast various complementary and alternative medical treatments.
9. Describe general health practices of Southeast Asian, African-American, and Latino cultures.

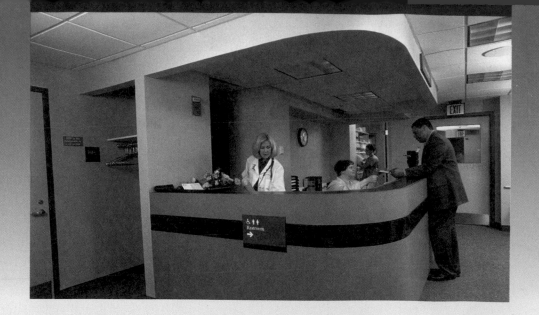

- Understand hereditary, cultural, and environmental influences on behavior
- Understand concepts of mental health and applied psychology

- Instruct individuals with special and specific needs

VOCABULARY

acting out (p. 40)	ego defense mechanism (p. 40)	palliative (p. 38)	projection (p. 40)
anxiety (p. 40)	empathy (p. 40)	physiologic needs (p. 39)	self-actualization (p. 39)
chronic (p. 39)	hierarchy (p. 38)	practice model (p. 44)	symptomatic (p. 38)
denial (p. 40)	holistic (p. 47)		

The World Health Organization (WHO) defines health as the absence of illness or disease, a state of being in which the individual feels well and is able to carry out the daily functions of life with no difficulties and no pain. In reality, no one reaches this optimum level of health. Everyone has aches and pains, psychological if not physical.

In our health care system, the doctor's function is to look at hundreds of people in the course of a week and try to zero in on particular problems that meet two criteria: they are causing or can cause severe difficulties in carrying out the daily functions of life and they can be treated, either by reducing the effects of the symptoms or by eradicating the problem altogether.

Each person the doctor sees presents the doctor with a different group of physical symptoms, as well as a different set of social circumstances and emotional issues. The doctor listens to the patient's description of his or her life, performs objective tests, and asks of each problem:

Is it serious?
Will it progress to become serious?
Is it going to interfere with any vital body processes (for example, circulation, breathing, elimination of waste)?

Doctors know that the vast majority of health problems do not pose a long-term threat to health. Most problems get better over time. Effective treatments are available to cure many problems; in many other cases the doctor can reduce the symptoms of the problem even if the underlying process is not significantly affected. This second kind of treatment is called **symptomatic** (responding to symptoms) or **palliative** (seeking to relieve or alleviate symptoms without curing the underlying condition).

Most treatments are grounded in scientific study; in the Western scientific tradition, as in no other medical tradition, medical approaches have been studied and tested. Doctors have large amounts of data about how effective medications, diagnostic tests, treatments, and procedures are at doing what they are supposed to do.

Even though scientific studies predict a certain response to a particular treatment or procedure, unless a doctor actually performs the treatment, the outcome is uncertain. The more the patient must cooperate with the procedure or treatment, or even perform the treat-

ment or procedure himself or herself, the less precisely it can be known what the outcome will be. This is because it is difficult to determine exactly how well patients are following the advice given to them. Motivating patients to comply with treatment is a responsibility of everyone in the office.

This self-contradiction in Western scientific medicine is very important for the medical assistant to understand. We know what medical science can deal with very well, pretty well, and not well at all.

The doctor focuses most on identifying medical problems and developing appropriate interventions and treatments. He or she wants to put the most energy into what can be dealt with very well, using procedures and treatments that are doctor controlled.

But patients have lots of personal feelings and beliefs that affect their response to health care and their cooperation. By establishing a warm and caring atmosphere, and by thoroughly explaining procedures and sometimes treatment regimens, medical assistants help foster any given patient's understanding and desire to become responsible for decisions affecting his or her health. Because medical assistants seem less like authority figures than do doctors, many patients will reveal their thoughts and feelings more readily to them.

This chapter discusses some basic psychological theory and explains in more detail what patients expect from health care. It discusses how these expectations often conflict with what doctors believe they are providing. It also discusses medical specialties and contrasts the Western scientific medical tradition with other medical traditions. Finally, the chapter concludes with a discussion of cross-cultural influences on patient behavior and expectations.

EFFECT OF BASIC NEEDS ON PATIENT BEHAVIOR IN THE HEALTH CARE SETTING

Maslow's Hierarchy of Needs

In his book, *Motivation and Personality*, the American psychiatrist Abraham Maslow defined what has come to be known as "Maslow's hierarchy of needs." The **hierarchy**, an arrangement in order of importance, describes the ascending ladder of human needs. This is shown as Figure 3–1. On the bottom of the pyramid

acute & chronic

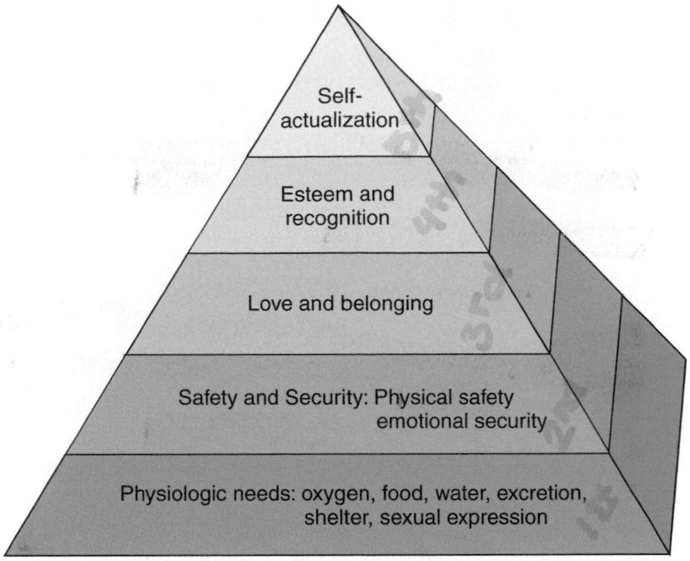

> **Figure 3–1** Maslow's hierarchy of needs

starts @ bottom then go UP

#1 (Level 1) are the **physiologic needs.** These are the basic biological needs for survival: oxygen, water, food, excretion, sleep, shelter, and sexual expression.

On the next level of the pyramid (Level 2) are the needs for *safety and security*. These include avoiding harm, attaining physical safety, and the emotional security that comes with freedom from fear and anxiety.

On the middle level of the pyramid (Level 3) are the needs for *love and belonging*. These include both receiving and giving personal affection, companionship with another individual, and identification with a group.

On the fourth level of the pyramid (Level 4) are the needs for *esteem and recognition*. These include self-esteem, the respect of others in one's peer group, success in work, and prestige in the community.

Finally, at the pyramid's pinnacle (Level 5) is the need for **self-actualization.** This is the fulfillment of each individual's potential.

Effects of Unmet Needs During Illness

It's important to understand that an individual cannot step up to the next level on Maslow's pyramid until his or her needs have been fully met on the current level. What does this mean in the context of medical office care?

An individual moves up or down in his or her place on the pyramid depending on what needs are currently unmet. Only when lower-level needs are met will the person be able to devote any significant amount of energy or concern for needs that are higher on the pyramid. In fact, a person has all the needs all the time but only becomes aware of higher-level needs once the lower-level needs are met.

This has a number of implications for the way patients relate to the medical care they receive.

First, many patients who come to the medical office are struggling to meet basic needs because they are ill. Health care professionals must recognize any difficulties in that area.

Second, the WHO definition of health cited at the beginning of this chapter implies that health requires more than just meeting basic needs. Part of health professionals' role is to foster the meeting of needs beyond physiologic needs. Some examples include:

1. Intervening for an abused child or battered woman helps meet needs for safety and security, as well as some sense of love and belonging, by knowing someone cares.
2. Teaching patients how to manage a **chronic** disease—one that continues to exist over time—helps a person's self-esteem by making the person feel competent in self-care.

Another area where understanding the hierarchy of need helps in the health care setting is the use of attention-getting behavior by patients to satisfy needs for love and belonging, or for esteem and recognition. Again, when people are ill, their usual means for meeting their attention needs (both for love and belonging, and esteem and recognition) may be interrupted.

Medical assistants must be able to recognize this and respond to these needs appropriately. Even if the medical assistant cannot directly meet the needs (the medical assistant is not a close friend and should not attempt to be one), by recognizing that the person feels a loss in this area, the medical assistant helps the person to identify his or her feelings and to cope with whatever need is not being met.

To be helpful in meeting an individual's needs, a person must not only be able to identify the individual's feelings of need, but also to understand those feelings, not in an intellectual way but in an emotional way. This understanding is called empathy. Empathy is the capacity to make an emotional connection with another person's feelings without allowing those feelings to become overpowering.

Illness, fear of certain diseases (such as cancer), loss of function associated with certain conditions, and impending death all can stir up strong feelings, including fear and anger, in a patient. An effective medical assistant must learn to be comfortable sharing some of these intense feelings with patients.

In many instances, the medical assistant may be the individual who identifies these feelings and explains them to a patient who is experiencing them but doesn't know what to call them. Many times in American culture, people are discouraged from experiencing strong emotions or at least from discussing them with others. A patient may feel embarrassed or ashamed by such emotions.

Reassure the patient that whatever he or she is feeling, a genuine emotional response to a situation, including the wish to avoid painful feelings, occurs spontaneously and can be accepted by others.

Often people do not know exactly what they are feeling. They may experience vague apprehension, uneasiness, or feelings of dread called anxiety. To reduce or avoid this feeling, they may adopt one of several ego defense mechanisms—unconscious mental processes and behavioral strategies that offer psychological protection. Instead of experiencing a feeling directly, they either say it is a feeling of someone else—called projection, fail to acknowledge the reality of the situation—called denial, or translate their feelings into an inappropriate activity—called acting out.

Through empathy, the health care professional should have some idea of what the underlying emotion is; by accepting it he or she can help the patient to become more aware that such feelings are normal and can be worked with. Medical assistants are often in a good position to do this because patients may feel more comfortable expressing emotion to them than to doctors. Patients may need support to adopt unfamiliar coping strategies in response to stress, including illness.

EGO DEFENSE MECHANISMS

Defense mechanisms are used by everyone at some time or another to protect against being overwhelmed by painful feelings. Although a person is sometimes aware of using these mechanisms, usually they operate on an unconscious level—that is, the person is not aware that he or she is disguising or blocking emotions or impulses.

Everyone tends to use defense mechanisms that have been effective in the past to reduce stress or anxiety. When a person first encounters a situation that would provoke strong feelings, such as a diagnosis of serious illness, a defense mechanism such as denial helps him or her avoid feeling overwhelmed and unable to cope. (Denial is unconsciously refusing to acknowledge something that is difficult to accept.) People say things like "It doesn't seem real to me" or "This must be a mistake."

Denial allows the truth to penetrate gradually, so the person has a chance to get used to the threat, to seek privacy to experience intense emotion, and to avoid total disorientation. However, if a person continues to use denial without attempting to accept the situation, negative consequences may occur.

The person may not take appropriate actions to respond to illness. Friends and family may respond negatively to the person's perceived lack of responsibility. And the person may miss the opportunity to grow and strengthen his or her sense of self-worth and ability to cope with adversity.

If a medical assistant can identify a patient's defense mechanisms and coping patterns, he or she can gain a better understanding of the patient's underlying fears and concerns. The medical assistant can try to respond to these concerns, but should not directly challenge the defenses or label them.

Any attack on defenses a person is using tends to increase the amount of energy the person invests in defending. On the other hand, supporting defenses perceived as necessary by another tends to promote a feeling of being understood and may decrease the need for rigidity in the defenses.

Example

Mr. Sykes has had to wait for about 45 minutes past his appointment time to see Dr. Lopez. When Kathy, the medical assistant, takes him back to the exam room, he says, "I think you should know that some of the people in the waiting room are really upset about how long they have been waiting."

Kathy may suspect that this is an example of projection—unconsciously identifying thoughts or feelings as originating in someone else when they really are one's own thoughts and feelings. She can be helpful to Mr. Sykes by responding in a way that reassures him that it is understandable for a person to be upset when there is an unusually long wait.

Responses that are not helpful (because they reinforce Mr. Sykes' fear that it would be dangerous to express a negative emotion directly) are:

1. Making it seem as if Mr. Sykes is overreacting and should not feel upset ("Oh, it hasn't been that long")
2. Labeling or challenging the defense mechanism ("Do you always project your own feelings on people around you?")
3. Trying to defend the doctor so the office will look good ("Dr. Lopez has been very busy with several sick patients.")
4. Talking negatively about the patients in the waiting room ("Some people are never happy, no matter how quickly they are seen.").

Below is a list of several other ego defense mechanisms, with examples that might occur in a medical office. Remember that using defense mechanisms usually helps people adapt to stressful situations.

Ego Defense Mechanisms

Mechanism	Definition	Examples
Selective inattention	Failing to hear or pay attention to information that may provoke anxiety	A patient expresses the belief that his cancer will definitely be cured if he has the primary tumor removed.
Regression	Returning to the emotional adjustment of an earlier stage of growth and development	An ill person who could be independent asks for assistance with personal hygiene.
Depersonalization	Removing feeling from something that is perceived as stressful	A medical assistant who is assisting with a lumbar puncture on a young child experiences the child as looking like a toy or doll.
Rationalization	Assigning logical reasons or excuses for actions which may have been motivated by self-interest or other emotions the person does not wish to acknowledge	A patient justifies not telling the doctor that he smokes by saying to himself, "The doctor isn't interested because he didn't ask about it."
Repression	Unconsciously excluding unacceptable ideas, impulses, or emotions from awareness	A diabetic patient who hates fingersticks continually forgets to test her blood sugar.
Suppression	Deciding to put uncomfortable or painful thoughts out of awareness	A patient says, "I don't want to think about my surgery until the day before."
Displacement	Shifting an emotion or behavior from the original object to a more acceptable substitute	A medical assistant who has just been given a poor evaluation is extremely rude to the next person she talks to on the telephone.
Undoing	Attempting to make amends for a feeling or behavior that makes the person feel guilty	A patient who notices that she hates the medical assistant's hairstyle and hair color immediately tells the medical assistant that she has beautiful eyes.
Compensation	Attempting to overcome a real or perceived handicap by developing some other ability or trait	A person who thinks that she is not very intelligent in school always offers to help the teacher.

EFFECTS OF PATIENT EXPECTATIONS

What Patients Expect from Health Care

Patient expectations are wrapped up in each patient's individual life circumstances, unmet physiological or psychological needs, and what kind of experiences the person has had in the past with the health care system.

Patients want to be seen by a doctor in a reasonable amount of time, and they want the doctor to "fix" whatever is wrong. Patients do not expect to have long-term problems. They want to be treated as if they were cars and doctors were mechanics—fix what's broken and get me back on the road of life!

In addition, people expect doctors to take care of them when they are really sick and not fuss too much over them when they are generally well. People certainly do not want doctors to nag them about changing their lifestyle to improve their health. But doctors, especially those who practice primary care adult medicine or pediatrics, tend to take a much more aggressive stance today when confronting patients about lifestyle issues such as eating healthy foods in reasonable portions, not smoking, reducing alcohol intake, and exercising. A healthy lifestyle can reduce the amount and intensity of medical care a person needs in the future.

Doctors know that people should get checked regularly to make sure nothing is going on that cannot be seen or felt by the patient. This is called "preventive medicine" or "wellness." Receiving health care even when one is not feeling bad can help detect a number of cancers, such as breast, testicular, prostate, and colorectal cancer; it can also help patients get early treatment in cases of diabetes, glaucoma, tuberculosis, heart disease, hypertension (high blood pressure), and scoliosis, to name just some of the conditions that can be detected by examination or diagnostic tests before the patient experiences actual symptoms.

One of the benefits of the managed care movement has been its increased emphasis on routine care and regular diagnostic testing for early detection of problems. Health professionals themselves have been teaching patients for years that it is important to have regular checkups, lab tests, and diagnostic procedures like mammograms and sigmoidoscopies.

Conflicts Between Patient Expectations and Provider Services

Conflicts between patient expectations and services provided by medical offices do arise. In some health maintenance organizations (HMOs), patients do not always see the same doctor for urgent problems, and they often feel that there is poor continuity of care, that the people caring for them do not know them, and that the treatment they receive is inconsistent. Often patients cannot obtain appointments with their primary care provider without waiting longer than they feel they should. This may be both waiting to get an appointment, then physically waiting to see the doctor once they are in the office.

Patients are sometimes so wrapped up in their primary aim—to get relief from pain or other symptoms—that they have difficulty accepting that doctors are often looking for the root cause of their illness, not just to alleviate symptoms. This can cause a lot of frustration for patients, especially if no significant relief can be given or if the doctor does not seem to think that alleviating the symptoms would be appropriate.

A common example is a viral illness such as the common cold. A patient may have a fever, muscle aches, weakness, vomiting, and diarrhea. But once the doctor establishes that the patient is not suffering from a more serious condition and is not dehydrated, he or she may recommend only rest, fluids, and over-the-counter medication such as acetaminophen or ibuprofen for fever reduction and relief of soreness.

This can be very frustrating for a patient, who wants to feel better and have a speedy recovery. Often patients turn to alternative medical treatments in place of,

or complementary therapies in addition to, their regular medical care. The popularity of alternative and complementary therapies has been surprising to the medical establishment, especially since they usually are not paid for by health insurance. Despite the scarcity of rigorous scientific studies of these therapies, many patients feel that they are often effective and that their practitioners are somehow more personal and empathetic than medical doctors.

STRUCTURE OF TRADITIONAL SCIENTIFIC MEDICAL CARE

Medical Specialties

Since the middle of the 20th century, the practice of medicine has been broken down into fields of specialty and subspecialty. In 1950 most Americans received their medical care from a general practitioner, who took care of adults and children, often delivered babies, and performed many general surgical procedures.

Today, Americans may see two, three, or more doctors routinely. Table 3–1 shows medical specialties and subspecialties.

Primary care doctors either specialize in internal medicine (treatment of the internal organs of adults by other than surgical means), pediatrics (general medical care of children and adolescents), or family medicine (general medical care of children, adolescents, and adults; today's equivalent of general practice).

Over the course of time, the activities of different types of doctors has shifted. For instance, fewer family practitioners deliver babies today than did general practitioners in the 1950s and 1960s, preferring to leave that task to obstetrician/gynecologists (OB/GYNs), due to the cost of malpractice insurance. However, although some women continue to see a gynecologist for an annual pelvic exam and Pap test, the primary care provider performs these activities more often today than in the past.

Because of the requirements for a primary care provider in managed care plans, some specialists—especially obstetrician/gynecologists—have taken over general care for some patients in their practice.

At a finer level of distinction are the subspecialists, also listed in Table 3–1.

All doctors participate in a period of training (called a residency) after medical school. Internal medicine, family practice, and pediatric residencies last 3 years; OB/GYN residencies last 4 years because of the need to learn surgery; psychiatric residencies last 3 years after 1 year of either internal medicine or pediatrics (total of 4 years); surgical residencies last 5 years or longer. In some states, it is possible to obtain a medical license without completing a residency program, but it is not

Table 3–1	**Medical Specialties and Subspecialties**

Specialties That Diagnose and Treat Using Medical Treatment

Allergy & Immunology (Allergist, Immunologist)
Treats adults and/or children with allergies and problems of the immune system *(hiv)*
   Subspecialty: Clinical and Laboratory Immunology

Emergency Medicine
Treats patients for emergency conditions, usually in the emergency room of a hospital
   Subspecialty: Pediatric Emergency Medicine

Family Practice (Family Practitioner)
Treats adults and children for routine care and complaints; often the primary care doctor for all family members
   Subspecialty: Geriatric Medicine (care of the elderly)

Internal Medicine (Internist)
Provides medical treatment for conditions of various body systems
Within the discipline of internal medicine are several subspecialties:
   Subspecialty: Adolescent Medicine (care of adolescents)
   Subspecialty: Cardiovascular Medicine (Cardiologist)
     Treats adults and/or children for conditions of the heart and circulatory system
   Subspecialty: Endocrinology (Endocrinologist)
     Specializes in the treatment of diseases of the endocrine glands, such as diabetes mellitus and thyroid problems
   Subspecialty: Gastroenterology (Gastroenterologist)
     Specializes in the treatment of diseases of the stomach and intestines
   Subspecialty: Hematology (Hematologist)
     Specializes in diseases of the blood and bone marrow, such as leukemia
   Subspecialty: Infectious Disease
     Specializes in the diagnosis and treatment of diseases caused by microorganisms
   Subspecialty: Medical Oncology (Oncologist)
     Specializes in the management of medical treatment for cancer
   Subspecialty: Nephrology (Nephrologist)
     Specializes in diseases of the kidney
   Subspecialty: Pulmonary Medicine
     Specializes in diseases of the lungs
   Subspecialty: Rheumatology (Rheumatologist)
     Specializes in medical treatment of rheumatic diseases that cause inflammation and pain of the muscles and joints
   Subspecialty: Sports Medicine
     Specializes in the prevention and treatment of conditions related to athletic activity

Neurology (Neurologist)
Treats adults and/or children with conditions of the nervous system such as epilepsy or Parkinson's disease

Occupational Medicine
Specializes in preventing, diagnosing, and treating conditions resulting from occupational hazards

Pediatrics (Pediatrician)
Specializes in the care of children. Many medical and surgical specialties have pediatric subspecialties:
   Subspecialties: Adolescent Medicine, Neonatal-Perinatal Medicine, Pediatric Cardiology, Pediatric Gastroenterology, Pediatric
   Hematology-Oncology, Pediatric Infectious Disease, Pediatric Nephrology, Pediatric Pulmonology

Physical Medicine & Rehabilitation (Physiatrist)
Specializes in the treatment and rehabilitation of patients with disabling conditions such as spinal cord injury and stroke

Psychiatry (Psychiatrist)
Specializes in diagnosing, treating and preventing mental illness
   Subspecialties: Addiction Psychiatry, Child & Adolescent Psychiatry, Clinical Neurophysiology

Specialties That Use Both Medical and Surgical Treatment

Dermatology (Dermatologist)
Specializes in conditions of the skin

Gastroenterology (Gastroenterologist)
Specializes in treatment of conditions of the stomach and small and large intestines

Obstetrics (Obstetrician) and Gynecology (Gynecologist)
Specializes in care during pregnancy and delivery (obstetrician); specializes in other care and surgery of the female reproductive
   system (gynecologist)

Ophthalmology (Ophthalmologist)
Specializes in the care of the eye, including surgery

Otolaryngology (Otolaryngologist or ENT)
Specializes in the care of the ear, nose, and throat, including surgery

Urology (Urologist)
Specializes in the care of the urinary system in males and females and the reproductive tract in males; also specializes in surgery
   of the urinary tract and male reproductive tract

Table continued on following page

Table 3–1	**Medical Specialties and Subspecialties** *(Continued)*

Specialties That Assist in Diagnosis and Treatment

Anesthesiology (Anesthesiologist)
Provides anesthesia during surgery and other procedures
Nuclear Medicine
Specializes in diagnosis using radionuclides, atoms that give off electromagnetic radiation
Pathology (Pathologist)
Examines cells, tissues, and other specimens to determine whether their structure is normal or abnormal; attempts to determine the nature or cause of disease
  Subspecialties: Blood Banking/Transfusion Medicine, Forensic Pathology, Immunopathology, Pediatric Pathology
Radiology (Radiologist)
Specializes in the use of X-ray and other ionizing radiation for diagnosis and treatment

Surgical Specialties

Colon and Rectal Surgery
Performs surgical treatment on the large intestine and rectum
General Surgery (General Surgeon)
Performs general surgical procedures
  Subspecialties: Pediatric Surgery, Surgical Critical Care, General Vascular Surgery
Neurological Surgery (Neurosurgeon)
Performs surgical treatment on the brain, spine, and nervous system
Orthopedic Surgery (Orthopedic Surgeon)
Performs surgical treatment on the musculoskeletal system
Plastic Surgery (Plastic Surgeon)
Performs surgical treatment to repair or reconstruct body structures
  Subspecialties: Hand Surgery, Maxillofacial Surgery

possible to be certified by any specialty board of examiners without completing a residency. Doctors who want to be subspecialists participate in an additional period of training after residency, called a fellowship, which usually lasts 2 or 3 years.

Subspecialties that perform surgery all have their own residency programs, which last 4 or 5 years. Some of these subspecialties are otorhinolaryngology—care and surgery of the ears, nose, and throat; ophthalmology—care and surgery of the eyes; and urology—care and surgery of the genitourinary tract.

Other specialties that have their own residency programs include:

Radiology—diagnosis using ionizing radiation (X-rays)
Pathology—study of diseased tissue via laboratory procedures and determination of cause of death
Nuclear Medicine—treatment of cancer using radiation and other substances.

Indeed, some of the subspecialties are being divided into even finer areas. For instance, some anesthesiologists work in the operating room keeping the patient anesthetized (asleep) during surgery; others focus on the treatment of post-surgical and other pain. Some cardiologists focus on treating problems of the heart using medications; others focus on such techniques as angioplasty, in which a catheter is threaded through a vein in the leg carrying a balloon that can be fastened to open up blocked arteries.

Practice Types

Fifty years ago most doctors who were not on full-time hospital staffs worked by themselves in a solo practice, and were "sole practitioners" for purposes of taxation and liability insurance. They paid their office expenses out of their income, and the difference was considered their "net income" from their practice. As their practice got busier their income increased.

Today, increasingly, doctors are employees working for a salary. Some of them have an ownership position in the company they work for, but others do not. When we talk about practice type, we are really talking about the combination of two variables:

One is the **practice model** under which the doctor

works, discussed here. The other is the business form the practice takes, discussed in chapter 40.

Solo Practice

It is still possible for a doctor to work in a solo practice. But to do so, he or she must make a number of trade-offs. Solo practices are limited in their size by the number of people one doctor can manage. When a doctor practices alone, the medical assistant is usually responsible for aspects of administrative and clinical support.

Even if a solo practitioner employs a nurse practitioner or physician's assistant to see additional patients, the doctor still must factor into his or her workday some time to oversee the work of these nondoctor professionals. In addition, the doctor, as the employer, is usually responsible for paying the malpractice insurance premiums for all of the licensed professionals in his or her office. Doctors in solo practice also must either be on call 24 hours a day, 7 days a week, or make arrangements with other doctors to share after-hours and weekend call.

Sometimes groups of doctors who practice alone share office space, equipment, and even a payroll for personnel (often each doctor pays his or her own nurse or medical assistant and a billing person, and the doctors share the salary of a receptionist). This type of arrangement is known as "expense sharing."

Multi-Practice, Single-Specialty

Most doctors today practice in a multi-practice, single-specialty model. In this model, a number of doctors who specialize in one area of medicine band together to share resources (office space, personnel). In these groups, medical assistants usually specialize in either clinical or administrative work.

Depending on the business form used, patients are either the responsibility of one doctor or "the group." In either case, if a patient's regular doctor is not available, another doctor in the office can see the patient. In addition, doctors who work in multi-practice, single-specialty groups usually share after-hours and weekend call responsibility. In addition, they usually split the cost of malpractice insurance, and the policy is written for the group rather than for each individual.

Multi-Practice, Multi-Specialty

Multi-practice, multi-specialty groups are becoming increasingly common throughout the country. This organizational form allows a sharing of resources that, in turn, allows each doctor in the group to provide a broader range of services. In the past, these groups have been more common in particular regions and in rural areas, where a single group of doctors has the responsibility both as the doctors in town and the staff of small, rural hospitals.

These practices often have separate administrative departments for billing, appointment scheduling, and referrals and separate clinical departments for phlebotomy, electrocardiograms, laboratory work, and X-ray. In such practices, medical assisting jobs can be limited in scope, depending on the department where the medical assistant works.

Community health centers, established by the federal government in the late 1960s, also usually operate as multi-practice, multi-specialty groups (with doctors as well as nurse practitioners, physician's assistants, and nurse-midwives all on salary). HMOs that provide all services in one building, so-called closed-panel HMOs, also operate as multi-practice, multi-specialty groups.

OTHER MEDICAL PRACTICES

A number of medical practice techniques are not part of the standard Western approach to medicine. For many years these were called "alternative" medicine. But since the early 1990s, scholars of medicine have begun to make finer distinctions among them. Studies from the early 1990s found that Americans annually spend literally millions of dollars on therapies that are not part of their doctor's standard approach. They often don't even tell their doctors about these other treatments. (See Eisenberg, David et. al., "Trends in Alternative Medicine Use in the United States, 1990–1997," *Journal of the American Medical Association,* Nov. 18, 1998 v.280 n.19 p.1720.)

Since then the federal government has established within the National Institutes of Health an Office of Alternative Medicine. The most well-respected medical journals, such as the *New England Journal of Medicine* and the *Journal of the American Medical Association,* have published a number of studies about the effectiveness of various nonstandard therapies, and numerous journals have been established to publish research about such therapies. More recently, doctors trained in the classical Western medical tradition are accepting nonstandard therapies as "complementary" rather than alternative and are even instituting some of these practices.

In late 1998, a newsletter called *The Integrative Medical Consult,* which bills itself as "the essential guide to integrating conventional and complementary medicine," began publishing. The distinction between complementary and alternative is somewhat fuzzy and open to interpretation. This book will define practices *as alternative* that expect their patients to be treated by that method alone rather than in addition to standard medical care. Table 3–2 shows the various groupings of practices.

Table 3–2	**Complementary and Alternative Medicine**

Complementary Medicine	Alternative Medicine	Non-Western Medical Systems (Traditional)

Acupuncture/Acupressure—technique for treating disease and inducing anesthesia by passing thin needles into specific points on the body (acupuncture) or by exerting pressure on those points (acupressure). Practitioner may be a doctor or acupuncturist.

Biofeedback—training program to develop a person's ability to control physiologic functions that are normally outside voluntary control by monitoring the target process and giving feedback in the form of sound or images. Practitioner may be a doctor or other trained professional.

Chiropractic—system of health care based on the importance of the relationship between the spinal column and the nervous system as a determinant of health. A chiropractor uses the initials DC (Doctor of Chiropractic). Medical assistants may work for chiropractors.

Herbal Medicine—use of herbal preparations, traditionally as infusions, to preserve health and treat illness. Currently this term is used for preparations regulated and sold as dietary supplements rather than medications. These preparations may also contain vitamins and minerals as well as animal or insect parts. Chinese or other foreign-trained doctors without credentials in the United States may practice as herbalists.

Hypnosis—use of an induced sleeplike state in which the subject is susceptible to the suggestions of the hypnotist.

Massage Therapy—use of manipulation, pressure, friction, and kneading of the skin and underlying tissue to relieve muscle tension, improve circulation, and (in traditional Chinese medicine) to treat disease processes.

Nutrition Therapy—dietary treatment often prescribed by a doctor with specific meal plans and food lists prepared by a registered dietitian.

Osteopathy—a system of medicine that emphasizes the importance of the interactions of the musculoskeletal system, environment, nutrition, and proper body function to produce health. An osteopath (DO, Doctor of Osteopathy) is licensed to practice medicine with all the privileges of an

Christian Science—a religious system that uses spirituality as the exclusive healing power for its practitioners.

Homeopathy—a medical system based on the practice of administering very small doses of the substances believed to cause illness to result in a cure.

Naturopathy—a therapeutic system that uses natural forces such as light, heat, air, water, and massage to cure illness.

Ayurvedic Medicine—traditional medical system of ancient India, which focuses on problems of circulation of the life force (*prana*). Ayurveda considers spiritual and physical well-being to be intertwined.

Traditional Chinese Medicine—traditional Chinese medicine has an ancient lineage based on manipulation of the circulation of *qi* (pronounced "chi"), or vital energy. The goal of Chinese medicine and spirituality is harmony and balance.

Folk Medicine of Various Cultures—medical practices exist in most non-Western countries, often based on a belief in "bad" spirits who enter human beings and cause illness. Various native healers, often called shamans in English, perform rituals to drive out bad spirits and promote health in an afflicted person.

Native American Traditional Medicine—each tribe of Native Americans has its own beliefs and practices to promote health and spiritual well-being. The English term for a traditional Native American healer is medicine man.

Table 3–2	**Complementary and Alternative Medicine** *(Continued)*	
Complementary Medicine	Alternative Medicine	Non-Western Medical Systems (Traditional)
MD. Medical assistants may work for osteopaths. **Podiatry**—the diagnosis and treatment of conditions of the foot. A podiatrist (DPM, Doctor of Podiatric Medicine) may use medical and surgical treatments. Medical assistants may work for podiatrists. **Postural Therapies**—various methods to improve health and well-being by aligning the musculoskeletal system. **Psychotherapy**—a method of treating mental disorders by means other than physical means, including talking therapies and behavior modification. **Prayer and Meditation**—a sharing or thoughts, feelings, or petitions with God or other deity (prayer) and focused contemplation (meditation). Prayer groups or meditation groups may focus attention on ill people. **Relaxation Techniques**—methods to attain deep relaxation as a means of coping with stress or chronic pain. **Therapeutic Touch**—a system that involves passing the hands above a patient's body to affect the patient's energy field. Practitioners are often registered nurses.		

Elsibeth Blackwore first nurse

Complementary Medicine

Osteopathy

Osteopathy is a mix of traditional scientific medicine and **holistic** medicine. This branch of medical practice seeks to balance the structure and function of the body through manipulation of muscles and joints. Osteopathy was started in the late 1800s by Andrew Taylor Still (1828–1917). Osteopaths see disease as the result of dysfunction in the skeletal and muscular systems. Pain, "asymmetry"—difference in anatomy between one side of the body and the other or differences in joint movement—and tissue tenderness are used to gauge symptoms. Osteopaths, who hold DO degrees, today are given all the privileges of those with MD degrees. Although they may practice as subspecialists, the majority of osteopaths practice as primary care doctors, where they believe their holistic and structural approach can be most effective.

Chiropractic

Chiropractic is the technique of spinal manipulation. Chiropractors believe that vertebral subluxations—partially dislocated spinal joints—cause nerve blockages, which in turn lead to pain in the back, neck, shoulders, and legs. Begun in 1895 by Daniel David Palmer (1845–1913), chiropractic holds that the body has its own ability to heal and maintain balance. According to chiropractic theory, the nervous system is the center of all disease and healing. Chiropractors disagree over the so-called subluxation disease theory, the theory that subluxation is the reason for all disease. Those who believe in this theory claim to cure everything from cancer to the common cold by vertebral manipulation. Most chiropractors today limit their treatment to discomfort clearly associated with the spine and integrate their practices into standard Western medical practice.

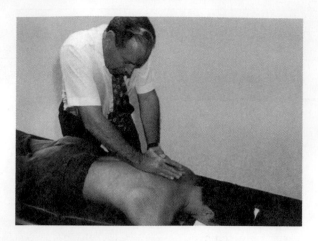

➢ **Figure 3–2** Spinal adjustment with patient in prone position (Courtesy of Gatterman MI: *Foundations of Chiropractic Subluxation*. St. Louis: Mosby, 1995)

Figures 3–2 and 3–3 demonstrate chiropractic adjustment.

Podiatry

Podiatrists use traditional medical and surgical techniques but are limited in their practice to treatment of disorders of the feet and ankles. Since the 1970s, podiatry has worked to enlarge its area of practice by focusing on surgery of the foot to alleviate such problems as bone spurs and bunions. This has put them into conflict with orthopedic surgeons, who traditionally did this work. Podiatrists are increasingly working closely with primary care doctors in the management of diabetic patients and the elderly, who tend to have many foot problems.

Psychotherapy

Psychologists, social workers, and other therapists, as well as psychiatrists, work with patients to treat their mental health. Psychiatrists have earned an MD degree and spent a period of residency training in psychiatry after an internship in internal medicine or pediatrics; psychologists have a degree in clinical psychology, usually a PhD. Other therapists may have one of a number of different degrees or certifications.

The only mental health practitioners allowed to prescribe medication are psychiatrists. All psychotherapists whether they use medication or not, also engage in various treatments, from "talking therapy" to behavior modification, to treat psychological conditions.

Acupuncture/Acupressure

Acupuncture and acupressure are traditional Chinese healing arts. They are based on the theory that there are 14 meridians, or channels, through which *qi* (pronounced "chi") is carried. *Qi* is usually translated into English as vital energy or energy of life. Disease or illness is characterized by an imbalance of *qi,* and acupuncture or acupressure is used to restore the correct flow of *qi*.

In acupuncture, extremely thin needles are inserted at various meridians, then twisted or twirled to stimulate the correct circulation of *qi* (see Figure 3–4). They are left in place for approximately 25 minutes. *Shiatsu, tsubu,* and *shin jyutsu* are common acupressure techniques, used to open channels for *qi* by stimulating

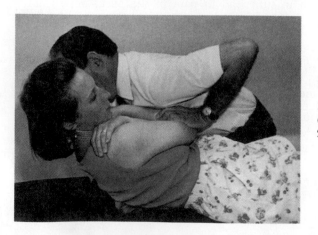

➢ **Figure 3–3** Spinal adjustment with patient in supine position (Courtesy of Gatterman MI: *Foundations of Chiropractic Subluxation*. St. Louis: Mosby, 1995.)

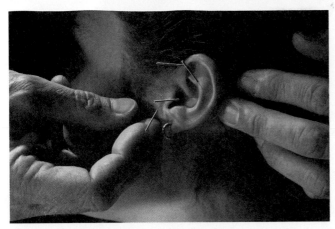

> **Figure 3–4** Acupuncture involves the placement of several extremely thin needles in various parts of the body.

meridians without the use of needles. In more than half the states and the District of Columbia, acupuncturists must be licensed and certified according to national board standards.

Many Chinese will go to traditional Chinese medicine practitioners, who use acupuncture or acupressure along with other techniques and traditional herbs; Westerners are increasingly using acupuncture or acupressure to alleviate chronic pain and headache. Acupuncture has recently been the subject of several scientific studies that provide evidence that it can be helpful in managing the pain of childbirth and assisting in the treatment of cocaine dependence.

Nutrition Therapy

Recognition of the link between good nutrition and health is becoming stronger and more widely accepted all the time. People's nutritional needs can change due to their health; for instance, fighting chronic inflammation or infection takes hundreds of extra calories of food energy per day. Illness can greatly affect nutritional intake; for instance, many digestive diseases damage the intestine's ability to absorb important nutrients.

We know that every person needs daily intake of vitamins A, B, C, D, E, and K, as well as the minerals magnesium, calcium, zinc, selenium, folic acid, and iron. Other nutrients have been researched, and some are today prescribed as treatments for certain conditions. For instance, antioxidants are believed to prevent cancer and also to enhance cardiovascular health. Essential fatty acids are thought by some to relieve pain.

Some practitioners prescribe "megadoses" of various nutrients. Diets have also been created that some practitioners argue enhance cardiac health, digestive health, and/or reduce the probability of cancer.

Biofeedback

In biofeedback, patients learn to control their body's physiologic responses to thought patterns. The technique was developed by Neal Miller in the 1960s. Patients are attached to a monitoring box and electrodes placed on strategic locations. Changes in muscle tension, skin temperature, brain waves, and breathing are most frequently measured. Patients use the monitoring box and electrodes to see if they are getting the desired changes in the body's involuntary responses such as heart rate, blood pressure, and voluntary muscle control.

Biofeedback is often used to treat tension headaches and chronic pain. Practitioners must be certified by the Biofeedback Certification Institute of America to receive reimbursement for the care from insurance companies. Most certified practitioners are doctors.

Hypnosis

Modern hypnosis, developed in the 1700s by Franz Anton Mesmer (1734–1815), is a technique in which the patient focuses concentration. In hypnosis, the patient becomes absorbed in the words or visualizations described by the hypnotherapist and is responsive to suggestions made by the hypnotherapist if they are in accordance with the patient's wishes. Hypnosis is actually self-hypnosis, and many hypnotherapists teach their patients the techniques. Hypnosis causes changes in body function that are similar to those caused by other relaxation techniques, including changes in brain wave activity, involuntary nervous system activity, oxygen and carbon dioxide metabolism, heart rate and blood pressure, and even changes in immune system function.

Hypnosis has been found to be helpful in treating phobias—abnormal fears—and addictions. The most current research shows it may also be helpful in treating anxiety and chronic pain. The American Board of Hypnosis and the American Council of Hypnotist Examiners both certify hypnotherapists, who must be certified by one or the other organization to practice. Doctors, dentists, registered nurses, and social workers are increasingly seeking certification in hypnosis.

Relaxation Techniques

Relaxation techniques include meditation, progressive muscle relaxation, and autogenic training.

Although many Westerners think of meditation as a part of Eastern religious practice, there are actually many different types of meditation. Dr. Herbert Benson, a cardiologist at Harvard Medical School and the director of the Mind/Body Medical Institute at Harvard's Beth Israel/Deaconess Medical Center in Boston, coined the term "relaxation response" to describe the lowering of blood pressure and other beneficial physiologic responses brought on by meditation when used by cardiac patients. Other researchers have found that meditation also helps relieve headaches, chronic pain, and stress.

Progressive muscle relaxation is a technique of slowly tensing and releasing each muscle group, starting at the toes and ending at the neck and head.

Autogenic training is a technique of putting a patient or oneself into a state of deep relaxation. The process begins with imagining a peaceful place, then focusing on physical sensations, moving from the feet to the head, with a special concentration on breath and heartbeat.

Meditation and relaxation techniques are increasingly being taught by Western medical practitioners and are sometimes covered by health insurance providers.

Therapeutic Touch

Therapeutic touch, most often practiced by nurses, actually does not involve touch. The technique, developed in 1972 by Dolores Krieger, a professor of nursing at the New York School of Nursing, and Dora Kunz, a medical clairvoyant, holds that each individual has an energy field that can be manipulated therapeutically by moving one's hands over an ill person to induce healing.

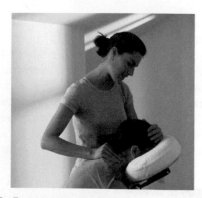

➤ **Figure 3–5** Massage techniques are used by massage therapists, chiropractors, physical therapists, and other health professionals.

Massage

Different massage techniques focus on different muscular groupings in the body. Massage has been shown not only to relieve muscle tension, but also to reduce stress and induce a feeling of calm. About 20 states currently license massage therapists, who must undergo training not only in their chosen massage specialty, but also in anatomy and physiology so they understand the workings of the musculoskeletal, cardiovascular, lymphatic, and nervous systems. They then must pass a national certification examination.

Neuromuscular massage focuses on specific muscle sets, using deep tissue massage to relieve pain, improve circulation, and loosen tight muscular knots that result from tension (see Figure 3–5).

The goal of lymphatic massage, developed by Dr. Emil Vodder, is to improve lymph flow, loosen connective tissue, and stimulate the lymphatic system.

Rolfing, also called structural integration, is based on manipulation of the fascia, the tissue sheaths that cover muscles. Developed in the late 1940s by Ida Rolf, a biophysicist, this strenuous massage is aimed at restoring proper muscular function by realigning the fascia away from gravitational pull.

Postural Therapies

Postural therapies seek to align the musculoskeletal system and alleviate discomfort through body movement and positioning. Three important postural therapies are the Alexander Technique, the Feldenkrais Method, and the Trager Method.

The Alexander Technique, commonly taught in acting school, was developed by F. M. Alexander, who believed that posture affects the voice quality. The technique is used today to reduce tension and lead to more efficient and less strained movement. Specific movements are performed both sitting and standing, sometimes accompanied by gentle pressure by a practitioner to muscle sites.

The Feldenkrais Method, developed by Moshe Feldenkrais, focuses on the conscious mapping of everyday movements, such as walking, combined with an awareness of the options in movement. A practitioner uses light touch to help an individual focus on specific areas of movement coordination.

The Trager Method, developed by Milton Trager, using shaking, rocking, and bouncing to loosen joints and release tension. Trager, a boxing trainer turned physical therapist, incorporated mental and meditative procedures into this series of directed movements aimed at increasing flexibility.

Herbal Medicine

In the United States, herbal (sometimes called botanical) preparations are considered dietary supplements, and are regulated as such by the federal Food and Drug Administration.

Americans are coming late to the herbal medicine game. Practitioners of traditional Native American medicine use herbal remedies, as do practitioners of traditional Chinese medicine and Eastern Indian medical practices (Ayurvedic medicine). Europeans never fully gave up the botanical basis for medical practice.

American medicine went completely to the scientific model beginning in the late 19th century, and development of medications in this century has been based primarily on synthetic chemical compounds.

Today, Americans are searching the traditional methodologies for appropriate use of botanicals in health promotion and the treatment of illness. The number of Americans who use herbal and vitamin therapies in addition to medicines prescribed by their doctor continues to rise sharply. Some of these herbal remedies can cause side effects; others can interact with prescription medications. Patients should be asked about any herbal preparations or vitamins they take regularly.

Prayer and Meditation

Doctors are increasingly recognizing that prayer is a form of meditation. In fact, Dr. Benson has extended his theory of the "relaxation response," and has said the combination of meditative relaxation technique combined with inner spirituality leads to what he calls "the faith factor." A number of studies throughout the 1990s have shown that people who have strong religious faith, people who participate in a strong religious community, and even people who know that others are praying for them (even people of other faiths) have better outcomes in controlled research studies.

Alternative Medicine

Homeopathy

The basic theory of homeopathy is that "like cures like," also called the "law of similars." This theory, which is ridiculed by most medical doctors, states that a substance that causes illness in a healthy person will cure a person sick with that illness, if given in the correct, infinitesimally small dose.

This theory was put forth by Samuel Hahnemann (1755–1843), an 18th-century German doctor, who noted that when he drank quinine he felt symptoms of malaria although he did not actually have the illness. Hahnemann believed that any remedy would become increasingly potent in its fight against disease as it was exponentially diluted.

Today, although anecdotal evidence exists that some homeopathic remedies work, there is no scientifically proven evidence to show this. Most doctors discount homeopathy because it purports to provide treatment using medications that appear to have no medical value. Homeopathy is not usually practiced by conventionally trained doctors, although some do. Most states do not require licensure or certification; however, Connecticut and Arizona license MDs or DOs as homeopaths.

Naturopathy

Naturopaths see disease as an outcome of stress and imbalance. Naturopathic doctors (NDs), use a broad range of therapeutic resources, some from Western scientific medicine and many from such diverse practices as traditional Chinese medicine, homeopathy, clinical nutrition, and behavioral medicine.

They strive to pinpoint the underlying cause of illness to treat it rather than simply treating symptoms. They recognize the body's ability to heal itself and use as many natural healing resources as possible, including herbal, dietary, and environmental treatments. They use holistic treatment methods, treating the entire person and not just the current complaint.

Herbs and nutritional therapy, as well as relaxation techniques, massage, and yoga are prescribed to address both the patient's physical and spiritual well-being.

Two schools of naturopathic medicine train naturopaths in the United States. Eleven states currently license naturopathic doctors.

Spiritual Healing (Christian Science, Jehovah's Witnesses)

The most famous of the American religious sects that believe in spiritual healing and often refuse medical treatment are the Christian Scientists. Called the Church of Christ, Scientist, the sect was founded by Mary Baker Eddy (1821–1910) in the 19th century. It holds that an important element of Christianity is healing through spirituality.

Christian Scientists believe that all disease and illness can be corrected through prayer and spirituality. They reject all scientific medicine, to the point of refusing blood transfusions in cases where they are medically necessary.

Jehovah's Witnesses and members of the Church of Jesus Christ of Latter Day Saints ('Mormons') also routinely seek exemptions to refuse transfusions and other medical procedures.

Courts have ruled that adults have the right to refuse medical treatment on religious grounds, but that they do not have the right to refuse medical treatment that might save the life of one of their children. The courts have ruled that there is a compelling public policy to have such children declared wards of the state for the duration of their treatment; the legal reasoning for this compromise is that this does not violate the parent's religious convictions, yet upholds society's belief that all citizens deserve the best medical care available to them.

Hospitals routinely seek court orders to make children whose parents refuse treatment on religious grounds wards of the state so as to treat children with conditions that can routinely be cured by scientific medical means. After treatment, the children are usually returned to the custody of their parents.

Non-Western Medicine (Traditional Medicines)

Traditional Chinese Medicine

The central tenet of Chinese medicine is the concept of *qi,* the life force that moves throughout the body and is the basis for all the body systems' functions.

Chinese medical practitioners look for the cause of illness in the imbalance of the three major components of life—*qi,* blood, and moisture, as well as an imbalance in heat and cold. Five organ networks—the liver, heart, spleen, lungs, and kidneys—manifest these imbalances, because each independently is capable of generating heat or cold, dampness or dryness, and wind. The five organ networks are also said to correspond to five phases, five cycles of development, five seasons, five climates, and five personality types.

Illness is caused by an organ system that is out of balance and/or functioning with insufficient *qi.* Treatment with herbs, acupuncture, or acupressure is performed to restore balance and promote the circulation of *qi* to organ networks where *qi* is currently insufficient.

Traditional Chinese practitioners believe that every disease has two phases, the invisible and the visible. The highest art is to treat the diseases in their invisible phase, when there is an energy imbalance that has not yet manifested itself as outward signs and symptoms.

Some of the treatment modalities used by Chinese practitioners, such as acupuncture and massage, are regulated, as discussed in the section on complementary medicine. Other treatment methods, including herbal medicine, meditation, and exercise such as t'ai chi and chi gong, are not regulated.

Ayurvedic Medicine (Ayurveda, Traditional Indian Medicine)

Ayurveda considers spiritual and physical well-being to be completely intertwined. The English translation of the two words *ayur* and *veda* is longevity and knowledge, the concept being that increased knowledge leads to increased longevity. In Ayurvedic practice, spirituality and consciousness are wound up in the environment, diet, work, and interpersonal relationships.

The concepts of anatomy and physiology in Ayurveda are similar to those in Chinese medicine. The life force—called *prana*—is centered in five organ centers—called *vayus*—located in the brain, throat, heart, small intestine, and lower abdomen. *Srotas,* conceptually like Chinese meridians, help circulate *prana.* Disease is caused by deficiency of *prana* and blockage of *srotas.*

Therapies include performing yoga—a form of movement and meditation—reciting certain mantras, rubbing the skin with oil, cleansing the body of toxins, and administering herbal remedies.

There is no regulation of Ayurveda in the United States.

Native American Traditional Medicine

Native Americans also use preparations of botanicals from their environment to treat a number of illnesses. In addition, folk medicine is provided by shamans—medicine men—who perform a number of spiritual ceremonies to purge the body of disease. In addition to the heavy use of herbs, Native American medicine uses fasting, meditation, heat, and massage therapy.

Among the over 400 Native American tribes, the most common belief is that man needs to be in harmony with nature. Native Americans accept the world as it is and do not try to mold it to their own will. They also believe in taking only what is needed to live from the world around them. This belief system is manifest in Native American folk medicine in many ways, and religion and medicine are practically indistinguishable. Much of the goal of singing, dancing, and other medical rituals is to restore the individual to harmony with the world around him or her.

The Indian Health Service of the U.S. Department of Health and Human Services began a program in the late 1990s of hiring medicine men to serve in clinics alongside Western-trained doctors.

THE INFLUENCE OF CULTURE ON PATIENT EXPECTATIONS OF HEALTH CARE PROVIDERS

As a medical assistant, you need to become sensitive to cultures that have some level of distrust of Western scientific medicine but do not have a strong medical tradition of their own. Although some patients who come to your office may also seek care from a practitioner of traditional Chinese medicine or Ayurveda, others will be complementing your care with care from practitioners whose methods are more based on folk wisdom, spiritism, faith healing, and various treatments that have not been studied scientifically.

In many traditional practices, religion and medicine are tightly interwoven. Both patients and practitioners hope to affect health by influencing spirits or gods in the unseen world. People from many cultures believe in the effectiveness of sacred words, tattoos, or amulets—objects worn to prevent injury or evil—as well as specific rituals that may involve chanting, fire, or even animal sacrifice.

Many cultures distinguish between illness caused by bad spirits or evil people and illness that has more physiologic origins. Many things that are fundamental to scientific medical practice are foreign to traditional practices, such as frequent handwashing to remove invisible organisms, taking medicine when you don't feel ill, and causing pain to healthy children by giving them immunizations.

When patients have different beliefs it is important that you do not dismiss them, but rather that you find a way to make the patient understand how important it is for him or her to communicate with you about other treatments that are being used. You also need to spend sufficient time with people who are using folk healers to get them to understand the importance of the treatments being offered by scientific medicine and to encourage compliance with standard medical treatment regimens in addition to their traditional practices.

In many cultures, the aged are held in high regard not only for their longevity, but also for their wisdom. This means that it is often difficult to make the transition from a folk-medicine-based culture to a scientific-medicine-based culture. Specific influences of various cultures you might encounter are discussed below.

Southeast Asian

Asians generally have a strong sense of self-respect, as well as a respect for authority, hard work, and age. Asians are generally oriented toward the welfare of the family as a unit above the welfare of the individual. Families are expected to share and to function closely as extended families. There is a strong emphasis on harmony and an attempt to avoid conflicts.

Disease is believed to be caused by an imbalance of energy and possibly by strong emotions. Herbs, diets, and application of hot or cold therapies are used to treat illnesses, according to their classification as hot or cold illnesses.

Throughout Southeast Asia, health care is crisis oriented, with alleviation of symptoms the goal. Much of the medical care takes its cue from traditional Chinese medicine, including acupuncture and acupressure, as well as herbal remedies. Small heated cups may be used to draw the "bad wind" out of the "sick area." Rubbing the skin with the side of a coin is a common treatment. Although this practice is done with enough pressure to bruise the skin, it does not break the skin and is not considered dangerous.

Southeast Asians often feel frightened by diagnostic tests and are uncomfortable responding to direct questioning for a medical history. If there is a misunderstanding, they often feel they have "lost face" by having caused the misunderstanding. In all Asian cultures, the head is believed to be the "seat of life," and touching someone's head, especially a child's head, is very frightening to an Asian.

African-American and African-Caribbean

Black Americans, whether in this country for many generations or more recently immigrated from Caribbean cultures, show many similar cultural traits. These include a strong family orientation, strong kinship bonds, and a strong sense of religion, mostly Protestant. The church has been an important focus for African-American aspirations.

African-American and African-Caribbean people are often said to be "present oriented," focused on what is happening now and not what will happen in the future. This has implications for health education, and a medical assistant working to educate such a person on the necessity to maintain compliance with health and medication regimens must understand how this outlook on life affects the patient's thinking.

African-American and African-Caribbean folk medicine includes a strong link between health and religion, including faith healers, root doctors, and spiritualists. Maintaining the balance between good and evil is also considered important to health, and voodoo doctors or conjurers cast out evil spirits and demons. Roots, minerals, and plant mixtures are also used extensively.

Latino Cultures

In Latino cultures, the family is the primary unit. A child's parents and grandparents have a special bond. Age is respected, and deference is given to men. The Roman Catholic church has a strong influence. Many Latinos hold the notion that God gives good health and can create illness as a punishment, for which proper atonement can provide a cure.

Latino folk medicine is based on the notion of "humors" or fluids common in ancient Greek medicine, which existed more than 2,000 years ago. This medical tradition was brought to Spain from the Arab lands by the Moors, who ruled southern Spain for about 500 years shortly after the beginning of Christianity. Spanish conquistadors brought this tradition to Central and South America during the age of European exploration from the 13th to the 16th centuries.

Humoral medical beliefs hold that all bodily functions are regulated by four bodily fluids, or "humors," each of which has a specific purpose. Each is also a combination of hot or cold, wet or dry. Blood is hot and wet, yellow bile is hot and dry, black bile is cold and dry, and phlegm is cold and wet. The key to good health is balance between the hot and cold humors. When these humors fall out of balance, they can be brought into balance through foods, medicines, herbs, or drinks that are either "hot" (*caliente*) or "cold" (*frio*).

Disease may be attributed to supernatural causes such as the evil eye (*mal ojo*), or magic.

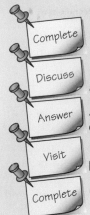

STUDENT STUDY PLAN

To reinforce your understanding of the material in this chapter . . .

Complete *Complete* the **Review & Recall** questions below.

Discuss *Discuss* the situation in **If You Were the Medical Assistant** with your classmates and answer the questions.

Answer *Answer* the **Critical Thinking Questions** below, and discuss them with your classmates.

Visit *Visit* **Web sites** suggested below and search for additional Web sites using **Keywords for Internet Searches**.

Complete *Complete* the exercises in chapter 3 of the **Student Mastery Manual**.

REVIEW & RECALL

1. Identify the types of needs people have at each level of Maslow's hierarchy of needs.

2. Why are needs for esteem and recognition placed higher in the hierarchy than needs for food, water, and shelter?

3. Identify three things that patients expect when they seek health care.

4. Describe the education a doctor receives in the United States.

5. List and define several medical specialties, surgical specialties, and specialties that provide both medical and surgical treatment.

6. What are the major differences between a solo practice, a multi-practice single-specialty group, and a multi-practice multi-specialty group?

7. List 10 types of complementary medicine. List three types of alternative medicine.

8. Give at least two reasons why patients choose to use complementary or alternative medicine.

9. Describe three types of non-Western (traditional) medicine.

10. Describe briefly beliefs about health or health practices a medical assistant may find in individuals from Southeast Asian, African-American or African-Caribbean, or Latino culture.

IF YOU WERE THE MEDICAL ASSISTANT

Mrs. Andrews is a 65-year-old patient of Dr. Lawler. The doctor has prescribed several medications for Mrs. Andrews because she has a heart condition and high blood pressure.

While you are interviewing her in the examination room, she tells you that 2 days earlier a burglar broke a window, got into her apartment, and stole some money and jewelry that her late husband had given her.

She says, "This has upset me terribly. I feel like such a baby. I can't eat. I can't sleep. I just don't feel safe in my apartment any more. I wasn't there when it happened, but I keep thinking, 'What if the burglar comes back?' "

Answer the following questions:

1. What kind of needs (according to Maslow's hierarchy) is Mrs. Andrews having trouble meeting?

2. Would today be a good day to start teaching Mrs. Andrews to take her own blood pressure at home? Why or why not?

3. Which of the following replies can you use to reassure Mrs. Andrews that strong feelings are appropriate in a situation like this?
   a. Did you call the police?
   b. Don't you think you are overreacting a little? I'm sure you have had the window fixed.
   c. It must feel like your home has been violated.
   d. This is the third burglary I have heard about this week. Where do you live?

As Mrs. Andrews continues to talk about the burglary, she says, "Normally, I don't take any medicine except what Dr. Lawler tells me to take. But I have been so upset that I have been taking a natural remedy that my mother used to take for her nerves. It's called Rescue Remedy; have you ever heard of it?"
Mrs. Andrews takes a bottle out of her handbag to show you.

Answer the following questions:

1. Would you assess that Mrs. Andrews is using complementary medicine, alternative medicine, traditional medicine, or none of these? Explain your answer.

2. Why should you instruct Mrs. Andrews to tell Dr. Lawler that she is taking Rescue Remedy?

3. Do you think Mrs. Andrews will want to tell Dr. Lawler about this? Why or why not?

CRITICAL THINKING QUESTIONS

1. What types of complementary, alternative, and traditional medicine are available in your community? Use the telephone book as a resource. Which types are most common? Discuss with your classmates how you can get information to answer this question.

2. How has your own cultural background influenced your attitudes about health and health care? To answer this question, you may want to first describe that cultural background, including country of birth, places lived, other family members, and your religion.

   Discuss why you think people get sick with a cold and why people get diseases like cancer. What happens in your family if someone gets sick? Give examples. How are the elderly members of your family treated? Does this affect their health care? Give examples if you can.

   How do the people in your family expect to have their babies? Are there any special things they do during pregnancy? After the delivery?

3. Do you agree that sometimes patient expectations are somewhat different from the priorities of the medical office? Why or why not?

4. Medical students must make a choice about the branch of medicine they wish to pursue before they can enter a residency program. What factors influence their decision?

   If you have watched the television series *ER* or *Chicago Hope*, you may already have some information to begin to answer this question. Where can you look for more information?

5. How would you get information about an herbal remedy such as Rescue Remedy? (Rescue Remedy is a real product.) Identify three different methods you might use to get information.

EXPLORE THE WEB

INTERNET WEB SITES

American Board of Medical Specialists (ABMS)
www.abms.org

Cultural psychology
www.socialpsychology.org/cultural.htm

National Center for Complementary and Alternative Medicine
nccam.nih.gov

Psychology web sites
www.socialpsychology.org

KEYWORDS FOR INTERNET SEARCHES

acupuncture	herbal medicine	naturopathy
alternative medicine	holistic medicine	osteopathy
anxiety	homeopathy	podiatry
biofeedback	hypnosis	prayer
chiropractic	Maslow, Abraham	psychotherapy
Christian Science	meditation	therapeutic touch
ego defense mechanisms		

Basic Concepts: Professionalism & Law, Communication, and Safety

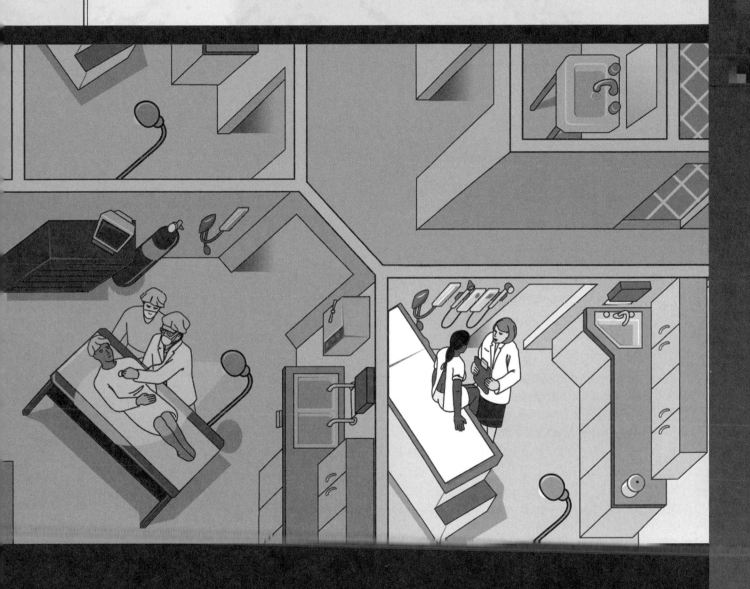

Chapter 4

Professionalism and Law: How Do You Behave in the Workplace?

Chapter Topics

Characteristics of Effective Health Care Workers
Character Traits
Personality Traits
Appearance and Behavior
Professionalism
Professionalism for Doctors
Professionalism for Medical Assistants

Introduction to Legal Concepts
Discussion of Law
State Regulation of Health Occupations
Credentials of Medical Assistants
Mandated Reporting
Patient Rights
Confidentiality and Privacy

The Doctor–Patient Relationship
Informed Consent
Background Checks
Personal and Professional Liability
Standard of Care
Measures to Avoid Lawsuits
Employee Rights

Instructional Objectives

After completing this chapter, you will be able to do the following:

1. Define and spell the vocabulary words for the chapter.
2. Describe the character and personality traits of effective health care workers.
3. Identify elements of a professional appearance for the medical assistant.
4. List examples of appropriate ways for a medical assistant to demonstrate initiative.
5. Identify ethical standards that influence the practice of medicine.
6. Differentiate among civil, criminal, and contract law.
7. Identify ways in which state law affects the medical office.
8. Discuss measures to maintain patient confidentiality and privacy.
9. Identify three intentional torts that could result from failure to protect a patient's privacy.
10. Identify the implications of the doctor–patient contract.
11. Describe measures to prevent lawsuits for abandonment.
12. Describe the medical assistant's role in obtaining informed consent.
13. Describe professional liability and the role of professional liability insurance.
14. Describe the appropriate standard of care for a doctor and a medical assistant.
15. Identify employee rights that are protected by federal and state laws.

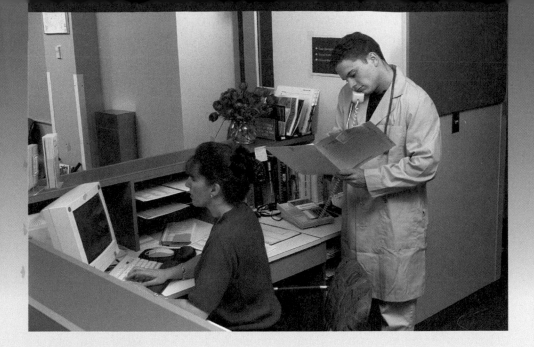

- Understand legal guidelines and requirements for health care
- Demonstrate the personal attributes of the professional medical assistant
- Understand workplace dynamics

- Identify and respond to issues of confidentiality
- Perform within legal and ethical boundaries

VOCABULARY

abandonment (p. 69)	endoscopy (p. 69)	libel (p. 67)	sexual harassment (p. 74)
act (p. 65)	expressed contract (p. 68)	licensure (p. 65)	slander (p. 67)
advocate (p. 64)	Good Samaritan Acts (p. 74)	malpractice (p. 72)	standard of care (p. 72)
arbitrary (p. 69)	implied contract (p. 68)	medical practice act (p. 65)	standards (p. 62)
brand image (p. 61)	informed consent (p. 69)	negligence (p. 70)	statute (p. 65)
certification (p. 66)	initiative (p. 61)	objectivity (p. 61)	tort (p. 67)
civil law (p. 65)	intimidation (p. 74)	plaintiff (p. 65)	verbal contract (p. 68)
contract (p. 68)	invasion of privacy (p. 67)	professional liability (p. 70)	written consent (p. 67)
criminal law (p. 65)	legislation (p. 70)	professionalism (p. 62)	written contract (p. 68)
defendant (p. 65)	legislator (p. 65)	prudent (p. 71)	
doctrine of *respondeat*	liability (p. 70)	reciprocal licensing (p. 66)	
superior (p. 73)			

Perhaps the most important thing to remember as a medical assistant is that you are a professional. Being a professional means that you have a number of responsibilities: to the patients you help care for, to the people you work for, and to the people you work with. It also means you have a number of rights; most important is the right to be treated with dignity and respect.

Professionalism is as much an attitude and a manner of being as it is a matter of education and training. In this chapter I'll discuss some of the ways you can project professionalism. Behaving like a professional can greatly enhance your work experience.

A medical assistant represents the doctor. Patients need to have the same kind of trust in the medical assistant that they have in the doctor. Acting in a professional manner provides a signal to a patient that the medical assistant is knowledgeable and can be trusted to do competently what the patient needs done.

A medical assistant needs to look and act like a competent, caring person. Neatness, cleanliness, good grooming, and a courteous and warm manner go a long way toward making the patient believe that his blood will be drawn properly or that her paperwork will be filled out without mistakes. It is especially important that patients feel the medical assistant is "old enough" to perform the necessary duties. By this I mean that the medical assistant must look and behave maturely. Neat hair and an appropriate uniform help even a very young medical assistant to project a mature appearance and an image of competence.

CHARACTERISTICS OF EFFECTIVE HEALTH CARE WORKERS

Good medical assistants have a number of characteristics that make them effective in their work. Although a person's character and personality have been shaped by heredity and environment, a medical assisting student can work to enhance the traits that are important to become an effective professional. Appearance and behavior are visible and are also important means of projecting competence in the medical field.

Character Traits

The most important character traits of a good medical assistant are honesty, organization, reliability, and dependability. The medical assistant is an integral part of the office practice, and as such must arrive at work on time and not take unplanned days off, except when ill or if a family emergency arises. A medical assistant must be able to organize the day's work and seem prepared for each patient interaction.

A medical assistant projects honesty by working within his or her "scope of practice"; that is, doing only what he or she is trained to do and being comfortable saying "I don't know" or "I don't know how to" when appropriate. Office staff must be able to count on the medical assistant to maintain confidentiality and behave ethically, even when not under direct supervision, because of the higher level of trust needed to provide excellent patient care.

Personality Traits

Many people who have the right character traits do not have the right personality traits to be successful medical assistants. A medical assistant needs to be genuinely interested in helping people, warm and caring, and able to put the needs of others first.

Medical practice is one of the "caring professions." Every professional in the medical office needs to have a serious interest in helping people. Although the medical assistant must know how to perform the necessary administrative activities effectively and efficiently, the first priority is the care of patients who come to the office.

The concepts of warmth and caring will be discussed in more detail in the next chapter, on communication. For now, it's important to say that caring is a key personality trait. Some aspects of caring can be learned and practiced. But if a person doesn't have a naturally caring personality, he or she will find it much harder to learn the necessary caring communication skills.

The ability to put the needs of others first is very important. This means not allowing your personal circumstances to interfere with the way you interact with patients, colleagues, or doctor(s). Later discussions of communicating with patients, and especially taking a medical history, will cover the importance of **objectivity,** and of not allowing what is going on in your life to distract you or change the way you understand and describe a patient's physical or emotional state.

Appearance and Behavior

If you possess the right character and personality traits, you will find it much easier to learn and practice the proper behaviors necessary for becoming a medical assistant and easier to understand why personal appearance is so important.

Psychologists have long known that we respond to other people's physical appearance. Being a patient is humbling. In a doctor's office, every patient is treated the same; whether the patient is a bank president, a bricklayer, or a stay-at-home mom in "real life," in the doctor's office that person is just another person, possibly a frightened one.

The way you look and how you behave sets an impression for the patient about the office in general. When you call a patient to come from the waiting room to the examination or treatment room, the patient immediately forms an impression of the quality of care you—and the doctor—are going to provide. If you are neat, clean, and well groomed, you project a sense of professionalism, authority, and high standards.

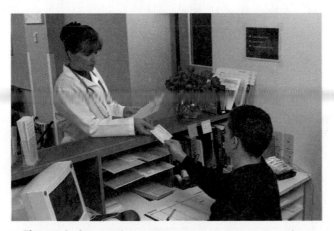

➤ **Figure 4–1** A medical assistant should present a professional appearance whether wearing a uniform, lab coat, or street clothes.

When you are courteous you project to the patient that you believe that a person has dignity, even when he or she is dressed only in underwear and an examination gown.

Most medical offices require that medical assistants wear some sort of uniform, usually white pants or scrub pants, white soft-soled shoes, and a lab coat or uniform top. These tops might be a hospital scrub-type shirt, a white shirt that matches the pants, or even a three-button golf shirt with the name of the practice embroidered on the front. The latter type of uniform is especially popular in pediatric practices, which often strive for informality, or in practices that are seeking to create a **brand image** in an increasingly competitive medical care environment. Brand image is the consumers' perception of the value they receive from a product or service, including medical care (Figure 4–1).

Neatness and good grooming are also important for health and safety reasons. Hair carries bacteria, even if regularly washed. Anyone performing clinical activities should not have "big hair"—that is, long, loose, and/or frizzy hair. People with long hair should pull it back from their faces and tie it, usually in a ponytail. A little bit of makeup goes a long way in making you look professional and healthy, but too much is not appropriate for a work environment. Dress, hair, and makeup should present a businesslike appearance.

Nails should be kept relatively short and should not be polished. Long nails are not functional for keyboard work, patient care, or laboratory procedures. Bacteria can collect under chipped nail polish.

Traditionally, health professionals were only allowed to wear "functional" jewelry—a wristwatch and a plain wedding band—because jewelry is not regularly washed and can become tangled in equipment. Today, most medical offices allow staff to wear "small" earrings, which don't dangle below the earlobe, and necklaces that can be tucked into the shirtfront. It's not a good idea to wear rings other than a wedding band; they can cut through protective gloves or scrape a patient. Also, they need to be taken off frequently for handwashing.

Initiative, the ability to begin or follow through on a plan without being supervised, is an important concept for a health care team member. When you are willing to take some initiative and perform a small task that may not normally be yours to do, you project to others that you are part of a well-functioning team.

Initiative, however, does not mean taking over. The office is the doctor's place of business and the doctor expects to run it. Initiative does not mean redecorating the waiting room without asking the doctor. It does mean doing things that need to be done without being asked, keeping up with current issues in practice without being told, and identifying helpful educational opportunities and asking permission to attend. It also means finding useful things to do when the office is slow, such as restocking supplies, ordering supplies, and cleaning out cabinets and cupboards.

Teachers sometimes hear from office managers who have students working for them in externships that medical assisting students do not take enough initiative. Taking initiative is something that, once you have learned it, should begin to come naturally. While in school, students often wait for someone to tell them what to do and how to do it. In the workplace, a medical assistant is expected to take initiative—even on an externship.

Over the first few days and weeks in a new job or externship, you need to create a mental file, or write note cards, of all the little tasks that must be done. If you see that they are not being done because other people are busy, you can do them. That's initiative. You also have to take the time to learn and understand office policies and procedures. If the office policy is to answer any phone within four rings and a line is ring-

ing while the receptionist is speaking with a difficult patient and cannot break away, pick up the telephone. Explain that the receptionist will be with the person in a moment and put the person on hold. Write the person's name and the phone line on a sticky note and put it on the table next to the receptionist's phone. That's initiative.

Initiative is one of the things employers look for in new employees, and they may even test your initiative by showing you how to do something—restocking an exam room at the end of the day, for instance. Then they will watch to see if you restock the exam room without being told or if someone has to remind you.

PROFESSIONALISM

Professionalism is behavior based on a body of knowledge and ethical **standards** (norms that are gen-

---

AMA Principles of Medical Ethics
Preamble

The medical profession has long subscribed to a body of ethical statements developed primarily for the benefit of the patient. As a member of this profession, a physician must recognize responsibility not only to patients, but also to society, to other health professionals, and to self. The following Principles adopted by the American Medical Association are not laws, but standards of conduct which define the essentials of honorable behavior for the physician.

I. A physician shall be dedicated to providing competent medical service with compassion and respect for human dignity.

II. A physician shall deal honestly with patients and colleagues, and strive to expose those physicians deficient in character or competence, or who engage in fraud or deception.

III. A physician shall respect the law and also recognize a responsibility to seek changes in those requirements which are contrary to the best interests of the patient.

IV. A physician shall respect the rights of patients, of colleagues, and of other health professionals, and shall safeguard patient confidences within the constraints of the law.

V. A physician shall continue to study, apply and advance scientific knowledge, make relevant information available to patients, colleagues and the public, obtain consultation, and use the talents of other health professionals when indicated.

VI. A physician shall, in the provision of appropriate patient care except in emergencies, to be free to choose whom to serve, with whom to associate, and the environment in which to provide medical services.

VII. A physician shall recognize a responsibility to participate in activities contributing to an improved community.

➤ **Figure 4–2** AMA code of ethics. (From *Code of Medical Ethics. Current Opinions of the Council on Ethical and Judicial Affairs.* Copyright 1995-1999. American Medical Association.)

The Oath of Hippocrates

I swear by Apollo, the physician, and Aesculapius, and Health, and Allheal, and all the gods and goddesses, that, according to my ability and judgment, I will keep this oath and stipulation, to reckon him who taught me this art equally dear to me as my parents, to share my substance with him and relieve his necessities if required; to regard his offspring as on the same footing with my own brothers, and to teach them this art if they should wish to learn it, without fee or stipulation, and that by precept, lecture, and every other mode of instruction, I will impart knowledge of the art to my own sons and those of my teachers, and to disciples bound by a stipulation and oath, according to the law of medicine, but to none other.

I will follow that method of treatment which, according to my ability and judgment, I consider for the benefit of my patients, and abstain from whatever is deleterious and mischievous. I will give no deadly medicine to anyone if asked, nor suggest any such counsel; furthermore, I will not give to a woman an instrument to produce abortion.

With purity and holiness, I will pass my life and practice my art. I will not cut a person who is suffering with a stone, but will leave this to be done by those who are practitioners of this work. Into whatever houses I enter I will go into them for the benefit of the sick and will abstain from every voluntary act of mischief and corruption; and further from the seduction of females or males, bond or free.

Whatever, in connection with my professional practice, or not in connection with it, I may see or hear in the lives of men which ought not to be spoken abroad, I will not divulge, as reckoning that all should be kept secret.

While I continue to keep this oath unviolated, may it be granted to me to enjoy life and the practice of the art, respected by all men at all times, but should I trespass and violate this oath, may the reverse be my lot.

➢ **Figure 4–3** The Oath of Hippocrates.

---

erally agreed on) to serve the public. The particular body of knowledge, and the ethical standards that must be met, are different for each profession.

Professionalism for Doctors

For medical doctors, professionalism means treating patients based on the body of scientific knowledge they have accumulated, and continue to accumulate, over their working lifetime. In addition, doctors are bound by a host of ethical standards and legal regulations.

One set of standards is the American Medical Association's (AMA) code of ethics, which is shown in Figure 4–2.

Other standards include state and federal regulations, as well as regulations of the hospital(s) to which the doctors admit patients, any open-panel health maintenance organizations or preferred provider organizations in which they participate, and standards or guidelines developed by the national medical board of their specialty or subspecialty.

Doctors also take guidance from the ancient Greek physician Hippocrates (c. 460–377 B.C.), the best known of the ancient physicians; he is especially well known for his Hippocratic Oath, shown in Figure 4–3.

Very few of today's doctors actually swear the Hippocratic Oath when they graduate medical school, but its philosophical underpinnings are still taught in medical school and adhered to by doctors, especially the key concept: "first, do no harm."

The Hippocratic Oath is the earliest written ethical standard for doctors. But much has changed in 2,500 years. When you compare the Hippocratic Oath to the AMA code of ethics, you notice a number of similarities and number of differences.

Similarities. The notion of doctor–patient confidentiality stems from the Hippocratic Oath. So does the idea that the doctor should not take advantage of the doctor–patient relationship, especially by initiating a sexual relationship with the patient.

The idea, now being challenged, that doctors heal but do not assist death, is also present in the Hippocratic Oath. The Hippocratic Oath is the basis for many doctor's arguments against doctor-assisted suicide, participating in capital punishment by pronouncing the time of death after an execution, and performing abortions, which the Hippocratic Oath specifically prohibits.

Changes. In Hippocrates' time, medical knowledge was secret, to be shared only with fellow doctors and medical students. There was a father-son type of relationship between teacher and student and a brotherly relationship among all doctors. The notion that a doctor cannot "inform on" a fellow doctor can be directly traced to the Hippocratic Oath.

Today's AMA code of ethics contradicts this directly, stating that doctors have an obligation to expose colleagues who are incompetent, have character defects, are incapacitated because of substance abuse, or engage in fraud or deception. Medical knowledge is no longer secret, and for a doctor to use a secret remedy is considered unethical. Treatments must have been studied scientifically, with results published and other studies duplicating the study results, to be considered effective.

Currently, controversy exists over whether drug companies should be able to obtain patents on biological therapeutic discoveries derived from genetic engineering. For example, parts of the human genome have been patented, which affects how the scientific community can use the knowledge. If a scientist were to find a way to conduct a procedure to correct a genetic defect, should he be allowed to collect payments from others using the technique?

Additions. Perhaps the most important additions in the AMA code of ethics are the obligation for remaining current with new knowledge and skills, the commitment to providing community service, and the freedom to practice as the individual doctor desires.

Professionalism for Medical Assistants

The American Association of Medical Assistants (AAMA) has a code of ethics that is similar to the AMA code in requiring respect for patients, patient confidentiality, continuing education, and community service. The AAMA Code of Ethics is shown in Figure 4–4.

The medical assistant's ethical responsibilities are to admit mistakes, stay within the personal limits of his or her training, maintain confidentiality, stay current, be an **advocate** (a person who speaks up) for the patient, and follow the law. This may mean having to confront a fellow worker who is not adhering to such principles.

Dealing with a coworker's inappropriate conduct is difficult, especially if you are a new employee, or if the coworker is someone above you in the organizational hierarchy. We live in a society that doesn't like "tattletales." On the other hand, unprofessional behavior in a medical office is disruptive to the concept of teamwork, and even if it does not pose an immediate threat

---

AAMA Code of Ethics and AAMA Creed

Code of Ethics

The Code of Ethics of AAMA shall set forth principles of ethical and moral conduct as they relate to the medical profession and the particular practice of medical assisting.

Members of AAMA dedicated to the conscientious pursuit of their profession, and thus desiring to merit the high regard of the entire medical profession and the respect of the general public which they serve, do pledge themselves to strive always to:

    A. render service with full respect for the dignity of humanity;

    B. respect confidential information obtained through employment unless legally authorized or required by responsible performance of duty to divulge such information;

    C. uphold the honor and high principles of the profession and accept its disciplines;

    D. seek to continually improve knowledge and skills of medical assistants for the benefit of patients and professional colleagues;

    E. participate in additional service activities aimed toward improving the health and well-being of the community.

AAMA Creed

I believe in the principles and purposes of the profession of medical assisting.

I endeavor to be more effective.

I aspire to render greater service.

I protect the confidence entrusted to me.

I am dedicated to the care and well-being of all people.

I am loyal to my employer.

I am true to the ethics of my profession.

I am strengthened by compassion, courage and faith.

➤ Figure 4–4 AAMA Code of Ethics and AAMA Creed. (Courtesy of the American Association of Medical Assistants.)

to a patient, any behavior that results in people not working well together can lead to a dangerous situation.

You should first confront the individual calmly, noting that you believe his or her actions or behavior is inappropriate. Give the person a chance to respond and to change the behavior or act in a different way. If the person does not correct the situation, it is appropriate for you to speak to that person's supervisor.

If the unprofessional behavior is by a doctor or nurse, it can be reported to the state authority that licenses that individual. These agencies have different names in different states, for example, Board of Registration (Massachusetts), Board of Medical Practice (Minnesota), or Board of Medical Examiners (Oregon). Before making any kind of report you must make sure you have firsthand evidence (not supposition). That means that you have been an actual witness or involved party. In most states, reports can be made online; information about professionals whose licenses have been revoked or suspended is also available online in many states. Also, in most states, these reports can be made anonymously.

INTRODUCTION TO LEGAL CONCEPTS

Discussion of Law

The legal system in the United States is primarily divided into two parts, criminal law and civil law. The term **criminal law** is used to refer to the set of laws that protect society in a large sense, such as laws against robbery, rape, and operating a motor vehicle while under the influence of alcohol or a controlled drug. **Civil law** is the set of laws that deals with disputes between two people or groups of people; between people and corporations, government, or other organizations; or between one corporate, government, or organizational entity and another such entity.

Contracts are considered a part of civil law; disputes about contracts that go to court are tried as part of the civil court system. In any civil court proceeding, there is a **plaintiff**, the person or entity that makes the complaint, and a **defendant**, the person or entity who is charged with violating the law.

A number of highly specialized areas of the law fall outside criminal and civil law. These include maritime law, international law, and administrative law, which has to do with federal government agencies such as the Social Security Administration and the Internal Revenue Service.

In criminal law, the criminal activity itself is held to be harmful or potentially harmful to society or individual members of society. The act itself is punishable, regardless of whether anyone was actually harmed by the act. In civil law, an injury or damage must result because of someone's wrongful act for liability to arise. The same misdeed can provoke both a criminal charge and a civil lawsuit—the criminal charge to determine if the person is guilty of committing a crime punishable by a fine paid to the government or imprisonment, and the civil suit to assess what liability the person has to the injured party.

The best example of this dual legal picture is possibly the O.J. Simpson case. Simpson was found not guilty by a jury of the murder of his ex-wife. However, her estate filed a civil suit against him on the grounds of "wrongful death," and a separate jury found him guilty of causing her death and ruled that he had to pay her estate many millions of dollars.

In the context of the medical office, most legal disputes will have to do with civil liability (malpractice) or breach of contract. This will be discussed in more detail in this chapter. For further discussion of criminal law, see chapter 40.

Laws are created either by common law, also called case law, which is laws that come about over time through court rulings, or by enactment of **statutes.** These statutes are written and voted on, by **legislators**, who are elected by popular vote to serve in either the state legislature or the federal House of Representatives or Senate. Statutes passed by the legislature are then signed into law by the President (for a federal law) or a state governor (for law applicable to one state). Towns and cities can also enact laws, called ordinances; these usually have to do with such issues as smoking in public places, parking, leash laws for pets, and curfews at parks.

Groups of laws on the same topic are called **acts.** All employees of the medical office must be aware of the federal and state laws that regulate business operations, and health professionals must also be knowledgeable of laws regulating the provision of health care. Legal issues will be discussed in more detail in chapter 40.

State Regulation of Health Occupations

Each state regulates medical care and certain other health professions through medical practice acts. **Medical practice acts** vary from state to state, but they generally contain most of the following elements:

1. Definition of the practice of medicine.
2. Limitation to qualified practitioners by **licensure**—the process by which the state examines a person's qualifications, in this case the qualifications to practice medicine, and issues permission to practice in the form of a license.

In most states, a doctor can be licensed after he or she has:

1. Graduated from an accredited U.S. 4-year postgraduate school of medicine and received an MD

degree, a 4-year postgraduate school of osteopathy and received a DO degree, or a recognized foreign medical school and received an MD degree

2. Passed parts I, II, and III of the United States Medical Licensing Examination (USMLE), as well as an English language competence examination if foreign born and foreign educated

3. Served at least 1 year of postdoctoral hospital-based training, called an internship. Many states will only license doctors after they have completed 2 years of postdoctoral training, an internship and another year of residency, also called the PG-2 year

4. Is found by the board of medical examiners to be of good moral character.

Doctors can also be licensed in most states if they have held a medical license in another state for more than 5 years. This is called **reciprocal licensing**. Usually this is simply a matter of requesting a license if a doctor is moving from one state to another. In some states with many doctors, such as Massachusetts, reciprocal licensing is more difficult to obtain. Florida severely limits reciprocal licensing in an effort to keep older doctors from "retiring" to Florida and then opening practices or taking hospital or clinic jobs.

State boards of medical examiners approve the original application for a license, then renew the license yearly or biannually—every 2 years. A board of medical examiners can revoke or suspend a doctor's license for conviction of a crime, unprofessional activity, and physical or mental incapacitation, including alcoholism, drug abuse, and senility.

Similar acts govern the licensure and revocation of licenses for such professions as registered nurses, nurse practitioners, and physician's assistants. These acts clarify what the member of the profession can and cannot do. For example, the law in a given state would allow or prohibit a nurse practitioner from writing prescriptions.

Many medical professions, such as medical assistants, are not licensed by the state, and most states do not specifically define the scope of practice of the profession. Certain activities, such as taking X-rays, may be limited to certain licensed professionals or those who have completed specific training and received certification. Some states also limit administering medication or giving injections to certain licensed professionals. It is the responsibility of the medical assistant to find out what legal restrictions apply in the state in which he or she is training or employed and to practice within those restrictions.

Credentials of Medical Assistants

Even though medical assistants are not licensed, they are encouraged to become certified. **Certification** is a process by which a professional organization verifies a certain level of education and training. Two national organizations provide certification for medical assistants: the American Association of Medical Assistants (AAMA) and the American Medical Technologists (AMT).

Both organizations are affiliated with other organizations that accredit medical assisting programs in colleges and proprietary schools. Graduates take a certification examination. Graduates of programs accredited by the Commission on Accreditation of Allied Health Education Programs (CAAHEP) are eligible to take the AAMA certification exam. Those who pass the exam are awarded the credential CMA (certified medical assistant). They must meet continuing education requirements or be retested every 5 years to maintain certification.

Graduates of programs accredited by the AMT are eligible to take the AMT exam. Those who pass this exam are awarded the credential RMA (registered medical assistant). In some parts of the country more schools of medical assisting are affiliated with the AAMA; in other parts of the country more are affiliated with the AMT. CMAs and RMAs maintain professional organizations with regular meetings, journals, continuing education programs, and other member benefits.

Mandated Reporting

For public health reasons and the good of society as a whole doctors are required to make certain reports. Some are required by law and cannot be refused because the patient does not want the information released. These are:

1. Records of births, stillbirths, and deaths.
2. Reports to the medical examiner or coroner (the name depends on the state).

   Under certain circumstances, a death must be reported to the medical examiner/coroner. The medical examiner then decides whether to investigate. These circumstances include:

   death occurring after patient is in the hospital less than 24 hours

   death occurring outside the hospital when the person has not been seen by a doctor within a reasonable time

   death from unknown causes

   death from violence or possible death due to a crime.

3. Reports of infectious disease cases.

   These have to be reported to the board of health. Each state has a list of reportable diseases, which include diseases that pose a public health risk such as rabies, measles, and acquired immunodeficiency syndrome (AIDS). Dog bites and human bites usually also have to be reported.

4. Reports of injuries that may have occurred as a result of violence.

These have to be reported to the police. Sometimes a patient asks that the report not be made. The injured person may not press charges, but the injury still must be reported. If there is a likely need for evidence to be collected from the injured person (for example, in the case of a rape), the person should be directed to an emergency room, which has personnel trained in the procedure. Because most doctors do not want police in their waiting room, if this kind of case seems likely when patients call to ask for an appointment, they should be politely and tactfully referred to the emergency room.

5. Reports of possible abuse or neglect.

State laws vary, but all states require that suspected child abuse or neglect be reported to the police or a particular state agency. Suspicion does not have to be backed up with evidence. Certain professions are mandated (legally required) to report; this varies from state to state.

Doctors and nurses are always required to make such reports, and in some states medical assistants, as allied health care professionals, are also included in the list of those mandated to make reports.

6. Other reports.

Various reports are mandated by the states. Some states require reports about diagnosis of epilepsy, some for PKU (phenylketonuria), and some for cancer.

PATIENT RIGHTS

As a member of the medical team, the medical assistant is responsible for maintaining the rights of all patients. Most important among those rights are the rights to confidentiality and privacy in the relationship between the patient and the doctor (and all of the doctor's staff, acting as the doctor's agents), the right to be safe and secure in the doctor–patient relationship, and the right to be fully informed and give consent to any medical procedure the doctor believes it is prudent to undertake.

Confidentiality and Privacy

Information about patients that is learned during treatment must be held in confidence by those who need the information to provide care. This includes the doctor and other staff in the office. The doctor needs **written consent** (an agreement in writing) from the patient before he or she can release information about the patient, even to another doctor who is providing treatment. The consent form will be discussed in more

detail later in this chapter, and the procedure for releasing medical records will be discussed in chapter 35.

You should not release any information to family, friends, or others who call. Patient problems should not be discussed except in relation to immediate care being given. Patients should never be spoken about in a negative way.

These are among the most frequently broken rules in the office. For some reason, office staff love to gossip about patients. The more private the patient's problems—sexually transmitted disease, for instance—the more likely the issue is to be a topic of conversation. Gossip is a natural human tendency, but it is inappropriate in a medical office setting.

If you find it necessary to speak about a patient with another staff member or with a doctor, do it in the privacy of an examination room or the doctor's private office.

Dealing with colleagues who like to gossip is one of those difficult situations. It is probably impossible to stop office gossip, but let colleagues know that you are uncomfortable with it. Use "I" statements, such as "I'm really uncomfortable talking about patients. I was trained not to talk about patients, except when necessary." (See "On The Job.")

Release of information about a person or release of photographs without that person's permission is called **invasion of privacy.** Allowing another person to be present at a procedure without consent is an invasion of privacy; patients should always be asked for their consent to have a student or trainee in the room during an examination. Giving information to an insurance company or to a journalist without consent is also an invasion of privacy. Every medical office has forms that patients sign giving the office permission to release medical information.

Slander and **libel** are terms for the release of false information about a person. Slander is when verbal information is given; libel is when written information is given. A person can commit slander or libel against doctors or other medical office workers in addition to patients. Medical assistants should never speak loosely about the doctors, other staff, or the office where they work or did an externship. If it can be shown that something a medical assistant said or wrote caused the medical practice to lose patients or lose business, that would be grounds for the practice to sue the assistant for slander or libel.

Invasion of privacy, slander, and libel are all intentional **torts.** Tort is a legal term that means a person was done an injury that can be compensated. Invasion of privacy, slander, and libel are not physical injuries; rather, they are injuries of reputation. A person's reputation has value, and a court can rule that an injury to reputation did damage that should be paid for. Tort cases are tried under civil law, the law that regulates interactions between individuals.

ON THE JOB: THE NOSY RECEPTIONIST

In the office of Blackburn Primary Care Associates Stacy, the medical assistant, comes out to the front desk after placing a patient in an exam room. The receptionist, Ellen, is looking through a patient's medical record and asks Stacy about the patient.

Ellen: You know that girl that was just here, Brittany? I know her.
Stacy: Oh, you do?
Ellen: Yes. Because we lived in the same neighborhood, and her mother and I used to carpool the kids. I can't believe what she looks like. She's lost, what, 10 pounds since the last visit? What does she eat, lettuce leaves, or grapes? She has one of those, what, eating disorders, right?
Stacy: That's the kind of information I can't really discuss with you.
Ellen: No, no.
Stacy: It's between me and the doctor.
Ellen: Oh, sure. No, no. I was just scanning here. I just can't believe it. She's dropped a lot, hasn't she?

Stacy knows that it is highly unprofessional to gossip about patients at the front desk. She also knows that patient confidentiality requires that office staff only read patient medical records when necessary for patient care, billing, or other administrative reasons.

QUESTIONS

1. Did Stacy do the correct thing by refusing to tell Ellen anything about the patient? Why or why not?

2. What is the next thing Stacy might say as the situation continues?

3. Who is behaving professionally in this situation: Stacy, Ellen, both, or neither? Justify your answer.

4. Why might Stacy be reluctant to report this situation to the office manager or doctor? Should she?

The Doctor–Patient Relationship

The doctor–patient relationship is a contractual relationship. It is governed by law, and each party has certain rights and responsibilities under the relationship. A **contract** is:

1. A mutual agreement
2. to do or refrain from doing
3. something that is legal
4. in exchange for a consideration (service or nonfinancial benefit) or for payment (money or goods).

A contract can be **implied** (not formally agreed to but obvious under the circumstances). If you take your clothes to the dry cleaners but do not ask how much it will cost to have them cleaned, you still must pay to retrieve the clothes. The same is true for a patient who visits a doctor's office.

A contract can be **expressed** (formally agreed to). If you ask a neighbor to baby-sit Saturday evening for $5.50 per hour and she agrees, you and she have a

verbal contract (one agreed to in words but not written). If you sign a loan agreement to borrow money to pay for a new car, you have a **written contract**. Signing a surgery charge sheet is also creating a written contract.

In all contract matters, it is important to understand that certain classes of people are not legally able to be a party to contracts, including most medical care contracts. These people are also not able to give informed consent.

These classes of people include children, mentally ill or retarded adults, those who are temporarily mentally incapacitated, those who are under threat or duress (fear of a threat), and those who have been found incompetent to handle their affairs. When with such people, all documentation should be signed and all implied contracts made with a competent party acting as a willing health care decision maker for the incompetent person.

Agreements between a doctor and patient are usually implied or verbal. The conditions of the doctor–patient contract are:

The Doctor. The doctor provides skillful care to the patient and continues to treat the patient unless he or she informs the patient that the relationship will be terminated and gives the patient time to make other arrangements. The doctor arranges for someone else to treat the patient if the doctor is unavailable (such as on nights, weekends, and vacations). The doctor informs the patient about treatments or procedures and only carries out those treatments and procedures that the patient consents to. The doctor informs the patient of test results, diagnoses, and medical conditions and gives the patient instructions for follow-up care and procedures to follow at home.

A doctor has the right to accept or decline to treat a patient, to choose to limit the medical practice to a particular size or certain specialty, and to decide where to practice and when to operate. Decisions not to treat particular patients may not be **arbitrary** (based on a whim or subjective judgment).

The Patient. The patient agrees to keep appointments, give accurate information about his or her medical condition, provide an accurate medical history, follow directions, and pay for the service.

The patient has the right to refuse treatment, receive complete information about procedures, select a doctor, receive continuity of care, receive confidentiality of verbal and written communication with the doctor and the doctor's agents, be treated with respect and dignity, and receive complete information about the treatment suggested, alternatives, and possible consequences of alternatives or no treatment.

To end a relationship with a patient, a doctor must notify the patient in writing, using certified mail and return receipt requested (types of mailing will be discussed in detail in chapter 35). The letter needs to be dated, must state the reasons for termination of care, and must describe how medical records will be made available. Copies of any correspondence regarding termination and receipts should be kept in the medical record.

Common reasons for a doctor terminating care of a patient include the following:

The doctor moves.
The doctor retires.
The doctor dies.
The doctor closes the practice for other reasons.
The patient regularly and continually breaks appointments.
The patient regularly and continually refuses to follow medical advice.

Doctors also send notification of termination of the doctor–patient relationship to confirm a telephone conversation with the patient in which the patient has notified that doctor that he or she wishes to terminate the relationship.

If a patient can convince a court that he or she was under the belief that a doctor–patient relationship still existed and because of such belief did not seek out another practitioner, and suffered injury, a successful case can be made for **abandonment.** This is rare and should never happen if the doctor keeps good written records about any termination notification. Figure 4–5 is a sample letter of termination.

Informed Consent

Like contract, consent is either implied or expressed. If a medical assistant says, "Roll up your sleeve so I can give you an injection," and the patient does, the patient has given implied consent to the medical assistant to administer the injection. Although the patient has not verbally agreed, the act of preparing for the injection suggests that the patient is willing to undergo the procedure.

Again, as with a contract, expressed consent can be verbal or written. We know, however, that simply expressing consent does not always represent understanding. Patients today have the legal right to completely understand what will be done to them or for them. For this reason, many medical offices now use written consent forms. This is called **informed consent.**

Written consent forms are now always used for surgery; for invasive procedures such as **endoscopy,** in which a thin, flexible glass tube with a light source and camera lens is put in the mouth and down the throat to visualize the esophagus or in the anus to visualize the rectum and colon; and for testing for human immunodeficiency virus, the virus that causes AIDS. Written consent forms are increasingly being used as well for immunizations, treatment with birth control pills, transfusions of blood or blood products such as plasma, and other treatments and procedures. A consent form for surgery is shown in Figure 4–6.

You should realize that legally it is not the form but the understanding by the person on whom the treatment or procedure will be performed that truly represents consent. It is the responsibility of the person performing the procedure, prescribing the medication, or performing the test or examination to inform the patient about the potential risks of the action, the discomfort it may cause, the common side effects, and why it is important to do and the probable results if the test or procedure is not done.

Often the medical assistant is asked to obtain the signature on the consent form and witness that signature. If the medical assistant believes that the patient does not fully understand what he or she is consenting to, the matter should be referred back to the doctor. This is a good example of the medical assistant acting as a liaison between the patient and the doctor and being an advocate for the patient.

Another kind of consent that must be obtained is a patient's consent to release medical records, either to other doctors or to insurance companies so the doctor can be paid for the services performed.

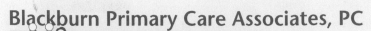

Blackburn Primary Care Associates, PC

1990 Turquiose Drive • Blackburn, WI 54937 • 608-459-8857

Howard M. Lawler, MD
Joanne R. Hughes, MD
Ralph Garcia Lopez, MD

October 28, 1999

James Winston
824 Arcana Road
Blackburn, WI 54937

Dear Mr. Winston:

This letter is to inform you I am withdrawing from providing medical service to you because you have consistently failed to keep appointments even though your condition requires medical care. Your medical conditions require frequent monitoring and adherence to prescribed regimens, but your failure to keep the last three appointments make it impossible for me to assume responsibility for your state of health or illness. I do agree to provide care to you, if you wish, up to December 31, 1999 which should give you adequate time to seek another primary care provider.

I encourage you to find another physician promptly, and I hope that you will find a practitioner with whom you can establish an effective relationship. Please feel free to call our office, your insurance company or the state medical society to obtain a referral to another physician.

Please notify us in writing when you have selected a new physician, and we will be happy to forward a copy of your medical record and a summary of your treatment.

Very truly yours,

Howard Lawler

Howard Lawler, MD

> **Figure 4–5** Sample letter notifying patient of doctor's withdrawal as primary care doctor.

Background Checks

In its Medicare legislation, the federal government requires that background checks be conducted for caregivers who work with the elderly, to prevent people with criminal records from being hired to take care of elderly patients. States have passed laws to comply with this regulation, and in those laws many states have also included a requirement for other types of health care facilities to perform background checks on all employees.

PERSONAL AND PROFESSIONAL LIABILITY

Liability means legal responsibility. A person is responsible for his or her actions and may be required to pay if those actions injure another person. In daily life we are required to act as a reasonable person would act in the same circumstances. The failure to act—or refrain from acting—as a reasonable person would act in similar circumstances is called **negligence**.

A common example of negligence relates to a wet floor. If someone spills water on the floor and does not

CONSENT FOR SURGERY

Date_____

Time_____

I authorize the performance of the following procedure(s) _____
_____on _____
                                                              (Name of patient)
to be performed by_____, MD.
                              (Name of physician)

The following have been explained to me by Dr._____
                                                              (Name of physician)

     1. Nature of the procedure (followed by exact description):

     2. Reason(s) for procedure (followed by reasons):

     3. Possible risks (followed by risks and likelihood, if known):

     4. Possible complications (followed by complications and likelihood, if known):

I understand that no warranty or guarantee of the effectiveness of the surgery can be made.

I have been informed of possible alternative treatments including _(description of possible alternative treatments)_ and of the likely consequences of receiving no treatment, and I freely consent to this procedure.

I hereby authorize the above named surgeon and his/her assistants to provide additional services including administering anesthesia and/or medication, performing needed diagnostic tests including but not limited to radiology, and any other additional service deemed necessary for my well-being. I consent to have removed tissue examined by a pathologist who may then dispose of the tissue as he/she sees fit.

Signed_____ Relationship to Patient _____
       (Patient/Parent/Guardian)

Witness_____

> **Figure 4–6** Sample consent form for surgery.

wipe it up, or if someone washes a floor, the floor becomes slippery. When an unsuspecting person comes along and is not aware that the floor is wet, that person could slip and be injured. The person responsible for making the floor wet will be expected to know that the wet floor is slippery and could cause someone to fall.

If a person falls, is injured, and files a lawsuit, the person who washed the floor could be found guilty of negligence and be responsible (liable) to pay for the injured person's medical care, lost wages, and any other costs caused by the fall on the wet floor.

Standard of Care

A person without any special training is held only to a standard of a "reasonably prudent person." The term **prudent** means careful or using common sense. For instance, if a person who doesn't know how to do cardiopulmonary resuscitation (CPR) performs CPR on someone who has a heartbeat and breaks some of the person's ribs, so that a lung is punctured, the person who gave CPR might be found in court to be not prudent.

A medical assistant is generally held to a professional standard, especially when performing procedures that are also or primarily done by a licensed health professional. The medical assistant must be especially careful to avoid offering advice or making decisions that may be interpreted as diagnosing illness or prescribing treatment.

If the medical assistant administers medication, he or she must do so correctly and must follow proper procedures and precautions to protect the patient from injury. A doctor must be on the premises (not necessarily in the room) any time medication is given by a medical assistant, because in most states the medical assistant can only perform the procedure under the authority and supervision of a doctor.

IMPORTANT: It is your obligation as a medical assistant to know what you are legally allowed to do in the state in which you work and the standard of care to which you are held.

In emergency situations, when no qualified professional is available, health care practitioners are allowed to give care for which they have been trained but at which they may not be proficient. For instance, a psychiatrist who performs a tracheotomy—an incision through the neck and into the windpipe to allow a patient to breathe—in his office would have to meet the same standard as a surgeon. But if that same psychiatrist performed an emergency tracheotomy at the scene of an accident where a trauma victim's airway is blocked, she will be held to a lower standard; this allows a doctor to extend himself or herself into an area in which he or she is less competent in order to save a patient's life without fear of a malpractice lawsuit.

Patients make an assumption that in a medical office they will receive medical treatment, even in the event of an emergency. All medical office personnel are expected to be able to give advice in an emergency or to activate the office's emergency medical system if they cannot handle the situation.

Many, if not most, medical offices, train all of their personnel in CPR and first aid. If a medical assistant, secretary, or receptionist tells any patient that a problem is not serious and it is, that person will most likely be liable if there is injury to the patient due to delay of treatment. Failure to respond correctly to an emergency can be considered a "breach of contract" because there is an implied contract between a patient and a medical office that any emergency will be handled by competent staff.

Health professionals are generally held to a high standard of care. The doctor's key legal obligation is to provide care to patients that meets an acceptable standard. For doctors and other health professionals, the term **standard of care** defines the level of appropriate care legally required of any health care professional, the care that would be given by any other practitioner providing the same care in the same geographic region. In general, if a legal question arises, a professional will be held to the standard of care of the professional who would normally perform the care in question.

For example, if a family practice doctor prescribes blood pressure medication, he or she has to do it as competently as another family practice doctor in the same area. If a nurse practitioner prescribes blood pressure medication, he or she has to meet the same standard as the family practice doctor. If a patient suffers injury from taking the medication, in either case, the court would look at the appropriateness of the medication for the particular patient, the dose, and the monitoring performed to see whether either practitioner has acted at an acceptable level.

Professional negligence is often called **malpractice.** To avoid lawsuits for malpractice, a health professional must be sure that he or she is acting within the limits of his or her profession, and must act (or refrain from acting) in a given situation as a reasonable and prudent person of the same profession would. When the medical assistant performs procedures that are usually performed by other professionals, such as nurses, the medical assistant will be held to the same standard as the professional who usually performs the procedure. No one always does everything perfectly, and both negligence and malpractice are assumed to be mistakes and unintentional. The legal term for such an occurrence is an unintentional tort, a wrongful act that results in injury to another person.

To prove that a professional is guilty of malpractice and liable for the outcome, four things must be proved "by a preponderance—a large majority—of the evidence." Sometimes these are called the 4 D's of malpractice.

1. The person who caused the injury has a *duty* to the person who was injured.
2. The person was *derelict* (neglectful) in performing that duty.
3. The failure to perform the duty was the *direct* cause of the injury and nothing could have intervened.
4. The failure to perform the duty caused *damage* or injury.

A doctor who gives casual medical advice at a party may not consider the person a patient he or she has a duty to take care of. But if the person fails to seek medical treatment based on the doctor's casual words, a court may have to decide if the doctor owed a duty to the person.

If a professional does exactly what any other professional would have done, and the patient has a poor outcome, the doctor is not necessarily derelict. For example, even with the best sterile technique it is possible to get a wound infection. A person with a wound infection must show that proper technique was not used. If the injured person does not follow directions to keep the wound dry and the wound gets infected,

FOCUS ON
LEGAL ISSUES

MEASURES TO PREVENT MALPRACTICE

The best way to protect against malpractice lawsuits is to use the following procedures to prevent mistakes:

1. Make sure all equipment is in good working order and that you have been properly trained to use it.

2. Make sure you know how to do procedures, and review them in the procedure manual if you have any doubts.

3. Be sure that patients understand the nature of procedures and surgery, and always obtain written consent for surgery and invasive procedures.

4. Always document accurately and completely. Promptly report any problems, and document your report.

5. Protect patients from injury by using equipment correctly. Transfer correctly to and from wheelchairs.

6. Don't leave patients alone if there is any question of their balance or mental status. Don't ever leave children unattended in an examination room or the waiting room.

7. Use care to identify any medication, medication dose, patient for specimen. Label all specimens correctly. Log and track all results so none slip through the cracks.

8. Never leave patients unattended with hot packs or where hot water or hot pipes are present.

9. Clean liquid spills promptly and put up signs if floors are wet.

10. Don't make promises about outcomes.

11. Keep current on procedures and equipment, and get training as necessary.

12. Notify a doctor of any patient complaints or requests for patient records.

13. Always follow up with post-surgical patients.

maybe the infection was not directly caused by the surgery, but because the patient did not follow directions.

If someone makes a mistake but there is no injury, the person who makes the mistake will not be liable and will not have to pay any damages. Many mistakes can be corrected if they are reported promptly.

Sometimes lawsuits do occur; these will be discussed in greater detail in chapter 40. To protect against financial loss, doctors usually have professional liability insurance (also called malpractice insurance).

This is for two reasons. One is to protect them for their own negligent actions. The second is to protect them if they are sued for the negligent actions of their employees while on the job.

If an injury occurs the law allows the injured person to sue both the person responsible for causing the injury *and that person's employer*, provided that the incident occurred while the person responsible was at work, under what is known as the **doctrine of *respondeat superior*.** The English translation of this Latin term is literally "let the master answer," meaning let the person at the head of the organization answer for the injuries caused by his or her underlings.

This legal doctrine provides an incentive for employers to be sure that their employees are careful and gives the injured person a better chance of collecting actual money for any injury, because the lower-level employee might not have insurance to cover such an incident or enough money to pay the amount received in judgment. Medical assistants who belong to the American Association of Medical Assistants have the opportunity to purchase their own inexpensive malpractice insurance; you should look into this when you begin working.

Laws that protect health professionals from being sued for giving emergency care are called **Good Samaritan Acts.** They vary from state to state, and may cover doctors, nurses, emergency medical technicians, anyone certified to perform CPR, and other professionals.

Measures to Avoid Lawsuits

There are two important elements to avoiding malpractice suits. The first is to implement proper procedures to prevent mistakes. These procedures are part of the overall process of risk management, a term that means measures taken to reduce risks within the medical office.

Safety plans, chemical hygiene plans, evacuation plans, and standard precautions are all part of risk management. So are measures to avoid theft by patients or staff, or fraud by financial staff. In addition, education and training of all staff helps each staff member provide proper care to patients.

A second element of risk management is to prevent patients from becoming angry about the care (or lack of care) they receive. This requires all staff who interact with patients to be courteous, give complete explanations, and treat patients and their families with respect and dignity. If the office maintains good relations with patients, patients will be more likely to understand when there is a poor outcome or a mistake is made. Demonstrating respect and concern for patients at all times is one of the most important ways to prevent malpractice lawsuits.

Although the owners of the practice are ultimately responsible, the job of developing and implementing risk management plans usually falls to the office manager and, in a small office, to the head medical assistant. See box "Measures to Prevent Malpractice."

EMPLOYEE RIGHTS

Your main role is in safeguarding patient rights, but you also need to make sure that your rights within the employment relationship are being recognized. You have the right to know and understand the personnel standards of your employer's office, the way and means by which you will be compensated and evaluated; the right to see your personnel records and challenge information that is in them; and the right to be free from sexual harassment or any other type of personal **intimidation** (deliberately making someone uncomfortable) that makes the workplace hostile. Sexual harassment is a legal term with a specific meaning.

Sexual harassment occurs when any person makes intentional and clearly understood statements, or takes intentional and clearly understood actions, that cause another person to feel that his or her job is at risk if the other person's sexual advances are not accepted. Intimidation can be sexual or racial, or can be based on a person's sexual orientation or ethnicity.

For instance, a doctor who insists on taking a medical assistant to dinner to discuss "opportunities for advancement in the office" even after she has said she would like to have the discussion in the office could be charged with sexual harassment. A nurse who continually comments to married colleagues about the new medical assistant's "cute girlfriend" when it is clear that the medical assistant can hear the conversation could be charged with harassment.

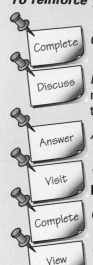

STUDENT STUDY PLAN

To reinforce your understanding of the material in this chapter . . .

Complete — *Complete* the **Review & Recall** questions.

Discuss — *Discuss* the situation in **If You Were The Medical Assistant** with your classmates and answer the questions. If possible, view scene 1.2A, "Antibiotic Reaction," from the Saunders video series.

Answer — *Answer* the **Critical Thinking questions** and discuss them with your classmates.

Visit — *Visit* the **Web sites** suggested and search for additional Web sites using the **Keywords for Internet Searches.**

Complete — *Complete* the exercises in chapter 4 of the **Student Mastery Manual.**

View — *View* the **Videotape:** *Ethical, Legal and Professional Issues.*

REVIEW & RECALL

1. List character and personality traits of an effective medical assistant.
2. Why does a professional appearance improve a medical assistant's effectiveness?
3. List several ethical standards that guide modern doctors.
4. What are the major differences between civil law and criminal law?
5. List the four elements of a contract.
6. Describe the concept of confidentiality as it applies to the medical office.
7. Give examples of three intentional torts.
8. Why should a doctor notify a patient in writing if he or she plans to terminate the doctor–patient relationship?
9. How does the term "standard of care" apply to the doctor and to the medical assistant?
10. List and define the four elements that must exist for malpractice to be present.

IF YOU WERE THE MEDICAL ASSISTANT

See Video: Ethical, Legal and Professional Issues, "The Mistake"

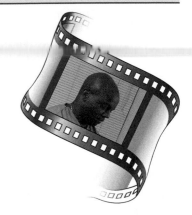

In the office of Blackburn Primary Care Associates, Kevin, a medical assistant has brought Mrs. McAllister into an examination room to tell her that her son Keith, a patient of Dr. Hughes, has had a reaction to an antibiotic he was given in the office that morning and that the doctor is working to stabilize Keith's condition. Mrs. McAllister becomes very upset during the discussion for several reasons.

Although Keith is 18 years old and therefore legally able to consent to medical treatment, Mrs. McAllister still considers him a child and states that she should have been consulted before the antibiotic was given. In addition, she states that in the past Keith had had a reaction to a similar antibiotic, and she feels that the doctor should have known that Keith should not receive this medication. She says that she isn't sure she trusts Dr. Hughes after this and demands to see the doctor at once.

1. Based on the information given here, would you say that a doctor–patient relationship exists between Keith McAllister and Dr. Hughes? Why or why not?

2. Keith might have given implied consent or verbally given informed consent to the injection. Which type of consent should have been obtained? If the doctor gave the injection, what might she have said to obtain implied consent? What else would have been necessary to obtain informed consent?

3. If the medical assistant had given the injection, could the doctrine of *respondeat superior* apply to the situation? What would that mean?

4. To bring a lawsuit for malpractice, four elements must exist. List these elements and identify further information you would need for any or all of them to decide if Keith's antibiotic reaction is a result of professional negligence (malpractice).

 ## CRITICAL THINKING QUESTIONS

1. Assess your own ability to demonstrate initiative: Do you ask questions about material you do not understand? Do you try to find answers to questions by looking up information in dictionaries, encyclopedias, books, or on the Internet? Do you ever do extra work to try to master a difficult topic or subject? Do you contribute to class discussions? Would you ever ask a teacher to discuss in more depth a topic that interests you? How do these questions help you assess your own level of initiative?

2. Compare and contrast the Hippocratic Oath and the AMA Principles of Medical Ethics in detail. Use this comparison to identify ideas about medical ethics that have persisted since the time of the Greeks, ideas that have changed, and new ideas that have developed. Do research if necessary to identify circumstances that have triggered any new ideas about medical ethics.

3. Discuss the following situations with your classmates and decide if you think the person was behaving as a "reasonably prudent person."
   A. A person parks his car under a tree where a workman is removing branches. The workman tells him not to park there because a branch may fall on his car. The person says, "You can see my car; you better be careful," and walks away. If a branch does fall on the car and damages it, did the car owner behave prudently to protect his property?
   B. A child spills water on a linoleum floor in the medical office playroom. The mother comes to the front desk and asks for a paper towel to dry the water. The medical assistant goes to get some paper towels but is called away to assist a doctor. The mother waits at the desk; after several minutes another child slips in the wet area and falls. Was the mother of the child who spilled the water reasonably prudent? Was the medical assistant?

   C. A medical assistant assists an elderly and apparently confused woman to the examination room, and has her sit on the end of the exam table. She closes the door and leaves the patient to wait for the doctor. After a short time she hears a crash from the exam room. She finds the woman lying on the floor. Did the medical assistant behave in a prudent way? Would this patient also be required to behave as a prudent person?

4. Identify individuals in your own experience who are professionals. Discuss the character and personality traits listed in this book that those people display. Are some more professional than others? Why do you say this?

5. Obtain examples of consent forms, either from your instructor or from medical offices in your area. Analyze them to determine if they contain complete information. Are there any additions you would recommend?

6. Discuss the standard of care for a medical assistant. What might happen if a medical assistant did not meet the appropriate standard (for example, did not apply a hot pack correctly)? What might happen if a medical assistant was not aware of the scope of practice for medical assisting and went beyond it (for example, by advising a patient with a high fever to take ibuprofen and wait 24 hours to see if the fever went down)?

7. Why do health professionals obtain professional liability insurance? Find out if you are covered by liability insurance as a student when you are doing an externship.

EXPLORE THE WEB

INTERNET WEB SITES

Physician licensing boards
www.fsmb.org/members.htm
www.docboard.org

Accreditation of medical assisting programs
American Association of Medical Assistants
(AAMA)
www.aama-ntl.org
Commission on Accreditation of Allied Health
Programs (affiliated with AAMA)
www.caahep.org
American Medical Technologists
www.amt1.org
Accrediting Bureau of Health Education Schools
(affiliated with AMT)
www.abhes.org

Summary of state malpractice law by state
www.mcandl.com/introduction.html

KEYWORDS FOR INTERNET SEARCHES

For the Web site of any state's department of public
health, find the state's Web site (name of state.gov)
then add DPH (or Department of Public Health). State
Web sites also usually have a heading for "state laws"
as well.

child abuse
patient rights
medical license
nursing license
medical malpractice

 ANSWERS TO "ON THE JOB"

1. Stacy did the correct thing by telling Ellen that the medical information about the patient was between herself and the doctor. This protects patient confidentiality.

2. This situation comes from the videotape "Ethical, Legal and Professional Issues," where a real medical assistant was placed in this situation. The next thing Stacy did say was,
   "I really can't discuss that with you. It's between me and the doctor and Brittany."
   She basically repeated what she had said before. This is a firm and direct response that avoids labeling the receptionist's behavior.

3. Stacy is behaving professionally in this situation by protecting the patient's confidentiality and by treating her coworker with respect. Ellen is behaving unprofessionally by reading a patient medical record for personal reasons and by asking for personal information about the patient from the medical assistant.

4. Stacy might be reluctant to say anything about Ellen's behavior because American society does not encourage "telling on" someone else, or "blowing the whistle." In the interview between the video producer and Stacy after the scene was shot, Stacy said that unless she was personally involved, she would not report a fellow employee who was "pushing the envelope of confidentiality." In this situation, she said, "I would report it, like I said, if I was involved in the situation like I was in the scene. I would probably just mention it to the office manager, or to the doctor, 'Listen, she shouldn't be going in the charts, and maybe you can handle it from there.' "

Communication: How Do You Speak in the Workplace?

Instructional Objectives

After completing this chapter, you will be able to do the following:

1. Define and spell the vocabulary terms.
2. Describe the steps in the communication process.
3. Differentiate between verbal and nonverbal communication.
4. Describe how nonverbal communication occurs.
5. Identify things that can interfere with effective communication.
6. Identify the elements of active listening.
7. Describe how eye contact can have different meanings based on cultural background.
8. Describe the appropriate use of the following interview techniques:
   - open-ended questions
   - closed questions
   - paraphrasing
   - translating into feelings
   - reflecting
   - summarizing
   - restating
   - silence
9. List measures to evaluate if communication has been effective.
10. List several reasons to establish caring relationships with patients.
11. Identify how empathy helps improve the relationship between the medical assistant and the patient.
12. List ways to adapt communication when barriers are present, such as impaired understanding, impaired sensation, impairment due to strong emotions, and language barriers.

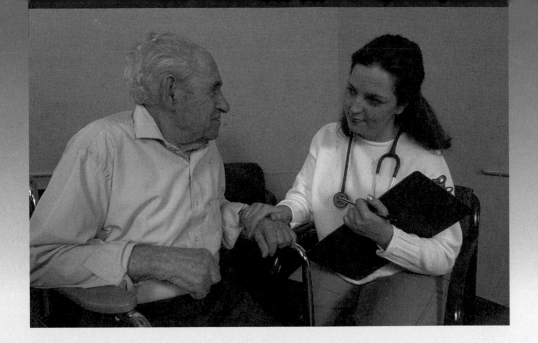

- Understand principles of mental health and applied psychology
- Understand cultural influences on behavior
- Understand principles of verbal and nonverbal communication

- Adapt method of communication to meet individual needs
- Recognize and respond to verbal communication
- Recognize and respond to nonverbal communication

VOCABULARY

active listening (p. 82)
autonomy (p. 86)
barriers to communication (p. 81)
body language (p. 81)
closed questions (p. 83)

empathy (p. 86)
judgmental (p. 83)
noncompliant (p. 86)
nonverbal (p. 80)

open-ended questions (p. 83)
oral (p. 81)
paraphrasing (p. 83)
perception (p. 80)

reflecting (p. 84)
summarizing (p. 84)
translating into feelings (p. 84)
verbal (p. 80)

The statement "illness is a state of mind" may seem silly or even harsh. To be sure, physical illness exists, it is real. But as we enter the 21st century, doctors in all areas of medical practice are coming to realize that people's **perception**—the way they believe things are—of their state of health is extremely important. Easing fear and anxiety, and helping people to understand their state of health and how to manage any illness they have is a major part of health care.

To assess patients' perception of their health and help them understand how to take care of themselves, a health care professional must be a good communicator. This means being effective at both sending and receiving messages.

In this chapter, I'll quickly review the fundamentals of communication, then put these fundamentals into the health care setting, explaining how to interview patients, how to establish caring relationships with patients, and how to adapt your normal communication style when barriers to communication exist.

COMMUNICATION SKILLS

Figure 5–1 shows in graphic form the basic theory of communication. A sender sends a message to a receiver. The message can be either **verbal** (using spoken or written words) or **nonverbal** (expressed without

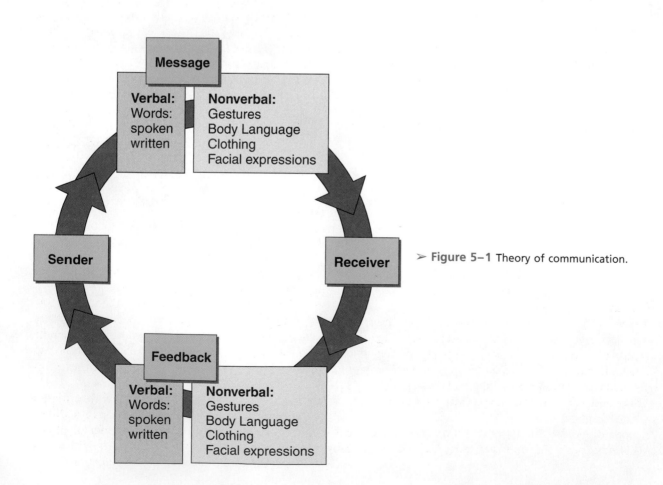

➤ **Figure 5–1** Theory of communication.

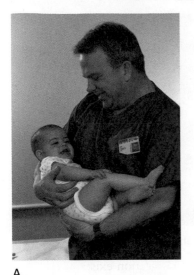
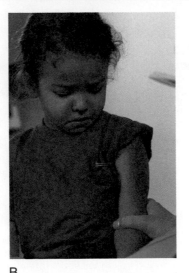
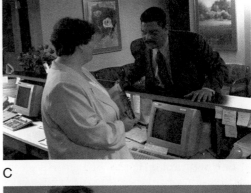

A   B   C

D

➢ **Figure 5–2** Most adults can easily identify the people in these photographs as expressing A—pleasure, B—uncertainty or lack of confidence, C—aggression, D—confusion.

words, using body language, facial expression, and other means).

Verbal and Nonverbal Communication

Verbal communication is either **oral,** meaning spoken, or written. Written communication has traditionally been thought of as more formal than oral conversation—a formal letter rather than a phone call. Today, however, with the increasing use of e-mail, written communication is often as informal as oral communication.

Nonverbal communication, often called nonverbal cues, refers to information that is received from **body language** (the way a person's body signals feelings or emotions; for instance, hands folded across the chest and a rigid posture may signal anger), tone of voice, anything other than actual words. Nonverbal communication is the secondary communication that goes on during oral conversation, including voice pitch, volume, and quality. These often provide more information than the words themselves.

If you ask a patient a simple question: "How are you feeling today, Mr. Jackson?" the oral response "all right" doesn't tell you much. But the quality of the voice—pinched, pained, flat, excited, spoken with a deep sigh—tells you more about Mr. Jackson's physical condition and can tell you an enormous amount about his state of mind.

Other types of nonverbal communication are facial expression, body position, and gestures used while speaking.

Between the sender and receiver any one of a number of elements can interfere with communication. These are sometimes called static. The best analogy for simple communication is listening to the radio. The radio station, the sender, broadcasts a signal. When you turn on the car radio to that station you become the receiver. Any number of outside elements can interfere with the radio station's signal: a storm that causes electrical interference in the atmosphere, air traffic controllers switching to a radio frequency that interferes with the broadcast frequency, driving through a tunnel or over a bridge with steel suspension.

In the medical office, interference often comes not from *outside* factors, but from factors *inside* the patient's physical and, more importantly, emotional condition. Pain, fatigue, fear, anxiety, and anger all create interference with communication. Sometimes we call these interfering elements **barriers to communication.** Other barriers arise because people's understanding is impaired or because their senses are impaired.

Psychologists and communication theorists have shown through research that most people are pretty good at reading nonverbal cues and that generally women are better than men. Their research also shows that emotions generally cross cultural boundaries (Figure 5–2).

What does not necessarily cross cultural boundaries well are gestures. Different cultures also have a different idea of personal space, as well as the act of physically touching another person. Cultural sensitivity is especially important in effective communication; nonverbal communication that is part of your general approach, such as smiling, looking straight into the speaker's eye, or lightly touching someone's shoulder to show concern may create interference if the gesture is not common to the listener's culture.

The four major components to being a good receiver of communication include:

listening skills
eye contact
response to body language
tact and diplomacy

Some people are naturally better listeners than others, but listening skills can be learned and practiced. The most important listening skill is called **active listening.**

Active listening means paying attention with your entire mind to what is being said, being "in the moment." By this I mean not thinking about anything else and focusing all of your attention on the person you are listening to in the time and place you are. To receive a message clearly, you need to examine your own attitudes and feelings, and put any aside that may interfere with your concentration on the speaker's message.

What a speaker says will naturally trigger responses. But often, you have to let go of the urge to respond verbally, grab the conversation, and air your own views. If you have successfully removed your mental focus from yourself and put the focus on the patient, you will not be tempted to let your mental responses become spoken responses, and you will be able to have your mental responses be a flicker that fades quickly as the patient says something else, rather than a response that gets stuck in your brain and inhibits you from receiving later messages.

Other important elements necessary for listening are:

1. Checking to make sure your interpretation of the message is correct. That may involve asking the patient to repeat what has been said by rephrasing a question. I'll discuss this further in the next section on interviewing techniques.
2. Listening for feelings. Be alert for key words or themes the patient uses frequently to describe the medical condition. These can often be important clues as to the patient's emotional state. Be aware of changes in your own feelings. They may mirror the patient's.
3. Be observant while listening. The flip side of being careful about the nonverbal cues you send is being diligent in picking up the nonverbal cues you are receiving. Facial expression, body language, tone of voice, and other nonverbal cues can tell a lot about the patient's emotional state.
4. Be patient and listen completely. Allowing patients to tell their story in their own time and in

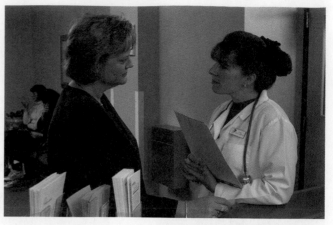

> Figure 5–3 Photograph showing comfortable talking distance in the United States.

their own way is important. Interruption interferes with this. You have questions you need to ask, but you should ask them in the way that least breaks the patient's natural storytelling flow.

In American culture, eye contact is very important (Figure 5–3). Maintaining eye contact is a sign of interest and involvement. But in many cultures it is not respectful to look directly at older people. This is especially true in Asian cultures and in Native American culture. Many Latinos also do not look directly at a person they respect, such as a teacher or a doctor.

If the patient looks away and you continue to seek eye contact with that person, he or she may perceive your attempt as aggression. Maintaining eye contact with someone who is culturally uncomfortable with that nonverbal communication creates a barrier.

We have far less control over our body movements than over our words, because control of body language is largely unconscious. But being aware of nonverbal messages allows the medical assistant to focus on trying to maintain an open, relaxed body posture. When a person's words and body language do not match, the body language often is a more genuine reflection of the person's feelings.

Be careful in responding to a patient's body language. If you respond to a patient's body language by saying "you look tense" or "you look tired," this may be interpreted as too much concern or even as criticism.

Touching a person, even gently, can also be interpreted in many different ways. Moving closer can indicate interest, but it may be seen by some people as aggressive. Many adults do not like to be touched by people they do not know well.

Again, cultural sensitivity is important. For instance, Asians do not like to have their own or their children's heads touched, even though they understand the importance of measuring an infant's head circumference. Reminding them in a reassuring tone of voice that this is an important medical activity and that there is no disrespect in the action may help.

If your own style is relaxed, a gentle pat on the shoulder can be very reassuring to some patients. Be sure to watch the patient for signs of tenseness or discomfort. If you notice the patient move back, wait until he or she relaxes. In the United States, people normally maintain a distance of about 4 feet for conversation with others; in other cultures, this comfort zone varies. Often, the medical assistant must come closer to perform a procedure.

Because the medical assistant's job is to make the person feel comfortable, you should avoid being too casual or familiar with a patient until you know him or her. If you think a subject may be sensitive, but it is important to ask about it, you can do so in a somewhat tentative way to make it easier for the patient to reply. Many people are not always aware of their feelings and may deny feelings that may be clear to you as the receiver of their nonverbal communication. Others are only too glad to have their feelings recognized.

Anger is a common emotion displayed by people who are ill. If you recognize this, you can say, "you seem angry about . . ." Do not be surprised if the response you get is delivered in an angry tone. In this case you need to allow the patient to vent and express his or her strong feelings without feeling personally attacked yourself. Remember that people often displace anger; this means expressing anger toward a different person or event than the one that is really triggering the feeling. Try very hard not to respond with anger yourself; buy time by leaving the room, counting to 10, or simply taking a couple of deep breaths.

Interviewing Techniques

When conducting an interview, you can ask two different types of questions. **Closed questions** are questions for which you are looking for a one-word or short answer, often even a "yes" or a "no." Examples of closed questions are:

What is your date of birth?
Are you sexually active?
Who referred you to our office?
What medications are you currently taking? What dosage?

Closed questions are especially effective when you need to get specific information.

Open-ended questions are questions that encourage the person being asked to open up and talk. Examples of open-ended questions are:

Describe your pain for me.
What has been going on with you for the past few days, since you were last here? How has your appetite been the past few days?
How have you been sleeping this past month?

When you are interviewing a person to see what is wrong, allow the patient to pick out what is important, express feelings, and give perceptions. You should express yourself honestly, without being **judgmental**, which means critical or negative. You can disagree with what a patient is saying, especially if that disagreement will get the patient to elaborate on what is being said. But you should not argue; arguing sets up a competitive situation. Because you represent medical authority, the patient can easily feel threatened and unworthy.

When the patient stops speaking, you want to encourage him or her to continue, but you do not always want to steer the conversation in a particular direction. The person who feels as if he or she is being listened to and understood feels validated and safe. Remember Maslow's hierarchy. The need for safety is one of the basic needs people have.

Active listening techniques are extremely important in doing an interview with a lot of open-ended questions, such as an interview to get a patient history or to determine the patient's chief complaint at this particular visit. Open-ended questions are especially good for getting a patient to tell you about a current problem, about the patient's perception of his or her condition, or about feelings.

Use closed and open-ended questions purposefully. Whichever type of question you use, try to avoid questions that ask "why" such as:

Why are you not taking your medication?
Why are you not staying with your diet?

"Why" questions tend to make people defensive. Rather than having the patient justify his or her actions, you want to get at the underlying reasons why the patient did not take the medication or stay on the diet. Ask open-ended questions, such as "How do you set up your meals and snacks?" or "What problems are you having taking your medication?" or "What do you think about having to take medication at school?" In answering any of these questions, the patient may give you some clues as to underlying reasons he or she is not staying with the medical regimen.

A number of techniques can be used to draw patients out and get them to talk more. Among them are:

paraphrasing
translating into feelings
reflecting
summarizing
repeating or restating
using silence

Paraphrasing means attempting to put the patient's meaning into your own words. Paraphrasing shows that you have been listening carefully. Give the patient an opportunity to confirm that your statement is correct.

Translating into feelings is an attempt to catch the patient's emotion and meaning, then reflect it back to the patient. You may reflect the emotion in the tone of voice you use. You may use the phrase "it sounds like . . ." at the beginning of the statement you make; for example, "It sounds like you're really angry that you couldn't reach your daughter this morning when you woke up not feeling well."

Reflecting turns a question or statement around to give the patient the opportunity to continue.

When you paraphrase, you attempt to include all information. When **summarizing**, you make your statement shorter and pull out the highlights of what the patient said previously. After the patient has been speaking for a long period, a summary may help make a transition to a new topic. After you summarize, leave time for the patient to respond and emphasize points you did not include or to add to the information he or she gave the first time.

Repeating or restating is a technique you can use to keep people talking when their statements seem to trail off. Repeating, or restating and changing slightly, the last few words often gets the person to add more information. See Table 5–1 for a full listing of communication techniques that demonstrate active listening.

Silence may not be golden, but it is often an effective interviewing technique. Most people are uncomfortable with silence and will speak to fill the hole. Silence also allows the patient to direct the conversation anywhere he or she wants to go. Notice, however, if the patient finds the silence very awkward; if so, silence is counterproductive.

At a number of times during the interview/conversation, you should evaluate the effectiveness of your

Table 5–1	Communication Techniques That Demonstrate Active Listening	
Technique	**Description**	**Example**
Using open-ended questions	Asking questions that do not require a particular answer, especially a yes or no answer	"What's been going on lately?" "Tell me about your stomach pain."
Repeating or rephrasing	Saying the same thing as the patient, either as a statement or question, to encourage agreement, disagreement, or clarification	*Patient:* "It feels like someone is stabbing me in the side." *Medical Assistant:* "Like a knife in your side . . ."
Translating into feelings	Translating patient's message into verbal expression of emotion	*Patient:* "All the doctor visits, the medication, the pain—it's really too much." *Medical Assistant:* "You sound like you feel overwhelmed."
Reflecting	Turning question or statement around to reflect back to patient, thereby giving patient confidence to continue	*Patient:* "Would you have this surgery if you were me?" *Medical Assistant:* "What do you think about having the surgery?"
Paraphrasing and summarizing	Putting patient's statement into medical assistant's own words (paraphrasing); restating meaning but leaving out some details (summarizing), to validate that medical assistant has understood and to encourage clarification	*Medical Assistant:* "So for the past week the pain has been getting steadily more intense and more frequent, and since this morning it hasn't let up at all."
Providing silence	Simply waiting for patient to continue; allows patient to choose whether to continue or move on to a new topic	(Silence)
Verbalizing the implied	Saying what patient seems to mean but has not expressed	*Patient:* "Usually I don't mind coming to see Dr. Hughes." *Medical Assistant:* "But you didn't want to come today . . ."
Asking for clarification	Asking for more detail or a clearer statement; lets patient know that medical assistant has not understood and may show patient how to make message clearer	*Medical Assistant:* "It's not clear to me how often you have been taking this medication. Do you take it before every meal, or just when you are at home?"

	Table 5–2	Blocks to Effective Communication

Technique	Description	Example
Offering false reassurance	Telling patient that everything will be all right; implies that patient should not feel anxiety or concern; especially inappropriate when the medical assistant does not know what will happen.	*Medical Assistant:* "Don't worry, your husband will come through this with flying colors."
Disapproving, blaming	Making negative value judgment about patient's thinking or behavior; implying or stating that patient is responsible for health problem, encourages patient to defend against attack rather than establishing trust	*Medical Assistant:* "You shouldn't be smoking anyway. No wonder you have trouble breathing."
Challenging	Insisting that patient prove a statement or belief	*Medical Assistant:* "Just show me something in writing that says people should never take a bath."
Defending	Protecting oneself or someone else from criticism; implies that patient does not have right to a different opinion.	*Medical Assistant:* "Dr. Lawler's patients never have to wait very long."
Asking for explanations of feelings or behavior	Asking why; may be frustrating and intrusive because patient may not know why they feel or act as they do	*Medical Assistant:* "Why don't you stick to your diet?" *Medical Assistant:* "Why are you angry?"
Belittling or negating feelings	Acting as if feelings are not present or are less intense than they are; implies that patient's feelings are not real or not justified.	*Medical Assistant:* "You are really making a big deal out of a little cut."
Changing the subject	Not responding to a statement, especially if it expresses feelings; medical assistant implies that patient's feelings are inappropriate or can't be accepted.	*Patient:* "Sometimes I am so down that I can't get out of bed." *Medical Assistant:* "Would you just sit over here so I can take your temperature?"
Stereotyping	Minimizing a person's unique experience by reducing people to generalized categories	*Medical Assistant:* "You are just feeling upset because you are pregnant."

communication with the patient. You want to evaluate both how well the patient is receiving messages you are sending and how well you are receiving messages the patient is sending.

To see how effectively you are receiving messages, you want to paraphrase, repeat and restate, possibly beginning your statement back to the patient with a phrase like, "If I understand you correctly, (repeat, restate, paraphrase) . . . Am I correct?"

Blocks to Effective Communication

To see how well you are sending messages, you can say something like "Have I been clear?" or "Can you repeat to me what I've just said? I realize they are complicated instructions."

Avoid communication techniques that are disapproving, blaming, challenging, or not genuine. These blocks to effective communication are summarized in Table 5–2.

ESTABLISHING CARING RELATIONSHIPS

Patients who have come to a doctor's office are often fragile, emotionally as well as physically. Remember our discussion of Maslow's hierarchy, and the notion that no matter where on the pyramid people are in their "real" lives, illness forces people to deal with basic needs. One of the primary roles of a medical assistant is to create and maintain a caring relationship with the patient. The medical assistant is often the patient's earliest, most frequent, and most consistent point of contact with the office's clinical staff.

Common Feelings of Patients

When creating a caring relationship with a new patient, remember three key feelings that patients may have.

First, patients may feel guilt about their illness. The amount of guilt they feel varies from one patient to another, and the amount of guilt they are willing to express, as opposed to the amount they repress, varies from one patient to the next.

Often it seems that the amount of guilt patients feel about their illness is related to how much their actions have contributed to their illness. The less their actions contribute, the more they may feel guilty, or at least the more they may be willing to express their feelings of guilt. The more their actions contribute to the illness, the less guilty they feel, or the more they repress their feelings of guilt. Individuals who engage in behaviors that are known to be risky to health, such as cigarette smoking, drinking, and drug abuse, may display a devil-may-care attitude about their disease.

People who engage in these risky behaviors know intellectually about the dangers of their actions. Smokers, for instance, have been bombarded with scientifically valid information for almost 40 years about the link between smoking and heart disease, lung cancer, and chronic obstructive pulmonary disease. Yet many continue to smoke without an outward sense of guilt. It seems as though they have convinced themselves that their risky behavior is not the cause of their disease.

On the other hand, patients with conditions totally out of their control are often terribly outwardly guilty. For instance, someone with rheumatoid arthritis will tell you that if he had taken better care of himself or changed the kind of work he did when the symptoms first began, somehow he could have avoided the disease's effects.

Second, patients are extremely impatient with disease or illness and with health care. They want the doctor to be able to "fix" their problem, if not immediately then certainly in a short time. As soon as the most troublesome symptoms are gone, they believe they are well or at least they consciously tell themselves they are well. And if they are well, that means they do not have to take the medications, stay on their diet, or show up for follow-up visits. Hence the huge problem with patients who are said to be **noncompliant,** meaning that they fail to follow a doctor's advice or regimen.

Third, in a doctor's office patients have a feeling of a loss of **autonomy,** a loss of control. They feel they are not able to make the decisions and therefore are not in control. They have to take their clothes off. People get physically close to them, sometimes even touch them. People tell them to do things they do not want to do. They are anxious and become defensive.

Empathy

You can help patients through these feelings by showing empathy. **Empathy** is the ability to put yourself mentally into another person's place and imagine how that person feels. Empathy is often thought of as a feeling, but it is more than that. You can show your empathy with another person by taking specific actions.

Empathy differs from sympathy. When you feel sympathy you feel sorry for someone. When you feel empathy you actually "feel the feeling" without allowing it to overwhelm you.

Because you are sensitive to the feelings people have when they go through the office routine, you can think of commonsense or even creative ways to ease their concerns.

I like to think of an empathetic person almost as a human lightning rod. An empathetic person is able to drain some of the emotional electricity from another person and carry it away into the ground rather than becoming electrically charged by it or passing it on.

Expressing Caring as a Professional

There are two ways you can appropriately express your caring as a professional. One way is through how you speak to patients. The other is through your body language.

Verbally, you express your caring as described earlier in this chapter in the section on interviewing techniques, by drawing patients out and letting them tell their story in their own way, in their own time. You accept and validate a patient's feelings, recognizing that the patient may be uncomfortable with them but can benefit by acknowledging them and having someone else acknowledge them.

You show your caring in a nonverbal way through your body language and through the way you position yourself during your conversations with patients (Figure 5–4). Typically, either the patient sits on the examining table while you stand, which has you about at equal height, or if the patient is more comfortable sitting in the examining room chair, you can sit on the doctor's stool, which again puts you at about equal height. This is much more friendly than if you stand while the patient sits in the chair.

Value of Effective Relationships with Patients

It is hard to say enough about how important the caring relationship is. The medical assistant is often the patient's most frequent, and long-term, point of contact with the medical office. A medical assistant who gets to know a patient well can be of invaluable assistance to both the patient and the doctor, a true liaison.

The experience of being understood and cared for is one of the important steps in beginning to heal or cope effectively with a chronic condition. Ideally, each person the patient comes in contact with at the office will convey this sense, but it is most important for those

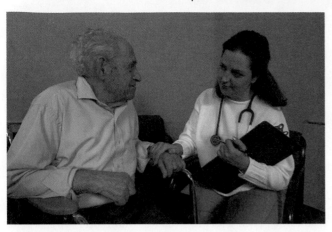

> **Figure 5–4** Photograph showing a medical assistant talking to a patient, expressing caring by looking directly at the patient and touching the patient's hand.

who are performing procedures. If the patient feels understood, he or she will also develop trust and be able to relax during procedures. This makes the procedure easier and less painful, and facilitates both the procedure and the response to the office visit.

ADAPTING COMMUNICATION WHEN THERE ARE BARRIERS TO EFFECTIVE COMMUNICATION

Four major barriers to effective communication between the medical office staff and the patient arise. Two of these involve patients who are impaired, either in their ability to understand or in their senses. The third is when the patient is temporarily impaired because of emotional trauma. The fourth is a language barrier.

Impaired Level of Understanding

In the case of an individual with an impaired level of understanding, you must simplify your communication. Use short sentences. Use simple words. Make strong and constant eye contact. Speak slowly, but do not raise your voice; being loud might help you to be heard, but it does not help you to be understood. Your tone of voice should express your concern and empathy, not imply that the patient is not intelligent.

It may be necessary to repeat what you have said. Saying the same thing in a few different ways is also often helpful. Use gestures and demonstration to reinforce your message.

Those with limited understanding of medical complexities—children, the elderly (especially those who suffer from some degree of dementia), and those who are mentally disabled—need constant reassurance. You must be very direct and complete in your explanation

of every procedure. Even young children need to be informed about what is going to be done to them. For instance, if you are going to draw blood, it is not enough to say, "I'm going to draw your blood. It's going to hurt for just a moment."

You may need to say something like, "I'm going to use this needle and syringe to take some blood from your arm. I'm going to put it through the skin, into where your blood is. It will feel kind of like someone is pinching you, but only for a second. Then I'll put a Band-Aid on it, and it will stop bleeding."

Remember, a young child or an individual with an impaired level of understanding cannot legally give informed consent. An individual who can legally give informed consent for the impaired patient must be present before you can proceed.

Impaired Sensation (Vision, Hearing)

For those with impaired sight, the medical assistant needs to be verbally descriptive. To get sight-impaired people from the waiting room to the examination room and to help them around the exam room, you may need to touch them gently and guide them. Usually people with impaired vision prefer to take your arm and follow your movements rather than having you try to steer them.

You need to explain exactly where things are; a clock image sometimes helps. For instance, you may say, "Directly in front of you, at 12:00, is the clothes hanger. To your left, at 9:00, is the exam table. There is a gown on the table."

For those who are hearing impaired, you should remember to speak clearly, slowly, and in short sentences. Again, do not raise your voice. Look at the person you are speaking to; even if he or she does not lip-read, most people who lose their hearing learn how to associate facial expression and mouth shape with words they know and continue to recognize.

You may need to touch the person gently to get his or her attention at the beginning of the conversation. If the person normally uses a hearing aid, it may be helpful to ask if the person has the hearing aid and if it is turned on.

Sign language is often used by the hearing impaired as a method of communication. Hand and finger positions are used to stand for letters (finger spelling) or words. Several different systems exist, but American Sign Language is the recognized language in the United States.

Because each sign can be an entire word, a person who uses sign language may be able to communicate as fast as, or faster than, a person who is speaking. Because sign language has its own grammar and structure, it takes a lot of practice to become fluent. However, you may develop an interest in learning it.

Usually, a person who uses sign language is brought into the office by someone who can interpret. If the patient does not have an interpreter, the law requires that the office provide one. Be sure to maintain eye contact with the patient, because you are speaking to the patient, not the interpreter. Do not assume that the patient cannot read lips.

STAGES OF RISING ANXIETY

Panic

Severe state of psycholgic stess. Person unable to focus or cope. May focus on small details which are totally blown out of proportion.

Manifestations: incoherent speech, ineffective communication, sweating, rapid pulse and breathing, muscle tremors, increased muscle tension, elevated blood pressure.

Interventions: The panic state usually subsides fairly quickly because the body cannot sustain it. Interventions are the same for severe anxiety. It may be necessary to make transportation arrangements for the patient.

Severe anxiety

Painful level of anxiety produces loss of abstract thinking and consumes almost all of a person's energy. The person cannot notice what is going on even if it is pointed out.

Manifestations: crying, confused speech, dry mouth, sweating, rapid pulse and breathing, muscle tremors, increased muscle tension, elevated blood pressure

Interventions: Provide a quiet area for the person to regain control. A calm manner is reassuring. Encourage the patient to take slow deep breaths. Seek guidance from the physician if the patient is breathing faster than 22-24 breaths per minute.

Moderate anxiety

Attention is restricted to a particular task or problem rather than entire situation (called selective inattention). Still able to think fairly clearly but focuses on only one thing at a time.

Manifestations: sweating, rapid pulse and breathing, muscle tension and possible stomach pain, frequent urination and/or diarrhea

Interventions: A calm manner is reassuring. Acknowledge that the patient appears anxious. Focus on one thing at a time. Encourage the patient to take slow deep breaths.

Mild anxiety

Manifestations: The body functions well in this state. The person may feel a little nervous.

➢ **Figure 5–5** Stages of anxiety.

Neither hearing nor visual impairment normally affects obtaining informed consent.

Effects of Emotions (Anxiety, Anger)

The two emotions that often leave people's ability to understand temporarily impaired are anxiety and anger.

Anxiety is a response to a perceived threat. All animals, including humans, have an instinctive set of responses to danger, called the "fight or flight response." Anxiety is the "flight" option.

A person who is moderately to severely anxious is not able to converse coherently and will not pick up nonverbal cues that he or she would normally notice. You have to get the person's attention, slow down the conversation, and help the person to focus on the conversation. Make sure to validate the person's concern, but try to get his or her anxiety level reduced and energy channeled in a more productive way.

You should assume that a very anxious person will not remember the conversation well. It is important to help the person create some memory aids and usually a good idea to write the instructions down as well. Figure 5–5 shows the various stages of increasing anxiety.

Severe anxiety can be medically problematic. Symptoms of a full-blown anxiety attack include the following. An overly anxious person hyperventilates, has an extremely rapid heart rate, and becomes unresponsive. Some people get numbness in their fingers and toes; others feel a sensation of fluid in their ears. Some people become intensely fearful or have a sense of dread.

An anxiety attack must be dealt with as a medical issue first. Try to get the person to acknowledge the anxiety, for two reasons. First, naming the emotion helps a person gain control. Second, having strong emotions accepted by another person decreases the sense of fear that many people have about their emotions.

You may begin with a statement such as "You seem really anxious" or "It's hard to concentrate when things seem really scary."

If the person is breathing rapidly, encourage slow, deep breaths. If he or she is breathing more rapidly than 22 to 24 breaths a minute, you can suggest breathing into a paper bag. Extremely rapid breathing allows a person to blow off too much carbon dioxide, which leads to some of the physical symptoms of anxiety.

Encourage the person to describe his or her feelings, and acknowledge that this is a real response. You may explain that any physical symptoms are the result of anxiety, but avoid downplaying the real and strong experience of being anxious. Stay with the person until the symptoms begin to subside, usually within 1 or 2 minutes.

After the person has returned to a level of relative calm, you can communicate about the business at hand. Later you can try to get the person to discuss the experience with anxiety, strive to understand it, then create mechanisms for handling anxiety in the future.

In many ways anger is the flip side of anxiety, the "fight" option in the natural response to a perceived threat. The main thing to remember in dealing with the angry patient is that although the anger is channeled to you, it is not directed at you personally. Because anger is part of the fight or flight response, it is a subconscious response. You just happen to be the person in the room with the patient who feels he or she is in a corner and must fight.

When dealing with an angry patient, you need to identify the emotion without feeling attacked. You need to help the angry person to identify the true source of the anger.

Anger is the more difficult of the incapacitating emotions to deal with. Anger tests your empathy and your ability to put aside private issues to help patients. Your first instinct—remember, you have a fight or flight response as well—is to fight back at the angry patient.

You need to accept that the person is angry, but not allow him or her to threaten others. It is perfectly all right to tell the person that he or she is acting inappropriately, that he or she is making it difficult for other patients, or that shouting will not be tolerated. To protect the confidentiality of the person who is temporarily out of control, try to move to a private area. It is also appropriate to ask your supervisor to help deal with the angry patient. Sometimes anger, like electricity, becomes diffused when the connection is broken.

Getting informed consent from an emotionally impaired patient is often difficult. A person in a highly charged emotional state cannot legally sign a consent form, nor can a person who is under the influence of a mind-altering drug. In either case, a procedure must be delayed if informed consent has not already been obtained.

Language (and Cultural) Barriers

The best way to work around language barriers is with translation assistance. Translators can be office staff, community volunteers, or patient family members. In cases such as this, you should find out when the appointment is made if a family member will translate or if the office's translation services will be needed.

When conversing with a patient through a translator, remember to speak to the patient not the translator. Let the translator translate, then go on. Speak slowly and carefully, using simple terms and short sentences. Many people who do not feel comfortable speaking English can understand English.

If you are working in an office without translation services, the translator is busy, or patient's family member is translating but the patient wants to converse with you alone, you may need to improvise. Use gestures and pantomime to get your ideas across.

When you need to get a patient's informed consent to a procedure, it is imperative that you have someone translate. Consent forms are usually written in English, but the explanation needs to be in the patient's native language. If a practice has a large number of non-English-speaking patients, it is a good idea to have common consent forms and instructional materials translated and available. Or use American telephone assist translators.

STUDENT STUDY PLAN

To reinforce your understanding of the material in this chapter . . .

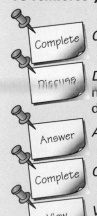

Complete the **Review & Recall** questions.

Discuss the situation in **If You Were the Medical Assistant** with your classmates, and answer the questions. If possible, view Scene 2.1C from the Saunders video.

Answer the **Critical Thinking Questions** and discuss them with your classmates.

Complete the exercises in chapter 5 of the **Student Mastery Manual**.

View the **Videotape:** *Communication and Caring:* Part One.

REVIEW & RECALL

1. Describe the differences between verbal and nonverbal communication.

2. Assume that a patient tells you the following:

   "It has been realy difficult dealing with arthritis the past few weeks. I have been in a lot of pain, but my kids don't help, and my husband still expects me to keep the house clean. I'm so depressed I can hardly get out of bed in the morning."

   How could the medical assistant answer to demonstrate each of the following communication techniques?
   Translating into feelings
   Reflecting
   Summarizing
   Restating
   Asking for clarification

3. Define empathy and give several examples from your own experience.

4. List ways to adapt communication in the following situations:
   a. a child or mentally retarded person
   b. a person with impaired hearing
   c. a person with impaired vision
   d. a person who speaks poor English
   e. a person who is very anxious
   f. a person who is very angry.

IF YOU WERE THE MEDICAL ASSISTANT

See Videotape: Communication and Caring, "Following Up"

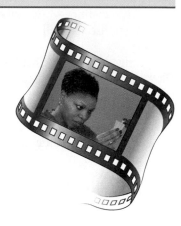

Kathy, a medical assistant in the office of Blackstone Primary Care Associates, is interviewing Mr. Costello, a patient of Dr. Lopez. Mr. Costello paid a visit to the office a few weeks previously complaining of stomach pain. The doctor ordered several tests, all of which were negative. Today, Mr. Costello has returned because he is still worried about the pain. Mr. Costello has asked if the X-ray could have missed something.

Mr. Costello: Not that I want bad news, but I want to do something, to just get a diagnosis and get it done with, over with, you know what I mean?
Kathy: I don't blame you.
Mr. Costello: Maybe the pain is lower down. Maybe if we could do—do they do like a lower GI, is that what they call it?
Kathy: Well, it would be up to the doctor to decide that, but . . .
Mr. Costello: I really am wondering whether it is lower or something, you know?
Kathy: You think it may be lower . . .
Mr. Costello: I mean that's where my brother's cancer was, lower.
Kathy: Your brother had stomach cancer? When was that?
Mr. Costello: You know, he had it like for the last year and a half or so.
Kathy: He's had stomach cancer for a year and a half?
Mr. Costello: Well, he died, he died 3 months ago. I know it's not the same, but I am still worried.
Kathy: I think that anybody that had something like that happen in their family would be very worried.

1. Identify several communication techniques that Kathy is using to encourage Mr. Costello to continue talking.

2. How does Kathy remain within the scope of practice of medical assisting?

3. What kind of nonverbal messages would Kathy use to express concern and acceptance of a difficult topic of conversation?

4. Does Kathy do or say anything to block communication? If so, what?

CRITICAL THINKING QUESTIONS

1. Watch part of a movie or television program with the sound turned off. Record nonverbal cues you see. Write down what you think is going on. How much of the meaning do you think you were able to get from nonverbal cues?

2. Working with a classmate, imagine that you are feeling a strong emotion such as anger, fear, joy, anxiety, or disgust. Talk to your classmate about what you did today from the time you got up. Have your classmate guess what emotion you were imagining. Discuss how well this worked. How is the emotion communicated?

3. How might an effective medical assistant respond to each of the following statements? Practice with a classmate, then switch roles. How do different types of responses influence the interaction?

   a. Do you think I should have the surgery Dr. Hughes recommended?

   b. I absolutely hate having a mammogram. It's so embarrassing.

   c. My husband has been away on business this week, and the kids are driving me crazy. They are hanging on me, I never get a break. It's really getting to me.

   d. I have been waiting for over an hour. My time is valuable too, you know. Is the doctor ever going to see me?

Chapter 6

Safety: How Do You Work Safely and Protect Patients?

Instructional Objectives

After completing this chapter, you will be able to do the following:

1. Define and spell the vocabulary words for this chapter.
2. Identify general safety measures recommended for use in the medical office.
3. List fire safety measures for the medical office.
4. Correlate principles of good body mechanics to lifting and carrying heavy objects.
5. Describe principles of ergonomics related to use of a computer and/or keyboard.
6. Identify the following stages of Hans Seyle's general adaptation syndrome: alarm reaction, stage of resistance, stage of exhaustion.
7. Describe seven measures to cope with stress.
8. Identify activities that a medical assistant can use to reduce stress.
9. Describe OSHA's requirements for employers to protect employees from diseases caused by blood-borne pathogens.
10. Identify the steps to take if a health professional is exposed to blood-borne pathogens and the follow-up.
11. Discuss the implications of OSHA's standard concerning occupational exposure to hazardous chemicals.
12. Describe the purpose of universal precautions, standard precautions, and isolation precautions.
13. Identify the specific recommendations of standard precautions.
14. Identify body fluids, secretions, and excretions to which standard precautions apply.
15. Identify specific situations in which gowns, gloves, masks, and protective eyewear are required.
16. List requirements for hazardous waste disposal.
17. Identify specific measures to prevent needle-stick injury.

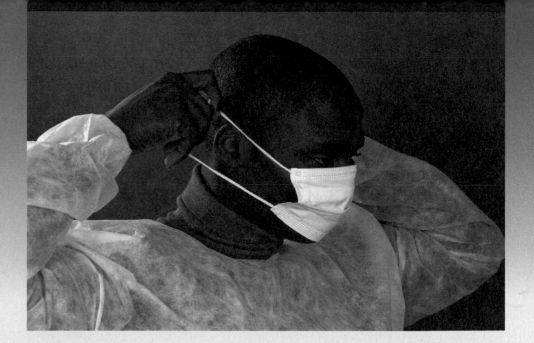

- Dispose of biohazardous materials
- Understand legal guidelines and requirements for health care
- Perform risk management procedures
- Practice standard precautions

Vocabulary

airborne precautions (p. 105)
biohazard (p. 100)
biohazard symbol (p. 104)
body mechanics (p. 95)

category-specific isolation precautions (p. 105)
contact precautions (p. 106)
droplet precautions (p. 105)

ergonomics (p. 95)
isolation precautions (p. 101)
personal protective equipment (p. 101)
sharps (p. 100)

standard precautions (p. 101)
stress (p. 96)
universal precautions (p. 101)

ABBREVIATIONS

CDC (p. 100)
GAS (p. 96)

HBV (p. 100)
HIV (p. 101)

MSDS (p. 101)
OSHA (p. 98)

PPE (p. 101)

GENERAL OFFICE SAFETY

Maintaining a safe office is not as difficult as maintaining a safe construction site. No hardhats or steel-toed boots are necessary in an office. But there are safety issues, and commonsense precautions need to be taken.

Removing Hazards

Throw rugs or scatter rugs should not be used in offices. They can slide or bunch up, causing people to fall. Floors in waiting rooms should be carpeted; floors in hallways and examination treatment rooms should be linoleum; floors in doctor's private offices are usually carpeted.

All walkways should be kept clear. Boxes should immediately be put in the storage room or behind a desk, even if they will be emptied later. Boxes should not be piled high on top of file cabinets, and no heavy boxes should be put on top of file cabinets.

All file cabinets should be weighted so they do not tip over when more than one drawer is open. If you cannot purchase this kind of file cabinet, bolt the file cabinets to the wall. File drawers, desk drawers, and cabinet doors should be closed except when someone is retrieving something inside.

If you must get to a high cabinet or to something on top of a file cabinet, use a step stool. Do not stand on chairs, especially those with adjustable seats or ball bearings on the bottom for rolling.

Instruments, scissors, and other sharp objects should be kept in drawers except when in use.

Electrical equipment should be kept in good working order. Cords should be checked regularly for fraying or wires that have been stripped of insulation and exposed. Make sure all electrical plugs are grounded. Computers and other equipment should be plugged into a surge-protector, not directly into the wall.

Routine office cleaning should be done when the office is closed. If there is a spill on a linoleum floor, clean it up immediately and put "wet floor" caution signs a few feet away from the wet area on all sides. Keep the signs up until the floor is completely dry and no longer poses a risk.

Maintaining an office to the highest level of safety is not only common sense and important, but it is also a legal requirement. By law, all public buildings, including medical offices, need at least two exits to the hallway; these should be labeled clearly with lighted exit signs. The exits should always be kept clear of boxes or other hazards.

Modern office buildings usually have smoke and heat detectors wired into the building's main electrical paneling, but older buildings do not. If your office does not have such hard-wired detectors, you should have a number of battery-powered detectors throughout the office. Batteries should be checked monthly using the alarm's self-test mechanism and should be changed twice a year, in spring and fall. Doing it at the same time you change the office clocks for the beginning and end of Daylight Savings Time is a good way to remember.

In the kitchen area, microwave ovens or toaster-ovens should never be left unattended, and coffee machines should never be allowed to boil dry. The person who drinks the last cup from the pot should start another pot or turn off the machine and wash out the empty pot.

Fire Safety

You need to have at least two fire extinguishers in the office—one in the laboratory and one in any room where oxygen may be used. If you have portable oxygen, a fire extinguisher should be part of the equipment cart on which the oxygen tank is placed. If your break/lunch room has kitchen facilities, a fire extinguisher should also be placed there. Many people also put fire extinguishers near exits to increase safety during an evacuation. All staff members should have an annual training session on fire safety, including use of the extinguishers, and that training should be documented.

Emergency Numbers and Emergency Plans

Every medical office needs to have clear emergency plans, and the staff must have training and regular reminders on how to execute the plan. Staff should be trained annually and new staff trained during orientation on the building's emergency evacuation plan. The building plan should be posted, with recommended evacuation routes, in the waiting area and next to all exits from the office.

Telephone numbers for fire, police, emergency medical services, and the regional poison control center should be posted by every telephone.

ERGONOMICS AND BODY MECHANICS

A typical working day in a medical office puts a lot of physical stress on personnel. Bending, lifting, reaching, squatting, having a telephone stuck in the crook of the neck, and repeatedly using a typing keyboard put stress on the body. The human body was not designed by nature to perform such activities so frequently.

In the past 25 years, doctors and scientists who study body mechanics have developed ways to reduce these physical stresses. Some of these ways have been incorporated into exercise regimens that are recommended for people who perform these activities; others have been designed into the physical structure of the office environment.

Ergonomics

We call this study ergonomics. The word *ergonomics* comes from the Greek root *ergon*, which means work. **Ergonomics** is the study of maximizing work efficiency by adapting the work environment for optimal physical and mental function. We most often encounter ergonomics in the form of office seating designed to provide maximum support for the back and computer keyboards designed to reduce repetitive motion injuries to the hands, wrists, and arms. But ergonomics does not have to be high tech; it can be as simple as placing a small footstool at the side of an examining table, not only so the patient can step up before sitting on the table, but also so the doctor, who stands and performs exams for hours a day, can rest a foot there and take pressure off his or her lower back.

Maintaining good posture can reduce backache and fatigue. To understand posture, you need to understand the physiology of the spine. The spine is a flexible stack of small bones called vertebrae. The back gets its flexibility because vertebrae are connected by fibrous ligaments containing gelatin-like tissue, called disks. To increase the strength of the back and neck, there are two primary curves in the spine, the cervical curve at the neck and the lumbar curve at the lower back.

The human head should sit above the pelvis, supported by the spine. People have a tendency to lean forward, both when walking and when sitting. This bad posture places extra strain on the back and neck muscles, and causes excess muscle tension. Over time, the vertebrae are pulled out of position and lose flexibility.

When using a typewriter or computer keyboard, an adjustable chair should be used to provide lower-back support. The keyboard should be about waist high, so the forearms are level. The forearms and wrists should be supported to lessen the chance for repetitive motion injury. Feet should be flat on the floor or resting on an inclined step stool.

Adequate lighting is important. The monitor should be placed at a height so that the user can look relatively straight ahead at the screen (shown in Figure 6–1). You should take frequent breaks, both to look away from the monitor and focus at a distance to relieve eyestrain, and to stretch muscles that can become bunched from sitting in one position for too long.

Using Good Body Mechanics

When working with patients, remember to use proper body mechanics. The term **body mechanics** is used to refer to ways for health professionals to maintain good body alignment and optimal use of the muscles, bones, and joints when lifting, pulling, or carrying weight. This helps prevent injury and allows efficient lifting, moving, and transfer of patients.

The seven steps to proper moving and lifting heavy objects are:

1. Keep feet shoulder-width apart to provide a good base of support.
2. Use large muscles of legs to push, pull, or lift; do not lean over from the waist and use the back muscles.
3. Pivot the body rather than turning the upper body.
4. Pull or push rather than lifting. If lifting is necessary, get help.
5. Avoid lifting objects above your head; use a step stool or stepladder to keep the objects below shoulder level.
6. Hold heavy objects close to your body.
7. Bend from the knees when lifting; do not stoop over.

Figure 6–2 shows good body mechanics for lifting. This is opposed to Figure 6–3, which demonstrates an incorrect lifting posture that places strain on the lower back.

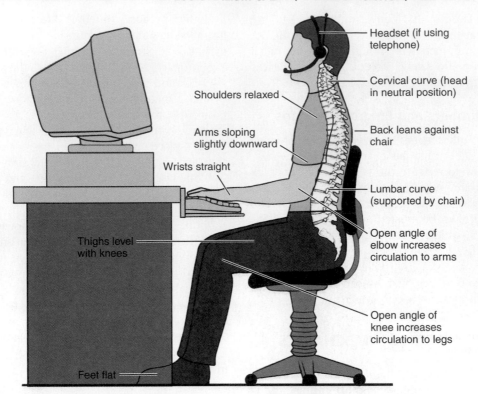

- Top of monitor at eye level
- Keyboard below elbows, sloped slightly away from user
- Chair supports lower back, height allows feet to rest on floor slightly ahead of knee on footrest if necessary
- Mouse within easy reach
- At least 2 inches from chair seat to back of knee

➤ Figure 6–1 Good posture at a computer workstation

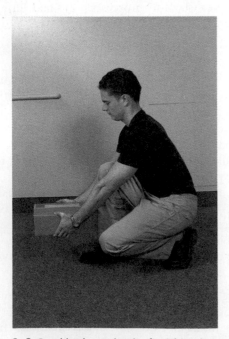

➤ Figure 6–2 Good body mechanics for lifting heavy objects

STRESS

Stress is the body's response to change. Some stress is good, because it pushes us to perform at our highest capabilities. Even some good things can be stressful, like a romantic relationship or a school or work project in which we are emotionally invested and wish to perform well. But too much stress, either in a concentrated period or over a long time, can be dangerous.

General Adaptation Syndrome

Hans Selye, an Austrian doctor who practiced in the middle of the 20th century, described the body's reaction to stress as a four-part general adaptation syndrome (GAS), also known as the fight or flight response, which is shown in Figure 6–4.

The four stages of the GAS are the alarm reaction, the stage of resistance, the recovery phase, and the stage of exhaustion.

In the first stage, the alarm reaction, the body senses

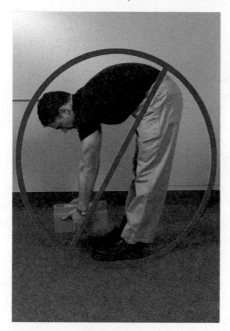

> **Figure 6-3** Poor body mechanics for lifting: Bending with straight legs places strain on the lower back.

a stress and begins to react. Epinephrine released from the adrenal medulla stimulates the sympathetic nervous system. The pupils dilate, the heart beats faster, respirations become faster and deeper, and the blood pressure rises. The body prepares to fight or run away. In a busy office, many people's bodies may be in a constant state of alarm.

In the second stage, the stage of resistance, the stress remains but the body adapts. Levels of adrenal hormones may remain slightly high or drop back to normal. More energy is required to maintain the stage of resistance than the normal state.

After the stress is removed, the body enters the recovery phase, and as the parasympathetic system begins to regain control, the body returns to its normal level of function.

If stress persists or is always present, it causes an increase in blood pressure, elevated glucose (blood sugar) level, increased metabolism, and increased intraocular (inside the eye) pressure. This is why constant stress leads to fatigue, hunger, and headaches.

Eventually, in a person subjected to chronic stress, the body is unable to maintain the response, becomes exhausted, and is more prone to a variety of illnesses. The person may also experience symptoms of anxiety.

Body Reaction When Stress Persists

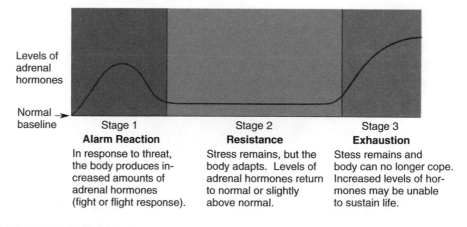

Levels of adrenal hormones

Normal baseline

Stage 1	Stage 2	Stage 3
Alarm Reaction	**Resistance**	**Exhaustion**
In response to threat, the body produces increased amounts of adrenal hormones (fight or flight response).	Stress remains, but the body adapts. Levels of adrenal hormones return to normal or slightly above normal.	Stess remains and body can no longer cope. Increased levels of hormones may be unable to sustain life.

> **Figure 6-4** Hans Selye's general adaptation syndrome (GAS)

Body Reaction When Stress is Removed

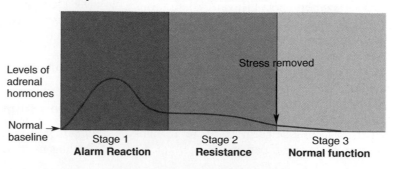

Levels of adrenal hormones

Stress removed

Normal baseline

Stage 1	Stage 2	Stage 3
Alarm Reaction	**Resistance**	**Normal function**

Eight important mechanisms for coping with stress have been identified:

1. Provide for adequate rest periods during the day. Do not keep going like the Energizer Bunny.
2. Avoid perfectionism. Do the best you can; realize that it is human to make mistakes in things that are not life-threatening.
3. Eat regular meals and avoid food high in sugar, which does provide a quick burst of energy but may result in rebound low blood sugar an hour later.
4. Get regular exercise, and take regular stretch breaks.
5. Plan daily work, set priorities, do not allow supplies to run out, and keep examination rooms restocked so you do not have to run to get something at the last minute.
6. When feeling overwhelmed, ask for help. Do not let stress build up.
7. Take breaks, get out of the office at lunchtime, even if just for a 5-minute walk around the block.
8. Tackle problems, and encourage office members to work with you in identifying specific problems to work on, goals to meet, and time frames to work within. Many problems that everyone has complained about for years can at least be reduced.

Stress Prevention and Reduction

You can perform some physical and mental exercises for a couple of minutes at a time, a few times a day, to reduce stress. These include the following five stress reducers:

1. Muscle relaxation exercises. These are best done lying down but can be done sitting or even standing against a wall. Close your eyes and relax your entire body as much as possible immediately. Then begin lightly bunching, then releasing, each muscle group, beginning with the muscles in your feet, working up your legs, buttocks, abdominal muscles, arms, back, then finally your neck and shoulders. Breathe smoothly and gently.
2. Breathing exercises. Again, get into the most comfortable position possible and close your eyes. Begin to breathe deeply and evenly. Feel your chest and diaphragm expand and contract with each breath. Feel any tingling in your extremities, and feel for muscle groups that slowly unbunch and relax. You may even feel your body twitch (which is sometimes a sign that you are about to fall asleep). Although a long nap may leave a person feeling sluggish, a 10- to 15-minute nap often revitalizes a person.
3. Visualization. In this exercise, close your eyes and create a pleasant scene in your mind—the ocean or mountains or fall colors on the trees in your own backyard. Fill in the details of your imaginary scene slowly, adding one element at a time—a person, a color, a sound such as waves or wind rustling leaves. Again, you should begin to feel your breathing regulating and becoming slow and deep, and feel your muscles unbunch and relax.
4. Focusing on the moment (meditation). Although most of us think of meditation as part of Eastern religions, anyone can meditate. Meditation involves separating yourself from all that is exogenous—meaning those stimuli that come from outside us—and turning inward to focus on your own physical and mental processes in the immediate moment. There are many formal meditation forms, some of which include following the breath, repeating a simple word or phrase—a mantra. Others involve some aspects of the exercises described above. Other people use music to assist their meditation, concentrating on simple melodies. Within many religious traditions, a growing number of singers are releasing CDs of "spiritual" music that are ideal as relaxation aids.

Before getting to the fifth technique, I'd like to note that if you find any of these techniques especially helpful in reducing your stress, you can in the course of your work teach them to patients who visit your office.

5. Physical exercise. This is also a terrific stress reducer. You may want to ask the doctor(s) you work for to get a bicycle or treadmill for staff to use during breaks. Five minutes of exercise can clear your mind, and 30 minutes at 10 to 12 mph on a stationary bike or at 6 to 7 mph on a treadmill is great for the cardiovascular system. (If you do this, you will probably need a shower facility and a change of clothes as well.)

OCCUPATIONAL SAFETY AND HEALTH ADMINISTRATION

The Occupational Safety and Health Administration (OSHA) is the federal agency responsible for the physical protection of employees in the workplace. OSHA regulates all workplace environments, but has two specific functions related to the medical office.

Protection from Exposure to Disease

One OSHA regulation relates to preventing exposure to pathogens that cause disease. Effective March of

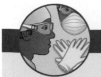

FOCUS ON
SAFETY

STANDARDS OF THE OCCUPATIONAL SAFETY AND HEALTH ADMINISTRATION

In 1970, the federal government passed the Occupational Safety and Health Act, which established the Occupational Safety and Health Administration (OSHA), the body that establishes safety regulations for employers and monitors compliance. OSHA has the right to inspect private and public work sites to be sure all protocols and guidelines are being followed.

The general health of the employee must be protected, and many standards require plans, training of employees, and monitoring of injuries with detailed records. In addition, the employer must provide general protective equipment (such as first aid kits and fire extinguishers) as well as specialized protective equipment as needed.

Fire Safety Plan. An OSHA-compliant fire protection plan must include written procedures. Exits must be marked and escape routes published. Fire extinguishers and fire alarm pull boxes must be present, and the employer must conduct fire prevention, fire drills, testing of the fire alarm and sprinkler system, and employee training.

Hazard Communication Plan. A hazard communication plan protects the rights of employees to know what types of hazardous chemicals are present in the workplace and what health risks are associated with those chemicals.

A Material Safety Data Sheet (MSDS) must be kept on file for all hazardous chemicals. An MSDS is a printed report describing the chemical and the hazards associated with it, as well as emergency and first aid procedures, and spill or leak procedures and preventions. These sheets are obtained from the chemical's manufacturer.

All hazardous chemicals must have warning labels, as shown in Figure 6-A.

The employer must have a plan in place to report accidents and injuries, to train employees about hazardous chemicals, and to notify employees of new hazardous chemicals.

Exposure Control Plan. The exposure control plan is designed to minimize risk of exposure to infectious material and blood-borne disease. The plan, which must be written and updated as necessary, includes nine elements:

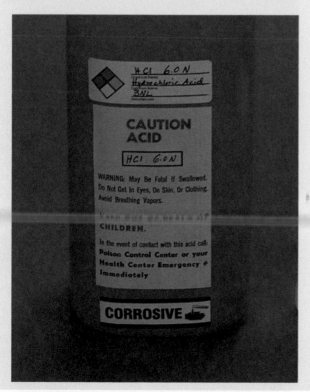

➤ Figure 6A This collection bottle for a 24-hour urine sample contains a warning label to identify the effects of hazardous chemicals.

Focus On continued on following page

1. Measures to determine which jobs have the potential for exposure to infectious materials.

2. Measures to show how the facility complies with regulations. All potential biohazardous materials must be clearly labeled.

3. Availability of vaccination against hepatitis B virus for all employees with potential for exposure.

4. Use of appropriate biohazard waste containers.

5. Measures to describe types of hazardous waste and the proper storage and removal of each type.

6. Laundry procedures for linen, lab coats, and other items that have come in contact with body fluids.

7. Procedures for follow-up for any incidents such as needle-stick injury or exposure to blood or body fluids.

8. Training of employees for proper use of personal protective equipment; handling of materials that contain, or have been exposed to, blood or body fluids; procedures to follow if exposure should occur; and disposal of hazardous waste.

9. Measures to keep records of training, exposure, and so on, as required.

Occupational Exposure to Tuberculosis. Measures must be taken to minimize danger of exposure and transmission of tuberculosis when employees have a potential for coming in contact with individuals infected with tuberculosis. There must be screening for tuberculosis before employment as well as during employment; training in the transmission of tuberculosis and use of appropriate preventive measures; and follow-up after known exposure or a positive Mantoux test.

OSHA also has regulations for or provides information about laser hazards, radioactive materials, and latex allergy.

1992, the Occupational Exposure to Blood-borne Pathogen Standard requires employers to have an exposure control plan, which identifies all employees who might come into contact with blood and other potentially hazardous materials. The plan must include safe handling procedures for specimens; contaminated sharps such as needles, glass slides, and scalpel blades; contaminated laundry; and hazardous disposable waste.

Employers are required to provide employees with immunization to the hepatitis B virus (HBV); to provide personal protective equipment for employees; to label biohazards (materials that may be able to transmit infection) waste containers and other hazards; and to provide medical care if an employee is exposed to blood-borne pathogens or other hazardous material.

Employees must receive initial training and have this training updated annually.

A plan for follow-up after an exposure also must be in place.

Direct contact with blood or other body fluids, and needle-stick injuries, make it possible for an employee to get AIDS, hepatitis B, or other diseases. Prevention of this exposure is the best way to avoid this. Nevertheless, as many as 800,000 needle-stick injuries occur annually, according to the federal Centers for Disease Control and Prevention (CDC).

Protection from Exposure to Chemicals

The second area of medical office practice that is of specific concern to OSHA relates to hazardous chemi-

Needle-Stick Procedure

The following procedure should be followed in the event of a needle-stick injury:

1. Document the exposure, including where on the body it occurred and how it happened.
2. If possible, identify the person who was the source of the exposure.
3. Immediately wash the area with soap and water; if the mouth, rinse it; if the eye, flush it with large amounts of water.
4. Report the exposure to your immediate supervisor, who is responsible for following up.
5. Test for HIV and HBV (the exposed person has the right to refuse to be tested).
6. Seek permission from the source of the exposure to test for HIV and HBV; if permission is received, test the source.
7. The exposed individual is offered immune serum globulin, a medication that provides temporary immunity against a large number of diseases, as well as HBV vaccine.
8. File a report with OSHA.
9. Information about a patient treated for a needle stick, including the medical record, is confidential and not available to the employer.

cals. OSHA maintains the Standard for Occupational Exposure to Hazardous Chemicals in the Laboratory.

Each employer must have a written plan and must designate a chemical safety officer. If potentially hazardous chemicals are in use, including stains, bleach, acetone, and isopropyl alcohol, any work site with employees is subject to regulation. Figure 6–5 is a sample hazardous Material Safety Data Sheet **(MSDS).**

All potentially hazardous chemicals must be inventoried. A Material Safety Data Sheet manual must be created for each laboratory and must be made available to every employee. Employees must be trained before handling any hazardous chemicals. Employees have a right to know of any hazardous chemicals in their environment.

If an employee is injured, the employer must provide medical care. An emergency eyewash station should be present in any area where there is a potential for splashes to the eyes, and an area that uses open flame or flammable chemicals should have an emergency shower, as shown in Figure 6–6.

Chemical spills should be cleaned according to guidelines for the specific chemical. Spill cleanup kits should be available; these have absorbent materials, a material to solidify liquid spills, gloves, and shovels to help remove hazardous material.

Physician office laboratories are also governed under the 1988 amendments to the Clinical Laboratory Act, which was discussed briefly in chapter 2, and will be discussed in more detail in the unit on working in the laboratory.

PREVENTION OF THE SPREAD OF INFECTIONS

A number of measures need to be put in place to prevent the spread of infection from patient to patient and/or employees. Initially, the focus of the CDC recommendations was on preventing the spread of blood-borne infection, especially the human immunodeficiency virus **(HIV)** and the hepatitis B virus (HBV). The CDC first described **universal precautions** (measures used to prevent health care workers from contact with pathogens) in 1987. Since then, it has revised its guidelines and issued updated guidelines for use in hospitals to prevent the spread of various infections. The new set of precautions, issued in 1996, incorporates elements of a system called body fluid isolation, which defines ways for health care personnel to avoid coming in contact with any body fluids (not just blood) using **standard precautions** (used in all situations) and specific **isolation precautions** (used when there is a high risk of exposure to specific diseases).

Standard Precautions

Standard precautions should be used in the medical office. The goal is to prevent any contact with body fluids that may transmit disease. (Universal precautions focused on avoiding contact with blood.) Standard precautions apply to blood, other body fluids containing visible blood, semen, vaginal secretions, cerebrospinal fluid, and synovial fluid, pleural fluid, and peritoneal, pericardial, and amniotic fluid. Even though some body fluids or secretions have not been shown to transmit HIV, a health care worker should also use standard precautions for the following: urine, feces, nasal secretions, sputum, breast milk, tears, saliva, and vomitus. In addition, a health care worker should use standard precautions when dealing with nonintact skin (broken skin) and the mucous membranes inside the mouth, nose, and body cavities.

Taking standard precautions means using appropriate **personal protective equipment (PPE)** (which protects from exposure to pathogens) and undertaking proper disposal of hazardous waste, all of which must be placed in containers marked to indicate its presence (Figure 6–7).

```
HUNT PRODUCTS, INC.- ISOPROPYL ALCOHOL 70% RUBBING-ISOPROPYL
RUBBING ALCOHOL, USP
MATERIAL SAFETY DATA SHEET
NSN: 6505006558366
Manufacturer's CAGE: 12334
Part No. Indicator: C
Part Number/Trade Name: ISOPROPYL ALCOHOL 70% RUBBING

================================================================================
                            General Information
================================================================================

    Item name: ISOPROPYL RUBBING ALCOHOL, USP
    Company's Name: HUNT PRODUCTS, INC.
    Company's Street: 625 Ridge Avenue
    Company City: Fairfield
    Company State: NJ
    Company's Country: US
    Company Zip Code: 08265
    Company's Emerg. Ph#: 201-343-2993
    Company's Info. Ph#: 201-343-2893
    Record No. For Safety Entry: 022
    Tot Safety Entries This STK#: 017
    Status: TE
    Date MSDS Prepared: 12Dec98
    Safety Data Review Date: 05Aug99
    Supply Item Manager: MP
    MSDS Serial Number: BJYXF
    Hazard Characteristic Code: F4
    Unit of Issue: BT
    Unit Of Issue Container Qty: 16
    Type of Container: Bottle
    Net Unit Weight: 12 OUNCES

================================================================================
                      Ingredients/Identity Information
================================================================================

    Proprietary: NO
    Ingredient: ISOPROPYL ALCOHOL (SARA III)
    Ingredient Sequence Number: 01
    Percent: 70%

================================================================================
                      Physical/Chemical Characteristics
================================================================================

    Appearance And Odor: Clear, Slight Odor, Colorless Liquid
    Boiling Point: Not Given
    Melting Point: Not Given

================================================================================
                        Fire and Explosion Hazard Data
================================================================================

    Flash Point: 72.5'F, 22.1'C
    Flash Point Method: TOC
    Lower Explosion Limit: 3
    Upper Explosion Limit: 13

================================================================================
                               Reactivity Data
================================================================================

    Stability: Yes
    Cond To Avoid (Stability): High Temperatures, Sparks, Flames
    Materials to Avoid: Strong Oxidizing Agents, Acetaldehyde, Chlorine

================================================================================
                             Health Hazard Data
================================================================================

    LD50-LC50 Mixture: Not Given for Product
    Route of Entry - Inhalation: Yes
    Route of Entry - Skin: Yes
    Route of Entry - Digestion: Yes
    breathing difficult. Obtain Medical Attention.  INGESTION: Do not induce vomiting if
    unconcious.  If within the first 15 min. induce vomiting immediately

================================================================================
                    Precautions for Safe Handling and Use
================================================================================
Steps In Matl Released/Spill: Flammable. Eliminate all ignition sources.  Ventilate Area.
Contain and remove with inert absorbent and non-sparking tools.
```

➢ Figure 6–5 Material Safety Data Sheet for isopropyl alcohol

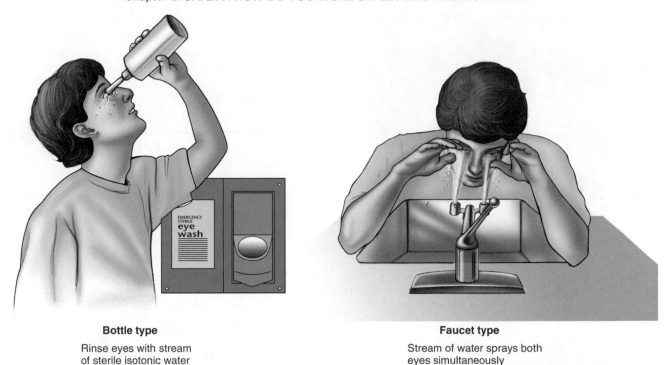

Bottle type

Rinse eyes with stream
of sterile isotonic water
from bottle

Faucet type

Stream of water sprays both
eyes simultaneously

➢ **Figure 6–6** Use of emergency eyewash station

Use of Personal Protective Equipment

PPEs include gloves, gowns or lab coats, aprons, masks, and protective eyewear. These should all be worn when the potential to come in contact with body fluids is present. Figure 6–8 shows a collection of personal protective equipment.

There are seven steps to proper use of PPEs.

1. Wash hands. Always wash hands after removing gloves and between patients. If you have come into contact with any body fluid, excretion, or secretion, wash hands immediately. Always wash hands after a break and after using the restroom.

2. Wear gloves. Do so whenever there is any chance of coming in contact with body fluids, excretions, secretions, nonintact skin, or mucous membranes and whenever there is a chance of touching an item that has been soiled with blood or body fluids to which standard precautions apply. Gloves should be used for any patient con-

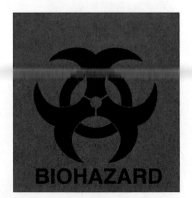

➢ **Figure 6–7** Biohazard logo must be on all containers of hazardous waste.

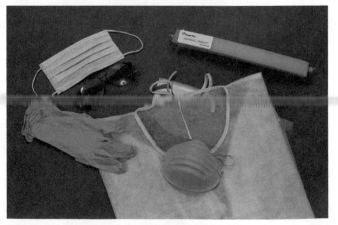

➢ **Figure 6–8** Items of protective equipment, including barrier gown, gloves, face masks, face shield, and protective eyewear

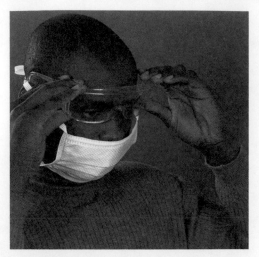

➢ **Figure 6–9** Protective eye and face protection

tact if the health care worker has breaks in his or her skin.

3. Change gloves between patients and wash hands whenever gloves are removed.

4. Wear an apron or gown that cannot be penetrated by fluid for any procedure that may generate splashes or sprays of blood or body fluids. If a gown or lab coat becomes soiled with blood or body fluids, launder it or discard it if disposable, as shown in Figure 6–8.

5. Wear a mask to protect the mucous membranes of your mouth and nose and protective eyewear to protect your eyes, if there is any chance of splashes or sprays of blood or body fluids to the face. Safety glasses must be made of plastic or safety glass-

and have side pieces to protect from splashes that come from the side. A protective face shield may be substituted for the mask and eyewear. Protective eyewear is shown in Figure 6–9.

6. For isolation precautions or handling contaminated specimens or spills, wear a barrier gown with knit cuffs, as well as mouth, nose, eye protection, and gloves pulled over the knit cuffs, as shown in Figure 6–10. See "On The Job" for practice choosing appropriate PPEs.

7. Take precautions to avoid needle-stick injuries. Do not recap needles that have been used on a patient; do not bend or break them. Discard used syringes and needles, scalpels, and other sharp objects into rigid, puncture-resistant sharps containers. Do not fill containers more than two-thirds full. Never reach into a sharps container with your hand. A rigid biohazard container for sharps is seen in Figure 6–11.

Disposal of Hazardous Waste

Some needles are reusable. Once these needles are used and contaminated with blood, they should be handled with a forceps (not by hand) and kept in a puncture-resistant container until they are sterilized. Any materials that have come into contact with blood or body fluids are treated as hazardous waste. Various containers are used to collect hazardous material. Waste containers are labeled with the **biohazard symbol** to ensure that all employees are aware of the contents. Plastic bags are used for gloves, paper towels, dressings, and other soft material; rigid containers are

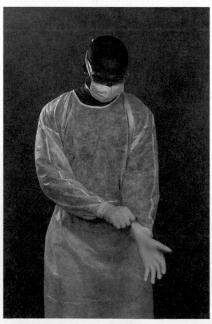

➢ **Figure 6–10** Medical assistant wearing barrier gown with knit cuffs, gloves, mask, and safety goggles

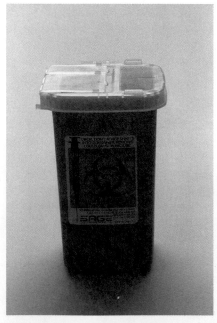

➢ **Figure 6–11** Rigid biohazard waste container for sharps

ON THE JOB

While working in the lab of Blackburn Primary Care Associates, you are given several tasks to perform. You may need to wear personal protective equipment. If you need PPE(s), choose the item(s) from the list below that you would wear to perform each of the following tasks. Give reasons for your choices.

Available PPEs
latex gloves
lab coat
barrier lab coat with knit sleeves
mask
safety glasses

Tasks
1. Taking a patient's blood pressure
2. Taking a filled urine specimen cup with the cover on from a patient
3. Taking a patient's temperature with a glass mercury thermometer
4. Wiping counter surfaces in the lab using a 10:1 bleach solution and paper towels
5. Collecting a sputum specimen from a patient who may have tuberculosis
6. Cleaning the inside of a microwave in the kitchen area with paper towels
7. Putting away equipment that has already been sterilized

used for sharps such as needles, glass slides, and scalpel blades (Fig 6–12).

This material may be incinerated or autoclaved—heated in a sterilizer—to make it harmless. Most facilities contract with a company that specializes in hazardous waste removal and disposal. Cleaning staff should be instructed not to empty hazardous waste containers. When health care workers change bags, they must wear gloves, masks, and protective eyewear; close the bags securely; and put the bag inside a second hazardous waste bag (that is, double bag) if there is any chance of leakage. The bags are then stored in a secure place until the hazardous waste removal contractor collects them.

If office staff wear cloth lab coats, or if the office uses cloth gowns and drapes for patient examination, these must either be laundered in the office or by a laundry able to handle contaminated material and should be stored in special leakproof bags until the laundry collects them. Lab coats should be changed and laundered whenever they come in contact with body fluids or are soiled.

Category-Specific Isolation Precautions

Category-specific isolation precautions are used in addition to standard precautions in particular situations. In the office setting they include the following:

Airborne precautions are used for patients with a known diagnosis of illnesses transported by airborne droplet nuclei. These include measles, chicken pox, and tuberculosis. The patient should wear a mask in the waiting room, and health care workers who are not immune to the disease should wear a mask.

Droplet precautions are used for patients known to have or suspected of having illnesses transmitted by particle droplets. These include meningitis or pneumo-

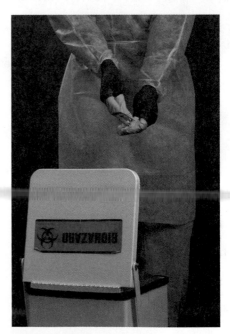

➤ **Figure 6–12** Disposing of soiled gloves in a wastebasket lined with a red plastic biohazard bag

nia caused by *Haemophilus influenzae* type b or *Neisseria* meningitis, diphtheria, pertussis, mumps, and influenza. The patient should wear a mask in the waiting room, and health care personnel should wear masks.

Contact precautions are used for serious skin and wound infections caused by a variety of microorganisms. Health care workers should wear disposable gowns and gloves; they should remove the gowns and

gloves before leaving the patient treatment room and wash their hands immediately. The hazardous waste should be disposed of immediately, and the hazardous waste bag should be double bagged.

A patient who requires any category-specific isolation should be placed in an examination room as soon as possible to prevent contact with other patients in the waiting room.

Student Study Plan

To reinforce your understanding of the material in this chapter . . .

Complete the **Review & Recall** questions.

Answer the **Critical Thinking Questions** and discuss them with your classmates.

Visit Web sites suggested, and search for additional Web sites using **Keywords for Internet Searches.**

Complete the exercises in chapter 6 of the **Student Mastery Manual.**

 REVIEW & RECALL

1. Identify four hazards that should be removed as part of a general office safety plan.
2. List four locations where fire extinguishers should be placed in the medical office.
3. What principles should be used to lift heavy objects safely?
4. Describe the proper position of the feet, arms, hands, back, and head when using a computer.
5. Describe the four stages of Hans Seyle's general adaptation syndrome.
6. List several specific areas regulated by the Occupational Safety and Health Administration (OSHA).
7. What is the purpose of using standard precautions?
8. List 10 body fluids, secretions, and excretions to which standard precautions apply.
9. Where can you find information about chemicals in the workplace that might be hazardous?
10. List four items of personal protective equipment and describe when each is used.

 IF YOU WERE THE MEDICAL ASSISTANT

While working in the laboratory of Blackburn Primary Care Associates, you are given several items to discard. Choose the proper waste disposal container from the following list for disposal of the items:

Ordinary waste basket
Plastic biohazard bag
Rigid biohazard waste container

1. paper towels used for drying hands
2. bandage after use on a bleeding wound
3. glass slide from microscope that has a sample of dried blood on it
4. gloves worn to practice applying and removing gloves
5. used plastic urine specimen container
6. needle used to give an injection
7. paper towels and gloves used to clean up blood spill on a counter

CRITICAL THINKING QUESTIONS

1. Discuss why it is important to use proper position when using a computer keyboard for several hours a day.

2. Give a general rule to follow if you are not sure what type of a waste container to discard an item in.

3. Describe how ergonomics can help to reduce repetitive strain injuries and back problems for individuals who use computers in the workplace.

4. Identify the six most important current sources of stress in your life. What are two things you could do to reduce the effects of each of these stressors?

5. If you had to develop a training plan for your employer related to chemical safety, where would you look for information? What would you include?

6. List the categories of information found on a Material Safety Data Sheet. Find at least three Material Data Safety Sheets as a basis for your list. Where will you look to find them?

7. Discuss exactly what should happen if a medical assisting student is stuck by a needle that had been used to draw blood from a classmate. What measures will help ensure that this does not happen in your training program?

8. Can you find out what happens to biohazardous waste after it is removed from the medical office? Research this question. (Hint: Find a company on the Internet that handles medical waste.)

9. Identify the specific muscle groups that are more prone to strain if heavy objects are lifted or carried using poor body mechanics. Describe why this is true.

10. Analyze a computer work station, your own if possible, and make specific suggestions to improve body position and reduce muscle, joint, and eye strain.

EXPLORE THE WEB

INTERNET WEB SITES

Centers for Disease Control and Prevention (CDC)
www.cdc.gov

Material Safety Data Sheets
siri.uvm.edu/msds

National Institute for Occupational Safety and Health (NIOSH)
www.cdc.gov/niosh/homepage.html

Occupational Safety and Health Administration (OSHA)
www.osha.gov

University of Wisconsin—Environmental Health, Safety & Risk Management
www.uwm.edu/Dept/EHSRM/EHSLINKS

KEYWORDS FOR INTERNET SEARCHES

blood-borne pathogens
chemical safety
ergonomics
medical waste
stress
stress reduction
hepatitis

ANSWERS TO ON THE JOB

1. You do not need any personal protective equipment for this procedure. If there were open skin lesions on the patient's arm or on your own hands, you would wear gloves.

2. You should wear gloves to handle a closed urine specimen cup because it is possible that there is urine on the outside of the container.

3. You should wear gloves to take a patient's temperature with a glass thermometer. Saliva is one of the body fluids that you should not come into direct contact with.

4. You should wear a lab coat and gloves to clean counter surfaces in the lab. If you see any spills on the counter, you should also wear a mask and safety glasses because they might contain hazardous chemicals or body fluids.

5. You should wear a barrier lab coat with knit sleeves, a mask, and safety glasses. You only need a mask to talk to the patient, but the sputum specimen is considered a body fluid that should not touch your hands or clothing.

6. You do not need any personal protective equipment for this procedure.

7. You do not need any personal protective equipment for this procedure.

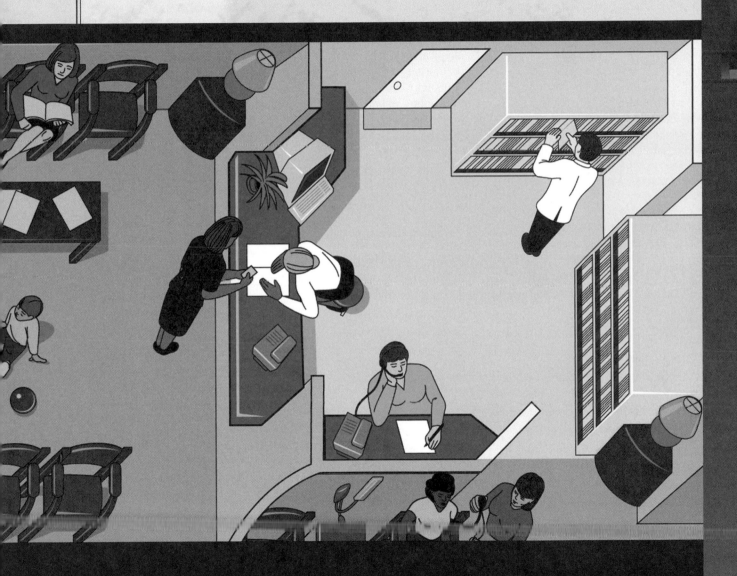

Chapter 7

Telephone Techniques

Instructional Objectives

After completing this chapter, you will be able to do the following:

1. Define and spell the vocabulary words for this chapter.
2. Describe the importance of the telephone for the medical office.
3. Explain the use of the following telephone technology:
   multi-line telephone
   facsimile (fax) machine
   pager
   voice mail.
4. Differentiate between telephone calls the medical assistant can handle and those that he or she should refer to others.
5. Describe the correct procedure for answering incoming calls.
6. Describe the correct procedure for taking messages.
7. Identify the correct steps to respond to a telephone call regarding an emergency or urgent medical problem.
8. Describe how to deal with problem calls.
9. Describe the correct procedure for placing outgoing calls.

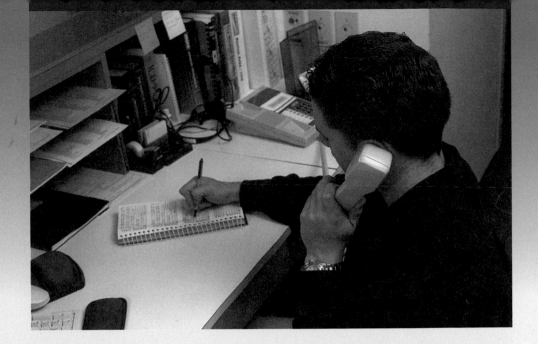

CMA/RMA CERTIFICATION
Content and Competencies

- Use the telephone
- Demonstrate telephone technique
- Identify and respond to issues of confidentiality

Performance Objectives

After completing this chapter, you will be able to do the following:

1. Demonstrate proper telephone technique (Procedure 7–1).
2. Demonstrate proper technique for taking a telephone message (Procedure 7–2).
3. Demonstrate proper technique for taking a message requesting medication or a prescription refill (Procedure 7–3).
4. Answer, screen, and respond appropriately to an emergency telephone call (Procedure 7–4).
5. Activate the emergency medical services system by telephone (Procedure 7–5).
6. Place an outgoing call using correct technique (Procedure 7–6).

111

VOCABULARY

answering service (p. 115)
cellular (wireless)
    telephone (p. 117)

e-mail (p. 115)
emergency medical services
    (EMS) (p. 123)

enunciation (p. 112)
facsimile (fax) (p. 115)
modem (p. 115)

pager (p. 117)
voice mail (p. 115)

IMPORTANCE OF THE TELEPHONE AS THE FIRST CONTACT WITH PATIENTS AND THE COMMUNITY

Contact with a patient takes many forms. In addition to face-to-face contact, medical assistants have much contact with patients over the telephone. The telephone is probably the most frequently used tool in the doctor's office. The telephone is often the first contact between the medical office and a patient. In addition, the telephone is used throughout the day to make and receive referrals, request laboratory results, call in prescriptions for patients, and respond to patient questions.

Managing the phone is one of the most important jobs in the office. It is the first chance you have to project a positive attitude and image to a patient. Remember: *You never get a second chance to make a first impression.*

Two important aspects of communicating using a telephone are:

1. Telephone courtesy
2. Telephone personality.

Telephone Courtesy

Telephone courtesy includes some basics:

Answer promptly. Some offices have a policy that every phone call should be answered within three rings.

Identify the office and give your own name.

Find out who is calling. If you are putting a call through to a doctor in the office, the doctor needs to know who will be on the other end of the call. Both the doctor and the caller will be uncomfortable if the doctor is unprepared for the call.

Speak before putting someone on hold. We have all called somewhere and been told "XYZ company, please hold" and then were left sitting with a dead telephone in hand. It is far more polite to obtain the caller's name and purpose for calling before putting the caller on hold. This way, when you come back to the call, you know who you are speaking with. Keep a written record of each caller's name, with the number of the line where he or she is holding.

Never put a doctor on hold if you can avoid it.

Check back about every 30 seconds or so with a person who is on hold. Let the person know you have not forgotten him or her, and try to give an idea of how long it will take before that person's call will be taken.

When someone comes off hold, apologize for the delay.

Do not do anything else while you are on the phone. The caller can tell that you are distracted.

Do not chew gum or eat while answering the telephone.

Telephone Personality

Because the caller can not see you, he or she is taking a number of cues from the quality of your voice. Your "telephone personality" is important; stay focused on the call and smile. Make sure to use the same volume as when speaking in person. Avoid developing an artificial telephone voice; it may come across as cold and unreal.

Enunciate clearly. **Enunciation** is the way you form the parts of words. Enunciating clearly may mean working to speak more slowly than you normally do or trying to soften a particular accent you have. Listen to the way television news readers speak; they enunciate clearly. If you need to practice speaking clearly and enunciating clearly, use a tape recorder. Listen to yourself; you may be surprised at the quality of your voice.

Qualities such as interest, friendliness, concern, and understanding are clearly communicated over the telephone. So too are boredom, anxiety, and lack of concern.

Guidelines for Effective Telephone Communication

The caller needs to have your complete attention. Try to complete the call without interruption. If you must put someone on hold or if someone in the office begins speaking to you while you are on the phone, apologize to the caller.

Be organized. Have information and materials available to handle the majority of phone calls. These include message slips, pen, the office appointment book or computer appointment screen, and a list of frequently used telephone numbers. Be sure to have a desk clock or wristwatch to note the time of messages.

Identify the practice and yourself when you answer

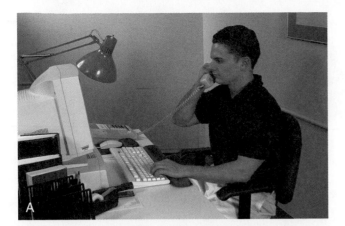

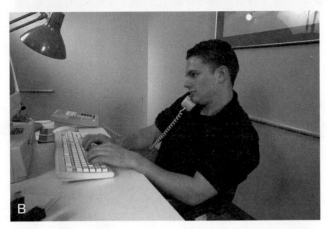

> **Figure 7–1 (A)** Good posture when answering the telephone improves voice quality and prevents muscle strain. **(B)** Leaning back in the chair and using the shoulder to hold the telephone result in poor voice quality and muscle strain.

piece that sits under your mouth, and a brace that holds the two components on your head. Your hands are free. Figure 7–2 shows such a headset.

Be clear with callers about when they can expect their calls to be returned. Many doctors return phone calls in the late morning or at lunch, then again at the end of the day between 5:00 and 7:00 PM, unless the call is urgent.

Avoid cutting into a person's replies, even if he or she rambles and repeats himself or herself. When you do get a chance to speak, try to give a focused answer that lets the caller know what you can do and what you are going to do.

Legal and Ethical Guidelines

You have three major legal/ethical responsibilities in telephone communications:

1. Maintain confidentiality.
2. Stay within the scope of your education and training, and within the policies and procedures of your office.
3. Follow through on what you agree to do.

Confidentiality

Maintaining confidentiality means that using a speaker phone is not appropriate. In a small office, you may need to answer the telephone where patients in the waiting room can overhear your conversations. If the office has a sliding glass window that can be closed

the telephone. For example, "Blackburn Medical Associates, Linda speaking." If the caller asks a question without identifying himself or herself, politely ask for the caller's name. "Who am I speaking with?" Use complete sentences, and avoid being abrupt, because it sounds like rudeness.

A multi-line telephone allows two or more telephone lines to be answered using one telephone. In addition, several extension telephones are usually located throughout the office.

For your own health, use good posture. Sit with your back supported and your head in a neutral position (not forward or to one side). Keep your feet flat on the floor. Do not make a habit of tucking the receiver between your head and shoulder; this places strain on your shoulder muscles and may change your breathing and voice quality. Figure 7–1 shows proper and improper body mechanics for answering the telephone.

If you work a lot at the telephone, talk to the office manager about getting a headset. The headset consists of an earpiece that fits over your ear, a little mouth-

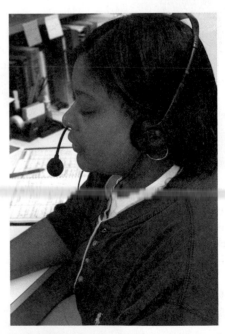

> **Figure 7–2** A telephone headset leaves the hands free and facilitates good body posture.

between the reception desk and the waiting room, it should be used when answering the telephone. If there is no glass partition, the medical assistant may need to move to another telephone for any discussion of a patient's personal information.

Scope of Education and Training

This is important especially when dealing with pharmacists, responding to questions about medical conditions, or taking laboratory reports and giving patients the results of their lab tests. As in any other phase of working in a medical office, medical assistants must always stay within the scope of their education and training.

Follow Through

Callers expect follow through. You need to make sure that you actually do pass along messages, call back if you are too busy to talk when the call comes in, or call back when you find the information you promised the caller.

TELEPHONE TECHNOLOGY

Twenty-five years ago, communicating by phone was easy. There was one telephone, maybe two, or possibly a phone with a "roll-over" line, a second telephone line that the calls rolled over to if the first line was busy.

Today's doctor's office phone system might include any or all of the following:

multi-line phone
voice mail boxes
modem for electronic information transfer
fax machine
direct dial to pagers or frequently called numbers
cellular phones.

Multi-line Phones

Most offices have a multi-line phone, with several extensions. Become familiar with your phone system. Learn how to determine which line is ringing, how to place calls on hold, and how to transfer calls to examination rooms and offices. Figure 7–3 illustrates a multi-line telephone with a headset and message pad.

A flashing light usually identifies a line that is ringing; it flashes at a different rate on a line where a person is on hold. To answer a call, press the button on the telephone that corresponds to the line that is ringing. If a second call comes in while you are speaking to a caller, tell the first caller that you need to place him or her on hold. Pressing the button corre-

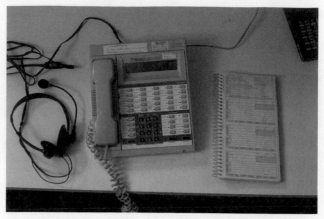

> **Figure 7–3** A multi-line telephone is commonly used in a medical office. A headset can be attached to the telephone.

sponding to the line you are speaking on puts the caller on that line on hold. Answer the second call, and respond as quickly as possible. Then return to the first caller and apologize for the interruption.

If the caller asks to be connected to another extension or person, you may ask, "Whom shall I say is calling?" To transfer a call, you may need to press another button and/or dial an extension number, depending on the type of telephone system your office uses. You may also ask the telephone number of the individual on the line, saying, "May I get your name and number in case we get cut off during the transfer?"

Keep the names of all callers who are on hold, as well as the number of the telephone line they are on, on a piece of paper. While a caller is on hold, the light on that line will flash. If the light continues to flash, pick up that line about every 30 seconds, and ask if the person is still holding. Sometimes transfers do not go through or the call is not picked up.

Other Features

Telephone systems also come with other features, including speed dialing and call forwarding.

Speed dialing allows you to put frequently called telephone numbers into the telephone system's memory, then call them by pressing a button or a one- or two-digit code.

Call forwarding allows you to have all incoming calls directed to another telephone number. This service is turned on and off by dialing a sequence of numbers and activity keys.

Call waiting is a service available only on single-line phones, which allows them to be used as two-line phones. When you are on the phone and another call comes in, you will hear a clicking. By depressing the receiver quickly one time, you can switch to the second caller without hanging up on the first caller. Because most medical offices have multi-line systems, they do not have call waiting.

Answering Machines and Voice Mail

Doctors have always needed to be available at all times. Most doctors' offices still use an answering service for getting messages to doctors during hours when the office is normally closed. This is an independent company that answers telephones for a number of clients.

Some offices also have an answering machine, which has a message with a number to call outside of office hours and gives people the option to leave a nonurgent message on the answering tape. Answering services and answering machines are activated whenever the office is closed, including during lunch break if no one is assigned to take phone calls during that time. The answering service should be notified if the office is closed, although they usually pick up phones after a predetermined number of rings.

Increasingly, doctors' offices are going to voice mail systems. Voice mail is a system provided by the office's telephone carrier that allows for messages to be left in a number of "mailboxes" for different people. Each doctor might have his or her own voice mail box, as well as each medical assistant; the business manager, and so on.

The message will have a number to call for urgent messages outside of office hours, but will also offer the caller the option of leaving a nonurgent message in any voice mail box. Each box has a two- to four-number extension. Many voice mail systems have a directory by which people can find voice mail box numbers by using their touch-tone phone to type in the first three letters of the last name of the person they would like to speak with.

Even if an office has a voice mail system, almost every medical office will still need to have a contract with an answering service. The answering service provides a medical office with coverage outside of normal business hours. The service either answers all of the office's telephone calls or takes calls that are forwarded to it by individuals who listen to the voice mail system message and press the appropriate message code for an urgent message. The answering service must be informed how to deal with urgent calls.

Faxes and E-Mails

Telephone lines are also used to send data rapidly. This is done either by facsimile (fax) or directly from one computer to another using e-mail. Both of these systems use the telephone lines. In the case of a fax, paper is placed in the machine, which translates the

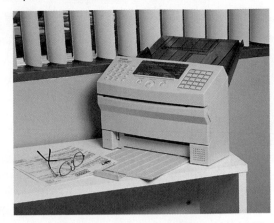

> **Figure 7–4** Facsimile (fax) machine. (From Kinn ME, Woods MA: *The Medical Assistant, Administrative and Clinical.* Philadelphia, WB Saunders, 1999.)

images on the paper into analog signals to be sent over the phone. In the case of e-mail, a modem in the computer translates the data in the e-mail file into an analog signal to send over the phone line. At the other end, a fax machine or computer with modem retranslates from analog into either image or computer data.

There should be dedicated telephone lines (lines used for only one purpose) for these pieces of data-transmission equipment. Figure 7–4 shows a fax machine.

The phone number for the fax machine should be listed next to every telephone, so you or anyone else can tell a caller how to fax information to the office.

Insurance companies are increasingly moving toward electronic transmission of claims, which will be discussed in more detail in chapter 38, which covers filing insurance claims. Some insurance companies are even making payments electronically directly into the office's bank account.

Security and confidentiality are issues when using e-mail or sending a fax. Assume that an e-mail message may be read by someone else (such as a member of the recipient's family). Assume also that the organization you work for may have access to e-mail messages, even if you have deleted them. Never use e-mail for information that should be kept private.

A fax is efficient for rapid transmission of information, but again security and especially confidentiality are issues. Anyone walking by the fax machine can see the pages that have just come through. The fax is useful for doing business—ordering supplies—and for sending out meeting agendas or receiving résumés when hiring. But avoid sending any direct patient information on the fax whenever possible. If you must send personal information, use a cover sheet that identifies that the fax is confidential for the person you are sending it to.

PROCEDURE 7-1

Answering Incoming Calls

Performance Objective: The student will demonstrate proper telephone technique.
Supplies and Equipment: Telephone, message pad, pen or pencil, appointment book or computer terminal, clock or watch.

Procedure Steps

1 Answer the telephone each time it rings within the first three rings.
Rationale: Callers become annoyed when their calls are not answered promptly.

2. Identify the practice and give your name. Each practice will have a preferred way for all employees to answer the telephone. Example: "Blackburn Primary Care Associates, this is Joanne speaking." Do not rush through the greeting. The caller needs to hear this first sentence clearly.
Rationale: Callers needs to know who they have reached and with whom they are speaking. Otherwise they will have to ask if this is Blackburn Primary Care Associates.

3. Listen carefully to what the caller says and decide as soon as possible if this is a call you can handle, if you need to take a message, or

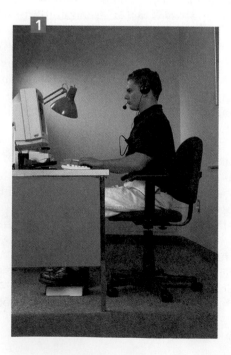

if the call should be transferred to someone else in the office.
Rationale: The caller does not want to have to repeat all the details if the call must be transferred. If you need to take a message, begin writing.

4. Ask for the caller's name. "May I ask who is calling?"
Rationale: You will need the caller's name either to address the caller by name, to take a message, or to identify the caller before transferring the call.

5. If you can handle the call, such as a call for an appointment, do so promptly.

6. If you need to take a message see Procedure 7-2, Taking a Telephone Message.

7. If you need to transfer the call to someone else in the office, place the caller on hold, noting the caller's name and the extension. Tell the person you are transferring the call to who is calling and what extension the call is on.
Rationale: It is a courtesy to tell the person you transfer a call to who is calling; he or she must be able to locate the call if more than one line has a call on hold.

8. If your telephone has more than two lines, it is helpful to keep a list of the names of callers and extensions. When a call is on hold, the light for that telephone line blinks. If you have transferred a call, but the call remains on hold, within 30 to 45 seconds you should determine if the caller is still holding; if so, you should try to transfer the call again or take a message.
Rationale: Sometimes transfer does not go through or the call is not picked up. The caller has no way to get back in contact with you to leave a message or ask to speak to someone else.

9. If the telephone rings for another call, ask if you may put the caller you are speaking to on hold and wait for the caller to agree. After pressing the hold button, answer the other call and explain that you are speaking to a caller on another line. Give the second caller the option to hold and wait for you or take their number and offer to call back as soon as you are finished. Never leave a call on hold for more than 45 seconds.

Rationale: You need to finish with the first caller before taking the second call. By asking for permission to put the caller on hold, you give the caller a chance to tell you if it is an emergency. Some callers prefer to hold; others prefer to be called back. Time passes slowly when a caller is on hold, and the caller may become tired of waiting and wish to leave a message.

10. At the end of the call you can repeat any information you have discussed (such as the date and time of an appointment). End the call by saying thank you (if appropriate) and good-bye.
Rationale: Confirmation helps avoid misunderstandings. You demonstrate courtesy by thanking the caller and closing the conversation.

Pagers and Cellular Phones

Pagers used to beep, and the doctors who wore them knew to call the answering service. Today, pagers are either numeric or alphanumeric. They beep or vibrate to signal a message.

A numeric pager's message is a telephone number (the answering service, the office, the emergency room, home, a colleague, and so on). The doctor then returns the call to the number on the display. An alphanumeric pager displays an entire message, so the doctor can return a phone call or act on the information that is relayed to the pager. The office staff should have the pager numbers for each doctor in the practice.

Increasingly, doctors are using **cellular (wireless) telephones,** which allow them to return calls at any time from wherever they are. Be sure you know each doctor's preference about whether to page or call on the cellular phone.

INCOMING CALLS

An incoming telephone call sounds like a routine event. And after you have handled a few thousand, it is indeed routine. But breaking down the process, it becomes clear that a number of different elements go into answering a routine call.

First is the issue of centralized versus electronic routing of calls. This is really a policy decision, but it is one that needs to be made so that staff know how to handle individual calls. In total, there are eight facets to the process of answering incoming calls:

1. Centralized or electronic routing
2. Answering incoming calls
3. Screening calls
4. Calls the medical assistant can handle
5. Calls where the medical assistant takes a message or refers the call to the doctor
6. Emergency or urgent calls
7. Referring calls to a specialist in the office or in the community
8. Problem calls.

Centralized or Electronic Routing

Many offices use a voice mail system to direct calls and take messages for office staff who are not available. By offering the caller several options (press 1 to schedule an appointment, 2 to speak to Dr. Hughes' medical assistant, 3 to speak to Dr. Lawler's medical assistant, 4 if you have a question about your bill, and so on), the electronic routing system directs the call to the appropriate part of the office, saving the expense of a staff person who would otherwise be answering the call. It also keeps patients from being put on hold, which some people appreciate.

However, other patients find electronic routing of messages confusing and frustrating, especially if the person they need to speak with is not available and does not return calls promptly.

If electronic routing is used, the message should be kept up to date and should be as clear and concise as possible.

Depending on the size of the office, the person responsible for routing calls may only answer the phones, may double as a receptionist, or may even be responsible for billing or other administrative work as well. Many patients appreciate the human touch, and this person can give a little more attention to individuals who might be confused by the technology of electronic routing.

Answering Incoming Calls

A medical assistant should be prepared to answer calls. This means having the right supplies—message pad, pen, clock or watch, and appointment calendar, either paper or computer based. He or she also must be familiar with the telephone and be able to juggle the office's phone lines.

The medical assistant must be able to appear to be paying complete attention to the caller (telephone courtesy) while in reality dividing his or her attention between the phone and other duties, such as checking patients in, directing patients to the lab, assisting with processing referrals, or taking insurance co-payments.

See Procedure 7–1, Answering Incoming Calls, for a step-by-step discussion of this task.

Screening Calls (How Important Is the Call, and Who Should Answer It?)

The purpose of screening calls is to find out how urgent the call is and who should answer it.

Most calls are routine and can be handled in the order in which they come in. However, there are some exceptions:

Calls from other doctors are put through at once.

Emergency calls are treated as urgent and receive top priority. They will be discussed in detail later in this chapter.

If the caller asks for a member of the office staff by name, transfer the call to that person after you get the caller's name. If the caller has a question, you decide who the best person to answer it is, using the guidelines discussed below.

Often, the caller asks to speak to the doctor. Most doctors do not take calls while they are seeing patients, except from other doctors or callers the doctor has told you to put through.

Calls the Medical Assistant Can Handle

The medical assistant can handle four kinds of calls.

Scheduling Appointments

One is scheduling appointments and tests, either in the office or at an outside laboratory or the hospital. This topic will be discussed in detail in chapter 9.

Billing Inquiries

Another is billing inquiries. For this type of call, pull the ledger card or computer ledger screen, and give the caller the information requested. If the caller's question is complicated, the call may be referred to a billing specialist or the office manager.

Diagnostic Test and Lab Results

The medical assistant can also take calls regarding diagnostic test and lab results. Many lab results today are sent to doctors' offices by fax or directly on the computer system. But if a laboratory calls in test results, the medical assistant needs to have a blank lab slip so that the results can be filled in, along with the patient's name and the date the tests were taken. After taking the results, you should pull the patient's medical record, clip the results to the front, and place the chart where the doctor can review it. Be sure to take the information accurately.

Requests for Information

Finally, the medical assistant can handle calls requesting information, such as directions to get to the

office, office hours, and the office's medical specialty. See the above box for examples of telephone calls the medical assistant can handle.

Examples of Telephone Calls the Medical Assistant Can Handle

EXAMPLE 1: BILLING INQUIRY

MA: Hello, Blackburn Primary Care Associates. Joanne speaking.

Caller: This is Donna Fuller. My last bill includes a co-payment that I made at the office.

MA: Just a minute, please. I need to get your account up on my computer. (Pause) Are we talking about your visit on June 6?

Caller: Yes. I wrote a check for $10 while I was in the office. But you billed me for that amount in the June bill.

MA: We do not show that payment. I'm sorry. We must have made an error. Could you send us a copy of the canceled check so we can credit your account? Send it to my attention, Joanne Cabot, and I'll take care of it.

Caller: The check hasn't come back yet. I'll send it as soon as I receive it. Thank you.

MA: Thank you.

EXAMPLE 2: REQUEST FOR INFORMATION

MA: Hello, Blackburn Primary Care Associates. Joanne speaking.

Caller: Hello. Do you have office hours on Saturdays?

MA: With whom am I speaking? Are you a patient of one of our doctors?

Caller: My name is John Finegold. I've just moved to Blackburn, and I need to find a doctor who can see me on Saturdays. I'm on the road during the work week.

MA: Mr. Finegold, one of our doctors is always in the office on Saturday morning. We also have office hours Thursday evenings. I could set up an appointment right now for one of those times.

Caller: Thank you. Let me look at my calendar.

When the Medical Assistant Takes a Message or Refers the Call to a Doctor

The best system for taking telephone messages is to use a message pad, as illustrated in Figure 7–5, with a carbon copy so that the office has a record of all messages. Some offices use noncarbon message pads and a telephone log.

See Procedure 7–2 for a fuller discussion.

The box on page 121 contains examples of telephone calls where the medical assistant takes a message.

Patients Requesting Test Results

When a patient calls requesting test results, the medical assistant should find out when and where the test was done and take a message for the doctor. Following the call, the medical assistant should locate the

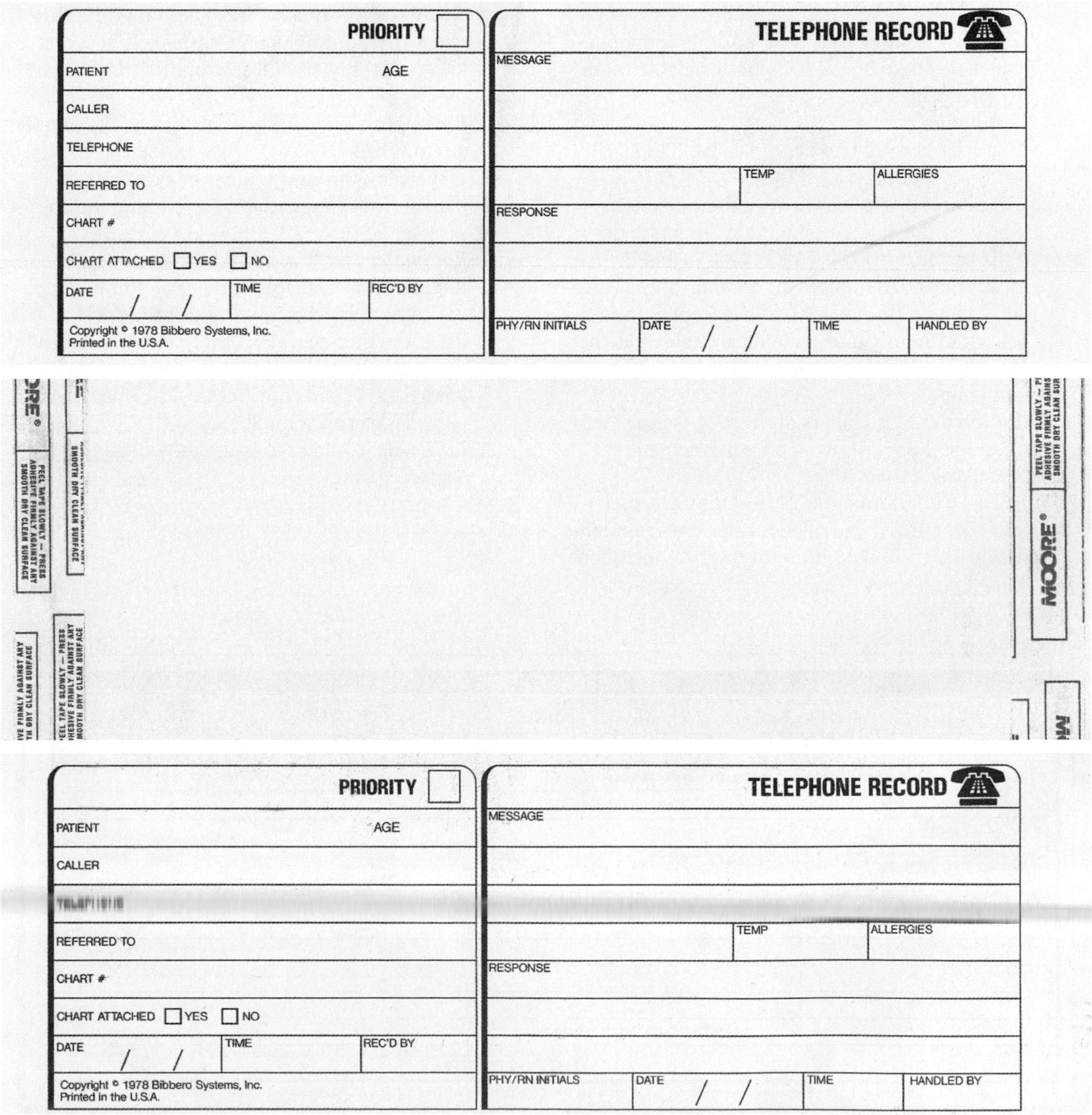
PRIORITY
PATIENT AGE
CALLER
TELEPHONE
REFERRED TO
CHART #
CHART ATTACHED YES NO
DATE / / TIME REC'D BY
Copyright © 1978 Bibbero Systems, Inc.
Printed in the U.S.A.

TELEPHONE RECORD
MESSAGE
TEMP ALLERGIES
RESPONSE
PHY/RN INITIALS DATE / / TIME HANDLED BY

PRIORITY
PATIENT AGE
CALLER
TELEPHONE
REFERRED TO
CHART #
CHART ATTACHED YES NO
DATE / / TIME REC'D BY
Copyright © 1978 Bibbero Systems, Inc.
Printed in the U.S.A.

TELEPHONE RECORD
MESSAGE
TEMP ALLERGIES
RESPONSE
PHY/RN INITIALS DATE / / TIME HANDLED BY

➢ **Figure 7–5** A message pad should contain an original and a copy. In this system, the original (white) contains an adhesive backing for mounting in the medical record. The copy (yellow) remains on the message pad to form a telephone log. (Courtesy of Bibbero Systems, Inc., Petaluma, CA; 800-272-2376, Fax 800-242-9330; www.bibbero.com.)

PROCEDURE 7–2

Taking a Telephone Message

Performance Objective: The student will demonstrate proper technique for taking a telephone message.
Supplies and Equipment: Message pad, pen or pencil, clock or watch.

Procedure Steps

1. If you determine that the person a telephone caller wants to speak to is not available, offer to take a message.
   Rationale: A message is a way of communicating to a person who is not available to speak on the telephone.

2. Give the caller a reason why the person cannot take the call. Acceptable reasons are as follows: busy with a patient, not at his or her desk, not in the office, on another line. Generally doctors do not take calls except during specified hours, and patients are told that the doctor is not in the office or is busy with patients.
   Rationale: Most callers are willing to leave a message if they understand why their call is not being answered.

3. Fill in the information on the message pad, including the name of the caller, business affiliation (if any), date, time of the call, telephone number including area code, and the information the caller wishes to leave about the reason for the call. Place your initials on the message in case there are questions.
   Rationale: Complete information is necessary to return a call.

4. Verify the information. If possible give a time when the call might be returned. If you don't know this, say "I will give him (or her) the message."
   Rationale: Callers like to know when to expect a return call.

5. If the call is from a patient or concerns a patient, pull the medical record and clip the message to it.
   Rationale: This ensures that information about the patient is available and the action taken on the call can be charted if necessary.

6. Place the message (with the patient record, if needed) where the person for whom it is intended expects to find messages. This may be on a desk or in a mailbox.
   Rationale: A message is useless unless the person receives it.

4

MESSAGE FROM								
For Dr. *Lawler*	Name of Caller *Anne Richards*	Ref. to pt. *mother*	Patient *Janice*	Pt. Age. *4*	Pt. Temp. *101°*	Message Date *10/13/XX*	Message Time *9:00 AM*	Urgent ☐ Yes ☐ No

Message: *Child has been on antibiotic for two days – still has fever. Should she come in again?*   Allergies *∅*

Respond to Phone # *814-322-6570*	Best Time to Call *any* AM PM	Pharmacy Name / # *West Side* *814-754-9817*	Patient's Chart Attached ☒ Yes ☐ No	Patient's chart #	Initials *KJ*

DOCTOR - STAFF RESPONSE

Doctor's / Staff Orders / Follow-up Action

	Call Back ☐ Yes ☐ No	Chart. Mes. ☐ Yes ☐ No	Follow-up Date / /	Follow-up Completed-Date/Time / /	AM PM	Response By:

Product # 78-9156-Pkg, #78-9157-Pads, Bibbero Systems, Inc., Petaluma, CA. To order, call toll free 800-BIBBERO (800 242-2376) OR FAX 800-242-9330.

medical record, be sure the requisition for and results of the laboratory or diagnostic test in question are in the record, and leave the message and medical record—with the applicable report highlighted—for the doctor.

Some offices choose to send patients letters about lab results, which cuts down on the number of telephone calls requesting information, especially for routine tests.

In some offices, the doctor permits medical assistants to tell patients if results of lab tests are within normal ranges. However, if patients know this, they may worry when the medical assistant refers a particular call to the doctor.

In addition, test results should never be given to family members unless the patient is a child.

Patients Reporting Satisfactory or Unsatisfactory Progress

Calls with patient reports of their condition always generate a message for the doctor. Doctors often tell a patient to call and check in after a visit, to report on how a condition is resolving after treatment.

Example of a Telephone Call Where the Medical Assistant Must Take a Message

MA: Hello, Blackburn Primary Care Associates. Joanne speaking.

Caller: Hi, this is Jason Chin. I had an ultrasound of my gall bladder at Memorial Hospital last Thursday. Dr. Lopez asked me to call today for the results.

MA: Let me take a message so Dr. Lopez can call you back. Do you spell your name "C-h-i-n"?

Caller: Can't you give me the results?

MA: Dr. Lopez always talks to his patients about test results. He usually does these calls in the late afternoon. Did I spell your name correctly?

Caller: Yes, you did.

MA: Can I have a telephone number where Dr. Lopez can reach you after 4:00 this afternoon, Mr. Chin?

Caller: 549-2222.

MA: Is that in area code 609?

Caller: Yes, it is.

MA: I'll give Dr. Lopez the message, and he'll call you about the results.

Caller: Thank you.

If the patient reports satisfactory progress, the medical assistant should take a brief message, put it in the chart, and leave it for the doctor. An unsatisfactory report should generate a more complete message, and the chart should be pulled and the message clipped to it so the doctor can call the patient.

Calls from Other Doctors

Calls from other doctors are usually put right through to the doctor. Tell the doctor who it is, because doctors should not be interrupted during patient visits except for other doctor's phone calls or for calls from whomever else the doctor specifies, such as a family member. Avoid telling the doctor who is calling in front of the patient; if possible, hand the doctor a slip of paper with the name of the person calling or tell the doctor over the phone before transferring the call.

Patients with Medical Questions

For patients with medical questions, take a message for a doctor or refer the call to a medical assistant or nurse designated by the office to handle such calls. The office should have written guidelines to follow if a medical assistant screens medical questions. The medical assistant should follow the written guidelines closely and take a message for the doctor about any concern or question that falls outside the preset guidelines.

Requests for Medication or Prescription Refills

Often patients or pharmacies call with requests to have prescriptions refilled (or renewed, with multiple refills). Patients are usually told to have the pharmacy call. If you take a message directly from the patient, make sure to get the pharmacy phone number, the medication, strength, amount, refills remaining on the prescription, and any other relevant information.

See Procedure 7–3.

Calls from Salespeople

Often a sales representative from a pharmaceutical company or equipment company calls before visiting the doctor's office. Salespeople are usually seen by the office manager, who gives the information to the doctor. Drug representatives usually drop by, but occasionally they call and ask for an appointment, especially if they have a new product to discuss. The doctor has to agree to see the representative before a medical assistant makes an appointment.

PROCEDURE 7–3

Taking Requests for Medication or Prescription Refills

Performance Objective: The student will demonstrate proper technique for taking a message requesting medication or a prescription refill.

Supplies and Equipment: Message pad, pen or pencil, clock or watch.

Procedure Steps

1. Identify the caller and telephone number.
   Rationale: This enables you to know where to return the call.

2. Identify if it is a patient or a pharmacy. If it is a patient, take the information about the medication or refill requested, and obtain the number of the patient's preferred pharmacy. In some offices patients are directed to have the pharmacy call the office because the doctor wishes to speak directly to the pharmacist.
   Rationale: It depends on whether the doctor wishes to speak to the pharmacist about refills or delegates the medical assistant to call refills or prescriptions to the pharmacy.

3. If it is a pharmacy usually the medical assistant takes a message, including the name and address of the patient, the medication re-

quested, and the dose and amount received before. Inform the pharmacy when the doctor is likely to okay the refill so the pharmacy can tell the patient.
   Rationale: Usually doctors have specific times when they review and respond to messages.

4. Pull the patient's medical record and place with the message where the doctor can review it. If the doctor responds directly to pharmacy calls, put the pharmacist on hold, pull the patient's medical record, and give it to the doctor before transferring the call.
   Rationale: The doctor will need to review information about the patient before agreeing to refill or prescribe medication.

5. Usually the doctor indicates on the message slip if the prescription may be refilled or writes a new prescription on the message slip. The medical assistant can then call the pharmacy with the information. Read the prescription from the message slip exactly as the doctor has written it.
   Rationale: The medical assistant functions as an agent of the doctor in this case. He or she must give the exact information the doctor has indicated.

5

MESSAGE FROM								
For Dr. *Hughes*	Name of Caller	Ref. to pt.	Patient *Roland Aiken*	Pt. Age *40+*	Pt. Temp.	Message Date *10/13/XX*	Message Time *3:00* AM PM	Urgent ☐ Yes ☒ No
Message: *needs more Aldactazide (25mg tabs) — takes 1 daily*							Allergies *∅*	

Respond to Phone # *814-798-2010*	Best Time to Call AM PM	Pharmacy Name / # *West Side* *814-754-9817*	Patient's Chart Attached ☒ Yes ☐ No	Patient's chart #	Initials *KJ*

DOCTOR - STAFF RESPONSE

Doctor's / Staff Orders / Follow-up Action

OK - call to pharmacy JH
#30
12 refills
Sig: 1 po qam

	Call Back ☐ Yes ☐ No	Chart. Mes. ☐ Yes ☐ No	Follow-up Date / /	Follow-up Completed-Date/Time / /	AM PM	Response By:

Product # 78-9156-Pkg, #78-9157-Pads, Bibbero Systems, Inc., Petaluma, CA. To order, call toll free 800-BIBBERO (800 242-2376) OR FAX 800-242-9330.

6. Document the refill or prescription in the patient's medical record. In some offices the message itself is filed in the medical record, in others the medical assistant writes the information in the progress notes of the medical record.
Rationale: Any treatment of the patient must be documented in the medical record as part of the continuous record of care given. See chapter 22 for specifics on documenting medications.

Charting Example	
Date:	
10/13/XX	4:30 PM Prescription called to
	Westside Pharmacy for Aldactazide
	25 mg tabs, #30, Sig: i po q am,
	12 refills.
	K. Anderson, CMA

Emergency or Urgent Calls

If a patient calls with an urgent medical problem, the medical assistant should remain calm and get the following information:

the caller's name
the caller's telephone number
who has the problem (the patient's name, age, and relationship to the caller)
the patient's symptoms and current condition
a brief history of the symptoms or the accident
any treatment that has already been given.

More complete details are found in Procedure 7–4.
After determining the nature of the emergency or urgent problem, the medical assistant or receptionist should follow office policy. If a doctor is in the office, he or she will want to take the call; in a multi-doctor office, one doctor may be assigned at all times to take urgent calls. If there is no doctor in the office, a nurse practitioner or physician's assistant may be assigned to take urgent calls. If no licensed professional is present in the office, the medical assistant must advise the caller or contact the on-call doctor. The following are the guidelines for dealing with such a call.

1. If the emergency is serious or life-threatening, tell the caller to call an ambulance (dial 911). In most areas dialing 911 gives access to a variety of services such as the police department, fire department, ambulance services, and so on. This is called the **emergency medical services (EMS)** system. If the caller is a child, or seems upset or confused, you can offer to call an ambulance for the caller. Be sure to get the caller's address and phone number before activating the EMS system. See Procedure 7–5.

PROCEDURE 7–4

Procedure for Emergency Calls

Performance Objective: The student will answer, assess, and respond appropriately to an emergency telephone call.
Supplies and Equipment: Telephone, message pad, pen or pencil, procedure manual, list of emergency telephone numbers (including local emergency rooms, poison control center, ambulance, and doctor's pager and cellular telephone).

Procedure Steps

1. When answering an incoming telephone call, if you need to put the caller on hold, always ask permission first.
Rationale: This allows the caller to tell you that there is an emergency.

2. If the caller states that a problem is an emergency or urgent, assess the situation at once. Remain calm.
Rationale: Time may be a crucial factor to saving someone's life or restoring normal function.

3. Write down the following information on a message pad:
   • caller's name
   • telephone number
   • who has the problem (patient's name, age, relationship to caller)
   • patient's symptoms and current condition
   • brief history of symptoms or accident
   • any treatment that has been given.

Procedure continued on next page

PROCEDURE 7-4 *(continued)*

Rationale: If you get disconnected, you need to know where to call back. You need enough information to assess the situation. Write the details down to avoid errors.

4. Confirm the details by reading them back to the caller.

5. Decide if the situation is:
   - very serious and potentially life-threatening
   - not life-threatening but requires the facilities of an emergency room for treatment
   - a poisoning, not life-threatening but requires immediate treatment
   - one that requires treatment that day
   - not urgent.

   Rationale: The more serious the emergency, the sooner treatment must be initiated. Your assessment guides your next actions.

6. If the situation is a medical emergency, transfer the call immediately to the doctor or any licensed health professional in the office.

   Rationale: Emergency situations are best handled by professionals with the most education and training.

7. If there is no one in the office to assist you and the emergency is serious or life-threatening, tell the caller to call an ambulance. If the caller is a child or seems too upset, you can offer to call an ambulance for the patient. Be sure to get the address from which the call is being made before activating the emergency medical services (EMS) System (See Procedure 7–5, Activating the EMS System). Remain on the line until the ambulance arrives if possible, but the caller may need to hang up to call an ambulance.

   Rationale: You want to be assured that the caller has received needed medical assistance.

8. If the emergency is a case of poisoning, instruct the caller to call the poison control center; the telephone number should be at all office telephones.

9. If the patient has a problem that requires

treatment at an emergency room but is conscious and able to walk (such as a fracture of an arm), instruct the caller to take the patient to the nearest emergency room.

10. After you have instructed the patient or if you are unsure how urgent the problem is, tell the caller that you will call the doctor for instructions, then page the doctor or place a call on the cellular telephone. Follow up as soon as possible.

    Rationale: Once the caller has spoken with you, he or she will assume that you are responding to the problem and will usually not seek other assistance. You and the doctor will be liable for any problems that result from unnecessary delay in response.

11. In any of the above situations, notify the doctor as soon as possible. Describe your actions in the patient's medical record, including the date, time, emergency, your action, and that you notified the doctor.

Charting Example	
Date:	
12/01/XX	11:15 AM Pt. called office complaining of severe chest pain radiating to the Ⓛ arm, nausea, and weakness. Pt. stated, "I think I am having a heart attack." A neighbor was with the Pt. Instructed Pt. to call an ambulance immediately. 11:25 AM Notified Dr. Lawler by telephone who said he would follow up with the emergency room at Memorial Hospital. ———————— ———————————— J. Cummings, RMA

2. If the emergency is a case of poisoning, instruct the caller to call the poison control center for your area; the telephone number of the poison control center should be placed next to every phone line in the medical office.

3. If the patient has a problem that requires treatment in an emergency room but is conscious and able to walk (such as a fractured arm), instruct the caller to take the patient to the nearest emergency room. If the patient is alone, have him or her call an ambulance.

4. If the patient's problem is usually treated in the office, give the patient an appointment for that day.

5. If you are unsure how urgent the problem is, tell the caller that you will call the doctor for instructions, then page the doctor or place a call on his or her cellular telephone.

Finally, if you do not know exactly what to do, protect the patient and protect yourself from liability by having the patient go to the emergency room.

Referring Calls to Specialists in the Office or Community

A patient may call to say he or she needs a referral (because of a particular insurance company's policy) to see a specialist outside the medical group or to have a laboratory test or diagnostic procedure done.

Take the necessary information (what type of referral, for what, to whom). Then check with the doctor to make sure he or she feels a specialist is indicated. If a

---

PROCEDURE 7–5

Activating the Emergency Medical Services (EMS) System

Performance Objective: The student will activate the EMS system by telephone.
Supplies and Equipment: Telephone, completed message form or written notes, pen or pencil.

Procedure Steps

1. Determine that you need to activate the EMS system, either following instructions from the doctor or another professional or based on your own assessment when no licensed professional is available to help you. The following are situations where you might need to activate the EMS system:
   a. You receive an emergency telephone call about a patient with a serious or life-threatening injury from a child or other person who appears too upset or nervous to call an ambulance.
   b. You receive an emergency telephone call from a patient who talks to you at first but either loses consciousness or becomes unable to talk coherently during the conversation.
   c. A patient in the office becomes seriously ill and needs to be moved to a hospital immediately.
   d. An accident occurs in your office or office building and someone who is administering first aid asks you to call an ambulance.
   e. An emergency situation occurs when you are not at work and you need to call an ambulance.
   Rationale: In a serious emergency, a person may be unable to activate the EMS system without assistance.
2. Dial the correct number for your location. In many communities the number 911 is used for all types of emergencies. Emergency numbers (including ambulance, fire, and poison control center) should be located near all telephones in the medical office.
3. Have the following information ready for the person who answers the telephone:
   • Nature of the emergency
   • Your name and address
   • Telephone number you are calling from
   • Who has the problem (patient's name, age, relationship to caller)
   • Patient's symptoms and current condition
   • Brief history of symptoms or accident
   • Any treatment that has been given
   • Medications that the patient has taken recently.
   Rationale: Knowledge about the emergency allows the dispatcher to send appropriate equipment and personnel to the scene of the emergency.
4. Arrange to have someone wait at the street entrance for the ambulance and direct the medical personnel to the patient's exact location.
   Rationale: Time can be saved by assisting medical personnel to find the patient quickly and efficiently.
5. If possible, stay on the telephone line until an ambulance and medical personnel have arrived. Otherwise follow up to be sure assistance was received. In the medical office, notify the patient's primary care doctor of the action taken.
   Rationale: You can provide emotional support while the caller is waiting for assistance. Notifying the doctor is necessary for prompt follow-up.
6. In the medical office, document actions taken in the patient's medical record, including date, time, emergency, your action, and that you notified the doctor.

FOCUS ON
LEGAL ISSUES

RECOGNIZING AND RESPONDING TO TELEPHONE EMERGENCIES

When a telephone call concerns a life-threatening or serious emergency, the medical assistant becomes legally responsible to provide appropriate assistance, even if the medical office is not equipped to provide the actual care needed. Once the medical assistant identifies an emergency, he or she must maintain contact with the caller, help the caller get assistance, and follow up to be sure that care was received.

State Good Samaritan laws generally do not apply to the medical office, because people expect to receive medical care and/or medical advice from doctors and medical offices.

The most desirable response is to refer an emergency or urgent call to a doctor or other licensed health care provider in the office (nurse practitioner, physician's assistant, or nurse). However, if no licensed professional is able to take the call, the medical assistant should assist the caller to assess the situation. Then the medical assistant should instruct (or assist if necessary) the caller to arrange transportation to an emergency room if the patient's health will be harmed by delayed treatment.

Use the following guidelines to respond to an emergency call:

1. Always ask if you may put the caller on hold. This gives the caller an opportunity to inform you that the call is truly urgent, or an emergency.

2. Keep an updated procedure manual near the telephone. The manual should list specific urgent problems and situations, specific questions to ask, and responses to the caller's questions. Keep emergency numbers near all telephones; these include the numbers for the EMS system, which for many areas is 911; the number for the local or regional poison control center; and the pager numbers or cellular phone numbers for all the doctors in the practice.

3. Write down the caller's name and telephone number as early in the call as possible, in case the call is interrupted. Avoid putting the caller on hold or transferring to another telephone if at all possible. If you must transfer or put the call on hold, be sure to have the caller's name and phone number before doing so.

4. If you believe delay in treatment poses a threat to the health of the ill or injured person, instruct the caller to call an ambulance. If the caller is a child or seems too confused or anxious to make the call, do it for the caller. Try to keep the line the caller is on open by picking up a second telephone to place the call to the ambulance. Before calling for an ambulance, be sure to get the caller's location. This is the best way to make sure qualified health care professionals evaluate the situation as quickly as possible.

5. Follow up by notifying the doctor (if you have not already done so), by calling the emergency room at the local hospital to inform them that a person will be coming in, and by describing the incident completely. If the injured or ill person is a patient of the practice, this should be noted in the patient's medical record. If the injured or ill person is not a patient of the practice, the incident should be reported in a memo entitled: "Report of Unusual Incident." Some practices will ask for such an incident report to be written even for a patient. Bring the written report to a doctor's attention as soon as possible.

referral is appropriate—or necessary because of an insurance company or health maintenance organization policy—fill out a referral form as completely as possible. Give it to the doctor to complete and sign. Be sure to fill out a message slip in case you need to call the patient back. If the patient is asking for a lab test, such as a throat culture, fill out the lab form for the patient to pick up when he or she comes in for the test, after verifying with the doctor that the requested test is appropriate.

Dealing with Problem Calls

You should always try to handle the difficult call on your own. But you should not put so much effort in that it upsets you; working with extremely difficult people is really the responsibility of the doctor and the office manager. Use empathy to help calm down an angry or very upset person.

The following are the three major types of difficult calls:

The Caller Who Refuses to Give Information

This is usually a salesperson who wants to speak to the doctor, but knows that if he or she gives a name, the doctor will refuse to talk. Explain politely that you need the caller's name and telephone number to leave a message. If the caller still refuses to give information, instruct the caller to write a letter to the doctor and to mark it personal.

Complaints

Listen carefully. Avoid getting angry yourself. Take specific information. Be professional, patient, and a good listener. Identify what you can do and tell the caller exactly what you plan to do. You may need to refer the matter to the office manager or the doctor, but try to get as much information as possible so that the person who ends up dealing with the problem can be prepared to handle it.

Avoid hanging up on an angry caller. Keep your voice at a normal speaking tone and suggest that the person call back when he or she is calmer. Inform the person what you plan to do and when the caller can expect to hear back from someone in the office.

Patients with Special Problems

If a patient calls who has a problem such as difficulty with English or confusion, listen carefully and try as hard as possible to understand. Always obtain the caller's name and telephone number. Speak at a normal volume (DON'T SHOUT), but try to speak more slowly. Use simple language. Ask if the caller understands what you are saying. If you believe the caller does not understand because of a language barrier, get a translator or say you will call back when you find someone who speaks the caller's language. If the person seems confused, ask if there is another person with whom you can speak. This may be a medical emergency.

OUTGOING CALLS

More calls come into the office than go out. But there are certainly enough outgoing calls. Medical assistants make many of them. Outgoing calls a medical assistant may make include calls to patients, suppliers, insurance companies, other medical offices, laboratories, pharmacies, and hospitals.

You should always avoid making calls about patients, whether the matter is medical or financial, from the front desk. Prepare any information you need before making the call.

You may need to call a patient about an overdue account. For this call, provide for privacy. Do not discuss billing information with anyone other than the person responsible for the bill.

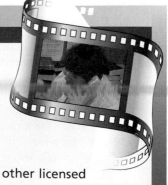

ON THE JOB

Videotape: Communication and Caring, "On the Telephone"

When Joanne, the medical assistant at Blackburn Primary Care Associates, answers the telephone, the caller begins the call by saying, "Please help me, I'm having chest pain. It might be a heart attack."

QUESTIONS:
1. What information should Joanne ask for immediately?
2. If there is a doctor in the office, what should Joanne do?
3. What resources can help Joanne respond to this caller if there is no doctor or other licensed professional in the office when she takes the call?
4. If Joanne determines that the patient's symptoms indicate a serious or life-threatening emergency, and she is the most experienced person in the office at the time, what four things should she do?

When ordering supplies, get your order information organized before placing the call.

If placing a call for one of the office's doctors, make sure the doctor is ready to talk before you place the call. The person who is making the call is expected to be on the phone when the call goes through.

See Procedure 7–6.

Personal Calls

Medical assistants and other office staff should not make or receive personal calls using the office telephone system except for emergencies, both to avoid tying up the telephone and because telephone calls take time away from work. Plan to make outgoing calls during breaks or at lunchtime using a pay phone or personal cellular phone. Although permission may be given to make an urgent call using the office telephone, a personal long-distance call is never appropriate.

Long-Distance Calls

Long-distance calls can usually be dialed directly. If you need to get a phone number for a long-distance call, information is available at (area code)-555-1212. In some parts of the country, you need to dial the number 1 before the area code. Be aware of different time zones, as shown in Figure 7–6.

Know the calling plan from your phone service provider, because the time when you call can make a difference in the rate you pay for long-distance calls. There should also be a telephone book handy. In addition to local telephone numbers, phone books contain area codes across the United States and Canada, as well as international codes.

To make an operator-assisted call (either person-to-person or collect) dial 0 then the area code and the telephone number. The operator will come on and assist you.

To make international calls, dial 1 then the country code then the telephone number.

PROCEDURE 7–6

Placing Outgoing Telephone Calls

Performance Objective: The student will place an outgoing telephone call using correct technique.
Supplies and Equipment: Telephone, scratch paper, pen or pencil, material necessary to place the call, such as a telephone book, order numbers, insurance information, patient record.

Procedure Steps

1. Organize all materials that may be needed during the telephone call. Schedule calls during business hours. Avoid calling doctor's offices between 12:00 PM and 1:30 PM because many close for lunch.
   Rationale: Preparation allows calls to be made more efficiently.
2. Write the telephone number on a piece of paper. Include the area code and a country code, if necessary.
   Rationale: It may be difficult to remember the number, especially if you do not reach the number on the first attempt.

3. Place the call. When it is answered ask for your party. If you do not know who to speak to, identify yourself with your practice name and your name (this is Joanne from Blackburn Primary Care Associates), and give a brief description of the reason for your call so that it can be routed to the proper person.
   Rationale: Identifying yourself allows the recipient of the call to route your call efficiently.
4. Conduct your business efficiently and professionally.
   Rationale: You represent your office and want to appear professional.
5. Repeat information for confirmation and thank the person for their assistance. End calls with "Good-bye."
   Rationale: You want to give a friendly closing.

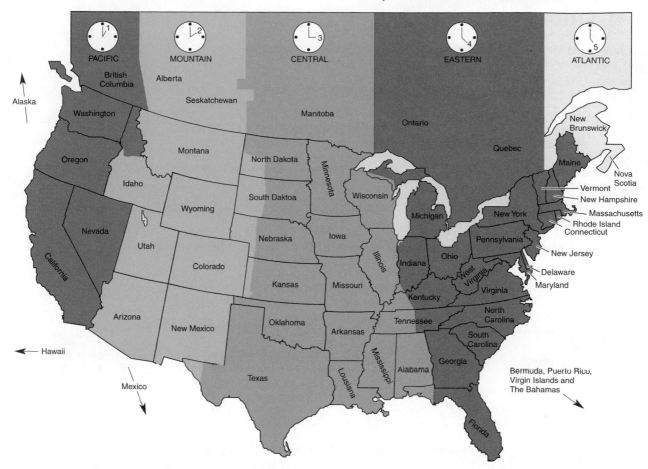

> **Figure 7–6** Time zones in the United States and Canada.

Conference Calls

Some phone systems allow you to make a conference call among three parties—your office, which is initiating the call, and two people who you are dialing at two different telephone numbers. If your system allows this, you should learn how to set up such calls for the doctors.

For conference calls where there will be many parties, most of the large long-distance carriers (such as MCI Worldcom, AT&T, and Sprint) will help you set up the call. In one method, all parties to the call will be asked to dial the same 1-800 number. You (the doctor in your office), as the host, will get a "host code." Other people on the call will get a "participant code."

At the appointed time for the call, the host and participants all dial the 1-800 number, enter their codes, and are connected to the call. If you are respon-

sible for putting such a call together, you need to work with your long-distance carrier to obtain the time, the 1-800 number to be dialed to, and all of the host and participant codes. Then you must call all of the participants (or their secretaries or medical assistants) and inform them of the time, the 1-800 number, and their particular participant code. A follow-up fax with the name information should be sent to each participant. You should write the instructions for each participant and for the doctor in your office in the following way:

Time:
Dial-in: ({1, if necessary}-800-XXX-XXXX)
Host or Participant Code: YYYYYYYYY

In the other method of conference calling, you provide the telephone numbers for all the parties to the conference call operator, who contacts each party and brings them into the call.

STUDENT STUDY PLAN

To reinforce your understanding of the material in this chapter . . .

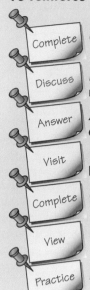

Complete the **Review & Recall** questions below.

Discuss the situation in **If You Were the Medical Assistant** with your class-mates, and answer the questions.

Answer the **Critical Thinking Questions** below and discuss them with your classmates.

Visit the **Web sites** suggested below, and search for additional Web sites using **Keywords for Internet Searches.**

Complete the exercises in chapter 7 of the *Student Mastery Manual.*

View the **videotape:** *Communication and Caring,* "On the Telephone."

Practice telephone activities in Case 1 and 4 on the **CD-ROM.**

REVIEW & RECALL

1. List three reasons why the telephone is of vital importance to the functioning of the medical office.

2. How are the following used in the medical office: multi-line telephone, facsimile (fax) machine, pager, voice mail?

3. List four types of telephone calls that the medical assistant can handle.

4. List five types of telephone calls where the medical assistant may need to take a message.

5. What information must be included in a telephone message?

6. Identify three types of problem calls.

7. Describe how to place an outgoing call.

IF YOU WERE THE MEDICAL ASSISTANT

Joanne: Blackburn Primary Care Associates. This is Joanne speaking.
Mary Carter: Hi, this is Mary Carter. I ran out of my blood pressure pills. I need some more.
Joanne: OK, Mrs. Carter. What are the pills?
Mary Carter: Hold on. I have to go get the bottle.

(While Mary is gone, another line rings. Joanne places Mary on hold to answer another call. When Mary returns to the telephone, she doesn't realize she has been put on hold, hangs up, and calls the office again.)

Joanne: Blackburn Primary Care Associates. This is Joanne speaking.
Mary Carter: This is Mary Carter. I found my pills.
Joanne: OK, Mrs. Carter. What are they?
Mary Carter: It's atenolol, 100 milligrams. I take one every day.
Joanne: What is the pharmacy?
Mary Carter: I get my prescription filled at the West Street Pharmacy, in Read-ville.
Joanne: West Street Pharmacy, Readville. What's the phone number there?
Mary Carter: Hold on. I need to get the bottle again.
Joanne: I need to put you on hold while you go get the bottle.
Mary Carter: OK.

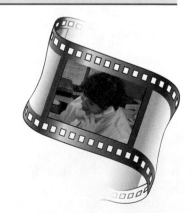

Answer the following questions about the scene above:

1. Identify at least three things Joanne did right.
2. Discuss the difference between the first and second time Joanne put Mrs. Carter on hold.

3. Write a suggestion for what Joanne could say to a patient asking for a prescription refill to help the patient provide the necessary information.

 ## CRITICAL THINKING QUESTIONS

Discuss what the medical assistant should say and/or do in each of the following situations.

1. The caller asks to speak to Kathy, another medical assistant. Kathy is taking a patient's blood pressure.
2. The caller asks for the results of a Pap test performed 2 weeks ago.
3. The caller identifies himself as Dr. Parks, and asks to speak to Dr. Lopez. Dr. Lopez is in an examination room with a patient.
4. The medical assistant returns from lunch. How can he or she find out if there were telephone calls during the absence?

5. A caller becomes very upset after being placed on hold. When the medical assistant returns to the call, the caller begins speaking loudly and calls the medical assistant a "jerk."
6. A caller asks for information about his wife's pelvic ultrasound, which was performed the previous day.
7. A caller asks the medical assistant to fax a copy of his medical record to another doctor.

 ## EXPLORE THE WEB

INTERNET WEBSITES

telephone directories
www.teldir.com

business listings
www.zip2.com

KEYWORDS FOR INTERNET SEARCHES

cellular telephone
     long-distance telephone
     telephone directories
     telephone systems
     yellow pages

 ## ANSWERS TO ON THE JOB

1. Joanne should immediately ask the caller's name, telephone number, and doctor's name.
2. If the caller's doctor is in the office, Joanne should refer the call to that doctor. If the caller's doctor is not in the office, but another doctor is present, Joanne should refer the call to that doctor. If possible, Joanne should ask the doctor to take the call on the main telephone without transferring the call or putting the caller on hold.

3. Joanne can use an office procedure manual to find specific questions to ask the patient about chest pain.
4. Joanne should instruct the caller to call an ambulance. She should have the caller repeat her instructions to be sure they are understood. She should page or call the patient's doctor. Finally, she should document the call in the patient's medical record.

Computers in the Medical Office

Instructional Objectives

After completing this chapter, you will be able to do the following:

1. Define and spell the vocabulary words for this chapter.

2. Describe the use of devices to provide input to the computer, including the keyboard, mouse, and modem.

3. Describe the function of the computer's central processing unit (CPU).

4. Distinguish between ROM (read-only memory) and RAM (random access memory).

5. Compare and contrast computer storage systems, including hard drive, floppy disks, CD-ROM, and backup storage systems.

6. Describe the uses of computer output devices, including the monitor.

7. List advantages and disadvantages of a computer network.

8. Describe two types of computer operating systems.

9. Differentiate between a computer operating system and application software.

10. Explain how practice management software, databases, and word processing software are used in the medical office.

11. Describe the necessary care and maintenance of a computer.

12. Explain how patient confidentiality is maintained when data is stored on a computer or computer network.

13. Describe federal legislation to protect patient confidentiality when data is transferred electronically.

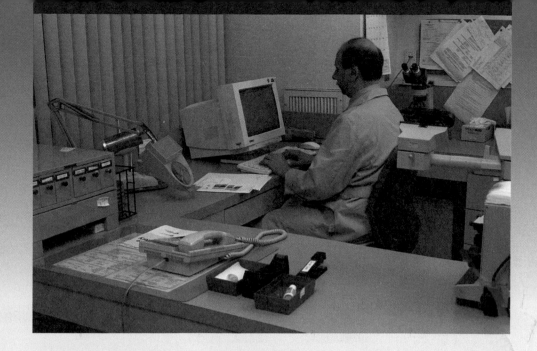

- Understand legal guidelines and requirements for health care
- Utilize computer software to maintain office systems
- Identify and respond to issues of confidentiality

VOCABULARY

application software (p. 136)
backup (p. 138)
boot (p. 140)
byte (p. 136)
central processing unit
   (CPU) (p. 136)
cursor (p. 136)
database (p. 140)
desktop (p. 140)

disk drive (p. 134)
e-mail (p. 141)
file (p. 140)
folder (p. 140)
gigabyte (p. 137)
hardware (p. 136)
icon (p. 140)
keyboard (p. 135)

log on (log in) (p. 143)
megabyte (p. 136)
memory (p. 136)
modem (p. 136)
monitor (p. 138)
motherboard (p. 136)
mouse (p. 136)
network (p. 136)

operating system (p. 139)
password (p. 143)
printer (p. 139)
random access memory (RAM) (p. 136)
read-only memory (ROM) (p. 136)
spreadsheet (p. 140)
template (p. 144)
word processing (p. 140)

ABBREVIATIONS

CPU (p. 136)
CD-ROM (p. 138)

DOS (p. 139)
GB (p. 137)

HIPAA (p. 143)
LAN (p. 136)

MB (p. 136)
RAM (p. 136)

ROM (p. 136)

WAN (p. 136)

After the telephone, the computer is probably the most frequently used and possibly the most important piece of equipment in the modern medical office. It is imperative that the medical assistant be familiar with the computer equipment used in the office and with all the different programs that he or she will be asked to use.

In this chapter, I'll give an overview of the physical parts of the medical office computer system as well as its uses, which range from sending out reminder notes, to billing and scheduling, to maintaining computerized medical records.

PARTS OF A COMPUTER SYSTEM

Computers come in all different sizes and shapes. As of early 1999, they also come in many colors, if you buy an Apple Computer Corporation iMac. Most medical office computers are still a dull beige or gray. Some have snazzy keyboards and some plain keyboards; some large screens and some smaller; some have the **disk drives** (where you put the floppy disk or CD-ROM) in a central processing unit that sits on the table; others in a "tower" that usually sits under the desk. Figure 8–1 shows a computer tower, with keyboard, monitor, and mouse.

The individual pieces of the computer system can be categorized according to their function, as illustrated in Figure 8–2. These functions are:

1. Input brings information into the computer. The major input components are the keyboard, mouse, and modem. The network is also considered an input component. Other input components that can be used are a scanner and microphone.

2. Processing is where the computer actually performs its calculations and data manipulation. Processing components are the central processing unit and the motherboard.

3. Storage is where data is stored for future use. Storage components are the hard drive, floppy disk drive, CD-ROM drive, and backup tape storage systems.

4. Output enables information to leave the computer to be used by a person. The major output components are the monitor and printer. Other output components are the modem and audio speakers.

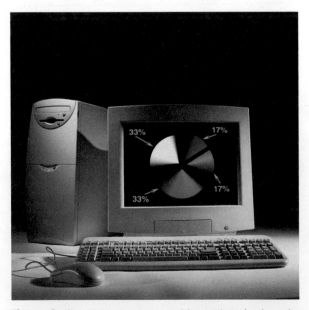

> **Figure 8–1** A computer tower with monitor, keyboard, and mouse are the basic components of a computer system.

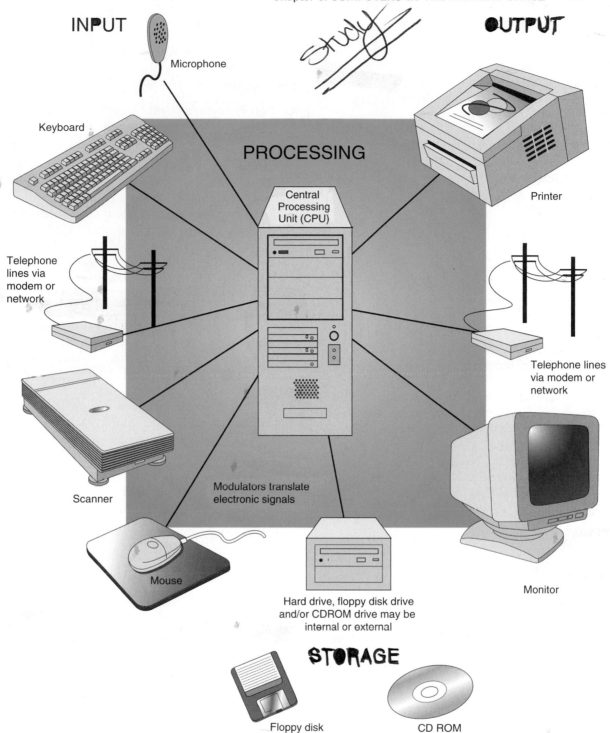

INPUT

Microphone

Keyboard

PROCESSING

OUTPUT

Printer

Central
Processing
Unit (CPU)

Telephone
lines via
modem or
network

Telephone lines
via modem or
network

Scanner

Modulators translate
electronic signals

Monitor

Mouse

Hard drive, floppy disk drive
and/or CDROM drive may be
internal or external

STORAGE

Floppy disk

CD ROM

➤ Figure 8–2 A computer system contains various devices for input, processing, storage, and output.

Input

Keyboard

➜ The letters on a computer **keyboard** are laid out in the same way as a typewriter, in the so-called QWERTY layout, named for the first six letters across the top row.

➜ In addition to alphanumeric characters, a computer keyboard also has a row of function keys across the top, above the letter rows. These functions are either preset in the computer's operating software or are set within particular application software. In either event, the function keys allow a computer operator to undertake tasks, such as moving text, with one keystroke that may take many commands if done another way.

Typewriter keyboards only allow left-to-right movement of the device that strikes the paper, a computer keyboard allows a user to manipulate the **cursor** (the flashing dot that appears where the next character will be written) up, down, left, or right.

Early desktop computer keyboards were essentially all alike. Beginning in the late 1980s, a number of computer keyboards have been designed to reduce the risk of repetitive stress injuries to users' hands and wrists. In addition, office furniture is increasingly being designed with keyboard shelves that have padded wrist guards to further reduce the risk of injury.

Mouse

A **mouse** is a device that allows a computer user to manipulate the cursor without using the up, down, left, or right cursor arrows. The mouse was developed by Apple Computer to manipulate its "graphic user interface" computer, the Macintosh. Today, most computers use a mouse, although the Windows operating system is used on most. The mouse allows a user to quickly move back and forth from inputting characters to accessing the function bar across the top of the screen, or to move from one file to another, from file to folder, and from one window to another. Files, folders, and windows will be discussed in more detail in the section on software below.

Modem

A **modem** (modulator-demodulator) is the device that translates the digital signals from a computer into an analog signal to transmit information over the telephone line, then retranslates the information into a digital signal to be accepted by the receiving computer. It can provide input to the computer and also is an output device from the computer to another computer.

A modem can either be a physical piece of equipment that is peripheral to the computer or simply a computer circuit inside the computer.

Network

A **network** is a group of computers that are connected. A network can be a local area network (**LAN**), in which case the computers are connected by hard wires running from machine to machine. LANs can be simple—many individual computers connected to a central printer and a central modem—or more complex "client-server" systems, in which a single computer holds all of the application software and serves it to the other computers, which act as clients, pulling the software from the server.

Another kind of network is a wide area network (**WAN**), which communicates over telephone lines across distances that cannot be hard wired. A company's intranet, which connects offices in many locations, is a type of WAN.

Processing

Central Processing Unit

The **central processing unit** (CPU) is the "guts" of the computer. This is where all the microcircuitry sits that allows a computer to do what it does. A CPU's power lies both in its speed and its **memory,** the amount of information it can store.

Speed is determined by the type of microprocessor, or chip, that powers the computer. A 300 megahertz (MHz) chip is faster than a 200 MHz chip, and so on. In 2001, Intel began shipping its fastest chip, the Pentium IV, to computer manufacturers.

Memory comes in two forms, **random access memory (RAM)** and **read-only memory (ROM)**. Memory is measured in terms of **megabytes**—millions of individual characters of information (called bytes)—that can be stored in the memory at any time. A computer with 64 megabytes **(MB)** of RAM can handle over 64 million **bytes** (characters) of information in its memory. Although many people believe that a megabyte is 1 million bytes, it is really 2^{20} (2 to the 20th power) bytes, or 1,048,576 bytes. That is why floppy disks always have a little more room than you think they will.

RAM is the type of memory that can store information while your computer is on (like what you have typed, where your margins are, how many spaces you want to tab over), but which is wiped clear as soon as your computer is turned off, even if it is only a momentary power loss. **ROM** controls the computer itself and does not allow you to discard information and write over it with new information.

The amount of memory in the computer is important, because increasingly sophisticated **application software** requires more memory to run properly. Application software are the programs that allow you to perform specific tasks, such as database management, desktop publishing, and insurance processing. When a program is being used, the application software is loaded from the storage into the computer's RAM for use.

Motherboard

The **motherboard** is the printed circuit board inside the CPU on which all of the computer's microcircuitry sits. It contains the physical components or **hardware** that make the computer work. It is akin to the computer's central nervous system. The individual chips or cards that sit on the motherboard are made of a bottom layer of silicon with layers of other materials above. Electrical circuits the width of human hairs are etched onto the material; the electrical impulses that

Hard Drive Storage Capacity

Hard drive storage was first measured in megabytes. In the early 1990s, most desktop computers had hard drive capacity of 40, 80, or possibly 120 megabytes. By the mid-1990s, computers came with 350, 500, or even 800 megabytes of hard drive capacity.

By 2000, even the least expensive desktop computers for home use (under $1,000) all came with at least 2 **gigabytes (GB)** (each gigabyte is 1,000 megabytes) of hard drive capacity. Just for an idea of how much storage capacity that is, an entire 26-volume encyclopedia, including color photographs, which take up huge amounts of memory, takes up less than one gigabyte.

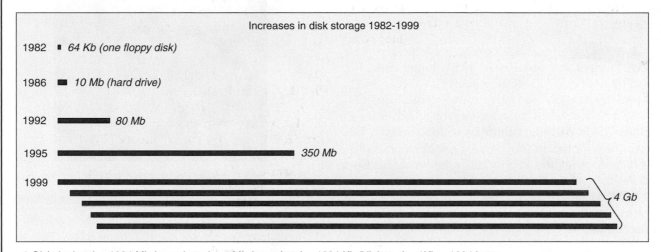

Increases in disk storage 1982-1999

1982	64 Kb (one floppy disk)
1986	10 Mb (hard drive)
1992	80 Mb
1995	350 Mb
1999	4 Gb

1 Gb(gigabyte) = 1024 Mb (megabytes)   1 Mb (megabyte) = 1024 Kb (kilobytes)   1Kb = 1024 bytes

carry messages to and from the computer travel through these circuits.

Storage

Among the computer's greatest virtues is its ability to store voluminous information, and the fact that its filing system is simple and intuitive. In most instances, the filing system is dictated by the application software used, so an office does not fall into the problem of having the person who set up a quirky filing system retire or otherwise leave, throwing the entire operation into disarray.

Hard Drive

The hard drive is the computer's main internal storage device. Hard drives were first developed in the mid-1980s. Before that, desktop computer users needed to insert a program, located on a floppy disk, into one floppy drive and store information on a second floppy drive.

Today, application programs are stored on the hard drive, and users can move from one application to another simply by clicking the mouse to open or close a window.

Floppy Disks

Floppy disks are no longer actually floppy. They used to be, in the early 1980s. They also used to be 5½″ across and hold about 250 kilobytes of memory (a kilobyte is 1,000 bytes; there are 1,000 kilobytes to a megabyte).

Today's floppy disks, like the one shown in Figure 8–3, are 3¼″ across, covered in rigid plastic, and store about 1.2 megabytes of information.

Some application software still comes on floppy disks and can be installed onto a computer's hard drive. However, most software currently comes on CD-ROMs or is downloaded directly from the Internet.

Floppy disks are used as backup storage for "small" amounts of information and to transfer information from one computer to another. For instance, if a doctor is using the office computer to write a report or an academic paper and wants to do some work on vacation, he or she can take the document off the office computer and put it on a floppy disk. Then he or she can insert the floppy disk into a laptop computer and work on the document, put it back on the floppy disk, insert it into the office computer on return, and print it out.

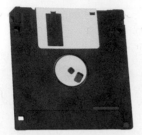

➤ Figure 8–3 3.25 inch floppy disk.

CD-ROM

CD-ROMs (compact disk, read-only memory) are storage devices that store more than floppy disks but are still portable. A CD-ROM is shown in Figure 8–4.

Most application software today comes on CD-ROMs, and is installed onto a computer's hard drive to operate. CD-ROMs hold hundreds of thousands of megabytes of information (but not a gigabyte). Sometimes, only a portion of the application program is installed into the computer's hard drive; the rest remains on the CD-ROM so as not to fill up the hard drive storage capacity. In this case, the CD must be in the CD drive to successfully run the program.

When the information on the CD-ROM is put into the computer's memory, it cannot be "written to" (hence the term read-only memory). This keeps the CD from accidentally being altered.

CD-ROMs can store enough information to enable programmers to write interactive programs, where the user can interact with the program. The CD-ROM that comes with this book is interactive; you are asked to respond to various prompts and answer certain ques-

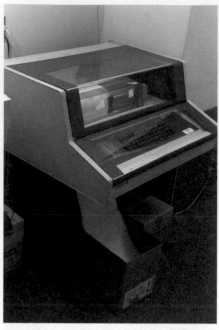

➤ Figure 8–5 Dot-matrix printer that feeds forms continuously from the box below the printer.

tions. In this program, your answers are stored either on a floppy disk or in the computer's hard drive.

Drives that allow a user to write to a CD-ROM disk have become more affordable. However, once created, the disk cannot be altered.

Backup Storage (Magnetic Tape and Zip Disks)

Another of the computer's great virtues is that information is stored in such a small space that it is practical to make **backup** (duplicate) copies of every piece of transactional and medical record information. This was impossible when records were all paper based.

Records are permanently stored on the computer's hard drive. But each computer's data should be backed up daily. This can be done easily, with a click of the mouse. Backup copies are stored on diskettes, magnetic tape, or a zip disk; tape and zip disks can store more than a gigabyte of information. The backup storage medium should be kept somewhere other than near the computers, preferably in a fireproof safe in the office or at another site.

Output

Monitor

The **monitor** is the screen on which information is displayed. Every time you press a key on the keyboard, electrical signals pass through the computer's circuitry, and the symbol on that key appears on the monitor. The important things to look for in a monitor are good

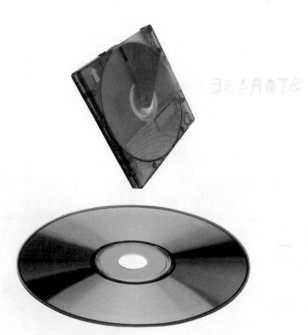

➤ Figure 8–4 CD-ROM.

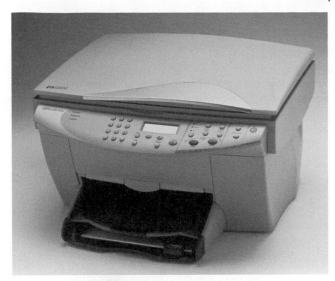

> **Figure 8–6** Laser printer.

resolution (sharp characters) and screen size. For people who will spend many hours a day at the computer keyboard, a good monitor is important, as it helps reduce eyestrain.

Printer

A **printer** allows you to make paper copies of the information stored in the computer. Increasingly, printers double as fax machines and photocopiers.

A printer can be dedicated to one computer or can be networked to a number of computers.

Printers come in many varieties: laser, which provides the sharpest clarity; ink jet, which are the most commonly used printers in homes; and dot-matrix, which are easiest to attach a continuous paper-feed carrier to.

Figure 8–5 shows a dot-matrix printer, the kind still in use in many medical offices. Figure 8–6 shows a laser printer.

SOFTWARE

Software is the instructions that make a computer do what it does. There are two types of software, the operating system and application software.

The Operating System

Almost all of today's medical office computers run on a Windows **operating system,** the program that controls the computer's basic functions and provides the interface for the user. However, a few offices might still be using computers that use the DOS operating system (**DOS** actually stands for disk operating system.)

DOS was designed before the advent of hard disk drives, when an application program was inserted into one floppy drive. DOS commands allow the user to move from the application program to the storage medium by designating which drive is in use at any particular time. The user calls the program from drive A into RAM, then begins operations, making sure to store data on drive B. Manipulating DOS takes much getting used to. Figure 8–7 shows an MS-DOS prompt.

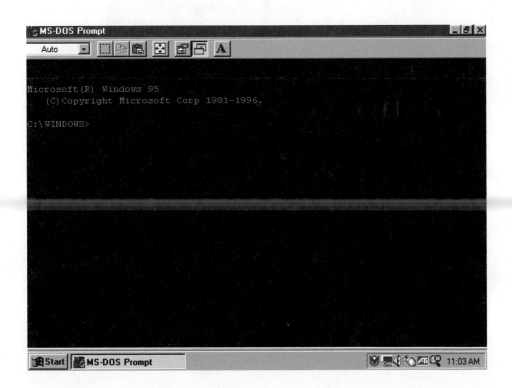

> **Figure 8–7** DOS screen, which requires the computer operator to use DOS commands.

The Windows operating system was designed in the early 1990s to mimic Apple's operating system designed for Macintosh computers. Windows and Mac OS are both operating systems based on the concept of the graphical user interface (GUI, pronounced gooey).

The theory behind this type of operating system is that it operates the way people think—it is intuitive. When you **boot**, or turn on, a computer that uses Windows or a Macintosh, you are presented with a **desktop**, the computer analogy of all the items you need to create and then store records. Arranged on the desktop screen are several **icons** (small graphics that link to files, folders, or applications), including a small computer (My Computer) and icons for the programs you use most often. At the bottom left is the start button. When you click on the start button once, a list of options rises from it. Many have small arrows pointing to the right; if you highlight one of these items, submenus appear. By clicking again, you can open the application you want to use.

An individual item, such as a patient record, a daily appointment list, or a medical record, is called a **file**. A file is a set of computer data that has been saved to disk—either the hard drive, a diskette, a CD-ROM, a zip drive, or a magnetic tape. Files are collected in **folders**, indicated by an icon of a file folder. Folders can be displayed individually either within a window or on the desktop.

If you open a folder, the folder opens as a window, and all the files that reside in the folder are in the window. If you want to move a file from one folder to another, you can remove it and place it in the correct folder, just as you would at your desk with papers, folders, and files. Figure 8–8 shows a Windows operating system screen, with My Computer open and application software folders on the hard drive (C drive).

Within the operating system are ever-more complex interactions between computer and human, between computer and peripheral equipment, and between computer and computer, utilizing modems, telephones, and mainframe computers that act as storage sites for information that can be transmitted using the Internet.

Application Software

Modern operating systems allow people to work with computers in a way that closely mimics the way they work with physical paper and records. It is truly brilliant.

This is carried down into the programs that allow the computer to perform specific manipulations, such as **word processing** (the computer version of typing), **spreadsheets** (data arranged in a matrix), and **databases** (sets of records of information).

Medical billing programs evolved from the pegboard accounting system, where the charges for each patient

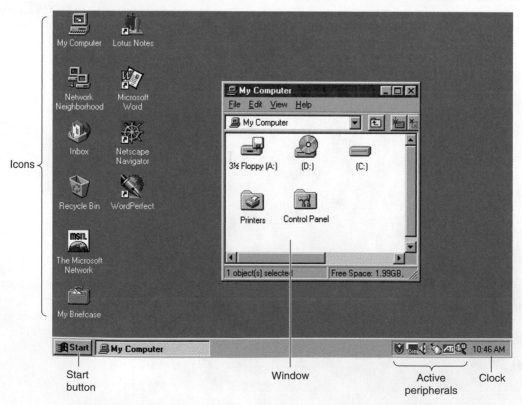

➢ **Figure 8–8** Windows desktop with open window for My Computer icon.

are entered at the time of the visit both in a patient account or ledger and the record of the day's financial transactions. Screen displays of appointment scheduling programs evolved from the traditional appointment book. In reality, the medical billing programs and appointment scheduling programs combine aspects of database programs (groups of records such as patient information records, lists of providers, lists of insurance companies, and diagnostic codes) with aspects of spreadsheets (charts with vertical and horizontal displays, such as appointment schedules). They perform computations like spreadsheets and update information in various records like databases.

The medical billing program can reference all of the stored information so you only have to enter it once. For example, once you have entered a patient's charges, you can print an insurance claim form or a receipt without entering additional information. When you enter a patient's name into an appointment time, the program finds the patient's telephone number and adds it to the appointment information automatically.

Application software is loaded onto the computer's hard drive and called upon when needed. When a particular application needs to be used, it is moved from storage on the hard drive into the computer's RAM for easy access.

This gets back to the earlier discussion about the importance of enough computer memory. (There is a saying that you can never be too wealthy, too good looking, or have too much computer memory.)

One of the main virtues of a Windows or Mac operating system—besides the intuitive ease of the display—is that many programs can reside in memory and be running simultaneously, even though the individual using the computer is only using one program at a time.

For instance, you can be writing a scientific paper using a word processing program such as Microsoft Word. To draw the graphs, you use a graphics program such as Microsoft Paint. These two different programs must both be moved out of hard drive storage and into memory to insert the graphic into the text.

Then, just to make it complicated, you are going to attach this document and graphic and send it to a scientific journal via **e-mail** (electronic mail), rather than sending it by paper mail (called snail mail by those who do everything via computer). This means that your e-mail software and your modem communications software both have to be in memory.

At some point, if you simply continue to open application windows without ever closing other application windows (in effect not putting the software away into hard drive storage) you may get a message that says: "Not enough available memory to run the application." It is important to keep your computer system updated, with enough memory to avoid this problem.

COMPUTER APPLICATIONS IN THE MEDICAL OFFICE

It is possible to computerize the entire set of medical office record-keeping. This information falls into six main categories:

1. **Databases.** These include sets of information about patients, insurance carriers, referrals, and procedure and diagnostic codes.
2. **Charges and payments for patient visits.** These records are a kind of database, but they also include instructions to do the math like a spreadsheet. Once the data has been entered from the day's charge sheets, you can see current information about individual patient accounts, day sheets for each primary care provider whose time is billable, day sheets for different insurance companies, and other financial data.
3. **Appointments.** These include patient appointments, lunch, breaks, meetings, and other regularly scheduled events.
4. **Other financial records.** These include payroll and bills paid by the office. These may be handled in special programs or a general spreadsheet program such as Microsoft Excel.
5. **Patient records.** If the patient record is kept on a computer, a separate program is usually used. It may use special software to interpret dictated materials, a handheld notepad, or other types of input. Medical data is usually kept separate from financial data to protect patient confidentiality.
6. **Word processing.** This type of program is used for correspondence, memos, and transcription of notes on patient visits.

Practice Management Software

Appointments

The next chapter discusses scheduling appointments in detail. For this discussion, we should simply say that computerized scheduling accomplishes three important goals.

First, it is easier to make a change on a computer than with pencil and paper. Using a computer, the name can simply be deleted and the space in the schedule template left open. Second, at the beginning of the day, the day's schedule can be printed out and does not have to be copied from pencil to pen (pencil for the advance schedule, to accommodate changes, ink—or typewritten—for the permanent record that must be maintained as a legal document). Third, if a patient needs to make regular weekly or monthly visits, a time of day and day of week can be chosen and the computer will automatically put the patient's name in that time slot for as many visits as are scheduled.

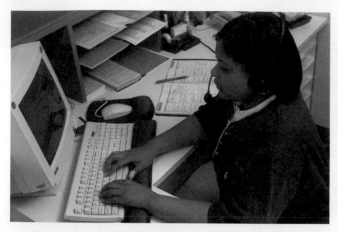

> **Figure 8–9** The medical assistant uses the computer to enter patient information.

Billing Information

Computerization of billing and insurance information saves literally hours of manual work each week for medical assistants and office managers. To set up the process of billing, the medical assistant keys into the computer information from the charge slip (encounter form) the doctor has filled in during the patient visit. The charge slip lists all of the things that were done during the visit. The computer has codes for all procedures in a database (discussed later) and knows how much should be charged for each procedure. The computer can thus create a bill. Figure 8–9 shows a medical assistant using a computer to enter patient information.

For instance, the visit might be an "extended visit," for a current patient, as opposed to a brief extended visit, a full physical, or a new-patient visit. Different charges are set for different length visits. During the visit, the doctor might have performed a rectal exam and a test for occult blood in the patient's stool; a fee is charged for each test. The medical assistant might have performed an electrocardiogram; a fee is charged for this.

Depending on the patient's type of insurance coverage, the patient may have a co-payment to make for the visit. The computer prints the bill, credits the co-payment, and lists the rest of the charges as pending reimbursement from the insurance carrier. From the same information, the computer is also able to generate an insurance claim form, which can be submitted to the insurance company.

Many insurance companies are moving to electronic filing of claims, especially with larger medical practices, clinics, and community health centers. In electronic filing, the insurance claim is sent using a computer protocol called electronic data interchange. Issues of data security in electronic transactions, and its effect on patient confidentiality (see Focus on Legal Issues: Security for Computer Systems), have been the biggest barrier to more rapid implementation of electronic claim submission.

With electronic claim filing comes electronic payment; that means that insurance companies transfer payment to the medical practice's bank account rather than issue paper checks.

Computerized Medical Records

A computerized medical record contains the same information as resides in a paper file. For most doctors, the expense of transferring old medical records to computer is probably too much to justify complete transfer. However, for new practices and for records going forward, computerization has significant advantages, including saving space, decreasing the cost of storage, and allowing easy access to records, often using terminals or laptop computers in each exam room.

With paper records, most doctors keep current patient files in the office, and after a patient has been inactive for a time (usually 3 to 5 years) they transfer the record to permanent storage, either at home or, more commonly, especially for large practices, in a commercial record-storage facility.

When records are computerized, medical offices can save the cost of the entire area currently rented for record-storage space in the office, as well as the cost of permanent commercial storage for old files. More importantly perhaps, they can transfer patient information among the entire network of health care providers who are caring for an individual.

Think of a patient with multiple medical problems, such as heart disease, diabetes, and progressive kidney failure. That person may see five or more different medical practitioners, such as an internist (or general practitioner), a cardiologist, a nephrologist (kidney specialist), a podiatrist to treat foot problems secondary to the diabetes, and a nutritionist. The patient may have an appointment every week with one or another practitioner.

All of the specialists must communicate with the internist who is the patient's primary care provider. This means either a copy of the provider's notes for each visit or a summary note in the form of a letter needs to be sent to the internist. Medical assistant time to coordinate the paper flow, paper, printer cartridges or ribbons, and postage—all to manage the paper flow of medical records for this one patient—is very costly each year. If each medical provider's notes, as well as test results, go into a patient medical record, then are e-mailed to the primary provider for insertion into the patient's primary electronic file, it can be an incredible saving of time and money. This kind of system is most efficient when all providers are part of the same network and share the same computer system.

Such a universal electronic record would also have enormous clinical benefit as well. If the patient had to

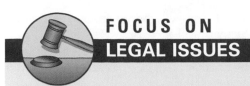

FOCUS ON
LEGAL ISSUES

COMPUTER AND NETWORK SECURITY

As more patient information is stored on computers, shared on computer networks that can often be accessed from a doctor's home, and sent electronically to third-party payers, security and privacy has become a national priority. Several legal and regulatory measures can have an impact on health care organizations and the way they maintain security of electronically recorded and stored patient information.

These include federal regulations, as well as guidelines from professional organizations and accrediting agencies such as the Joint Commission on Accreditation of Healthcare Organizations. The most comprehensive regulation is provided by the Health Insurance Portability and Accountability Act of 1996 (HIPAA). Among HIPAA's many parts is one intended to protect patient privacy by requiring creation of uniform standards for electronic transmission of health information. Standards will address a number of issues.

The process of developing and adopting standards has progressed more slowly than expected. Standards have been developed in several areas. Once they are formally adopted, organizations have 24 months to demonstrate compliance. Five standards have been adopted:

1. Electronic transmission of financial (claims processing) information

2. Use of standard code sets

3. Use of national provider identifiers (NPIs)

4. Use of employer identification numbers (EINs)

5. Confidentiality and security protection measures to establish and enforce security within an organization, measures to maintain security of the physical parts of a computer system where data is stored, measures to control access to data, and measures to protect information and restrict access to electronically transmitted data.

Health providers must become aware of these standards and be sure that their facilities conform to them.

In addition, within a medical office, each individual who uses the computer should have a unique **password,** which should be changed on a regular basis. The password is a set of alpha numeric characters that allow the user to **log on** (enter) the system or specific parts of the computer system. Individuals should not share their passwords with others.

Each individual should have access to only the types of information and applications that fall within his or her scope of work and responsibility. System security should be designed in such a way that each security level permits access to only the applications and databases each individual needs to perform his or her tasks. Each specific application should know which individuals are authorized to use it.

If a practice uses a service bureau to prepare documents, at the end of the contractual period, all documents, in paper or electronic media, should be returned to the practice.

---

be hospitalized, the doctors at the hospital would have access to the patient's entire record of treatment rather than just the information gathered from the hospital intake process.

We are not far from this being a reality. Larger practices, hospitals, and public clinics will have fully computerized medical record systems soon (some already do), and smaller practices will become fully computerized in the near future as equipment costs continue to drop and as new doctors and other medical professionals begin practice fully computer literate and

want to be completely linked with their network of peers and referral providers.

Word Processing

Word processing refers to writing with a computer. This book was written with word processing software.

But word processing is more than just typing. Word processing software allows the user to manipulate text in nearly innumerable ways.

You can move words, sentences, or entire paragraphs, what used to be called "cutting and pasting" when it was done with scissors and glue. You can **bold face**, *italicize* and underline simply by clicking on icons on the function bar.

You can save sample documents as a **template**, which provides the proper formatting and maybe some general language that is always used. Information can be added to personalize letters, reports, and other documents. Documents can be shared by more than one person. You can add graphics and charts.

Correspondence and Memos

Word processing makes routine correspondence truly routine, because you can store as a set of files all of the basic letters the office will need. When you need to send a particular letter, you simply call up the file, put the appropriate greeting on the top, add any particular information that is necessary, put the appropriate closing on, and print the letter out.

The same can be true of routine memos that must go into the file or that are issued to office personnel.

Transcription

Computerized transcription is another rapidly advancing area. Doctors record the substance of their patient encounters in what are called "notes." In some offices, doctors hand-write their notes on lined chart-note paper. Many doctors have, for some time, dictated their notes for later word processing.

A few doctors on the cutting edge of computer technology are beginning to use voice recognition software to skip the transcription phase altogether. Voice recognition software, or "speak and write" software, allows you to speak into a microphone connected directly to the computer. Using "artificial intelligence" programming, the computer then types out the dictation in close to real time. The speaker can read the dictation over and, using the keyboard, change any words the computer might have misunderstood.

The effect voice-activated/voice recognition transcription will have on medical transcriptionists and medical assistants is unknown. Pessimists believe computer transcription will be one more example of machines taking over jobs formerly done by people—the doctor will read over the computer-written transcript and sign off on it. Optimists see computer transcription as an opportunity for transcriptionists and medical assistants to become true "knowledge workers."

Doctors will still dictate in a sort of medical shorthand, which will have to be translated. Because the transcript itself will be generated by the computer, this translation from "doctor speak" to English will take place in the post-transcript editing process rather than in the process of listening to the tape and typing the transcript. In the optimistic view, transcription will become a more high value-added medical editing job, the drudge work of typing will be taken out, and transcription productivity will increase.

Databases

A database is a collection of individual pieces of data that can be manipulated using particular application software, called database management software.

The record of information about each patient is part of a database. The record of information about each specialist to whom the doctor refers patients is part of a database. The office holiday card list is a database. Information may be entered into an existing record or a new record can be created in an existing database. A new database can also be created, depending on the information needs.

Using Application Software in Tandem

If you know how, you can use your database software, word processing software, and patient record software to keep a strong communication link with your patients. This is good for health promotion and for marketing as well.

The simplest form of this is sending out reminder cards when it is time for people to schedule a physical. You can code your patient record and database software to "flag" names when they should come in, even taking into account the different time frames that certain insurance companies use for how frequently they will cover well care visits. In some large clinics, appointments for routine tests are simply scheduled for you at the appropriate time.

Or it can be a little more sophisticated. For instance, the doctor you work for is a pediatrician. You maintain a database of patient families, with the ages and school years of all children. It's September. The doctor wants to send letters to all of his patients who have just started kindergarten, congratulating them on starting school and reminding them of some safety tips, such as wearing a bicycle helmet, looking both ways before crossing the street, and so on.

If you have been keeping your database up to date, you have recorded each child who has been to the office in the prior 6 or 8 months for the mandatory kindergarten registration physical and have marked in the family record that the child was starting school in the fall.

Database management software will allow you to pull out a subset of your database, the families with children who had kindergarten physicals in the past year.

Word processing software will allow you to write a letter. The "mail merge" function in your word processing software will allow you to individually address each letter with the child's proper name. "Dear Jimmy" is certainly nicer than "Dear Patient."

CARE AND MAINTENANCE OF THE COMPUTER

Computers are sophisticated equipment. A medical office computer system, with input and output devices and sufficient terminals for the staff, can cost many thousands of dollars. Remember, this is a business system; it is not ever to be used for personal use, playing games, or surfing the Internet for fun.

Although large computers were developed as early as the 1950s, the first desktop computers (or personal computers—PCs) began to appear in the late 1970s and were hobbyist toys. Many early users built their own or altered early commercial versions. They added memory and microchips that allowed the computer to produce graphics or sound.

Just as most people are incapable of fixing cars, most people are incapable of fixing computers. But everyone can learn maintenance techniques that can keep their computers running better longer.

Care of Equipment

There are four important things to remember about keeping the computer running properly.

First, the computer should be protected from electrical surges. This is done simply by purchasing a surge protector, which plugs into a regular wall socket. The protector is a strip of outlet plugs into which all of the computer equipment can be plugged. Inside the protector is a circuit breaker. In the event of an electrical surge, the protector shuts off, just like a circuit breaker in the office's power electrical circuit box.

Second, the computer should be kept as free of dust as possible. The keyboard, CPU, monitor, and any other input or output devices should be dusted regularly. Most components have vents to cool them; unfortunately, dust collects in these vents. The computer should be covered with a plastic dust cover at night to prevent the buildup of dust in the vents.

Third, don't eat or drink while using the computer. Liquid spilled on the keyboard can cause a short circuit. And fingers sticky with food leave residue that is difficult to remove.

Finally, clean the monitor regularly with solution such as eyeglass cleaner or mild soap and water. Use a soft cloth to clean the monitor.

Service Agreements

One of the medical assistant's responsibilities in most offices is maintaining the service agreements for the office's computer systems. These agreements include maintenance agreements for the hardware, as well as what is known as system support agreements for the software and training of personnel on the software.

You should keep all of the manuals that come with the computer and printer, as well as those that come with application software. One person in the office should be designated to be responsible for all the computers. This person is responsible for being the liaison with any companies providing service to the hardware, or maintenance, upgrade, and consulting for the software.

System Maintenance

Someone needs to be responsible for setting up and overseeing the system. There are three aspects of system maintenance:

1. Disk cleanup
2. Disk defragmentation
3. System administration

Disk Cleanup

The "ScanDisk" program can be run to find and fix errors. In addition, the person responsible for system maintenance should remove old files that may slow down system performance, especially if the Internet is being used frequently. Outgoing e-mail messages and incoming messages that have been read and deleted actually continue to reside in the system after being removed from what is seen on the screen. They must be eliminated from the system by the system maintenance manager.

Disk Defragmentation

Defragmentation rearranges information on the hard disk so files and programs are stored together. On today's hard disks, which often measure their storage capacity in gigabytes (thousands of megabytes), this can take a long time. It is usually performed at night or on a weekend.

System Administration

The system administrator is the person designated to maintain the computer system, especially a large network system. He or she is responsible for overall system/network function. The system administrator is usually a computer specialist. Small offices often use a consultant, sometimes from the company that provided the practice management software. Practices with several sites, health maintenance organizations, and community health centers often have a specialist, or even a department, that handles both administration of the current system and planning for future computer needs.

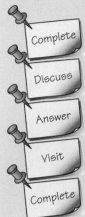

STUDENT STUDY PLAN

To reinforce your understanding of the material in this chapter . . .

Complete — *Complete* the **Review & Recall** questions below.

Discuss — *Discuss* the situation in **If You Were the Medical Assistant** with your classmates, and answer the questions.

Answer — *Answer* the **Critical Thinking Questions** below, and discuss them with your classmates.

Visit — *Visit* the **Web sites** suggested below and search for additional Web sites using the **Keywords for Internet Searches.**

Complete — *Complete* the exercises in chapter 8 of the **Student Mastery Manual.**

 REVIEW & RECALL

1. Compare the use of the keyboard and mouse as input devices for a computer.

2. What does *modem* stand for? How is a modem used?

3. In what part of the computer is the actual "computing" done?

4. What does the term *computer memory* refer to?

5. What type of memory is used to store programs for use when the computer is being used for word processing?

6. What are two differences between a floppy disk and a CD-ROM?

7. Describe two types of printers, and give advantages and disadvantages of each.

8. Describe a computer network.

9. What is the function of a computer's operating system?

10. Identify several functions of practice management software.

11. What type of software program would a medical assistant use to write a letter? To store procedure codes? To write a report? To make patient appointments?

12. How are passwords used to provide security for a computer?

 IF YOU WERE THE MEDICAL ASSISTANT

Discuss each of the following situations and describe how the medical assistant should proceed to solve his or her problem.

Situation 1

Kathy, a medical assistant at Blackburn Primary Care Associates, has been entering data into the computer for at least 2 to 4 hours each day for several days when she notices that her right elbow and shoulder are tense and uncomfortable by the time she leaves work.

1. What should she consider related to her work at the computer? (You may need to review the section on good body position in chapter 6.)

2. Find out what devices are available to reduce strain while using a computer keyboard.

Situation 2

One afternoon when Paul, a medical assistant, is reviewing patient lab results at a computer terminal in an area where patients pass by on their way to the exam room, he is called away to answer the telephone, which is at the medical assisting desk about 10 yards away.

1. What should he do before taking the telephone call?
2. Identify several possible consequences if Paul goes to take the phone call and leaves patient data in place on the computer.

CRITICAL THINKING QUESTIONS

1. If you were working for a medical office that wanted to implement a computer billing system or change to different billing software, how would you plan the process to decide which software to buy?

2. Do research via the Internet to identify at least three practice management software programs, and identify features they incorporate.

3. List tasks necessary for computer care and maintenance, and decide how often you think they should be performed. Discuss with your classmates how an office manager should decide who should be responsible for these tasks.

4. If you have access to a computer, make a list of all methods of obtaining help that are located on the computer itself. Locate methods for obtaining help that can be accessed from the computer via the Internet. Use the Internet to locate at least two Web sites that you could use as resources.

5. Locate a computer either in your home, in the computer lab at school, or in another location, and evaluate if the chair provides proper support, if the keyboard allows the forearms to be level or sloping slightly downward, if the wrists are supported when using both the keyboard and mouse, and if the monitor can be viewed without eyestrain. What suggestions would you make for improvement?

6. Discuss the issue of confidentiality of patient information stored on computer with your classmates, and make a list of potential problems.

EXPLORE THE WEB

INTERNET WEB SITES

American Health Information Management Association (AHIMA)
www.ahima.org

Computer Security Institute
www.gocsi.com

Department of Health and Human Services HIPAA Web Site
aspe.hhs.gov/admnsimp/index.htm

HIPAA Implementation Guides
hipaa.wpc-edi.com/HIPAA_40.asp

Microsoft Windows
www.microsoft.com/windows

Microsoft Office
www.microsoft.com/office

KEYWORDS FOR INTERNET SEARCHES

computer or printer manufacturer's name
computerized medical record
Health Insurance Portability and Accountability Act (HIPAA)
medical billing software
medical record software
medical software
practice management software

Chapter 9

Scheduling Appointments

Learning Objectives

After completing this chapter, you will be able to do the following:

1. Define and spell the vocabulary words for this chapter.
2. Describe the importance of an efficient way to schedule appointments.
3. Identify several types of scheduling, including clustering, wave, modified wave, fixed appointment, double booking, and open hours.
4. Describe the correct use of appointment books and computer scheduling programs to make appointments.
5. Describe the legal implications of maintaining and updating the daily schedule.
6. List the steps in setting up the appointment matrix.
7. Identify information needed to make appointments for new patients and established patients.
8. Differentiate between medical conditions that require emergency care, urgent care, and routine care.
9. Describe the method for changing or canceling appointments.
10. Identify three methods to remind patients to make or keep appointments.

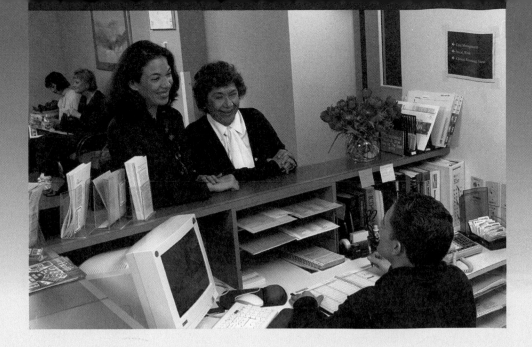

- Schedule and manage appointments
- Perform within legal and ethical boundaries

- Perform telephone and in-person screening

Performance Objectives

1. Set up an appointment matrix, incorporating office guidelines (Procedure 9–1).
2. Make an appointment for a patient (Procedure 9–2).

VOCABULARY

blocked (p. 153)
clustering (p. 152)
double booking (p. 152)

fixed scheduling (p. 152)
matrix (p. 153)
modified wave (p. 152)

no-show (p. 151)
suture (p. 158)

triage (p. 158)
wave (p. 152)

Scheduling appointments is one of the most important administrative activities a medical assistant carries out. Up until the 1960s, people went to a doctor's office expecting to wait, often for an hour or two. Most doctors liked to see a full waiting room; it reassured them that their practice was healthy.

But going into the new century, people have little tolerance for waiting in a doctor's office. They have busy lives. Many have to take personal time away from work to go to the doctor, and they feel that their time is as valuable as the doctor's.

The person responsible for scheduling appointments plays a very important role in making the office run smoothly. The patient who has made an appointment weeks or months ahead of time wants to be seen within 15 to 20 minutes of arriving at the office. The doctor wants a smooth flow of patients during the time set to see patients. Patients who are ill or have accidents want to be able to see their own doctor on the day of the illness or injury. They prefer to be given a specific time, even if it is later in the day, rather than come into the office and wait for an open moment.

Satisfaction or dissatisfaction with the person who makes the appointment and the amount of time a person has to wait to see the doctor are major factors in whether an individual remains a patient of the practice or finds another doctor. This means that the medical assistant's demeanor while making the appointment is extremely important. There are six things to remember when making an appointment, either by telephone or in person at the end of a current visit:

1. Speak clearly, and know what information to ask for.
2. Avoid the appearance of being rushed.
3. Repeat information given to you to avoid errors.
4. Concentrate on the person to whom you are speaking, and speak in a friendly, courteous, and interested way.
5. Obtain and record complete and correct information.
6. Schedule the correct amount of time for the type of appointment you are making.

METHODS OF SCHEDULING

Appointments are scheduled either manually, using appointment books, or by computer, using scheduling software. Some offices use both.

Appointment Books

An appointment book is usually spiral-bound, so it will lie flat. Each doctor usually has his or her own book. Choose a book that suits the practice. It may have pages for a single day, pages that show a week when open (over two pages), or pages with two or three doctors' schedules for a single day. The page may be set up in 10- or 15-minute intervals.

Appointment books are usually kept in pencil so they can be changed if necessary, as shown in Figure 9–1. In preparing for a day's visits, a list of patients is created in pen or on a word processor. This list is kept as the permanent record.

Computer Programs

A computerized appointment schedule, like the one shown in Figure 9–2, shows the same information as is in an appointment book. Usually, each doctor has a screen for each day, which is printed out to provide the daily appointment sheet.

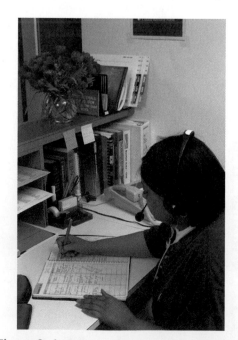

➤ **Figure 9–1** Medical assistant making appointment.

Schedule for 10/13/XX   For Dr. Howard Lawler

Time	Patient	Phone	Comments
8:00a	HOSPITAL ROUNDS		
8:20a	↓		
8:40a	↓		
9:00a	Wayne Harris	452-8117	New Patient; Complete Physical
9:20a	*****************		
9:40a	~~Ella Jones~~	~~932-8174~~	~~recheck~~ *cancel 8am 10/13*
10:00a	Fred Linstatt	452-0667	recheck
10:20a	Mary Higgens	731-8241	recheck; URI 2 weeks ago
10:40a	Tina Leggett	931-0451	PE
11:00a			
11:20a	Tracey Jones	462-0157	2yr PE; father Robert
11:40a	Keth Jones		3 yr PE
12:00p	LUNCH		
12:20p	↓		
12:40p	↓		
1:00p	↓		
1:20p			
1:40p			
2:00p	Winston Hill	648-0791	PE
2:20p			
2:40p			
3:00p			
3:20p			
3:40p			
4:00p	Meeting at hospital		
4:20p	↓		
4:40p	↓		
5:00p			
5:20p			
5:40p			

➢ **Figure 9–2** Computer-generated appointment schedule.

The appointment interval can be adjusted to 10, 15, or 20 minutes depending on the practice's needs. Patients can be double booked as desired.

It is easy to set up repeating appointments, change appointments, and set up a recall system so that patients can be contacted when it is time for them to schedule an appointment.

Daily Appointment Schedule

Each day a list should be created from the appointment book or printed from the computer schedule for each doctor, so the medical records can be pulled and to serve as a daily schedule. This list should be typed or printed from a computer; additions and corrections must be made in ink, because this list is usually an official legal record of patients seen on a given day.

Corrections in Ink

No-shows (people who simply do not show up for their appointment) and those who call to cancel on the day of the appointment are marked in red on the daily schedule. That information is also noted on the patient medical record. The reason for this is to have a permanent record if the patient becomes more ill and claims the office did not see him. A list of cancellations may also be kept on the computer.

Most offices have a policy of reviewing records of patients after three missed appointments in a row. If the patient is not motivated to keep to the treatment plan, the doctor may wish to terminate the relationship with the patient. This requires that a letter be sent by certified mail, with a return receipt to the doctor, informing the patient of the reasons for concern and offering assistance in finding another health care provider.

(See chapter 35 for a discussion of correspondence and a sample termination letter.)

Legal Document

The office is required to keep a list of patients seen. This is a legal record. Because the appointment book is usually kept in pencil, the daily appointment sheet is usually maintained as the legal record, which is why additions and corrections must be done in ink.

The Internal Revenue Service can also ask for records to validate tax returns. These appointment sheets should be kept for a minimum of 5 years, but many practices keep them indefinitely.

TYPES OF SCHEDULING

Scheduled Appointments

Most offices schedule appointments at specific times. The goal is to minimize waiting time for the patient while keeping a steady flow of patients during the times when the doctor is seeing patients.

The schedule needs some free time to accommodate ill or injured patients, or urgent telephone calls, without becoming backed up. The doctor expects to spend about 30 minutes with a new patient, about 15 minutes with an established patient, and 30 to 45 minutes for a full physical examination. Some practices, especially specialty practices, allow longer appointments for new patients or consultation visits. There are several systems for scheduling patients. These include:

clustering
wave
modified wave
stream
double booking.

Clustering

Many offices group patients with similar problems or conditions on certain days or at certain times of the day. This method of scheduling is called **clustering**. Examples of conditions that can easily be clustered into a portion of each day are:

pregnant women in an OB/GYN practice
injections in an internal medicine practice
kindergarten physicals, camp physicals, or routine physicals in a pediatrics practice.

Special tests such as proctosigmoidoscopies might be done one morning a week.

Wave

In the **wave** system, three or four patients are scheduled every half hour, and they are seen in the order in which they arrive at the office. Sometimes, ill patients are taken before those with routine appointments.

This system assumes that some patients will need to be worked into the schedule. Sometimes patients become uncomfortable when they realize that another patient was given the same appointment time, but a simple explanation can usually reassure that person.

Modified Wave

The wave system may be changed in several ways, creating a **modified wave** schedule.

For instance, the office can schedule patients at intervals during the first half of each hour and leave the second half hour open for working in patients, seeing patients who came late, or finishing up with patients from the first half hour.

Another method involves scheduling appointments that are expected to take longer (such as physical exams) on the hour, and three or four rechecks or follow-up appointments on the half hour.

Fixed Scheduling

The most common scheduling method, **fixed scheduling**, divides each hour into intervals of 10 or 15 minutes and assign a patient to a fixed appointment time, filling in one or more intervals, depending on how long the appointment is expected to last.

Double Booking

When two patients are given the same appointment time, the practice is called **double booking**, the practice of booking two people into a single time slot. This may occur when one patient can be fitted in around a patient who may need diagnostic tests such as an electrocardiogram or having blood drawn, or when a patient is added to a full schedule because of injury or acute illness.

Open Hours

Sometimes a patient is not given a specific time to see the doctor but is told to come in during a time range, such as 9:00 to 11:00 AM, or 1:30 to 3:00 PM. The patients are then seen in the order in which they arrive. This is often done with patients who call that day, feeling ill, and are told the set appointments are all booked. This method is also often used in clinics.

In an open-hours system, those with an injury or an acute illness are often seen ahead of those with less significant complaints.

Open hours works best when there is a constant stream of patients. But on busy days, patients often have to wait a longer time.

PROCEDURE 9–1

Setting Up the Appointment Matrix

Performance Objective: The student will set up an appointment matrix incorporating office guidelines.

Supplies and Equipment: Appointment book or computer program, pen, doctor's schedule, office calendar.

Procedure Steps

1. Mark an X through times when the office is not open to see patients. This includes times in the book before office hours begin, lunch and/or breaks, afternoons or days when the office is closed, and holidays when the office will be closed. Some offices set up the appointment matrix 6 months in advance, others for a year in advance. If the office uses a computer program, is should be possible to limit the available hours to those when the office is open and mark the different reasons for office closure.

   Rationale: To create an appointment schedule where only open appointment times are unmarked.

2. For each doctor, mark an X through times in the appointment book when the doctor is not available to see patients, including vacations, conferences, hospital rounds, or other anticipated absences. If the doctor has regular meetings or other regular commitments (such as nursing home visits), mark these in also. If the office uses a computer program, enter the reason (such as Meeting, Vacation, Conference) into all times when the doctor is not available to see patients.

Rationale: To create an appointment schedule for each doctor in which only open appointment times are unmarked.

3. For each doctor, mark times when the doctor does certain types of examinations or procedures (such as physical examinations or obstetric visits). In an appointment book these are often highlighted with marker or given a written title at the beginning of the time block. In a computer program these times may be set up as if for a separate doctor (such as Dr. Lopez and Dr. Lopez—OB visits).

   Rationale: Because more than one person may make appointments, any system used for clustering appointments must be clear and easy to understand.

4. Depending on office policy, block out as much time as anticipated for emergency visits and reserve times for unexpected needs. Depending on the practice this may be 15 minutes in the morning and afternoon for each doctor or longer for all or one particular doctor on a rotating basis. These times can be marked in various ways as long as office staff understand that they must be saved until the scheduled day.

   Rationale: Experience in the practice will dictate how much time is usually needed for urgent appointments and patients who must be worked in. Having the time blocked out in preparation leaves time available and avoids cranky patients who are waiting longer than they want to.

Multiple Offices

Many doctors see patients in different offices, with appointments booked through a central system. In this case, you need to clarify with the patient which office he or she wishes to visit. It is also necessary to move the medical record from office to office.

SETTING UP THE APPOINTMENT MATRIX

Appointments are usually scheduled up to 6 months in advance. Before scheduling can begin, the appointment book or computer software must be set up to

show the times when each doctor will take appointments. Meetings, surgery, vacations, and other activities are also recorded.

Times when each doctor is not available are **blocked** (crossed out). The resulting page is sometimes called an appointment **matrix** (*matrix* means form or arrangement). See Procedure 9–1, Setting up the Appointment Matrix.

Figure 9–3 shows an appointment matrix.

Scheduling System

The matrix will take into account two variables. One is the scheduling system, which is chosen to meet the

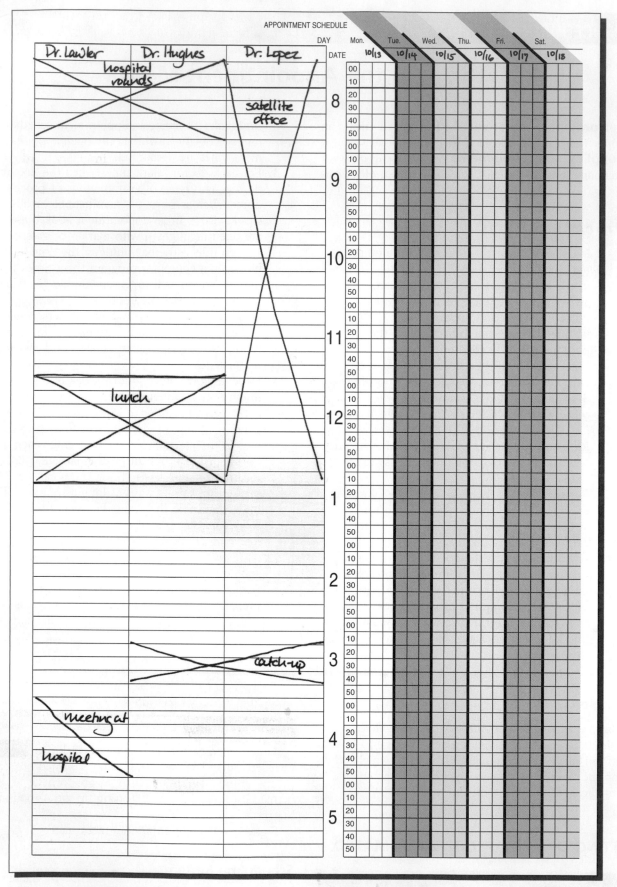

> **Figure 9–3** The appointment matrix using an appointment book for three doctors.

needs of the practice. The scheduling system also involves the amount of time in an appointment unit, days or times set aside for specific types of visits (such as follow-ups or physicals), and how much time is set aside to see sick patients who call in that day. A sample schedule is shown in Figure 9–4.

Doctor's Preference and Needs

The other variable is the doctor's preference and needs. This has to do with the times during the day that the doctor is available to see patients. When one doctor or another has an obligation such as hospital rounds, nursing home visits, days or parts of days at different offices, and days or parts of days for clustering or procedures, this is entered into the schedule. Days are also blocked out of each doctor's schedule for vacation, days off, attendance at conferences, giving lectures, or any other professional activities.

GUIDELINES FOR SCHEDULING

When you set up an appointment, you need to get the proper information from the patient, legibly print it in the schedule, and confirm it with the patient. If the patient is in the office, fill out an appointment reminder card and hand it to the patient. Figure 9–5 shows an appointment reminder card.

When scheduling appointments, be sure you know if the patient is an established patient or a new patient.

Established Patient

An established patient has been seen in your office within the past 3 years and has a current medical record. Patients who have not been seen within the past 3 years are usually treated as new patients.

If the patient is scheduling a return appointment, the doctor has probably stated a specific time period before the patient should return (i.e., 1 week, 1 month, 6 months). The appointment should be set up for the appropriate amount of time (usually one unit— 10 to 15 minutes—for a recheck) for that date in the future.

If the patient needs an appointment for a date later than the appointment book is set up for, either ask the patient to call for an appointment or keep the name in a list to be scheduled and call the patient when the new appointment book is set. Offices vary on how long in advance their doctors' schedules are set.

New Patient or Referral

You need to get a lot of information from a new patient. (See Procedure 9–2, Making an Appointment, for more detail.)

The information you need to get includes the name of the doctor who made the referral, the patient's full name, daytime telephone number, and the reason for the visit or type of visit (sick visit, physical exam, test, and so on).

Most offices schedule new patients for 30 to 45 minutes.

You should ask the patient what type of insurance he or she has, and you may need to get the patient's date of birth, the name on the insurance card (if the patient is a spouse or child of a person covered through a group insurance plan). You should tell the patient how much to expect to be charged.

There are three different possible scenarios for payment. One is that the patient must pay at the time of service, then submit a claim for reimbursement from the insurance company. The second is that the doctor's office bills first to the insurance company, then to the patient if the insurance company refuses the claim, or if the patient has not met the plan's deductible yet. The third is that the patient belongs to a managed care plan, or health maintenance organization in which case the doctor takes a co-payment from the patient, then submits the bill for the remainder of the fee to the insurance company.

When the patient has been referred by another doctor, try to get the patient an appointment as soon as possible, especially if the patient has urgent symptoms or if the patient's primary care provider's office is calling to make the appointment.

SICK AND URGENT VISITS

Although a majority of appointments are made well in advance of the date a patient will see the doctor, urgent situations do occur. These are actually the most challenging for the medical assistant responsible for making the appointment. It is important to give any caller a chance to tell you that it is an urgent or emergency situation before putting the call on hold.

Urgent Medical Problems

A life-threatening or serious medical problem should be immediately referred to one of the office's doctors or the office's triage nurse, if there is one. This person will make the decision about the appropriate course of action to take. If neither is present, the caller should be referred to the emergency room as outlined in Procedure 7–4.

The following problems usually require care in an emergency room as soon as possible:

1. Medical problems that can result in damage to the body structures if not treated as soon as possible. This is especially important for prob-

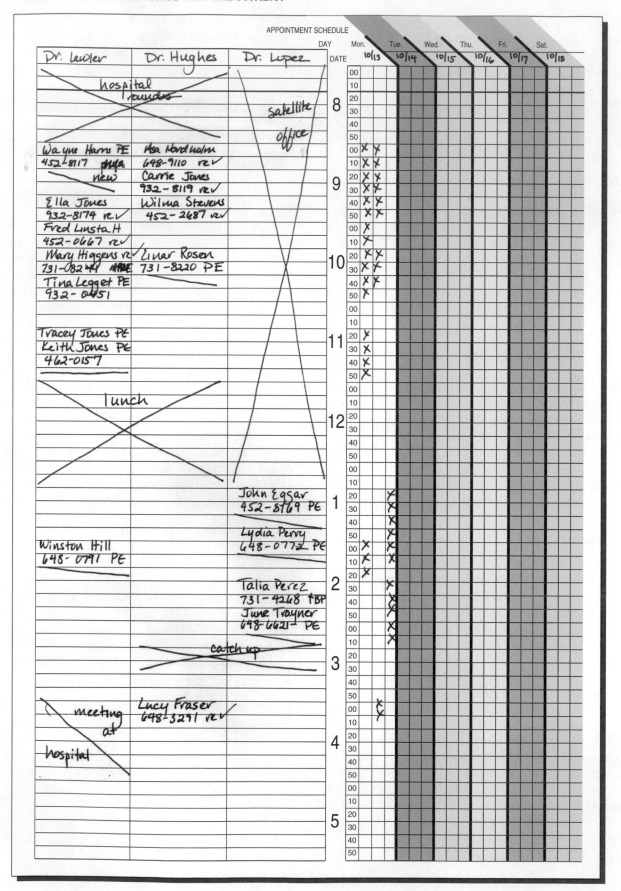

➤ **Figure 9–4** Sample appointment schedule.

Blackburn Primary Care Associates, PC

1990 Turquiose Drive • Blackburn, WI 54937 • 608-459-8857

_____   _____
has an appointment on   provider

_____   _____
date   time

Please telephone one day in advance if you will be unable to keep the appointment

➤ **Figure 9–5** Appointment reminder card.

PROCEDURE 9–2

Making an Appointment

Performance Objective: The student will make an appointment for a patient.
Supplies and Equipment: Appointment book or computer program, pencil.

Procedure Steps

1. Obtain information from the patient: which doctor to book the appointment with, the purpose of the appointment, and any scheduling preference. Referrals are usually offered the first available appointment. If you do not recognize the patient's name, ask if the patient has been seen before. New patients may be encouraged to choose a doctor who has joined the practice recently and is not as busy as the more established doctors. Established patients are usually booked with their primary care doctor, but if it is an urgent problem they may accept an appointment with another provider in the practice.
   Rationale: You need to locate an appropriate appointment for the patient of the needed length.

2. Offer the patient a date and time for the appointment. Keep locating appointments until you and the patient agree on a date and time. The more urgent the appointment, the more the patient must adapt to the office schedule.
   Rationale: The more particular the patient is about a specific day and time for the appointment, the more likely it is that the appoint-

ment cannot be scheduled for a few weeks or longer. The more urgent the patient's condition, the more the patient is expected to accept the time you offer.

3. Obtain the information to fill in the appointment book. For an established patient this includes the patient's name, reason for the visit, daytime telephone number, and in many practices date of birth (to avoid confusion with other patients of the same name). Enter the information in pencil and block out the correct amount of time.
   Rationale: You need enough information to identify and contact the patient.

4. If it is a new patient, you also need the name of the patient's insurance company and you may need to obtain the patient's insurance group number and ID number, a referral number, or other information related to insurance. Be sure to discuss the cost of the visit if the patient does not have insurance and inform the patient if a referral form from the primary care doctor is necessary.
   Rationale: New patients must be oriented to your billing methods. In some cases you may need to confirm ahead of time that the patient's insurance will cover services in your office.

5. Repeat the information to the patient before ending the call. Offer directions to a new patient.
   Rationale: Repeating the information about the appointment helps prevent misunderstandings.

TRIAGE

Triage is the process of sorting patients according to their need for care. When a disaster occurs, health care workers choose which patients to treat first, depending both on the severity of their injuries and the likelihood the person will survive.

Victims are sorted into three groups—hence the word *triage*—from the French meaning to sort into three groups. There are those whose injuries are minor and can wait for treatment; those whose injuries are so severe they will probably not survive whatever effort is put into their treatment; and those whose injuries are severe but will probably survive if prompt treatment is given.

This system has been adapted to the office and appointment scheduling to decide if a patient can wait for the next available appointment, if the patient should be seen immediately, or if the patient should be sent to the emergency room. Triage in the medical office setting is rarely a case of life or death, and the term "triage" is usually reserved for screening performed by licensed health care personnel with the education needed to assess the medical needs of ill patients.

The medical assistant does screen calls and make decisions based on guidelines established by the doctors where he or she works. The medical assistant must remember that if there is any question about a patient needing immediate care, either the telephone call should be referred to a qualified person in the office or the patient should be directed to an emergency room or other facility where care can be obtained. The medical assistant should be familiar with the policies of his or her employer and should work within them to avoid injuring the patient and to protect against liability in a potential lawsuit.

lems that can cause significant decrease in oxygen in the blood due to interference with breathing or circulation. Such conditions include:

breathing problems, or respiratory arrest
severe chest pain, or cardiac arrest
bleeding that cannot be controlled
large open wounds
any suspicion of internal bleeding
potential accidental poisoning
bleeding in, or injury to, a pregnant woman.

2. Medical problems that result in very low blood pressure, such as:

shock
serious burns
severe bleeding.

3. Medical problems that result in continued change in the level of consciousness, onset of disorientation, confusion, and/or loss of alertness. Any head injury in which even a momentary loss of consciousness occurs should be treated in the emergency room.

4. Serious injuries such as fractures or large wounds that do not significantly affect breathing, circulation, or consciousness but require the equipment found in an emergency room.

The office procedure manual should help you respond to emergencies.

Treat in the Office Quickly

The following problems are usually treated in the medical office and should be scheduled as soon as possible:

1. Wounds without fracture or dislocation. The doctor may suture the wound (use stitches to hold the skin edges in place.)
2. Sprains, strains, and sometimes undisplaced fractures (cracks in the bone or partial fractures where the bone ends stay in position), especially if the upper body is affected and the patient can walk.
3. Nausea, vomiting, or diarrhea that persists over 2 to 3 days.
4. High fever (over 101° Fahrenheit, tympanic [temperature taken in the ear] for children, over 103° for adults).
5. Sudden illness or severe pain without bleeding, fainting, or loss of consciousness.
6. Sore throat, especially with fever.
7. Burning, frequency, or urgency on urination, especially if accompanied by fever or blood in the urine.
8. Vaginal bleeding in a pregnant woman (may also be sent to the emergency room).

Patients with these types of conditions may need to be scheduled with a practitioner who has a more flexible schedule if the individual's primary care doctor is completely booked. In many multi-practitioner offices, one doctor's schedule is left unfilled for a block of time to accommodate urgent visits. See "On The Job."

Walk-In Patients

Sometimes patients walk into the office without an appointment and ask to be seen. If such a patient is

ON THE JOB

Assume that Craig takes the following telephone calls requesting appointments with Dr. Hughes on a day when her schedule is completely booked. Which of the following patients should be seen that day, even if they have to be fitted in around patients who already have appointments, or should be offered an appointment with one of the practice's other doctors? Justify your answers.

1. A 41-year-old established patient with a fever of 101°F, who also complains of nausea and diarrhea during the previous night and that morning.
2. A 12-year-old established patient who fell that morning at school, injuring his right arm and shoulder. He is complaining of pain in his shoulder. He is able to move his arm and shoulder but was sent home from school. The pain has become more severe during the afternoon.
3. A 72-year-old man who has been referred to Dr. Hughes because of episodes of forgetfulness and difficulty speaking, which occur every few weeks and last for about 10 to 15 minutes.
4. A 25-year-old woman with a large, hard, red, swollen area on her right breast that she describes as "like a huge pimple." This woman is not pregnant or breastfeeding. She does not think she has a fever.

experiencing an emergency or urgent problems, or is following up from an emergency, the doctor may work the patient into the schedule. But in routine cases, the person is offered an appointment and told to return. If the doctor does see such a patient, the patient should be tactfully informed of the office's usual method of scheduling appointments.

MANAGING THE APPOINTMENT BOOK

Changing Appointments

If a patient needs to change an appointment, be sure to erase the original appointment and enter all the information in the new time slot. Some computer appointment programs allow you to cut and paste appointments; they can also set up repeating appointments on a weekly, biweekly, or monthly basis.

If there is a change in the doctor's schedule or if the doctor knows he or she will be delayed because of a particular commitment or an emergency, you may be asked to call a block of patients to reschedule. Every effort must be made to accommodate these patients by giving them a new appointment as quickly as possible.

If the doctor is running seriously behind schedule, patients often become impatient. Some may wish to reschedule; others may wish to go and have coffee or a snack. Usually the doctor is willing to stay late to finish the day's appointments, but if the doctor must leave at a particular time, appointments set for late in the day may need to be rescheduled.

Appointment Reminders

Patients who make appointments while in the office are usually given an appointment card. These cards help patients remember the exact date and time of their next appointment.

Most offices also call patients 1 or 2 days before the appointment. The medical assistant or another office employee uses the appointment book to call each patient who is scheduled for an appointment.

Patients have a right to confidentiality regarding the appointment, so new patients should be asked if it is all right to leave a message about the appointment on an answering machine or voice mail system when you get the daytime phone number.

Computer appointment programs usually allow you to flag patients who need a physical exam or other appointment at a time beyond the current schedule, in order to send them reminders. Such reminders are usually sent out once a month to patients who need to make an appointment. These reminders are usually form letters generated by the computer.

Storing Appointment Books and Daily Schedules

In some offices, the appointment book is kept in ink and used as the office record of appointments. Be sure the official book or schedule is updated as described earlier in the chapter and is stored in a secure area.

STUDENT STUDY PLAN

To reinforce your understanding of the material in this chapter . . .

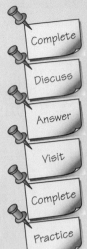

Complete the **Review & Recall** questions below.

Discuss the situation in **If You Were the Medical Assistant** with your classmates, and answer the questions.

Answer the **Critical Thinking Questions** below and discuss them with your classmates.

Visit **Web sites** suggested in searching **Keywords for Internet Searches**.

Complete the exercises in chapter 9 of the **Student Mastery Manual**.

Practice scheduling appointments in Case 1 on the **CD-ROM**.

REVIEW & RECALL

1. Describe and contrast the following types of appointment scheduling systems: cluster, wave, modified wave, fixed appointment, and open hours.

2. What is double booking? When is it used?

3. What determines the medical assistant's selection of an appropriate appointment for a patient?

4. Why is the daily schedule typed or computer generated?

5. What information must be added to the daily schedule as the day progresses?

6. What must be documented if a patient does not keep an appointment?

7. What information is recorded when a new patient makes an appointment?

8. What are the advantages and disadvantages of a computerized appointment schedule?

9. Identify the steps in setting up the appointment matrix.

10. Describe three methods to remind patients to make or keep appointments.

IF YOU WERE THE MEDICAL ASSISTANT

You are the medical assistant at Blackburn Primary Care Associates. Dr. Lopez is the only doctor scheduled to be in the office this afternoon. It is very important that he leave promptly at 3:45 because he is scheduled to give a lecture to medical students shortly after 4:00.

Dr. Lopez has been running behind because two extra patients have been worked into the schedule. At 2:30, you notice that in addition to three patients in the waiting room, he still has four established patients scheduled, as well as one new patient scheduled for 3:15, the last appointment of the day. What should you suggest to Dr. Lopez as a possible way to deal with this problem?

CRITICAL THINKING QUESTIONS

1. Discuss advantages and disadvantages of using the appointment book instead of the daily schedule as the permanent record of appointments.

2. Patients sometimes arrive at the office believing they have an appointment, but they are not listed on the schedule. What policy should an office develop to deal with this situation? Give your reasons.

3. If you were a medical assistant working in a practice where patients often sat in the waiting room for 30 to 40 minutes, describe what you would analyze to identify the reason(s) for such long waits.

4. What factors influence a medical practice's choice of appointment scheduling method? What is the best choice?

5. If you notice that one day of the week is especially likely to result in prolonged waits for patients, what could you suggest to adjust the appointment schedule for that day?

6. Gather information about how long appointments are for new patients and established patients at various practices. What pressures encourage doctors to see patients for shorter periods of time? What pressures encourage longer appointments?

 EXPLORE THE WEB

KEYWORDS FOR INTERNET SEARCHES

medical appointment software
    practice management software

 ANSWERS TO ON THE JOB

1. Unless symptoms intensify, this patient can be given an appointment for tomorrow, with advice to call again if the fever becomes higher or if blood is seen in the stool.

2. This patient should be seen to be sure there is no upper arm fracture or shoulder dislocation.

3. This patient should be given the first open appointment. The history given by the patient indicates he is stable. As a new patient, he requires a 45-minute appointment. Dr. Hughes would prefer to see him herself.

4. Unless this woman develops a fever or other symptoms of distress, she also can wait for an appointment tomorrow. If she were pregnant or breastfeeding, it would be important for her to be seen today.

Chapter 10

Medical Records and Filing Systems

Instructional Objectives

After completing this chapter, you will be able to do the following:

1. Define and spell the vocabulary words for this chapter.
2. Differentiate between source-based and problem-oriented medical records.
3. Describe proper methods of documenting in patient records.
4. Identify the parts of a SOAP progress note.
5. Describe the proper method for making corrections in the medical record.
6. Describe the contents of a typical medical record.
7. Identify supplies and equipment needed to create and store medical records.
8. List principles of alphabetic and numeric filing.
9. Compare and contrast advantages and disadvantages of alphabetic and numeric filing systems.
10. Describe the process of filing reports and patient records.
11. Differentiate between storage of active and inactive records.
12. Identify legal implications of retention of medical records.

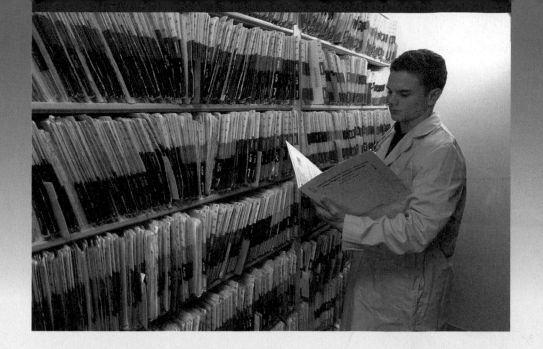

CMA/RMA CERTIFICATION
Content and Competencies

- Organize a patient's medical record
- File medical records

- Establish and maintain the medical record

Performance Objectives

1. Prepare a medical record for a new patient (Procedure 10–1).
2. Prepare a monthly tickler file (Procedure 10–2).
3. File reports, correspondence, and other material in a patient record (Procedure 10–3).
4. File patient records correctly (Procedure 10–4).

VOCABULARY

acronym (p. 176)
assessment (p. 166)
continuity of care (p. 164)
cross-index (p. 175)
database (p. 165)
demographic (p. 164)
guides (p. 174)
indexing units (p. 175)

litigation (p. 168)
objective (p. 166)
out guides (p. 174)
plan (p. 166)
problem list (p. 165)
problem-oriented medical record
  (POMR) (p. 164)
progress notes (p. 165)

SOAP charting (p. 165)
sorter (p. 168)
source-oriented medical record
  (SOMR) (p. 164)
statute of limitations (p. 181)
subjective (p. 165)
subpoena *duces tecum* (p. 164)
terminal digit filing (p. 177)

tickler file (p. 177)
treatment plan (p. 165)

ABBREVIATIONS

POMR (p. 164)   SOAP (p. 165)   SOMR (p. 164)

INTRODUCTION TO MEDICAL RECORDS

Medical records are written documentation of all aspects of a patient's health care. Medical records help doctors and other health care professionals to provide patients with **continuity of care** (continuing care based on knowledge of previous care). They are also necessary legal records of the care given and are also needed for creating statistical information about the practice.

With so many patients in most practices, it is impossible for a doctor or other professional to remember every detail of care, such as the results of a physical examination or doses of particular medications. Many people in the primary care doctor's office have contact with a patient, as well as with consulting professionals, laboratories, and hospitals involved in the care of that patient. It is important that each document is stored in the patient's medical record filed in chronological order, with the most recent medical service in the front. This is the ongoing record of both the patient's state of health and the service provided by the medical office.

Medical records are legal documents, used by the doctor if questions arise about the care given. If a patient sues a doctor, the court may issue a **subpoena** *duces tecum* for the patient's medical record as evidence of the care the patient received. This type of subpoena legally requires documentary evidence such as a medical record to be presented in court. The court will take the position that whatever is documented in the record is the care that was given. If something is not charted, officially it never happened.

Lack of completeness in the medical record, such as missing laboratory test results, prescription refills, visits without doctor's notes, *never happened* because there is no evidence that they did. To protect the legal interests of the doctor's office, you need to keep complete medical records.

Types of Records

Two systems are commonly used for keeping medical records.

One is the **source-oriented medical record (SOMR),** in which the record is organized by what types of services were performed. The second is the **problem-oriented medical record (POMR),** in which information is grouped in the record according to the patient's particular problem.

Some offices use the POMR format in the patient progress notes (the ongoing record of care given in the office) and the SOMR format for other records, such as reports from laboratories, hospitals, and other outside agencies or doctor's offices.

Source-Oriented Medical Records

The SOMR is the format traditionally used by hospitals. Records received from the same source, such as the laboratory or the radiology department, are grouped together. They are arranged in reverse chronological order, with the oldest information in the back. Some information groupings are:

1. **Demographic** information, such as name, address, telephone number, and insurance information.
2. Progress notes.
3. History and physical exam.
4. Lab reports.
5. Reports of diagnostic tests, such as X-rays, ultrasound, or magnetic resonance imaging.
6. Consultation reports.
7. Reports from any hospitalization.
8. Correspondence.
9. Miscellaneous papers related to the patient but not to treatment, such as insurance-related re-

cords, transfer forms, and legal forms such as a power of attorney, living will, or health care proxy.

The medical record found in the hospital may have additional sections, including doctors' orders, surgical and anesthesia reports, and admission and discharge summaries. After a hospitalization, copies of the discharge summary and any operative report for surgery are sent to the primary care doctor's office and are filed in the patient's medical record there.

Problem-Oriented Medical Records

The POMR is the more popular of the methods to document and arrange patient records. Developed in the 1960s by Dr. Lawrence Weed, charting in the POMR is based on a problem list, with each problem numbered. Flowcharts are used to keep track of information about a particular problem.

Components of the POMR System

In the POMR system, the chart is divided into four sections:

1. **Database.** Information about the patient, including the history and physical exam, laboratory data, and reports of diagnostic tests.
2. **Problem list.** A list of each physical, social, or psychological problem the patient has or has had

in the past, with the date it was identified and a number that is used to cross-reference the problem with the progress notes. The sheet containing the list of problems usually identifies allergies, medications, immunizations, and/or other data about the patient. Some problems are eventually resolved; others become chronic and must be addressed at each office visit.

3. **Treatment plan.** A written description of the plan for the patient, including diagnostic testing, treatments, and follow-up. In the medical office, this usually is not a separate section but is found in the progress notes.
4. **Progress notes.** Health professionals chart problems in so-called SOAP format (named after the four components: subjective impressions, objective data, assessment, and planning). Each entry is given the number of the particular problem being discussed.

SOAP Charting

The **SOAP charting** system has four main components, described below. Figure 10–1 shows SOAP notes. In the first example (Figure 10–1A), there is a note related to each specific problem. The second example (Figure 10–1B) uses one SOAP note to chart an entire patient visit.

(S)ubjective. Impressions the patient has about his or her own condition, the things the patient describes

➢ Figure 10–1A SOAP charting related to a problem list.

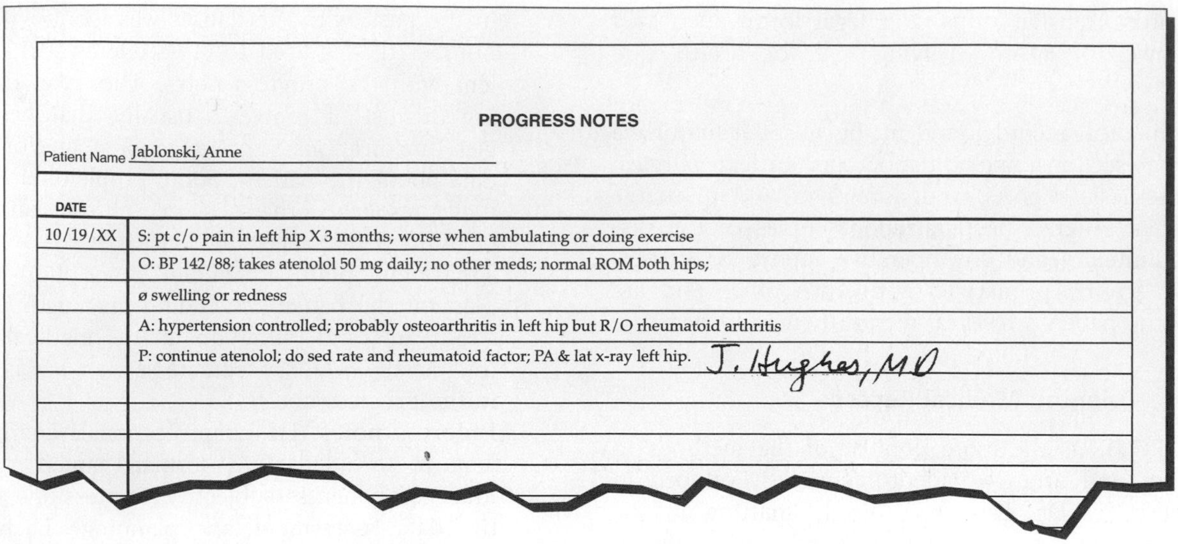

PROGRESS NOTES

Patient Name Jablonski, Anne

DATE	
10/19/XX	S: pt c/o pain in left hip X 3 months; worse when ambulating or doing exercise
	O: BP 142/88; takes atenolol 50 mg daily; no other meds; normal ROM both hips;
	ø swelling or redness
	A: hypertension controlled; probably osteoarthritis in left hip but R/O rheumatoid arthritis
	P: continue atenolol; do sed rate and rheumatoid factor; PA & lat x-ray left hip. *J. Hughes, MD*

> **Figure 10–1B** One SOAP note relates to a patient visit, although the patient has more than one problem.

that only he or she can experience, such as nausea, headache, pain, or itching, as well as feelings such as anger, depression, and confusion. These are often noted in the patient's own words, using quotation marks. For example, "I feel like someone is pounding nails into my head."

(O)bjective. Information that can be observed or measured. It includes results of diagnostic and laboratory tests, as well as vital signs.

(A)ssessment. A summary of what the subjective impressions and objective data mean. In the doctor's charting, this is often written as an impression of the preliminary diagnosis. Other health professionals must avoid using a medical diagnosis in their charting.

(P)lan. A written description of the diagnostic tests the patient will undergo, medications that will be prescribed, treatments that will be given, and follow-up the patient will receive.

Even when the medical record is not totally problem-oriented, the SOAP format is often used for charting. In the medical office, all information related to a particular office visit may be included in a SOAP note.

The Computerized Record

In some hospitals and clinics, part or all of the medical record is maintained on computer. Documentation is recorded directly into the computer system, using a computer terminal, handheld device, or voice recognition system. There are a number of advantages to this, including that the note is always legible and the information is easy to retrieve. Access to laboratory data and test results is quick and easy. It results in less time spent filing (and reduced costs for filing clerks and others) and easy storage.

The disadvantages of a computer-based patient record system have mostly to do with data security (and hence patient confidentiality) as well as the possibility of computer crashes and the need for more equipment and training to use the equipment. Many offices have a computer terminal in each examination room to facilitate access to patient information.

Some facilities print out a full or partial record for office visits and then enter new information during the visit or immediately after the patient has been seen. The system needs to be set up so that only authorized people have access to the record. Once data is accepted, it should not be available to be altered or deleted.

Legal Implications of the Medical Record

The medical record is initiated by the medical office and belongs to the person or group who produced it. The doctor or office owns the physical record.

However, the information in the record belongs to the patient, and the patient controls access to the information. Any request to release copies of records must come from the patient or someone who is authorized to act for the patient.

The original record must never be released. If the original record is subpoenaed by a court, an employee of the office should travel with the record to safeguard it and be sure that no part is lost or tampered with. A copy of the record should be left at the office.

The office should have a form for patients to sign that gives permission to release the medical record, similar to the one shown in Figure 10–2.

The release must be signed by the patient or by a

guardian if the patient is a minor. In some states, information regarding human immunodeficiency virus (HIV)/acquired immune deficiency syndrome (AIDS) must be requested on a separate consent form and should not be released unless this special form is signed.

When a patient begins a new relationship with a doctor's office, the patient routinely signs a release form allowing the doctor to send necessary information to an insurance company. One of the standards being developed under the Health Insurance Portability and Accountability Act legislation concerns a standard format for electronic signatures.

Another time records are usually released is when a patient moves away or begins a relationship with another doctor. If the purpose of copying records is for such continuity of care, offices do not charge. Sometimes they do charge a copying fee, a handling fee, and postage, especially if the record is requested by a lawyer for litigation.

AUTHORIZATION FOR RELEASE OF MEDICAL INFORMATION
please complete in ink

Date _____

PATIENT IDENTIFICATION   Name _____

                              Address _____

                              _____

MEDICAL FACILITY   Telephone _____

                              Doctor _____

                              Address _____

                              _____

I hearby authorize and request you to release the complete medical records in your possession, concerning my illness and/or treatment during the period from _____ to _____

I understand that if my medical record contains information in reference to drug and/or alcohol abuse, psychiatric, venereal disease, social service and/or sensitive information, hepatitis testing/treatment, I agree to its release.

_____   _____
Signature of patient/legal guardian   Date

Note:
In ADDITION to the signature above, if you want your HIV/AIDS testing/treatment records released you MUST sign and date below.

I agree to the release of HIV/AIDS testing/treatment information found in my medical record:

_____   _____
Signature of patient/legal guardian   Date

➤ **Figure 10–2** Form to authorize release of the medical record.

Documentation

Making Accurate and Complete Entries

When documenting in a patient chart, entries must be accurate and complete. A note must be dated and signed with the first initial, last name, and credentials, although some offices use just initials and credentials. Documentation is supposed to be performed at the time the care is provided or immediately after. If the notation is handwritten, it should be in blue or black permanent (not erasable) ink. If it is dictated and transcribed, the transcriber may correct using ordinary methods, and the note is then signed by the person who dictated it. Although it may make the entries look crowded, if there are no blank lines it is much more difficult to alter entries later.

When charting, be sure you have the correct record. The patient's name should be on each sheet of the record. Document any missed appointments and if you called the patient about the appointment. Telephone calls and pharmacy refills should also be documented.

A medical assistant may not use a medical diagnosis in charting and should not make judgmental statements. Use the patient's own words in quotations if possible. When noting a situation, describe it rather than drawing conclusions. For instance, the note should say "the patient is quiet, not making eye contact," rather than "patient appears depressed."

Corrections

If you need to correct an entry, do so by drawing a single line through any mistake, adding the correction, then initialing the crossed out portion. If you are correcting on a different date than the mistake was made, date and initial the correction. Do not use liquid correction fluid to correct handwritten notes. The original note should not be obscured or erased (i.e., do not use whiteout).

Legal Implications

The medical record is a legal document. It is the chronological record of the care given. If the doctor becomes involved in **litigation** (a court case), the judge will assume, and will instruct a jury to assume, that only what is in the medical record actually occurred, and that alterations where the original entry cannot be read are intended to cover up a problem. Figure 10–3 shows the proper way to correct a note.

PREPARING A MEDICAL RECORD FOR A NEW PATIENT

Equipment and Supplies

Most offices use file folders with prong fasteners and various index dividers to form separate sections for information. The office usually has a two-hole punch to prepare folders and/or papers to fit over the prong fastener.

A system of color-coded labels is usually used for letters in the patient's name or numbers in the patient's clinic number. Some offices use colored folders. I will discuss both alphabetic and numeric filing systems below.

Additional labels or colored folders may be used to indicate the year, the doctor, allergies, insurance information, or information to cluster certain records (for example, pregnant patients in an OB/GYN practice). A **sorter** is a device that facilitates placing documents in alphabetic or numerical order. It has pockets or dividers for each letter or number.

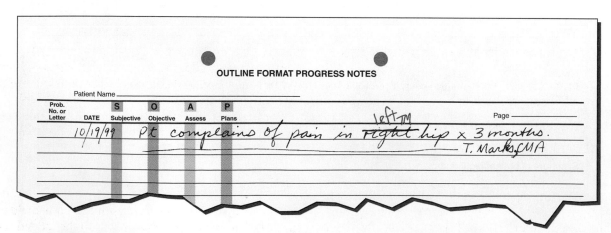

➤ **Figure 10–3** To correct an entry in the medical record, draw a single line through the incorrect information, correct it, and initial. Date the correction if made on a different day from the original entry.

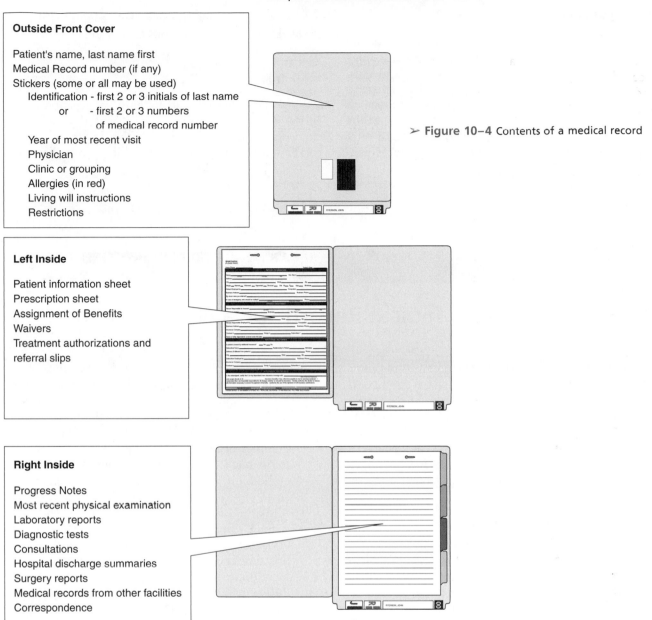

Outside Front Cover

Patient's name, last name first
Medical Record number (if any)
Stickers (some or all may be used)
    Identification - first 2 or 3 initials of last name
      or   - first 2 or 3 numbers
           of medical record number
    Year of most recent visit
    Physician
    Clinic or grouping
    Allergies (in red)
    Living will instructions
    Restrictions

➤ Figure 10-4 Contents of a medical record

Left Inside

Patient information sheet
Prescription sheet
Assignment of Benefits
Waivers
Treatment authorizations and
referral slips

Right Inside

Progress Notes
Most recent physical examination
Laboratory reports
Diagnostic tests
Consultations
Hospital discharge summaries
Surgery reports
Medical records from other facilities
Correspondence

The contents of a patient record are listed in Figure 10-4.

See Procedure 10-1, Preparing a Medical Record for a New Patient, for details.

Contents and Organization

Patient Information Sheet

Every new patient fills out a patient information sheet at the first visit, with demographic, billing/insurance, and health information. This is usually filed on the left inside of the folder, so that the medical assistant can verify the address, telephone number, and insurance information at each visit. Figure 10-5 is a sample patient information sheet. Offices—especially specialty practices—often develop their own forms to obtain the specific information the doctor prefers.

The sheet is given to the patient to fill out before seeing a doctor and is mounted in the chart after the visit.

Problem List

The problem list may be preprinted on a divider of the medical record or may need to be added as a separate sheet. These documents have several formats. Figure 10-6 shows a problem list.

History and Physical Examination

Most offices use a printed questionnaire to obtain information about the patient history. These questions can differ, depending on the particular office's medical specialty. The questionnaire is given to the patient to fill out before seeing the doctor, along with the patient information sheet, and mounted in the record after the visit. Notes on the physical exam may be entered on a particular form or dictated by the doctor. This is usually done for a new patient. See chapter 16 for a detailed description of the physical exam.

Flow Sheets

Flow sheets are used to monitor information over a period of time. An example is a growth chart for a child. Each time the child visits the doctor, the child's height and weight are plotted on the growth chart. The

---

PROCEDURE 10–1

Preparing a Medical Record for a New Patient

Performance Objective: The student will prepare a medical record for a new patient.

Supplies and Equipment: Record folder, forms used by the office (problem list, physical exam form, flow sheets, progress notes, lab report form), label for name, color-coding labels, label for year, labels for special information (allergies, insurance information, and so on), pen (or typewriter, computer), hole punch.

Procedure Steps

1. If the office uses an alphabetic filing system (using the letters of the patient's name) write, type, or key in a label with the patient's name in the same order as the folder will be filed (e.g. Jones, Mary A.) If the office uses a numeric filing system (each patient assigned a number), create a label with the patient's number.

   Rationale: This label will be used to identify the folder. It will be easier to file if it presents the information in the same order as the folder will be filed.

2. Select a folder. If the office uses color-coded folders, select the correct color for the first letter of the patient's last name or the patient's number. Mount the label on the tabbed edge of the folder. Depending on the type of folders used, the tabbed edge may be on the top or end of the folder.

   Rationale: The name or number should be visible when the medical record has been filed. For standard file cabinets, top tabs are visible. For lateral filing cabinets, end tabs are visible.

3. Add color-coding labels according to office practice. These usually include color-coded labels for alphanumeric files (the first two letters of the last name and sometimes the first letter of the first name) or the first two or three numbers of the patient's number.

   Rationale: Color-coded labels facilitate filing and finding lost charts because misfiled charts stand out from their neighbors.

4. Add a year label to the end or top tab. The current year is used for a new patient and to update the chart of an established patient the first time the patient comes in for an appointment during the current year.

   Rationale: Year labels make it easy to see which patients have been seen in the current or previous year. They also facilitate removing charts of inactive patients.

5. Apply any additional labels your office uses, such as allergies, insurance or other information.

   Rationale: These special labels help identify patients who fall into selected categories.

6. Insert blank forms used by your office into the record. Label each sheet with the patient's name by writing it or using computer-generated labels. In some offices the forms for several records are compiled at once, and you only need to enter the patient's name on the sheets. Punch holes in the sheets if necessary.

   Rationale: If pages fall out of a record, you have to be able to identify the proper record to refile them.

REGISTRATION
(PLEASE PRINT)

Home Phone: _____   Today's Date: _____

PATIENT INFORMATION

Name _____   Soc. Sec.# _____
       Last Name   First Name   Initial

Address _____

City _____ State _____   Zip _____

Single ___ Married ___ Widowed ___ Separated ___ Divorced ___   Sex M___ F___   Age ___   Birthdate _____

Patient Employed by _____ Occupation _____

Business Address _____ Business Phone _____

By whom were you referred? _____

In case of emergency who should be notified? _____ Phone _____
                         Last Name   Relationship to Patient

PRIMARY INSURANCE

Person Responsible for Account _____
                      Last Name   First Name   Initial

Relation to Patient _____ Birthdate _____   Soc. Sec.# _____

Address (if different from patient's) _____ Phone _____

City _____ State _____ Zip _____

Person Responsible Employed by _____ Occupation _____

Business Address _____ Business Phone _____

Insurance Company _____

Contract # _____ Group # _____ Subscriber # _____

Name of other dependents covered under this plan _____

ADDITIONAL INSURANCE

Is patient covered by additional insurance?   ____ Yes ____ No

Subscriber Name _____ Relationship to Patient _____ Birthdate _____

Address (if different from patient's) _____ Phone _____

City _____ State _____ Zip _____

Subscriber Employed by _____ Business Phone _____

Insurance Company _____

Contract # _____ Group # _____ Subscriber # _____

Name of other dependents covered under this plan _____

ASSIGNMENT AND RELEASE

I, the undersigned, certify that I (or my dependent) have insurance coverage with _____

and assign directly to Dr. _____ insurance benefits, if any, otherwise payable to me for services rendered. I understand that I am financially responsible for all charges whether or not paid by insurance. I hereby authorize the doctor to release all information necessary to secure the payment of benefits. I authorize the use of this signature on all insurance submissions.

_____   _____   _____
   Responsible Party Signature   Relationship   Date

ORDER# 58-8426 • © 1996 BIBBERO SYSTEMS, INC. • PETALUMA, CALIFORNIA • TO REORDER CALL TOLL FREE: (800) 242-9330

➤ **Figure 10–5** New patient information sheet (Courtesy of Bibbero Systems, Inc., Petaluma, California, (800) 272-2376; Fax (800) 242-9330; www.bibbero.com.)

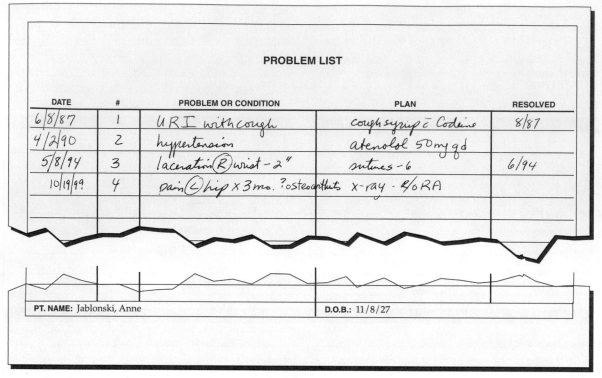

PROBLEM LIST

DATE	#	PROBLEM OR CONDITION	PLAN	RESOLVED
6/8/87	1	URI with cough	cough syrup c̄ Codeine	8/87
4/2/90	2	hypertension	atenolol 50mg qd	
5/8/94	3	laceration (R) wrist - 2"	sutures - 6	6/94
10/19/99	4	pain (L) hip x 3 mo. ?osteoarthritis	x-ray - R/O RA	

PT. NAME: Jablonski, Anne   D.O.B.: 11/8/27

➤ **Figure 10–6** Problem list.

doctor can see the pattern of the child's growth at a glance, because all the data is in one place. Other examples of flow charts are records of blood pressure or lab tests, such as blood sugar for a diabetic. Although there are several different kinds of flow charts, they all provide information over time on a single sheet. Figure 10–7 is a completed growth chart.

Progress Notes

Progress notes are ongoing records of patient visits. One or two sheets are used for a new record. The notes may be written in SOAP format or in a narrative that summarizes the patient visit.

Diagnostic Test Results

Diagnostic test reports, such as electrocardiogram, X-ray reports, and ultrasound reports, may be kept together in a section for tests or different types of tests may be in different sections. All test results should be initialed by a doctor before being filed.

Laboratory Reports

Lab test reports are usually filed in a format called shingling, in which several lab reports can be mounted on the same sheet. The oldest test is on the bottom, the most recent on top. Figure 10–8 shows a lab report form. Place a blank lab report form in a new chart.

Hospital Reports

A separate section of the medical record is reserved for surgical reports and discharge summaries from hospitals.

Consultation Reports

When a patient is seen by a specialist, the specialist sends a brief report of the visit to the patient's primary care doctor. In the case of surgery for a medical problem that is being taken care of by a specialist, the surgeon's consultation report and the operation report will go both to the primary care doctor and the specialist.

Correspondence

The file may contain one or more miscellaneous correspondences, either to the patient from the doctor or to the doctor from the patient.

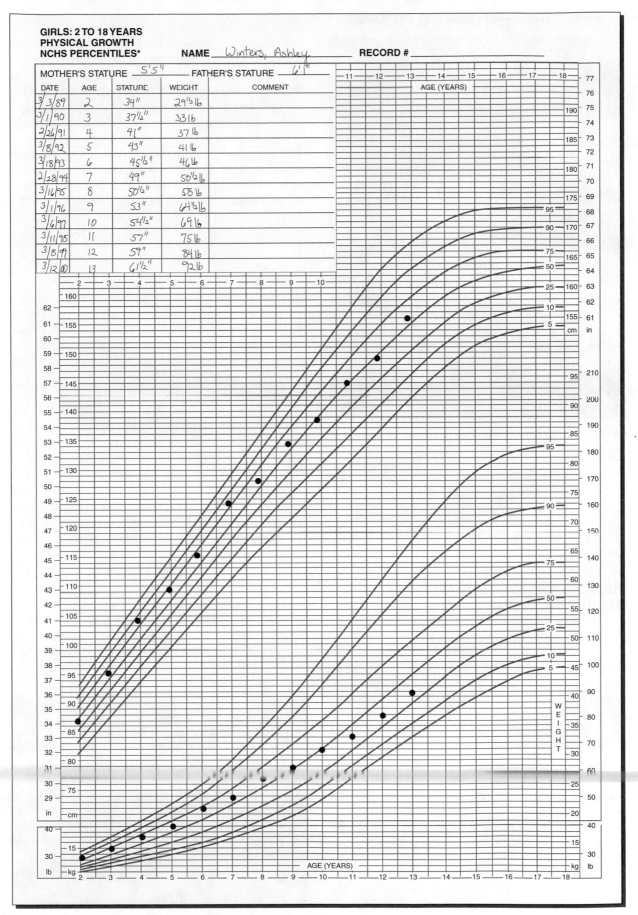

GIRLS: 2 TO 18 YEARS
PHYSICAL GROWTH
NCHS PERCENTILES*   NAME __Winters, Ashley__   RECORD # _____

MOTHER'S STATURE __5'5"__ FATHER'S STATURE __6'1"__

DATE	AGE	STATURE	WEIGHT	COMMENT
3/3/89	2	34"	29½ lb	
3/1/90	3	37½"	33 lb	
2/26/91	4	41"	37 lb	
3/8/92	5	43"	41 lb	
3/18/93	6	45½"	46 lb	
2/28/94	7	49"	50½ lb	
3/16/95	8	50½"	58 lb	
3/1/96	9	53"	64½ lb	
3/6/97	10	54½"	69 lb	
3/11/98	11	57"	75 lb	
3/8/99	12	59"	84 lb	
3/12/00	13	61½"	92 lb	

➤ **Figure 10–7** Completed growth chart shows data about the height and weight of a child over time. Used with permission of Ross Products Division, Abbott Laboratories, Columbus, OH 43216. From NCHS Growth Charts, © 1986 Ross Products Division, Abbott Laboratories.

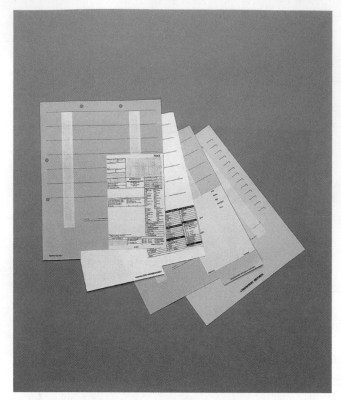

> **Figure 10–8** Lab reports are often mounted one above the other so the most recent is visible on top. (Courtesy of Bibbero Systems, Inc., Petaluma, California, (800) 272-2376; Fax (800) 242-9330; www.bibbero.com.)

RETRIEVING OR FILING A MEDICAL RECORD

Equipment and Supplies

Medical records are kept in various types of file cabinets, including standard drawer files that pull out, lateral files (the drawer holds files side to side and two deep), or shelf files (the files are stored side to side and are retrieved from the side). The door to a shelf file system can be used as a countertop on which to view or work on the file. Large offices may even use an automated system, which stores more records and brings the record to the operator, or may keep files in a separate room.

Whatever type of file cabinet is used, it should always be of heavy construction, with proper weighting on the bottom so that if a top drawer is pulled out the cabinet does not tip over. The file drawer runners should be heavy gauge, and should contain a center trough in which file dividers can be placed. The file cabinet should have a locking system, or the room where the files are kept should be able to be locked.

Figure 10–9 shows a lateral file system.

In addition to the records to be filed, some other equipment is frequently used. **Guides** (heavy sheets made of pressboard or plastic, with tabs) may be used to separate folders into sections. The guides may have tabs with letters, numbers, or words to identify the various sections.

These tabs should extend beyond the file folder, so that they can be seen easily. **Out guides,** shown in Figure 10–10, are placed in the file to mark the place where a folder has been removed. They usually have a pocket to insert a card to indicate who checked out the record.

Color Coding

A variety of file labeling systems are available that use colored labels printed with letter or numbers and/or folders. Such a system is used so that a misfiled chart stands out from its neighbors because the colors are incorrect. Such a system also allows a person filing a record to quickly find the proper area for filing.

If you are ordering supplies for the office, make sure you order new labels that are compatible with the system already in use. Figure 10–11 shows color-coded labels and sample folders.

If the office uses an alphabetic system, several colors may be used; a given color may be used more than once. The letters of the alphabet are printed on labels, and the first two or three letters of the first filing unit (usually the patient's last name) are coded on the edge of the folder. If a numeric system is used, each number has a different color, and labels for some or all of the numbers are placed on the edge of each patient folder.

Basic Guidelines for Filing

The purpose of a filing system is to organize records so that one individual record can be efficiently located.

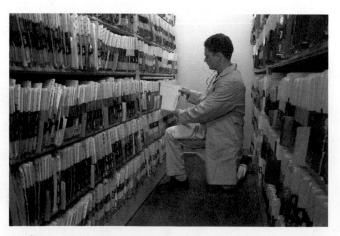

> **Figure 10–9** Lateral file system; numeric filing system using three colored labels on each record.

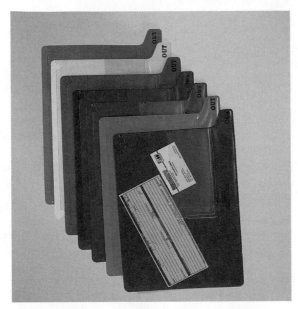

> **Figure 10–10** Out guides. (Courtesy of Bibbero Systems, Inc., Petaluma, California, (800) 272-2376; Fax (800) 242-9330.)

In both systems, it is necessary to identify and agree on a method of filing. This is done by identifying and ordering **indexing units,** or pieces of information used to identify the correct filing location.

Alphabetic

This method of filing uses legal names as the basis. When used for patient records, the files are arranged alphabetically, using standard rules. Each part of the name is considered a filing unit. The records are arranged alphabetically based on the first unit.

All units that have exactly the same first unit are then arranged by the second unit, then the third unit, etc. Unusual names or unclear names (unclear which is the surname [last name]) may be **cross-indexed.** To cross-index means to file under one unit and to file a guide or card referring to the primary filing location under another unit.

Rule 1: Individual Names

In a person's name, the surname (last name) is the first unit, the given name (first name) is the second unit, and the middle name or middle initial is the third unit. A name with only two units is filed before a name with three units. A unit with only an initial is filed before a unit with a full name beginning with that initial. Business names are indexed in the order of the names in the business (excluding "a," "an," and "the").

Example:

Unit 1	Unit 2	Unit 3
Stede	Mary	Ann
Stedman	Alan	
Stedman	Alan	C.
Stedman	Alan	Charles
Stedman	Medical	Supply
Stedson	Craig	H.

Rule 2: Prefixes

If the last name has a prefix, such as Mc, Mac, Van, de, Des, or D', the prefix is considered part of the last name. Therefore, it begins the first indexing unit. Mc

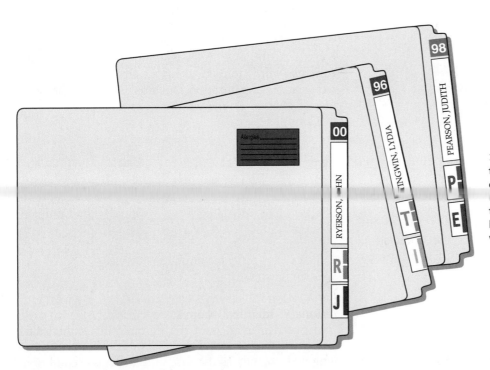

> **Figure 10–11** Color labels facilitate filing. In an alphabetic system, one label indicates the first letter of the last name, and another indicates the first letter of the first name; labels for the year of the patient's last visit are also color-coded.

and Mac may be filed in regular order, or either or both may be grouped separate from the M's.

Example:

Name	Unit 1	Unit 2	Unit 3
Lyndon A. De Larosa	Delarosa	Lyndon	A.
Stephen P. Dennis	Dennis	Stephen	P.
Mary Ann D'Entremont	Dentremont	Mary	Ann
Joanne McCarthy	Mccarthy	Joanne	
John Vanderbilt	Vanderbilt	John	
Joel P. van Twisk	Vantwisk	Joel	P.

Rule 3: Abbreviations and Nicknames

Abbreviated names are filed as if the name were written in full. If a nickname is used on the record, it is indexed as if it were the legal name (often it is). If abbreviation is part of the last name (such as St., which is indexed as Saint), it is part of the first indexing unit. Acronyms or initials in business names are indexed as one unit.

Example:

Name	Unit 1	Unit 2	Unit 3
Alex M. St. Croix	Saintcroix	Alex	M.
Dottie A. Settland	Settland	Dottie	A.
SSI Transport Service	SSI	Transport	Service
Jas. Charles Ryan	Ryan	James	Charles
Wm. van der Post	Vanderpost	William	

Rule 4: Hyphenation

Hyphenated names are indexed as one unit, whether first names, last names, or names of children using both parents' last names.

Example:

Name	Unit 1	Unit 2	Unit 3
Eustace F. Brightfellow	Brightfellow	Eustace	F.
Claire Bryant-Litson	Bryantlitson	Claire	
Annabelle Smith	Smith	Annabelle	
Ann-Marie Smith	Smith	Annmarie	

Rule 5: Titles

Disregard titles unless the complete name is not given. Seniority terms, such as Jr., may be indexed as the last unit. Numeric seniority terms are indexed in numerical order before alphabetical terms. If a male child has exactly the same name as his father, he is called "Jr." until his father dies. He is a "III" if his father is a "Jr." In this case, he has the exact same name as his father and his grandfather. If he is named exactly for his grandfather, who is still living, but not for his father, he is called "II."

Example:

Name	Unit 1	Unit 2	Unit 3
Samuel Jolson Jr.	Jolson	Samuel	Jr.
Samuel Jolson Sr.	Jolson	Samuel	Sr.
Dr. Patricia A. Roy	Roy	Patricia	A.

Rule 6: Marriage

A married woman may take her husband's surname, but she retains her own first and middle names. Her legal name may be:

1. Her own first and middle names, and her husband's surname
2. Her own first name, her family's surname as middle name (her maiden name), and her husband's surname
3. Her own first name, middle name, and her family's surname.

Sometimes her married surname is formed by hyphenating her family's surname and her husband's surname, or the hyphenated surname may be reserved for the couple's children with the woman using either the second or third option above.

Example:

Name	Unit 1	Unit 2	Unit 3
Mrs. Arlene Sandra Trim	Trim	Arlene	Sandra
Mrs. Joan Walker Trim	Trim	Joan	Walker
Mrs. Ann Walker	Walker	Ann	
Mrs. Ann R. Walker	Walker	Ann	R.
Mrs. Diane A. Walker-Trim	Walkertrim	Diane	A.

Rule 7: Companies and Businesses

The names of companies and businesses are indexed in the same order as written. Numbers are indexed as though written out and are filed as one unit. Disregard punctuation such as commas, apostrophes, or hyphens. Disregard articles such as *a*, *an*, and *the*. Disregard prepositions such as *up* and *out*, and conjunctions, such as *isn't* or *didn't*. In a name that begins with *the*, such as The New York Times Company, *the* must be considered the final indexing unit. When indexing **acronyms** (words formed using the first letters of all the words in an organization, such as NYNEX), the acronym is indexed as one word.

Example:

Company Name	Unit 1	Unit 2	Unit 3
Edson's Pharmacy	Edsons	Pharmacy	
The Redline Supply Company	Redline	Supply	Company (The)
Rent-A-Computer Service	Rentacomputer	Service	

Rule 8: Identical Names

If two names are exactly the same, index them first under the name, and then under the location, beginning with the city as the first unit, state as second unit, street as third unit, and street number from lowest to highest. This applies to names of patients and businesses.

Example:

Name	Unit 1	Unit 2	Unit 3
Finedrug Pharmacy	Reading	MA	Salem30
Finedrug Pharmacy	Reading	MA	Salem120
Finedrug Pharmacy	Wakefield	MA	Main280
Jones William M.	Lansing	MI	Hillcrest30
Jones William M.	Lansing	MI	Hinsdale85

Numeric or Alphanumeric

In many practices, patients are given numbers. There are two major advantages to a numeric system:

1. It is easier to preserve confidentiality.
2. In a large practice, it is easier to deal with a number of patients who have the same surname.

This method works much better in offices that have computerized their records. If the practice uses paper-based files, a separate file is required to cross-reference the name and number.

In consecutive filing systems, numbers are arranged and filed from the lowest to the highest. In such a system, zeroes are assigned or assumed as the first unit, so that each number has the same number of digits.

Example:

Number	Unit 1	Unit 2	Unit 3	Unit 4	Unit 5
02642	0	2	6	4	2
11853	1	1	8	5	3

In nonconsecutive filing systems, numbers are arranged in groups (such as Social Security numbers). Each group of numbers is considered a unit, with the final or terminal group filed as unit 1. This filing method is also called **terminal digit filing.**

With terminal digit filing, index the numbers by group, working back from the final to the first group. Then arrange the numbers from lowest to highest within each group. The advantage of nonconsecutive filing is that it mixes up active and inactive records in a large institution, so everyone is not trying to file in the area of most recently assigned numbers.

Examples:

Using terminal groups of two digits:

Number	Unit 1	Unit 2	Unit 3
89-25-68	68	25	89
48-31-69	69	31	48
48-35-69	69	35	48

Using uneven groups arranged like Social Security numbers:

Number	Unit 1	Unit 2	Unit 3
894-63-3925	3925	63	894
618-52-4880	4880	52	618
781-52-4880	4880	52	781
527-63-4880	4880	63	527
017-30-5945	5945	30	017

Another way to provide nonconsecutive filing is to assign each patient a combination of both letters and numbers. The records are then filed under the letters alphabetically, followed by the numbers, using one of the systems described above. The letters may be used to group patients in several ways (i.e., by which doctor in the group primarily sees the patient, by specialty, by insurance carrier, and so on).

Subject

Filing systems for documents (such as invoices, purchase orders, and service agreements) are arranged according to subject. With the subject category, documents may be arranged alphabetically or chronologically. In the medical office, subject filing is often used for insurance, bills, research, or other documents related to running the practice rather than the patient records.

Chronological

A chronological record is a record using dates, such as appointment records or a **tickler file,** which is a special file used to remind people about things that need to happen at a future time. Reports within the patient record are filed in reverse chronological order in each section.

Tickler Files

A tickler file is a reminder system. You can set up a tickler file in the computer or you can create a paper-based tickler file using a calendar, index cards, or file folder.

Each time you notice a need to do something on a certain date, make an entry in the tickler file on that date. The entry in the tickler file should contain:

1. Date for the action to be taken
2. Type of action to be taken (for example, send a reminder about a checkup visit)
3. Other information needed to take the action, such as the patient's name, address, and telephone number.

Procedure 10–2 takes you through the details of creating a tickler file.

PROCEDURE 10-2

Setting Up a Tickler File

Performance Objective: The student will prepare a monthly tickler file.

Supplies and Equipment: 12 file folders or dividers for an index card storage box, 12 labels, pen or typewriter, paper or index cards.

Procedure Steps

1. Type and label folders for each month. With this file you will be able to work for 1 year in advance. For a smaller file, type and label 12 dividers for an index card storage box.
   Rationale: The folders allow you to file reminders for the next 12 months in the appropriate folder.

2. Place upcoming responsibilities on separate pieces of paper or separate index cards. Each piece of paper or index card should contain a task or responsibility, a description of activities to complete it, a date to begin work on it, and a date for final completion.
   Rationale: Separate sheets facilitate filing and making notes.

3. Sort the sheets by month and file chronologically in the appropriate folders. If using index cards, arrange in the same way and file in the appropriate section of the storage box.
   Rationale: Each month it is easy to identify tasks which must be begun and/or completed.

4. At the beginning of a month, organize all activities for that month in chronological order. Many people use an expanding folder with 31 pockets and check the file each day. If you make your notes on index cards, you can use an additional index card storage box with 31 numbered dividers for the current month. If your file does not contain daily activities, you can keep all pages in the monthly folder and check it weekly.
   Rationale: The purpose of the file is to remind you of activities you must set it up so it will be most helpful to you.

5. When activities are completed, discard the sheets. At the end of the month move the empty folder to the back of the stack and move on to the next month.

Retrieving Patient Records

A patient record has to be removed from its proper location in the file whenever someone in the office wants to look at it (i.e., for an appointment or when a patient leaves a message).

The record is located using the filing guidelines of the particular office. If an alphabetic system is used, find the areas in record storage where the patient's last name is stored, then the first name and, if necessary, the middle initial. Medical records needed for patients with appointments on a particular day are usually pulled the afternoon before the appointments using the printed appointment list. Then they are arranged by appointment time, with the record of the patient with the earliest appointment on top. Each time a record is taken from storage, an out guide is placed exactly where the record was removed, as illustrated in Figure 10-12.

The person removing the record fills in a card with the name or number on the record and the name of the person who will have the record. Although it seems cumbersome to fill in a card for every record removed, in the long run it is much less frustrating

than searching the entire office for a record when the patient is in the waiting room.

Filing Reports and Correspondence

All reports, letters, and other materials that come into the office should be reviewed by the doctor, initialed, and then filed in the patient record. A date stamp is often used to identify exactly when a report or letter was received. There is no end to the filing, and when there is a time crunch, it is the last thing to get done. Sometimes doctors even come into the office on the weekend to go through these mountains of paper. Because of this, there is often a stack of material to be filed, especially on Monday.

Filing goes quicker when you follow these six steps, which are described in detail in Procedure 10-3:

1. Remove all clips, pins, or other extraneous material; tape any tears and punch holes as necessary.
2. Make sure the doctor has initialed every report.
3. Sort the reports alphabetically or numerically using the sorter.

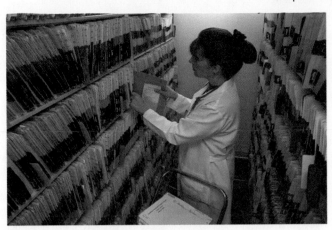

> **Figure 10–12** Placing an out guide.

4. Take all the material for one patient, find the patient's record, and file the material in the correct places in the patient's file.
5. Put the record back together if necessary.
6. If the record is not in the files, place the report back in the sorter, or in the out guide pocket.

Filing Records

Each day, several records need to be returned to the file. First be sure that the doctor or other person who has seen the patient is finished with the record. In most offices, records ready for filing are placed in one location. See Procedure 10–4 for details about filing.

PROCEDURE 10–3

Filing Reports or Other Material in a Patient Record

Performance Objective: The student will condition and file reports, correspondence, and other material in a patient record.

Supplies and Equipment: Medical records of established patients, assorted reports, letters or other material to be filed, hole punch, tape, stapler, sorter.

Procedure Steps

1. Assemble materials to be filed and necessary supplies to assist in the filing process.
2. Condition the material to be filed. To condition means to remove extraneous materials such as paper clips or pins, to mend any tears with tape, and to staple related pages together. Punch holes if necessary.
   Rationale: Preparation before filing allows all materials in the record to be maintained in good condition.
3. Verify that each report is ready to be filed. In most offices the doctors initial reports after they have seen them. If the doctors initials are missing, the report should go back to him or her.
   Rationale: The doctor must see each report that comes to the medical office. A procedure verifying that the doctor has seen it before filing prevents reports from being accidentally overlooked.
4. Sort the reports using the sorter alphabetically or numerically, depending on the filing system. Sort by letters, numbers, or number groups first, then sort within each letter or number group.
   Rationale: Even in a small office large numbers of reports need to be filed in patient records. It is more efficient to file in order, especially since some patients have more than one report to be filed.
5. Take all reports for a particular patient, find the correct record, and insert the report(s) into the record in the correct location. In any section, reports are filed chronologically with the most recent reports at the front of the section. When several reports are shingled on a page, the oldest report goes at the bottom with newer reports progressing up the page and in front of the older reports. You may need to place a divider in the record if you are filing the first report in a given section.
   Rationale: There are usually several sections within the record in a specific order. Reports need to be in the correct section to be easily located.
6. Put the record back together if necessary and refile.
   Rationale: It is easier to file records in the wrong record when several records are out.
7. If the record is not in the file, place the report back in the sorter or in the pocket of the outguide.
   Rationale: It is more efficient to file reports in records you can find easily than to hunt for records just to file reports.

Measures to Ensure Accuracy or Locate Misplaced Records

These seven steps can ensure accuracy in filing or locating a misplaced record. A missing record creates multiple problems; working carefully can help avoid lost records.

1. Work slowly and carefully when filing records.
2. Use out guides, and always note where the record has gone.
3. Return records to storage. Do not just pass a record to someone else in the office. If you do, your out guide will be wrong. If you do not refile the record, update the out guide.
4. Discourage doctors or other personnel from hoarding records. Encourage them to finish their dictation each day, review lab reports, and sign off on them. Take action on records as needed.
5. Encourage office personnel to keep records in orderly piles. When you are looking for a record, identify the color code you are looking for and scan the piles for possible matches.
6. Always remove misfiled records from the files when you notice them; then file them correctly.
7. Keep lists of "missing" records, and be alert to find them in unexpected places. After all measures to locate a missing record have been taken, it may be necessary to create a second record for a patient. This would create a difficult situation in the event of a lawsuit.

STORING MEDICAL RECORDS

Records should be stored using the principle that the more likely you are to need it, the closer it should be.

Active Records

Active records—of patients who have been seen within the past 2 to 5 years, depending on the practice—are stored in the office, in the active patient filing system, as described above.

PROCEDURE 10–4

Filing Patient Records

Performance Objective: The student will file patient records correctly.
Supplies and Equipment: Patient records, file cabinet.

Procedure Steps

1. Gather the records that are ready to be filed and remove any elastic bands or paper clips.
   Rationale: Paper clips, elastic bands, and so on prevent the record from sliding easily in and out of the file.
2. Check the records to be sure that no loose sheets of paper are present. If loose sheets are found, insert them in the record (see Procedure 10–3, Filing Reports or Other Material in a Patient Record).
   Rationale: Until reports or other papers are permanently filed into the record, they can easily fall out and be lost or misplaced.
3. Sort the records according to the indexing units of the file system used in your office. For example, if an alphabetic system is used, arrange the records alphabetically by last name.

Rationale: It is more efficient to file records in order, especially if you have many records to file.
4. Find the correct location in the file, pull the out guide halfway out, slide the record in front of the out guide in the correct location in the file, and finish removing the out guide. If your office does not use out guides, use your hand to make a space between the record before and the record after the one you are filing.
   Rationale: You must remove the out guide every time you file a record.
5. Remove the index card that showed who had the record from the out guide and place the out guide with other unused out guides. Some offices keep index cards for the doctors in separate boxes so that new cards do not need to be written; some offices cross out the name and reuse the index cards; some offices use slips of paper that are discarded after each use.
   Rationale: If stored out guides are empty, they cannot contain misleading information.

Inactive Records

Inactive records—of patients who have not been seen within the time period specified by the practice—are usually kept in the office in closed storage. If there is not enough space in the office to store inactive records, they are sometimes stored at a doctor's home, in a storage room in the office or clinic, or in rented storage space.

In some practices, a patient who has not been seen in more than 5 years is treated as if he or she were a new patient and is given a new record. However, the old record may still need to be consulted. At regular intervals (usually once a year), inactive files are removed from the active file area by pulling all records with the inactive-year sticker. For instance, at the end of 2000, most doctors will remove from their active files any patient record with a last-year sticker for 1996.

Retention of Records

The length of time that a medical record must be retained is difficult to determine. Each state has a law limiting the time period for beginning a lawsuit for malpractice. This is known as the **statute of limitations** for medical malpractice. In most states, the statute of limitations for medical malpractice is 2 or 3 years.

Normally the period begins at the time the alleged incident of malpractice took place or when a person should have discovered the incident (if it is not immediately obvious). For example, in the case of a surgery in which a metal clamp was left in the patient, the time begins when the patient finds the clamp.

But there are exceptions. For instance, in the case of children who suffered birth injuries, most states begin the statute of limitations from the time when a diagnosis is made that the child's disability may have been caused at birth. When a child reaches age 18, he or she also has the opportunity to see his or her medical record.

For these reasons, doctors need to retain even inactive files for many years. Most doctors retain their medical records indefinitely. Records that are closed (it is known that the patient will not return) and records inactive longer than 7 years may be transferred to microfilm or microfiche. They can also be copied using a laser beam and stored on laser disks. These options are expensive and time consuming, but may be worthwhile for larger practices.

Other records that should be kept indefinitely, are insurance policies, licenses, and Drug Enforcement Administration (DEA) controlled-substance records. All tax records should also be kept for 7 years; after that, background records used to determine taxes can be destroyed, but copies of tax forms should be kept indefinitely.

Storing Computerized Records

Many offices keep medical records on computer. This simplifies storage, because inactive records can be transferred to tape storage or packed files. Precautions must be taken to prevent access to both active and inactive records by unauthorized individuals. In addition, records should be regularly backed up and a copy stored off-site.

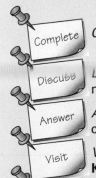

STUDENT STUDY PLAN

To reinforce your understanding of the material in this chapter . . .

Complete — *Complete* the **Review & Recall** questions below.

Discuss — *Discuss* the situation in **If You Were the Medical Assistant** with your classmates, and answer the questions.

Answer — *Answer* the **Critical Thinking Questions** below, and discuss them with your classmates.

Visit — *Visit* **Web sites** suggested below and search for additional Web sites using the **Keywords for Internet Searches**.

Complete — *Complete* the exercises in chapter 10 of the **Student Mastery Manual**.

REVIEW & RECALL

1. Compare and contrast the arrangement of the medical record using the problem-oriented medical record and the source-oriented medical record.
2. Describe the four parts of a SOAP progress note.
3. Identify the proper form for documenting in the patient's medical record.
4. How should a correction be made in the medical record? Why is it important that the incorrect information be visible and not completely obscured?
5. List eight different types of reports that are filed in the medical record.
6. Identify some common methods of storing records.
7. Compare and contrast the advantages and disadvantages of alphabetic and numeric filing systems.
8. Describe two different methods of numeric filing.
9. How is the medical record prepared for filing?
10. Why are active and inactive medical records often stored in different places?
11. How long should health care facilities retain medical records? Why?

IF YOU WERE THE MEDICAL ASSISTANT

1. Arrange the following list of names in correct order for filing, using an alphabetic filing system.

   Mrs. Elaine F. Salisbury
   Dr. Peter E. Salcer
   Peter E. Salcer Jr.
   Reginald St. Croix
   Gerald R. Salisbury-Williams
   Ruth Jones Santis
   Mrs. Sandra B. Sanderson
   Annette May Sanderson
   Joan Sanders
   Ryan T. Sandelman

2. Arrange the following list of medical record numbers in the correct order for filing, using terminal groups of two numbers.

   01-64-22
   72-55-20
   44-41-20
   17-41-20
   56-42-21
   91-88-21
   15-24-22
   82-49-20
   08-94-21
   24-42-22

CRITICAL THINKING QUESTIONS

1. If a medical record is not found in the correct place in the file, what are at least four ways you could try to locate it?
2. Describe appropriate filing systems for each of the following: a list of telephone numbers, a list of e-mail addresses, 20 bank statements, all of your mother's favorite recipes, your personal library of books and magazines, the procedures in a procedure manual, and your notes from all medical assisting classes.
3. Discuss the advantages and disadvantages of the problem-oriented medical record. Why do you think many offices use it primarily for progress notes instead of for the entire record?
4. Discuss methods to maintain confidentiality when storing papers and electronic medical records.

EXPLORE THE WEB

INTERNET WEB SITES

American Health Information Management Association
www.ahima.org

Medical Records Institute
www.medrecinst.com

KEYWORDS FOR INTERNET SEARCHES

health records systems
  medical records
  medical records privacy
  medical records software
  POMR
  tickler files

Chapter 11

Maintaining the Medical Office

Instructional Objectives

After completing this chapter, you will be able to do the following:

1. Define and spell the vocabulary words for this chapter.
2. List the equipment and supplies needed in various areas of the medical office.
3. Describe routine maintenance activities in the medical office.
4. Identify five methods of fire protection for the medical office and its records.
5. Describe an efficient system of maintaining equipment inventory lists and operator manuals.
6. Compare service contracts to service calls for equipment in the medical office.
7. Describe the process of obtaining new equipment.
8. Explain what is necessary for an effective office security system.
9. Explain procedures for taking inventory, ordering, receiving, and storing supplies.
10. Describe how incident reports should be used to protect the medical office.
11. List types of liability protection for doctors, the medical office, and medical assistants.
12. Describe the various components of risk management in the medical office.
13. Identify the components of a quality improvement plan.

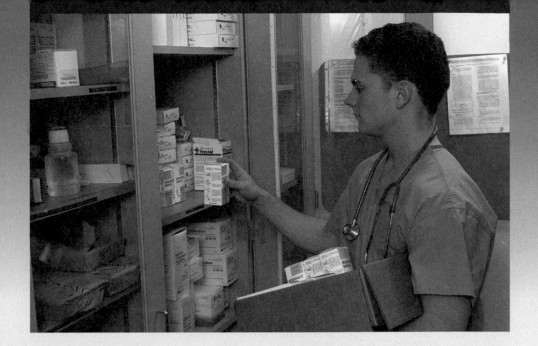

- Understand legal guidelines and requirements for health care
- Manage the health care facility
- Perform risk management procedures

- Perform an inventory of supplies and equipment
- Perform routine maintenance of administrative and clinical equipment

Performance Objectives

After completing this chapter, you will be able to do the following:

1. Take a supply inventory (Procedure 11–1).
2. Stock supply cabinets and dispose of expired supplies (Procedure 11–2).
3. Prepare a purchase order (Procedure 11–3).

VOCABULARY

back order (p. 195)   Mayo stand (p. 187)   reorder point (p. 192)   service contract (p. 191)
inventory (p. 190)   purchase order (PO) (p. 195) risk management (p. 195)   vendor (p. 195)

ABBREVIATIONS

CQI (p. 198)   PO (p. 195)   TQM (p. 198)

THE OFFICE ENVIRONMENT

In many medical practices, a medical assistant acts as the office administrator. Office administration entails a number of activities regarding maintenance of equipment and supplies. Much of this maintenance is not performed by office staff, but rather by contractors; thus, office administration involves managing the relationship between the office and contractors or vendors of services, as well as medical, pharmaceutical, and office supply companies.

The Administrative Area

A medical assistant acting as receptionist must be able to effectively and efficiently answer two or three calls coming in quickly, as well as to greet patients and handle paperwork. To do this, the reception area needs to be stocked with:

message pads
each doctor's appointment book or the office's master schedule
reminder cards for follow-up appointments
pens and pencils
date stamp
stapler.

Depending on the size of the administrative staff, the receptionist may also handle office correspondence and billing. In addition to the telephone (discussed in detail in chapter 7), the reception area usually contains a personal computer or terminal attached to the office's computer network and may contain a calculator or adding machine. Materials for creating new patient folders should be at hand, including:

folders
labels
patient information forms
consent forms
other forms used in the medical record
paper
pens.

If the receptionist also does office correspondence, the area will also have stationery and envelopes. If the receptionist also handles billing, billing forms and coding reference books will also be kept at the receptionist's station.

The administrative area needs to have enough room to perform the required activities without the patient files and other papers becoming mixed up and it must also allow you to maintain patient confidentiality. See Figure 11–1.

Again, depending on the size of the office, business operations will either take place in the front office close to the reception area or in a separate area in the office. In the business office are the rest of the pieces of equipment necessary for administering the office, including the photocopy machine, fax machine, and postage meter/electronic mailing system. In some offices, an all-in-one printer/copier/fax is used.

Patient billing records are available either in hardcopy files in the business office or on the computer. If computers are used to print encounter forms or bills, the printer is usually a dot-matrix type, with the ability to handle continuous-feed forms, which have little holes along each side and ride along a tractor.

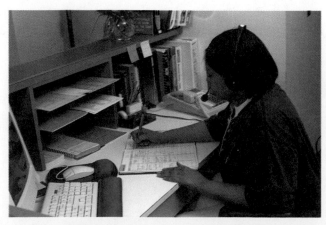

➤ **Figure 11–1** Well-organized front office.

Whoever is responsible for the business office is also responsible for the maintenance of the equipment. This person should be familiar not only with the equipment's operation, but also with the maintenance responsibilities, such as reloading paper and adding toner or printer cartridges, as well as the maintenance agreements and when to call for maintenance or repair.

Generally, the administrative area needs about 76 to 100 square feet of floor space for every desk in the space. This allows room for a wastebasket and wastepaper-recycling bin for each desk, as well as for the necessary file cabinets and other supply cabinets necessary. (One hundred square feet is an area about 10 feet by 10 feet, or 12 feet by 8 feet.)

Many offices also have a paper shredder for disposing of confidential documents. Although medical records must be maintained indefinitely, old telephone logs, old payroll records, canceled checks more than 7 years old, and minutes of practice management meetings should all be shredded rather than simply thrown away in the wastebasket or in a wastepaper-recycling bin. Shredded paper can still be recycled, and there is no danger that sensitive personal or business information will be seen by anyone who should not have access to it.

Examination and Treatment Rooms

Each examination or treatment room also needs approximately 100 square feet of floor space to hold an examination or treatment table, cabinets and countertop, patient chair and doctor stool, and a small surface for the doctor to write on. The room should be laid out so a doctor and a medical assistant can move freely about the room. Equipment and supplies should be within easy reach or stored in drawers or cabinets easy to get to.

Each exam or treatment room needs to have a sink, as well as soap and paper towel dispensers. Each has three waste containers: a regular wastebasket; a rigid container for the disposal of sharps such as needles, scalpel blades, or other dangerous objects that are used once and discarded; and another container for biohazards, materials that contain body fluids such as blood, mucus, or pus. Containers for hazardous waste must be covered, except when adding waste. A foot pedal to open the cover facilitates use.

Usually, each exam room, whether or not treatments and procedures are performed there, has a blood pressure cuff and gauge (sphygmomanometer), which is often attached to the wall; an otoscope/ophthalmoscope for ear and eye examinations, also often attached to the wall, with a supply of disposable ear pieces; and glass or metal containers for items such as Band-Aids, tongue blades, gauze, alcohol wipes, and cotton swabs.

Cabinets and drawers contain a host of other items. Patient gowns, drape sheets, and exam-table paper are stored in each exam room, usually in drawers or the cabinet part of the exam table.

If treatments and procedures are conducted in the room, instruments also need to be stored in the room. Equipment such as an electrocardiograph or a flexible sigmoidoscope may also stay in the room in which those procedures are performed.

A Mayo stand should be available to hold the particular instruments used in a procedure. A **Mayo stand** is a small table with a removable tray top which can be positioned beside the patient or over the patient's legs. If procedures are being performed, overhead lighting needs to be supplemented by one or more gooseneck lamps or a light source that can be attached to instruments or the doctor's head. If vital signs are not taken in a patient preparation area, each exam room must also have a scale.

If doctors in the practice dictate their patient notes, a dictation machine may be in each exam room, or each doctor may have a portable tape recorder in his or her office for dictation.

Finally, each exam room needs at least a small space for writing and for storing one or two reference books.

In addition, examination/treatment rooms in a pediatric office or a family practice office that has a lot of young patients will also have children's books and plastic toys available. These are used both as a way to occupy a child while a doctor is talking to a parent and as tools to aid the doctor in testing the child's motor skills and developmental stage.

For safety reasons, exam rooms should not contain syringes, needles, or medication samples. Cleaning materials and chemical solutions should never be stored under the counter in an exam room, especially if it is used for children.

Exam tables have an adjustable back that can be raised and an extension that can be pulled out to support the legs. The patient usually sits on the end to begin the examination and is instructed to move into various positions during the exam. The table has drawers or cabinets on the side to store gowns and drapes, as well as drawers at the end to store supplies used during the exam, especially supplies for a Pap test. Standard exam tables have a pull-out step under the drawers at the end. The table is covered with paper from a roll, which is changed between patients. Modern exam tables are electrically powered so the back, foot, or entire table can be raised or lowered by pressing various buttons.

Treatment tables are full-length and the backs usually are not adjustable. They have open storage on a shelf under the table. Treatment tables are used in the exam rooms of many pediatricians and orthopedic surgeons, and in the treatment rooms of other doctors. They are also covered with paper from a roll, which is changed between patients.

Examination/treatment rooms in surgeons' offices or family practice offices where minor surgical procedures are performed will also have an operating table and surgical lighting, a Mayo stand on wheels, and specimen collection jars. Just outside this room there may be a small scrub room with a special surgical scrub sink.

Waiting Room

The waiting room makes a first impression on a new patient. It must be neat and welcoming. The waiting room needs two to four chairs for each doctor in the office at one time, current magazines, and a table or magazine stand to hold them. If the practice sees children, some toys should be available in a separate play area. One person should be assigned to tidy up the waiting room a couple of times during the day.

A waiting room should have signs that inform patients about office policies. Common signs include:

No Smoking.
Co-payments are expected at the time of service, (or some other language regarding the expectation of payment).
Credit cards that are accepted.
No eating or drinking.

Some offices have a display rack with health information brochures. A number of companies produce patient-education materials that they "brand" with the office's logo or the doctor's name.

Sometimes there is a television and videocassette recorder in the waiting room. In practices that see children, children's videos are often playing. In some practices, health information videos are playing. Other practices have a radio tuned to an easy-listening station, or a CD player with quiet pop or light classical music.

ROUTINE MAINTENANCE

Depending on the size of the office, many if not most routine maintenance activities are undertaken by staff. These include controlling the temperature, cleaning cabinets and drawers, changing light bulbs and replacing batteries in battery-powered equipment, turning the security system on and off, making sure fire protection equipment is in working order, and daily cleaning.

Temperature and Ventilation

The reception area should be kept warmer than working areas. People who are ill are sensitive to cold and drafts. The reception and patient waiting areas should be about 70° to 72° F. The temperature in the exam/treatment rooms and in doctors' offices should be

about 68° to 70°F. A room used for minor surgery can be kept a little cooler, because the doctor and assistant will be wearing gowns, masks, and hair covers.

Ventilation is also important. Keeping air circulating is important both to dissipate odors and to allow germs to escape from the office atmosphere.

General Cleaning

Larger offices may contract for cleaning services, or office cleaning may be included in the monthly rent, especially in buildings that are dedicated to medical offices. Contracted cleaning is usually done one or two times a week, so even if the major cleaning is contracted out daily cleaning tasks still must be performed.

Daily cleaning includes tidying up all areas of the office—reception and waiting rooms, administrative space, doctors' offices, exam and treatment rooms, and the lab.

Sinks should all be toweled dry, and rest rooms should be checked to make sure ample toilet and facial tissue, soap, and paper towels are available. Rest room sinks should be toweled dry, and any spills or puddles on the floor should be mopped up. If these contain urine, feces, or vomitus, they should be treated as a biohazard and cleaned using standard precautions.

Wastebaskets and wastepaper-recycling bins should be checked daily and emptied as necessary. Sharps containers should be checked daily and replaced before they are full, and biohazard baskets should be emptied and rebagged daily. Contracted cleaning services will usually not empty biohazard containers. These should be double-bagged by an office staff member wearing a gown, gloves, and face protection.

If the office staff must do more intense cleaning, this should be done at least weekly. These tasks include mopping linoleum floors and vacuuming carpets, cleaning the glass at the reception area, polishing furniture and accessories, dusting, and thoroughly cleaning the rest rooms.

It is important to try to avoid a "medical smell" in the office. This is done by maintaining proper ventilation, as well as by cleaning up spills and accidents immediately, using light or unscented air fresheners in rest rooms and exam rooms, and keeping disinfectants and cleaning materials closed tightly when not in use and out of patients' reach. The disinfectants used in a medical office must be effective against tuberculosis and human immunodeficiency virus. These will be discussed in chapter 13.

Cleaning Cabinets and Drawers

Storage cabinets, drawers, and bookcases are cleaned less frequently, often on a day when the doctor or some of the doctors in the practice are absent so the room is not in use.

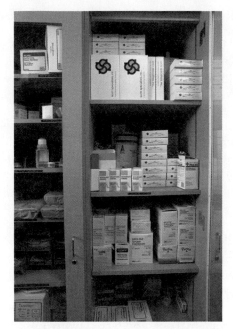

➤ **Figure 11–2** Well-organized supply closet.

Whether cleaning an open set of bookshelves or a closed cabinet with shelving or drawers, the process is essentially the same.

First, if possible, remove all the items from the bookcase or cabinet, and place them on a table. If there are too many items, remove all the items from at least two shelves at a time. Always work from the top of the shelving or cabinet, so that dirt and dust will not fall on shelves that have already been cleaned.

For metal cabinets or shelving, wash the shelf with warm water and soap. Rinse and dry thoroughly. Then dust the items from the shelves and replace them in their proper place. Wooden bookcases should be washed with extreme care, and some will need to be done with furniture cleaner rather than soap and water.

Check labels on all items before putting them back on shelves. Secure labels that are becoming unstuck. Check for the expiration date on supplies and make a list of any items that need to be ordered or restocked from the general supply area to the cabinet. Outdated supplies must be disposed of properly in accordance with information found on Material Safety Data Sheets. Check all instruments for faults; clean and polish them before replacing them on the shelf. See Figure 11–2.

Miscellaneous Tasks

Among the miscellaneous tasks that have to be performed daily by the office staff are rearranging the waiting room chairs and replacing magazines in their racks (as well as toys if toys are available); cleaning mirrors in the rest rooms and exam rooms; and cleaning the tops of cabinets and undersides of towel, tape, and exam paper dispensers. Toys must be cleaned and

disinfected on a regular basis, because they can harbor microorganisms.

The staff is responsible for replacing light bulbs in gooseneck lamps and other special lighting. Ceiling lighting is usually a responsibility of the maintenance staff employed by the building owner; if the space is owned by the practice, this may be a staff responsibility or may be covered by the cleaning/maintenance contract with an outside service.

Security Systems

A medical office maintains a number of different security systems.

First, if the office is entered from a corridor in an office building, the building owner or office condominium association most likely has an electronic security system for the building itself.

Second, regardless of whether the office is entered from a corridor or directly from the outside, the practice should maintain an electronic security system against break-ins to the office itself.

The office's security/safety alarm system is monitored by an alarm company and may or may not also be tied to the local police and fire departments. Whether or not the system is tied into police and fire, the alarm company will call the practice's liaison to the company whenever the alarm goes off.

This designated person is often the practice administrator or "managing partner." However, two or three people are always listed as backups in case the liaison is not available.

Third, various places within the office require another layer of security. Medication cabinets—with all medications and prescription pads inside—should be locked, and a limited number of people should have keys to the medication cabinet lock. The laboratory, doctors' private offices, the medical records cabinet or room, and the business office are other areas that often have a lock and limited access.

If controlled substances are stored in the office, they should be "double-locked"—in a locked drawer within a locked cabinet. Two separate keys should open the two different locks.

Fire Protection

Fire protection for the building is the responsibility of the landlord or office condominium association. But fire protection for the contents of the office is the responsibility of office staff.

Many states require sprinklers in commercial and office buildings. Some states that require sprinklers for larger office buildings do not require them for smaller offices, such as a doctor's office that has been converted from a house.

In addition to the health hazards smoking presents, there are also potential fire hazards related to smoking.

Smoking should not be permitted in a doctor's office, and signs advising patients and visitors that the office is a smoke-free environment should be clearly posted in the waiting area.

Exits should be clearly marked, and if the office is in a multi-office building, an emergency evacuation map should be posted near the door to the waiting room. Lighted exit signs should be tested by shutting off the lights in the room; bulbs should be replaced if necessary.

In a large office or free-standing clinic, there may be fire doors at certain points in corridors. These doors are designed to contain any fire on one side of the door from going into another area of the building. Fire doors should never be propped open but should be allowed to shut to their naturally closed position.

Fire extinguishers should be placed in each room near the exit. These fire extinguishers are important not so much for putting out a fire but for giving a person in the room the ability to clear an exit path. They are placed near the door so the fire does not get between the person and the exit.

Whenever possible, records should be stored in fire-resistant file cabinets. Computer data backup disks should be stored in a fire-resistant file cabinet or fire-resistant box-type safe with a copy at another location.

Smoke detector laws vary by state, in terms of how many must be in an office and where they must be placed. In many buildings, smoke detectors are wired into the building's security and safety alarm system, and are tied to the sprinkler system.

If the office has battery-operated smoke detectors, these should be tested monthly by pressing the test button. Batteries should be changed and the detectors labeled every 6 months.

MAINTAINING EQUIPMENT

Every doctor's office has a number of pieces of equipment, both for medical purposes and for business purposes. The medical assistant who manages the office is responsible for relationship management with the individuals or companies that sell and maintain the equipment, as well as with those who provide supplies for the equipment.

Inventory

An **inventory** of the equipment should be maintained. This inventory lists each piece of equipment, the serial number, the date it was purchased, the length of the warranty, the name of the provider who services it, the manufacturer's suggested service schedule, and the last date of service.

An inventory is important for two reasons.

First, there are tax consequences. The cost of larger pieces of medical and office equipment must be de-ducted from the practice's income over 5 years (called depreciation of the capital purchase); smaller pieces of equipment can be fully deducted as an expense in the year in which they are purchased.

Second, in case of theft or damage, an inventory is necessary to make a complete report to the police and/or claim to the office's insurance company.

Operation manuals for the equipment can either be stored centrally with the inventory list, or each manual can be stored with the piece of equipment it is used for. Many pieces of equipment come with a plastic pouch on the side of the item or storage unit in which manuals and maintenance schedules can be kept.

Monitoring Equipment Function and Readiness for Use

Always be on the lookout for equipment problems, especially problems that could lead to a dangerous situation. Check all instruments when preparing them for sterilization. Look for frayed wires, bent or damaged instruments, and machines that are not functioning properly.

The decision whether to repair or replace a piece of equipment belongs to the office manager. That decision will usually be made taking into account the equipment's age, how expensive a new piece of equipment is, the level of use the equipment gets, and if any important features have been added to newer models of the equipment.

If there is no service contract for the piece of equipment and the decision is made to repair it, a repair service must be located and a repair arranged. The manufacturer usually has a list of authorized repair services by region. In larger organizations, a purchase order is usually necessary for an equipment repair.

Emergency equipment must always be ready for use. Because it may be required only once in a long time, this equipment must be checked at least monthly and more often in many larger facilities. The contents of the emergency box or crash cart (discussed in detail in chapter 31) should be checked for completeness by a designated person, who will initial a form to verify the presence of each item on the checklist.

Oxygen tanks are checked at the same time and are sent to be refilled when the level falls to a predetermined level. Expiration dates of emergency medications are checked at the same time.

Service Contracts

Most pieces of medical office equipment are purchased with a **service contract.** Such contracts usually allow for unlimited repair calls for a specific time period. Service contracts go into effect after the manufacturer's warranty expires. Contracts usually call for larger pieces of equipment to be serviced at the doctor's office. Smaller pieces of equipment often have a two-price contract: one price if the item is brought to a service center for repair and another price if repair is carried out on site.

Service Calls

Before calling in a service technician, check the equipment thoroughly. A plug accidentally removed from a socket or a disconnected wire is often the cause of what seems like a machine breakdown.

Make sure to conduct the necessary routine maintenance or call for a technician to perform it if covered by the service contract.

Document all service calls, the reason the call was made, the response, whether there was a service charge, and the suggested follow-up.

New Equipment Purchases

Although the doctors in the practice or the clinic administrator is responsible for purchasing equipment, the medical assistant may be asked to help research options.

Manufacturers will be glad to send you information about the piece of equipment in question. Many companies now have Web sites that can be browsed to see product features and costs. Some sites even have video demonstrations.

Some practices look for used equipment or furniture. Companies that sell equipment from a number of manufacturers often have used equipment in inventory. Used equipment can also be found from doctors who are buying new equipment or retiring.

The medical assistant may be asked to research the "lease vs. buy" decision, whether to purchase the equipment or lease it over a period of time. Most medical and office equipment can be leased. Leasing and buying each have advantages and disadvantages, mostly in terms of tax treatment. The practice lawyer should be consulted on this decision.

The availability of leasing also means that more used equipment is now coming "off lease" that is only 2 to 3 years old and may have a number of years of useful life left.

When new equipment is received in the office, it is a good idea to note replacement part numbers, such as bulbs, batteries, and cartridges, and add them to the supply-ordering system.

Telephone and Answering Services

Arrangements must be made with a telephone company for the number of telephone lines and the type of service. Depending on the size of the practice, these arrangements can be made with the business user portion of the major telephone company that services the area or with one of numerous companies that market complete telephone systems for large offices.

The office may own its own telephones and answering machines or it may lease a complete system, which may be referred to as a PBX, for private branch exchange. Many local phone companies, as well as system providers, provide voice mail inside the system software, so there is no need for a separate answering machine.

Telephone problems can originate in the inside-office equipment, the inside lines, or the outside lines. Since the breakup of AT&T in the 1980s, the user must pay the local phone company for service to any inside lines. If telephone service is being provided by a system provider, service to inside lines should be part of the service contract. Problems with lines outside the office or building are the responsibility of the local phone company.

SUPPLIES

A busy medical office goes through an enormous amount of supplies—both clinical and administrative—in a month. Managing the purchase and stocking of supplies is a task that often falls to a medical assistant.

The number of supplies that can be ordered at one time is dependent on the amount of storage space in the office. A practice can usually get a better price by ordering large amounts, but many offices are limited in the amount they can store. Sometimes it is possible to get extra storage space in the basement of the building where space is being rented.

Also, many doctors receive discounts on supplies by virtue of membership in some sort of a buying group or independent practice organization. Other practices are beginning to move toward Web-based purchasing of medical supplies. The savings to suppliers from their customers ordering over the Internet can sometimes be so large (no need for the orders to be rekeyed into the supplier's computer system by order-entry clerks) that they offer enormous discounts.

It is important to develop a good system of tracking supplies, usage, and storage capacity. In this way, reordering is not done too early when there is no room or too late when the practice may actually run out of important supplies.

When planning a new office or office move, it is important to plan for adequate supply-storage space.

Supply Inventory

A supply inventory is a listing of all the supplies regularly used in the office. This inventory can be kept in a notebook with a separate page for each supply, or it can be a set of cards—one for each supply. Notebook pages or cards can be grouped either by the type of supply (i.e., surgical disposable, photocopier, and so on) or by the supplier.

ITEM NAME	SUPPLIER	ITEM #	COST	REORDER AT	# TO ORDER
Bandages & Dressings					
nonsterile sponges 2" x 2"	H Medical	XY 2544	$3.50/pkg/200	5 pkg	10 pkg
nonsterile sponges 4" x 4"	H Medical	XY 7812	$8.25/pkg/200	5 pkg	10 pkg
sterile sponges 4" x 4"	H Medical	XY 5540	$22.00/box/00	2 box	5 box
non-sterile conforming bandage 2"	Winscott	49J265	$5.25/pkg/12	10 pkg	10 pkg
non-sterile conforming bandage 4"	Winscott	49J266	$8.62/pkg/12	10 pkg	10 pkg
paste bandage 4"	Winscott	57J381	$4.10 each	10	10
					10

➤ **Figure 11–3** Sample supply inventory.

The supply list should contain the following information:

1. The item's name
2. Any specific size used
3. The usual supplier
4. The cost per a standard quantity (i.e., $3.50 per 100) if known
5. The **reorder point**. The reorder point marks when the number of items remaining is low enough that it must be reordered. The reorder point is calculated by determining the number of items used per day or week, and the number of days or weeks it takes for an order to be received. For instance, if the office uses 100 pairs of gloves per day, there are 50 pairs in each box, and it takes 5 working days to receive a new order of gloves, the reorder point would be when fewer than 15 boxes (750 gloves) are in the supply room (7 1/2 days' worth).
6. The quantity ordered each time.

Figure 11–3 shows a sample supply inventory. Information related to specific items is often main-

➤ **Figure 11–4** Form for inventory control. (Courtesy of Colwell Systems, Champaign, IL)

PROCEDURE 11–1

Taking a Supply Inventory

Performance Objective: The student will take a supply inventory, using an inventory card system or inventory notebook.
Supplies and Equipment: Inventory cards or notebook, supplies, pen.

Procedure Steps

1. Obtain list of items in inventory—either an inventory notebook, computer file, or box of inventory cards.
   Rationale: You will need a master list of supplies to compare it to what you see.

2. Consider the supplies on hand in both examination rooms and storage, checking expiration dates and disposing of those that are expired.

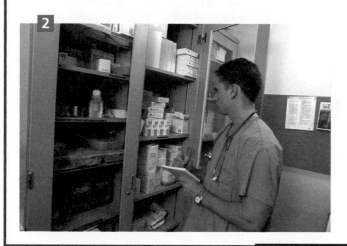

Count the remaining supplies. Enter this number in the appropriate place on inventory card or notebook.
Rationale: Expired items should be thrown away and not counted as part of the inventory. The point of taking inventory is to keep track of the number of items on hand.

3. Check the number of supplies on hand against the number listed as the reorder point. If the number of items on hand is close to the reorder point, flag the item as one that needs to be reordered per the custom of your office (e.g., colored paper clips or a clip over a certain part of the card).
   Rationale: This will prevent you from running out of an item.

4. Check that the information on the inventory card or list is correct and complete. There should be a description of the size, color, and price, as well as the usual supplier of the item.
   Rationale: You will need this information when reordering supplies.

5. Be sure that your storage space is tidy and that items can be found when needed.
   Rationale: Supplies are useless unless they can be found.

6. Place inventory cards, computer printout sheet, or inventory book in the proper location for follow-up, including placing orders or updating computer information and storage until needed again.

---

tained on cards or a sheet with the items ordered. This usually contains additional information about order dates and dates of receipt, initialed by the person who placed and/or received the order, as shown in Figure 11–4.

Most offices routinely order supplies on a monthly basis. Some supplies are routinely reordered each ordering period, but others are ordered only on an "as needed" basis. For these items, inventory control can be managed using a set of three "flags" that can be three different-colored paper clips.

When the item is getting low and should be ordered in the next ordering period, one colored clip is put on the card in the box or on the notebook page for that item. When the item has been ordered, a different-colored clip is put on, so that someone seeing that the item is low does not think it needs to be ordered. When the order has been received but the billing has not been reconciled yet, a third colored clip is put on.

Computerized inventory record-keeping can be maintained on a spreadsheet.

Procedure 11–1 describes taking a supply inventory in detail.

Even if the office has been using the same supplier for a long time, it is a good practice to check other suppliers at least annually to see if a better relationship can be established. This might involve discounts for the volumes purchased, faster delivery, better prices

PROCEDURE 11–2

Stocking the Supply Cabinet

Performance Objective: The student will stock supply cabinets and dispose of expired supplies.

Supplies and Equipment: Inventory cards or notebook, new supplies, invoice or packing list, pen or pencil.

Procedure Steps

1. When supplies are delivered, bring them to the area where they are going to be placed (i.e., the supply closet, copy room, or staff area).

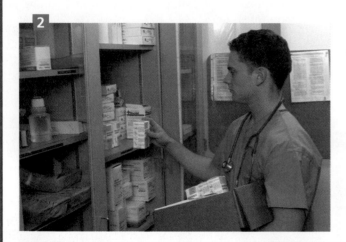

Rationale: Medical supplies should not be left unattended in the office.

2. Unpack the supplies and check what is received against the packing slip.
   Rationale: For billing and legal purposes, what is received should be what was ordered. If they do not match, you or your accounts payable department will have to follow procedures for alerting the vendor to discrepancies.

3. Shelve the supplies, making sure to place older supplies in front of the new. Always check the expiration date on older supplies to be sure that they are still good.
   Rationale: Placing the oldest supplies in front assures that they will be used first; expired supplies must be disposed of.

4. Note in the inventory card or notebook the amount of supplies received. If using a card system that has flags to alert staff when items are on order, be sure to switch the flag to the received signal (i.e., change paper clip color or move clip off ordered section of card).
   Rationale: This will avoid confusion over stock numbers and billing.

5. File invoice/packing slips in the the proper file (i.e., the received file and/or the to be paid file).
   Rationale: Vendors must be paid and paperwork must not be lost.

---

overall, or an availability of more product from one supplier than is currently available. If you think you have the possibility of switching suppliers, always give the current supplier the opportunity to "meet or beat" the current offer in terms of price, product range, service, delivery reliability, and overall quality of the relationship.

When storing supplies in the main supply area, make sure to review the expiration dates of all items remaining before shelving the new items. Discard outdated supplies. Move the supplies with the expiration date closest to the current date to the front of the area so they are used first. Put new supplies behind the older supplies. Any sterilized packs more than 30 days old must be resterilized.

Moving supplies from the central supply area to the place where they will be used is called restocking.

Exam rooms should be restocked daily; administrative areas are usually restocked weekly (the exception being the photocopy and fax machines, which may need paper restocks daily, depending on the volume of work done). Procedure 11–2 describes restocking in more detail.

Ordering Supplies

A supply order is created by combining the list of supplies that are routinely ordered with the items that have been "flagged" using the inventory control system. When this list is complete, the supplier for each item must be identified, and orders for that supplier created. Most offices will try to have one or two suppliers for clinical supplies and one or two for administrative supplies. Medications may be purchased from the same company as the one used for clinical supplies or from a pharmaceutical supplier.

For each supply on each order, make sure all of the variables are correct, such as quantity, size (or quantity for each of a number of different sizes), and color.

It is a good idea to put the order aside for a moment, then recheck it or have a colleague do so, before sending. This avoids time-consuming errors.

After placing the order, make sure to properly note on the inventory and in the inventory control flag system that the supplies have been ordered.

Supplies are usually ordered in one of three ways: by telephone, fax, or mail. Some medical supply companies are beginning to offer computer-based purchasing via their Web sites. Even when using the telephone or computer, you should maintain a paper record of the transaction to reconcile against receipt of the supplies and for proper accounting. If ordering by fax, it is a good idea to make a follow-up phone call to make sure the fax has come through clearly and that the order-entry person at the supply house has no questions.

You can use either a purchase order unique to the office or an order form supplied by the **vendor**, the company that sells the supplies or equipment. A **purchase order (PO)** is the form used to order supplies and the order itself.

In large organizations, authorization to place orders may be limited to one or two people. In either case, place a "tracking number" on any paperwork, again for the purpose of reconciling receipt of supplies and payment of the invoice. When the vendor cannot ship the item immediately, the item is said to be on **back order**. Flag the order to be sure it arrives when promised. A back-ordered item is billed separately unless prepaid.

In some states, ordering of any prescription-based supplies requires an authorization from a doctor and a copy of the doctor's state medical license for purchase. For purchase of controlled substances such as narcotics, a doctor authorization and a copy of the doctor's federal Drug Enforcement Administration certificate is necessary.

Procedure 11–3 describes how to prepare a purchase order.

Receiving Supplies

Different suppliers ship their supplies different ways: either through the U.S. Postal Service; a large national package delivery company like United Parcel Service, FedEx Ground, or a local courier service.

You need to become familiar with the way different suppliers ship goods, so you know when to expect delivery and who to expect making the delivery.

The delivery service will ask for a signature to confirm that the delivery was made. When supplies are received, they should immediately be brought to the storage room. At the first convenient opportunity, the packing slip should be inspected and reconciled with the order to make sure all items have been received or that items that are to be received in a separate delivery are noted on the packing slip. If the packing slip is incorrect, note the missing items and notify the supplier.

The packing slip should be clipped to the order form. When all items have been received, the order form with all the packing slips attached should be marked "okay to pay" and delivered to the business manager, who will make payment against the invoice. The invoice should arrive within a few days of delivery of the final items on the order.

RISK MANAGEMENT

Risk management is the process of assessing risk and putting in place policies and procedures that minimize it. Risk in a medical office comes in a number of forms.

There is physical risk: the risk of injury or illness, both to employees and patients. There is also business risk: the risk of reduced patient visits because of poor "customer relations," as well as the risk of liability, which may lead to a lawsuit.

A medical office can have liability—meaning it is legally responsible for an event that causes harm to someone else—because of patient care that leads to a malpractice claim or because of injury or illness to someone that occurs because the office neglected to take reasonable and adequate precautions.

The office manager or a medical assistant is often responsible for maintaining the risk management program, in close consultation with the doctor or the managing partner among the doctors. In larger clinics or hospitals, there may be a full-time risk manager or risk management may be a part of the duties of one of the clinic's top administrators. Policies and procedures are designed by the doctors and the office's top administrator, who work closely with an attorney, an insurance professional, and a risk management professional. When a new policy is adopted, a copy is given to each employee covered by the policy. Policy and procedure manuals, once developed, should be accessible to all employees when questions arise.

Incident Reports

Whenever something happens in the office for which the office could be considered liable, an incident report should be filled out. An incident can be as simple as a staff member or patient tripping over a chair or it could be as serious as a staff member sticking himself or herself with a needle that has just been used to give an injection.

PROCEDURE 11–3

Preparing a Purchase Order

Performance Objective: The student will prepare a purchase order.

Supplies and Equipment: Inventory list, purchase order form, pen, list of "flagged" or low quantity items, copier, and phone, fax, or computer.

Procedure Steps

1. Collect a list of regularly purchased items and any supplies that have been flagged on their inventory cards or otherwise noted as being low.
   Rationale: You must know what items are needed.

2. Using either a form provided by the vendor or an office-generated form that has been approved by the vendor, create a list of the needed supplies, noting quantity, size, color, and price. This form should have a purchase order number on it that allows you to track the order.
   Rationale: Each vendor will have a different ordering system; you will need to accommodate them as well as keep track of the order for receiving and billing purposes.

3. For some medical supplies you will need a doctor's signature, a copy of their medical license, and/or a copy of the doctor's DEA cer-

2

PURCHASE ORDER   No. **1554**

Bill to: **Ship to:**

Blackburn Primary Care Associates. PC   Blackburn Primary Care Associates, PC
1990 Turquoise Drive   1990 Turquoise Drive
Blackburn, WI 54937   Blackburn, WI 54937

Vendor: _____

_____

_____

Terms: _____

ORDER #	DESCRIPTION	QTY.	COLOR	SIZE	UNIT PRICE	TOTAL PRICE
					SUBTOTAL	
					TAX	
					SHIPPING	
					TOTAL	

tificate. Have these available to include in your fax or mailing.

Rationale: Different types of supplies will require different authorizations and you should be able to access any needed identification for your office.

4. To place your order, different vendors will have you call, fax, mail, or submit your order electronically. If you fax either your order or medical authorization information, be sure to also call and check that the fax went through. Whether faxing, mailing, phoning, or submitting an order by computer, be sure to keep a copy for your records.

Rationale: If anything happens to your order in transmission or shipping, you want to be sure that you are able to resubmit the order.

5. If your inventory system has flags to indicate when items are on order, indicate on the inventory cards that you have done so.

Rationale: This prevents duplicate ordering.

6. Place copies of submitted orders in the appropriate file.

Rationale: You will need to be able to access this order when the supplies have come in.

The incident report should be initiated by the staff member who is injured or who is closest to the patient or visitor when he or she is injured. A supervisor should review the report before giving it to the individual who manages the risk management program. See Box 11–1, "Information Included in an Incident Report."

Incident reports should always be filled out if a patient, employee, or visitor slips or falls, if a medication error is made, if blood is drawn from the wrong patient, if the number of surgical instruments counted after a procedure does not match the number counted before the procedure, or if an employee is stuck with a needle.

Information that needs to be on an incident report includes the name, address, telephone number, date of birth, and gender of the injured person; the time of day, day, date, and exact location in the office where the incident happened; a brief narrative of exactly what

happened; and what if any diagnostic procedures or treatments were performed to assess the injury. These items are applicable whether the injured person was a staff member, patient, or visitor.

Any witnesses to the incident should be asked for their name, address, and phone number, so the office's insurance provider can call and investigate the incident further if necessary. The report should be dated and signed by the person filling it out. A doctor and/or supervisor's signature also goes on the form, according to the office's policy for incident reports.

Liability Coverage

Every office should have adequate insurance protection against liability, both professional liability (commonly called malpractice) and liability for any accident that might occur in the office.

Professional liability insurance covers a medical pro-

ON THE JOB

Assume you have been asked to find information to place an order for the following supplies: Adhesive bandages (3/4" × 3" plastic strips) and alcohol prep pads. The adhesive bandages and alcohol prep pads are routine items used regularly by your office.

1. How can you determine the reorder point and the amount to order for the items?

2. Where will you check to find out if the supply of adhesive bandages and alcohol prep pads actually is low and if they need to be ordered? Why might this be more difficult than it seems?

3. Assume that the office manager has asked you to try less expensive bandages and pads. Identify three specific steps you might take to do this.

4. After you have located the supplies you want to buy, what steps are necessary to place the order?

5. When the supplies arrive, what should you do with them?

fessional for patient claims that diagnostic procedures, tests, or treatments either caused an injury or failed to detect an existing medical condition that should have been detected using good medical practice.

Some doctors purchase insurance in their own name only and have professional staff members purchase their own professional liability policies. If this is the case, the medical assistant can purchase a professional liability policy through a professional organization such as the American Association of Medical Assistants.

In other cases, a practice purchases professional liability insurance for the entire staff. If this is the case, every professional staff member should be named on the policy.

Box 11–1   Information Included on Incident Reports

Incident report forms vary widely, but usually ask for the following information.

■ When did the incident occur?

Date
Time

■ Who was involved?

Full name (Last, First, Middle or Initial)
Social Security Number
Age and/or birthdate
Address
Telephone numbers (home and work)
Sex
Employee, Student, Visitor, Patient?

■ Where did the incident occur?

Address
Building, room

■ How did the incident occur?

Equipment involved
Activity the person was engaged in
Describe exactly what occurred

■ Describe any injury or potential injury.

Exact body part involved
Extent of injury

■ Who witnessed the incident?

Name
Telephone number

■ Plans to treat injury or follow up

Name, address, telephone number of doctor or health professional providing follow-up

■ Name of person in organization to whom incident was reported
■ Date of receipt/follow-up by supervisor

The office should also have adequate insurance to cover property damage to the office because of fire, storm, or flooding (similar to homeowner insurance). In addition, the practice should have adequate coverage against personal injury sustained on the office's property by a patient or employee. Many patients are ill and/or fragile, and a fall can occur at any time. The policy should cover any injury sustained on the property controlled by the practice. If the practice is in an office building, the public hallways are the responsibility of the landlord or medical office condominium association. If the office is in a freestanding building, the practice is responsible for any occurrences that happen on walkways, in the parking lot, or other outdoor areas up to the public road or sidewalk.

Managing Safety Plans

As discussed in chapter 6, the Occupational Safety and Health Administration (OSHA) creates regulations to protect the safety and health of American workers and monitors employers to be sure they comply with these regulations. Of course, these safety plans also protect patients as well.

Every employer is required to have several written plans to protect workers' safety and health, and to designate a specific employee or employees to develop and implement those plans. Managing safety plans involves five sets of activities:

1. Providing equipment and supplies needed to meet all OSHA standards
2. Developing and implementing written policies and procedures
3. Keeping records of incidents and changes made as a result of incidents
4. Training new employees and updating skills of current employees
5. Providing access for employees to OSHA standards and information about potential health and safety hazards.

QUALITY IMPROVEMENTS

Making quality improvements involves developing a plan to identify problems and improve service. A quality improvement plan utilizes a specific, scientific format to measure the quality of the output of its processes. In the medical office, this is based on validated outcomes of treatment and patient satisfaction with the services provided by the medical office. Different terms may be used to identify these programs, such as continuous quality improvement (CQI) or total quality management (TQM).

Improvements should be sought in identification and correction of any system failures in the provision of care, service to patients and their families, patient outcomes, employee efficiency and productivity, em-

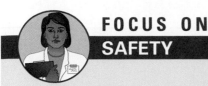

FOCUS ON
SAFETY

USING THE INTERNET TO DEVELOP SAFETY TRAINING PROGRAMS FOR EMPLOYEES

Many large educational institutions have their safety training programs, chemical hygiene plans, hazard communication plans, and risk management manuals on Web sites on the Internet. This can be a valuable resource for medical offices or clinics when developing their own plans. As a student, you can supplement your education by visiting one of these Web sites to review information or to take a quiz to test your knowledge.

RESOURCES FOR BLOOD-BORNE PATHOGEN TRAINING

www.pp.okstate.edu/ehs/modules/bbp.htm
www.fpm.wisc.edu/bbp
ehs.clemson.edu/BBP/index.htm

GENERAL SAFETY RESOURCES

www.pp.okstate.edu/ehs
www.fpm.wisc.edu/safety
ehs.clemson.edu

LAB SAFETY

www.pp.okstate.edu/ehs/hazmat.htm

ployees' ability to work as an effective health care team, and employees' satisfaction with the conditions under which they work.

In addition to quality control efforts required under federal legislation such as CLIA '88, quality improvement in health care facilities is being pushed by organizations that accredit health care facilities. One such organization is the Joint Commission on Accreditation of Healthcare Organizations (JCAHO), established to evaluate hospitals, rehabilitation centers, and nursing homes. More recently, it has expanded the scope of its accreditation to federally chartered community health centers, public clinics, freestanding health maintenance organizations, doctors' offices, and managed care organizations.

An organization that accredits managed care plans is the National Committee for Quality Assurance (NCQA). As with the JCAHO, accreditation is voluntary and requires a program of quality assurance. The NCQA rates its members on their compliance with quality standards (called HEDIS measures) and issues a report so consumers can determine how well different managed care organizations perform.

In a medical office, quality improvement programs seek to solve problems in all three major areas—administrative, clinical, and laboratory. There are seven steps to implementing a quality improvement program:

1. Identify each specific problem.
2. For each problem identified, create a task force to study it.
3. Assign an expected threshold—a numerical goal—for each problem. The threshold is the number of times a problem should be expected to occur after the improvement is made.
4. Explore each problem in depth, and propose solutions to reduce the incidence of the problem from the current level to the expected threshold.
5. Implement a solution or solutions to each problem.
6. Establish a monitoring program to obtain data about results.
7. Review the data and compare actual occurrences for each problem to the expected threshold for that problem over the specified time.

CONCLUSION

Maintaining a medical office, even a small office, can be complex. Many systems need to be in place to keep the office functioning smoothly. The payoff for all of this effort is an office that is clean, safe, appealing, and prepared to care for patients.

STUDENT STUDY PLAN

To reinforce your understanding of the material in this chapter. . . .

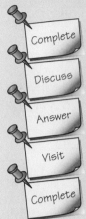

Complete the **Review & Recall** questions.

Discuss the situation in **If You Were the Medical Assistant** with your class-mates, and answer the questions.

Answer the **Critical Thinking Questions,** and discuss them with your class-mates.

Visit **Web sites** suggested below and search for additional Web sites using the **Keywords for Internet Searches.**

Complete the exercises in chapter 11 of the **Student Mastery Manual.**

 REVIEW & RECALL

1. List equipment and supplies needed in the following areas of the medical office: reception area, billing office, examination room.

2. What tasks have to be done daily to keep the medi-cal office clean and neat? Weekly? Less frequently?

3. Describe three parts of an adequate security system for the medical office.

4. List two reasons why it is important to maintain an inventory of equipment in the medical office.

5. Describe how each of the following fire safety mea-sures should be implemented in the medical office: sprinklers, fire doors, fire extinguishers, smoke de-tectors, exit signs.

6. Compare and contrast general liability insurance and malpractice insurance.

7. Identify the components of a risk management pro-gram in the medical office.

8. List the components of a quality improvement plan.

 IF YOU WERE THE MEDICAL ASSISTANT

Using a catalog for medical supplies or an on-line catalog find two different types of adhesive bandages (plastic strips 3/4″ × 3″). Obtain the catalog number and price information to order one box of 100 of each of these types. Obtain the price per box if a larger quantity is ordered (usually 12 boxes for this item). Assume your office uses 144 boxes of adhesive bandages in 6 months.

Calculate and compare the cost of the less expensive brand to the more expensive brand, both for orders of one box at a time and for 12 boxes at a time. Discuss the implications for office cost over 6 months.

(Because Internet searches are not efficient at identifying medical supply stores with on-line catalogs, two are provided here as a means for answering this question: www.mooremedical.com and www.emsproducts.com)

 CRITICAL THINKING QUESTIONS

1. Research the advantages and disadvantages of leas-ing versus buying expensive medical equipment, such as ultrasound and X-ray equipment.

2. Obtain blank copies of forms discussed in this chap-ter from medical offices or clinics (incident reports, lease agreements, supply or equipment inventory, purchase order) and discuss how they are similar or different.

3. Inventory the supplies in your medical assisting school practice area. Create an inventory supply list and establish reorder points and amounts to order for at least 20 items, assuming that you want to keep a 6-month supply on hand.

4. What are the advantages and disadvantages of ordering monthly as opposed to every 6 months? Identify at least three advantages and three disadvantages for each system.

5. Make a list of at least 10 types of events that could occur in a medical office for which an incident report should be filled out. Discuss appropriate follow-up for each incident.

6. Discuss the process of locating information about particular pieces of equipment or particular supplies to be ordered for the medical office. Assume that your office wants to buy a three-channel EKG machine. Get information about one particular model, including price and warranty information. Compare this to information gathered by your classmates. How would you decide which model to buy?

7. Discuss the advantages and disadvantages of accreditation for a health care provider. Research the process by which an organization becomes accredited.

EXPLORE THE WEB

INTERNET WEB SITES

Centers for Disease Control and Prevention (CDC)
www.cdc.gov

Joint Commission on Accreditation of Healthcare Organizations (JCAHO)
www.jcaho.org

Material Safety Data Sheets
siri.uvm.edu/msds
www.msds.pdc.cornell.edu/msdssrch.asp

National Committee for Quality Assurance
www.ncqa.org

National Institute for Occupational Safety and Health (NIOSH)
www.cdc.gov/niosh/homepage.html

Occupational Safety and Health Administration (OSHA)
www.osha.gov

KEYWORDS FOR INTERNET SEARCHES

blood-borne pathogen standard
chemical hygiene plan
continuous quality improvement (CQI)
fire protection
hazardous waste
liability insurance
malpractice insurance
medical equipment
medical incident report
medical office supplies
total quality management (TQM)

ANSWERS TO ON THE JOB

1. You can determine the reorder point for adhesive bandages and alcohol prep pads by checking the sample supply inventory sheet, the list of all supplies used by the office, or the card for inventory control for each of the individual items. Each of these forms will also tell you how many to order.

2. You should check the supply cabinet to find out if the supply actually is low. Ideally, all boxes of adhesive bandages and all boxes of alcohol prep pads will be stored in one place in the supply cabinet, with a label to show clearly where the item would be if it were in stock. In practice, space limitations and lack of time to organize may result in a disorganized supply cabinet, with boxes of the same item stored in different places, or behind other items where they are not clearly visible.

3. To find a less expensive product: 1) Obtain catalogs from several suppliers and compare prices. 2) Ask medical assistants or office managers in other practices for names of suppliers. or 3) Search for a new supplier on the Internet. Many office supply companies sell house brands of common items such as adhesive bandages or alcohol prep pads that are less expensive than brand-name products. Inexpen-

sive alcohol prep pads may be smaller or thinner than more expensive ones. The office must decide whether the less expensive type meets the office's needs.

4. To place the order, make a list that includes the following information for each item: 1) description of the product, 2) the supplier's (or manufacturer's) catalog number, 3) the quantity to purchase, 4) the color and/or size if needed, and 5) the unit price. Assign a purchase order number to the order according to the system used in the office. Fill out a written purchase order, including total price and tax, to either send or fax to the supplier, telephone the order, or order on-line using the Internet.

5. When the supplies arrive, check and note on the packing list to be sure all items are included. Place the new items in the supply cabinet behind the old items, so that old stock is used first. Update the card for inventory control or the supply list to note that supplies ordered have been received and process the bill for payment. Be sure that items on back order are not included on the current bill (unless the order was prepaid) and follow up to be sure they are received when promised.

Chapter 12

Opening the Office and Checking Patients In

Instructional Objectives

After completing this chapter, you will be able to do the following:

1. Define and spell the vocabulary words for this chapter.
2. Describe how to open the office and prepare for the day's activities.
3. Discuss measures to protect the confidentiality of patients in the reception areas.
4. List information that must be given to a new patient about the practice.
5. List information that must be obtained from new patients.
6. Discuss procedures that are necessary to validate that a patient's insurance will pay the bill.
7. Describe the proper procedure to check a patient in.

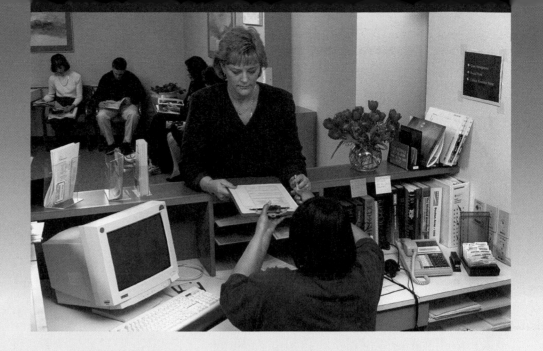

CMA/RMA CERTIFICATION
Content and Competencies

- Check patients in
- Explain general office policies

- Identify and respond to issues of confidentiality

Performance Objectives

After completing this chapter, you will be able to perform the following activities correctly:

1. Retrieve, record, and assess the importance of messages from an answering machine (Procedure 12–1).
2. Retrieve, record, and assess the importance of messages from an answering service (Procedure 12–2).
3. Check patients in for office visits (Procedure 12–3).

VOCABULARY

assignment of benefits (p. 209)
call in times (p. 208)

co-payment (p. 212)
encounter form (p. 206)

Medicaid (p. 212)
point-of-service device (p. 212)

superbill (p. 206)

ABBREVIATIONS

POS (p. 212)

OPENING THE OFFICE

Office staff need to arrive at the office at least 15 to 20 minutes before the first patient is scheduled. This allows time to make sure the office is prepared for the patients.

The first person into the office (often the office manager or the head medical assistant) is responsible for the following organizing activities:

1. disarming the alarm system (if the office has one)
2. turning on the lights
3. unlocking the door through which patients enter
4. unlocking file cabinets and medicine cabinets
5. turning on all of the office equipment that will be used, such as computers and copy machines.

Depending on the way the office is organized, various people may be responsible for some or all of the following activities:

1. checking for messages and/or faxes
2. reviewing the day's activities
3. making sure patient charts are prepared
4. checking the waiting room.

PROCEDURE 12–1

Taking Messages from an Answering Machine

Performance Objective: The student will retrieve, record, and assess the importance of messages from an answering machine.
Equipment and Supplies: Answering machine, telephone message pad, pen, clock or watch.

Procedure Steps

1. Whenever the office has been closed, someone must check for messages as soon as the office reopens.
   Rationale: Callers to a business expect calls to be picked up as soon as the business opens. There may be an urgent message on the machine.
2. Listen to the messages in order, writing down the pertinent information for each message on a message pad. Fill in the information, including the name of the caller, business affiliation (if any), date, time of the call, telephone number including area code, and the information the caller wishes to leave about the reason for

the call. Place your initials on the message in case there are questions.
   Rationale: Complete information is necessary to return a call.
3. After you have obtained all the messages, reset the answering machine to the day message and be prepared to answer the telephone if it rings.
   Rationale: It is more efficient to answer calls than to listen to messages again in 5 or 10 minutes.
4. Arrange the messages in order of importance. Deal with any urgent calls at once, then work through other calls. Pull medical records for calls from patients and place the messages in the appropriate locations for various office staff to review.
   Rationale: It is more efficient to deliver all messages together than to make individual trips. Urgent calls should be responded to as soon as possible.

PROCEDURE 12-2

Taking Messages from an Answering Service

Performance Objective: The student will retrieve, record, and assess the importance of calls from an answering service.

Equipment and Supplies: Answering machine, telephone message pad, pen, clock or watch

Procedure Steps

1. Whenever the office has been closed, someone must check for messages as soon as the office reopens.
   Rationale: Callers to a business expect calls to be picked up as soon as the business opens, and the answering service needs to know that someone is in the office.

2. Call the answering service, identify yourself, and give the name of the office. State that you are in the office and would like to pick up messages for the practice.
   Rationale: The answering service will only release message information to authorized personnel. Once the service knows you are in the office, they will wait until the fourth ring or after to take a call.

3. Write down the pertinent information for each message on the message pad. Fill in the information, including the name of the caller, business affiliation (if any), date, time of the call, telephone number including area code, and the information the caller has left about the reason for the call. Place your initials on the message in case there are questions.
   Rationale: Complete information is necessary to return a call.

4. Repeat all information to be sure you have written it correctly. If you have any instructions for the answering service, give them now.
   Rationale: You want to be sure you have the correct information for each message.

5. Arrange the calls in order of importance. Deal with any urgent calls at once, then work through other calls. Pull medical records for calls from patients and place the messages in the appropriate locations for various office staff to review.
   Rationale: It is more efficient to deliver all messages together than to make individual trips. Urgent calls should be responded to as quickly as possible.

Checking for Messages and/or Faxes

Someone must review messages and prepare the telephone system for the day's activities. If the office uses an answering machine, a new message may need to be recorded each day. However, nearly all modern voice mail systems can handle multiple messages. So for most offices it is simply a matter of switching from the night/weekend message (which states that the office is closed and directs the caller to leave a message for nonurgent matters or to call another number for urgent matters) to the day message (which states that the receptionist is busy with another call).

Procedure 12-1 describes how to get messages using an automated system.

If your office uses an answering service, you need to call the service to say that the office is open and to get any messages that have not already been forwarded to the doctor who was on call overnight.

Procedure 12-2 describes how to properly interact with answering service personnel to get messages.

The person who checks for messages usually also checks for faxes that have arrived overnight, routes them to the appropriate person, and makes sure the fax machine's paper tray is full.

Reviewing the Day's Activities

It is helpful to take a minute at the beginning of the day to mentally organize the day's tasks, review appointment lists, and note deviations from the routine schedule, such as doctors who are out of the office for various engagements, all-doctor meetings, full staff meetings, or staff training. If the office uses a manual bookkeeping system, you need to be sure that the pegboard is prepared with a new day sheet and charge slips.

Making Sure Patient Charts Are Prepared

Patient charts are usually pulled the evening before the appointment and arranged with an appointment schedule for each doctor. In most practices, a charge slip—sometimes called an **encounter form**, or **superbill**—is printed for each person before the visit. Figure 12–1 shows the charge slip. The charge slip may be entered by hand or printed from information stored in the computer. This information includes the patient's name, address, birth date, telephone number, and insurance information.

The charge slip may be placed with the record in the morning or when the patient arrives. If the medical record or charge slips have not been prepared the night before for some reason, that is the first thing that must be done.

Charts for the day are usually kept at the front desk, but some doctors like the full day's charts on their private desk when they start to see patients.

As patients are added to the appointment schedule, their records must be pulled and their names added to all copies of the schedule.

The entire appointment schedule for the office needs to be posted in a designated location, and a copy of each doctor's individual schedule should also be placed in his or her office.

Checking the Waiting Room

The waiting room, as well as the reception area, and the examination/treatment rooms, all need to be checked for:

cleanliness
neatness
correct temperature
correct equipment
patient-education materials.

You may need to add office supplies to the reception area or medical supplies to the exam rooms, although some offices make this part of the afternoon closing routine. You may need to turn on or set up equipment used for clinical procedures, run controls in the laboratory, and/or remove items from a battery charger. You may need to empty the autoclave and put away equipment that was sterilized the evening before.

WHEN PATIENTS OR VISITORS ARRIVE

Greeting Patients or Visitors

It is important to acknowledge everyone who enters the office as soon as possible to prevent that person from feeling awkward. In larger offices, someone sits at the reception desk at all times. This person should greet everyone who enters the office. If another patient

is at the window, ask the new person's name and then politely instruct him or her to have a seat until you can finish with the current patient.

In smaller offices, a buzzer or bell may be connected to the door that notifies staff in other rooms that someone has entered the office.

Some offices have patients sign in on a sheet. Usually, a sign instructs patients what to do. Although this system may be overlooked by new patients, established patients become used to it. It can relieve pressure on the staff in a small office.

Whatever the system, once the patient has been identified, you need to locate the medical record and the charge slip.

Maintaining Confidentiality

Many offices have a sliding glass window that prevents people in the waiting room from hearing telephone conversations or other discussions in the reception area, as shown in Figure 12–2.

In many modern facilities, patients approach an island without any means of providing confidentiality. In such settings, patients should be instructed to sit down so that only one person is at the desk or window at a time, as shown in Figure 12–3.

If it becomes apparent that sensitive information will be discussed, ask the patient to step inside the reception area behind the partition so the conversation can be completed in a private area.

Orienting Patients to Policies, Procedures, and the Physical Aspects of the Office

New patients and prospective patients often have many questions about a practice. Part of the medical assistant's job may be to answer them and inform the patient of office policies and procedures. The medical assistant should be familiar with all of the following information and be able to discuss it with patients.

Necessary Information

1. A description of the practice: This includes a brief description of the doctors, how long each has been in practice, what each doctor's specialty is and his or her credentials, and if each doctor is accepting new patients.

   A doctor might not be accepting new patients for a few reasons. A doctor may have so many patients that he or she can't in all fairness accept new patients. After several months, the doctor may begin again to accept new patients. The doctor may be returning from a maternity, family, or personal disability leave and be working a reduced schedule. Or the doctor may be easing back before retiring. If a doctor joins a

Blackburn Primary Care Associates, PC
1990 Turquoise Drive
Blackburn, WI 54937
(608) 459-8857

Howard M. Lawler, MD 11
Joanne R. Hughes, MD 21
Ralph Garcia Lopez, MD 31
TAX ID NO. 00-00000000

GUARANTOR NAME AND ADDRESS	PATIENT NO.	PATIENT NAME	DOCTOR NO.	DATE

	DATE OF BIRTH	TELEPHONE NO.	INSURANCE			
			CODE	DESCRIPTION	CERTIFICATE NO.	

OFFICE - NEW

X	CPT	SERVICE	FEE
	99201	Prob Foc/Straight	
	99202	Exp Prob/Straight	
	99203	Detailed/Low	
	99204	Compre/Moderate	
	99205	Compre/High	

OFFICE - ESTABLISHED

X	CPT	SERVICE	FEE
	99211	Nurse/Minimal	
	99212	Prob Foc/Straight	
	99213	Exp Prob/Low	
	99214	Detailed/Moderate	
	99215	Compre/High	

OFFICE - CONSULT

X	CPT	SERVICE	FEE
	99241	Prob/Foc/Straight	
	99242	Exp Prob/Straight	
	99243	Detailed/Low	
	99244	Compre/Moderate	
	99245	Compre/High	

PREVENTIVE CARE - ADULT

X	CPT	SERVICE	FEE
	99385	18-39 Initial	
	99386	40-64 Initial	
	99387	65+ Initial	
	99395	18-39 Periodic	
	99396	40-64 Periodic	
	99397	65+ Periodic	

GASTROENEROLOGY

X	CPT	SERVICE	FEE
	45300	Sigmoidoscopy Rig	
	45305	Sigmoid Rig w/bx	
	45330	Sigmoidoscopy Flex	
	45331	Sigmoid Flex w/bx	
	45378	Colonoscopy Diag	
	45380	Colonoscopy w/bx	
	46600	Anoscopy	

CARDIOLOGY & HEARING

X	CPT	SERVICE	FEE
	93000	EKG (Global)	
	93015	Stress Test (Global)	
	93224	Holter (Global)	
	93225	Holter Hook Up	
	93227	Holter Interpretation	
	94010	Pulm Function Test	
	92551	Audiometry Screen	

INJECTIONS & IMMUNIZATION

X	CPT	SERVICE	FEE
	86585	TB Skin Test	
	90716	Varicella Vaccine	
	90724	Flu Vaccine	
	90732	Pneumovax	
	90718	TD Immunization	
	90782	Injection IM*	
	90788	Injection IM Antibiot*	
		Injection joint*	

REPAIR & DERMATOLOGY

X	CPT	SERVICE	FEE
	17110	Warts: #	
		Tags: #	
		Lesion Excis	
		Lesion Destruct	
SIZE CM:		SITE:	
MALIG:		PREMAL/BEN:	
		(Check One Above)	
		Simple Closure	
		Intermed Closure	

OTHER

SUPPLIES/DRUGS*

DRUG NAME:	
UNIT/MEASURE:	
QUANTITY	

SM	MED	MAJOR
	(circle one)	
FOR ALL INJECTIONS, SUPPLY DRUG		
INFORMATION		

SIZE CM:	SITE:
10060	I&D Abscess
10080	I&D Cyst

DIAGNOSTIC CODES: ICD-9-CM

☐ 789.0 Abdominal Pain	☐ 782.3 Edema	☐ 614.9 Pelvic Inflammatory Disease	☐ 474.0 Tonsillitis, Chronic
☐ 795.0 Abnormal Pap Smear	☐ 492.8 Emphysema	☐ 685.1 Pilonidal Cyst	☐ 465.9 Upper Respiratory Infection, Acute
☐ 706.1 Acne Vulgaris	☐ V16.0 Family History Of Diabetes	☐ 462 Pharyngitis, Acute	☐ 599.0 Urinary Tract Infection
☐ 477.0 Allergic Rhinitis	☐ 780.6 Fever of Undetermined Origin	☐ 627.1 Postmenopausal Bleeding	☐ V03.9 Vaccination/Bacterial Dis.
☐ 285.9 Anemia, NOS	☐ 578.9 G.I. Bleeding, Unspecified	☐ 625.4 Premenstrual Tension	☐ V06.8 Vaccination/Combination
☐ 281.0 Pernicious	☐ 727.41 Ganglion of Joint	☐ 782.1 Rash	☐ V04.8 Vaccination, Influenza
☐ 411.1 Angina, Unstable	☐ 535.0 Gastritis, Acute	☐ 569.3 Rectal Bleeding	☐ 616.10 Vaginitis, Vulvitis, NOS
☐ 427.9 Arythmia, NOS	☐ V72.3 Arythmia, NOS	☐ 398.90 Rheumatic Heart Disease, NOS	☐ 780.4 Vertigo
☐ 440.9 Arteriosclerosis	☐ 748.0 Headache	☐ 431.9 Sinusitis, Acute, NOS	☐ 787.0 Vomiting, Nausea
☐ 714.0 Arthritis, Rheumatoid	☐ 550.90 Hernia, inguinal, NOS	☐ 782.1 Skin Eruption, Rash	☐ ____ _____
☐ 414.0 ASHD	☐ 054.9 Herpes Simplex	☐ 845.00 Sprain, Ankle	☐ ____ _____
☐ 493.90 Asthma, Bronchial W/O Status Ast.	☐ 053.9 Herpes Zoster	☐ 848.9 Sprain, Muscle, Unspec. Site	☐ ____ _____
☐ 493.91 Asthma, Bronchial W/Status Ast.	☐ 708.9 Hives/Urticaria	☐ 785.6 Swollen Glands	☐ ____ _____
☐ 466.1 Bronchiolitis, Acute	☐ 401.1 Hypertension, Benign	☐ 246.9 Thyroid Disease, Unspecified	☐ ____ _____
☐ 466.0 Bronchitis, Acute	☐ 401.0 Hypertension, Malignant	☐ 463 Tonsillitis, Acute	
☐ 727.3 Bursitis	☐ 402.90 Hypertension, W/O CHF		
☐ 786.50 Chest Pain	☐ 244.9 Hypothyroidism, Primary		
☐ 574.20 Cholelithiasis	☐ 380.4 Impacted Cerumen		
☐ 372.30 Conjunctivitis, Unspecified	☐ 487.1 Influenza		
☐ 564.0 Constipation	☐ 564.1 Irritable Bowel Syndrome		
☐ 496 COPD	☐ 464.0 Laryngitis, Acute		
☐ 692.9 Dermatitis, Allergic	☐ 454.9 Leg Varicose Veins		
☐ 250.01 Diabetes Mellitus, ID	☐ 424.0 Mitral Valve Prolapse		
☐ 250.00 Diabetes Mellitus, NID	☐ 412 Myocardial Infarction, Old		
☐ 558.9 Diarrhea	☐ 715.90 Osteoarthritis, Unspec. Site		
☐ 562.11 Diverticulitis	☐ 620.2 Ovarian Cyst		
☐ 562.10 Diverticulosis			

RETURN APPOINTMENT

_____ Days

_____ Weeks

_____ Months

Authorization Number:

▶ _____

BALANCE DUE

DATE OF SERVICE	CPT CODE	DIAGNOSIS CODE(S)	CHARGE

Place of Service:
( ) Office
( ) Emergency Room
( ) In Patient Hospital
( ) Out-Patient Hospital
( ) Nursing Home

TOTAL CHARGE	$
AMOUNT PAID	$
PREVIOUS BAL	$
BALANCE DUE	$

Check #: _____

(Circle Method of Payment)
CASH   CHECK   MC   VISA

Physician's Signature

▶ _____

> **Figure 12–1** A charge slip (superbill or encounter form) is prepared for each of the day's patients. The top two lines are filled in by hand or by computer before the patient visit.

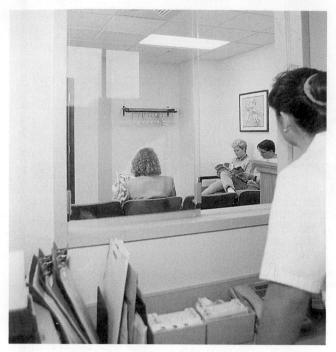

➤ **Figure 12–2** A sliding glass window can be used to provide privacy for the receptionist. (From Chester, GA. *Modern Medical Assisting.* Philadelphia: Saunders, 1998)

new health maintenance organization (HMO), he or she usually has to agree to reopen to new patients; sometimes the doctor can negotiate to take a particular number of patients from the plan.

2. Specialties of doctors in the practice and the rights of patients in the practice: Describe the specialties and special interests of the doctors in the practice, types of patients seen, and if there is an emphasis on preventive care. Some practices include information about languages spoken, if the doctor practices alternative therapies such as acupuncture, or if the doctor insists that patients stop smoking.

3. Location of the main office and satellite offices: Include directions to any office and a description of available parking and access to public transportation, if applicable.

4. The types of insurance that the practice accepts: This includes which open-panel HMOs the practice belongs to, as well as whether referrals are needed and how to get them.

5. Payment policy: The patient needs to know whether the doctor submits the insurance claim or expects the patient to pay and then file for reimbursement from the insurance company. This is especially important for the first visit.

The medical assistant should also be able to tell prospective patients how much time to allow for a first (new patient) visit and, in a primary care practice, the time for a standard

physical exam (as well as the cost for each). Most doctors only see new patients on certain days and times, and medical assistants should be sure to remind patients to bring all of their medications to the initial appointment, as well as a written list of concerns.

6. How to make appointments: Include the policy regarding canceling appointments. Patients are normally asked to give 24 hours notice if possible for a cancellation.

7. The telephone procedure: This includes **call in times** (when the doctor takes phone calls) and/or when during the day the doctor usually returns phone calls.

8. What hospitals the doctor(s) is affiliated with, what nursing homes the doctors make visits to, and when the doctors make house calls.

9. How medication refills are handled.

10. What to do when the office is closed.

The Patient Information Booklet

An increasing number of practices today have a booklet or brochure that contains the above information. If the practice you work for puts out a first-time booklet or a new booklet, you should encourage every patient to take one at the end of a visit. New patients should be given one at the beginning of the first visit, when they are given their new patient forms to fill out.

The patient information booklet must be kept up to date. If new doctors, nurse practitioners, or physician's

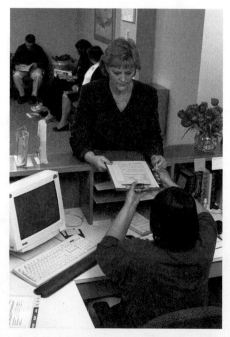

➤ **Figure 12–3** If an open desk is used for reception, the waiting room should be large enough to prevent other patients from overhearing the conversation at the desk.

assistants join the practice; if the doctors affiliate with a new hospital; or if the doctors open a new satellite office or procedure suite (such as an endoscopy suite for gastroenterologists), an updated patient information booklet should be prepared.

Patient information booklets are very successful marketing and public relations tools. They are greatly appreciated by patients. However, they often receive low priority on the list of things to do in the crush of day-to-day patient care.

A study published in *The Professional Medical Assistant* of May/June 2000 revealed that many practices were not prepared to present themselves professionally on the telephone or in published material (Bowell, "Presenting the Practice to the Public—Are You Ready?" *PMA* May/June 2000: 26–28).

CHECKING PATIENTS IN

Checking patients in for an appointment is a straightforward process, but one that demands attention to detail and involves a number of different steps. See Procedure 12–3 for details on checking patients in.

Obtaining Information from New Patients

When a new patient arrives, he or she is usually given one or more forms to fill out.

New Patient Information Form

The new patient information form, as discussed in chapter 10, requests demographic information from the patient.

Consent For Treatment/Release of Information

The patient is usually asked to sign a statement that allows the office to release information to the insurance company for billing purposes. This consent may be part of the patient information form or may be a separate sheet.

Assignment of Benefits

If the office accepts payments directly from the insurance company (called accepting **assignment of benefits**) the patient also must sign a form authorizing this. The assignment of benefits statement is usually included with the consent to release information to insurance companies. Figure 12–4 shows an example of a new patient information form that has been completed by a patient.

Note that by signing the bottom section, the patient authorizes Blackburn Primary Care Associates to release information to the insurance company and authorizes the insurance company to pay the medical practice directly. In addition, the patient has agreed to be responsible for charges not covered by insurance.

Patient History Form

Most offices also have a history form for the patient to fill out before being seen by the doctor. The medical assistant goes over this form with the patient in the exam room to be sure that all of the relevant information has been included. Medical information should not be discussed at the front desk if it can be avoided.

Verifying Data for Established Patients

If the patient has been seen in the office before, it is only necessary to verify that the billing information is still correct. When checking a patient in, the medical assistant should ask if the address and telephone number are still the same and if the patient has the same insurance as the last time he or she was seen.

If there are changes, the updated information needs to go both into the computer billing system and into the medical record, whether paper or computer based.

Verifying Insurance and/or Referral

After a new patient has filled out the patient information sheet, or if an existing patient has a change in insurance carrier, the medical assistant should ask for the insurance card and photocopy both sides. This is then placed in the patient's medical record. It verifies the information given by the patient and sometimes gives additional information needed for billing. In addition, it provides expiration data about current insurance. When the expiration date arrives, you must verify that the patient has continued the insurance or has switched to another insurance carrier (Fig. 12–5).

If the patient has been referred to your office by another doctor through a managed care plan, be sure the patient has a completed referral form from the primary care doctor. Sometimes the referring doctor has sent it in advance, but often the patient brings it personally to the visit. If there is no referral form, the insurance company may not pay for the visit.

The written referral will state how many visits are allowed (how many will be paid for by the managed care plan) and the problem for which the patient is being referred. Depending on the patient's insurance or managed care plan, you may also need to have the patient sign a statement promising to pay any charges that the insurance does not cover.

Managed care plans usually do not allow doctors who accept referrals to bill for excess charges to the

PROCEDURE 12–3

Checking Patients In

Performance Objective: The student will check patients in for office visits.

Equipment and Supplies: Charge slip, medical record, pen, appointment schedule; for new patients: patient information form, authorization to release information to insurance company, assignment of benefits form; patient information booklet, photocopy machine.

Procedure Steps:

1. When someone enters the office waiting room, make eye contact and greet them. If you are assisting someone at the desk or window, ask the newly arrived person to have a seat until you are free.
   Rationale: Many people find it awkward to enter an unfamiliar office. To be greeted at once is reassuring and helps a person feel comfortable. To ensure privacy, only one person should be speaking with the medical assistant at the desk or window.

2. When you speak with the newly arrived person, establish if he or she is a patient. If so, find the charge slip and medical record (or print the charge slip if this is only done after the patient arrives). You should already be familiar with the names of patients expected for the day.
   Rationale: You need to prepare the medical record and charge slip before the patient can be examined.

3. Ask a new patient to fill out the forms used by your office, which may include a new patient information sheet, patient history, and consent forms for billing the insurance company and assigning benefits. If the patient has been referred by another doctor, ask for a referral form. If your office has a patient information booklet, give it to the patient.
   Rationale: Before the examination, you need to collect necessary information and consents for billing.

4. When the patient returns the completed forms, review them for completeness and accuracy. Make a photocopy of both sides of the patient's insurance card.
   Rationale: Correct information facilitates collections.

5. Confirm patient eligibility for insurance coverage if necessary, and confirm that any referral is correctly filled out. If the visit will not be completely covered by insurance, discuss the patient's financial responsibility.
   Rationale: The patient has a right to know what his or her financial obligation will be before receiving service.

6. If the patient is an established patient, ask if there have been any address, telephone, or insurance changes; document any new information in the computer and the medical record. If you ask your question while reading the information on file ("Do you still live at 20 Oak Park Drive in Woodville?"), the patient will know easily you have the most current information.
   Rationale: Patients may not remember to tell you about changes in personal information.

7. Collect the co-payment, if any, and enter the amount on the charge slip.
   Rationale: Co-payments are usually collected before the visit because they do not change no matter what service the patient receives, but it is also correct to collect them after the visit. By law an office must collect co-payments and may not "forget about them." Medical offices attempt to avoid sending bills, especially for small amounts, in order to reduce overhead costs.

8. Use a pen to check off the patient on the master appointment list.
   Rationale: The office must keep an official record of patients seen for financial purposes.

9. Insert any new forms into the medical record and place it with the charge slip. Ask the patient to have a seat and tell him or her approximately how long before the examination.
   Rationale: When the paperwork is complete, it will help the patient feel more in control to know how long he or she can expect to wait before the examination.

10. Place the chart and charge slip in the designated place to indicate to the doctor or clinical assistant that the patient is in the waiting room and ready to be seen.
    Rationale: All paperwork is completed before the patient is placed in an examination room.

REGISTRATION
(PLEASE PRINT)

Home Phone: 608-297-1349   Today's Date: 1/5/05

PATIENT INFORMATION

Name: SHAPIRO   IVAN   R.   Soc. Sec.# 591-23-1971
Last Name   First Name   Initial

Address: 3242 Kentucky Lane

City: Blackburn   State: WI   Zip: 54938

Single ___ Married X Widowed ___ Separated ___ Divorced ___   Sex M X F___ Age 59 Birthdate 3/6/45

Patient Employed by: SELF   Occupation: CARPENTER

Business Address: as above   Business Phone: as above

By whom were you referred? _____

In case of emergency who should be notified? MARYANNE SHAPIRO (WIFE) Phone 6082971349
Last Name   Relationship to Patient

PRIMARY INSURANCE

Person Responsible for Account: SHAPIRO   IVAN   R
Last Name   First Name   Initial
591-23-1971

Relation to Patient: SELF   Birthdate 3/6/45   Soc. Sec.# 591-23-1971

Address (if different from patient's): Same   Phone _____

City _____   State _____   Zip _____

Person Responsible Employed by: SELF   Occupation CARPENTER

Business Address: as above   Business Phone _____

Insurance Company: Blue Cross Blue Shield

Contract # none   Group # none   Subscriber # 591-23-1971A

Name of other dependents covered under this plan MARYANNE SHAPIRO

ADDITIONAL INSURANCE

Is patient covered by additional insurance? ___ Yes X No

Subscriber Name _____ Relationship to Patient _____ Birthdate _____

Address (if different from patient's) _____ Phone _____

City _____ State _____ Zip _____

Subscriber Employed by _____ Business Phone _____

Insurance Company _____

Contract # _____ Group # _____ Subscriber # _____

Name of other dependents covered under this plan _____

ASSIGNMENT AND RELEASE

I, the undersigned, certify that I (or my dependent) have insurance coverage with Blue Cross Blue Shield
and assign directly to Dr. Blackburn Primary Care Associates insurance benefits, if any, otherwise payable to me for services rendered. I understand that I am financially responsible for all charges whether or not paid by insurance. I hereby authorize the doctor to release all information necessary to secure the payment of benefits. I authorize the use of this signature on all insurance submissions.

Ivan Shapiro   Self   01/05/05
Responsible Party Signature   Relationship   Date

ORDER# 58-8426 • © 1996 BIBBERO SYSTEMS, INC. • PETALUMA, CALIFORNIA • TO REORDER CALL TOLL FREE: (800) 242-9330

➤ **Figure 12–4** When the new patient information form is complete, the patient's signature authorizes release of information to the insurance company and assignment of benefits.

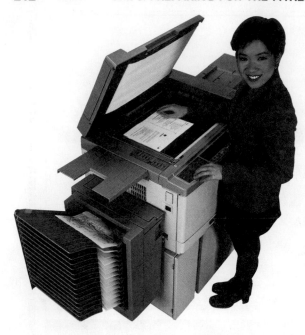

➤ **Figure 12–5** The medical assistant uses the photocopy machine to obtain copies of the patient's insurance card and sometimes the referral form or other information.

patient (a practice known as balance billing). Medicare also does not allow balance billing from providers who agree to accept Medicare patients. However, if the patient receives a service not covered by insurance or Medicare, he or she can be billed.

See Figure 12–6 for a typical referral form.

If the patient has not yet obtained a referral form, or if it is uncertain that the insurance will cover the services, the patient needs to understand that he or she will be responsible for payment of the bill.

Obtaining Authorizations

Some types of insurance require authorization every time the patient visits the primary care doctor. Patients with Medicaid must usually have their coverage verified and/or must receive prior authorization for each visit. **Medicaid** is an insurance program established by the federal government that pays for low-income patients' medical needs. Each state administers Medicaid, and the program has a different name in each state. The cost is split between the state and the federal government, which mandates that certain medical services be covered. Other services are optional, and the federal government funds a larger percentage of optional services than basic services.

In some states, some patients on Medicaid receive new identification cards each month; in other states patients can be verified by telephone, fax, or an electronic **point-of-service (POS) device**, a small machine in the doctor's office that is connected via telephone to

the insurance company's database and can verify insurance benefits while the patient is in the office. A POS device is shown in Figure 12–7.

For other types of insurance, it may be necessary to call the patient's insurance company to obtain authorization for treatment. This may be done when the patient makes the appointment, when the patient checks in, or after the first visit, when the doctor has identified what treatment is needed and how many visits are anticipated.

Each office has its own procedure for verifying insurance. In general, if there is a question whether the patient has insurance coverage, or whether the service will be covered, call before the doctor sees the patient. If the service is routine, and the patient has a valid insurance card or referral, verify after the visit.

Taking Co-payments

A **co-payment** is a fixed amount of money that the patient is required to pay each time he or she receives medical treatment. The amount of the co-payment is printed on the patient's insurance card, sometimes on the back (one reason it is important to photocopy both sides of the card).

Many offices collect the co-payment before the visit because it is a fixed fee, although it can also be done at the end of the visit. The amount paid is entered on the patient's charge slip. A receipt should be given to the patient at the time the co-payment is made.

Health Plan Referral Form

REFERRAL NUMBER: A06

WRITTEN REFERRALS ARE REQUIRED FOR ALL SERVICES, EXCEPT FOR ROUTINE YEARLY EYE EXAMS, ORAL SURGERY, LAB, DIAGNOSTIC & RADIOLOGICAL SERVICES.

(1) Patient Name: _____

(2) Date of Referral: _____ / _____ / _____

(3) Patient Identification Number: _____ (4) [SUFFIX # REQUIRED]

(5) Date of Birth: _____ / _____ / _____

(6) Referred From: _____
NAME OF PERSONAL CARE PHYSICIAN   Provider ID #

(7) I.P.A. No. [   ]

(8) _____
ADDRESS OF PERSONAL CARE PHYSICIAN

Referred To: _____
NAME OF SPECIALTY CARE PHYSICIAN/PROVIDER/EMERGENCY   Provider ID #

(10) _____
ADDRESS OF SPECIALTY CARE PHYSICIAN/PROVIDER/EMERGENCY

REFERRAL STATUS:
(CHECK ONE)   In I.P.A. ☐   ☐   ☐   ☐

REASON FOR REFERRAL (STATE DIAGNOSIS): _____

SERVICES REQUESTED (CHECK ONE)   **REFERRAL VALID FOR TWELVE MONTHS FROM DATE OF REFERRAL.**

☐ Consultative OPINION. (One (1) visit only) CONTACT PCP PRIOR TO INITIATING TREATMENT.

☐ SECOND SURGICAL OPINION ONLY (Surgery is not to be performed by this provider)

☐ Consultative OPINION and NECESSARY DIAGNOSTIC STUDIES. (Not to exceed three (3) visits)

☐ Consultative OPINION and NECESSARY DIAGNOSTIC STUDY AND TREATMENT. **Indicate number of visits** [   ]

☐ Mental Health EVALUATION: Circle one (1) or two (2) visits only. (FOR PCP USE ONLY)

☐ Substance Abuse Outpatient EVALUATION: Circle one (1) or two (2) visits only. (FOR PCP USE ONLY)

☐ Mental Health/Substance Abuse Treatment (PSYCHIATRIC REVIEWER USE ONLY) subsequent visits, indicate number [   ]

AUTHORIZATION FOR MENTAL HEALTH OR SUBSTANCE ABUSE OUTPATIENT SERVICES DOES NOT OVERRIDE BENEFIT MAXIMUMS.

☐ Therapies (type of therapy: _____). **Indicate number of visits** [   ] (PT not to exceed six (6) visits per referral)

☐ Obstetrical Treatment. Designate duration of care: _____

☐ Emergency Room Treatment. Date of service: _____ / _____ / _____
SEPARATE REFERRAL FORM REQUIRED FOR EACH EMERGENCY ROOM DATE OF SERVICE

Note: Only those services included in the Health Plan Description of Benefits will be covered. If you have any questions contact your Professional Relations Coordinator.

I have enclosed a clinical document summary, have performed the followingt diagnostic studies and arm supplying the information to assist you.

DIAGNOSTIC PROCEDURES	DATE OF SERVICE	RESULTS

INSTRUCTIONS

PCP:	SPECIALIST:	ER AUTHORIZATION
Complete Form	Fax Referral to another Specialist Consult W/ PCP	• Send Health Plan Copy to Appropriate Address (see above)
• Send Health Plan Copy and Specialist Copy to Specialist	• Send Health Plan Copy to Appropriate Address (see above)	• Retain Copy for your file
• Retain PCP Copy for your file		• Be sure to notify

X _____   _____ / _____ / _____

X _____   _____ / _____ / _____
SIGNATURE OF PHYSICIUAN REVIEWER*   AUTHORIZATION DATE
*ALL OUT OF PLAN REFERRALS REQUIRE PHYSICIAN REVIEWER SIGNATURE

➤ **Figure 12–6** A typical patient referral form.

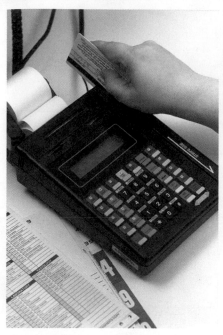

> Figure 12–7 Point-of-service device used to validate insurance coverage for Medicaid and other insurance plans.

Indicating That the Patient Is in the Waiting Room

After the patient has been checked in at the front desk, the medical record is placed in the designated space for patients who are ready to be seen. If a computerized record is used, a routing slip is generated.

The forms that the patient filled out are inserted in the medical record. The charge slip is usually attached to the front of the record for the doctor to fill in.

If there are several doctors in the practice, each one uses a separate cubby or box to hold the charts of patients who have been checked in and are waiting to be seen.

STUDENT STUDY PLAN

To reinforce your understanding of the material in this chapter . . .

Complete *Complete* the **Review & Recall** questions below.

Discuss *Discuss* the situation in **If You Were the Medical Assistant** with your classmates, and answer the questions.

Answer *Answer* the **Critical Thinking Questions** below and discuss them with your classmates.

Visit *Visit* **Web sites** suggested below, and search for additional Web sites using **Keywords for Internet Searches.**

Complete *Complete* the exercises in chapter 12 of the **Student Mastery Manual.**

REVIEW & RECALL

1. Where do you get messages and/or faxes when you first open the office?

2. How should you record messages from an answering machine?

3. Before a patient enters the office, what is prepared for the visit?

4. What should be done to prepare the waiting area for patients each day?

5. What are some ways to maintain patient confidentiality at the reception window or desk?

6. What information about the practice should be available to new patients, either verbally or in a printed brochure?

7. What must a new patient usually consent to?

8. What should the medical assistant ask an established patient who is checking in for an appointment?

9. Why does the medical assistant photocopy a new patient's insurance card?

10. Describe the nature and purpose of a referral form.

11. How can you obtain authorization for a procedure from an insurance company?

12. How is the doctor made aware that a patient is in the waiting room, waiting to be seen?

 IF YOU WERE THE MEDICAL ASSISTANT

Assume that you are opening the office at Blackburn Primary Care Associates. Identify what you must do:

1. To turn on equipment

2. To get messages

3. To prepare to see patients.

During the first hour you are in the office, three patients call for appointments. Identify each step you must take to prepare for these appointments.

When the first patient arrives in the office and steps to the window, what would you say to him or her? What should happen before this patient is placed in an examination room if the person is an established patient? If he or she is a new patient?

 CRITICAL THINKING QUESTIONS

1. Discuss how a new patient feels if he or she enters the waiting room in a medical office and there is no one in the reception area. How does he or she feel if there is a line of two or three people at the reception desk?

2. Work with your classmates to gather patient information books from various medical offices in your area. Compare them for layout and content. Based on the examples you have, which medical practice would you choose if you needed to find a new doctor? Give your reasons.

3. Call your own (or your parents') insurance company to find out if one of the following three services is covered:

   Surgery to remove impacted wisdom teeth
   Treatment of acne by a dermatologist
   Treatment by a chiropractor for acute back pain.

   Obtain information about whether a written referral and/or telephone preauthorization is necessary to receive coverage for the service and how you would obtain such a referral.

 EXPLORE THE WEB

INTERNET WEB SITES

Medscape—medical office manager
www.medscape.com/Home/network/MOM/MOM.html

Sample medical office information on line
www.physicianweb.net

4 The Patient Visit

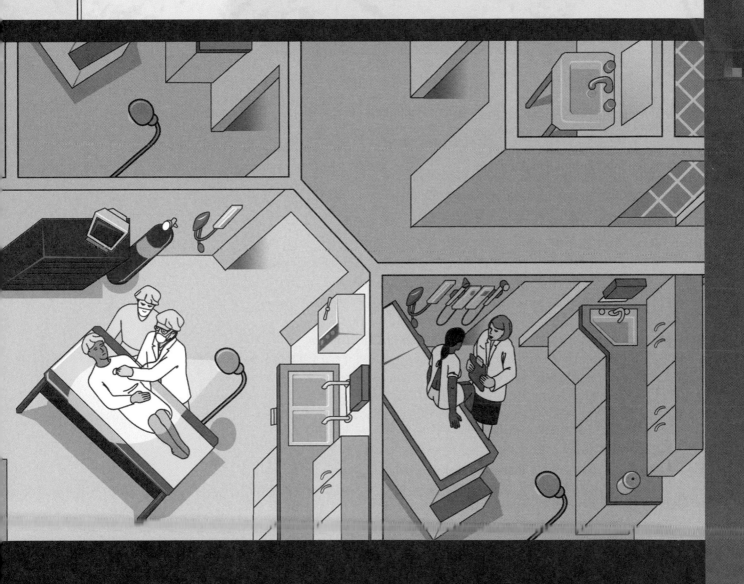

Chapter 13

Medical Asepsis and Infection Control

Instructional Objectives

After completing this chapter, you will be able to do the following:

1. Define and spell the vocabulary words for this chapter.
2. List seven reasons for preventing the transmission of infectious disease.
3. Describe five types of microorganisms that can cause disease.
4. Identify six conditions that promote growth of microorganisms.
5. Differentiate between microorganisms that are normal flora and those that are pathogens.
6. Describe physiologic responses that are natural defenses against infection.
7. Differentiate between the cellular immune response and the humoral immune response.
8. Differentiate between natural and artificial immunity, and give examples of active and passive types of both.
9. Discuss the five links in the infection cycle.
10. Describe the purpose and methods of medical asepsis.
11. Describe the procedure for medical aseptic handwashing.
12. Compare methods of sanitizing, disinfecting, and sterilizing equipment, and discuss when each is appropriate.
13. Identify three levels of disinfection.
14. Identify four methods of sterilization.
15. Describe the procedure for wrapping instruments for steam sterilization.
16. Discuss the purpose of sterilization indicators and culture tests.
17. Identify principles of loading the autoclave for effective sterilization.
18. Describe the procedure for steam sterilization of instruments using an autoclave.

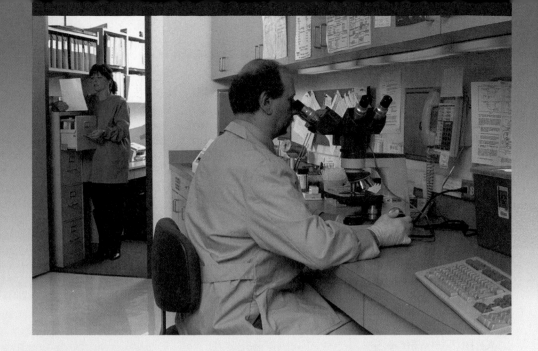

Performance Objectives

After completing this chapter, you will be able to do the following:

1. Perform a medical aseptic handwash (Procedure 13–1).
2. Remove soiled gloves and dispose of them properly (Procedure 13–2).
3. Sanitize soiled instruments following standard precautions (Procedure 13–3).
4. Wrap instruments for sterilization (Procedure 13–4).
5. Operate an autoclave to sterilize instruments and/or equipment (Procedure 13–5)

VOCABULARY

acquired immunity (p. 227)
active immunity (p. 227)
aerobic (p. 225)
anaerobic (p. 225)
antibodies (p. 226)
antigens (p. 226)
artificial immunity (p. 227)
asepsis (p. 229)
bacillus (p. 223)
bacteria (p. 222)
B cells (p. 227)
cell-mediated immune
   response (p. 226)

coccus (p. 222)
colonization (p. 225)
cytotoxic (p. 227)
disinfection (p. 234)
epidemic (p. 221)
fomite (p. 228)
fungi (p. 224)
gamma globulins (p. 226)
genetic immunity (p. 227)
humoral immune response
   (p. 227)
immunoglobulins (p. 226)
infectious disease (p. 220)

inflammation (p. 226)
medical asepsis (p. 229)
metazoa (p. 224)
mold (p. 224)
natural immunity (p. 227)
normal flora (p. 225)
passive immunity (p. 227)
pathogen (p. 220)
pH (p. 225)
protozoa (p. 224)
resistance (p. 220)
sanitizing (p. 234)

spirochete (p. 223)
spore (p. 223)
sterile (p. 229)
sterile technique (p. 229)
sterilization (p. 237)
surgical asepsis (p. 229)
T cells (p. 227)
vector (p. 228)
virulent (p. 221)
virus (p. 223)
yeast (p. 224)

ABBREVIATIONS

OSHA (p. 233)   PPE (p. 232)

PURPOSE OF INFECTION CONTROL SYSTEMS

One of medicine's traditional efforts has been to prevent and treat **infectious disease.** Infectious diseases are those caused by pathogenic microorganisms—bacteria, viruses, parasites, and fungi—which can be spread from one person to another.

Effects of Infectious Disease

Throughout history, larger organisms such as humans have been at the mercy of diseases caused by smaller organisms. Infectious disease has been the cause of much suffering and death.

Microorganisms are present everywhere. The vast majority do not kill; in fact, they do not cause any adverse symptoms at all. The majority of microorganisms coexist with other beings, large and small, in a constant competition for resources.

In the last part of the 19th century, scientists such as Joseph Lister and Louis Pasteur began to understand this fact. They discovered ways to reduce the mortality (death) and morbidity (disease) caused by **pathogens,** the microorganisms that can cause disease. Throughout the 20th century, as the result of doctors and scientists developing more effective prevention and treatment, the effects of infectious disease have been greatly reduced, especially in the industrialized world.

We cannot become complacent, however. Our ability to treat infectious disease may be turning around as a consequence of our overuse of antibiotic medications. Those bacteria that survive after antibiotic treatment

are often resistant to medication (some newspapers have called them "superbugs").

The life cycle of bacteria and viruses is very short, and genetic mutation occurs frequently. This allows microorganisms to adapt very quickly (as compared to humans and other large animals) to changes in their environment. Bacteria that survive antibiotic treatment begin to multiply rapidly, resulting in a new strain that is immune to the drugs faster than scientists can develop new antibiotics. This immunity is called **resistance.**

During 1999 alone, strains of bacteria developed that resist all antibiotics except vancomycin. The medical community fears that it is only a matter of time before even this powerful antibiotic will be ineffective on some bacteria. In addition, resistant strains of bacteria once only found in hospitals now seem to be present in individuals in the population at large. Because of their ability to multiply rapidly, these antibiotic-resistant bacteria pose a serious threat.

But this chapter is not about treatment. Rather, it is about prevention and the role of the medical assistant in controlling potential infection in the medical office setting.

Reasons Prevention Is Important

A number of methods are used in the medical office to prevent microorganisms from infecting patients and workers. Preventing the transmission of infectious disease reduces the incidence (number of cases) of specific diseases. There are a number of reasons why prevention is important, especially in the outpatient setting of the doctor's office.

Easier and Cheaper to Prevent Than Treat

Overall, it is far easier, less time consuming, and less expensive to take precautions against contracting infectious diseases than it is to treat them. When people become sick with an infectious disease, they must receive additional medical attention, must often take a course of medication, and either miss work or are less productive.

Contagious Patients Are Present in the Medical Office

People are spending less time in hospitals. Shorter hospital stays are one way insurance companies and health maintenance organizations are trying to reduce the cost of health care.

Because of these short hospital stays, patients with complex needs must often be managed with office visits. They are also more likely to be seen in a doctor's office shortly after a hospital stay, when their ability to fight off infectious disease is reduced. It is important to use measures to prevent these patients from becoming ill.

Increasing Resistance

An increasing number of organisms are resistant to antibiotics. People infected with these organisms continue to suffer even after being treated with standard antibiotics, and new classes of antibiotics are necessary to successfully treat them.

The most visible of these is otitis media, the common ear infection that many children suffer with. Research shows that overtreatment of fluid buildup in the ear can lead to infection by organisms that are resistant to standard antibiotics; also, if the patient's parents do not complete the treatment for the full time prescribed, even after the child feels better, the possibility of developing antibiotic-resistant infection increases. The most dangerous antibiotic-resistant bacteria is tuberculosis, which was once thought to be all but wiped out in the United States. Today, however, tuberculosis is on the increase, and many cases are resistant to antibiotics.

This has occurred primarily because the antibiotics that are so successful in fighting tuberculosis must be taken for a long time. But those medications have side effects such as nausea, and many people stop taking them as soon as the symptoms and discomfort from the disease begin to get better. In addition, tuberculosis is also on the increase because it flourishes in areas of crowding and where people have decreased immunity, due to acquired immune deficiency syndrome (AIDS) or other chronic illnesses. These conditions are often found in this country in prisons and homeless shelters.

Outwardly, these people may appear well, at least for a time. However, they still have some of the pathogens in their bodies. In fact, the tuberculosis bacteria that still exist in a person who has taken a short course of antibiotics are the strongest bacteria. As they multiply, the individual then becomes host to enough antibiotic-resistant tuberculosis bacteria to infect a number of people. This progression is also evident in diseases less deadly than tuberculosis.

Lack of Effective Treatment for Viruses

Medicine has developed no ability to neutralize viruses once they have infected the host. Most treatment for viral infections is done to reduce symptoms. These infections last a few days to a few weeks, until the body's defenses destroy the attacking viruses; more serious viral infections, such as the human immunodeficiency virus (HIV), polio, and rabies, can have deadly consequences. Preventing the spread of viral infections in the medical office is a prime goal.

Epidemic of Blood-Borne Diseases

Much of the world is now in the grip of three widespread blood-borne diseases; AIDS, hepatitis B, and hepatitis C. These three diseases are transmitted only by direct contact with blood or body fluids, including during unprotected sex and intravenous drug use where needles are shared. However, it is possible for these diseases to be passed during medical procedures during which staff come into contact with the blood or other body fluids of an infected patient (rarely, a patient may come in contact with blood or other body fluids of an infected staff member).

Encroachment on Formerly Inaccessible Habitat

The human encroachment on rain forest and formerly isolated areas increases the possibility of animal diseases spreading to humans. These diseases, if formerly unknown or rare, may become especially **virulent** (able to cause serious illness) once they enter the human population. Such diseases include the Ebola and Marburg viruses, which kill almost all people who become infected. In addition, some scientists believe that HIV, the virus that causes AIDS, is a genetic mutation of a disease that has long affected gorillas, chimpanzees, and other apes; it is believed to have begun affecting humans after mutation in the 1970s. The eastern United States has since 1999 been witnessing the spread of West Nile virus in many species of birds and in some humans as well.

Global Travel

High rates of travel make any **epidemic** (disease that attacks many people at one time) an instant worldwide problem. Scientists fear the spread of antibiotic-resistant tuberculosis to industrialized countries by

Table 13–1	Types of Bacteria			
Group	Shape	Grouping	Specific Examples	Diseases Caused
Diplococcus	Spheres	Pairs	*Neisseria gonorrhoeae*	Gonorrhea
Staphylococcus	Spheres	Clusters	*Staphylococcus aureus*	Boils, abscesses
Streptococcus	Spheres	Chains	Group A beta-hemolytic streptococci	Strep throat, scarlet fever
			Streptococcus pneumoniae	Pneumonia
Bacillus	Rod-shaped	Singles, pairs	*Mycobacterium tuberculosis*	Tuberculosis
		Chains	*Escherichia coli (E. coli)*	Normal resident of gastrointestinal tract; can cause diarrhea and urinary tract infections
Spirochetes	Comma-shaped	Singles	*Vibrio cholerae*	Cholera
	Flexible spirals		*Treponema pallidum*	Syphilis

immigrants from third-world countries, where they were not told of the necessity to take their medication after they felt better, or where the health care system has so few resources that antibiotics are used only for short periods to alleviate symptoms. A person with an infection spread by droplets from the respiratory tract traveling on an airplane where air is recycled throughout the cabin can potentially infect several people during a relatively short flight.

DISEASE-CAUSING MICROORGANISMS AND THEIR GROWTH

Microorganisms vary in size and characteristics. They also vary in how they pass from one person to another—through "casual contact" such as touching or sneezing or through "intimate contact" during which blood and fluids are exchanged.

Organisms That Cause Disease

Five types of microorganisms cause human disease:

bacteria
specialized bacteria
viruses
fungi
single-cell parasites.

If a virus such as polio is magnified to the size of a typewritten period, a bacteria like *E. coli* would be the size of an oval about 1/2″ inch by 1/4″, and a human red blood cell would be a circle almost 3″ in diameter.

Larger organisms, such as insects and worms, can also cause disease.

Bacteria

Bacteria (single, bacterium) vary in size, but are usually at least 1 micrometer (one millionth of a meter)

long. They are not visible to the naked eye, but can be seen under a microscope. There are three major groups of bacteria:

Coccus (pl. cocci, pronounced cox-eye). Cocci are spheres. They include staphylococci, streptococci, and diplococci. Staphylococci, which live in clusters on skin and mucous membranes, usually do not cause disease (nonpathogenic) unless they reach areas that are usually sterile, where they can cause large pustules or abscesses. Streptococci form chains and can cause sore throats, scarlet fever, pneumonia, and skin infections. Diplococci, which appear in pairs, cause bacterial meningitis, gonorrhea, and pneumonia.

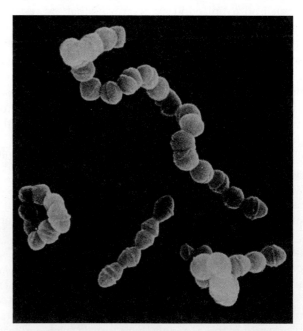

➤ **Figure 13–1** *Streptococcus* bacteria form pairs, clusters, or chains, as in this photograph taken by an electron microscope. (From Thibodeau G, Patton K: *The Human Body in Health and Disease.* St. Louis: Mosby, 1992)

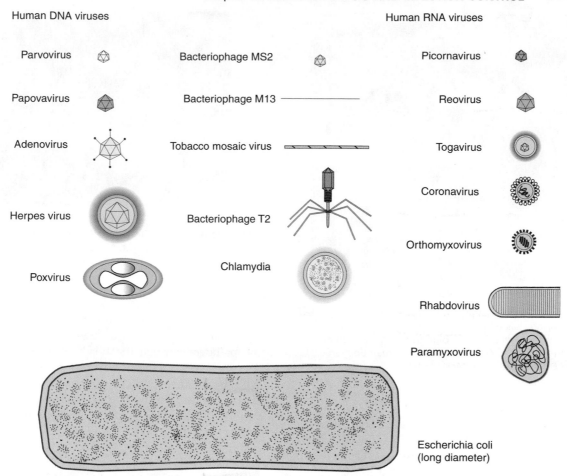

> **Figure 13–2** Viruses contain either DNA or RNA, which allows them to be smaller than bacteria such as *E. coli* or *Chlamydia*. Their elaborate shape usually includes a protein coat, which they shed as they enter human cells. (From Stepp CA, Woods MA: *Laboratory Procedures for Medical Office Personnel.* Philadelphia: WB Saunders, 1998)

Bacillus (pl. bacilli). Bacilli are rod shaped and cause tuberculosis, tetanus, and otitis media.

Spirochetes are long, spiral, flexible bacteria. They cause syphilis and Lyme disease.

Table 13–1 lists types of bacteria; Figure 13–1 shows a streptococcus bacteria.

Bacteria can grow outside a living host. They reproduce by cell division. Except for spirochetes, bacterial infections are diagnosed by culture (growth in a substance containing nutrients). Many bacteria produce spores to protect themselves under adverse conditions. A **spore** is a dormant form that has formed a thick capsule around itself that is highly resistant to heat or chemicals. It may be the adult or a reproductive form of the organism, depending on the species. Spore producers include organisms that cause tetanus, botulism, gas gangrene, and anthrax.

Specialized Bacteria

Specialized bacteria are smaller than most bacteria and cannot survive or reproduce outside a human host. They include rickettsia (ri-ket-see-a) and chlamydia (kla-mid-e-a). Rickettsia causes Rocky Mountain spotted fever. Chlamydia causes a common form of vaginitis (infection of the vagina) and trachoma, an eye disease that causes blindness in some parts of the world. They can be seen under a microscope.

Viruses

Viruses are the smallest of infectious agents; they contain only DNA or RNA, but not both. Viruses average about 100 nanometers (100 billionths of a meter) and were discovered long after bacteria because of their small size. Viruses reproduce by taking over cells and directing the cell to produce copies of the virus-infected cells. Viruses cannot grow outside a living cell.

The shape of viruses varies. But all contain an outer protein coat, which may have various complex shapes, as seen in Figure 13–2.

Viruses can only be seen under an electron microscope and can only be grown in tissue culture. The most definitive test for the presence of a virus is a blood test for antibodies to the virus. Because of the difficulty both seeing and growing viruses and the ex-

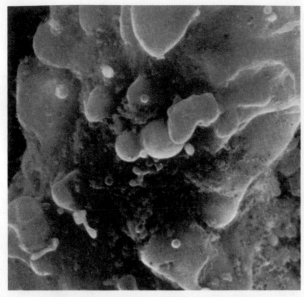

> **Figure 13–3** Human immunodeficiency viruses (HIV) spread over neighboring cells when released from an infected white blood cell. They are seen here in blue using an electron microscope. (From Thibodeau G, Patton K: *The Human Body in Health and Disease.* St. Louis: Mosby, 1992)

pense of blood tests, viruses are often assumed to be present based on the clinical presentation of illness. Figure 13–3 shows the virus that causes AIDS.

Fungi

Fungi (pronounced funge-eye, singular fungus) vary in size from microscopic to visible with the naked eye. Fungi are at least 10 times as large as bacteria.

They are single-celled or multicellular. If single-celled, they are usually about 0.01 millimeter long (10 millionths of a meter).

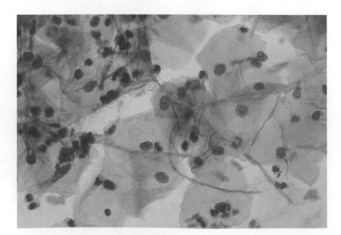

> **Figure 13–4** *Candida albicans*, a yeast, is seen in tissue. (From Stepp CA, Woods MA: *Laboratory Procedures for Medical Office Personnel.* Philadelphia: WB Saunders, 1998)

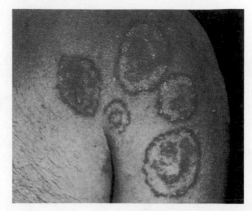

> **Figure 13–5** Ringworm can be seen as a circular discoloration on the skin. (From Thibodeau G, Patton K: *The Human Body in Health and Disease.* St. Louis: Mosby, 1992)

Fungi can grow outside a living host on organic material. They can be grown in artificial growth media. Usually, fungi do not cause disease, but they can become pathogenic when the host's normal defenses are weakened. Fungi include yeasts and molds.

Yeasts are single-celled organisms that reproduce by budding, an asexual method of reproduction in which a budlike process develops into a microorganism. They cause candidiasis, vaginal infections, and infections in the mouth called thrush. Figure 13–4 shows yeast cells in tissue.

Molds grow by extending tentacle-like projections. Mold colonies are visible to the naked eye. Molds include ringworm, nail fungus, and athlete's foot. See Figure 13–5.

Parasites

Parasites are larger organisms that live in or on another organism. They vary from single-celled organisms to worms and insects.

Single-celled parasites are **protozoa.** These include species of *Entamoeba* and *Giardia*, which cause diarrhea and dysentery; species of *Trichomonas,* which cause urinary tract and vaginal infections; and several species of *Plasmodium*, which cause malaria.

Multicellular parasites are called **metazoa.** These parasites often have complicated life cycles, which may include multiple hosts.

Worms (helminths and nematodes) can infest various organs. These include tapeworms, which live in the intestines; flukes, which live in the liver; pinworms, which live in the anus; and various species of *Trichinella,* which can spread throughout the body, causing trichinosis. *Trichinella spiralis* normally infest pigs and are spread to humans through uncooked or undercooked pork.

Insects (arthropods) include fleas, mites, lice, and ticks. In some cases, insects such as mites and lice live on the body, causing skin irritation, itching, and inflammation. In other cases, insects transmit disease-causing microorganisms. This is the case with Lyme disease, spread by bites from a deer tick. Figure 13–6 shows a tick as seen under a microscope.

Some insects that are not parasites can also transmit diseases. Mosquitoes, for instance, can transmit any number of diseases depending on where they live. Examples include eastern equine encephalitis, malaria, West Nile virus, or Rift Valley fever.

Conditions for Optimal Growth of Microorganisms

Six conditions are necessary for microorganisms to grow and thrive:

1. A moist environment; the body is very moist.
2. Nutrients; within the body are plenty of nutrients for parasites.

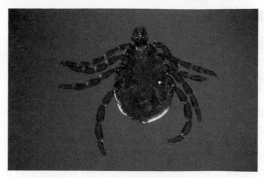

> Figure 13–6 A tick seen under a microscope.

3. Temperature of around 98.6°F; normal body temperature.
4. Darkness; inside the body's cavities and organs there is little if any light.
5. Neutral to slightly alkaline **pH.** pH is a measure of the amount of acid (hydrogen ions) in anything; a slightly alkaline pH is one with minimal acidity. The pH of blood and body tissue is normally neutral.
6. Either an oxygen source, for **aerobic** organisms, or an absence of oxygen, for **anaerobic** organisms. Most disease-causing microorganisms are aerobic, meaning they must have oxygen to continue to live. Anaerobic disease-causing microorganisms, which can live where no oxygen is present, thrive in a closed wound that has not been kept sterile. Examples include tetanus and gas gangrene.

DEFENSES AGAINST INFECTION

The body has a host of defenses against infection. The four major defenses are normal flora, physical factors, physiologic responses, and the immune systems.

Normal Flora

Normal flora are those microorganisms that normally live on the skin, in the gastrointestinal (GI) tract, and in the respiratory tract. Millions of normal flora live in the human body. These microorganisms do not cause disease unless the person's immune system is compromised or the organisms invade other parts of the body. Many, especially those in the gastrointestinal tract, are actually necessary for proper body function. By their presence, they prevent the **colonization** (taking over space and growing) of harmful microorganisms.

Physical Factors

Three normal physical factors help the body fight off harmful microorganisms:

LATIN NAMES

Many times the Latin name is used for organisms. For bacteria and larger organisms, two Latin names are used. The first is the genus, and the second is the species. The genus name is Capitalized; the species name is not. *Italics* are used, because the word is in a foreign language.

For instance, humans are *Homo sapiens.* This means that all humans on earth belong to the same genus and species.

You must remember that there is significant variation in bacteria, fungi, and so on, which belong to several different genera (genera is the plural of genus).

Bacteria of the same genus but different species, such as *Streptococcus pyogenes* and *Streptococcus viridans,* are related, but do not usually interbreed. The situation is analogous to that of a wolf (*Canis lupus*) and a dog (*Canis familiaris*), which belong to the same genus but different species.

When talking about members of a genus, sometimes only the initial of the genus is used, such as *E. coli* for *Escherichia coli* or *S. aureus* for *Staphylococcus aureus.*

Just as dogs have different breeds within their species, microorganisms also have subgroups. These are often given numbers.

Sometimes viruses are categorized into genus and species (*Herpes simplex* and *Herpes zoster*). But more commonly, viruses are given names that identify only the genus, such as adenovirus or poxvirus. Virus names are usually not italicized or capitalized.

Intact Skin. If the skin is intact, harmful microorganisms cannot penetrate and invade the warm, moist, nutrient-rich tissue underneath. Any time skin is cut, scraped, or scratched, it becomes open to infection. That is why thoroughly washing and putting a sterile covering on any open wound is important.

Mucous Membranes. These are the linings of the nose, mouth, GI tract, and respiratory tract, all of which secrete mucus. The linings of the lungs and respiratory tract, to the nose, contain cilia (small, hairlike projections), which move mucus up the airway and out of the body, carrying harmful microorganisms and small particles with it.

Secretions. Teary eyes and a moist mouth are natural ways the body expels harmful microorganisms. Tears flush the eyes and contain an enzyme that can destroy bacteria. Saliva prevents growth of bacteria. Hydrochloric acid in the stomach destroys most harmful microorganisms that are swallowed. Urine and vaginal secretions are slightly acidic, both of which create an unwelcoming environment for pathogens. See the box on this page, which lists the body defenses against microorganisms by body system.

Physiologic Responses

Physiologic responses are the mechanical responses the body makes to remove harmful irritants and pathogens.

Coughing and sneezing out mucus is a natural way of expelling as many harmful microorganisms as possible from the respiratory tract. Crying cleans the eyes. Vomiting and diarrhea remove pathogens from the gastrointestinal tract.

Fever raises the body's temperature above the level at which microorganisms thrive. (The traditional Native American practice of sweat lodges for maintaining health helps to prevent microbial growth.) Urinating flushes bacteria from the urethra.

Inflammation, which is the reaction of any tissue to injury, is characterized by four classic symptoms—redness, swelling, pain, and heat. When tissue is injured, chemicals are released that cause the capillaries to dilate and small gaps to occur in the capillary walls. This brings more blood into the area. The increased pressure of the blood pushes fluid into the tissues. Slowed blood flow allows white blood cells to move from the center of the blood vessel to the edges, and from there into the tissues. Once in the tissues, white blood cells engulf and destroy microorganisms and debris (in effect, cleaning up the battlefield).

Immune System and Immunity

In addition to the body's general defensive measures that protect against microorganisms, the body also has a specific immune system that develops throughout

The Body's Defenses Against Microorganisms

Eyes	Produce tears, which contain enzyme that destroys bacterial wall
Mouth	Saliva is slightly bactericidal
	Good oral hygiene prevents bacterial growth on gums
Respiratory tract	Produces mucus, which is moved toward the throat by cilia
	Irritants trigger coughing
	Macrophages are present in the alveoli
Digestive system	Gastric secretions are highly acidic
	Enzymes digest proteins, including microorganisms
	Normal flora occupies potential sites for colonization
Blood	White blood cells attack microorganisms
Skin	Normal flora prevents colonization
	When intact, cannot be penetrated by microorganisms
Urogenital tract	Urine is highly acidic
	Urination flushes entrance to urinary bladder
	Vaginal secretions are slightly acidic
Lymph nodes	Macrophages destroy microorganisms transported by lymphatic system

life. The immune system recognizes, attacks, and destroys pathogens.

Recognition is based on the ability of immune system cells to decide if any protein present in the body is "self" (part of the body) or "foreign" (not part of the body). These proteins are called **antigens.** When recognized as foreign, antigens stimulate the immune response. Once the body has learned to recognize these antigens, it can produce **antibodies,** specific proteins that attach themselves to the antigens, immobilize them, and target them for destruction. Antibodies, also called **immunoglobulins** or **gamma globulins,** make up about 15 percent of proteins in a person's blood.

The body has two types of responses to antigens:

The first is the **cell-mediated immune response.** This is effective against viruses, fungi, cancerous cells, and grafts of foreign tissue (such as an organ transplant). This reaction does not involve production of antibodies.

In the cell-mediated immune response, macrophages, evolved from monocytes (a type of white blood cell) that have left the bloodstream and live in tissues, as well as helper T cells, recognize pathogens. **T cells** are a type of lymphocyte (another type of white blood cell) that are produced by the thymus gland or have passed through the thymus gland to mature.

T cells can become activated and specialized into one of three different kinds:

1. **Cytotoxic** T cells that destroy foreign antigens; they are sometimes referred to as "killer" T cells.
2. Cells that remember foreign antigens for future encounters are called memory T cells.
3. Cells that stop the response when the invaders have been destroyed are called suppressor T cells.

Chemicals from the T cells attract macrophages and phagocytes, which then engulf the immobilized microorganisms and tissue debris.

The second type of immune response is the **humoral immune response**. This involves a mechanism for production of antibodies. Again, pathogens are recognized, not only by macrophages and T cells, but also by **B cells**, another type of lymphocyte produced in bone marrow and found in the spleen and lymph nodes. Activated B cells specialize into memory B cells, which will remember the specific antigen, and plasma cells, which produce antibodies specific to the target antigen.

These antibodies bind to the antigen and either destroy or immobilize it. This process may take place in the bloodstream or in the tissue. When the threat from the foreign substance passes, levels of T cells and B cells return to normal.

Once the cells have learned to recognize the antigen, if it is encountered again, large amounts of antibody can be produced quickly to prevent the microorganism from causing disease. This explains why people develop short- or long-term immunity to diseases they have had, such as chicken pox. This process is also the basis for immunizations.

Types of Immunity and Immunizations

An individual can have two types of immunity, **genetic immunity** or **acquired immunity.**

Genetic Immunity

Genetic immunity is based on a person's genetic resistance to many diseases. Each species of plant and animal can only be infected by certain pathogens. Tobacco plants, for instance, get tobacco mosaic viruses, but humans are immune to these pathogens. Humans get measles, but dogs and cats have genetic immunity to this viral disease.

Potential problems arise when certain pathogens jump from one species to another. This can happen in two ways. One is through new contact with a species that is genetically susceptible to the disease but previously had not been exposed to the disease. The second way is by the pathogen mutating, changing its own form in some way so that a species that had genetic immunity is no longer immune.

It is also possible that, within a species, some individuals are genetically immune to certain pathogens while others are not. A number of scientists today believe that most diseases are caused by pathogens, even such conditions as coronary artery disease; and that the reason some people get heart attacks and others do not is because some people have genetic immunity to the pathogen that causes the underlying problem, a buildup of fatty deposits in the arteries that supply blood to the heart muscle.

Acquired Immunity

Acquired immunity results from the presence of antibodies. If the person developed his or her own antibodies, we say that person has **active immunity.** If antibodies are introduced from the outside, we say the person has **passive immunity.** Table 13–2 shows the various types of immunity.

If the antibodies have been formed as a response to contracting a disease, we call this **natural immunity.** If the immunity is developed as an outcome of immunization, we call this **artificial immunity.**

So, a person who has had measles and develops his or her own antibodies to the measles virus, develops natural active immunity to measles.

When babies are born, they have the same antibodies in their blood as the mother; these antibodies have passed through the placenta during gestation. If the baby is breastfed, he or she continues to receive antibodies in the breast milk. These antibodies were developed naturally but not by the baby. This means that in the first few months of life, all babies have natural passive immunity to diseases their mothers have had.

Sometimes people are given injections of antibodies or gamma globulin when exposed to a serious disease to provide temporary immunity. Immune globulin injections are available for specific diseases such as rabies and in a general form that contains antibodies to several diseases (called immune serum globulin). This provides an artificial passive immunity. The person does not produce his or her own antibodies but is protected for a few months by the injected antibodies.

Most immunizations stimulate a person to produce antibodies because they contain killed organisms or live organisms that have been made weaker in the laboratory so that they no longer cause disease. (This strain of an organism is called *attenuated.*) After a tetanus or hepatitis B immunization, a person develops an artificial active immunity.

Table 13–2	Types of Immunity	
Natural	Acquired
Natural genetic immunity — species immune to disease that affect other organisms	Acquired genetic immunity — through bioengineering, immunity introduced into DNA; to date mainly in plants to prevent diseases that normally occur
Example: Human beings do not get distemper, a viral disease of animals.	Example: Genetically engineered corn may not be affected by certain parasitic diseases that can usually grow on corn plants.
Natural active immunity — occurs when an organism produces antibodies to a disease after exposure to the disease	Acquired active immunity — occurs after immunization; after injection with killed or weakened microorganisms a person produces antibodies that protect from the disease
Example: A person who has had chicken pox has natural active immunity to chicken pox.	Example: A child who has been immunized with the vaccine to prevent chicken pox has an acquired active immunity to chicken pox.
Natural passive immunity — occurs when antibodies are passed from mother to child, either before birth or during breastfeeding	Acquired passive immunity — occurs when antibodies (immune globulin) from another person or animal are injected to provide temporary immunity or sometimes to prevent the formation of antibodies (RhoGam)
Example: A child who is breastfeeding is immune to chicken pox if the mother has antibodies to the disease.	Example: A person may be given immune serum globulin to prevent viral hepatitis when making a trip to an area where the disease is common.

THE INFECTION CYCLE

For an infection to occur, five conditions must be met:

1. There must be a reservoir or reservoir host, a place where the disease-causing microorganism makes a home. This can be a human, an animal, a pool of stagnant water, or even medical equipment on which microorganisms remain from a previous procedure.
2. There must be a portal of exit. This is a way for the organism to get out of the host. If the host is a person, the portal of exit can be excretions, such as mucus coughed up; secretions, such as saliva; the skin itself; or droplets, such as the microscopic droplets that are expelled every time we exhale. (A person with tuberculosis can infect a room full of people simply by breathing.)
3. There must be a means of transmission. This can be direct, such as contact with the skin or with body fluids such as blood, feces, or urine that contains the pathogens. It can also be indirect, such as breathing in infected droplets or eating or drinking food or water that contains pathogens. The means of transmission can also be a

fomite, an inanimate object such as a piece of medical equipment that can pass microorganisms from one host to another. Disease can also be transmitted through vectors, insects or other animals that can pass disease, such as mosquitoes or fleas.
4. There must be a portal of entry. This is the way microorganisms can enter a new host, such as mucous membranes, GI tract, genitourinary tract, respiratory tract, or broken skin.
5. Finally, there must be a susceptible host. This must be a living being that can be infected by the microorganism. Several factors influence whether a potential host can be infected. These include how many organisms the individual is exposed to, how long the exposure lasts, how virulent the organism is, and the individual's general health, nutritional status, and the presence of any other diseases that can lower resistance.

Some microorganisms, such as the Ebola virus, cause disease in healthy individuals even if present only in very small amounts. Other organisms are normally resisted by healthy people, such as those that cause Hanson's disease (leprosy) or yeast (Candida).

All microorganisms have preferred hosts. But some that normally infect animals can pass to humans. Tuberculosis, for instance, affects both cows and humans and was often spread this way before routine pasteurization of milk.

Figure 13–7 depicts the infection cycle.

INFECTION CONTROL (ASEPSIS)

Because people who come to the doctor's office have infectious diseases, health care personnel use methods to prevent spreading pathogens from one person to another. Although the infection cycle can be interrupted at any point, the most effective way to eliminate transmission of disease from one host to another is through **asepsis.** Asepsis literally means **sterile** (free from microorganisms). In practice, it means an environment in which microorganisms are controlled and eliminated to the greatest degree possible.

Medical asepsis, also called clean technique, is aimed at removing pathogens and reducing transfer of microorganisms by cleaning any body part or surface that has been exposed to them. Medical asepsis benefits both the patient and the health care worker, so they are not exposed to pathogens from other patients, from each other, or from other staff.

Surgical asepsis, also called **sterile technique,** is the destruction of *all* microorganisms, pathogenic and nonpathogenic (including spores), on an object and uses measures to keep sterile objects from coming into contact with nonsterile objects. The goal is to prevent any microorganisms from entering the patient's body through an open wound, especially during surgery. Surgical asepsis is used whenever the skin is broken. It is also used when an object such as a needle is inserted under the skin or when a sterile body cavity is entered. Sterile body cavities include the thoracic, abdominopelvic, spinal, and cranial cavities. Surgical asepsis is also maintained when examining or catheterizing the urinary bladder.

The gastrointestinal tract, whether entered through the mouth or the anus, is not considered sterile. Although the lungs themselves are not considered sterile, sterile technique is always used when introducing instruments into the trachea (windpipe) and the lungs because of the danger of introducing microorganisms into the lungs.

Medical office personnel are trained to carry out procedures using the appropriate aseptic measures. All personnel use standard precautions, as already described in chapter 6, to prevent the spread of disease. Measures including proper handwashing technique and cleaning of instruments and equipment are discussed here.

Handwashing

The single most important means of preventing the spread of infection is frequent and effective handwashing by all medical office personnel. Medical aseptic handwashing removes dirt and pathogens from the hands. Special attention needs to be paid to the fingernails, because the area under the fingernails and around the cuticles tends to collect dirt and resist cleaning. Soap and the friction of rubbing the hands together loosens dirt so it can be rinsed away. It is best to have a sink where the water and the soap are controlled by foot pedals, so the hands do not pick up pathogens from shutting off the faucet.

After washing, the hands are not sterile, because skin cannot be sterilized. Normal flora remain. But most pathogens have been removed; the hands are considered clean up to the wrists.

You should avoid wearing jewelry or rings when performing procedures, because microorganisms often remain in crevices even after the hands have been washed. (You can review chapter 6 for guidelines on when hands should be washed.)

See Procedure 13–1, Medical Aseptic Handwashing.

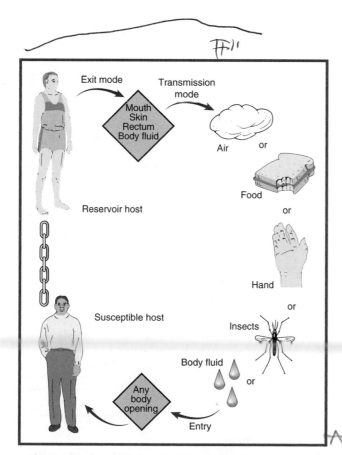

➤ **Figure 13–7** Infection cycle: Microorganisms that cause disease may pass directly from one individual to another susceptible host or may cycle through a nonhuman reservoir. (From Kinn ME, Woods M: *The Medical Assistant, Administrative and Clinical,* 8th ed. Philadelphia: W.B. Saunders, 1999)

SMALLPOX

Until the middle of the 20th century, when smallpox was eradicated, it was one of the most feared diseases in the world. A massive effort of vaccination by the World Health Organization (WHO) and national health organizations throughout the industrialized world ended smallpox as a contagious disease.

Smallpox is one of the most virulent diseases known to mankind. Before it was eradicated, it killed up to 500 million people in the 20th century alone. A single smallpox virus can cause disease.

People today have no immunity against smallpox. Smallpox vaccination has been discontinued around the world. In the United States, those born after 1972 do not have the telltale pockmark on their upper arm. For those who were vaccinated, immunity has worn off.

Today, the smallpox virus exists only in scientific and military laboratories in the United States and Russia. Only a small amount of vaccine is available today, and increasing vaccine production over the short term would be very difficult. Under these circumstances, scientific experts fear that, if the United States or Russia decided to utilize smallpox as a weapon of mass destruction, or if the virus were stolen by a terrorist group, the world's entire population might be at risk.

For years, both the United States and Soviet governments planned to destroy their smallpox repositories. However, in 1999, those who control the remaining smallpox stores decided not to destroy them. The reasoning was that there may, in some remote part of the world, be some smallpox virus left. If there is, and if there should ever come a time when an outbreak occurs, the only way to make sure the most effective vaccines can be made to fight any possible epidemic is if the material is available in the laboratory.

Smallpox has a long and well-documented history.

In 1350 B.C., the first recorded outbreak of smallpox occurred, during the Egyptian-Hittite war. Nearly 200 years later, the Pharaoh Ramses V died as a young man, apparently of smallpox.

Smallpox appeared in China in 48 A.D. By the late 6th century, the disease had spread from China to Korea and Japan. It spread to Europe and northern and western Africa in the 8th to the 11th centuries.

One person accompanying the Spanish explorer Hernando Cortes in 1520 carried smallpox to the Americas. By the 18th century, smallpox was killing upwards of 400,000 Europeans a year, from all strata of society, including members of the royal families of Spain, England, France, Russia, and Sweden.

The first use of smallpox as a biological weapon occurred from 1754 to 1767, when British forces under the control of Lord Jeffrey Amherst (for whom Amherst College is named) distributed smallpox-infected blankets among Native Americans in New England and New York.

Just 30 years later, in 1796, Edward Jenner created the first smallpox vaccination, injecting a young English boy with vaccine made from the pus of a dairy maid's cowpox lesion. The vaccination was successful because immunity to cowpox (a milder disease) also provided immunity to smallpox.

Within 5 years, vaccination against smallpox had become increasingly common for infants born in Europe, North America, and Russia. President Thomas Jefferson initiated smallpox vaccination among Native Americans in 1801.

Despite increasing vaccination rates, outbreaks of smallpox continued to occur, and in countries where no vaccinations occurred epidemics continued to kill millions. Medical historians believe President Abraham Lincoln was suffering from the early symptoms of smallpox when he gave the Gettysburg Address in 1863 at the dedication of the Civil War Cemetery in Gettysburg, Pennsylvania.

The last reported case of smallpox in the United States occurred in 1949. The disease was declared eradicated from Europe, North America, and Central America during the 1950s. In 1972 the United States ended its requirement for mandatory vaccination against smallpox. The disease was eradicated from India and Bangladesh in 1975, and declared by the WHO to be eradicated worldwide in 1980.

Smallpox is one of the greatest examples of a successful worldwide public health intervention.

Other Ways to Maintain Asepsis

There are five other means to maintain asepsis: general cleaning, using personal protective equipment (PPE), proper disposal of hazardous waste, cleaning and disinfecting of contaminated surfaces, and proper cleaning and sterilization of equipment.

General Cleaning

The office, including examining rooms, break room, lab area, waiting area, and administrative areas, should be cleaned regularly to keep it free of dirt and dust. If toys are kept in the waiting room, they also need to be cleaned and disinfected regularly.

PROCEDURE 13–1

Medical Aseptic Handwashing

Performance Objective: The student can perform a medical aseptic handwash correctly.

Supplies and Equipment: Sink, liquid soap, paper towels, nail stick or brush, and a wastebasket. It is desirable to have the water and soap controlled by foot pedals. Bar soap should be avoided because studies have shown that microorganisms grow on the soap and in the moist soap dish.

Procedure Steps

1. Remove rings, watch, or bracelets or push watch well above the wrist.
   Rationale: Hands cannot be properly cleaned under jewelry or watches. Because jewelry can harbor microorganisms, all items must be removed or pushed well above the wrist before washing hands. Rings and bracelets, with the exception of a plain wedding band, should not be worn during procedures.

2. Standing near the sink but not touching it, turn on water to a comfortable temperature. If the water is not controlled by foot pedals or a knee control, use a dry paper towel to turn the faucets and discard it.
   Rationale: The sink and faucets are considered contaminated and you do not want to touch them with your clothing or your hands. Water temperature is adjusted before washing hands so that it will not be necessary to touch the faucets during the procedure. Water should be warm but not hot for effective

cleaning and comfort but to avoid excessive drying of the skin.

3. Wet hands, pump about a tablespoon of liquid soap into hands, and work into a lather. Rub the hands and wrists briskly in a circular motion to create friction.
   Rationale: Soap lathers better on wet hands. Friction loosens soil and microorganisms.

4. Clean hands, fingers, and wrists using a circular motion and interlacing the fingers at least 10 times. Wash for 1 to 2 minutes. Use the longer time if hands are dirty from contact with soil, food, dust, etc. *15 to 30 sec*
   Rationale: All parts of the hands and fingers must be cleaned thoroughly.

5. Use a clean orangewood stick or stiff brush to clean under the fingernails and around the cuticle.
   Rationale: The area around the fingernails retains the most dirt and must be cleaned carefully, especially each time the hands are washed after being out of the office or if the hands have been contaminated. Avoid using a nail file or other sharp object, which can break the skin.

6. Holding the fingers below the wrists, rinse hands, fingers, and wrists completely under the running water.
   Rationale: Running water will rinse away any dirt, debris, and pathogens. After the procedure the hands will be clean from the wrists

Procedure continued on following page

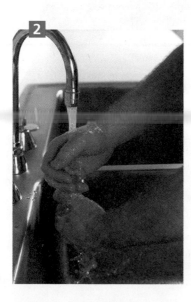

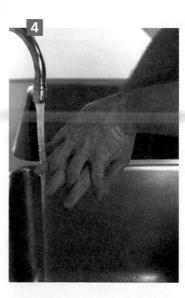

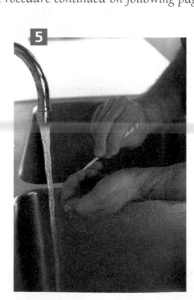

PROCEDURE 13-1 *(continued)*

down to the fingers. Keeping the fingers below the wrists prevents water from running to the arms (which have not been cleaned) and then back to the hands, possibly contaminating the hands with dirt or microorganisms from the arms.

7. The first time the hands are washed each day, anytime hands or fingernails are visibly dirty at the beginning of the handwash, and after contamination of the hands with body fluids, repeat steps 3, 4, 5, and 6.
   Rationale: A second application of soap, friction, and rinsing is more effective at removing pathogens and is used when hands are assumed to be dirtier.

8. Still holding fingers below wrists, dry the hands with paper towels. Use at least one paper towel for each hand. Drop used towels directly into a wastebasket.
   Rationale: Until the hands are dry, water that flows to an unwashed area of the arm and

back to the hands may reintroduce dirt or pathogens to the hands. Drop used paper towels directly into a wastebasket to avoid having to pick them up from a surface that is not as clean as your hands after washing.

9. Using a clean, dry paper towel, turn off the faucets. Dry the inside of the sink and any areas where water has splashed with a paper towel, being careful not to touch the sink directly with your hands or allowing the towel to rewet hands.
   Rationale: Using a paper towel prevents recontamination of the hands from the faucets or sink. Drying wet areas prevents growth of microorganisms in the sink.

10. Apply mild hand lotion as needed to prevent cracking of skin on hands.
    Rationale: Frequent handwashing dries skin. Lotion helps prevent breaks in the skin; which could be a portal of entry for microorganisms.

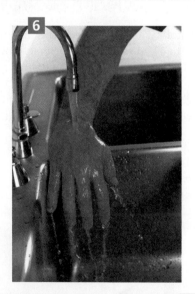

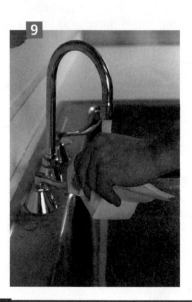

Use of Personal Protective Equipment

PPE should be used whenever there is a chance of coming into contact with body fluids. These are items that protect the body from contact with microorganisms, and include face shields or goggles and mask to protect the eyes, nose, and mouth; a lab coat, apron, or barrier gown to protect the uniform; and gloves to protect the hands. See the box on page 234 for information on choosing the correct glove size.

Unfortunately, there is an increasing incidence of sensitivity among health care workers to latex, a fluid produced by the rubber trees that are used to make gloves and other medical products. Other people are allergic to the powder used in gloves to make them easier to put on.

Proper Disposal of Hazardous Waste

Dispose of hazardous waste and sharps promptly and appropriately. All items that have come in contact with any body fluid, feces, or secretion should be treated as hazardous waste.

Clean and Disinfect Contaminated Areas

Clean surfaces in examination rooms with disinfec-

FOCUS ON
SAFETY

OSHA STANDARD FOR CLEANING TO PREVENT THE TRANSMISSION OF INFECTION

The Federal Occupational Safety and Health Administration (OSHA) has set standards for cleaning and sterilizing medical facilities. The standards are set in the context of the health and safety of the personnel who work in the facility, although it certainly applies to patient health and safety as well. They are designed to minimize the risk of contamination due to blood-borne pathogens.

The standards are comprised of six main points:

1. Immediately decontaminate and disinfect every area where an accidental spill of blood or other body fluid has occurred. Also, work surfaces should be disinfected immediately after each procedure.

2. Clean and disinfect all reusable containers on a regular basis.

3. Maintain sharps containers in an upright position, as close as possible to the work area. Replace sharps containers regularly; do not allow them to become more than three-quarters full. Be sure the lid is securely closed before disposing of the sharps container.

4. Do not pick up spilled material or broken glassware with hands. Use a broom or brush, a dustpan, and forceps or tongs to pick up the material. Use a spill clean-up kit if necessary, and call a hazardous spill clean-up company if the spill is too large to decontaminate effectively with the equipment in the office or if the spill contains mercury.

5. Double-bag linens soiled with blood or other body fluids. Handle soiled linens with gloves only and as little as possible. Transport soiled linens in a bag that does not leak.

6. Dispose of all biohazardous waste in impermeable biohazard bags or containers. These polyethylene or polypropylene bags or containers must then be disposed of according to all federal, state, and local regulations.

OSHA also mandates that every medical facility, including doctors' offices, have a written exposure control plan and an exposure control officer. The plan should set forth procedures for the staff to minimize staff exposure and exposure by patients to blood-borne pathogens.

The plan must be updated at least once a year and must be immediately available to all staff as a reference. Mandatory training must be part of the plan, both as part of a new-employee orientation and as inservice training for all staff, including doctors.

The directive, *CPL 2-2.60: Exposure Control Plan for OSHA Personnel with Occupational Exposure to Blood-borne Pathogens,* can be obtained from the OSHA Web site, http://www.osha-slc.gov/OshDoc/ Directive_data/CPL_2-2_60.html. OSHA is an office of the U.S. Department of Labor.

The directive details requirements for:

1. Use of standard precautions

2. Work practice controls

3. Personal protective equipment

4. Regulated waste.

In addition, the document outlines requirements and suggestions for immunization of health care workers, as well as postexposure evaluation and follow-up. There are also detailed instructions on training and record-keeping.

Choosing the Proper Gloves

Different kinds of protective gloves are worn by medical assistants and other personnel for different purposes.

Nonsterile Gloves are used to protect the medical assistant. They should fit snugly so the medical assistant can pick up small or narrow instruments and can do procedures. They should not be so tight, however, that they will rip or be too uncomfortable.

Nonsterile gloves come in sizes extra-small, small, medium, and large. There are also "one-size-fits-all" gloves that stretch to fit most hand sizes. Many offices use one-size-fits-all gloves because then they only need a single box of gloves in each examination room.

For procedures in which finger dexterity is important or for a person who wears gloves all day, gloves that are sized may be more comfortable.

Latex gloves are more supple than vinyl gloves and are preferred, unless the user has an allergy to latex. Nonlatex gloves that fit well and are supple are available, but often cost more than latex gloves. Many offices use powder-free gloves because powder is both an allergen in itself and it suspends molecules of latex in the air, which may induce a reaction in a latex-sensitive individual even if that individual is not coming into contact with the latex item.

Sterile Gloves are used to protect the patient whenever the medical assistant is touching something sterile that will penetrate a sterile body cavity. Sterile gloves have a longer cuff than nonsterile gloves. The cuff goes up over a sterile gown when assisting with surgery.

Sterile gloves should be worn when assisting with sterile procedures, administering or changing sterile dressings, touching sterile items, or adjusting sterile items on a sterile field.

Sterile gloves come in calibrated sizes: 6, 6½, 7, 7½, and so on. It is important for each person to experiment to find the correct size.

tant solution daily and whenever they become contaminated with body fluids or secretions.

Clean and Sterilize Equipment

Proper cleaning and sterilization of equipment is the subject for the rest of this chapter. Equipment may be treated in several different ways, depending on how "clean" you want to make it. Cleaning and sanitizing means washing with soap and water. Disinfection means treating with chemicals or heat to kill pathogens. Some methods are more effective than others at destroying hardy bacteria such as the tuberculosis bacteria. There are different classifications for disinfectants.

Cleaning and Sanitizing

Instruments and equipment need to be cleaned promptly after every use to remove visible residue. Organisms can hide under residue and survive the disinfection or sterilization process if residue is not removed. In addition, the longer residue remains on the instrument, the more difficult it is to get off. Blood is especially hard to remove after drying.

Items that cannot be cleaned at once are usually rinsed with cold water and placed in a soaking solution to prevent anyone from touching them and to prevent the residue from hardening. Because items in need of cleaning may be highly contaminated, the medical assistant should wear protective equipment, including an apron or lab coat to protect the front of the uniform, disposable gloves, and eye, mouth, and nose protection to protect against being splashed in the face.

See Procedure 13–2, Removing Soiled Gloves, and Procedure 13–3, Sanitizing Soiled Instruments.

Disinfection

Measures taken to kill microorganisms on a surface are called disinfection. Disinfection can be accomplished by use of a chemical disinfectant or by boiling.

Disinfection is used for items that enter body cavities, such as the mouth or anus, which are not sterile. It is used for items that are sensitive to heat such as glass thermometers, for synthetic materials such as rubber, and for items that will rust if exposed to heat. Disinfection is also used· for large equipment and counter surfaces, which cannot fit into an autoclave for sterilization.

Chemical disinfectants are most commonly used. Follow the manufacturer's directions carefully regarding the length of time to soak items in the disinfectant solution.

Boiling kills many microorganisms, but does not kill bacterial spores and is not used as a disinfection method in the medical office because chemicals are effective and easier to use.

The ability of a disinfection method to destroy the bacteria that causes tuberculosis (*Mycobacterium tuberculosis*) and bacterial spores determines the level of disinfection, which is described as low, intermediate, or high.

Low-level disinfection kills most bacteria and viruses, but not *M. tuberculosis* or bacterial spores. This level of disinfection is used to decontaminate surfaces that have not been exposed to blood or body fluids. Disinfectant soaps, for example, provide low-level disinfection.

Intermediate-level disinfection kills bacteria and viruses, including *M. tuberculosis,* but does not kill bacterial spores. Disinfectant solutions provide directions on the label as to how to use them properly to provide this level of disinfection, including the proper length of time to soak items.

Many medical offices use commercial solutions or prepare solutions containing household bleach. A 1:10 solution of household bleach (1 part bleach to 10 parts water) provides intermediate-level disinfection. This solution, which must be prepared fresh daily, can be used to clean surfaces and equipment that touch intact skin, such as stethoscopes.

Small spills of blood or body fluids on counter surfaces can be cleaned with bleach solution and paper towels. The medical assistant should wear personal protective equipment to protect against splashes. Soiled paper towels and personal protective equipment that have come in contact with blood or body fluids should be discarded into a plastic biohazard bag. The treated area should be allowed to air-dry; drying time is an essential part of the disinfection process.

High-level disinfection requires soaking in a chemical disinfectant that kills all microorganisms except large numbers of bacterial spores. The items should be soaked for between 10 and 45 minutes, depending on the solutions used. Instruments that come in contact with intact mucous membranes, such as laryngoscopes, can be disinfected this way.

■ LATEX ALLERGY

The increasing use of personal protective devices made of latex has highlighted awareness of those who suffer from allergic reaction to this substance. Latex is a fluid produced by rubber plants that is used as a primary material in protective gloves and many other medical supplies and equipment. Both patients and staff may be allergic to latex.

An allergic reaction to latex can be mild, a localized skin reaction on itching. It can be a more severe, but still localized, reaction such as hives. A more severe reaction would be swelling of the throat that makes it difficult to breath, heart arrhythmia, or hypotension (low blood pressure). At its most severe, an allergic reaction can cause anaphylaxis, a condition of respiratory failure and vascular collapse.

Staff who are allergic to latex can wear vinyl gloves that provide the same protection against contamination from blood-borne pathogens. Any person with a latex allergy should wear a medical alert bracelet or other identification to notify emergency personnel of the situation.

Because the powder used to make gloves easier to put on disperses latex molecules throughout a room, latex-sensitive individuals may experience symptoms even if they are not in contact with latex gloves. Many offices use powder-free or nonlatex gloves, especially if one or more employees is latex sensitive.

Patients also may be allergic to latex. This fact should be clearly labeled on their medical record. The office should stock latex-free alternatives for syringes, tourniquets, and gloves and have a supply of cloth towels to wrap any item (such as a blood pressure cuff) that may contain latex.

List of Medical Office Supplies That Contain Latex

Emergency Equipment

Blood pressure cuff
Stethoscope
Disposable gloves
Oral and nasal airways
Endotracheal tubes
Tourniquets
Intravenous tubing
Syringes
Electrode pads

Personal Protective Equipment

Gloves
Surgical masks
Goggles
Respirators
Rubber aprons

Other Hospital/Office Items

Anesthesia masks
Catheters
Wound drains
Injection ports
Rubber tops of multidose vials
Dental dams

FOCUS ON
SAFETY

USING A SPILL KIT

Spill kits are used for decontaminating large spills of blood, other body fluids, or hazardous chemicals. Before beginning, put on a gown or lab coat that is impervious to liquid, face protection, and protective gloves. The clean-up is a five-step procedure.

1. Sprinkle the powder in the kit over the spill. The powder makes the liquid congeal.

2. Scoop up the spill with the cardboard paddles in the kit. (Do not touch the spill, even with gloved hands.)

3. Place the material in a red biohazard bag.

4. Disinfect the area with germicide.

5. Dispose of the cleaning materials in the biohazard bag.

At this point, the biohazard bag should be sealed and disposed of according to the office's standard procedures, taking into account all federal, state, and local regulations.

PROCEDURE 13-2

Removing Soiled Gloves

Performance Objective: The student will demonstrate proper procedure for removal and disposal of soiled gloves.

☑ Wash hands
☑ Gloves
☐ Eye and Face Protection
☐ Lab Coat or Apron
☑ Plastic Biohazard Bag
☐ Rigid Biohazard Container

Supplies and Equipment: Gloves, hazardous waste container.

Procedure Steps

1. While wearing sterile or nonsterile gloves that have become soiled, grasp the outside of the soiled glove near the cuff with the other gloved hand. (If both gloves are soiled, remove the dirtiest glove first.) Be careful not to touch the skin above the glove.
Rationale: Neither hand should touch your skin or uniform to prevent the transfer of microorganisms from the glove.

2. Pull the soiled glove inside out as you remove it.
Rationale: This contains the contaminated area inside the glove.

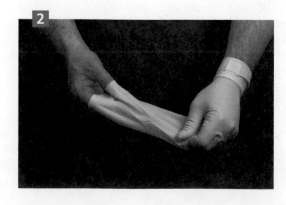

3 Grasp the glove you have removed in the gloved hand and contain it completely with your fingers.
Rationale: When you remove the second glove, you want it to have the first glove completely inside it.

4 Using your ungloved hand, grasp the cuff of the remaining glove and pull it off inside out over the soiled glove.

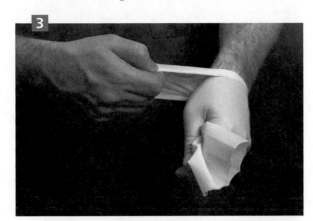

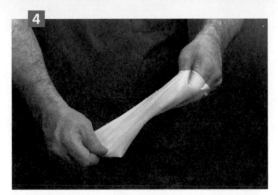

Rationale: The inside of the second glove is the cleanest area and can be held with your ungloved hands.

5 If the gloves have been exposed to body fluids, dispose of the soiled gloves in a waste container lined with a plastic biohazard bag.
Rationale: Although the soiled part of the gloves is now inside, they are still considered hazardous waste. Gloves may be disposed of in a plastic biohazard bag because they have no edges to puncture the plastic.

6. Wash hands promptly.
Rationale: You should always wash your hands after removing gloves as a further precaution against transferring microorganisms. Washing also removes the powder residue from the inside of the gloves.

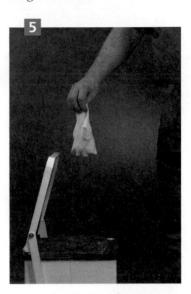

Disinfection by Boiling

Boiling water has been used in the past as a means of disinfection. Water reaches the boiling temperature of 212° F at sea level (lower temperature at higher altitude), and then turns to water vapor.

Most bacteria are destroyed after 15 minutes at a rolling boil. However, bacterial spores and some viruses can survive. Therefore, boiling is only effective for instruments that will not enter sterile body cavities (such as nasal specula). Because of these limitations, boiling is rarely used in the medical office today.

Sterilization

Sterilization refers to the killing of all microorganisms, including bacteria, viruses, and bacterial spores. There are four means to provide sterilization: chemical, gas, dry heat, and steam.

Chemical Sterilization

Chemical sterilization requires submersion in a sterilizing solution for a period sufficient to kill bacterial spores. This is usually 12 to 24 hours. After sterilization, the item must be removed from the solution using sterile forceps, rinsed with sterile water, and dried with a sterile towel. In the medical office, this process is used for equipment that cannot be exposed to the heat or corrosive action of steam sterilization.

Gas Sterilization

Exposure to ethylene oxide gas also provides effective sterilization. This method is commonly used in hospitals that have room-size gas sterilizers. The process is toxic, time-consuming, and expensive. Because of this, medical offices do not usually use gas sterilization.

PROCEDURE 13-3

Sanitizing Soiled Instruments

Performance Objective: Wearing appropriate PPE, the student will sanitize one or more soiled instruments before disinfection or sterilization.

☑ Wash hands

☑ Gloves

☑ Eye and Face Protection

☑ Lab Coat or Apron

☑ Plastic Biohazard Bag

☐ Rigid Biohazard Container

Supplies and Equipment: Basin, gloves, PPE, detergent, scrub brush, paper towels.

Procedure Steps

1 Put on lab coat or apron, eye and face protection, and gloves. You may use heavy-duty cleaning gloves, especially if you must clean sharp objects.
Rationale: Begin all procedures by putting on appropriate PPE to protect from contact with microorganisms. In this procedure there is a potential for splashes to the face and front of the uniform.

2. Collect soiled instruments and rinse under cold water.
Rationale: The mechanical action of the water will remove surface soil. Blood is most easily removed with cold water.

3. Add detergent to a basin and fill with warm water. There should be visible suds.
Rationale: Soap will loosen debris or residue on the instruments.

4 Scrub all surfaces of each instrument with a scrub brush and rinse under running water. Be especially careful not to puncture your gloves with sharp tips of scissors or forceps. Do not allow water to splash out of the sink.
Rationale: All visible debris must be removed before disinfection or sterilization. Debris tends to collect in hinges or ridged surfaces of instruments.

5. Rinse thoroughly with hot water and place clean instruments on paper towels; repeat the process with other soiled instruments.
Rationale: Hot water dries more quickly and helps avoid water spots on instruments. All residue and soap must be removed before disinfection or sterilization.

6. Dry the clean instruments using paper towels.
Rationale: Prompt drying prevents rusting. Instruments must be dry before further processing.

7. If using heavy-duty cleaning gloves, wash the outside of the gloves, rinse, remove, and store. If using disposable gloves, follow procedure for removing soiled gloves. Wash hands promptly.
Rationale: You should always wash your hands after removing gloves as a further precaution against transferring microorganisms.

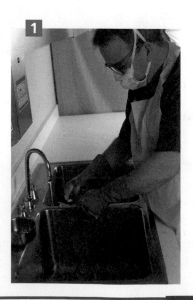

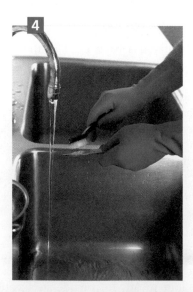

ON THE JOB

Paul Dean, one of the medical assistants at Blackburn Primary Care Associates, is preparing to sanitize instruments. In the sink there is a bowl containing a mild disinfectant and the instruments used during the day for several procedures. Paul has been asked to clean the instruments and lay them on paper towels to air-dry before further processing.

Questions
1. Why does Paul need to clean the instruments if they are going to be sterilized or disinfected later?
2. What PPE should Paul put on before cleaning the instruments?
3. Describe how Paul should clean the instruments.
4. If Paul has used heavy-duty gloves, what should he do with them after cleaning the instruments?

Dry-Heat Sterilization

Exposure to dry heat for a long period provides effective sterilization. This technique requires higher heat and a longer time than steam sterilization, but it is less corrosive to many instruments. Some offices use both a dry-heat sterilizer and a steam sterilizer.

Steam Sterilization

Although water can only be heated to its boiling point of 212° F, steam can become much hotter when contained in a small place. The pressure that builds up when steam continues to be heated allows not only a higher temperature, but more effective destruction of microorganisms. In the medical office the autoclave is used to safely sterilize using steam that has been heated to 250° F and maintained under about 15 pounds of pressure for a period of time. Microorganisms and bacterial spores cannot survive in this environment.

Wrapping Equipment for Sterilization

Wrapping keeps equipment sterile after sterilization. The wrap is sterilized with the item. After sterilization, the inside of the package remains sterile while the outside can be touched.

Items to be used in surgery are often wrapped twice. This allows the inside wrapping to be touched by a person wearing sterile gloves.

First, an inner package is made. The inner package is then covered with an outer wrapping. After the pack has been sterilized, the outer package can be opened in the usual way and the inner package can be placed on a sterile field. Because both the inside and the outside of the inner package remain sterile, the inner package can be touched by a person wearing sterile gloves.

Material used in wrapping must prevent microorganisms from entering the wrapped package. If paper or cloth wrap is used, two sheets are needed. Surgical packs are wrapped as described above, but single instruments, bowls, and so on may be wrapped once using two sheets of wrap. This is called double wrapping. All packages must be dated, and if the wrapping material is opaque (not clearly seen through), the contents of the package must be described. (See Procedure 13–4, Wrapping Instruments for Sterilization.)

Most instruments need to be wrapped for both dry-heat and steam sterilization.

Cloth is often used for wrapping, especially large packs containing all equipment and instruments needed for a procedure such as surgical packs. Everything wrapped in cloth needs to be labeled carefully, because you can't see through cloth. If a cloth wrapping becomes torn or frayed, it should be thrown away.

Paper wrap can be purchased in several sizes. After use the paper is discarded. Large wraps allow packs to be created that contain a set of instruments and supplies for specific procedures. Like cloth wraps, you cannot see through paper, and careful labeling is necessary.

Sterilization pouches consist of paper or transparent wrap that allows steam to penetrate. They come in various sizes and are usually transparent on at least one side. Some pouches require both ends to be sealed; others only need to have one end taped and the other end peeled open when needed.

The medical assistant selects an appropriately sized pouch for the instruments, inserts the instruments handles first (so when the pouch is opened the instru-

PROCEDURE 13–4

Wrapping an Instrument for Sterilization

Performance Objective: Using paper or cloth wrap and autoclave tape, the student will wrap a previously sanitized instrument for autoclaving and will label it correctly.

Supplies and Equipment: Paper or cloth wrap, autoclave tape, instrument to wrap, pen with waterproof ink, sterilization indicator.

Procedure Steps

1. Wash hands.
2. Select a piece of wrap of an appropriate size. Paper wrap can be cut if too large. The square of wrap should be approximately twice as long on each side as the object to be wrapped.
   Rationale: If the wrap is too small, the object to be wrapped will not be completely covered and microorganisms will be able to get into the wrapped package. If the wrap is too large, it becomes unwieldy and difficult to use. Two layers of wrap make it more difficult for microorganisms to penetrate the pack. Two layers of wrap can be folded as one for extra protection.
3. Place the wrap on a flat, dry surface with a corner facing you and lay the object(s) to be wrapped about one-third of the way up the wrap, long ends toward the corners. Instruments should be wrapped open so the maximum surface area is exposed. If paper wrap is used, sharp tips should be protected by gauze squares.
   Rationale: Steam needs to penetrate to each surface of each item to be sterilized. Gauze is used to protect sharp tips so that the instru-

ment will not pierce the wrap and allow contamination by microorganisms.

4. Lay a sterilization indicator in the middle of the pack if it is large.
   Rationale: It is most difficult for steam to penetrate to the center of the pack. The sterilization indicator changes color to show that the steam has penetrated for effective sterilization.
5. Fold the corner facing you toward the instrument. Then fold the corner back toward yourself. The corner flap should be 1″ to 2″ in depth.
   Rationale: The flap will be used to pull the edge of the pack open without touching more than the outside edges.
6. Fold each side toward the center at the ends of the object being wrapped and fold 1″ to 2″ back toward the side to make small flaps on each side.

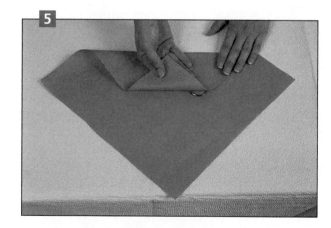

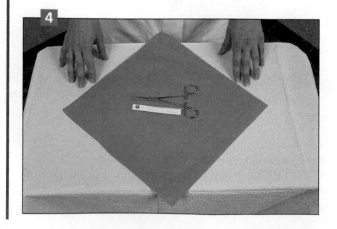

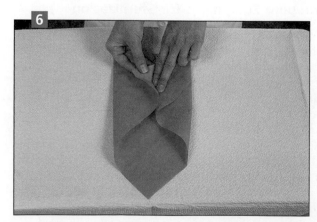

Rationale: The flaps will be used to open the pack without touching more than the outside edges.

7 Then wrap the instrument toward the final corner until you have formed a neat package.

Rationale: The instrument must be wrapped tightly enough so that microorganisms cannot penetrate the wrap.

8. If you are preparing a surgical pack, repeat steps 2 through 7 to create a second layer of wrap, which can be opened to provide a sterile inner package.

Rationale: For surgical procedures all instruments and supplies are often wrapped in a single pack. The outer wrap forms the sterile field and the sterile inner wrap can be touched by someone wearing sterile gloves during surgery. Instruments and sterile bowls often do not require this additional step, because they will be opened and added to an existing sterile field.

9. Secure the final corner with autoclave tape, which should extend at least 1″ beyond the corner on either side. It is helpful if you make a tab by turning one end of the tape back on itself for 1/4″ to 1/2″.

Rationale: The autoclave tape will hold the package closed and will also change color after autoclaving.

10 Write the contents of the package, date, and your initials on the tape using a pen with waterproof ink (not a felt-tipped pen) to label the package.

Rationale: Unless labeled, it will be difficult to determine what is in the package. The date allows you to know when an item is no longer considered sterile. Items in paper or cloth wraps must be resterilized after 1 month. Items wrapped in paper should be rewrapped, because some types of paper wrap become brittle after resterilization. Items wrapped in cloth should be taped and labeled again but do not need to be rewrapped.

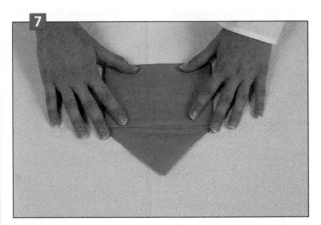
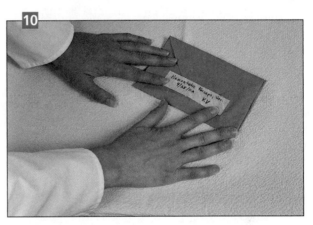

Photos from Bonewit-West, K: *Clinical Procedures for Medical Assistants* (5/e). Philadelphia: W.B. Saunders, 2000.

ments will drop from the pouch onto the handles instead of the delicate tips), tapes the pouch closed, and labels the sealed end.

Sterilization Indicators

Various methods are used to indicate that sterilization has occurred. The two most common are color-change indicators and culture tests.

Color-Change Indicators. Sterilization tape is all one color before sterilization. During sterilization, brown stripes appear.

Sterilization pouches have arrows that turn from pink to brown during steam sterilization and from blue to yellow during gas sterilization.

Sterilization strips may be placed inside large packs to be sure that steam has penetrated. Color arrows appear after effective sterilization.

Culture Tests. Various types of culture tests for bacterial spores are also placed inside packs. These strips or ampules contain bacterial spores. They are autoclaved with the load, and then placed in an incubator or sent to a lab to see if any spores have survived. It is important to test autoclaves regularly for

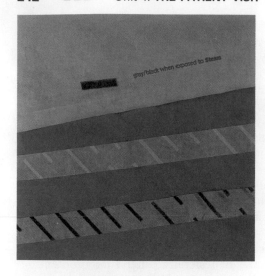

> **Figure 13–8** After effective sterilization the rectangle on the sterilization pouch changes from tan to black and sterilization tape changes from plain beige to beige with diagonal stripes.

the ability to kill all spores effectively. Figure 13–8 shows sterilization indications.

Using an Autoclave for Steam Sterilization

The autoclave is the most common method of sterilization in the medical office. Both wrapped and unwrapped items can be sterilized.

Most medical instruments are wrapped. Metal vaginal speculums are usually not wrapped; they are sterilized to destroy microorganisms that may adhere to them after use, but they are then stored as clean instruments, because they are used in a nonsterile body cavity.

How long items must remain in the autoclave depends on the temperature, the pressure, the amount of wrapping, and how full the autoclave is. The following principles apply:

The higher the temperature, the shorter the time necessary to sterilize.
The higher the pressure, the shorter the time necessary to sterilize.
The more wrapping is used, the longer the time necessary to sterilize.
The fuller the autoclave is, the longer the time necessary to sterilize.

An autoclave consists of an outer portion and an inner chamber. The inner chamber is sealed, steam is generated, and pressure builds. Controls allow regulation of temperature and pressure so they do not build to unsafe levels.

After the correct levels of temperature and pressure are reached, a timer allows the operator to know how long the items have been in the autoclave. When enough time has passed, room air is allowed into the inner chamber to release the pressure, a process known as venting the autoclave. The temperature falls rapidly, and the door to the autoclave can be opened. Figure 13–9 shows an autoclave.

Length of Sterilization

The length of time an item should be autoclaved depends on the temperature reached by the particular

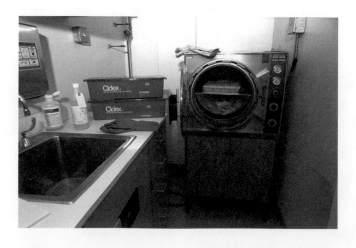

> **Figure 13–9** An autoclave with the door open and articles to autoclave inside.

Wrong method

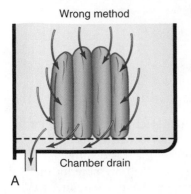

Chamber drain

A

Right method

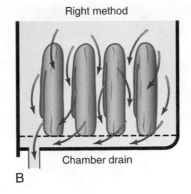

Chamber drain

B

> **Figure 13–10** Within the autoclave items should be arranged so that steam can circulate to all sides of each item. (A) Items packed so closely that steam cannot penetrate from side to side. (B) Items loaded correctly so that steam circulates around each item. (Courtesy of STERIS Corporation, Mentor, Ohio)

autoclave. Once the temperature reaches 250° F (121° C) at 15 pounds of pressure, items should be autoclaved as follows:

unwrapped items	15 minutes
wrapped instrument packages	30 minutes
large double-wrapped packs	45 minutes or longer

Some autoclaves reach a higher temperature and require a shorter time to sterilize equipment. The manufacturer's directions offer guidelines for each particular model.

Loading the Autoclave

Items are placed on trays in the autoclave. Because steam must be able to circulate throughout the autoclave, the trays have holes in them. When placing wrapped or unwrapped items on the trays, place the packages or items beside each other, or stand packages on their sides so steam can circulate freely around each package or item.

Bowls or other containers should be upside down, so water will not condense in the bottom and prevent drying. There should be at least an inch between trays, and some trays can be left out if packages are tall. Figure 13–10 shows correct loading of an autoclave.

Operating the Autoclave

Follow the manufacturer's directions for the particular autoclave model being used. Never try to open the autoclave until the pressure has dropped. The door seal is supposed to prevent accidental opening, but if the seal fails a serious accident could occur. Always keep face and hands away from hot steam when the door is open. Open the door slightly to allow steam to escape; after the drying cycle is complete, open the door fully to remove instruments. Procedure 13–5 discusses operating an autoclave in detail.

Removal and Storage of Sterilized Items

Sterilized items must be left in the autoclave until they are completely dry. Microorganisms can penetrate wet wrappings. In many offices, the autoclave is run in the late afternoon and the articles are left to dry overnight.

Once dry, wrapped packages can be removed by hand because only the inside needs to remain sterile. Packages should be stored in a clean area, with the most recently sterilized items behind items that were sterilized earlier.

Monitor dates, and resterilize as needed. Items wrapped in paper or cloth can be stored for 1 month before they need to be resterilized. Items wrapped in sterilization pouches can be stored for 3 months.

Unwrapped containers and their covers that will be used to hold clean items, such as tongue blades or horizontally placed, are removed by touching only the outside of the container and lid.

PROCEDURE 13-5

Operating the Autoclave

Performance Objective: The student will load and operate an autoclave according to the manufacturer's directions, and will use sterilization tape or indicators to show effective sterilization.

Supplies and Equipment: autoclave, distilled water, items to sterilize (such as wrapped packages and unwrapped items), manufacturer's direction manual.

Procedure Steps

1. Fill the reservoir to the correct level with distilled water. The reservoir is a tank, usually accessible from the top of the autoclave.
   Rationale: Distilled water is used to produce steam to avoid buildup of minerals in the reservoir.

2. Load the autoclave so that there is room for steam to circulate. Packages or items to be sterilized should not touch each other, and containers should be on their sides or upside down to prevent condensation.
   Rationale: Steam needs to penetrate to each surface of each item to be sterilized.

3. Using the valve on the autoclave, allow water to flow into the sterilization chamber to the level recommended by the manufacturer. Monitor the flow of water and stop as soon as it reaches the correct level.
   Rationale: A measured amount of water is needed in the sterilization chamber for effective sterilization.

4. Close and tighten or lock the door to create a seal.
   Rationale: The door must be closed tightly enough to create a seal or the autoclave will not operate properly.

5. Turn on the autoclave, set controls, and allow the heat and pressure to rise to the level recommended by the manufacturer. Set the timer for the approximate time to reach this level.
   Rationale: The manufacturer has determined the optimum temperature and pressure for the autoclave. It usually takes 10 to 15 minutes to reach this level. The timer will remind you to check back and adjust the temperature if needed.

6. When the correct temperature and pressure have been reached, adjust the controls if necessary to maintain the desired level. Set the timer again for the amount of time to sterilize the load.
   Rationale: Sterilization time is calculated from the time when correct temperature and pressure have been reached.

7. When the timer informs you that sterilization is complete, vent the autoclave. Allow the pressure to drop completely, then open the door carefully a small amount so that the steam can escape. This is called "cracking" the door.
   Rationale: When the autoclave is vented, air escapes and both pressure and temperature drop, but the air in the autoclave is still hot.

8. Allow the sterilized items to remain in the autoclave until fully dry. The autoclave may have a drying cycle. If you use it, set the timer so that you will remember to turn the autoclave off after the drying cycle.
   Rationale: Microorganisms can penetrate wet wrap so it is important to leave wrapped articles in the autoclave until completely dry.

9. When you remove sterilized items from the autoclave, check sterilization tape to be sure the colors have changed, indicating effective sterilization.
   Rationale: Effective sterilization must occur to kill all microorganisms and spores.

STUDENT STUDY PLAN

To reinforce your understanding of the material in this chapter . . .

Complete the **Review & Recall** questions.

Discuss the situation in **If You Were the Medical Assistant** with your classmates, and answer the questions.

Answer the **Critical Thinking Questions** and discuss them with your classmates.

Visit the **Web sites** suggested and search for additional sites using **Keywords for Internet Searches.**

Complete the exercises in chapter 13 of the **Student Mastery Manual.**

 REVIEW & RECALL

1. Why are medical asepsis and surgical asepsis used in the medical office?

2. Compare and contrast bacteria, specialized bacteria, viruses, fungi, and parasites in respect to size, shape, what kind of equipment (if any) are required to see them, and whether they can grow outside a living host.

3. List six conditions that are necessary for microorganisms to grow and thrive.

4. Describe what is meant by the term "normal flora."

5. What are six normal physical factors and physiologic responses that help human beings fight off harmful microorganisms?

6. Describe antigens and antibodies, and correlate them to the body's immune response.

7. Differentiate between genetic immunity and acquired immunity, active immunity and passive immunity, and natural immunity and artificial immunity.

8. What are the five conditions necessary for the infection cycle to occur?

9. When is medical asepsis used? Surgical asepsis?

10. Describe how an item can be disinfected. What is the difference between low-level, intermediate-level, and high-level disinfection?

11. Identify four methods to perform sterilization.

12. Describe the procedure for steam sterilization of instruments using an autoclave.

 IF YOU WERE THE MEDICAL ASSISTANT

Paul Dean has been asked to load an autoclave and sterilize four small packages wrapped with paper wrap and two metal containers the office uses to hold tongue depressors and cotton balls. The metal containers are being sterilized to kill all pathogens that might be on them. After sterilization, Paul can touch the outsides and they can be refilled with fresh supplies.

1. Why should Paul check the reservoir on the autoclave before beginning the sterilization cycle?

2. Should Paul load the packs closely together or spaced apart? Why?

3. Should Paul position the metal containers right-side up, upside down, or on their sides? Why? How should he position the covers?

4. How long should the temperature of 250° F at 15 pounds of pressure be maintained to sterilize all the articles in the load completely?

5. Describe what Paul should do to vent the autoclave and open the door after the sterilization cycle is complete.

6. Why should Paul allow the load to dry completely (or run the dry cycle if the autoclave has one)?

7. How long are paper-wrapped packages considered sterile?

 ## CRITICAL THINKING QUESTIONS

1. What factors are important if an office is considering purchasing a new sterilizer?

2. Discuss why the resistance of bacteria to antibiotics is of great concern to doctors and scientists. Do research to find information about how doctors are trying to prevent further resistance from emerging.

3. What are the possible consequences to patients if proper procedures for preventing infection are not followed? Imagine several specific problems that could arise.

4. If you noticed that a coworker did not use personal protective equipment when cleaning and handling contaminated instruments, what would you say to that person? Develop an argument to persuade the person that he or she should always use personal protective equipment.

5. Identify several different problems that could cause an individual to have a decreased resistance to disease. Do research to get more information if necessary.

 ## EXPLORE THE WEB

INTERNET WEB SITES

Asepsis game
www.quia.com/jg/47715.html

CDC hospital infection program
www.cdc.gov/ncidod/hip/Sterile/sterile.htm

Virtual library of microorganisms
www.microbiol.org/vl_micro/index.htm

KEYWORDS FOR INTERNET SEARCHES

asepsis
bacteria
microorganisms

 ## ANSWERS TO ON THE JOB

1. The instruments must be cleaned to remove any body fluid, blood, or other residue before further treatment. This residue might be baked on during steam sterilization; potentially, microorganisms could be protected from destruction.

2. Paul should put on face protection (such as a mask and goggles or face shield), gloves, and clothing protection such as an apron, lab coat, or barrier gown. Paul may choose to use heavy-duty rubber gloves.

3. Using detergent, water, and a brush, Paul should clean and scrub each instrument until it is free of visible dirt or debris. He should then rinse each item completely and place them on paper towels to drain. The instruments must be allowed to air dry or be dried with paper towels.

4. Paul should wash the outside of the gloves with soap and water before he removes them. He should then leave them to dry in the designated location (often under the sink). He should then wash and dry his hands, using the medical aseptic handwash.

Chapter 14

Preparing the Patient for Examination

Instructional Objectives

After completing this chapter, you will be able to do the following:

1. Describe how to prepare an examination room for a patient.
2. Describe how to call a patient from the waiting room.
3. Identify steps to assist a weak patient to ambulate and sit on the examination table.
4. Describe how to assist a patient to transfer to and from a wheelchair.
5. Describe an appropriate location to obtain the medical history.
6. Identify information that must be included in the assessment of the chief complaint.
7. Differentiate between information obtained from a new patient and an established patient.
8. Identify information contained in the following parts of the medical history:
   current medical problems
   past history (PH)
   family history (FH)
   social history (SH)
   occupational history (OH)
   review of systems (ROS).
9. Identify appropriate measures to help you decide when a patient cannot safely be left alone in an examination room.

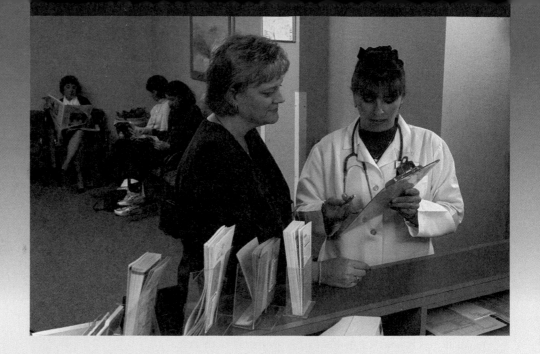

- Obtain and record patient history
- Prepare and maintain examination and treatment areas

- Assist with transfers of weak patients and patients in wheelchairs
- Maintain patient safety

Performance Objectives

After completing this chapter, you will be able to do the following:

1. Assist a patient to transfer safely between a wheelchair and an examination table (Procedure 14–1).
2. Obtain and record a patient history or information about a patient's current medical problem (Procedure 14–2).

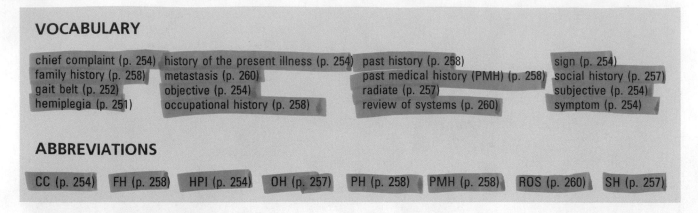

VOCABULARY

chief complaint (p. 254) history of the present illness (p. 254) past history (p. 258) sign (p. 254)
family history (p. 258) metastasis (p. 260) past medical history (PMH) (p. 258) social history (p. 257)
gait belt (p. 252) objective (p. 254) radiate (p. 257) subjective (p. 254)
hemiplegia (p. 251) occupational history (p. 258) review of systems (p. 260) symptom (p. 254)

ABBREVIATIONS

CC (p. 254) FH (p. 258) HPI (p. 254) OH (p. 257) PH (p. 258) PMH (p. 258) ROS (p. 260) SH (p. 257)

PREPARING THE EXAMINATION ROOM

The examination room needs to be prepared both at the beginning of the day and for each new patient.

Daily preparation includes making sure that all necessary item are stocked and in their proper place. This includes items as diverse as patient gowns, tongue depressors, cotton balls, bandages, and blood pressure cuffs. Exam rooms are often prepared at the end of the day for the next day's patients. Items that need to be recharged, such as battery-powered otoscopes, should be plugged into wall sockets at the end of the day to charge overnight.

Cleaning the Examination Room

Cleaning is done between patients, preferably before the patient is called in from the waiting room. Four activities are involved in cleaning the exam room for a new patient:

1. Pick up.
2. Clean surfaces.
3. Put clean paper on the examination table.
4. Wash hands.

Pick Up

Any supplies used for the previous patient need to be picked up. Disposable supplies are thrown away, either in the trash or in the hazardous wastebag. If necessary, the sink and countertops should be wiped with a dry paper towel.

Clean Contaminated Surfaces

Wearing gloves, clean any surface that has come into contact with blood or body fluids, using a 1:10 solution of household bleach (1 part bleach to 10 parts water) or other approved disinfectant. Allow the surface to air-dry.

Put On Clean Paper

Pull out a short length of clean table paper from the roll at the head of the table, tear off the used paper, and throw it away. Then pull enough clean paper from the roll to cover the entire table surface, and fold it under or tuck it under the end of the table.

Wash Hands

When you are done cleaning the room, wash hands using guidelines for medical asepsis, as described in Chapter 13.

Replacing Table Paper If Needed

Each roll of table paper accommodates approximately 75 patients. Unfortunately, you always seem to run out of table paper in the middle of a busy day, so it needs to be changed between patients.

To change the roll, raise the backrest so you can see the metal rod that holds the cardboard cylinder from the old roll of paper. Remove the old cardboard, and insert the metal rod into a new roll of paper. Place the roll back into position under the backrest, and bring the paper up over the end of the table. Pull the paper down to cover the table.

BRINGING THE PATIENT INTO THE EXAMINATION ROOM

Calling the Patient from the Waiting Room

The medical assistant who brings patients back to be examined is often greeting the patient for the first time that day; he or she may not have checked the patient in. The medical assistant wants to create in the patient a feeling of security and confidence in the office medical staff. This is accomplished by appearing confident, speaking clearly, and knowing as much about the patient as possible.

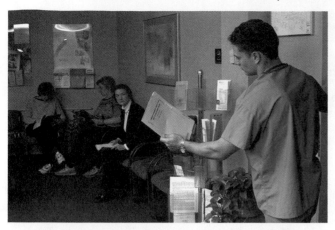

➤ **Figure 14–1** The medical assistant calls the patient from the waiting room.

If the medical assistant has any questions about pronouncing the patient's name, he or she should ask the receptionist before going into the waiting room. To be polite, a medical assistant should address a patient as Mr., Mrs., Miss, Ms., or Dr., followed by the last name, unless the patient has said at a previous visit that he or she wishes to be addressed by a first name.

If the waiting room is full, as is usually the case in a clinic, the medical assistant can avoid confusion by addressing the patient by his or her full name; for instance, Mr. Ivan Shapiro rather than Mr. Shapiro.

During this short interaction, the medical assistant wants to establish eye contact, smile, and make the patient feel welcome. She or he should look confident and competent, and clearly direct the patient to the exam room or to the cental area for height, weight, and vital signs. Calling a patient is illustrated in Figure 14–1.

The Patient with Limited Mobility

The kind of practice and the patient population will determine how many patients with limited mobility the medical assistant will encounter. Patients with limited mobility are defined as those who are either very weak, who need assistance moving about or those who use a wheelchair and need assistance in transferring from the wheelchair to the examination table and back again.

Weakness

A patient who comes to the office with an ambulatory aid (a walker, cane, crutches) needs to have all doors held open. The medical assistant should stand to the side of the door, leaving the entrance totally free. If necessary, anything that may block the patient's path should be moved.

The medical assistant should avoid any demonstration of impatience and tell the patient to take his or her time. A weak or slightly unsteady patient may be supported by a family member or the medical assistant. But if the patient cannot manage to walk to the exam room, most offices keep a wheelchair handy.

A weak or unsteady patient may need assistance to step up to the exam table. If the person has a walker or crutches, he or she supports the body weight on the equipment and steps up with the good (or better) foot first. The medical assistant can help support the patient's body weight by standing on the weaker side and holding the patient firmly under the armpit. The medical assistant can help the person balance while turning around, once the person is standing on the step of the exam table. If the table does not have a built-in step, a sturdy portable step can be used.

Wheelchair

When a patient needs assistance getting from a wheelchair to the exam table, safety, for both the patient and the medical assistant, is very important. If a patient has had a cerebrovascular accident, also called a stroke (bleeding inside the skull that affects the brain) he or she may be paralyzed or have **hemiplegia**—paralysis on one side of the body. In this case, the transfer must accommodate the patient's disability. There are nine steps to making a safe transfer from a wheelchair to an exam table, as described in Procedure 14–1.

To get a patient off the exam table and into the wheelchair, reverse the process. Often, the person who brings the patient to the office will be familiar with the patient's usual mode of transfer and can direct the medical assistant in ways to modify this basic approach to best help the patient. When making a wheelchair transfer, remember to lock the brake before the patient attempts to lift himself or herself out of the chair.

Many older patients who are confined to a wheelchair because of stroke are fearful of their limits and of changes in their routine. You should try to work in a way that is most comfortable for the patient, as long as it is consistent with maintaining safety.

INTRODUCTION TO THE PATIENT INTERVIEW

The patient interview is perhaps the most important aspect of a medical assistant's job. By obtaining a clear medical history and statement of the patient's chief complaint, the medical assistant can save the doctor valuable time. And, because the medical assistant is

PROCEDURE 14–1

Assisting a Patient to Transfer to and from a Wheelchair

Performance Objective: The student will assist a patient to transfer between a wheelchair and the examination table safely.

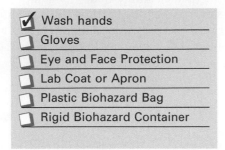

- ☑ Wash hands
- ☐ Gloves
- ☐ Eye and Face Protection
- ☐ Lab Coat or Apron
- ☐ Plastic Biohazard Bag
- ☐ Rigid Biohazard Container

Supplies and Equipment: Wheelchair, examination table.

Procedure Steps

1. Wash hands.
2. Explain the procedure to the patient.
   Rationale: The patient will be more comfortable and cooperative if he or she knows what to expect.
3. Pull out the step of the examination table. If the table does not have a step, position a step stool beside it.
   Rationale: The exam table is usually higher than the seat of a chair or wheelchair.
4. Place the wheelchair next to the exam table or other table you wish to transfer the pa-

tient to, with the patient's stronger side immediately beside the exam table and step.
   Rationale: The patient will be able to provide more help when transferring toward his or her strong side.
5. Move both footrests out of the way if possible, or move the footplate up and have the patient put his or her feet on the floor.
   Rationale: This enables the patient to stand with assistance.
6. Lock both wheels of the wheelchair.
   Rationale: This will prevent the wheelchair from moving.
7. Ask the patient to move forward in the wheelchair. Hold the patient to prevent him or her from falling.
   Rationale: It is easier to stand from the edge of a chair.
8. Instruct the patient to push up with the arms and assist the patient to stand, providing enough support to prevent the patient from falling. It may be necessary to use a **gait belt** (a strong cloth belt) around the patient's waist so that you have something to grab to support the patient's weight.
   Rationale: Pushing with the arms will help raise the patient's body from the wheelchair.
9. Assist the patient to step up on the step of the exam table using his or her strong leg and pushing up on the table with his or her arm.

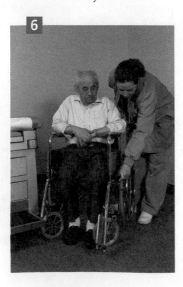

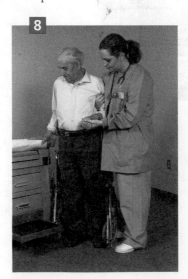

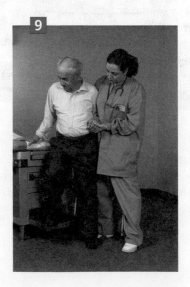

Rationale: Leading with the strong leg allows the patient to assist as much as possible.

10. While continuing to provide support, assist the patient to shift the entire body weight up onto the step and pivot until his or her back is toward the table.

11. Assist the patient to sit on the end of the table.

12. Move the wheelchair out of the way.

13. Reverse the sequence of steps to help the patient get off the table and return to the wheelchair.

Note: If the patient is unable to support his or her own weight, two people may be needed to hold the patient during the transfer. It may be easier for one to hold the upper body and one to hold the legs while lifting the patient to the table over the arm of the wheelchair.

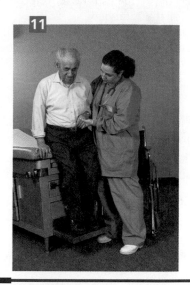

often able to spend more time with a patient than a doctor can, he or she is often able to get the patient to open up and discuss some of the underlying issues beyond the immediate medical problem.

To do this, however, the medical assistant must learn to conduct an effective patient interview and to document the interview thoroughly and clearly.

Effective Interviewing Technique

There are two important aspects of interviewing the patient. The first is maintaining privacy in the discussion of private topics. The second is communicating clearly with the patient.

Privacy

Although the patient has been asked questions about his or her billing and insurance at the front desk, and often has filled out a written health history questionnaire while waiting to be seen, the medical assistant should take the patient to a private area to discuss the medical history and current health problem.

Sometimes a patient is taken directly to an exam room, where the medical interview takes place before or after height, weight, and vital signs are taken. If the office has a central area for taking height, weight, and vital signs, the patient interview will take place afterward.

The order in which things are done does not matter. Making sure the medical interview takes place in private does matter.

Communication

One important reason the medical assistant or other health professional goes over the health history before the patient sees the doctor is to help the patient organize his or her thoughts and to focus on problems or symptoms that the patient may consider unimportant. Although the doctor will try to identify problems or symptoms that are significant, these are not always the most important things to the patient.

An analogy to think of as to why the medical assistant interviews the patient before the doctor is that of a lawyer and witness. The lawyer will always interview a witness before the witness appears before a judge or jury, to make sure the witness is articulating the real issues clearly.

When conducting the medical interview, a medical assistant must do three things:

1. Avoid distractions and interruptions whenever possible. This allows both the medical assistant and the patient to focus on the matter at hand.

2. Be familiar with the forms being used. Know how to pronounce all of the words on the forms.

3. Utilize the techniques for effective communication presented in chapter 5. These include speaking directly to the patient, making eye contact, and listening closely and "actively" to the patient's responses.

A new medical assistant must undertake two self-learning goals during the first few interviews he or she performs:

1. Learn how to manage an interview so that all of the relevant items can be covered in the time allotted for the interview.
2. Learn how to summarize findings from the interview in a way that is helpful to the doctor. Learn how to be concise yet complete in these summaries.

Documentation

Remember that everything in a patient's medical record is a legal document. (Review chapter 10 for information about charting and correct entries.) If the patient's own words are used to describe something, make sure to use quotation marks around the statement. (Example: "My legs itch so much I could scratch them off.")

A medical assistant may be expected to write a continuous note, or to use a note in SOAP format, as described in chapter 10. It is important to always use medical terminology and to organize information properly when charting, even if writing a temporary note that will be incorporated into the doctor's dictation.

(Remember, different offices have different methods for medical assistants to record the findings of patient interviews. In some offices, the medical assistant documents directly onto the medical record. In other cases, the medical assistant writes notes on a sheet of paper and clips it to the chart, and the doctor incorporates the information from these notes into his or her dictation after seeing the patient.)

OBTAINING THE MEDICAL HISTORY

The medical history is all of the information a patient can give about previous health care, medical problems and potential medical problems, and previous and current treatments. This information is necessary for the doctor to decide what medical problems the patient has and how to treat them.

Usually, a new patient fills out a questionnaire; in other instances the medical assistant fills in the questionnaire using the patient's answers to verbal questions. If the patient is illiterate, the medical assistant must ask appropriate questions and record the answers. A complete medical history is taken for a new patient; an established patient only needs to have the present health history updated. Figure 14–2 shows a health history questionnaire.

The Chief Complaint

The main problem that has brought a patient to see the doctor is called the **chief complaint (CC)**. For a new patient, the chief complaint will be the first item on the health history questionnaire.

Assessing the Chief Complaint

The medical assistant should ask an established patient: "What brings you to see the doctor today?" or "What is the reason for your visit today?" If the patient has come for a routine physical exam, there may not be a chief complaint.

A change in the body that indicates altered function or disease is called a **symptom.** The word *symptom* is often reserved for those changes that the patient experiences through the senses (touch, vision, hearing) or experiences as a sensation (pain, nausea, itching) or feeling (sadness, anger). These are called **subjective** complaints, because they cannot be measured or validated.

A **sign** is the term for changes that can be observed and/or measured, such as redness, swelling, or weight gain. Such changes are called **objective,** which means they can be observed and measured by other people.

In SOAP charting, symptoms are included under S(ubjective) and signs under O(bjective).

Additional Information to Describe the Chief Complaint

Information to expand the chief complaint is sometimes called the **history of the present illness (HPI).** Seven categories of information are usually included:

1. Location
2. Quality
3. Severity
4. Chronology
5. How it began
6. What makes it better or worse
7. Associated symptoms

Location asks about where exactly on the body the symptom is located. A patient often refers to a general location, but determining the specific location is helpful. For instance, the patient might say "My arm hurts." Questions such as "Where exactly does it hurt?" or "Can you show me where it hurts?" can help the patient pinpoint the area of pain to the outer elbow or forearm.

Quality of a symptom or a sign refers to how one would characterize the symptom or sign as fully as possible. The quality of pain can be described as sharp and sudden, throbbing, dull and constant, or burning; intestinal pain is often crampy; and the pain of a heart attack is often characterized as "viselike pressure."

The medical assistant needs to both get the patient to describe subjective symptoms and fully describe

---

➤ **Figure 14–2** Sample health history questionnaire form. (Courtesy of Bibbero Systems, Inc., Petaluma, California, (800) 272-2376. Fax (800) 242-9330; www.bibbero.com.)

ANDRUS/CLINI-REC® HEALTH HISTORY QUESTIONNAIRE

Chart No. _____

Identification Information

Today's Date _____

Name_____ Date of Birth_____

Occupation _____ Marital Status _____

PART A – PRESENT HEALTH HISTORY

I. CURRENT MEDICAL PROBLEMS

Please list the medical problems for which you came to see the doctor. About when did they begin?

Problems	Date Began
_____	_____
_____	_____
_____	_____

What concerns you most about these problems?

_____

_____

If you are being treated for any other illness or medical problems by another physician, please describe the problems and write the name of the physician or medical facility treating you.

Illness or Medical Problem	Physician or Medical Facility	City
_____	_____	_____
_____	_____	_____

II. MEDICATIONS

Please list all medications you are now taking, including those you buy without a doctor's prescription (such as aspirin, cold tablets or vitamin supplements).

_____ _____ _____

_____ _____ _____

III. ALLERGIES AND SENSITIVITIES

List anything that you are allergic to such as certain foods, medications, dust, chemicals or soaps, household items, pollens, bee stings, etc., and indicate how each affects you.

Allergic To:	Effect	Allergic To:	Effect
_____	_____	_____	_____
_____	_____	_____	_____

IV. GENERAL HEALTH, ATTITUDE AND HABITS

How is your overall health now? . . . . Health now: Poor _____ Fair _____ Good _____ Excellent _____

How has it been most of your life? . . . . Health has been: Poor _____ Fair _____ Good _____ Excellent _____

In the past year:

Has your appetite changed? . . . . Appetite: Decreased _____ Increased _____ Stayed same _____

Has your weight changed? . . . . Weight: Lost _____ lbs. Gained _____ lbs. No change _____

Are you thirsty much of the time? . . . . Thirsty: No _____ Yes _____

Has your overall 'pep' changed? . . . . Pep: Decreased _____ Increased _____ Stayed same _____

Do you usually have trouble sleeping? . . . . Trouble sleeping: No _____ Yes _____

How much do you exercise? . . . . Exercise: Little or none _____ Less than I need _____ All I need _____

Do you smoke? . . . . Smokes: No _____ Yes _____ If yes, how many years? _____

How many each day? . . . . _____ Cigarettes _____ Cigars _____ Pipesfull

Have you ever smoked? . . . . Smoked: No _____ Yes _____ If yes, how many years? _____

How many each day? . . . . _____ Cigarettes _____ Cigars _____ Pipesfull

Do you drink alcoholic beverages? . . . . Alcohol: No _____ Yes _____ I drink _____ Beers _____ Glasses of wine

_____ Drinks of hard liquor - per day

Have you ever had a problem with alcohol? . . . . Prior problem: No _____ Yes _____

How much coffee or tea do you usually drink? . . . . Coffee/Tea: _____ cups of coffee or tea a day

Do you regularly wear seatbelts? . . . . Seatbelts: No _____ Yes _____

DO YOU:	Rarely/Never	Occasionally	Frequently	DO YOU:	Rarely/Never	Occasionally	Frequently
Feel nervous?	_____	_____	_____	Ever feel like committing suicide?	_____	_____	_____
Feel depressed?	_____	_____	_____	Feel bored with your life?	_____	_____	_____
Find it hard to make decisions?	_____	_____	_____	Use marijuana?	_____	_____	_____
Lose your temper?	_____	_____	_____	Use "hard drugs"?	_____	_____	_____
Worry a lot?	_____	_____	_____	Do you want to talk to the			
Tire easily?	_____	_____	_____	doctor about a personal matter? No _____ Yes _____			
Have trouble relaxing?	_____	_____	_____				
Have any sexual problems?							

CONFIDENTIAL

IV. GENERAL HEALTH, ATTITUDE AND HABITS (continued)

Have you recently had any changes in your: If yes, please explain:

Marital status?   No_____ Yes_____ _____

Job or work?   No_____ Yes_____ _____

Residence?   No_____ Yes_____ _____

Financial status?   No_____ Yes_____ _____

Are you having any legal problems
or trouble with the law?   No_____ Yes_____ _____

PART B – PAST HISTORY

I. FAMILY HEALTH

Please give the following information about your immediate family:

Relationship	Age, if Living	Age At Death	State of Health Or Cause of Death
Father	_____	_____	_____
Mother	_____	_____	_____
Brothers and Sisters	_____	_____	_____
	_____	_____	_____
	_____	_____	_____
Spouse	_____	_____	_____
Children	_____	_____	_____
	_____	_____	_____
	_____	_____	_____

Have any **blood relatives** had any of the following illnesses? If so, indicate relationship (mother, brother, etc.)

Illness	Family Members
Asthma	_____
Diabetes	_____
Cancer	_____
Blood Disease	_____
Glaucoma	_____
Epilepsy	_____
Rheumatoid Arthritis	_____
Tuberculosis	_____
Gout	_____
High Blood Pressure	_____
Heart Disease	_____
Mental Problems	_____
Suicide	_____
Stroke	_____
Alcoholism	_____
Rheumatic Fever	_____

II. HOSPITALIZATIONS, SURGERIES, INJURIES

Please list all times you have been hospitalized, operated on, or seriously injured.

Year	Operation, Illness, Injury	Hospital and City
_____	_____	_____
_____	_____	_____
_____	_____	_____

III. ILLNESS AND MEDICAL PROBLEMS

Please mark with an (X) any of the following illnesses and medical problems you have or have had and indicate the year when each started. If you are not certain when an illness started, write down an approximate year.

Illness	(x)	(Year)	Illness	(x)	(Year)
Eye or eye lid infection	___	___	Hernia	___	___
Glaucoma	___	___	Hemorrhoids	___	___
Other eye problems	___	___	Kidney or bladder disease	___	___
Ear trouble	___	___	Prostate problem (male only)	___	___
Deafness or decreased hearing	___	___	Mental problems	___	___
Thyroid trouble	___	___	Headaches	___	___
Strep throat	___	___	Head injury	___	___
Bronchitis	___	___	Stroke	___	___
Emphysema	___	___	Convulsions, seizures	___	___
Pneumonia	___	___	Arthritis	___	___
Allergies, asthma or hay fever	___	___	Gout	___	___
Tuberculosis	___	___	Cancer or tumor	___	___
Other lung problems	___	___	Bleeding tendency	___	___
High blood pressure	___	___	Diabetes	___	___
Heart attack	___	___	Measles/Rubeola	___	___
High cholesterol	___	___	German measles/Rubella	___	___
Arteriosclerosis (Hardening of arteries)	___	___	Polio	___	___
Heart murmur	___	___	Mumps	___	___
Other heart condition	___	___	Scarlet fever	___	___
Stomach/duodenal ulcer	___	___	Chicken pox	___	___
Diverticulosis	___	___	Mononucleosis	___	___
Colitis	___	___	Eczema	___	___
Other bowel problems	___	___	Psoriasis	___	___
Hepatitis	___	___	Venereal disease	___	___
Liver trouble	___	___	Genital herpes	___	___
Gallbladder trouble	___	___	HIV test	___	___
			AIDS	___	___

CONFIDENTIAL

> Figure 14–2 Continued

signs himself or herself. Is a patient's cough "productive," with the patient bringing up phlegm, or is it dry and hacking? If a patient vomits, what color is it? Is it liquid or particulate? What is the odor? Is there any blood present?

Severity gets at the quantitative aspects of the illness. Are symptoms intense, moderate, or mild? Are nosebleeds frequent or sporadic? What is the volume of blood, or vomitus, or stool, produced on each incident?

When discussing the severity of pain, the patient should be asked to rate severity on a scale of 1 to 10, with 1 being least severe and 10 most severe. It is also necessary to ask if the pain **radiates** (extends to anywhere else).

Chronology asks when the illness began and how long is has lasted, whether symptoms have been constant or intermittent, whether it is getting better or getting worse. On some forms, these issues are listed as date of onset, duration, frequency, and change over time.

How it began is self-explanatory. But it is important to determine what the patient was doing when the symptom began, to see if the activity or a specific location could have had anything to do with the illness.

What makes it better or worse gets at what the patient has done to try to relieve symptoms or if there are certain activities the patient undertakes on a regular basis that make the symptoms worse. Certain symptoms are often relieved by exercise, sitting or lying in a particular position, or bowel movement or urination. Also, outside factors such as weather sometimes affect symptoms.

Associated symptoms gets at the "minor" symptoms that occur around any disease process. Knowing what to ask about is a process of learning for any new medical assistant. Sore throats or ear pain are often accompanied by fever and/or stuffy nose. A stuffy nose and no fever may mean the sore throat is due to a virus, whereas fever and no stuffy nose may signal a bacterial infection.

A patient with a rash should not only be asked about allergies, but also about any changes in medication or even laundry detergent (as from sleeping in a hotel while away from home on business or pleasure).

A patient with shortness of breath needs to be asked if he or she has chest pain, ankle swelling, or weight gain.

Documenting the Chief Complaint

The chief complaint is usually documented along with the length of time the patient has had the complaint. Documentation is done using abbreviations as shown in Figure 14–3.

It is important for the medical assistant to document

accurately and precisely. She or he should use medical terminology to describe location on the body (e.g., medial aspect of inner thigh) and symptoms (e.g., dyspnea), but should avoid diagnostic terms.

Figure 14–4 shows a sample charting of a chief complaint.

Present Health History

The present health history is comprised of five items:

1. Ongoing medical problems
2. Medications currently being used
3. Allergies
4. Social history
5. Occupational history.

If the patient has completed the history questionnaire before the interview, the medical assistant asks questions to fill in missing sections or clarify anything that is unclear. The medical assistant may also ask questions and complete the form for the patient, as seen in Figure 14–5.

Ongoing Medical Problems

For a new patient, this pertains to medical problems for which the patient is being treated. A doctor needs to know the date each problem began, what kind of treatment the patient is receiving, and how effective the treatment has been.

Medications Currently Being Used

Many medications affect other medications, a process called drug interactions. It is important to get as complete a list as possible of medications being taken as well as the dose being used. Some offices ask new patients to bring all of their medications with them to a first office visit.

Allergies

Allergies, especially allergies to medications or foods, must be noted. Allergies to eggs and/or shellfish are especially important. Eggs are used to prepare vaccines. Allergy to shellfish may indicate potential problems with certain contrast media used for diagnostic tests. Be sure to complete an orange allergy sticker for the front of the chart at the time of the patient's visit.

Social History (SH) and Occupational History (OH)

The **social history** covers general health, attitudes, and habits. This includes appetite, sleeping, stamina, and nervousness or worrying. It also includes exercise habits, daily caffeine intake, smoking, and use of alcohol, street drugs, and over-the-counter medications.

Parts of the history and physical examination

H & P	history and physical examination
PE	physical examination
CC	chief complaint
HPI	history of present illness
FH	family history
SH	social history
OH	occupational history
ROS	review of systems

General

c̄	with	<	greater than
dc, D/C	discontinue	>	less than
DOB	date of birth	Δ	change
Dx	diagnosis	↑	increase
Hx, H/O	history of	↓	decrease
ETOH	alcohol intake	°	degree
NKA	no known allergies	Ø	without
pt	patients	@	at
Rx, Tx	treatment	♂	male
s̄	without	♀	female
SP, S/P	status post (has had in the past)	×	times (used with a time measurement, as in 2 weeks)
stat	immediately		

Body locations

lt or Ⓛ	left
rt or Ⓡ	right
LA	left arm
RA	right arm
LL	left leg
RL	right leg
abd	abdomen
LLQ	left lower quadrant of the abdomen
LUQ	left upper quadrant of the abdomen
RLQ	right lower quadrant of the abdomen
RUQ	right upper quadrant of the abdomen

Signs and symptoms

S & S	signs and symptoms
c/o	complains of
BM	bowel movement
LMP	last menstrual period
mod	moderate
N & V	nausea and vomiting
sl	slight
SOB	shortness of breath

➤ **Figure 14–3** Common abbreviations used in charting the chief complaint and medical history.

Some forms include an additional section for **occupational history** (history of jobs the patient has had). If the patient's chief complaint is a work-related problem, this area may need to be included in greater depth.

Past Health History (PH) or Past Medical History (PMH)

There are three elements to the **past history:**

1. Family history
2. Previous hospitalizations, surgeries, and injuries
3. Illnesses or medical problems.

Family History (FH)

The discussion of **family history** is undertaken in an effort to understand the general health status of family members and diseases that run in families. The questionnaire may ask about current age or age at death.

This is an area where the patient may ramble. It is important to try to get the patient to focus on diseases or conditions that might run in the family, such as arthritis, diabetes mellitus, heart disease, seizures, kidney disease, and cancer. If the patient states that a family member has or has had cancer, find out what type of cancer and the individual's current status.

Previous Hospitalization, Surgeries, and Injuries

Include the date (month and year, if known) and reason for each hospitalization, or the date and type of injury. An elderly person may not remember the exact year, but may be able to tell you about how old he or she was at the time. For women who had hospital-based childbirths, include the year and whether the birth was vaginal or by caesarean section.

If the medical assistant works in a gynecology practice, the history form will include a separate section for the obstetrical history. The obstetrical history will be discussed in chapter 29.

Illnesses or Medical Problems

Include when the problem began. A medical assistant may ask the patient if he or she has had any serious medical problems that are not listed on the form. Procedure 14–2 describes the process for completing and recording the patient's health history.

Patient Interview #1

Medical Assistant: What is the reason for your visit today?
Patient: My throat has been sore since Tuesday.
Medical Assistant: That's three days now isn't it? Have you had any fever?
Patient: I don't know. I don't think so.

Sample charting

6/12/99	c/o sore throat x 3 days---------------------------S. Williams, CMA

Patient Interview #2

Medical Assistant: Why have you come to see the doctor today?
Patient: I have had terrible stomach pain all morning.
Medical assistant: Can you show me where it hurts?
Patient points to area 3 inches below belly button in the middle.
Medical assistant: Have you taken anything to relieve the pain?
Patient: I took Maalox but it didn't help.
Medical assistant: When did you take it?
Patient: At 9:30 this morning.

Sample charting

6/12/99	Pt. c/o severe midline abdominal pain since this AM. Took Maalox at 9:30
	AM s̄ relief.--S. Williams, CMA

> **Figure 14–4** Sample patient interview and charting of the chief complaint.

Patient Interview #3

Medical Assistant: What is the reason for your visit today today?
Patient: I have been having really bad headaches.
Medical Assistant: When did the headaches begin?
Patient: Well, I always have headaches occasionally, but lately I've had two or three a week, like for the last two weeks.
Medical Assistant: Are they in the front or back, can you show me?
Patient: They are all over. It feels like someone is hammering my head.
Medical Assistant: On both sides?
Patient: Yes.
Medical Assistant: What do you do when you have one?
Patient: I have to lie down. I've been taking ibuprofen but it doesn't help. When I have one I'm too sick to do anything.
Medical Assistant: Do you have any nausea or see flashing lights?
Patient: No
Medical Assistant: Have you been sick or had any other problems?
Patient: Not really.

Sample charting

6/12/99	Pt. c/o severe generalized headaches x two weeks, about 2-3 per week.
	Describes as "it feels like someone is hammering my head." Pain is not
	relieved by ibuprofen. Denies other symptoms or illness.--------------------
	--S. Williams, CMA

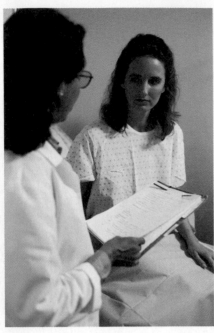

> Figure 14–5 The medical assistant reviews the health history questionnaire or fills it out while interviewing the patient.

Review of Medical Systems (ROS)

The **review of systems** is a series of questions that take in the patient from head to toe, to identify symptoms or problems that the patient may have experienced. Usually the doctor does the review of systems just before examining the patient. But when the questions are included on a health history questionnaire, the medical assistant goes over the form with the patient to explain anything that is unclear, and to be sure the patient has answered all of the questions.

Questions often identify symptoms that the patient does not think are very important. Groups of symptoms occurring together help the doctor focus and look for specific medical problems. Figure 14–6 shows a sample questionnaire.

Before the physical examination, the doctor will review the entire health history questionnaire with the patient and will usually dictate a report that summarizes the information obtained. Figure 14–7 shows a sample doctor's report. Instead of dictating, some doctors today use a computer program to record informa-

FOCUS ON:
COMMUNICATION

Following are two examples of patient–medical assistant conversations about family history issues:

EXAMPLE 1

Patient: My mother died of cancer 2 years ago.
Medical Assistant: That must have been very difficult for you. How old was she when she died?
Patient: 55.
Medical Assistant: She was young. Do you know what kind of cancer it was?
Patient: Stomach cancer.

If the patient had answered bone, liver, or brain cancer, it is appropriate to ask if the doctors who treated the patient's mother believed the cancer started there, or spread from somewhere else, since these are common sites of **metastasis,** or spread of cancer cells from one part of the body to another.

EXAMPLE 2

Patient: My sister has a lot of problems with her joints, and she has had surgery several times.
Medical Assistant: Does she have arthritis?
Patient: Yes, and she had to have her hip replaced, and she is going next month to have some plastic joints put into her fingers.
Medical Assistant: Do you know what kind of arthritis? Is it rheumatoid arthritis?
Patient: Yes.

In example 2, the medical assistant wants to direct the patient to pertinent information—namely, that the sister has rheumatoid arthritis—and avoid spending time to hear the sister's entire health history.

PROCEDURE 14–2

Obtaining and Recording a Patient History

Performance Objective: The student can obtain a complete and accurate medical history or information about a patient's current medical problem(s) and record the information.

Supplies and Equipment: Health history questionnaire, pen, medical record or progress note sheet.

Procedure Steps

1. Become familiar with the questionnaire. Before beginning the interview be sure you can pronounce every medical term and that you can give additional information to explain the meaning of each question.
   Rationale: Hesitation or uncertainty during the interview decreases patient confidence in your ability.

2. Ask the patient to accompany you to an area where you can speak privately. This may be an office or an exam room with a small table for you to write on.
   Rationale: Medical information is confidential. The patient will give more complete information in a relaxed and private area.

3. Seat the patient and yourself so that you are comfortable and can converse with good eye contact. You should be at the same eye level as the patient.
   Rationale: A comfortable conversation distance is 3 to 4 feet with both people at the same level. If the interviewer is too close, the patient may feel that his or her personal space has been threatened. If the interviewer is too far away, rapport will be decreased. If the interviewer stands while the patient sits, the patient may feel intimidated. If the patient sits on the exam table while the interviewer sits at a table, it may be difficult to maintain eye contact.

4. Explain the procedure. Explain that your purpose is to be sure that the doctor has needed information about the patient's health history. If the patient seems reluctant to discuss the form, explain further that it is helpful to the doctor when a patient has organized his or her thoughts and has called to mind dates and other aspects of the medical history and current problems.
   Rationale: Patients are more comfortable and cooperative when they understand the reason for procedures.

5. If the patient is a new patient, begin to go through the health history questionnaire. It is most efficient if the patient has filled in as much as possible before the interview, but you may also fill in the entire questionnaire.

6. Look for any omissions or incomplete answers, and explain any questions the patient does not understand.
   Rationale: This helps the patient understand the information the doctor needs to make a diagnosis.

7. If you are interviewing an established patient, ask the patient the reason for the visit, current medications, and additional questions related to the current problems according to the policy in your office.
   Rationale: Because the medical history does not change, after the first visit only current problems and treatment need to be discussed. For subsequent physical examinations the doctor asks questions for the review of systems just before examining the patient.

8. Use appropriate communication techniques to convey interest and understanding. Use open-ended questions if you want the patient to talk freely. Use questions asking for a specific answer if you want specific data or a yes or no answer. Look at the patient often to show interest and empathy.
   Rationale: The more comfortable the patient feels, the more likely he or she is to give complete and honest answers to your questions.

9. Patients may be embarrassed when discussing habits such as smoking or drinking alcohol, and especially sexual activity and drug use. If the doctor wants you to discuss these areas, ask questions in a neutral tone and avoid responding in a judgmental manner. If the patient does not wish to discuss any topic with you, leave the answer blank.
   Rationale: Patients have a right to refuse to give information. It is better to leave an answer blank than to pressure a patient and either create an uncomfortable atmosphere or encourage the patient to give an inaccurate answer. The doctor will have another opportunity to obtain the information.

10. Make additions to the medical history questionnaire in ink. Chart the chief complaint and other information for established patients

Procedure continued on following page

PROCEDURE 14–2 *(continued)*

according to the policy of your office. You may be expected to document the chief complaint and other information in the medical record or on a temporary page attached to the medical record. If the doctor dictates progress notes, he or she may want to incorporate all information about the current medical problems of an established patient into the dictated progress note.

Rationale: Anything in the patient's medical record is a legal document and must be re-

corded permanently. The medical history questionnaire will be filed in the patient record.

11. When the interview is complete, instruct the patient what clothing to remove and where to sit. Give the patient a realistic idea of how long he or she will have to wait for the doctor.

Rationale: Patients feel more comfortable when they know what is going to happen and how long they will be waiting.

---

tion about the patient's history. This type of computer program generates a report similar to the type a doctor would dictate to place in the patient's medical record.

THE PATIENT WHO CANNOT SAFELY BE LEFT ALONE

A medical office is legally responsible for the health and safety of patients while they are in the office. To meet this responsibility, office staff must keep in mind both general safety measures, which were discussed in chapter 6, and additional measures, which may be required because of an individual patient's problems and things the patient is asked to do as part of an examination or treatment.

Safety problems can occur because the exam table is relatively high and narrow, and patients are usually left in the exam room alone to wait for the examination. Therefore, it is important to assess a patient to see if he or she can be left alone in the exam room. If a patient cannot be left alone, the medical assistant or the patient's companion should remain in the exam room until the doctor arrives.

Assessment Criteria

Three types of patients should not be left alone in an exam room:

1. A child
2. An individual with decreased mental ability or poor judgment
3. An individual too ill to care for himself or herself.

Children are never left alone in an examination room. Adolescents often prefer to be examined without a parent present. By age 12 or 13, an adolescent can safely be left alone in the exam room, provided that both the child and parent are comfortable about it.

Individuals with decreased mental ability or poor judgment could include a retarded adult, a mentally ill adult, or an elderly individual with dementia. When the medical assistant interviews the patient, it is important to notice childlike speech, rambling speech, or a mood that does not match the circumstances (for instance, the patient makes a joke when he or she loses balance).

The medical assistant may observe certain things about the individual's physical appearance, such as bruises on the arms or legs, and notice also that the individual bumps into things in the exam room. The individual may act impulsively.

Patients who are too ill to care for themselves include patients who have a high fever, dizziness, bleeding, or vomiting. The patient may be faint or drowsy. A patient with any of these symptoms should be supervised carefully in case a crisis develops.

Legal Responsibilities

The office has a legal responsibility to protect patients and anyone else in the office. If a person is injured on the premises of a business (such as a medical office), the business usually will be legally liable. In the case of a patient with a medical condition, office personnel may have a greater responsibility to protect the patient from injury. Proper precautions help avoid lawsuits for negligence.

In addition, if children accompany the patient and they cannot be adequately supervised by the patient during the exam or treatment, someone in the office must be responsible.

➤ **Figure 14–6** Same questionnaire for body systems review (Courtesy of Bibbero Systems, Inc., Petaluma, California, (800) 272-2376. Fax (800) 242-9330; www.bibbero.com.)

PART C – BODY SYSTEMS REVIEW

Please answer all of the following questions.

Circle any questions you find difficult to answer.

__MEN:__   Please answer questions 1 through 12, then skip to question 18.
__WOMEN:__ Please start on question 6.

MEN ONLY

1. Have you had or do you have prostate trouble? . . . .   No _____   Yes _____
2. Do you have any sexual problems or a problem with impotency? . . . .   No _____   Yes _____
3. Have you ever had sores or lesions on your penis? . . . .   No _____   Yes _____
4. Have you ever had any discharge from your penis? . . . .   No _____   Yes _____
5. Do you ever have pain, lumps or swelling in your testicles? . . . .   No _____   Yes _____

Check here if you wish to discuss any special problems with the doctor . . . . [ ]

MEN & WOMEN

	Rarely/Never	Occasionally	Frequently
6. Is it sometimes hard to start your urine flow?	_____	_____	_____
7. Is urination ever painful?	_____	_____	_____
8. Do you have to urinate more than 5 times a day?	_____	_____	_____
9. Do you get up at night to urinate?	_____	_____	_____
10. Has your urine ever been bloody or dark colored?	_____	_____	_____
11. Do you ever lose urine when you strain, laugh, cough or sneeze?	_____	_____	_____
12. Do you ever lose urine during sleep?	_____	_____	_____

WOMEN ONLY

Do you:

	Rarely/Never	Occasionally	Frequently
13. a. Have any menstrual problems?	_____	_____	_____
b. Feel rather tense just before your period?	_____	_____	_____
c. Have heavy menstrual bleeding?	_____	_____	_____
d. Have painful menstrual periods?	_____	_____	_____
e. Have any bleeding between periods?	_____	_____	_____
f. Have any unusual vaginal discharge or itching?	_____	_____	_____
g. Ever have tender breasts?	_____	_____	_____
h. Have any discharge from your nipples?	_____	_____	_____
i. Have any hot flashes?	_____	_____	_____

14. How many times, if any, have you been pregnant? . . . . _____
15. How many children born alive? . . . . _____
16. Are you taking birth control pills? . . . .   No_____   Yes _____
17. Do you examine your breasts monthly for lumps? . . . .   No_____   Yes _____
17a. What was the date of your last menstrual period? . . . .   Date _____

Check here if you wish to discuss any special problem with the doctor . . . . [ ]

MEN & WOMEN

	Rarely/Never	Occasionally	Frequently
18. In the past year have you had any:			
a. Severe shoulder pain?	_____	_____	_____
b. Severe back pain?	_____	_____	_____
c. Muscle or joint stiffness or pain due to sports, exercise or injury?	_____	_____	_____
d. Pain or swelling in any joints not due to sports, exercise or injury?	_____	_____	_____

19. Do you have dry skin or brittle fingernails? . . . .   No_____   Yes _____
20. Do you bruise easily? . . . .   No_____   Yes _____
21. Do you have any moles that have changed in color or in size? . . . .   No_____   Yes _____
22. Do you have any other skin problems? . . . .   No_____   Yes _____

23. In the last 3 months have you had:
    a. A fever that lasted more than one day? . . . .   No_____   Yes _____
    b. Sores or cuts that were hard to heal? . . . .   No_____   Yes _____
    c. Any cold sores (fever blisters)? . . . .   No_____   Yes _____
    d. Any lumps in your neck, armpits or groin? . . . .   No_____   Yes _____
    e. Do you ever have chills or sweat at night? . . . .   No_____   Yes _____

24. Have you traveled out of the country in the last 2 years? . . . .   No_____   Yes, Traveled in: _____

25. Write in the dates for the shots you have had: . . . .
    { Measles _____   Smallpox _____
      Mumps _____   Tetanus _____
      Polio _____   Typhoid _____

26. Have you had a tuberculin (TB) skin test? . . . .   No_____   Yes _____   Date _____
    If so, was it negative or positive? . . . .   Neg _____   Pos _____
27. Have you had an HIV test for AIDS? . . . .   No_____   Yes _____   Date _____
    If so, was it negative or positive? . . . .   Neg _____   Pos _____

CONFIDENTIAL

28.	Do you wear eyeglasses?	No___	Yes___
29.	Do you wear contact lenses?	No___	Yes___
30.	Has your vision changed in the last year?	No___	Yes___

31.	How often do you have:	Rarely/ Never	Occasionally	Frequently
a.	Double vision?	___	___	___
b.	Blurry vision?	___	___	___
c.	Watery or itchy eyes?	___	___	___
32.	Do you ever see colored rings around lights?	___	___	___
33.	Do others tell you you have a hearing problem?	___	___	___
34.	Do you have trouble keeping your balance?	___	___	___
35.	Do you have any discharge from your ears?	___	___	___
36.	Do you ever feel dizzy or have motion sickness?	___	___	___
37.	Do you have any problems with your hearing?	No___	Yes___ Hearing Problems	
38.	Do you ever have ringing in your ears?	No___	Yes___ Ringing in ears	

39.	How often do you have:	Rarely/ Never	Occasionally	Frequently
a.	Head colds?	___	___	___
b.	Chest colds?	___	___	___
c.	Runny nose?	___	___	___
d.	Stuffed up nose?	___	___	___
e.	Sore/hoarse throat?	___	___	___
f.	Bad coughing spells?	___	___	___
g.	Sneezing spells?	___	___	___
h.	Trouble breathing?	___	___	___
i.	Nose bleeds?	___	___	___
j.	Cough blood?	___	___	___

40.	Have you ever worked or spent time:	No	Yes
a.	On a farm?	No___	Yes___
b.	In a mine?	No___	Yes___
c.	In a laundry or mill?	No___	Yes___
d.	In very dusty places?	No___	Yes___
e.	With or near toxic chemicals?	No___	Yes___
f.	With or near radioactive materials?	No___	Yes___
g.	With or near asbestos?	No___	Yes___

		Rarely/ Never	Occasionally	Frequently
41.	Do you get out of breath easily when you are active (like climbing stairs)?	___	___	___
42.	Do you ever feel light-headed or dizzy?	___	___	___
43.	Have you ever fainted or passed out?	___	___	___
44.	Do you sometimes feel your heart is racing or beating too fast?	___	___	___
45.	When you exercise do you ever get pains in your chest or shoulders?	___	___	___
46.	Do you have any leg cramps or pain in your thighs or legs when walking?	___	___	___
47.	Do you ever have to sit up at night to breathe easier?	___	___	___
48.	Do you use two pillows at night to help you breathe easier?	___	___	___
49.	Would you say you are a restless sleeper?	___	___	___
50.	Are you bothered by leg cramps at night?	___	___	___
51.	Do you sometimes have swollen ankles or feet?	___	___	___

52.	How often, if ever:	Rarely/ Never	Occasionally	Frequently
a.	Are you nauseated (sick to your stomach)?	___	___	___
b.	Do you have stomach pains?	___	___	___
c.	Do you burp a lot after eating?	___	___	___
d.	Do you have heartburn?	___	___	___
e.	Do you have trouble swallowing your food?	___	___	___
f.	Have you vomited blood?	___	___	___
g.	Are you constipated?	___	___	___
h.	Do you have diarrhea (watery stools)?	___	___	___
i.	Are your bowel movements painful?	___	___	___
j.	Are your bowel movements bloody?	___	___	___
k.	Are your bowel movements dark or black?	___	___	___
53.	Have you ever had a sigmoidoscopy?	No___	Yes___ Date___	

➤ **Figure 14–6** Continued

MEDICAL HISTORY AND REVIEW OF SYSTEMS

Ivan Shapiro
07/14/00

HISTORY OF PRESENT ILLNESS	This 55 year-old white male presents with a history of chest tightness when exercising for the past month which has increased in frequency during the last week. The tightness across the chest was first noticed when mowing the lawn. The episodes have been increasing in frequency until there are about one or two episodes per day, usually associated with exercise and all relieved by rest. Has taken antacids once or twice thinking that the pain might be due to indigestion without noticeable relief. Otherwise in good health.
MEDICATIONS	Not taking any prescription medications, but occasionally uses ibuprofen for relief of muscle pain; takes multivitamin daily.
ALLERGIES	Allergic to penicillin which results in urticaria. Has not taken penicillin for past thirty years.
PAST HISTORY	Had usual childhood diseases including mumps, measles, German measles, chicken pox. T&A when six years old. Fracture of left fibula at age 13, healed without problems. No other surgeries or medical problems.
FAMILY HISTORY	Father died at age 64 of MI. Mother living, has NIDDM, also being treated for hypertension. Siblings living and well. Has three children, all in good health. No other significant family history.
SOCIAL HISTORY	Smokes 20 cigarettes per day for the past 25 years. Social drinker. Drinks two cups of coffee daily.
OCCUPATIONAL HISTORY	Has been a carpenter for about 20 years. Worked on a farm for a few years after high school. No significant injuries due to occupation.
REVIEW OF SYSTEMS	Denies radiation of chest pain, has occasional indigestion, increasing in the past six months. Other than occasional muscle pain following physical exertion and recent chest pain, denies physical symptoms.

Joanne Hughes, MD

➤ **Figure 14–7** Sample medical report, including the patient history and review of systems.

Precautions

A number of precautions can be taken to avoid problems. These include:

Signs directing parents how to supervise children. The office should have signs advising parents to supervise children in any designated play area, as well as signs in exam rooms directing parents not to let infants or children play with medical equipment on the wall above the exam table used for examining eyes, ears, or blood pressure.

Whoever brought patient to the office must wait with patient. It should be policy that the person who brought the patient to the office wait in exam room with the patient. Parents always should wait with children. A person who brings a mentally retarded adult or fragile elderly person should wait with the patient.

Do not put patient in the exam room until the doctor is ready to examine. This should be done if there is any doubt that the individual can be safely left in the exam room and if there is no one accompanying the individual who can stay in the room with him or her.

Have the patient lie down on the examination table. This should be done if there is any chance that the individual will faint or lose balance sitting up. If the patient is weak, but judgment is good, the patient may be left alone.

Make frequent checks. Frequent checks should be made on patients who feel ill, dizzy, nauseous, or have a high fever. Avoid having patients who feel ill wait in the waiting room because they will be more comfortable in an exam room. Be sure to give a container to any patient with nausea in case the patient vomits. This may be a kidney-shaped basin or an oversize paper or plastic cup.

STUDENT STUDY PLAN

To reinforce your understanding of the material in this chapter . . .

Complete the **Review & Recall** questions below.

Discuss the situation in **If You Were the Medical Assistant** with your classmates and answer the questions.

Answer the **Critical Thinking Questions** below and discuss with your classmates.

Visit **Web sites** suggested below and search for additional Web sites using **Keywords for Internet Searches**.

Complete the exercises in chapter 14 of the **Student Mastery Manual**.

View **Videotape**: *Communications are Caring*, "Discovering the Chief Complaint."

Practice taking the history in Cases 1–4 on the **CD-ROM**.

 REVIEW & RECALL

1. Describe how to clean and prepare the examination room at the beginning of the day and between patients.

2. Describe how the medical assistant calls the patient from the waiting room.

3. How should the medical assistant assist a patient with weakness onto the examination table?

4. Describe how the medical assistant assists a patient to move safely from a wheelchair to the examination table.

5. Define each part of the medical history and review of systems.

6. Identify when the medical assistant obtains the complete medical history and when he or she obtains only the history of the present illness.

7. List seven areas that the medical assistant should ask about to obtain more information about the chief complaint.

8. Describe how the medical assistant decides that a patient cannot safely be left alone.

9. List measures to ensure the safety of patients in the examination room while waiting for the doctor to examine them.

 IF YOU WERE THE MEDICAL ASSISTANT

Read the following interview. Kathy Anderson is a medical assistant at the office of Blackburn Primary Care Associates.

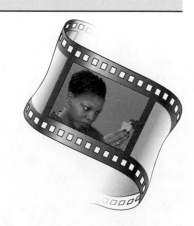

Kathy: What's the problem you're having today that brings you in?

Mr. Costello: I just got a little gas, you know what I mean? It's no big deal. My wife wants me to come in, so I figured I'd come in and get it done.

Kathy: How long have you had the gas?

Mr. Costello: Well, it's hard to say. A few months. This is really kind of a situation where—I mean, this is great, I don't mind doing what we have to do here, but it was hard to get the time off. I don't want to be here anyway, so . . .

Kathy: So, whereabouts are you experiencing the pain?

Mr. Costello: Oh, I thought you meant the wife being the pain.

Kathy: No, no.

Mr. Costello: It's right in here (pointing to the epigastric area). It's really nothing, it's a little gas. I get a little burning . . .

Kathy: Is it every day, that you get the gas?
Mr. Costello: It's off and on, it's, you know . . .
Kathy: Have you tried anything at all to relieve the symptoms?

1. Give specific examples of times when Mr. Costello started repeating himself or rambling and Kathy asked a question to refocus the conversation.

2. Are there any more questions that Kathy should ask as the conversation continues?

3. Do you think Mr. Costello was reluctant to see the doctor? Why or why not?

4. Can you tell from the excerpt given above if this is a new patient or an established patient? Are Kathy's questions appropriate for each type of patient?

CRITICAL THINKING QUESTIONS

1. How do you feel when you must talk with a person in a wheelchair, a person who wears one or two leg braces, or a person with a cast and crutches? Are your feelings different if you think the person has a permanent disability?

2. Interview someone who has limited mobility and must use crutches, a walker, or a wheelchair. Or interview a parent of a child with a mobility disability. Ask open-ended questions to get the person talking about the following issues:

How would you like people to respond to you?
How would you like them to feel when they meet you?
What are your pet peeves (what annoys you) about how people treat you?
When people try to help you, what kinds of awkward things happen?

3. Describe how you will try to treat a person with limited mobility when you are a medical assistant.

EXPLORE THE WEB

INTERNET WEBSITES

Interactive patient
medicus.marshall.edu/medicus.htm

KEYWORDS FOR INTERNET SEARCHES

patient medical history

Chapter 15

Taking Measurements and Vital Signs

Instructional Objectives

After completing this chapter, you will be able to do the following:

1. Define and spell the vocabulary words for this chapter.
2. State the purpose for measuring height, weight, and vital signs.
3. Explain the procedures for measuring a patient's height and weight.
4. Explain the physiology underlying normal and abnormal values for each of the vital signs: temperature, pulse, respiration, and blood pressure.
5. List the variables affecting each of the vital signs, and describe how each of these is influenced.
6. Discuss factors that affect the choice of site and method of measuring temperature.
7. Compare normal values of oral, rectal, axillary, and tympanic temperatures.
8. Discuss the care and cleaning of various types of thermometers.
9. Define a) the rate, rhythm, and volume of pulse, and b) the rate, rhythm, and depth of respirations.
10. Name and locate eight common arteries where pulses may be palpated.
11. Describe the procedure for measuring the radial pulse.
12. Describe the procedure for counting respirations accurately.
13. List factors that raise and lower blood pressure.
14. Identify the normal range of blood pressure for adults.
15. Describe the usual blood pressure changes throughout the life span.
16. Correlate the numbers used to describe blood pressure to body physiology.
17. Identify causes of errors in blood pressure readings.
18. Describe proper documentation of vital signs and anthropometric measurements.

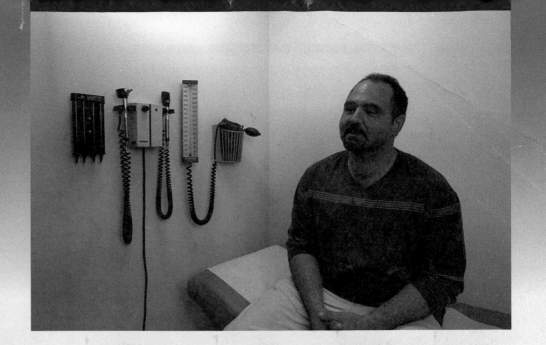

Performance Objectives

After completing this chapter, you will be able to do the following:

1. Measure a patient's height (Procedure 15–1).
2. Measure a patient's weight (Procedure 15–2).
3. Measure oral temperature using a glass mercury thermometer (Procedure 15–3).
4. Measure oral temperature using an electronic thermometer (Procedure 15–4).
5. Measure oral temperature using a disposable thermometer (Procedure 15–5).
6. Measure aural temperature using a tympanic thermometer (Procedure 15–6).
7. Measure rectal temperature (Procedure 15–7).
8. Measure axillary temperature (Procedure 15–8).
9. Measure the radial pulse (Procedure 15–9).
10. Measure the apical pulse (Procedure 15–10).
11. Measure respirations (Procedure 15–11).
12. Measure blood pressure (Procedure 15–12).
13. Document all measurements accurately.

VOCABULARY

aneroid (p. 296)
anthropometric (p. 270)
apex (p. 289)
apnea (p. 292)
arrhythmia (p. 290)
aural (p. 281)
auscultatory gap (p. 299)
axillary (p. 283)
baseline (p. 270)
bradycardia (p. 290)

bradypnea (p. 292)
Cheyne-Stokes respirations (p. 292)
continuous fever (p. 278)
diurnal (p. 277)
dyspnea (p. 294)
hyperpnea (p. 292)
hyperpyrexia (p. 278)
hyperthermia (p. 278)
hyperventilation (p. 293)

hypopnea (p. 292)
hypothermia (p. 278)
intermittent fever (p. 278)
oral (p. 279)
orthopnea (p. 294)
orthostatic hypotension (p. 295)
palpate (p. 298)
pyrexia (p. 277)
rectal (p. 279)

relapsing fever (p. 278)
remittent fever (p. 278)
sphygmomanometer (p. 296)
stethoscope (p. 290)
tachycardia (p. 290)
tachypnea (p. 292)
tympanic (p. 281)

ABBREVIATIONS

BP (p. 270)
C (p. 277)
F (p. 277)

ft (p. 273)
ht (p. 273)
in (p. 273)

lb (p. 275)
mm Hg (p. 296)

oz (p. 275)
P (p. 270)

R (p. 270)
SOB (p. 294)

T (p. 270)
wt (p. 275)

Taking the vital signs of patients who are about to be examined is one of the important activities a medical assistant will carry out in the course of a day's work. The care and professionalism with which this is done helps set the tone for the patient's entire encounter with the medical staff.

PURPOSE OF MEASUREMENTS

Vital signs (the Latin *vita* means life), sometimes called cardinal signs, are measurements of temperature (**T**), pulse (**P**), respiration (**R**), and blood pressure (**BP**). These measurements generally fall within certain average ranges (called normal values) when a person is in a state of well-being or good health. One or more of the measurements may fall outside the normal values when a person is ill, even if the person is not experiencing symptoms.

Accurate measurement of vital signs gives an early indication about a patient's health. Although normal values do not absolutely mean that a person is in a state of good health, abnormal values indicate that a person has a health problem.

Measurements recorded at a person's first visit provide a **baseline** to compare measurements from subsequent visits. A baseline is a known, or initial, value to which later measurements can be compared.

Height and weight are also important for accurate diagnosis. Weight fluctuations can be a sign of disease, and the height-to-weight ratio gives information about a person's nutritional status.

HEIGHT AND WEIGHT

Height and weight are so-called **anthropometric** measurements (measurements about the physical size of an individual). Measurement of height and weight can take place in the patient screening area, which should be private, or in an examination room. Figure 15–1 shows height and weight being measured in a patient screening area.

Purpose

Anthropometric measurements have four main purposes:

1. Provide information for diagnosis, treatment, and prevention
2. Determine a child's growth pattern
3. Serve as a guide for medication dosage
4. Adjust a machine for diagnostic tests.

Measurements Provide Information for Diagnosis, Treatment, and Prevention

Obesity is one of the most common health problems in America. Obese people are at higher risk for heart disease, stroke, and diabetes, and excess weight puts extra stress on knees, hips, and the lower back. On the other end of the spectrum, anorexia nervosa and bulimia are diseases in which individuals deprive themselves of nutrients in the quest for a "perfect" body.

In addition, a number of chronic illnesses require

close and constant monitoring of weight and nutritional condition. For example, patients with cancer often notice weight loss as a presenting symptom and may continue to lose weight due to loss of appetite and the disease process. Patients with heart disease or kidney problems may retain water, and sudden weight gain may indicate kidney or heart failure.

A person whose height declines regularly can be suffering from osteoporosis, a loss of bone density, which can put the person at increased risk for fractures.

Measurements Determine a Child's Growth Pattern

Chapter 27 covers the topics important in pediatrics. Here we will only point out that it is important to monitor every child's growth in both height and weight, charting those measurements against the average height and weight for children of that age.

Children who are not consuming enough nourishment to grow properly may also not be consuming enough for proper brain development. Children who are missing meals, especially breakfast, may not be alert enough to concentrate on school activities. On the flip side of this issue, obesity is increasingly becoming a problem in school-age children who are eating high-calorie, low-nutrition junk food, watching television or playing video games, and not getting enough exercise.

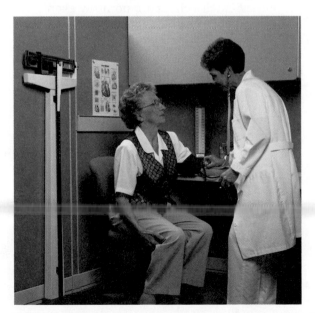

> ➤ **Figure 15–1** A private patient screening area may be used for vital signs before the patient is placed in an examination room.

General Guidelines for Analyzing a Measurement Scale or Graph

1. Establish the unit of measurement the graph or scale uses (inches, pounds, centimeters, etc.).
2. Count how many divisions there are in each unit on the figure being looked at. Inches are commonly divided into 2 (halves), 4 (quarters), 8 (eighths), 16 (sixteenths), and 32 (thirty-seconds). Pounds are commonly divided into 2 (half-pounds), 4 (quarter-pounds), 16 (ounces), or 32 (half-ounces). Metric measuring scales are divided into 10, so each division represents one-tenth of the unit being measured.
3. Find the value being measured, and record it using correct abbreviations.

Measurements Serve as a Guide for Medication Dosage

Many medication dosages are determined according to an individual's weight. This is especially true for children, but is also true for some classes of medication prescribed for adults.

Measurements Are Needed to Enable a Machine to Be Adjusted for Diagnostic Tests

Some diagnostic testing equipment, such as magnetic resonance imaging (MRI) machines, need to be adjusted to the patient's weight. With some machines (such as spirometers), height and weight must be entered for the machine to calculate accurate results.

Height

For adults, height is measured only on a patient's first visit to a new doctor's office unless the patient has a condition such as osteoporosis that can affect height. Medical offices need to be consistent about whether shoes are to be worn during the measurement for height. Older height/weight charts were standardized for a person wearing shoes, but today patients are generally weighed and measured without shoes. See Procedure 15–1, Measuring Height.

Height may be measured in one of two ways, either using the bar on the back of a balance-beam scale or using a chart or measuring stick mounted to a wall.

PROCEDURE 15-1

Measuring Height

Performance Objective: Using the measuring bar on a scale, the student can measure the height of an adult safely and accurately, and can convert the measurement of height from inches to feet and inches and document accurately.

☑ Wash hands
☐ Gloves
☐ Eye and Face Protection
☐ Lab Coat or Apron
☐ Plastic Biohazard Bag
☐ Rigid Biohazard Container

Supplies and Equipment: Balance scale with a height bar, paper towel.

Procedure Steps

1. Wash hands.
2. Assemble supplies and equipment.
3. Identify patient.
4. Explain procedure to patient.
5. Ask the patient to remove his or her shoes.
   Rationale: A more accurate height will be obtained without shoes.
6. Place a paper towel on the scale for the patient to step on.
   Rationale: A paper towel will prevent the patient's feet from touching the scale. If the patient's feet touch the scale, clean it after the procedure.
7. Raise the height bar to a level well above the patient's anticipated height and lift the measuring bar.
   Rationale: The measuring bar must be above the patient's head to avoid injury to the patient's head.
8. Ask the patient to step on the scale with his or her back to the measuring bar. Assist the patient if necessary.

Rationale: It is easier to measure height with the patient facing away from the bar. Because the weight platform is movable, the patient may need assistance for balance.

9. Lower the measuring bar to the top of the patient's head. Be sure to compress the hair. The patient should be standing as straight as possible.
   Rationale: To obtain an accurate measurement.
10. Leaving the measuring bar in place, ask the patient to step down from the scale. Read the height where the top part of the measuring bar rises away from the lower part.
    Rationale: The height scale is calibrated to be read where the top bar separates from the bottom bar.
11. Lower the measuring bar.
    Rationale: When the measuring bar is raised, it could easily injure a patient who steps on the scale. It is always kept lowered unless in use.
12. Discard paper towel used under patient's feet.
13. Wash hands.
14. Convert the measurement into feet and inches. Adult heights are normally expressed to the nearest 1/2″.
    Rationale: Heights are normally expressed in feet and inches. (Example: Ht: 5′ 4 1/2″)
15. Record the measurement in the patient's medical record.
    Rationale: The medical record provides the ongoing record of procedures performed and care given to the patient.

Charting Example	
Date	
6/7/xx	9:48 AM Ht 5′ 4 1/2″ ————
	———— S. Dellarosa, RMA

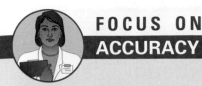

FOCUS ON
ACCURACY

READING HEIGHT MEASUREMENT

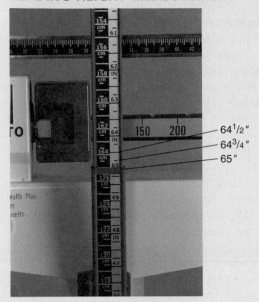

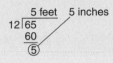

Height **(ht)** is usually expressed using feet, inches, and fractions of an inch (1/2, 1/4, 1/8, 1/16, 1/32). To change inches to feet and inches, divide the number of inches by 12 to obtain a whole number and remainder. (Do not calculate to a decimal.) The whole number is the number of feet, and the remainder is the number of inches. The abbreviation for feet is **ft** or ′ and the abbreviation for inches is **in** or ″. Measurements for height on a balance-beam scale are divided into fourths and read exactly where the top part pulls up from the bottom part. The numbers on the top half of the height indicator increase downwards until they reach the separation point.

The height in the example above is 65 inches. This is expressed as 5 ft 5 in or 5′ 5″.

$$\begin{array}{r} \underline{\quad 5\ \text{feet} \quad 5\ \text{inches}} \\ 12\overline{)65} \\ \underline{60} \\ \textcircled{5} \end{array}$$

Balance-Beam Scale Bar

When measuring height using the bar on the back of a balance-beam scale, be sure to pull the bar up over the patient's head, then ease it down onto the head. Measuring should be done with the patient's back to the balance beam. This is both more accurate and safer—the patient cannot be hit in the face or eye with the measuring bar.

Read the height at the point where the top part (the moving part) of the measuring bar comes away from the stationary lower part, as shown in Figure 15–2. Immediately after taking the measurement, be sure to lower the bar to its "closed" position so no one gets hurt.

Wall Chart

A height measurement chart may be mounted on a wall. A chart is most accurate if it has a measuring bar. If it does not, a ruler or even a book may be used to establish height.

Weight

Weight is usually recorded at every office visit, be it a routine physical, sick visit, or follow-up visit. See Procedure 15–2, Measuring Weight Using a Balance-Beam Scale.

Most people are very sensitive about their weight and about weight measurement. Because of this, the scale should be in a private place, either in each exam/treatment room or in a central patient intake area that is private.

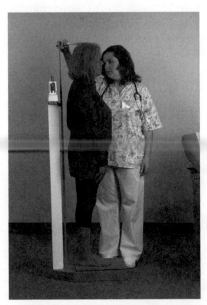

> **Figure 15–2** Measuring height.

PROCEDURE 15–2

Measuring Weight Using a Balance-Beam Scale

Performance Objective: The student can measure the weight of an adult using a balance scale and record the measurement accurately in pounds.

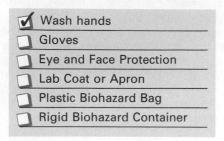

- ☑ Wash hands
- ☐ Gloves
- ☐ Eye and Face Protection
- ☐ Lab Coat or Apron
- ☐ Plastic Biohazard Bag
- ☐ Rigid Biohazard Container

Supplies and Equipment: Balance scale, paper towel.

Procedure Steps

1. Ask the patient to remove his or her shoes, coat or jacket, and put down anything he or she might be carrying (such as a purse).
   Rationale: A more accurate weight will be obtained without shoes and heavy clothing. Patients usually prefer to be weighed without shoes.

2. Place a paper towel on the scale for the patient to step on.
   Rationale: A paper towel will prevent the patient's feet from touching the scale platform. If the patient's feet touch the scale, clean the scale after the procedure.

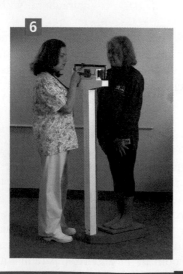

3. To balance the scale, move all the weights to zero and adjust the balance screw on the left of the scale so that the weight indicator is level (i.e., is balanced) and does not touch the top or bottom guard at the right of the scale.
   Rationale: The scale must be balanced before weighing the patient to give an accurate weight. The adjustment can easily be altered so that the scale becomes unbalanced.

4. Ask the patient to step on the scale facing the scale. Assist the patient if necessary.
   Rationale: The patient will be steadier facing the scale and is probably interested to see the weight. The weight platform is movable and the patient may need assistance.

5. Move the 50 pound counterweight to the notch nearest to the patient's weight but still less than the weight.
   Rationale: The weight will be read as a multiple of 50 plus a multiple of 1.

6. Slide the 1-pound counterweight along the top bar until the weight indicator balances (floats freely pointing at the balance line). Read the weight by adding the number indicated on the top bar to the number indicated on the bottom bar.
   Rationale: The weight indicator must balance for an accurate weight.

7. Ask the patient to step off the scale. Assist the patient if necessary.
   Rationale: Because the platform moves slightly, the patient may need assistance.

8. Discard the paper towel, return the counterweights to zero, and wash hands.
   Rationale: To reduce pressure on the scale, the counterweights should be kept at zero unless the scale is in use to maintain calibration.

9. Record the weight in the patient's chart in pounds.
   Rationale: Adult weights are expressed in pounds. (Example: 254 lb or 254 #)

Charting Example	
Date	
6/7/XX	9:52 AM Wt 254 lb
	S. Dellarosa, RMA

FOCUS ON
ACCURACY

READING WEIGHT MEASUREMENT

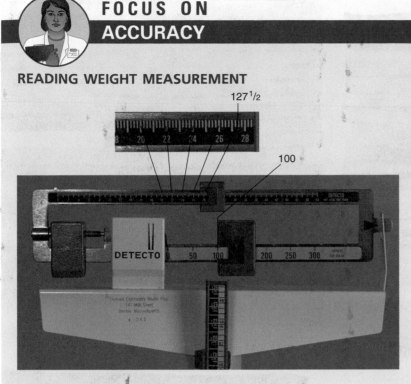

Weight **(wt)** in pounds is expressed using pounds and fractions (1/2, 1/4) or pounds and ounces. The abbreviation for pound(s) is **lb** or **#**. The abbreviation for ounce(s) is **oz** or ℥. (The symbol is usually only used for medication measurements.) When reading weight, read the number from the bottom counterweight (a multiple of 50) and add the number from the top counterweight indicator to the nearest half pound.

Weight should be measured without shoes for the greatest accuracy. Weight can be measured in either pounds or kilograms, but is usually measured in pounds because this gives a more meaningful measurement for patients. However, weight may be recorded in kilograms because some medication dosage formulas are based on kilograms. Both pounds and kilograms are found on some scales. Moving from one to the other is usually done by flipping a bar on the scale that reveals or hides the metric scale.

A balance-beam scale (shown on Figure 15–3) is the most common weight measurement device used in doctors' offices, but some offices have digital scales.

Height and Weight

For new patients, height and weight should be recorded on the history and physical examination form. For established patients, weight is recorded as part of a progress note.

TEMPERATURE

The usual temperature of adults is between 98.6°F and 99.4°F. The core temperature (the temperature within body cavities) is maintained within a narrow range, but temperature on the skin can fluctuate widely. Although higher or lower temperature can occur without the presence of disease, this is not usually the case. Temperature in infants is not as well regulated and fluctuates, depending on the infant's state of health, clothing, and the environment.

Regulation of Body Temperature

Body temperature represents a balance between heat produced and heat lost. Regulation is controlled by the hypothalamus, a section of the brain just above the brain stem. Information from temperature sensors throughout the body allows the hypothalamus to trigger mechanisms to raise temperature, conserve heat, or lower temperature. Normally, the temperature is maintained at a fairly constant value, called the temperature set point.

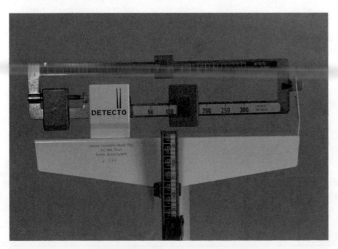

➤ **Figure 15–3** Balance-beam scale.

Heat Production and Conservation

The body produces and conserves heat through three mechanisms: metabolism, muscle activity, and constriction of superficial blood vessels.

Metabolism. Metabolism involves the chemical processes of the body that produce heat, especially digestion, respiration, ovulation, pregnancy, and changes in emotional state. A person at rest produces about 70 calories of heat per hour from normal metabolic processes; this is called the basal metabolic rate. When the level of thyroxine, a thyroid hormone, increases, the metabolism of the body cells speeds up and more heat is produced.

Muscle Activity. Both voluntary and involuntary muscle movement produces heat. Not only does exercise warm the body (voluntary muscle movement), but so does the movement of the jaw muscles when a person who is cold has chattering teeth (involuntary muscle movement).

Constriction of Superficial Blood Vessels. Superficial blood vessels are the ones on the surface of the body. When these blood vessels constrict (get smaller), they keep the heat in the interior of the body.

Heat Loss

Heat is lost from the body in three ways: through perspiration, elimination, and dilation of the superficial blood vessels.

Perspiration. When the internal body temperature is high, sweat glands begin to secrete fluid to the skin. The evaporation of water to vapor cools the skin. Evaporation occurs more rapidly when air is circulating freely; evaporation occurs less rapidly when air is highly saturated with moisture (for example, on a humid day). Because sweating is regulated by the autonomic nervous system, it is associated with certain conditions that stimulate a generalized response, such as a heart attack, fainting, and shock.

Elimination. Some heat is lost through normal body functions of elimination from the intestinal, urinary, and respiratory systems.

Dilation of Superficial Blood Vessels. Dilation (enlargement) of the superficial blood vessels allows more heat to be lost to the air through normal heat transfer. The skin becomes flushed as these blood vessels open wider. Heat radiates from the warmer body to the cooler air in the form of infrared rays. It is also conducted to the surrounding air from the skin and through the clothing.

Variations in Body Temperature

Although the normal core temperature of an adult is 98.6°F to 99.4°F, it is difficult to measure the core temperature directly. The routes used to measure temperature in the office may result in measured values that vary from the core temperature, even if the proce-

Table 15–1	**Comparison of Methods for Taking Temperature**		
Method	**Time Needed**	**Normal Temperature**	**Special Considerations**
Axillary	10 minutes	≈97.6°F; may be as much as 2.2°F below core temperature	Assist patient to hold arm tightly against side
Oral—glass mercury	3–5 minutes	≈98.6°F; may be as much as 0.8°F below core temperature	Do not use for children under age 5; not suitable for mouth breathers, patients receiving oxygen, inaccurate after recent eating, smoking, chewing gum, drinking
Oral—electronic	10–60 seconds	≈98.6°F; may be as much as 0.8°F below core temperature	May be used safely for children who can hold probe under tongue; other considerations same as oral glass mercury thermometer above
Oral—disposable	60 seconds–3 minutes	≈98.6°F; may be as much as 0.8°F below core temperature	May be used for children who can hold under tongue; other considerations same as oral glass mercury thermometer above
Tympanic—electronic	2 seconds	≈98.6°F	May be inaccurate if tip does not point to eardrum or if patient has excessive wax in the ear
Rectal—glass mercury	3–5 minutes	≈99.6°F; may be as much as 1°F above core temperature	Patient must lie still to avoid breaking bulb or stem of the thermometer or perforation of rectum
Rectal—electronic	10–60 seconds	≈99.6°F; may be as much as 1°F above core temperature	Patient must lie still to avoid perforation of the rectum

Data from Web article by Knies, Robert at *Emergency Nursing World: http://enw.org/Research-Thermometery.htm.* visited 2/13/00

Table 15–2	**Conversion Table: Fahrenheit and Centigrade**

Fahrenheit to Centigrade. Subtract 32 from the number of Fahrenheit degrees and multiply the difference by 5/9.

Centigrade to Fahrenheit. Multiply the number of Centigrade degrees by 9/5 and add 32.

Fahrenheit	Centigrade	Fahrenheit
32	32 − 32 = 0 (9/5) = 0	0 (9/5) = 0 + 32 = 32
50	50 − 32 = 18 (5/9) = 10	10 (9/5) = 18 + 32 = 50
68	68 − 32 = 36 (5/9) = 20	20 (9/5) = 36 + 32 = 68
86	86 − 32 = 56 (5/9) = 30	30 (9/5) = 56 + 32 = 86
104	104 − 32 = 82 (5/9) = 40	40 (9/5) = 82 + 32 = 104
122	122 − 32 = 90 (5/9) = 50	50 (9/5) = 90 + 32 = 122

dure is done accurately. (See Table 15–1, Comparison of Methods for Taking Temperature.)

In hospitals, temperature is often measured and recorded on the metric system, using the centigrade, or Celsius scale (°C). The normal core temperature in Celsius is between 36°C and 37.4°C. In the medical office, temperature is usually measured and recorded using the Fahrenheit scale (°F). (See Table 15–2, for conversions between Fahrenheit and Centigrade.)

Any of the following factors may cause body temperature to vary: age, gender, exercise, diurnal (daily) variation, emotions, high or low environmental temperature, or illness.

Age

The elderly often maintain a lower core temperature because of slower metabolism. Infants and younger children have greater variation in temperature set point, and more temperature fluctuation.

Gender

Women usually have a slightly higher core temperature than men, especially during ovulation.

Exercise

Muscle activity increases body heat production. The metabolic processes needed for energy produce heat. Muscle activity may be voluntary or an involuntary response to cold, such as chattering teeth or chills.

Diurnal Variation

Diurnal means daily. Everyone has normal diurnal variation in body temperature. Temperature is lowest in the morning (between 3:00 AM and 5:00 AM) and highest in the late afternoon and evening.

Emotions

Body temperature increases during times of stress or anger. When a person is depressed, the body temperature tends to be lower.

High or Low Environmental Temperature

People are mammals, and therefore warm blooded, meaning that our body temperature does not adjust to mirror the outside temperature. However, long exposure to high or low environmental temperature can raise or lower core body temperature enough to be dangerous.

Illness

Temperature can increase or decrease, depending on the disease or condition. When the disease is caused by a microorganism, the resulting rise in temperature is called a fever. When the disease depresses metabolism, as, for example, happens in hypothyroidism—decrease in thyroid gland function—the temperature set point may be low.

Abnormal Temperature

Although body temperature varies among people, at different times of the day for everyone, during ovulation for women, and possibly because of environmental temperatures, excessively high or low temperatures can affect health. Abnormally high temperature is called fever, abnormally low temperature hypothermia.

Fever

In response to infection or injury, the hypothalamus may raise the body's core temperature set point and maintain a core temperature that is higher than normal. This is **pyrexia,** commonly known as fever. Shivering or chills produces heat, which is retained by the constricting surface blood vessels.

The higher temperature is believed to improve the body's ability to fight off infection, but temperatures above 101° to 102°F (39.3° to 39.9°C) are usually treated, especially in infants, to avoid the possible adverse effects a high body temperature can cause.

Acetaminophen or ibuprofen is used for fevers over 101°F. These agents can be given in liquid form to infants and young children; as chewable tablets for older children; as pills for adolescents and adults; and as rectal suppositories for a patient who is vomiting or who is not allowed anything by mouth.

Fevers are graded as follows:

Low fever	99°F–101°F	(37.2°C–38.3°C)
Moderate fever	101.1°F–103°F	(38.4°C–39.4°C)
High fever	103.1°F–105°F	(39.5°C–40.6°C)
Hyperpyrexia	Over 105°F	(over 40.6°C)

Hyperpyrexia (fever over 105° F) is a serious condition, which may cause convulsions, brain damage, and/or death. Hyperpyrexia or **hyperthermia** (excessive body heat) may occur in infants and young children with a fever due to infection or in people of any age who exercise vigorously in hot, humid weather, especially if they do not replace fluids lost by sweating. The skin may be hot, flushed, and dry; the pulse rapid; and the person may experience headache, dizziness, confusion, and visual disturbance.

As soon as hyperpyrexia is recognized, begin to sponge the patient's skin with tepid water and fan the skin to facilitate evaporation. Do not immerse the patient in ice water, because if the patient begins to shiver, the body temperature may actually increase. If the temperature does not begin to fall, call for emergency assistance.

Hypothermia

Hypothermia is a lowering of the core body temperature below 95°F (35°C). Hypothermia is usually the result of long exposure to cold temperatures and occurs more quickly when a person is wearing wet clothing. Hypothermia can also happen more rapidly in a person with poor circulation, a high blood-alcohol level, and/or the presence of drugs that dilate peripheral blood vessels (these can either be prescription, over-the-counter, or street drugs).

Early signs and symptoms of hypothermia include shivering, blue skin, mental confusion, numbness, and slurred speech.

In cases of mild hypothermia, dry clothing, several dry blankets, and a warm environment facilitate rewarming. In cases of severe hypothermia, the person should be transported to an emergency center for monitoring and treatment.

Assessing the Pattern of a Fever

The pattern of a fever may help a doctor to determine its cause. The medical assistant should ask a patient who reports a fever a number of questions to try to get at the fever's pattern.

Questions to Ask

Six key questions should be asked when assessing a fever's pattern:

1. How high has the fever been?
2. Did it start suddenly or gradually?
3. Has it stayed high or does it go up and down?
4. Since the fever began, has your temperature been normal at times, or has it remained above normal?
5. Have you taken any medication such as acetaminophen or ibuprofen for the fever?
6. If yes, what happens after the medication wears off?

Fevers are characterized as either continuous, intermittent, remittent, or relapsing.

Continuous Fever

A **continuous fever** stays at about the same elevation all the time or returns to the same level about 4 hours after being treated with medication.

Intermittent Fever

An **intermittent fever** rises and returns to normal in a regular pattern. The fever rises are sometimes called spikes.

Remittent Fever

A **remittent fever** rises and falls, but always remains above normal.

Relapsing Fever

A **relapsing fever** appears to go away, and then returns. This may happen once or several times.

Types of Thermometers

Thermometers (instruments that measure temperature) can be either glass-mercury thermometers or electronic thermometers.

Glass-mercury thermometers may be used to take an oral temperature (in the mouth), a rectal temperature (in the rectum), or an axillary temperature (in the armpit).

An electronic thermometer measures temperature electronically and provides a digital readout. Oral, rectal, and tympanic thermometers may measure temperature electronically.

Glass-Mercury Thermometers

Glass-mercury thermometers have been used for many years. The thermometer consists of a long glass tube, marked with a temperature scale, and a bulb filled with mercury. When the mercury in the bulb is heated, it expands in the tube.

Once the mercury has risen, it stays at the highest level until it is shaken back down into the bulb. Thermometers with a long, slender bulb or a pear-shaped

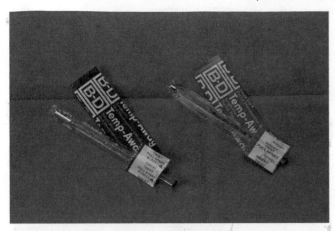

> **Figure 15–4** Glass-mercury thermometers with disposable sheaths. A blue sheath is used for the oral thermometer, which has a long and thin bulb; a red sheath is used for the rectal thermometer, which has a short and stubby bulb.

tip marked blue are intended for oral use. Thermometers with a rounded bulb marked red are intended for rectal use. If there is no color marking and the bulb is round (sometimes called a "stubby" thermometer), the thermometer can be used to take the temperature by any route, but after it has been used as a rectal thermometer, it should only be used for that purpose in the future.

In medical offices, a thin disposable plastic sheath is used to cover the thermometer to help prevent the spread of infection, as shown in Figure 15–4. Despite this, the thermometer must be sanitized after each use.

To read the thermometer, hold it at eye level with the right hand. Avoid touching the mercury bulb. Rotate the thermometer slowly until you can see the mercury line widen. Read up to the nearest two-tenths degree (Fahrenheit) or one-tenth degree (Celsius), as shown in Figure 15–5.

If a mercury thermometer breaks, treat it as a hazardous spill. **NEVER TOUCH MERCURY.** Call a hazardous waste disposal company to remove a mercury spill.

Electronic Thermometers

An electronic thermometer is a metal and plastic device with a probe on the end; a disposable cover fits over the probe. After the thermometer has taken the temperature, a digital readout shows. When not in use, the thermometer sits in a charger attached to a wall plug (home versions often have a battery inside). Figure 15–6 shows electronic thermometers.

Oral and Rectal. When using an electronic thermometer that registers temperature either orally or rectally, a new disposable probe cover should be used for each patient. The **oral** probe (to be used in the mouth) may be blue and the **rectal** probe (to measure temperature via the rectum) red. Plug the correct probe into the thermometer before using, for two reasons:

1. This will prevent transfer of organisms from the rectum to another person's mouth.
2. Each probe is calibrated to read the temperature as a glass thermometer.

Tympanic. When using an electronic thermometer that registers temperature via the tympanic membrane (eardrum), a new disposable plastic ear tip must be used for each patient. The manufacturer's instructions need to be followed closely. Once the thermometer is in place in the ear canal, press the button. An infrared signal bounces off the eardrum, and a digital readout shows. Remember to straighten the ear canal so the signal reaches the tympanic membrane and does not bounce off the wall of the ear canal. Taking temperature via the tympanic membrane is faster than taking an oral electronic temperature and is safe for all ages.

When a very high reading shows on a temperature taken electronically, a doctor may want to confirm it with a rectal temperature, especially when the patient is an infant.

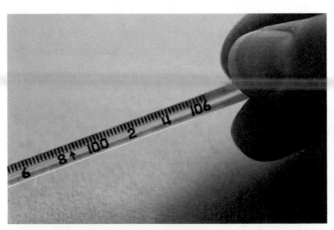

> **Figure 15–5** To read the temperature on a glass-mercury thermometer, rotate the thermometer until the line of mercury can be visualized.

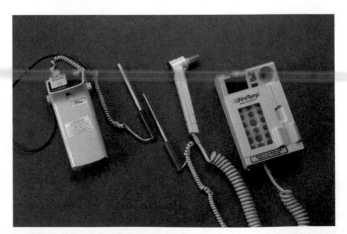

> **Figure 15–6** Electronic thermometer with blue oral probe and red rectal probe; tympanic thermometer.

Disposable Thermometers

There are two types of disposable thermometers. One, used orally, is a paper strip with dots that change color as the temperature rises. The other is a strip that is placed on the forehead, and temperature readings illuminate as the temperature rises. The oral thermometers are considered relatively accurate but not as accurate as glass or electronic thermometers. The forehead strips can only give a rough estimate; they are often used in day-care centers because they are not invasive and can be used by day-care teachers who are not trained medical personnel.

Disposable thermometers are most hygienic, because they are used once then thrown away.

Choosing the Site and Measuring Temperature

The choice of a site for temperature taking is made based on a patient's age, medical condition, or simply practice style. Whichever technique is used, care must be taken to get the most accurate reading.

Oral

Adult patients, teenagers, and older children are generally comfortable with this technique. However, taking a temperature orally may give an inaccurate reading if the patient is mouth breathing (because of nasal congestion or some other reason) or if the patient has been chewing gum, eating, or smoking recently.

Do not use a glass thermometer for children under age 5, because they tend to bite down hard on it and can break it. Pacifier thermometers with digital readouts are often used by parents, but should not be used in an office setting, because they are difficult if not impossible to properly clean and can transmit infection.

A person receiving oxygen should not have an oral temperature taken.

PROCEDURE 15–3

Measuring Oral Temperature Using a Glass-Mercury Thermometer

Performance Objective: The student will take and record an individual's oral temperature using a glass-mercury thermometer.

☑	Wash hands
☑	Gloves
☐	Eye and Face Protection
☐	Lab Coat or Apron
☑	Plastic Biohazard Bag
☐	Rigid Biohazard Container

Supplies and Equipment: Glass-mercury thermometer, disposable plastic sheath, gloves, biohazard waste container.

Procedure Steps

1. Explain procedure to patient. Ask if the patient has had anything to eat or drink or has smoked in the past 15 minutes.
   Rationale: The patient will be more comfortable and cooperative knowing what to expect. Hot or cold food, beverages, or smoking may cause an oral temperature to be inaccurate.

2. Select a clean, dry glass thermometer. Read the mercury level. If it is above 96°F, hold the thermometer firmly in one hand and shake using a snap of the wrist until the mercury level reaches 96°F or below.
   Rationale: The mercury level must be lower than the patient's temperature before beginning the procedure.

3. Insert the thermometer into the paper holder of a disposable plastic sheath. Grasping the paper cuff on the top of the sheath, twist and remove the paper from the part of the sheath that extends along the thermometer.
   Rationale: Even though the thermometer is

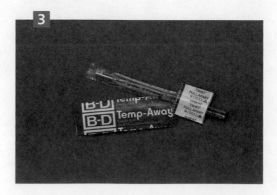

clean, the plastic sheath is an additional safe-guard to prevent the spread of microorganisms.

4. Put on gloves.
   Rationale: Begin all procedures by putting on appropriate PPE to protect from contact with microorganisms. In this procedure there is a potential to come in contact with the patient's saliva.

5. Ask the patient to open his or her mouth and hold the thermometer under the tongue.
   Tell the patient not to talk or bite the thermometer.
   Rationale: The thermometer must rest firmly under the tongue beside the frenulum with an airtight seal for 3 to 5 minutes, long enough to register the same temperature as the area under the tongue.

6. After 3 to 5 minutes, remove the thermometer. Holding the paper part of the plastic sheath, slide the sheath off the thermometer and discard in a biohazard container.

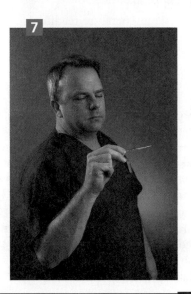

Rationale: The plastic sheath has been exposed to saliva and could transmit microorganisms.

7. Holding the thermometer at eye level, rotate until you can see the mercury column. Read the temperature. If the reading is between marks, read up to the nearest two-tenths of a degree if a Fahrenheit thermometer and to the nearest tenth of a degree if a Celsius thermometer.
   Rationale: You can only read accurately to the scale marked. The convention is to read up to the nearest mark.

8. Wash the thermometer using soap and cool water. Rinse it and dry with a paper towel. Place in soaking solution or in a container clearly marked "Used Thermometers" for later disinfection.
   Rationale: Even though a plastic sheath protected the thermometer, it must still be disinfected before being used again.

9. Remove soiled gloves and discard in a biohazard waste container. Wash hands.
   Rationale: Gloves may have come in contact with body fluids. Always wash hands after using gloves.

10. Record temperature, including location, in the patient's chart.
    Rationale: The doctor uses the site the temperature was taken to help assess the temperature.

Charting Example	
Date	
6/7/XX	9:54 AM T: 98.2°F orally ———————
	——————— S. Dellarosa, RMA

When taking an oral temperature, using either a glass or electronic thermometer, place the tip of the thermometer under the tongue and keep in place for 3 to 5 minutes. Procedures 15–3, 15–4, and 15–5 discuss measuring temperature using glass, electronic, and disposable thermometers, respectively.

Tympanic

Taking the temperature in the ear (**aural** temperature or **tympanic** temperature), using an electronic tympanic thermometer is rapidly becoming the most popular method of temperature measurement. It is fast and safe. However, accuracy has been questioned, especially in infants under age 3 months.

When using an electronic tympanic thermometer, make sure to follow the manufacturer's directions so the tip of the thermometer points toward the eardrum. If this is done, and a new disposable ear probe cover is used for each patient, the results are considered accurate, although they fluctuate when repeated measurements are made on the same person. Procedure 15–6 discusses measuring body temperature using a tympanic thermometer.

PROCEDURE 15–4

Measuring Oral Temperature Using an Electronic Thermometer

Performance Objective: The student will take and record an individual's oral temperature using an electronic thermometer.

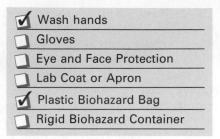

☑ Wash hands
☐ Gloves
☐ Eye and Face Protection
☐ Lab Coat or Apron
☑ Plastic Biohazard Bag
☐ Rigid Biohazard Container

Supplies and Equipment: Electronic thermometer, disposable plastic probe cover, biohazard waste container.

Procedure Steps

1. Explain procedure to patient. Ask if the patient has had anything to eat or drink or has smoked in the past 15 minutes.
   Rationale: The patient will be more comfortable and cooperative knowing what to expect. Hot or cold food, beverages, or smoking may cause an oral temperature to be inaccurate.
2. Remove thermometer probe from holder. Insert the probe firmly into a disposable plastic probe cover. A plastic sheath may be used for a small electronic thermometer.
   Rationale: A new probe cover must be used for each patient to prevent the transmission of microorganisms.
3. Turn on the thermometer. Wait for the electronic display to signal that you may begin

taking the temperature (often a beeping sound). Consult the manufacturer's directions to determine how this signal is given.
   Rationale: The thermometer must be ready to take the reading before the medical assistant begins to take the temperature.
4. Ask the patient to open his or her mouth and hold the thermometer under the tongue. Tell the patient not to talk or bite the thermometer.
   Rationale: The thermometer must rest firmly under the tongue beside the frenulum with an airtight seal long enough to register the same temperature as the area under the tongue. The amount of time varies according to the model of thermometer.
5. When the temperature reading is displayed (often accompanied by a beeping sound), remove the probe from the mouth. Discard the probe cover in a biohazard waste container.
   Rationale: The reading occurs almost immediately. A new probe cover must be used for each patient. Because it has been exposed to saliva, it is considered hazardous waste.
6. Return the thermometer unit to the base or to storage.
   Rationale: The thermometer may be rechargeable; in that case it needs to be fully charged to operate accurately. Smaller electronic thermometers contain batteries and should be stored in a clean location.
7. Wash hands.
8. Record temperature, including location, in the patient's chart.
   Rationale: The doctor uses the site the temperature was taken to help assess the temperature.

Rectal

Rectal temperature is considered to be the most accurate temperature measure because the rectum is a closed body cavity. Although this site is commonly used in the hospital, especially for patients with a decreased level of consciousness, it is rarely used in the medical office, except for infants.

When taking a rectal temperature, extreme care must be taken. The glass tip or electronic probe cover must be lubricated, and the thermometer inserted gently in the rectum. Avoid forcing the thermometer or inserting too deeply; the tip can cause injury to or even perforate (make a hole in) the rectal wall.

The patient must lie still to avoid injury. Temperature reading may be inaccurate if there is stool in the rectum. Rectal thermometers are not used in individuals who have recently undergone rectal surgery. Procedure 15–7 discusses measuring temperature using a rectal thermometer.

PROCEDURE 15–5

Measuring Oral Temperature Using a Disposable Thermometer

Performance Objective: The student will take and record an individual's oral temperature using a disposable thermometer.

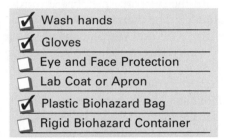

- ☑ Wash hands
- ☑ Gloves
- ☐ Eye and Face Protection
- ☐ Lab Coat or Apron
- ☑ Plastic Biohazard Bag
- ☐ Rigid Biohazard Container

Supplies and Equipment: Disposable thermometer, gloves, biohazard waste container.

Procedure Steps

1. Explain procedure to patient. Ask if the patient has had anything to eat or drink or has smoked in the past 15 minutes.
   Rationale: The patient will be more comfortable and cooperative knowing what to expect. Hot or cold food, beverages, or smoking may cause an oral temperature to be inaccurate.
2. Select a disposable thermometer, peel back wrapper to expose thermometer, put on gloves, and pick up disposable thermometer.
   Rationale: Begin all procedures by putting on appropriate PPEs to protect from contact with microorganisms. In this procedure there is a potential to come in contact with the patient's saliva.
3. Ask the patient to open his or her mouth and hold the thermometer under the tongue. Tell the patient not to talk.
   Rationale: The thermometer must rest firmly under the tongue beside the frenulum with an airtight seal to register the same temperature as the area under the tongue.
4. Wait as long as directed by the manufacturer, 60 seconds for some brands.
   Rationale: The thermometer must remain in place long enough to give an accurate reading.
5. Remove the thermometer, wait as long as directed by the manufacturer, and read by looking at the colored dots.
   Rationale: Some dots may return to their original color within a few seconds. These should not be included in the temperature reading.
6. Discard thermometer in the biohazard waste container.
   Rationale: The thermometer has come in contact with saliva.
7. Remove soiled gloves and discard in a biohazard waste container. Wash hands.
   Rationale: Gloves may have come in contact with body fluids.
8. Record temperature, including location, in the patient's chart.
   Rationale: The doctor uses the site the temperature was taken to help assess the temperature.

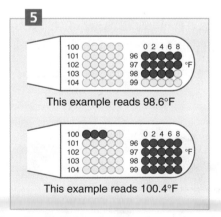

This example reads 98.6°F

This example reads 100.4°F

*Figure from Bonewit-West K: *Clinical Procedures for Medical Assistants,* 5th ed. Philadelphia: W.B. Saunders, 2000.

Axillary

Although the **axillary** temperature (in the armpit) is considered to be the least accurate method of temperature measurement, it has the advantages of being safe, posing little risk of transferring microorganisms. The thermometer must be held under the arm for a full 10 minutes to get a relatively accurate measurement. Procedure 15–8 discusses taking an axillary temperature.

PROCEDURE 15–6

Measuring Aural Temperature Using a Tympanic Thermometer

Performance Objective: The student will take and record an individual's aural temperature using a tympanic thermometer.

✔	Wash hands
☐	Gloves
☐	Eye and Face Protection
☐	Lab Coat or Apron
✔	Plastic Biohazard Bag
☐	Rigid Biohazard Container

Supplies and Equipment: Tympanic thermometer, disposable plastic probe cover, biohazard waste container.

Procedure Steps

1. Explain procedure to patient.
   Rationale: The patient will be more comfortable and cooperative knowing what to expect.
2. Remove thermometer unit from holder. Insert the probe firmly into a disposable plastic probe cover.
   Rationale: A new probe cover must be used for each patient to prevent the transmission of microorganisms.

3 Turn on the thermometer. Pull back on the patient's ear to straighten the ear canal, and insert the tip of the probe into the ear canal to form a tight seal. The probe must point toward the tympanic membrane (eardrum).
   Rationale: The thermometer bounces an infrared signal off the tympanic membrane to read the temperature. An airtight seal prevents air from cooling the membrane.
4. When the temperature reading is displayed, remove the probe from the ear. Discard the probe cover.
   Rationale: The reading occurs almost immediately. A new probe cover must be used for each patient.
5. Return the thermometer unit to the base.
   Rationale: The thermometer may be rechargeable; in that case it needs to be fully charged to operate accurately. It may use batteries, but it should still be stored in a base to prevent accidental dropping of the thermometer unit.
6. Wash hands.
7. Record temperature including location in the patient's chart. The abbreviation TM is used to indicate the tympanic membrane. It is also correct to write "aurally."
   Rationale: The doctor uses the site the temperature was taken to help assess the temperature.

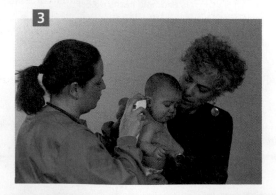

3

Charting Example	
Date	
7/19/XX	9:15 AM T: 99.2°F TM ————
	———————— S. Dellarosa, RMA

PROCEDURE 15–7

Measuring Rectal Temperature

Performance Objective: The student will take and record an individual's rectal temperature using a thermometer.

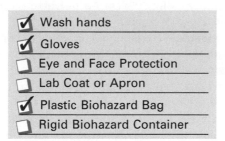

- ☑ Wash hands
- ☑ Gloves
- ☐ Eye and Face Protection
- ☐ Lab Coat or Apron
- ☑ Plastic Biohazard Bag
- ☐ Rigid Biohazard Container

Supplies and Equipment: Thermometer, lubricant, disposable plastic sheath or probe cover, gauze square, tissue, gloves, biohazard waste container.

Procedure Steps

1. Explain procedure to patient.
   Rationale: The patient will be more comfortable and cooperative knowing what to expect.
2. Position an adult patient on left side with right leg slightly forward (Sims' position). The patient needs to be undressed from the waist down with a drape for privacy. An infant can be positioned on back or on stomach but must be held firmly.
   Rationale: Sims' position gives easiest access to the rectum in an adult. The prone or supine position gives adequate access to the rectum in an infant.
3. Prepare either a rectal mercury thermometer with a plastic sheath (see Procedure 15–3) or an electronic thermometer with the red (rectal) probe and a disposable plastic probe cover.

Rationale: Thermometers or probes used for oral temperatures should never be used for rectal temperatures. The rectal mercury thermometer has a round end to prevent accidental breakage. The rectal probe of an electronic thermometer is calibrated to deliver a temperature comparable to a mercury thermometer.

4. Squeeze about 1″ of lubricant on a gauze square and lubricate the first 2″ inches of the thermometer or probe cover.
   Rationale: Lubrication facilitates insertion of the thermometer.
5. Put on gloves.
   Rationale: Begin all procedures by putting on appropriate PPE to protect from contact with microorganisms. In this procedure there is a potential to come in contact with the patient's stool.
6. Gently insert the thermometer or probe into the rectum (about 1/2″ for an infant or 1″ to 2″ for an adult). Try a different angle if you meet resistance. Instruct the patient not to move. Hold an infant firmly.
   Rationale: Avoid injury to the rectal wall by gentle insertion and having the patient lie still.
7. Leave a glass-mercury thermometer in place for 5 minutes. Follow the same procedure as for an oral temperature with an electronic thermometer. Remain with the patient throughout the procedure.
   Rationale: The thermometer must remain in the rectum long enough to register the same temperature as the rectal blood vessels. If the patient moves sharply or turns over, the tip of the thermometer may damage the rectal mucosa; a mercury thermometer may break.
8. Remove the thermometer. Remove the plastic

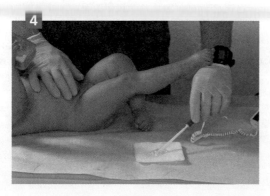

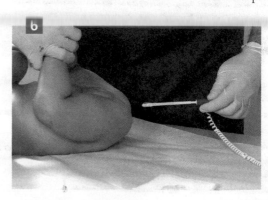

Procedure continued on following page

PROCEDURE 15–7 *(continued)*

sheath or the plastic probe cover and discard in a biohazard container. If necessary, wipe a mercury thermometer from shaft to bulb.

Rationale: The plastic sheath has been exposed to bacteria in the rectum and could transmit microorganisms. If lubricant or stool has penetrated the plastic sheath, you must wipe the thermometer to see the reading. The shaft is considered cleaner than the bulb, and you should wipe from the cleaner to the more contaminated area.

9. Read the temperature. On a glass thermometer, read up to the nearest two-tenths of a degree if a Fahrenheit thermometer and to the nearest tenth of a degree if a Celsius thermometer.

Rationale: You can only read accurately to the scale marked. The convention is to read up to the nearest mark.

10. Wipe the anal area of an infant with a tissue. Ask the parent to put on a clean diaper and supervise the child.

Rationale: You need to take care of soiled equipment before removing gloves.

11. Dispose of a rectal probe cover or plastic sheath in a biohazard container.

Rationale: The probe cover or plastic sheath may be contaminated with stool.

12. Wash a mercury thermometer using soap and cool water. Rinse it and dry with a paper towel. Place in soaking solution or in a

container clearly marked "Used Thermometers" for later disinfection.

Rationale: Even though a plastic sheath protected the thermometer, it must still be disinfected before being used again. After washing with soap and water, thermometers are soaked in a solution such as isopropyl alcohol 70% for at least 30 minutes.

13. Remove soiled gloves and discard in a biohazard waste container. Wash hands.

Rationale: Gloves may have come in contact with microorganisms. Always wash hands after using gloves.

14. Assist an adult patient to sit up. Offer a tissue and privacy for the patient to dress.

15. Record temperature, including location, in the patient's chart. A capital R, usually circled, is the common abbreviation for rectally.

Rationale: The doctor uses the site the temperature was taken to help assess the temperature.

Charting Example	
Date	
4/3/XX	10:00 AM T: 102.4°F ® ———————
	——————————— S. Williams, CMA

Care of Thermometers

Glass-Mercury Thermometers

Oral and rectal glass-mercury thermometers must be sanitized separately, and stored separately as well. After using a glass-mercury thermometer, following the principle of working from a cleaner area to a more soiled area, wipe from the stem to the bulb with a cotton ball or tissue. Wear gloves to wipe the thermometer.

Wash with soap and cool water, then rinse with cool water. Do not use hot water, because if a thermometer goes above its highest measurement level, it may not be possible to shake it down again.

After drying the thermometer, place it in disinfectant, such as Cidex or 70 percent alcohol, as seen in Figure 15–7, for 30 minutes to 1 hour. The solution should completely cover the thermometer.

Rinse with cold water and store dry. Shake the thermometer down to 96°F before using. Do not touch the bulb after sanitizing.

Electronic Oral/Rectal and Tympanic Thermometers

These are usually stored in an electronic charger, although some have batteries in them. It is important to return the thermometer to the charger after each use, so there is enough charge when the thermometer is needed.

Electronic thermometers need to be tested for accuracy regularly, following the manufacturer's directions. Electronic thermometers have a calibration device, which is inserted into the probe connector. When the unit is turned on, the calibration device produces a test

PROCEDURE 15-8

Measuring Axillary Temperature

Performance Objective: The student will take and record an individual's axillary temperature using a thermometer.

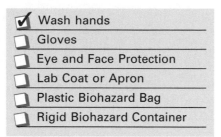

- ☑ Wash hands
- ☐ Gloves
- ☐ Eye and Face Protection
- ☐ Lab Coat or Apron
- ☐ Plastic Biohazard Bag
- ☐ Rigid Biohazard Container

Supplies and Equipment: Thermometer, disposable plastic sheath or probe cover, paper towel.

Procedure Steps

1. Explain procedure to patient.
   Rationale: The patient will be more comfortable and cooperative knowing what to expect.
2. Have patient undress so that underarm (axilla) is accessible. Provide a gown if the patient desires.
   Rationale: The thermometer must come in contact with the skin of the underarm for an accurate temperature reading.
3. Prepare either a glass-mercury thermometer with a plastic sheath (see Procedure 15–3) or an electronic thermometer with the blue (oral) probe and a disposable plastic probe cover

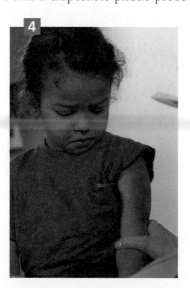

(see Procedure 15–4). Wipe the axilla with a paper towel.
Rationale: The axilla must be dry for an accurate reading.

4. Place the thermometer under the patient's arm, and instruct the patient to hold the arm tight against the side so that the thermometer remains in place. The patient may hold the forearm across the front of the body.
   Rationale: The skin of the axilla must prevent air from reaching the thermometer.
5. Leave a mercury thermometer in place for 10 minutes. Follow the same procedure with an electronic thermometer as when taking an oral temperature.
   Rationale: The thermometer must remain in the axilla long enough to register the same temperature as the skin of the axilla.
6. Remove the thermometer. Discard the plastic sheath or probe cover. Read the temperature. On a glass thermometer read up to the nearest two-tenths of a degree if a Fahrenheit thermometer and to the nearest tenth of a degree if a Celsius thermometer.
   Rationale: You can only read accurately to the scale marked. The convention is to read up to the nearest mark.
7. Wash a mercury thermometer using soap and cool water. Rinse it and dry with a paper towel. Place in soaking solution or in a container clearly marked "Used Thermometers" for later disinfection.
   Rationale: Even though a plastic sheath protected the thermometer, it must still be disinfected before being used again.
8. Wash hands. Offer privacy for the patient to dress. Record temperature, including location and scale (Fahrenheit or Celsius) used, in the patient's chart. The abbreviation "ax" may be used for axillary temperatures.
   Rationale: The doctor uses the site the temperature was taken to help assess the temperature.

Charting Example	
Date	
8/16/XX	4:44 PM T: 97.2°F ax ————————
	——————————— S. Williams, CMA

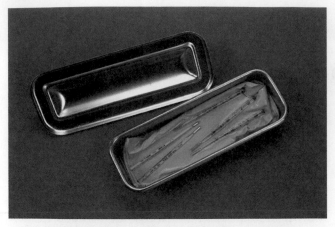

➤ Figure 15–7 Mercury thermometers in soaking solution.

temperature, which indicates if the unit is measuring correctly.

To clean these thermometers, wipe with a damp cloth. Avoid using chemicals or spilling solution on the thermometer. Do not handle a charger with wet hands to avoid an electric shock.

Documentation

Document the temperature reading, including the degree symbol (°) promptly in the patient's medical record, on the physical examination sheet for a new patient and in the progress notes for an established patient. Do not try to adjust any temperature readings to core temperature; simply document the reading obtained.

In most offices, the temperature reading is charted without specifying a route for the usual method of measuring temperature (traditionally oral). Medical assistants should specify if the temperature was measured using any other method, as follows: R for rectal; TM for tympanic, and AX for axillary.

PULSE

Pulse rate is an important measurement and one that will often vary among individuals, as well as in a single individual, depending on a number of factors.

Factors Affecting Rate of Heartbeat

When the heart beats, the beating can be felt as a throbbing at places in the body where an artery can be partially compressed against a bone. Pulse rate varies constantly in an individual for many reasons.

Increase

Women generally have a faster heartbeat than men; short, stocky people generally have a faster heartbeat than taller, thinner people. In addition, heartbeat often increases in the later part of the day. Emotions such as anger and excitement can cause the heartbeat to in-

ON THE JOB

Craig Johnson, a medical assistant at Blackburn Primary Care Associates, has called John Caswell, a 58-year-old established patient of Dr. Lopez, to the examination room.

Craig: What brings you to see Dr. Lopez today?
John Caswell: I have had a cold or the flu or something for a week. I can't breathe through my nose at all.
Craig: Have you had any other symptoms?
John Caswell: I ache all over and I don't feel like eating.
Craig: Have you had a fever?
John: I don't know. Probably. I've been having chills this morning and I really feel lousy.

QUESTIONS
1. Should Craig measure Mr. Caswell's height on this visit?
2. Should Craig measure Mr. Caswell's weight on this visit?
3. Which ways of measuring temperature may be used for Mr. Caswell?
4. Of the possible ways to measure Mr. Caswell's temperature, which is the best choice in this situation? Give reasons for your answer.
5. Why is it important to measure this patient's temperature?

crease, as can physical activity, fever, pain, stress, and infection. Even the stress of the doctor visit may cause the pulse to become more rapid.

Decrease

The opposite is also true; men have a slower heartbeat than women. Tall and thin people have a slower heartbeat than shorter, stocky people. The heart usually beats slower in the early part of the day. Among emotional and physical causes of short-term decrease in heartbeat are mental depression, chronic illness, and loss of body fluid due to dehydration or hemorrhage (bleeding).

Either Increase or Decrease

Heart disease or other diseases can cause either an increase or decrease in heart rate. So can recreational drugs or prescription medications such as digoxin, a common medication taken by the elderly that usually decreases the heart rate.

Locating Pulses

Eight places are commonly used to locate a pulse, as shown in Figure 15–8.

1. Temporal: about 1/2″ in front of the opening of the ear
2. Carotid: to right and left of Adam's apple in neck
3. **Apex** (pointed end) of the heart: at the fourth intercostal space to the left of the sternum
4. Brachial: inner aspect of arm at bend of elbow
5. Radial: on the thumb side of the wrist
6. Femoral: at the top of each leg, in the middle of the groin
7. Dorsalis pedis: upper surface of the foot
8. Popliteal: at the back of the knee.

Characteristics of the Pulse

Pulse rate is usually measured on the radial artery, on the thumb side of the wrist. When taking a pulse measurement, three characteristics are looked for: rate, rhythm, and volume.

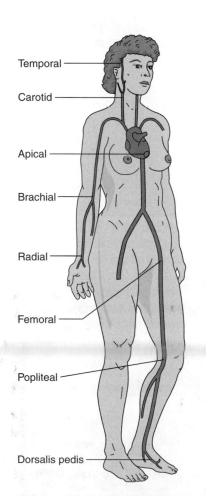

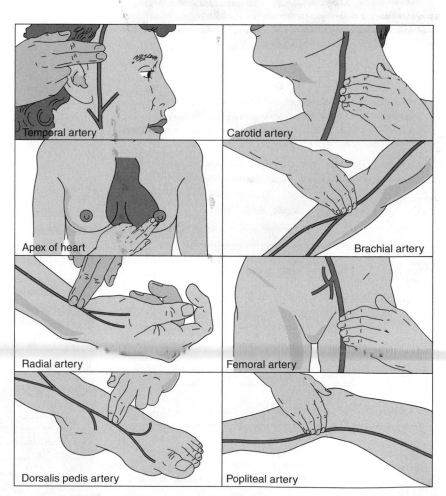

➤ **Figure 15–8** Common sites where a pulse can be located. (From Kinn ME, Woods M: *The Medical Assistant: Administrative and Clinical*, 8th ed. Philadelphia: WB Saunders, 1999.)

Rate

Pulse rate refers to the number of beats in 1 minute.

Rhythm

Pulse rhythm refers to the spaces between the pulsations. If the rhythm between pulsations is even, the pulse is regular. The pulse may skip beats or even have an overall irregular pattern. If irregular, count for 1 minute and note in the chart.

Volume

Pulse volume refers to the strength of each contraction of the heart. Normally, the volume is strong, or full. A very strong pulse is called bounding; a weak pulse is called weak, thready, or feeble; a pulse in which weak beats alternate with strong ones is called alternating.

Usual Values

Pulse rate gradually decreases from infancy to adulthood. See Table 15–3 for normal range of pulse rate and respiratory rate. The normal range for adults is between 60 and 100 beats per minute.

Measuring Pulse

The radial pulse at the thumb side of the wrist is usually measured for 60 seconds, especially if it is irregular, to obtain the most accurate measurement. If the pulse is regular, it is acceptable to count the number of beats in 30 seconds, and double the number, to obtain the number of beats per minute. Procedure 15–9 discusses measuring the radial pulse.

If the radial pulse is weak or some beats are weak, a more accurate measurement should be obtained. The most accurate measurement is the apical pulse, at the apex of the heart using a stethoscope.

The **stethoscope** is a device used to listen to body sounds. It consists of a circular chest piece that is placed on the body. The chest piece is connected to earpieces by a Y-shaped rubber tubing. To measure the apical pulse, the chest piece (called the diaphragm or bell) of the stethoscope is placed over the apex of the heart, and heartbeats are counted for a minute. Figure 15–9 shows a variety of stethoscopes.

When listening to the heart through a stethoscope, one hears two sounds for each heartbeat. These are the sounds of the heart values opening and closing. They are often referred to as "lubb" (the first sound) and "dubb" (the second sound).

Apical pulse should be measured in an infant or toddler (under age 2) and in any individual with a weak or irregular radial pulse. Procedure 15–10 discusses measuring the apical pulse.

Abnormal Pulse and Arrhythmias

A pulse rate below 60 beats per minute is termed **bradycardia,** and a pulse rate of over 100 beats per minute is termed **tachycardia.** However, these terms are considered a diagnosis and can only be used by the doctor, advanced-practice nurse, or physician's assistant. When charting, a medical assistant can only note the actual number of beats per minute and cannot give the pulse rate a diagnostic description.

An irregular heartbeat is termed an **arrhythmia.** Again, the medical assistant can use the term *irregular* (abbreviated irreg.) when charting, but not the term *arrhythmia,* which is a diagnostic term.

Pulse rate is usually recorded after the temperature. If the rhythm is regular and the volume is strong, only record the number of beats per minute. Note if the pulse is irregular or the volume, excessively strong, weak, or varying from weak to strong.

RESPIRATION

Respiration refers to the breaths per minute (a cycle of inhalation and exhalation). The respiratory center in the brain stem (the medulla oblongata) responds primarily to the carbon dioxide (CO_2) level of the blood. When the CO_2 level rises, the respiratory rate increases and respirations become deeper. When the CO_2 level falls, the respiratory rate decreases and respirations become slower and shallower.

Some patients with chronic obstructive pulmonary disease such as emphysema have high CO_2 levels at all times and breathe only in response to low oxygen levels. Note that it is dangerous to give these people too high a flow rate of oxygen, because the unaccustomed high blood levels of oxygen may prompt them to stop breathing.

Table 15–3	Normal Range of Heartbeat and Respirations at Various Ages	
Age	Normal Range of Pulse Rate	Normal Range of Respiratory Rate
Infants	110–170	30–60
Children (1–7 years)	80–120	18–30
Older children (7–12 years)	60–110	20–26
Adult	60–100	14–20

PROCEDURE 15–9

Measuring the Radial Pulse

Performance Objective: The student will measure and record the radial pulse of an individual and describe the rhythm and volume of the pulse.

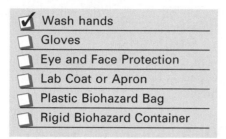

☑ Wash hands
☐ Gloves
☐ Eye and Face Protection
☐ Lab Coat or Apron
☐ Plastic Biohazard Bag
☐ Rigid Biohazard Container

Supplies and Equipment: Watch with sweep second hand.

Procedure Steps

1. Explain procedure to patient.
   Rationale: The patient will be more comfortable and cooperative knowing what to expect.
2. Wash hands.
   Rationale: Hands should always be clean before touching a patient or handling equipment.
3. Position the patient so that the arm is supported and relaxed.
   Rationale: Holding the arm up is uncomfortable for the patient and can even raise the pulse rate.

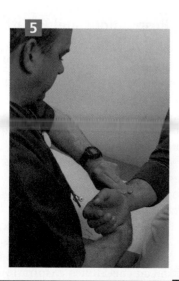

4. Locate the radial pulse with the first three fingers pressing hard enough to feel the pulse clearly but not hard enough to occlude the artery. The forearm may be turned up or down.
   Rationale: The pulse is felt by compressing the radial artery against the bone of the lower arm (radius). If there is too little compression, the pulse cannot be felt. If there is too much compression, the artery will be completely blocked. The thumb cannot be used to feel the pulse because it has its own pulse, which may be confused with the patient's.
5. When the pulse is located, begin to count heartbeats. Continue counting for 60 seconds. Note the quality of the pulse (regular, irregular, weak, strong, etc.).
   Rationale: The goal is to determine how many times the heart is beating each minute. The most accurate measurement is obtained by counting for a full minute. If the pulse is regular and strong, it is acceptable to count the number of beats in 30 seconds and multiply by 2 to obtain the number of beats per minute.
6. If respirations will be measured, leave fingers on pulse and count respirations immediately (see Procedure 15–11, Measuring Respirations).
   Rationale: Respirations are measured without informing the patient because the respiratory pattern often changes when patients are aware of being observed.
7. Wash hands and record the pulse in the patient's chart. Only the number of beats per minute is required if the rate is regular and the pulse is strong. If variation in the volume or rhythm are discovered, describe the variation.
   Rationale: It is most common for the pulse to be regular and strong. (Example 1: P: 80, Example 2: P: 68 irreg)

Charting Example	
Date	
6/7/XX	10:00 AM P: 80 irreg ————————
	———————— S. Dellarosa, RMA

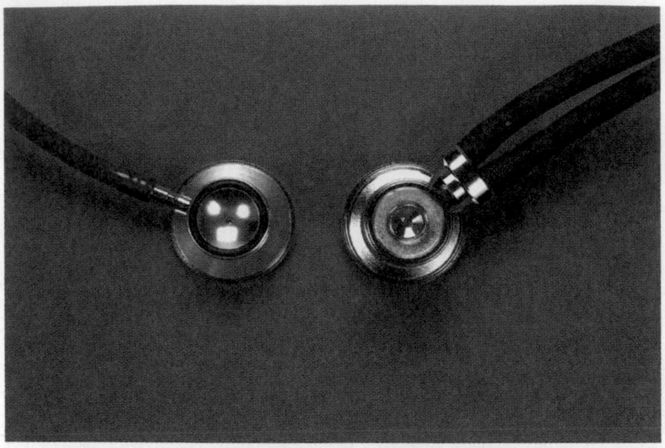

> Figure 15–9 The bell of the stethoscope may be attached with one tube or two tubes (Sprague-Rappaport type). The large side of the bell is used to measure blood pressure. Both the large and small sides may be used to listen to heart sounds.

Factors Affecting Respiration

A number of factors can increase or decrease respiration.

Increase

Factors that increase respiration include fever; exercise; excitement or nervousness; anything that increases the body's demand for oxygen; some medications, especially stimulants such as epinephrine; and recreational drugs such as cocaine.

Decrease

Factors that decrease respiration include sleep; relaxation; pressure on certain brain centers from head injury; some medications, especially those that depress the central nervous system such as narcotic analgesics (Percodan, morphine, codeine); and street drugs such as heroin.

Characteristics of Respiration

The three characteristics of respiration are rate, rhythm, and depth.

Rate

Rate refers to the number of respirations per minute, described as normal, rapid, or slow. For an individual with no respiratory problems, it is usually adequate to count the respirations for 30 seconds and double, to find the rate per minute. If the patient has respiratory symptoms, count respirations for a full minute.

Rhythm

Rhythm refers to how even or uneven the breathing is. Normally, people's respiratory rate is even, and each breath is about the same depth. An abnormal rhythm may be caused by an abnormal rate or abnormal depth. If the rhythm is irregular, count respirations for a full minute.

Depth

Depth refers to the amount of air inhaled and exhaled on each breath. It is described as normal, shallow, deep, or gasping.

Some abnormal rhythms are shallow breaths interspersed with deep breaths or a pattern of apnea, a time where the person does not breathe, followed by several gasping breaths.

Usual Values

The respiratory rate of a healthy adult is between 14 and 20 breaths per minute. Any rate below 12 or above 40 breaths per minute may be a serious symptom.

Infants and children have a high respiratory rate, which gradually decreased as they get older, to the adult rate. In general, the faster the heart rate, the faster the respiratory rate.

Counting Respirations

Because the respiratory rate is likely to change if the person knows he or she is being observed, respirations are usually measured immediately after taking the pulse, before the wrist is released. If respiration seems very shallow, they may be measured with a stethoscope. Procedure 15–11 discusses measuring respirations.

Abnormal Respirations and Breath Sounds

Respiratory changes in rate, rhythm, or depth may signal abnormalities.

There are various types of irregular rate. Respirations may be slower (**bradypnea**) or more rapid (**tachypnea**) than normal. They may also be slow and shallow (**hypopnea**) or rapid and deep (**hyperpnea**). Absent respirations are called **apnea.**

Of course, prolonged apnea requires resuscitation, or death results. But short periods of apnea occur in certain disorders, such as sleep apnea, in which the tongue blocks the airway until lack of oxygen causes the individual to wake up slightly and begin to breathe again.

Patterns of intermittent apnea occur in a respiratory pattern called **Cheyne-Stokes respirations,** in which a short period of apnea is followed by gradually increas-

PROCEDURE 15–10

Measuring the Apical Pulse

Performance Objective: The student will measure and record the apical pulse of an individual.

- ☑ Wash hands
- ☐ Gloves
- ☐ Eye and Face Protection
- ☐ Lab Coat or Apron
- ☐ Plastic Biohazard Bag
- ☐ Rigid Biohazard Container

Supplies and Equipment: Stethoscope, watch with sweep second hand.

Procedure Steps

1. Explain procedure to patient.
   Rationale: The patient will be more comfortable and cooperative knowing what to expect.
2. Wash hands.
   Rationale: Hands should always be clean before touching a patient or handling equipment.
3. Instruct the patient to remove clothing from the waist up. Provide a gown.
   Rationale: You must be able to visualize the correct area of the chest.
4. The patient may be in the sitting or supine position. Locate the apex of the heart by palpating the fifth intercostal space and moving laterally to the midclavicular line.
   Rationale: The pulse will be heard most clearly over the apex of the heart.
5. Clean the stethoscope diaphram with alcohol and place it over the apex of the heart and the eartips in your ears.
   Rationale: The stethoscope diaphram should be cleaned between each patient to prevent the spread of microorganisms.

6. When the pulse is located, begin to count heartbeats. Each lubb-dubb counts as one heartbeat. Continue for a full minute.
   Rationale: Each time the heart beats two sounds are heard, commonly expressed as "lubb-dubb." If it is necessary to measure the pulse apically, you can assume that it will be necessary to count heartbeats for a full minute.
7. Instruct the patient to dress. Wash hands and record the pulse in the patient's chart. Only the number of beats per minute is required if the rate is regular and the pulse is strong. If variation in the volume or rhythm is discovered, describe the variation.
   Rationale: It is most common for the pulse to be regular and strong

Charting Example	
Date	
6/7/XX	10:00 AM AP: 66, reg and strong
	S. Dellarosa, RMA

Apical-Radial Pulse. On some occasions two people take the pulse simultaneously to determine if all beats heard through the stethoscope can also be palpated at the radial artery. The two people must be sure to start and stop taking the pulse together. Normally the apical pulse rate is identical to the radial pulse rate. If fewer beats are heard at the radial pulse, there is a pulse deficit (decreased number of heartbeats at the wrist compared to the apex of the heart). This may indicate cardiac abnormality. Each measurement is charted (e.g., RP: 68; AP: 68, regular).

ing rate and depth, and then gradually decreasing rate and depth, of respirations, until another period of apnea is reached. The cycle may take up to a minute. This pattern occurs in some people during sleep (especially the elderly). But it can also indicate brain dysfunction and sometimes occurs when a person is close to death.

In certain conditions, respirations are very rapid and deep, such as is seen in **hyperventilation,** in which rapid, deep respirations result in excessive loss of carbon dioxide. Hyperventilation is often associated with severe anxiety. A low level of carbon dioxide in the blood can cause a feeling of light-headedness, tingling, and even muscle cramping, which only adds to the patient's anxiety. The patient may be instructed to breathe into a paper bag (to allow him or her to rebreathe air containing carbon dioxide). Attempts should be made to help the patient slow his or her breathing rate and relax.

A patient may complain of shortness of breath (**SOB**), especially when exercising, or difficulty breathing (**dyspnea**), which also occurs most frequently after exertion such as climbing stairs.

A person with a serious breathing problem such as an asthma attack or pulmonary embolism (blood clot in the lung) may have difficulty breathing while sitting still. The doctor may call this respiratory distress, to indicate that the person subjectively feels that he or she cannot get enough air. Patients may also describe a feeling of being unable to breathe when lying flat, which is relieved by sitting up or using extra pillows to sleep. This condition, called **orthopnea**, is usually seen in patients who are retaining fluid, such as those with congestive heart failure or renal (kidney) failure.

Documenting Pulse and Respirations

For a new patient, pulse and respirations are documented on the physical examination sheet. For an established patient, the heart and respiratory rates are charted in the progress notes. Any irregularity in rate,

---

PROCEDURE 15–11

Measuring Respirations

Performance Objective: The student will measure and record the respirations of an individual and describe the rhythm and depth of the respirations.

- ☑ Wash hands
- ☐ Gloves
- ☐ Eye and Face Protection
- ☐ Lab Coat or Apron
- ☐ Plastic Biohazard Bag
- ☐ Rigid Biohazard Container

Supplies and Equipment: Watch with sweep second hand.

Procedure Steps

1. Observe patient while he or she is sitting or lying in a comfortable position. Respirations are often counted immediately after the radial pulse is measured while the medical assistant holds the patient's wrist.
   Rationale: If a patient is aware that you are counting respirations, the respiratory pattern may change.
2. Watch the patient's chest rise and fall; each cycle of inhalation and exhalation is counted as one respiration. This may be more easily seen at the neck edge of the clothing.
   Rationale: The chest rises as the lungs fill with air and falls as air is exhaled.
3. If the respiratory rate is regular and strong, count for 30 seconds and multiply by two. If the respiratory rate is irregular, continue counting for a full minute.
   Rationale: The goal is to determine the respiratory rate per minute. For most people, you can establish that respirations are normal within 30 seconds.
4. Record the respiratory rate in the patient's chart. Only the number of respirations per minute is usually charted if the rate and depth are regular. If there is variation in the volume or rhythm, describe the variation.
   Rationale: It is most common for the respirations to be regular and deep.

Charting Example	
Date	
6/7/XX	10:05 AM R: 34, shallow ———————
	——————— S. Dellarosa, RMA

rhythm, or depth must be noted. If normal and regular, only the number of beats per minute (heart rate) and breaths per minute (respiratory rate) are recorded.

The medical assistant may use terms such as dyspnea (difficulty breathing) and orthopnea to document patient complaints, because these are subjective findings (e.g., the patient complains of dyspnea). But the medical assistant should not use diagnostic terms such as hyperventilation. Instead, medical assistants should describe breathing patterns (i.e., rapid, shallow respirations).

BLOOD PRESSURE

Blood pressure (**BP**) is the pressure of blood against the walls of arteries, which carry blood from the heart to the lungs for oxygenation, and then throughout the body. *Systole* refers to the pressure against the artery walls when the heart's ventricles contract; *diastole* refers to the pressure against the artery walls when the ventricles relax between heartbeats and indicates the resistance of the arteries to blood flow. Both systole and diastole are measured in millimeters of mercury (mm Hg—the height in millimeters that the pressure will raise a column of mercury).

Blood pressure may vary in different arteries; it is usually measured in the brachial artery of the arm, and is recorded as the systolic pressure over the diastolic pressure. Blood pressure is expressed as two numbers, separated by a slash, the systolic pressure first and the diastolic pressure second (e.g., 120/80 mm Hg).

Physiologic Control of Blood Pressure

Blood pressure results from the pumping action of the heart, which pushes blood out to the arteries. Various physiologic mechanisms control blood pressure. The kidneys are important in regulating blood pressure because they control the amount of fluid in the body and also because they secrete hormones that regulate the constriction or dilation of arteries and arterioles.

Five factors are important in the physiologic control of blood pressure:

1. blood volume
2. constriction or dilation of arterioles (known as peripheral resistance)
3. elasticity of arterial walls
4. the heart's pumping action
5. blood viscosity.

Blood Volume

Blood volume refers to the amount of fluid circulating in the body. The more there is, the higher the pressure. As known from experience, to raise the pressure of a gas or liquid, one must either increase the amount of gas or liquid in the same space or put the same volume in a smaller space. Increased volume increases pressure.

Peripheral Resistance

Peripheral resistance is the amount of constriction or dilation of the arterioles, the smaller arteries. The more constricted they are, the higher the blood pressure. When small arterioles are constricted, we say that the peripheral resistance has increased (peripheral resistance is decreased when the arterioles are dilated). They may be constricted due to nerve impulses, or they may simply be less able to dilate.

Elasticity of Arterial Walls

The elasticity of arterial walls has an impact on the arteries' and arterioles' ability to constrict or dilate. Elasticity may be impaired due to atherosclerosis, a condition of fatty deposits in the arteries.

Pumping Action

The heart must be able to pump effectively to maintain adequate blood flow (cardiac output). Pumping action can be impaired by damage to the heart muscle, damage to the valves, or impaired conduction of electrical impulses through the heart.

Blood Viscosity

Viscosity refers to the thickness of the blood. An increase in red blood cells makes blood thicker and tends to increases blood pressure. This happens at high altitudes and in some diseases.

Factors Affecting Blood Pressure Readings

Blood pressure readings vary constantly, depending on patient activity, position, and other factors. Blood pressure is usually measured at rest and can be affected by recent activity (such as being stuck in traffic on the way to the doctor's office) or even anxiety about the medical exam itself. For this reason, blood pressure is sometimes taken twice, at the beginning of the exam, then again at or near the end.

Blood pressure can also be affected by the patient's position when blood pressure is measured. Blood pressure tends to be higher when lying down, lower when sitting up, and lowest when standing. Blood pressure may fall rapidly when a person stands up, called postural hypotension, or **orthostatic hypotension.** An individual may even become dizzy because of this rapid change in blood pressure.

Increase

Factors that can cause an increase in blood pressure include exercise, stress, anxiety, excitement, arteriosclerosis, increased weight, smoking, and pain.

Decrease

Factors that can cause a decrease in blood pressure include hemorrhage (bleeding), depression, dehydration, sleep, and relaxation.

Effects of Medication

Many medications affect blood pressure; some cause it to rise, others cause it to fall.

Measurement of Blood Pressure with a Sphygmomanometer

The most common method of measuring blood pressure is to pump air into a blood pressure cuff wrapped around the upper arm until the brachial artery is totally compressed.

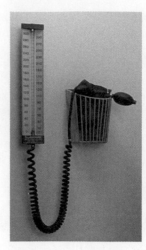

➢ **Figure 15–10** Mercury sphygmomanometer.

Medications for High Blood Pressure

Diuretics or beta-adrenergic blockers (commonly called beta blockers) are usually the first choice for combating high blood pressure, either alone or in combination. If blood pressure remains high or other cardiac symptoms appear, the doctor will usually add a vasodilator and/or a calcium channel blocker.

Diuretics reduce water absorption by the kidneys. The most commonly used diuretics are acetazolamide (trade name Diamox), chlorothiazide (Diuril), hydrochlorothiazide (Hydro-Diuril), spironolactone (Aldactone), and furosemide (Lasix).

Beta-adrenergic blockers block the response of beta receptors in the heart, arteries, and blood vessels, resulting in lower blood pressure and lower heart rate. Beta blockers are atenolol (Tenormin), metoprolol (Lopressor), and propranolol (Inderal).

Vasodilators relax the smooth muscles of the arteries and reduce peripheral vascular resistance. The drugs used are hydralazine (Apresoline) and minoxidil.

Calcium channel blockers create systemic vasodilation, resulting in lower blood pressure; they also reduce the pain of angina and arrhythmias. Drugs used are diltiazem (Cardizem), nifedipine (Procardia), and verapamil (Calan).

The instrument used to measure blood pressure is called a **sphygmomanometer** (literally, an instrument to measure pulse). The equipment is simple, consisting of the following:

1. A cloth cuff that contains an inflatable rubber bladder and is secured around the arm with Velcro or clips
2. A bulb to inflate the rubber bladder in the cuff, with a screw valve to control inflation and deflation
3. A manometer, or instrument to measure pressure

While listening with a stethoscope over the artery, the examiner gradually decreases cuff pressure. The heartbeat can be heard when the blood begins to enter the artery against resistance provided by the cuff, until the cuff no longer provides resistance and the blood flows freely.

Pressure in the artery is indicated either as a column of mercury on a mercury manometer, or on a dial calibrated to the mercury scale on an **aneroid** manometer, one that operates without fluid. In either case, blood pressure is expressed as millimeters of mercury (**mm Hg**). Figure 15–10 shows a mercury sphygmomanometer, and Figure 15–11 shows an aneroid sphygmomanometer.

The pressure when the blood first enters the artery (the first sound heard through the stethoscope) is the systolic pressure. The pressure when the cuff is no longer providing any resistance (the last sound of the heartbeat heard through the stethoscope) is the diastolic pressure.

Korotkoff Sounds

Sounds heard through the stethoscope while taking blood pressure are called Korotkoff sounds. As the cuff deflates, the quality of the sounds changes. There are five phases to the Korotkoff sounds.

Phase I. Faint tapping sounds, which begin as sharp sounds. The first sound is recorded as the systolic pressure, the tapping sounds become . . .

Phase II. Soft swishing sounds, which in turn become . . .

Phase III. Sharp, distinct, rhythmic tapping sounds; the tapping sounds get . . .

Phase IV. Fainter and more muffled, sounds that gradually . . .

Phase V. Disappear as blood flows freely through the artery. The absence of sound is recorded as the diastolic pressure.

Pulse Pressure

If the diastolic pressure is subtracted from the systolic pressure, the resulting number is called the pulse pressure. The most common pulse pressure is between 30 and 50 mm Hg. If the number is larger, the pulse pressure is said to be widened; if it is smaller, it is said to be narrowed, as occurs in shock.

Electronic Measurement

Electronic measurement uses a cuff, attached to an electronic device or computer that measures the blood pressure. The machine controls deflation of the cuff and provides a digital or computer readout of the blood pressure. Improvements in accuracy have made these devices more popular. The cuff may be designed for the finger or the arm.

Usual Values

Blood pressure is low at birth and gradually rises until adulthood. At birth, systolic blood pressure is

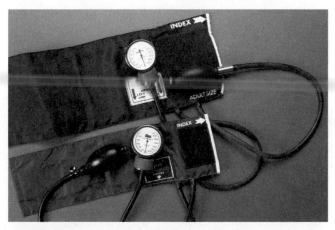

> **Figure 15–11** Aneroid sphygmomanometers: adult and child sizes.

Table 15–4	Average Blood Pressure at Various Ages	
Age		**Average Blood Pressure**
Infant (birth to 1 year)		90/50
Toddler (1–3 years)		90/50
Preschool (3–6 years)		94/56
School-age (6–13 years)		110/70
Adolescent (13–19 years)		120/80
Adult		120/80

about 80 mm Hg. By age 10, normal blood pressure ranges from 100/60 to 120/80. By about age 20, a person will have reached his or her level of "normal" adult blood pressure. Normal range for adults is between 90/60 and 140/90. Table 15–4 shows blood pressure at various ages.

As a person ages, blood pressure often continues to rise, especially the systolic pressure. By age 60, the normal values are between 140/92 and 170/100. But there is increasing agreement that older individuals remain healthier if measures are taken to keep the diastolic pressure at 100 mm Hg or lower.

Measuring Blood Pressure

Measuring blood pressure requires precision. If the procedure, outlined in Procedure 15–12, is not followed carefully, inaccurate findings will result.

In the medical office, blood pressure is normally measured on the brachial artery, with the patient sitting. Five major activities are involved in taking blood pressure:

1. Selecting the cuff
2. Applying the cuff
3. Palpating for systolic pressure
4. Listening for the auscultatory gap
5. Determining systolic and diastolic values.

Selecting Cuff

The width of the blood pressure cuff should be one-third larger than the diameter of the patient's arm. Figure 15–12 shows selection of the correct blood pressure cuff. The office should have a selection of cuffs appropriate for the patient population: infant, toddler, child, adult, and obese adult.

Applying Cuff

The rubber bladder inside the cuff, which fills with air, should be centered over the brachial artery of the arm, about 1″ to 2″ above the antecubital space (the

FOCUS ON
INSTRUCTION

TEACHING PATIENTS ABOUT HYPERTENSION AND ITS TREATMENT

Hypertension (high blood pressure) is probably the most frequently diagnosed chronic condition in the American population. Untreated hypertension can have a number of health consequences over time. But treatment is often difficult, for a number of reasons.

Causes. Primary hypertension, also called essential hypertension, has no known cause. Secondary hypertension is a complication of another condition, such as an adrenal tumor or kidney disease.

Diagnosis. Sustained blood pressure elevation, with systolic pressure over 140 mm Hg or diastolic pressure above 90 mm Hg in adults, is necessary for a diagnosis of hypertension. Sustained means at least two consecutive readings, days apart, at these levels.

Signs and symptoms. Hypertension often has no symptoms, even when blood pressure is severely elevated. Sometimes patients experience nosebleeds or headaches, but these usually only occur when blood pressure is severely elevated.

Treatment. For slight elevation, a patient may be instructed to lose weight, stop smoking, adhere to an exercise program, and/or avoid added salt in the diet. If these measures are inadequate, treatment is extended to include medications that help the patient to lose fluid as urine (diuretics) or help to dilate blood vessels (antihypertensives).

Treatment challenges. Many patients resist lifestyle changes necessary to reduce hypertension. Others may adhere to lifestyle changes, but fail to take medication regularly or stop taking medication once the blood pressure is brought under control.

Risks of untreated hypertension. Hypertension is a contributing factor to stroke, heart attack, heart failure, kidney failure, and blindness. The higher the blood pressure, the greater the risk of complications. Even a 5 mm Hg reduction appears to reduce the occurrence and severity of serious problems.

Helping patients understand blood pressure. The medical assistant plays a primary role in helping patients understand the consequences of high blood pressure and assisting them with maintaining their lifestyle changes and medication regimen. Some of the things medical assistants can do in this regard include:

1. Explain to patients clearly and concisely what blood pressure is and what each number means.

2. Suggest that patients who are concerned about blood pressure keep a record for comparison.

3. If the doctor wants the patient to monitor his or her blood pressure at home, discuss with the patient or a responsible family member what equipment to buy and how to obtain the BP reading.

4. Provide the patient with handouts about blood pressure or other recommendations the doctor has made, such as weight loss, low-salt diet, smoking cessation, and exercise programs.

bend in the elbow). If possible, the patient should push the sleeve of his or her shirt up. If this would constrict the arm, the arm should be removed from the sleeve.

If the patient has had a radical mastectomy, do not use the arm on that side for blood pressure measurement. Also, never take the blood pressure in an arm that has an ateriovenous fistula or shunt for dialysis.

Palpating for Systolic Pressure

Before measuring the blood pressure with a stethoscope, identify the approximate systolic pressure by palpation. It is possible to **palpate** (use a finger to feel the pulse) the systolic pressure by placing a finger on the radial artery while inflating the cuff. The systolic pressure is the point at which the pulse can no longer be felt.

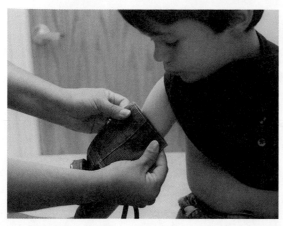

➤ **Figure 15–12** The patient's arm should be approximately two-thirds the width of a blood pressure cuff of the correct size. (From Kinn ME, Woods M: *The Medical Assistant: Administrative and Clinical*, 8th ed. Philadelphia: WB Saunders, 1999.)

There are several reasons for palpating the systolic pressure.

The blood pressure measurement is most accurate when the cuff has been pumped up to about 30 mm Hg higher than the systolic pressure before measuring and when the pressure is released from the cuff at about 2 to 3 mm Hg per second. Palpating the systolic pressure before measuring allows the medical assistant to know how high to go to get 30 mm Hg higher than the point noted for the systolic pressure.

Listening for the Auscultatory Gap

In some patients, Korotkoff sounds disappear between the beginning of sounds (Phase I) and the first change in sound quality (Phase II). This disappearance of sound is called an **auscultatory gap.** If the cuff is not pumped up high enough, the medical assistant may first hear sound at Phase II, below the gap, and mistake the first sound heard for the systolic pressure. Palpating the systolic pressure before listening with the stethoscope avoids a mistaken reading.

Determining Systolic and Diastolic Values

The scale on the manometer is marked in even numbers from 0 to 300 mm Hg. After pumping the cuff up about 30 mm Hg higher than the anticipated systolic pressure, listen through a stethoscope whose diaphragm is placed over the brachial artery.

Note the place on the scale where the first two consecutive tapping sounds are heard. The location of the first sound is the systolic pressure. Listen for the location where the sounds stop, as the air is released from the cuff. This is the diastolic pressure. The blood pressure is expressed as a fraction (120/80), with the first number the systolic pressure and the second number the diastolic pressure.

Because aneroid and mercury blood pressure scales only measure every two points, blood pressure measurements should be expressed in even numbers. Procedure 15–12 describes in detail measuring blood pressure.

Common Reasons for Inaccurate Blood Pressure Measurements

If any one of the following eight activities or problems occur, inaccurate blood pressure measurement could result.

1. Incorrect body posture
2. Incorrect cuff size
3. Incorrect arm position
4. Excessive pressure on head of stethoscope
5. Deflating cuff too quickly
6. Incorrectly calibrated equipment
7. Talking during measurement
8. Inadequate time for arm to rest and refill between readings

Incorrect Body Posture

The patient should be relaxed, with back and arm supported. If the patient has no back support or has to hold the arm up, the pressure may be artificially elevated.

Incorrect Cuff Size

A too-small cuff causes artificial elevation in blood pressure. A too-large cuff causes less distortion in the measurement but may result in a low reading.

Incorrect Arm Position

The cuff and arm should be at the level of the heart. The arm must not be held up, and the cuff should be applied 1″ to 2″ inches above the antecubital fossa (bend of the elbow).

Excessive Pressure on Head of Stethoscope

The stethoscope should be held tightly enough to seal it against the skin. However, additional pressure may cause a low diastolic pressure or cause the sounds to be heard below the diastolic, even all the way to 0 mm Hg.

Cuff Deflated Too Quickly

Deflating the cuff too quickly results in missed sounds and low readings.

PROCEDURE 15-12

Measuring Blood Pressure

Performance Objective: The student will measure and record the blood pressure of an individual.

- ☑ Wash hands
- ☐ Gloves
- ☐ Eye and Face Protection
- ☐ Lab Coat or Apron
- ☐ Plastic Biohazard Bag
- ☐ Rigid Biohazard Container

Supplies and Equipment: Stethoscope, alcohol wipe, sphygmomanometer.

Procedure Steps

1. Explain procedure to patient.
   Rationale: The patient will be more comfortable and cooperative knowing what to expect.
2. Wash hands.
   Rationale: Hands should always be clean before touching a patient or handling equipment.
3. Ask the patient to roll up his or her sleeve at least 5″ above the bend of the arm. If the sleeve is too tight, have the patient put on a gown.
   Rationale: The arm should be bare to apply the cuff with extra room for the head of the stethoscope.
4. Position the patient so that the lower arm is supported on a flat surface and the arm is relaxed. The part of the arm where blood pressure will be measured must be at the same level as the heart.
   Rationale: Holding the arm up is uncomfortable for the patient and can raise the blood pressure. Tense muscles can change the blood pressure reading and/or make it difficult to hear the blood pressure. If the arm is not at heart level, an inaccurate reading may be obtained.
5. Place the blood pressure cuff on the arm with the section of the cuff containing the rubber bladder centered over the brachial artery.
   Rationale: The rubber bladder must be centered over the artery to obtain an accurate measurement.
6. Wrap the cuff snugly around the arm and fasten.
   Rationale: The cuff must be fastened snugly around the arm to obtain an accurate measurement.
7. Hold the bulb in your dominant hand with the control valve between your thumb and first finger. Turn the screw clockwise to tighten and counterclockwise to loosen. As you begin the procedure, the screw should be tight but not so tight that it will be difficult to open.
   Rationale: If you always hold the bulb the same way, it will be easy to remember which direction to turn it to open or close the control valve.
8. Locate the radial pulse with your nondominant hand. Inflate the blood pressure cuff by squeezing the bulb until just above the point where you stop feeling the radial pulse. Take note of the reading, which is the systolic blood pressure.
   Rationale: If you know the systolic pressure, you are prepared to obtain the most accurate

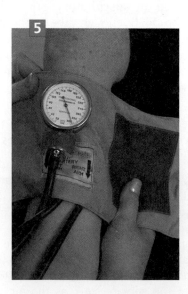

reading when listening through the stethoscope. This will also help you to avoid missing an auscultatory gap.

9. Deflate the blood pressure cuff quickly by opening the control valve. Clean the stethoscope diaphram with alcohol and place the head of the stethoscope over the brachial artery at the bend of the artery. Wait at least 30 seconds.
   Rationale: The head of the stethoscope should be cleaned between each patient to prevent the spread of microorganisms. Waiting 30 seconds allows the artery to rest between readings and the blood pressure to return to normal.

10. Inflate the blood pressure cuff again to 30 mm Hg higher than the reading at which the radial pulse disappeared on palpation.
    Rationale: The most accurate reading is obtained when the cuff is inflated to about 30 mm Hg higher than the systolic pressure.

11 Immediately open the control valve slightly so that the blood pressure indicator (mercury level or needle) decreases about 2 to 4 mm Hg per second.
   Rationale: The level needs to decrease slowly enough so that you hear the sounds clearly but fast enough to prevent excessive discomfort to the patient's arm.

12. Note the exact level when you hear the first sharp tapping sound. This is the systolic pressure.
    Rationale: The first sound occurs when the pressure of the heart's contraction is strong

enough to begin to force blood through the artery.

13. Continue to deflate the cuff at 2 to 4 mm of Hg per second. Listen as the Korotkoff sounds continue and change. Note the exact level at which the sound disappears. This is the diastolic pressure.
    Rationale: When the blood flows freely through the artery without pressure from the cuff, you cannot hear any sound through the stethoscope.

14. As soon as you have identified the diastolic pressure, open the control valve and allow the cuff to deflate quickly.
    Rationale: Rapid deflation after the diastolic pressure has been measured minimizes discomfort to the patient.

15. If you are satisfied with the reading, remove the cuff from the patient's arm. If you need to take another reading, wait a full minute to allow the artery to recover. **Never pump the cuff back up during the measurement.** If you do not hear the Korotkoff sounds clearly, deflate the cuff, wait a minute, and begin the measurement again.
    Rationale: If the cuff is reinflated too soon or remains inflated for too long a time, falsely elevated readings can occur.

16. After removing the cuff, wash hands and record the blood pressure in the patient's chart. Note the arm on which you took the blood pressure. If the patient was lying down or standing, note the position.
    Rationale: Normally the blood pressure varies slightly from arm to arm. The arm with the higher pressure is usually followed. In the doctor's office, the patient is assumed to be sitting for blood pressure unless otherwise noted.

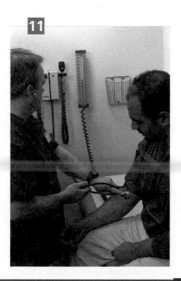

11

Charting Example	
Date	
6/7/XX	10:12 AM BP: 138/82 Ⓡ arm ———
	S. Dellarosa, RMA

Incorrectly Calibrated Equipment

Equipment that is improperly calibrated can cause an artificially high or low reading; tubing that contains leaks usually leads to a low reading.

Talking During Measurement

Talking by the patient during the measurement usually leads to an artificially high reading. In addition, it is difficult for the medical assistant to distinguish the Korotkoff sounds if he or she is being disturbed by the patient. Ask the patient not to talk during BP measurement.

Inadequate Time Between Readings

Sometimes, one inaccurate reading can lead to another.

Inadequate time for the arm to rest and the arteries to refill between readings can cause another bad reading. The arm needs to be at rest for at least 1 full minute to avoid an artificial elevation in blood pressure. A partially deflated cuff should never be reinflated because an accurate reading is unlikely. The cuff should be fully deflated and the patient allowed to relax for 1 to 2 minutes.

Care of Blood Pressure Equipment

Clean the stethoscope ear tips with alcohol if someone else has used it before you to prevent transmission of external ear infections. Clean the diaphragm with alcohol before each use, because it will touch each patient's skin.

Check the sphygmomanometer regularly for leaking tubing. Sphygmomanometers should be calibrated regularly to be sure they are accurate. Cuffs can be removed for laundering. Usually this is only done occasionally, but if the cuff has become soiled with body fluids such as blood, it must either be replaced or laundered with the contaminated laundry.

Documenting Blood Pressure

Note the blood pressure in the patient's chart as soon as possible after the measurement to avoid forgetting. Blood pressure is noted for a new patient on the physical examination sheet and on the progress notes for an established patient.

Note the arm on which the measurement was taken. For a new patient, both arms should be measured and the higher pressure followed over time. The measurement is assumed to be from a sitting patient. Note if the patient was lying down or standing up when the blood pressure was measured.

Sometimes a doctor will want to know the blood pressure in all three positions. If this is the case, measure in the following order: lying, sitting, standing. Do not remove the cuff in between; move directly from position to position.

Discussing Blood Pressure Measurements

Patients often ask about the results of BP measurements. Medical assistants can tell a patient the results of measurements, but should refer the patient to the doctor or doctor-approved educational materials for explanations of the meaning of the reading.

STUDENT STUDY PLAN

To reinforce your understanding of the material in this chapter . . .

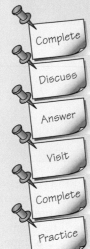

Complete — *Complete* the **Review & Recall** questions.

Discuss — *Discuss* the situation in **If You Were the Medical Assistant** with your classmates and answer the questions.

Answer — *Answer* the **Critical Thinking Questions** and discuss with your classmates.

Visit — *Visit* **Web sites** suggested and search for additional Web sites using **Keywords for Internet Searches.**

Complete — *Complete* the exercises in chapter 15 of the **Student Mastery Manual.**

Practice — *Practice* clinical activities on the **CD-ROM:** temperature, pulse, respirations, blood pressure, weight, and height.

 REVIEW & RECALL

1. What is the purpose of taking measurements such as height, weight, and vital signs?
2. Describe how height and weight are measured.
3. Compare and contrast normal body temperature variations with fever and hypothermia.
4. Discuss various types of thermometers and how they are used to take oral, aural, rectal, and axillary temperatures.
5. Identify factors that affect heart rate.
6. Describe eight places where a pulse can be palpated.
7. Describe the procedure for measuring the radial pulse.

8. Discuss factors that can influence the rate and depth of respirations.
9. Describe how blood pressure is controlled in the body.
10. Describe how blood pressure is measured with a sphygmomanometer.
11. Identify factors that can result in accurate blood pressure readings.
12. List equipment needed to measure height, weight, temperature, apical pulse, and blood pressure.

 IF YOU WERE THE MEDICAL ASSISTANT

Kathy Anderson, medical assistant to Dr. Hughes, is taking vital signs and preparing Shelby Curran, a 40-year-old woman, for a physical examination. Kathy has just taken Shelby Curran's blood pressure and obtained a value of 144/96.

Ms. Curran: How was my pressure?
Kathy: It was 144/96.
Ms. Curran: About 100 is normal, isn't it?

Questions

1. Does Shelby Curran appear to understand the meaning of her blood pressure measurement? Give reasons for your answer.

2. Is Ms. Curran's systolic blood pressure within normal limits for adults of her age? Identify the normal range of systolic pressure.

3. Is Ms. Curran's diastolic blood pressure within normal limits for adults of her age? Identify the normal range of diastolic pressure.

4. In your own words, describe what both the systolic and diastolic blood pressure measurements mean.

5. How should Kathy respond to Ms. Curran's question?

 ## CRITICAL THINKING QUESTIONS

1. Make a chart to compare methods of taking temperature by the oral, aural, rectal, and axillary routes, for the following age groups:

    infants
    children under age 5
    school-age children
    adolescents
    adults (including the elderly).

    Compare the various routes for safety, accuracy, ease of obtaining measurement, and cost of equipment.

2. In what situations would you avoid taking an oral temperature? A rectal temperature?

3. If a patient refuses to allow you to measure her weight, what would you do?

4. Identify situations that might occur in the medical office that would result in temporary elevations of heart rate, respiratory rate, and/or blood pressure. What should the medical assistant do if he or she thinks that such a situation is occurring to a patient?

5. Why might the doctor ask you to teach a patient to measure his or her pulse at home? Take and record his or her blood pressure?

6. Discuss with your classmates the information you would have to provide to teach a patient to monitor blood pressure at home. What equipment would you recommend? How would you schedule teaching sessions?

 ## EXPLORE THE WEB

INTERNET WEB SITES

American Heart Association
www.americanheart.org/hbp

Hypertension Network
www.bloodpressure.com

National Heart, Lung & Blood Institute
www.nhlbi.gov

KEYWORDS FOR INTERNET SEARCHES

blood pressure
    fever
        hypertension

ANSWERS TO ON THE JOB

1. It is not necessary to measure the height of an established patient for a sick visit.

2. Although many offices measure the weight of each patient on every visit, nothing in the patient's symptoms makes a weight measurement necessary.

3. Because Mr. Caswell is breathing through his mouth, an oral temperature will be inaccurate; he cannot keep his mouth closed around the thermometer. A tympanic, rectal, or axillary temperature could be measured for this patient.

4. A rectal temperature is the most accurate, but most offices do not like to take rectal temperatures on adults. A tympanic temperature is the best method for this situation, because it is more accurate and can be taken more quickly than an axillary temperature.

5. This patient reports chills, which may indicate that he has a fever.

Chapter 16

Assisting with the Patient Examination

Instructional Objectives

After completing this chapter, you will be able to do the following:

1. Define and spell the vocabulary words for this chapter.
2. List and describe six methods of examination used by doctors when performing a physical examination.
3. List the essential parts of a physical examination.
4. Identify and state the function of the instruments and supplies used for the physical examination.
5. Describe the proper preparation of the patient for the physical examination.
6. Identify and describe the following examination positions: erect, sitting, supine, lithotomy, dorsal recumbent, Sims' position, prone, knee-chest, Fowler's, and semi-Fowler's.
7. Describe the responsibilities of the medical assistant during the physical exam.
8. Discuss the special instructions that must be given to a patient before a Pap smear is taken.
9. Describe the procedure for assisting with a pelvic examination with a Pap smear.
10. Identify the instruments and equipment used for a Pap smear and pelvic examination.
11. List the information that should be included on a laboratory requisition when sending a specimen for cytologic examination.
12. Describe the procedure for a rectal examination.
13. Describe the procedure for measuring visual acuity at a measured distance.
14. Explain the significance of the numbers used to describe visual acuity.
15. Discuss measures to test color perception and near-distance vision.
16. Identify measures to test hearing acuity.
17. Describe the procedure for assisting a doctor to examine the rectum.
18. Discuss measures to examine the rectum and sigmoid colon.
19. Describe the procedure for testing stool for occult blood.

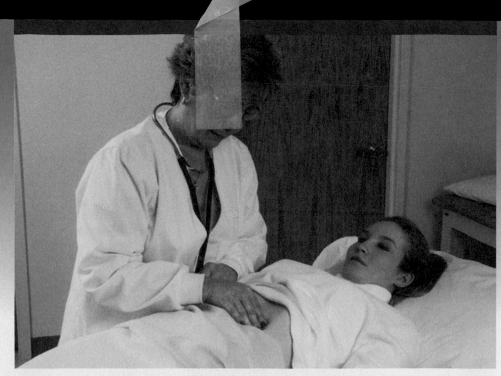

(From Kinn ME, Woods M: *The Medical Assistant, Administrative and Clinical,* 8th ed. Philadelphia: W.B. Saunders, 1999)

Performance Objectives

After completing this chapter you will be able to do the following:

1. Prepare the equipment and the patient for the physical examination, and assist the doctor with the physical examination (Procedure 16–1).
2. Prepare the equipment and the patient for a Pap test and pelvic examination, and assist the doctor with the examination (Procedure 16–2).
3. Measure visual acuity using a Snellen chart (Procedure 16–3).
4. Assess color vision using a book with Ishihara plates (Procedure 16–4).
5. Measure hearing using a manual audiometer, and record results (Procedure 16–5).
6. Test stool for occult blood (Procedure 16–6).
7. Set up for a flexible sigmoidoscopy, and assist the doctor with the examination (Procedure 16–7).

VOCABULARY

audiometer (p. 327)
auscultation (p. 308)
blood chemistry (p. 315)
bruit (p. 309)
carcinoma in situ (p. 325)
cerumen (p. 327)
cervical intraepithelial
    neoplasia (p. 325)
cytology (p. 320)
decibel (p. 327)
differential diagnosis (p. 320)

dysplasia (p. 325)
electrocardiogram (p. 316)
endoscope (p. 333)
guaiac (p. 333)
hernia (p. 310)
hyperopia (p. 325)
inspection (p. 308)
manipulation (p. 309)
menopause (p. 321)
mensuration (p. 309)
myopia (p. 325)

obturator (p. 333)
occluder (p. 326)
occult blood (p. 333)
palpation (p. 308)
percussion (p. 308)
postmenopausal (p. 323)
postpartum (p. 323)
presbyopia (p. 326)
quadrant (p. 310)
rales (p. 309)
refraction (p. 325)

rhonchi (p. 309)
speculum (p. 310)
spirometry (p. 316)
squamous cell carcinoma
    (p. 325)
squamous intraepithelial lesion
    (p. 325)
urinalysis (p. 315)
visual acuity (p. 325)

ABBREVIATIONS

CBC (p. 315)
CIN (p. 325)
dB (p. 327)

ECG (p. 316)
EKG (p. 316)
ENT (p. 327)

HEENT (p. 309)
LMP (p. 321)

OD (p. 326)
OS (p. 326)

OU (p. 326)
PERRLA (p. 309)

SIL (p. 325)
UA (p. 315)

During the course of the physical examination of the patient, which may include one or more diagnostic tests, the medical assistant will be asked to assist the doctor in many different ways. This chapter is designed to help the medical assisting student understand how best to assist the doctor, to improve efficiency of the exam, and to support the patient. Of course, each doctor has his or her own preferences for what assistance should be provided, and these preferences can only be learned on the job. But the more the medical assistant is able to anticipate the doctor's needs, the easier the doctor's job is.

THE PHYSICAL EXAMINATION

Purpose and Description

The physical examination is a systematic examination of the body, from head to toe. Its purpose is for the doctor to gather data from actually examining all parts of the patient's body. It is usually performed after the patient's vital signs, height, and weight have been obtained and after the medical history has been reviewed.

A physical examination requires the patient to be undressed, wearing a gown. Special equipment is required, and the patient needs to be placed in particular positions for the doctor to conduct the exam. The doctor uses six particular means to conduct the exam:

1. inspection
2. palpation
3. percussion
4. auscultation
5. mensuration
6. manipulation.

Inspection

Inspection is the visual observation of the body and its parts, including color, shape, rashes, scars, swelling, or injuries.

Palpation

Palpation is use of the fingers and hands to feel or touch body parts or organs. Palpation is used especially on the extremities, the abdomen, and the pelvic area.

Figure 16–1 shows examination of the abdomen using palpation.

Percussion

Percussion is the tapping of the body with an instrument or the fingers (by placing two fingers of one hand on the part and tapping on the fingers with the other hand). Percussion using fingers is used to determine hollowness, as of the lungs or abdomen. The percussion hammer is used to test reflexes of the arms, legs, and feet.

Auscultation

Auscultation is listening with a stethoscope and is used in examining the heart, lungs, and abdomen.

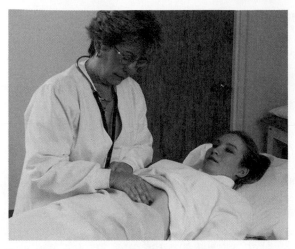

> ➤ **Figure 16–1** The doctor palpates the abdomen using gentle pressure of the hand. (From Kinn ME, Woods M: *The Medical Assistant: Administrative and Clinical,* 8th ed. Philadelphia: W.B. Saunders, 1999.)

Mensuration

Mensuration is measuring height, weight, blood pressure, temperature, head circumference, chest circumference, and leg or ankle diameter, to determine changes in measurements.

Manipulation

Manipulation is the passive movement of body parts to determine range of motion.

Essential Parts of the Physical Examination

The physical exam usually has nine parts. The exam begins with a general visual overview, then proceeds to body systems and regions, working from the top to bottom, leaving the extremities (arms and legs) for last. These nine parts include:

1. general
2. HEENT (head, eyes, ears, nose, and throat)
3. neck
4. chest
5. breast exam
6. abdomen
7. genitalia
8. rectum
9. extremities.

Sometimes skin is included with each section, or it may be examined separately. Sometimes the doctor does not examine areas of the patient that do not affect the chief complaint on an initial visit, preferring to wait for a scheduled physical exam.

On the physical exam report form, the medical assistant documents height, weight, vital signs, and blood pressure. He or she also documents the results of vi-sion and/or audiometric testing, which will be discussed in greater detail later in the chapter. The remainder of the exam is performed by the primary care provider (doctor, nurse practitioner, or physician assistant).

General

The doctor looks at the patient's general appearance, including how the patient walks (gait), posture, stature, nutritional status, appearance of the skin, speech pattern, and hair distribution.

HEENT

HEENT stands for head, eyes, ears, nose, and throat. First the doctor looks for suspect blemishes on the head and face. Examination of the eyes includes examining the retina and optic disk with an ophthalmoscope. The doctor also looks at external eye movement and pupils, which should be equal in size, round, and equally reactive to light and accomodation (**PERRLA**). The ear exam consists of looking at the eardrum (tympanic membrane) with an otoscope, to see if there is fluid behind the ear or a buildup of cerumen (wax). This is done with the otoscope with the ear speculum attached. Examination of the mouth, using a tongue depressor, includes looking at the gums, teeth, palate, and throat.

Neck

The neck examination looks for ease of motion (suppleness), as well as lumps and swelling. Using the stethoscope, the doctor listens over the carotid artery for **bruit** (pronounced brew ee: a rushing or blowing sound that can indicate narrowing due to atherosclerosis). The doctor also feels the thyroid gland for enlargement or nodules at rest and as the patient swallows.

Chest

A chest exam includes visual inspection for abnormalities, and palpation for swelling or masses, especially in the armpits. The doctor percusses the chest, listening for a hollow sound; if the sound is dull there may be fluid in the lungs. The doctor also listens to breath sounds from the back, where he or she may hear **rales** (small crackling sounds) or **rhonchi** (rattling sounds), then listens to the heart from the front. Any abnormal heart sounds may be caused by abnormalities in valves, holes in the heart, or arrhythmia.

Breast Examination

Breasts are examined for symmetry (similar size and shape). Each breast and armpit is examined for masses and for discharge from the nipples.

Abdomen

The doctor inspects the abdomen for visual abnormalities. Then he or she listens for bowel sounds, using the stethoscope; bowel sounds should include gurgling and high-pitched noises, and the stethoscope should pick up sounds of blood flow through abdominal blood vessels. The doctor also palpates each **quadrant** (quarter) of the abdomen. The naval is considered the midpoint, with right and left quadrants above and below. This palpation can reveal guarding (muscle tension to avoid pain), tenderness, masses, or increased size of internal organs. Percussion is also used to identify the size and location of internal organs.

Genitalia

The male genital exam consists of an examination of the penis and testes for discharge or masses and insertion of a gloved finger into the inguinal ring to assess for **hernia** (protrusion of an organ through the wall of the cavity that normally holds it, in this case protrusion of the intestine through the inguinal ring). The inguinal ring is the remains of the opening through which the testes descended from the abdomen into the testes.

The female genital exam will be discussed in detail later in this chapter.

Rectum

A rectal exam consists of insertion of a gloved finger into the rectum to palpate for masses and hemorrhoids. In examining a male, the doctor will also palpate the prostate gland, looking for enlargement or masses. In examining a female, the doctor also checks for herniation of the rectum through the rectal wall, a condition known as a rectocele. Stool on the glove is used for testing for the presence of occult (hidden) blood.

Extremities

The doctor looks for poor circulation, especially of the ankles or feet; this is done by feeling for temperature, looking at color, observing any swelling, and possibly listening with the stethoscope for blood flow in the vessels. The doctor also checks for strength of hands, arms, and legs; coordination; range of motion (ROM); and a person's ability to move an extremity in all normal ways. Reflexes are tested using the percussion hammer.

Instruments and Supplies

A number of instruments and supplies are needed for the physical examination. The medical assistant is responsible for making sure all are available before the examination begins.

General

For the general exam, two items are necessary: the gooseneck lamp or headlight, and the tape measure.

The lamp provides proper lighting for the doctor, and the tape measure is used to measure head circumference (in infants), calf circumference (a common site of swelling), and the size of the liver if necessary.

HEENT

For the HEENT exam, the doctor needs a number of instruments.

To examine the ears, the doctor needs an otoscope and an ear **speculum** (plural specula: an instrument to view). Ear specula are the tips for the end of the otoscope, which are either disposable or disinfected after each use. To examine the eyes, the doctor needs an ophthalmoscope. Figure 16–2 shows a wall-mounted ophthalmoscope and otoscope, with specula.

The same scope without attachment can be used to look in the nose and throat, or a penlight or flashlight can be used to examine the nose and throat. A nasal speculum of the appropriate size, shown in Figure 16–3, is used to examine the nose.

Also, a head mirror or other light source is used to examine the throat, as is a tongue depressor. If the larynx is being examined, a laryngeal mirror allows the doctor to see the vocal cords.

A tuning fork, as shown in Figure 16–4, is used to do a hearing test.

Chest and Abdomen

For the chest and abdomen, the only piece of equipment necessary is a stethoscope.

Rectal Examination

For the rectal exam, the doctor needs an exam glove and lubricant, a gel that reduces friction of the glove against the sensitive rectal tissue.

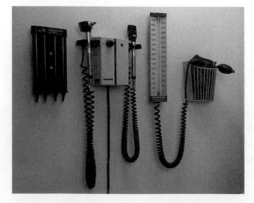

➤ **Figure 16–2** Most exam rooms contain a wall-mounted opthalmoscope and otoscope with ear specula.

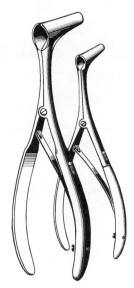

➤ **Figure 16–3** A nasal speculum of the appropriate size is used to examine the nose. (Courtesy of Sklar Instruments, West Chester, PA)

Extremities

The doctor needs a percussion hammer, as shown in Figure 16–5, to test reflexes in the extremities.

Preparing the Patient for the Physical Examination

After the medical assistant has taken vital signs and reviewed the medical history form, he or she must prepare the patient to be seen by the doctor. Some doctors complete the history before the patient undresses; others do both the history and physical exam after the patient has undressed.

The medical assistant should place a fresh gown (either a laundered cloth gown or a disposable paper gown) on the exam table, and instruct the patient how to put the gown on after he or she has undressed. A step stool or the pull-out exam-table step should be put in place for the patient to safely get onto the exam table after changing into the gown. Usually the patient is instructed to leave the gown open in the back, but for some examinations the doctor may prefer the opening to be in the front.

For a complete physical exam, the medical assistant instructs the patient to remove all clothing, including underwear, and put on a gown. Then the patient should sit on the end of the exam table, with a drape over his or her lap and legs.

Depending on the doctor and the patient, the medical assistant may or may not be present during the physical exam. If the medical assistant is present, she or he may assist the patient to assume various positions, as well as assist the doctor by providing certain equipment and supplies when requested.

When a medical doctor is examining a female pa-

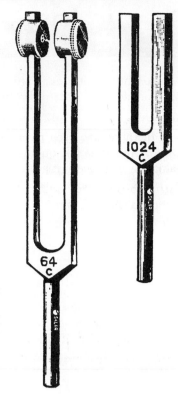

➤ **Figure 16–4** Tuning forks are used to test hearing. (Courtesy of Sklar Instruments, West Chester, PA).

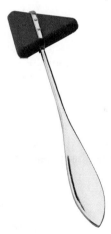

➤ **Figure 16–5** Percussion hammer used to test reflexes during the physical examination.

tient, it is recommended that he always have a female medical assistant present for the pelvic exam, so there can be no question of improper conduct by the doctor.

Positions Used for the Physical Examination

During the course of the physical exam, the doctor may ask the patient to move into one of a number of positions. The six most common positions are:

1. sitting
2. supine

ON THE JOB

Sandra Morse, the medical assistant at Blackburn Primary Care Associates, is preparing John Hilton, a 35-year-old male patient of Dr. Lopez, for his annual physical examination.

QUESTIONS

1. Sandra needs to be sure that Dr. Lopez has all equipment and supplies necessary to perform this examination. What equipment should be present in the exam room? What additional equipment or supplies should Sandra prepare for Dr. Lopez?
2. What instructions should Sandra give to Mr. Hilton after she has taken vital signs? What supplies should she give him?
3. Will Sandra usually be present when Dr. Lopez performs the physical exam? Why or why not?

3. semi-Fowler's position
4. dorsal recumbent position
5. Sims' or left lateral position
6. lithotomy position.

Other, less common positions the doctor may request that the patient move into include:

1. prone
2. standing
3. knee-chest.

The Trendelenburg position is used to improve blood flow to the brain or to prevent swelling in the legs. It is rarely used for the actual examination.

Sitting

The patient sits on the end of the table for the HEENT and chest exams. The drape is over the patient's knees, as shown in Figure 16–6. Reflexes are also usually tested in this position. Testing reflexes is shown in Figure 16–7.

(Note: The drape in the following photographs is transparent so students can see the patient and the proper position of the drape. However, in the office setting, opaque drapes that cannot be seen through are used.)

Supine

The patient lies on his or her back for the abdominal exam. As the patient lies back, the medical assistant (or doctor) raises the exam table extension so the patient's legs are supported. Before the patient lies down, the drape should be repositioned so it continues to cover the patient's legs, as well as the lower abdomen. The doctor will raise the gown to examine the abdomen, and the drape will cover the genital area. The doctor will lower the gown to examine the breasts. Figure 16–8 shows the supine position. While the patient is supine, the doctor also tests reflexes in the feet and the strength of the lower extremities.

Semi-Fowler's

A patient who is short of breath and/or has cardiac (heart) problems may find it difficult to breathe in the supine position. For such a patient, semi-Fowler's position can be used. The head of the exam table can be raised 45 degrees, with the table extension supporting

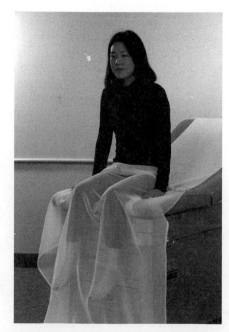

➤ **Figure 16–6** Sitting position.

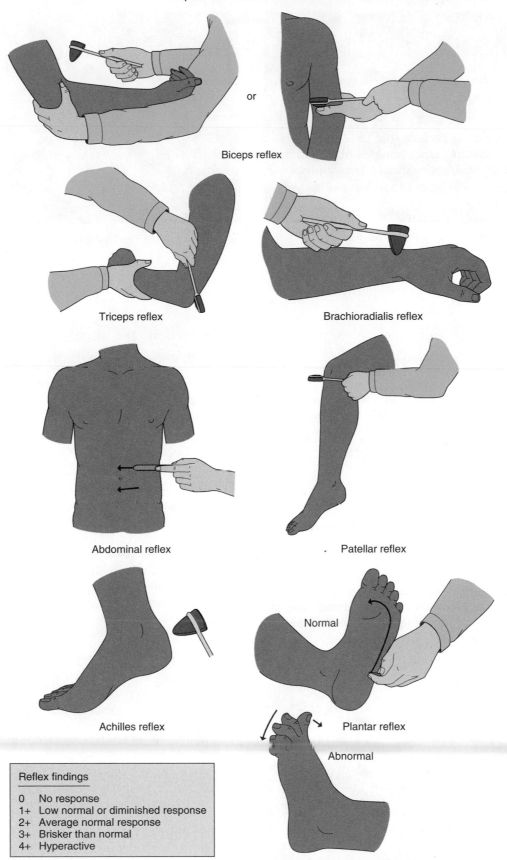

or

Biceps reflex

Triceps reflex

Brachioradialis reflex

Abdominal reflex

Patellar reflex

Achilles reflex

Normal

Plantar reflex

Abnormal

Reflex findings

0	No response
1+	Low normal or diminished response
2+	Average normal response
3+	Brisker than normal
4+	Hyperactive

➢ **Figure 16–7** Testing reflexes. (From Leahy J, Kizilay P: *Foundations of Nursing Practice*. Philadelphia: W.B. Saunders, 1998.)

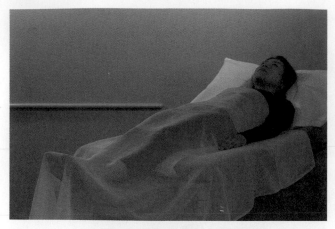

➤ **Figure 16–8** Supine position.

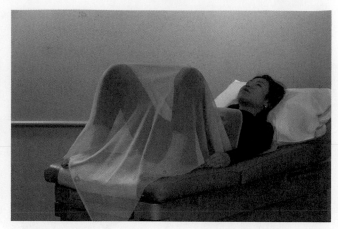

➤ **Figure 16–10** Dorsal recumbent position.

the legs, as shown in Figure 16–9. (When the head is up 90 degrees and the knees are extended, the position is called Fowler's position.)

A patient in need of being examined in semi-Fowler's position may be placed in this position as soon as he or she is brought into the exam room, because the additional support it provides the patient's body is less tiring. The drape is placed over the patient's legs and lower abdomen.

Dorsal Recumbent

In the dorsal recumbent position, the patient lies on his or her back with knees bent and feet on the end of the exam table. This position can be used for the rectal exam, or the rectal exam may be included with the examination of genitalia in another position (lithotomy for females, standing or bent over the exam table for males). The drape covers the legs and lower abdomen, and is raised by the doctor to examine the genitalia

and/or rectum. The dorsal recumbent position is shown in Figure 16–10. The medical assistant may be asked to squeeze a little lubricant onto the index finger of the doctor's gloved hand. The medical assistant can also give the patient a tissue after the rectal exam to wipe away excess lubricant.

Sims', or Left Lateral

For better access to the rectal area and lower back, the patient may get into Sims' position. The patient should be instructed to turn over onto the stomach from the supine position and bend the right knee up to almost 90 degrees. A medical assistant can stand so the patient turns toward her or him (for safety) and can hold the drape behind the patient's buttocks, allowing it to fall over the patient's lower body once he or she has turned over. Sims' position is shown in Figure 16–11.

Lithotomy

The patient lies on her back, with her feet in stirrups. The drape covers the lower abdomen and legs, and is lifted by the doctor to examine the female genitalia and pelvis. Just before the exam, the patient is instructed to move down toward the foot of the table until her buttocks reach the end of the table. The lithotomy position is shown in Figure 16–12.

Other Positions

Three other positions may be used for special examinations or for special patient needs.

Prone. The patient is on his or her abdomen, with legs extended. This position, shown in Figure 16–13, allows the doctor the best view of the back or the back of the legs.

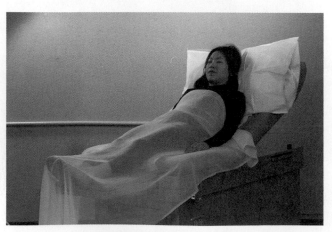

➤ **Figure 16–9.** Semi-Fowler's position.

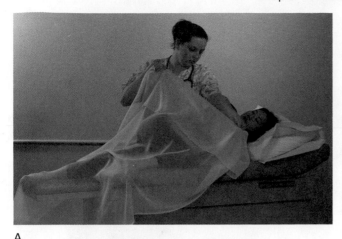

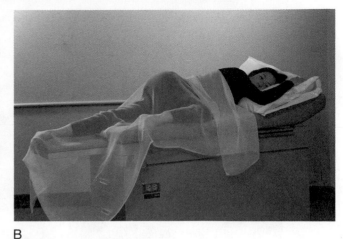

A

B

> **Figure 16–11** (A) Patient turning to Sims' position with medical assistant holding drape. (B) Patient in Sims' position.

Standing. This position is used to check balance and may be used for male testicular, hernia, and rectal exams.

Knee-Chest. The patient stands on the step of the exam table or a step stool, then kneels on the end of the exam table and bends forward to support his or her weight on the chest, elbows, and arms. If the patient holds the drape behind his or her back while getting into the position, the drape covers the back and buttocks until the examination begins. This position, shown in Figure 16–14, is used to examine the anus and rectum.

Trendelenburg. The patient lies on his or her back with head lower than the body. This position is used for patients with hypotension or patients in shock, to increase blood pressure. A modified position, using the examination table, is shown in Figure 16–15. In an emergency, a treatment table might be raised at one end using wooden blocks or even books, so the patient can lie head down. This position would not be used during an examination.

Routine Diagnostic Tests

Several diagnostic tests are done as part of the routine physical examination to screen for common medical problems.

A urine sample is obtained for **urinalysis (UA)**—physical, chemical, and microscopic analysis of the urine. The patient is usually asked to give this sample before the physical examination because it is more comfortable to be examined with an empty bladder.

Routine blood tests include a complete blood count **(CBC)** and **blood chemistry**, a screening test of sev-

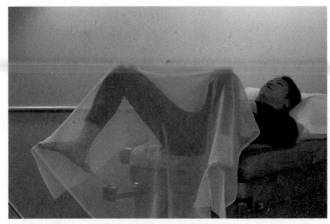

> **Figure 16–12** Lithotomy position.

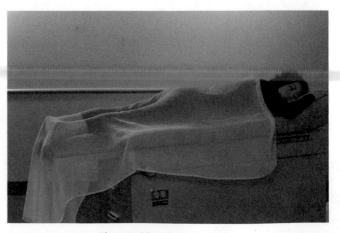

> **Figure 16–13** Prone position.

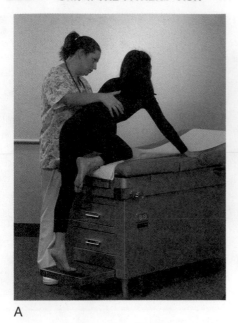

A

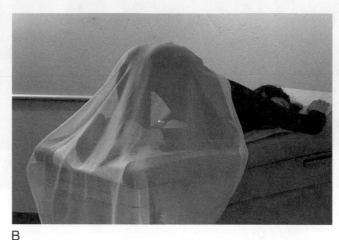

B

➤ **Figure 16–14** (A) Patient getting into knee-chest position. (B) Patient in knee-chest position.

eral chemicals in blood serum (Chem 7 tests for seven such chemicals, Chem 20 for 20 such chemicals). Blood is usually drawn after the physical exam in case the doctor wants additional blood studies beyond the routine, in which case more blood must be taken. Blood must be drawn into particular tubes for different tests. Hematology is covered in Chapter 25. Blood chemistry is discussed in Chapter 26.

Patients receiving employment physicals, patients over age 50, and patients with cardiac disorders usually get an **electrocardiogram** (a test to record the electrical activity of the heart; this test is known as either an **ECG** or an **EKG**).

Patients receiving employment physicals and patients with respiratory disorders such as emphysema and asthma may be given a **spirometry** test to measure breathing.

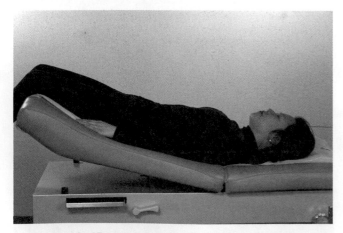

➤ **Figure 16–15** Modified Trendelenburg position, placing a patient with the legs on the raised backrest of an examination table.

It is best if all these tests can be performed before the exam, so the doctor has the results before examining the patient. After the exam, the patient over 40 years old will usually be sent home with additional kits to take stool samples and instructions to return them to the office to be tested for occult blood.

Procedure 16–1 discusses assisting with the physical exam.

The Physical Examination as the Basis for Treatment

After performing the exam, the doctor will either chart in the medical record or dictate a report summarizing findings. Figure 16–16 illustrates an example of a dictated report. At the conclusion of the report, if problems are found, the doctor writes his or her determination of the patient's diagnosis (or diagnoses, if more than one). Different terms are used for this:

Primary diagnosis. —The most important problem
Secondary diagnosis. —Additional problem
Differential diagnosis. —A process of determining which of several conditions the patient has, based on examination and lab tests.

SPECIAL EXAMINATIONS

Special examinations may be part of a complete physical examination performed by a primary care doctor, or may be done by a specialist. The special examinations are:

1. Pap smear and bimanual pelvic exam
2. Examinations of special senses
3. Examination of the rectum and sigmoid colon.

PROCEDURE 16–1

Assisting with the Physical Examination

Performance Objective: The student will prepare the equipment and the patient for a physical examination and will assist the doctor with the physical examination.

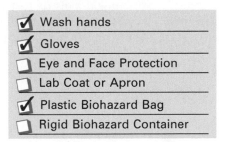

- ☑ Wash hands
- ☑ Gloves
- ☐ Eye and Face Protection
- ☐ Lab Coat or Apron
- ☑ Plastic Biohazard Bag
- ☐ Rigid Biohazard Container

Supplies and Equipment: Scale, thermometer, watch with second hand, stethoscope, sphygmomanometer, gown, drape, ophthalmoscope, otoscope with new or clean ear speculum, tongue depressor, percussion hammer, gloves, lubricant, hemoccult test kit, gauze square, paper towels, and biohazard waste container. The doctor may routinely use additional equipment, such as a tuning fork, nasal speculum, anoscope, tape measure, safety pins, or cotton balls.

Procedural Steps

1. Wash hands.
2. Assemble supplies and equipment.
3. Identify patient.
4. Explain procedure to patient.
5. Instruct the patient to remove shoes and heavy clothing and weigh the patient (Procedure 15–1). Measure the height of a new patient or a child (Procedure 15–2). Record findings.
   Rationale: The height of an established adult patient will already be recorded in the chart.
6. Seat the patient and take vital signs (Procedures 15–3 through 15–12). Select the most appropriate method of taking temperature. Record measurements.
   Rationale: Pulse, respirations, and blood pressure are routinely measured with the patient seated. The medical assistant assesses the patient to decide the most appropriate way to measure temperature and other vital signs.
7. Perform vision and hearing screening tests if needed (see Procedure 16–3).

Rationale: The results of these tests will assist the doctor to assess the patient. Vision testing is routinely done on children. Vision and hearing screening are performed as part of school and employee physical examinations. They may be done at any stage of the physical exam.

8. Review or take the patient history (Procedure 14–1).
   Rationale: The medical assistant goes over the patient history form to be sure it is as complete as possible and to help the patient organize information.
9. Instruct the patient how to obtain a urine specimen, label a urine specimen cup with the patient's name, give it to the patient, and bring the patient to the bathroom. If there is a window to pass the specimen to the lab, show the patient how to do this. Otherwise instruct the patient where to leave the specimen.
   Rationale: The physical examination will be most comfortable for the patient with an empty bladder. Urinalysis (physical, chemical, and microscopic examination of the urine) is considered part of the physical examination. You do not need to wear gloves to label the specimen cup before it is used but should wear gloves to handle the specimen cup after the specimen has been obtained.
10. Bring the patient back to the exam room and instruct him or her to remove all clothing, put on a gown, and sit on the end of the exam table when ready to be examined. Leave the room to provide privacy. Assist the patient if necessary.
    Rationale: Patients prefer to undress in privacy. The medical assistant assesses the patient's ability to be left alone and get on the exam table safely.
11. Perform an electrocardiogram if needed (Procedure 18–1).
    Rationale: The electrocardiogram is done for all patients with cardiac complaints and is usually part of the physical exam for patients over age 40. The chest must be bare for this exam. If done before the doctor examines the patient, the results will be available to help the doctor assess the patient.

Procedure continued on following page

PROCEDURE 16–1 *(continued)*

12. When the patient is again sitting on the exam table, place a drape sheet over the patient's lap and legs. Notify the doctor that the patient is ready to be examined. Place the medical record outside the exam room for the doctor to review before the exam.
Rationale: Having the patient in the sitting position allows the doctor to begin the exam efficiently. The drape sheet is available to provide privacy during the exam by covering body parts that are not being examined.

13. Assist the doctor during the examination as needed. Hand instruments in the order the doctor expects to use them with the handle toward the doctor. Assist the patient to assume the correct positions. When the doctor needs to dispose of used equipment, position the hazardous waste container so that he or she can reach it easily. Below is a list of equipment that may be used.
Rationale: Handing needed instruments allows the doctor to perform the examination efficiently. Positioning the instrument with the handle toward the doctor allows the doctor to grasp the instrument ready for use.

Position　Part Examined　Instrument

Position	Part Examined	Instrument
Sitting	Head and neck	Stethoscope
	Eyes	Ophthalmoscope, penlight
	Ears	Otoscope with disposable ear speculum, tuning fork
	Nose	Penlight, nasal speculum, substances to smell
	Mouth	Glove, tongue blade, penlight
	Chest	Stethoscope
	Arm reflexes	Percussion hammer
Supine	Abdomen	Stethoscope, tape measure
	Leg reflexes	Percussion hammer
	Sensation	Safety pin, tubes of hot and cold water
Standing	Hernia (male)	Glove
	Prostate (male)	Glove and lubricant
	Rectum (male)	Glove and lubricant
Lithotomy	Pelvis (female)	Gloves, vaginal speculum, slide or ThinPrep solution, cervical brush, cervical spatula, fixative
	Rectum (female)	Glove and lubricant

14. After the examination, assist the patient to sit up and instruct the patient to dress. Leave the room while the patient dresses.
Rationale: Patients prefer to dress in privacy. The medical assistant assesses the patient's need for assistance in dressing.

15. When the patient is dressed, provide any needed instructions and accompany the patient to the front desk.
Rationale: This gives the patient a final opportunity to ask questions and clarify instructions.

16

	VISION				AUDIOMETRIC TESTING			BLOOD PRESSURE		
HEIGHT __5'10"__	Without Glasses				250	500	1000	Sitting		
	Far	R 20/20	L 20/30	R	25dB	25dB	25dB			
WEIGHT __172 lb__	Near	R 20/	L 20/	L	25dB	25dB	25dB	R 126/84	L 122/80	
BUILD _____	With Glasses				2000	4000	8000	Standing		
		R 20/	L 20/	R	25dB	50dB	50dB			
PULSE __80 reg__		R 20/	L 20/	L	25dB	25dB	25dB	R /	L /	
RESP. __16 reg__	Tonometry R _____ L _____							Lying		
	Colorvision __all plates correct__			Gross Hearing _____						
TEMP. __97.8° F__	Peripheral Fields R ____ L ____							R /	L /	

16 For this procedure you will document height, weight, vital signs, results of urinalysis, results of eye tests, results of hearing tests, and/or any part of the procedure you have performed. To avoid forgetting results, it is best to document as you do each procedure and review the chart after the exam to be sure you have not forgotten anything. *Rationale:* The medical record provides the ongoing record of procedures performed and care given to the patient.

17. Before cleaning the exam room put on disposable gloves if body fluids or contaminated equipment are present.

Rationale: Adhere to standard precautions.

18. Discard disposable gown, drape, used table paper, and contaminated supplies or disposable equipment in appropriate biohazard container(s).

19. Remove instruments to the area where they will be cleaned and sterilized.

20. Clean contaminated surfaces with 10:1 household bleach solution and allow to air-dry.

21. Remove gloves and wash hands.

22. Cover exam table with clean paper and prepare exam room for the next patient.

PHYSICAL EXAMINATION

Ivan Shapiro
07/14/00

VITAL SIGNS: Pulse is 88 and regular, respirations 12 and regular, blood pressure 140/94.

GENERAL: This is a well-developed male complaining of chest pain during exercise.

HEENT: Head is normocephalic. PERRLA. Tympanic membranes clear. Nose and throat clear.

NECK: Neck is supple. No carotid bruits noted.

LUNGS: Clear to percussion and auscultation.

HEART: Normal sinus rhythm. Heart appears to be somewhat enlarged.

ABDOMEN: Without masses or tenderness. Bowel sounds normal

EXTREMITIES: No clubbing or cyanosis, but 1+ edema present in both lower extremities. Peripheral pulses intact.

NEUROLOGICAL: Reflexes equal and intact. Appears physiologically intact.

GENITALIA AND RECTAL: Prostate gland soft and slightly enlarged on digital exam.

IMPRESSION: 1. Angina pectoris probably due to ASHD
2. Hypertension
3. Cardiomegaly with possible slight congestive heart failure.

PLAN: 1. Obtain blood work to identify lipid and cholesterol levels.
2. EKG followed by stress test
3. Begin antihypertensive therapy, mod Na restriction, evaluate need for cholesterol lowering medication.
4. Continue workup for cause and control of angina pectoris.

➤ **Figure 16–16** Physical examination report.

DIFFERENTIAL DIAGNOSIS

The procedure called **differential diagnosis** is a determination of the cause and nature of a person's illness, based on comparison of symptoms of two or more similar diseases to determine, by a process of elimination, which disease the patient is suffering from. Engaging in a differential diagnosis is a three-step process.

1. *Interview:* Discussion of the present illness, history, symptoms, and lifestyle factors. The patient's complaints are called symptoms or subjective findings. Subjective means that they are known directly only to the patient (i.e., "my head hurts").
2. *Physical examination:* Examination of the body from the head down, including all body systems that may be relevant to the patient's problems. Observations made by the doctor are called signs, and are considered objective findings. Objective means they can be verified by a person other than the patient (i.e., the skin appears dry and red).
3. *Diagnostic tests:* Examination of specimens from the patient or of parts of the patient's body, using diagnostic procedures.

Based on the subjective data from the interview, the objective data from the physical examination, and the data from diagnostic tests that have been done, the doctor establishes an initial impression of the major manifestations of the patient's problem and all of the things that could possibly be causing the patient's symptoms. We say that the doctor attempts to "rule out" (eliminate as a possible cause) all conditions that the patient does not have, proving that he or she does have some particular condition. This is done through diagnostic testing and trial of various treatments.

For example, Ivan Shapiro comes to see Dr. Hughes because of chest pain he experiences during exercise. On physical examination (as described in Figure 16–16), Dr. Hughes notes that Mr. Shapiro has an enlarged heart, elevated blood pressure, and slightly swollen ankles.

Dr. Hughes orders diagnostic tests to determine if Mr. Shapiro has elevated lipid and cholesterol levels (indications of arteriosclerotic heart disease [ASHD]) and cardiac tests to determine if he is experiencing decreased blood flow to the myocardium at rest and/or during exercise, a common result of ASHD.

She begins to treat his hypertension right away with medication and diet, and after obtaining the results of the other tests, may prescribe cholesterol-lowering medication. If Mr. Shapiro's blood tests reveal a normal lipid profile and do not show elevated cholesterol, Dr. Hughes will return to the diagnostic process to try to find other reasons for his symptoms. Her treatment depends on the diagnosis.

If the cardiac tests show decreased blood flow to the heart, Mr. Shapiro may need medication to dilate the coronary arteries. Or he may need an additional test (cardiac catheterization) to identify the exact location(s) of blockages in the coronary arteries. Each additional test helps refine the differential diagnosis so the doctor can prescribe effective treatment.

PAP SMEAR AND BIMANUAL PELVIC EXAMINATION

With managed care, the trend is for this exam to be included as part of the female patient's physical exam done by the primary care doctor, instead of a separate exam performed by a gynecologist.

The Pap smear is used specifically for diagnosis of cancer of the cervix. It is recommended that the Pap smear be done each year until three consecutive normal Pap smears have been found. After that, the exam may be performed less frequently, depending on the doctor's assessment of the woman's risk of cervical cancer.

For a traditional Pap smear, a doctor collects up to three specimens. The cervical specimen is collected using a cervical spatula. The endocervical specimen is collected using a cervical brush or swab. After a hysterectomy, the vaginal specimen is collected using a spatula. Smears of the specimens are put on one to three slides and sent to a laboratory for examination, looking for cells that are abnormal or cancerous. Because the examination obtains cells, the specimen is sent to a cytology lab (**cytology** means the study of cells).

A recent innovation in Pap tests is the so-called ThinPrep® Pap Test. Instead of using a slide, the cells are placed in a liquid medium to be sent to the lab. The cells may be clearer for the pathologist to examine using this method.

The medical assistant has five specific roles in the Pap smear and bimanual pelvic exam:

1. providing instruction before the test
2. assisting the patient to move into the correct positions
3. assisting with equipment
4. preparing the patient and the lab form
5. assisting with the examination.

Instruction

The medical assistant provides the patient with a set of instructions at the time the appointment is made for a Pap smear or for a full physical exam that will include a Pap smear.

A patient who will undergo a Pap smear may not use a douche or vaginal medication within 24 hours of the test. She may not engage in intercourse for 2 days before the test. And she cannot have the test done if she is menstruating. The appointment should be set for 1 week after the menstrual period.

Position

A Pap smear is usually performed with the patient in the lithotomy position, with feet in stirrups. It may be done in the dorsal recumbent position. The patient wears a full gown and is covered by a drape. Because the breasts are usually examined at the same time, the patient must be completely undressed.

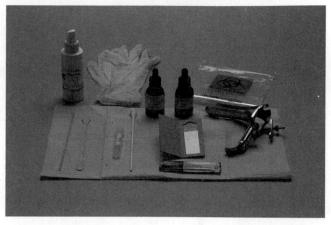

➢ **Figure 16–18** Equipment used for the Pap test and pelvic examination.

Equipment

Necessary equipment includes a gown and drape, a light source for the doctor, a vaginal speculum, water-soluble lubricant, gloves, slide or ThinPrep® solution, fixative, spatula, and swab or cervical brush.

Equipment should be prepared either on the counter near the exam table, in the drawer, or on a special cart that can be wheeled from room to room. This depends on the doctor's preference or on office procedure. Figure 16–17 shows a vaginal speculum used for the exam. An appropriate size should be chosen (small for girls or teens, extra large for women who have had multiple deliveries). Figure 16–18 shows equipment necessary for the Pap test and pelvic exam.

Preparation of Patient and Form

The cytology lab form, shown in Figure 16–19, is usually filled out before the exam so information can be obtained during the patient interview.

The medical assistant needs to ask the patient for the date of the first day of her last menstrual period **(LMP)** and her age. If the patient's LMP is not within the past month, the patient must be asked if she is pregnant or has gone through **menopause** (end of menstrual activity), and the appropriate box needs to be filled. The medical assistant also needs to note if the patient is on hormonal therapy—either birth control pills or estrogen replacement—if the patient has had previous surgical treatment of the cervix, and if the previous Pap smear was normal or abnormal. The patient's name is written in pencil on the end of the slide for identification.

The patient is asked to undress completely, put on a gown, and sit on the end of the exam table with the drape across her legs.

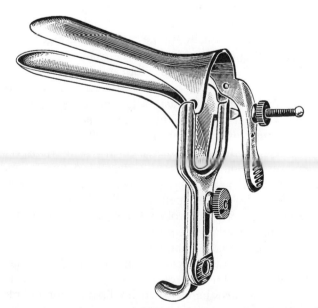

➢ **Figure 16–17** Vaginal specula come in various sizes. (Courtesy of Sklar Instruments, West Chester, PA)

CYTOLOGY REQUISITION   Please Print Clearly

PATIENT INFORMATION

Name_____   Medical Record #_____   Sex M____ F____
         Last Name   First Name   Initial

Birthdate _____   Social Security #_____   Phone _____

Address _____

       _____

       _____

Physician ___Blackburn Primary Care Associates_____

         ___1990 Turquoise Drive, Blackburn WI 54937_____

SPECIMEN

_____ Cervical   _____ Vaginal   _____ Vaginal with M.I.   _____ Endo Cervical   _____ Biopsy

_____ Fluid/Washing/Brushing   _____ Fine Needle   _____ Buccal   _____ Other

Source _____

Pre-Op DX _____

CLINICAL INFORMATION/REASON FOR PAP

Date collected _____   Date of LMP _____

Previous smear (Assession #/Date) _____

_____ Screening for CA Cervix _____ Hysterectomy _____ Post Abortion _____ Laser RX _____ PMB

_____ Spotting _____ Post Menopausal _____ Previous Abnormal _____ Radiation RX _____ Cervicitis

_____ Pregnant _____ Hormone Rx _____ Cervical Dysplasia _____ Chemo RX _____ STD

_____ Post Partum _____ BCP's _____ Cryotherapy _____ DES exposure _____ Smoker

_____ Nursing _____ IUD _____ Conization _____ Yeast Candida

➤ **Figure 16–19** The lab slip must be completed to accompany the Pap test.

Examination

The female genital exam has three parts. The Pap smear is performed first, followed by the bimanual pelvic exam, and finally by the rectal exam. Figure 16–20 shows the doctor performing the exam.

For the Pap smear, no lubricant is used on the vaginal speculum, which may be disposable plastic or metal. Metal specula must be sterilized between patients. A metal speculum may be warmed for comfort by keeping it on a heating pad in the drawer.

As soon as the doctor has finished placing the specimens on the slide, spray the slide with a fixative and allow to air-dry. If the doctor performs the ThinPrep procedure, hold the open container into which the doctor will insert the cytology brush or swab.

During the taking of specimens, the medical assistant may be asked to hand instruments to the doctor. Instruments should be picked up with the handle facing the doctor for him or her to grasp. The medical assistant may also be asked to hold a light or redirect the angle of a gooseneck lamp.

It the doctor suspects any vaginal infection, he or she will collect and culture a smear for analysis. If an

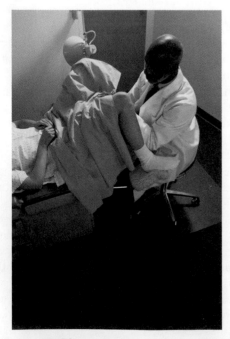

➤ **Figure 16–20** The doctor performing a Pap test.

active infection is clearly present, the doctor may prefer to treat the condition before doing the Pap test.

For the bimanual pelvic exam, the doctor uses water-soluble lubricant on gloves. He or she inserts two fingers of the gloved hand into the vagina and uses the other hand on the abdomen to feel the ovaries and uterus, palpating for masses and/or abnormal position.

Procedure 16–2 discusses assisting with the Pap test and pelvic exam.

For the rectal exam, the doctor then places one gloved finger in the rectum to feel for hemorrhoids, fissures, and possible herniation of the rectum through the rectal wall into the vagina (rectocele). If the doctor needs more information about the pelvic organs, he or

---

PROCEDURE 16–2

Assisting with the Pap Test and Pelvic Examination

Performance Objective: The student will prepare the equipment and the patient for a Pap test and pelvic examination and will assist the doctor with the examination.

- ☑ Wash hands
- ☑ Gloves
- ☐ Eye and Face Protection
- ☐ Lab Coat or Apron
- ☑ Plastic Biohazard Bag
- ☐ Rigid Biohazard Container

Supplies and Equipment: Gloves, water-soluble lubricant, tissues, patient gown, drape, vaginal speculum, slide and fixative or ThinPrep® transport solution, cytobrush, vaginal spatula, and cotton-tipped applicators (or broom-type cervical sampling device for ThinPrep® test).

Procedure Steps

1. Wash hands.
2. Assemble supplies and equipment. The equipment and supplies may be arranged in the examination table drawer, on a table, on a counter, or on a Mayo stand near the examination table. Position the light source so that it can easily be adjusted. Position the stirrups about 6″ to 12″ from the end of the examination table and angled slightly outward if possible.
   Rationale: The doctor will expect to find equipment and supplies in a customary position.
3. Identify patient.
4. Explain procedure to patient.
5. Instruct the patient to empty her bladder. Obtain a urine specimen if required.
   Rationale: This examination is most com-

fortable for the patient if the bladder is empty.

6. Fill out the lab slip for the cytology lab, including date of last menstrual period (LMP) or if the patient is pregnant, **postpartum** (having recently had a baby), or **postmenopausal** (no longer menstruating). Include any treatment with hormones, such as birth control pills or estrogen. In addition, include previous Pap smear results or surgery or treatment for cervical cancer.
   Rationale: The lab slip requires information that may not be found in the patient's medical record. It is usually easier to obtain this information before the examination, filling in the lab slip at the same time.
7. If the doctor performs a breast exam with the pelvic examination, instruct the patient to undress completely. For a pelvic exam without breast exam, the patient should undress from the waist down. In both cases the patient should put on a gown with the opening in the back.
8. Instruct the patient to sit on the end of the examination table with a drape over her lap after she is undressed.
9. Leave the room while the patient undresses.
   Rationale: Patients prefer to undress in privacy. The medical assistant assesses the patient's ability to be left alone and get on the exam table safely.
10. When the doctor is ready to perform the examination, assist the patient to the lithotomy position. Place the drape so that it covers the patient's legs. Tell her to place her feet in the stirrups and slide down to the end of the table. Be sure the drape covers her legs completely.
    Rationale: The optimal position for the examination brings the patient's buttocks to the very edge of the table. The drape is used to provide privacy until the examination begins.

Procedure continued on following page

PROCEDURE 16–2 *(continued)*

11. Prepare to assist the doctor as needed. This may include adjusting the light source, handing instruments or supplies, and raising the lid of the biohazard waste container. If the doctor does not want assistance, stand beside the patient and offer support or speak quietly with the patient. If the patient seems uncomfortable, you can instruct her to breathe evenly and deeply.
    Rationale: The individual preferences of each doctor must be respected. Many women find this examination embarrassing and sometimes uncomfortable. Focusing on beathing may serve as a distraction; deep breaths may reduce discomfort.

12. Before a breast examination, assist the patient to untie the gown and remove her arms to expose the breasts. After the breast examination assist the patient to put her arms back into the gown.
    Rationale: For warmth and privacy, only the area actually being examined is exposed.

13. For the Pap test, the doctor inserts a vaginal speculum made of metal or disposable plastic without lubricant. Metal speculums are sometimes stored on a heating pad to warm them for patient comfort.
    Rationale: Lubricant cannot be used because it affects test results. A warm metal speculum is more comfortable on insertion than a cold one.

14. The doctor may use one to three slides for the Pap smear. Mark the slide(s) with the patient's name or clinic number before use. Spray the slide(s) with fixative immediately or place in a fixative solution immediately. If the doctor uses the ThinPrep® method, the cytobrush and spatula (or broom-type collection device) are placed into the vial containing transport solution and rotated at least ten times before the collection implement is removed and discarded.
    Rationale: Cells must be preserved with fixative while alive (within seconds) for adequate examination by the pathology lab.

15. Be sure the doctor has a container easily accessible to receive a used metal vaginal speculum or a biohazard waste container for a disposable speculum.
    Rationale: Contaminated equipment must be kept separate from clean equipment to prevent the spread of infection.

16. Apply water-soluble lubricant to the doctor's gloved fingers.
    Rationale: Lubricant facilitates entry of the doctor's fingers into the vagina for the bi-manual pelvic examination. The doctor will palpate the abdominal organs against the fingers in the vagina to feel the uterus, vagina, and ovaries. Immediately after the pelvic examination, the doctor may progress to a rectal examination and obtain a stool specimen to be examined for occult blood (Procedure 16–6).

17. After the examination, assist the patient to remove her feet from the stirrups and sit up. Offer tissues and a sanitary pad if needed.
    Rationale: The patient may wish to remove excess lubricant from the perineal area.

18. Instruct the patient to dress and provide privacy unless the patient needs assistance.
    Rationale: Patients prefer to dress in privacy. The medical assistant assesses the patient's need for assistance in dressing.

19. Put on disposable gloves to handle slides, culture tubes and/or vials containing transport medium. Slides must air-dry for 10 to 15 minutes. Place any specimen in a plastic container for transport to the lab.
    Rationale: Gloves prevent contact with microorganisms that may be on smears or in cultures. Plastic bags prevent contact with body secretions during transport.

20. When the patient is dressed, provide any needed instructions and accompany the patient to the front desk.
    Rationale: This gives the patient a final opportunity to ask questions and clarify instructions.

21. Before cleaning the exam room put on disposable gloves if body fluids or contaminated equipment are present.
    Rationale: Adhere to standard precautions.

22. Discard disposable gown, drape, used table paper, and contaminated supplies or disposable equipment in appropriate biohazard container(s).

23. Remove instruments to the area where they will be cleaned and sterilized.

24. Clean contaminated surfaces with 10:1 household bleach solution and allow to air-dry.

25. Remove gloves and wash hands.

26. Cover exam table with clean paper and prepare exam room for the next patient.

27. Complete all lab slips, including those for any cultures for gonorrhea, chlamydia, yeast, or other vaginal infections.

28. Insert lab slips in the pocket of transport bag for pickup or mailing.
    Rationale: Complete lab slips must be sent with all procedures to lab.

she inserts a second gloved finger into the vagina at the same time, then palpates the abdomen again with the other hand.

After the exam, specimens are sent to the appropriate labs, with completed lab forms. Gloves should always be worn when handling slides during collection and preparation for transport.

The Pap smear is sent to the cytology lab. A record is kept in the office to be sure that lab reports are received, and patients are notified if follow-up is needed. (See "Pap Test Results and Recommended Follow-up.")

Vaginal cultures are sent to a microbiology lab. Slides containing vaginal smears may be examined under the microscope by the doctor in the office or may be sent to the lab for analysis. All vaginal specimens should be handled with gloves.

EXAMINATION OF SPECIAL SENSES

This refers to examinations of vision and hearing. The primary care provider is responsible for screening patients for problems with their eyes and ears.

Vision

In addition to examining the interior of the eye with the ophthalmoscope, as seen in Figure 16–21, many offices screen for **visual acuity** (the ability to see clearly) and for color blindness.

Although eye diseases are treated by an ophthalmologist, and corrective lenses are generally prescribed by an optometrist, it is important for primary care doctors to identify any patient who may have vision problems or eye disease. Table 16–1 is a list of common eye diseases and conditions.

Vision screening consists of three parts:

1. measuring distance visual acuity
2. measuring near-distance acuity
3. testing color vision.

Distance Visual Acuity. The ability of the eye's lens to bend light is called **refraction**. If the light rays reach a focal point in front of or behind the retina (the part of the eye where the image is formed), objects will be blurred. This condition is called **myopia** (near-sightedness). If the focal point is behind the retina the condition is called **hyperopia** (farsightedness). Farsightedness is common in young children. (See "Errors of Refraction and Conditions that Can Be Corrected.")

To test distance visual acuity, a patient is asked to read letters, either on a chart on the wall or through a machine. Children or non-English speakers may be asked to tell which way the capital letter E is pointing, and younger children may be asked to identify pictures of common items such as a star or boat. The charts used are called Snellen eye charts, and an example is shown in Figure 16–22.

Pap Test Results and Recommended Follow-up

Pap test results are usually reported according to the Bethesda System, following a 1988 National Cancer Institute-sponsored workshop. This system uses descriptive diagnostic terms instead of Class numbers, which had been used previously. In addition, the cytology report describes the adequacy of the specimen for evaluation.

The following terms may be used to describe abnormal changes in the cells that are seen on the Pap test.

PRECANCEROUS CHANGES

Dysplasia. A term used to describe abnormal (but not cancerous) cells. The cells look abnormal under the microscope but do not invade surrounding tissues. There are three degrees of dysplasia: mild, moderate, and severe.

Squamous intraepithelial lesion (SIL). A term used to describe abnormal changes of the outer cells of the cervix. Low-grade SIL is the term used when the change in the size, shape, and number of cells is early and only affects some cells. High-grade SIL is the term used when there are a large number of precancerous cells, with a marked change in appearance from normal cells.

Cervical intraepithelial neoplasia (CIN). Another term used to describe the presence of abnormal cells from the outer layers of the cervix. Numbers from 1 to 3 are used with the abbreviation CIN to describe the number and appearance of abnormal cells.

Mild dysplasia may be classified as low-grade SIL or CIN 1.

Moderate dysplasia may be classified as high-grade SIL or CIN 2.

Severe dysplasia may be classified as high-grade SIL or CIN 3.

CANCEROUS CHANGES

Carcinoma in situ. Cancerous changes of the surface cells that have not spread to surrounding tissues.

Squamous cell carcinoma. Cancerous changes of the surface that may have invaded the surrounding tissues or spread to distant sites.

Carcinoma in situ may be classified as high-grade SIL or CIN 3.

Abnormal findings on a Pap test indicate that further testing should be done. Additional procedures include colposcopy, cervical biopsy, and cryosurgery (freezing of the cervix).

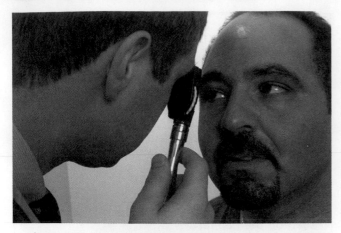

➤ **Figure 16–21** Examining a patient's eyes with an ophthalmoscope.

The medical assistant tests each eye using a device to cover the other eye called an **occluder**. The patient should have both eyes open during testing, because squinting or closing one eye improves vision in the other eye artificially. Procedure 16–3 discusses how to measure distance visual acuity using a Snellen chart.

On the side of a Snellen eye chart are sets of two numbers, one over the other like fractions. The top number is always 20, indicating the number of feet between the chart and the person taking the test (if being done in real space, using a wall chart, or its equivalent if the test is being done using a machine). The bottom number indicates the number of feet away at which a normal eye can see a letter that size.

For instance, the large E at the top of a Snellen chart is labeled 20/200, meaning that the normal eye can see a letter that size at 200 feet. If the bottom number is greater than the top number, it indicates that the individual being tested needs a corrective lens

to be able to see at 20 feet what a normal eye can see at 20 feet. Occasionally, a person has better than normal vision—20/15 or 20/10, meaning that the normal eye would need to be at 15 or 10 feet to see what that person can see at 20 feet.

Legal blindness is defined as vision of 20/200 or worse in both eyes when wearing corrective lenses.

The results of the distance visual acuity test are recorded using the abbreviations **OD** for right eye, **OS** for left eye, and **OU** for both eyes. If the patient reads the letters in a line, the fraction describing the line is given as the measurement. Up to two missed letters may be marked as -1 or -2. If the patient misses more than two letters in a line, record the vision using the fraction of the line above, which the patient was able to read correctly or with only one or two missed letters.

Near-Distance Acuity. As people age, the eyes' lenses become less supple and may focus poorly on near objects. This condition is called **presbyopia** (difficulty with near vision associated with aging). Presbyopia begins to appear in most people between ages 40 and 50.

Near-distance visual acuity can be tested by asking a patient to read letters from a near-distance visual acuity card. Like the Snellen test, each eye is tested separately, and the patient is asked to read until he or she reaches the smallest line that can be distinguished.

Color Vision. Although color vision is not tested routinely in the medical office, some employee physical examinations may ask for a screening test.

The Ishihara test, shown in Figure 16–23, uses a book with circles that have different color dots. People with normal color vision can see numbers in the circles; people with impaired color vision cannot read the numbers. Record the number of any plate that the patient cannot read. Procedure 16–4 describes using the Ishihara test of color vision.

Table 16–1	Common Eye Diseases	
Disease	Description	Treatment
Cataract	The crystalline lens becomes opaque, causing clouding of vision or blurred vision; more common in the elderly	Surgical removal of the lens with lens implant or use of corrective contact lens or glasses
Conjunctivitis	Inflammation of the cornea, caused by irritation or bacterial infection resulting in redness, itching, and irritation	Various medications depending on the cause: antihistamine, antibiotic, corticosteroid ointments, or eyedrops
Glaucoma	Increased pressure within the eyeball due to excess fluid; may have no symptoms but will cause blindness if untreated	Medication therapy with eyedrops or ointments to relieve pressure; surgery
Stye	Infection of one of the sebaceous glands of the eyelid, causing redness and swelling	Antibiotic ointment; warm compresses

Errors of Refraction and Conditions that Can Be Corrected

Astigmatism	Failure of image to form clearly on the retina because of curve in the surface of the cornea
Hyperopia (hypermetropia)	Farsightedness, or lack of ability to see near objects clearly because the image focus lies behind the retina
Myopia	Nearsightedness, or lack of ability to see distant objects clearly because the image focus lies in front of the retina
Presbyopia	Failure of the eye to accommodate for near vision, usually found as a person ages
Strabismus	Poor muscle coordination so that eyes cross or turn outward instead of working together

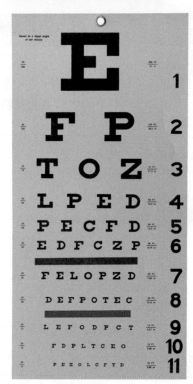

> **Figure 16–22** Snellen eye chart.

Hearing

The doctor examines the inside of the ear with the otoscope during the physical exam. Excessive **cerumen** (earwax), middle ear infections, foreign bodies in the ear, and holes or scarring of the tympanic membrane (eardrum) can be identified. The ear exam is shown in Figure 16–24.

In addition, the doctor can test general hearing using a tuning fork and can compare how the patient hears sound through air and through the bones of the skull by holding the tuning fork next to the ear (air conduction) and placing the base of the tuning fork against the mastoid bone directly behind the ear (bone conduction). The tuning fork test is shown in Figure 16–25.

Hearing Loss. Decreased hearing acuity is common, especially in the elderly. Conductive hearing loss occurs when a problem in the ear itself interferes with the transmission of sound through the ear bones and into the cochlea (the snail-shaped organ in the inner ear where sound waves are transformed into nerve impulses).

If the problem is in the nervous system (in the cochlea; on the auditory nerve, which transmits impulses to the brain, or in the brain itself), it is called perceptual hearing loss.

Many patients have a combination of conductive and perceptual hearing loss. Screening tests identify patients with significant hearing loss who need to be referred to an audiologist for more specialized testing

and/or to an ortorhinolaryngologist (a specialist who focuses on conditions of the ears, nose, and throat—or **ENT**). Table 16–2 is a list of diseases and conditions of the ear.

Measuring Hearing. Hearing may be screened in the office using an **audiometer** (an instrument that measures hearing). The audiometer tests for hearing loss at various degrees of intensity or loudness, measured in **decibels (dBs)**, as well as at low, middle, and high pitches, or frequency of sound vibrations. Hearing loss is usually more severe at some frequencies than others.

The patient is placed in a quiet area or soundproof cubicle, wearing earphones, and is instructed to raise his or her hand when a sound is heard. The patient's

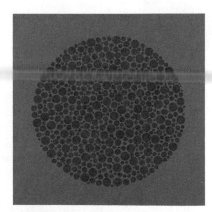

> **Figure 16–23** An Ishihara plate used for testing color vision.

PROCEDURE 16-3

Measuring Distance Visual Acuity Using a Snellen Chart

Performance Objective: The student will measure visual acuity accurately using the Snellen eye chart.

☑	Wash hands
☐	Gloves
☐	Eye and Face Protection
☐	Lab Coat or Apron
☐	Plastic Biohazard Bag
☐	Rigid Biohazard Container

Supplies and Equipment: Snellen chart, pointer, occluder or paper cup, alcohol wipes.

Procedure Steps

1. Wash hands.
2. Assemble supplies and equipment. The Snellen chart should be appropriate for the reading ability of the patient—pictures for preschool children, large Es for children in kindergarten or first grade, and letters for children or adults who can read.
3. Identify patient.
4. Explain procedure to patient.
5. Position the patient 20 feet from the eye chart. The room should be well lighted, and the patient should wear glasses or contact lenses normally used for distance vision.
   Rationale: The test screens to determine the patient's usual vision. It is designed to test vision at 20 feet.
6. Instruct the patient to keep both eyes open and cover the left eye with the occluder or a paper cup.
   Rationale: Only one eye is tested at a time. Both eyes are open to prevent squinting, which may alter vision.
7. Point to the 20/40 line and ask the patient to read each letter. (For children, ask the child to name the pictures or position the hand with the fingers pointing in the direction of the fingers of the Es.)
   Rationale: If the patient can see the letters, he or she will be able to verify by reading them out loud.

8. If the patient reads the letters correctly, ask the patient to read the line below and continue until the patient can no longer read a line with two or fewer mistakes.
   Rationale: As the patient progresses down the chart, the letters get smaller and harder to read.
9. If the patient cannot read the 20/40 line, ask him or her to read the line above it. Continue up the chart until the patient can read a line with two or fewer errors.
   Rationale: As the patient progresses up the chart, the letters get larger and easier to read.
10. When the patient has read a line correctly, ask him or her to cover the right eye and repeat the process. You may ask the patient to read the lines from right to left.
    Rationale: Each eye must be tested.
11. Ask the patient to read the lowest line he or she can see clearly with both eyes.
    Rationale: Both eyes are tested last to minimize the impact of the patient memorizing the chart.
12. Wipe the occluder with alcohol to remove microorganisms and allow to air-dry before reusing.
13. Wash hands.
14. Record the number of the smallest line the patient was able to read. If the patient missed one or two letters in the line, record the number as -1 or -2. Use the abbreviations OD (right eye), OS (left eye), and OU (both eyes).
    Rationale: The medical record provides an ongoing record of procedures performed and care given to the patient.

Charting Example	
Date	
7/5/XX	11:25 AM OD 20/30 −1; OS 20/20;
	OU 20/20 ————————————
	——————— S. Dellarosa, RMA

PROCEDURE 16-4

Ishihara Test of Color Vision

Performance Objective: The student will assess color vision using a book with Ishihara plates.

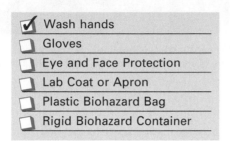

- ☑ Wash hands
- ☐ Gloves
- ☐ Eye and Face Protection
- ☐ Lab Coat or Apron
- ☐ Plastic Biohazard Bag
- ☐ Rigid Biohazard Container

Supplies and Equipment: Book of Ishihara plates.

Procedure Steps

1. Wash hands.
2. Assemble book of Ishihara plates.
3. Identify patient.
4. Explain procedure to patient.
5. Seat the patient and hold the book of Ishihara plates approximately 30″ from the patient with the plate at right angles to his or her line of vision. The room should be well lighted, and the patient should wear glasses or contact lenses normally used for distance vision.
   Rationale: The test screens to determine the patient's color vision. It is designed to have the plates about 30″ from the patient's eyes.
6. Instruct the patient to tell you what number he or she sees in the first plate.
   Rationale: The plates are designed so that people with ordinary color vision see a number in one color with a background of dots in another color. People with abnormal color vision may not see the number as a different color from the background dots.
7. Continue through the book until the patient has read all plates.
   Rationale: Different plates test for different color combinations.
8. Record the plate number with an X for each plate the patient could not read. Example: Plate 5: X, Plate 7: X. All other plates read correctly.
   Rationale: The medical record provides an ongoing record of procedures performed and care given to the patient.

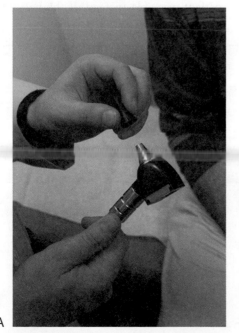

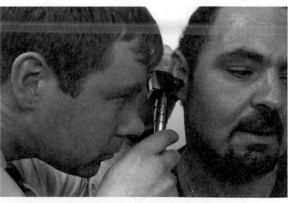

> **Figure 16–24** (A) Placing ear speculum on otoscope. (B) Examining a patient's ears with an otoscope.

A   B

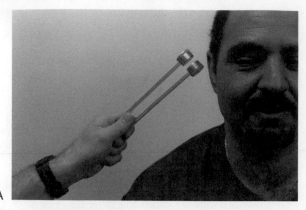
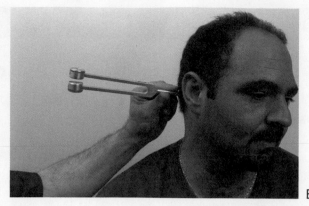

A   B

➤ **Figure 16–25** (A) A patient's ability to hear sound conducted through the air is tested by holding the tuning fork near the patient's ear. (B) A patient's ability to hear sound conducted through the bone of the skull is tested by holding the tuning fork against the skull behind the ear.

performance may be recorded through the audiometer or by hand. General screening may be done with a manual audiometer.

If the office tests hearing for employment physicals, a more accurate instrument is needed, and only specially trained personnel usually conduct the exam. Procedure 16–5 describes measuring hearing using a manual audiometer.

Table 16–2	Common Ear Diseases and Conditions	
Disease or Condition	**Description**	**Treatment**
Ceruminosis	Excess wax in the ear; can cause a feeling of fullness in the ear or impair hearing	Ear irrigation or eardrops to oxidize cerumen
Hearing loss; deafness	May be caused by congenital or acquired interference with sound conduction	Hearing aid; surgery
Otitis externa (swimmer's ear)	Infection of the external ear canal, causing pain and swelling in the canal	Antibiotic therapy; ear irrigation; use ear plugs when swimming or drops to dry ear canal after swimming
Otitis media (middle ear infection)	Infection of the middle ear that often accompanies an upper respiratory infection; during acute phase contains pus and causes severe pain and fever; fluid buildup may become chronic	Oral antibiotics; decongestants; occasionally tubes placed surgically to allow fluid to drain to the external ear canal (myringotomy)

PROCEDURE 16–5

Measuring Hearing Using a Manual Audiometer

Performance Objective: The student will measure hearing using a manual audiometer and will record the results accurately.

☑ Wash hands
☐ Gloves
☐ Eye and Face Protection
☐ Lab Coat or Apron
☐ Plastic Biohazard Bag
☐ Rigid Biohazard Container

Supplies and Equipment: Manual audiometer with headphones, alcohol wipes.

Procedure Steps

1. Wash hands.
2. Assemble audiometer and alcohol wipes.
3. Identify patient.
4. Explain procedure to patient.
5. Seat the patient in a soundproof cubicle or quiet room. Instruct the patient to raise his or her hand every time a sound is heard. If the machine has a device to record the patient's answers, instruct the patient to press the button every time a tone is heard. Have the patient put on the headphones and adjust for comfort. Be sure that the patient cannot see you press buttons.
   Rationale: The test screens for hearing at specific frequencies (highness or lowness of pitch) and loudness. The sound is delivered to each ear through headphones. It is important to avoid giving the patient visual cues that sound is being produced.
6. Press the correct button(s) to begin the test and if necessary to change frequencies and loudness. Test each ear.
   Rationale: Audiometers vary in design and function. The medical assistant should be trained to use the specific machine being used for testing.
7. Record how loud the tone needed to be for the patient to hear it at each pitch. If the machine records the results, print the results at the end of the test.
   Rationale: The purpose of the test is to determine how loud the sound must be at each frequency for the patient to hear it.
8. Wash hands.
9. Fill in a graph showing the loudness required for each frequency tested. If the machine records the patient's answers and prints results, label the printout with the patient's name and date.

HEARING LOSS AND HEARING AIDS

Best estimates are that there are approximately 28 million Americans (roughly 10 percent of the population) who suffer from a hearing loss severe enough to interfere with their daily activities. In addition, another 2 million Americans are profoundly deaf.

The number of Americans suffering hearing loss has been increasing steadily since the 1970s. One reason is the rapid increase in the number of older Americans, because the elderly suffer from hearing loss in far greater numbers than the younger adult population. Another reason is the increasingly noisy environment in which we live. It is believed that with the oncoming aging of the Baby Boomers, many of whom have enjoyed loud popular music since their teens and 20s, the number of older Americans with hearing loss will continue to increase.

Many school systems in the United States conduct an annual hearing screening and refer children who may be suffering a hearing loss to doctors and audiologists for further tests. Children with a family history of deafness; whose mothers contracted rubella during pregnancy; who were premature and/or low birth weight; or who suffered from measles, mumps, high fevers, meningitis, or recurrent or chronic ear infections are at increased risk of hearing difficulties.

Most hearing-impaired Americans suffer from conductive hearing loss. Children with conductive hearing loss most often have fluid in the middle ear that prevents the tympanic membrane from vibrating freely. In adults, conductive hearing loss is usually caused by otosclerosis, in which calcium deposits on the tiny bones in the ear cause them to become fixed and unable to pass on vibration when sounds enter the ear.

Some Americans, especially Baby Boomers, suffer from sensorineural hearing loss, caused by the constant bombardment of sounds louder than 75 to 100 decibels, the unit of measure for sound. Sensorineural hearing loss is seen in professional musicians, sound technicians, highway and road construction workers, factory workers, and those who work with heavy machinery.

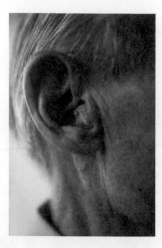

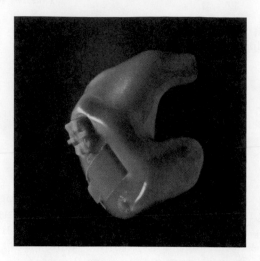

Hearing aids are of most benefit to individuals who suffer from mild to moderate conductive hearing loss. Those with sensorineural hearing loss obtain less satisfactory results from hearing aids.

The choice of a hearing aid must take into account two factors:

1. Size and type of the device
2. Type of circuitry.

Size and Type of Device

There are four types of hearing aids. Each fits in a different way, and they vary in size and convenience.

Behind the Ear (BTE). These devices are best for individuals with any fine-motor disability, who have difficulty handling small objects. They are large units that fit behind the ear. Newer units offer "mega power" and can help even those with profound hearing loss.

Eyeglass. Very few people use hearing aids attached to the temples of eyeglasses, and there is little research currently into improving them. They were developed for ease of use for individuals who wore both glasses and a hearing aid, because BTE units are difficult to maintain in the proper position while wearing glasses.

In the Ear. These hearing aids first appeared in the 1970s. They are custom molded to the individual's ear. They come in two subtypes—in the ear and in the canal.

The instrument case of an in the ear hearing aid fills the entire outer bowl (concha) of the ear and fits into the ear canal. In the canal units are smaller, filling about half the concha. With both units, all sound comes through the hearing aid rather than being mixed with ambient sound.

Problems include excessive wind noise and difficulty getting good sound while using a telephone.

Completely in the Canal (CIC). These are also custom fit and are placed deeply in the ear canal. They are the smallest units available. They have a nylon string used to remove them from the ear canal. CIC units are the most popular type of hearing aid used in the 21st century.

Because they are small, CIC units use less power, which means less distortion of noise. This is especially beneficial when using the telephone and in places where there is a lot of background noise, such as a party.

Type of Circuitry

In early generation hearing aids, circuits were typically analog Class A, which provided quality linear amplification, meaning they added the same amount of amplification to all levels of sound intensity.

Today, advanced technology circuitry allows for nonlinear, or compression, amplification. As a result, hearing aids are "smart", in that they amplify different types and intensities of sound to different degrees and magnitudes. This provides a more natural level of loudness or softness across an individual's listening range.

Programmable hearing aids contain a computer chip that can be programmed by the hearing specialist to accommodate an individual's amplification needs. This technology separates incoming sounds into bands and processes each band independently, so the individual can vary volume, adapt frequency response, and adjust the instrument for input and output compression. Such a hearing aid provides more volume for soft, high-frequency sounds, and less volume for more intense, low-frequency sounds. It can be reprogrammed over time as the individual's natural hearing changes.

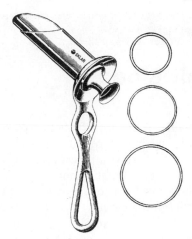

> **Figure 16–26** Hirschman anoscope used for examination of the rectum. (Courtesy of Sklar Instruments, West Chester, PA)

EXAMINATION OF THE RECTUM AND SIGMOID COLON

The rectal exam has been discussed earlier in this chapter, but only as it affects the examination of sexual organs (prostate cancer or enlargement for men and rectovaginal complications for women).

Another reason for examining the rectum is to detect signs of gastrointestinal disease, such as colon cancer or inflammatory bowel disease. Instrumentation allows the doctor to visualize not only the rectum, but also the sigmoid colon, the first 30 or so centimeters of the colon above the rectum.

Rectal Examination

If the doctor wants to visually examine the rectum, he or she asks the patient to move into Sims' position and introduces an anoscope into the rectum. An anoscope, shown in Figure 16–26, is a hollow instrument that looks like the barrel of a telescope. On the front end is an **obturator,** a smooth, rounded end that allows better comfort while the anoscope is being inserted.

After the instrument is in place, the obturator is removed. The doctor can then see the rectum through the opening.

After the doctor completes the manual rectal exam, a small amount of stool that usually adheres to the glove is tested for **occult blood** (hidden or invisible blood in the stool). This is a simple test that requires only a small sample of stool. After the stool is applied to the test paper, a drop of developer is placed on it. If a blue color is seen, the test is positive, as seen in Figure 16–27.

If a small amount of blood is present in the stool, it may be an early sign of colon cancer. This test may be called a stool **guaiac,** a chemical commonly used as a developer. After the exam, patients over age 50 are given three cards, instructed to obtain stool specimens, and return the cards in an ordinary envelope to the office for testing. They should not mail the cards because of the presence of stool. Procedure 16–6 describes testing stool for occult blood.

Proctosigmoidoscopy

The rectum and sigmoid colon can be examined with a sigmoidoscope, a type of **endoscope** (an instrument inserted into a body cavity to view an internal structure). All endoscopes have a light, a tube to introduce water or air, and blades to remove a piece of tissue for biopsy.

The doctor can either look directly through the tube or indirectly through mirrors or a video camera.

Sigmoidoscopy (viewing the rectum and sigmoid colon) is recommended beginning at age 50 and every 3 years thereafter, for early detection of colon cancer and for removal of precancerous lesions such as polyps.

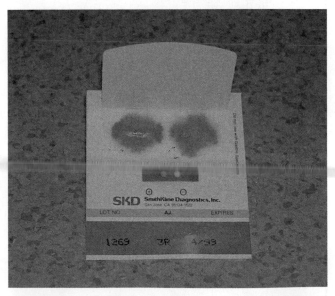

> **Figure 16–27** Hemoccult II testing card showing positive results. (From Stepp CA, Woods MA: *Laboratory Procedures for Medical Office Personnel.* Philadelphia: W.B. Saunders, 1998.)

PROCEDURE 16-6

Testing Stool for Occult Blood

Performance Objective: The student will test a stool specimen for occult blood.

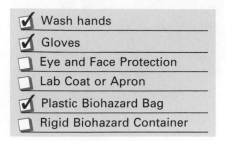

☑ Wash hands

☑ Gloves

☐ Eye and Face Protection

☐ Lab Coat or Apron

☑ Plastic Biohazard Bag

☐ Rigid Biohazard Container

Supplies and Equipment: stool specimen, wooden spatula or tongue depressor, gloves, test kit for occult blood, including developer.

Procedure Steps

1. Wash hands.
2. Assemble supplies and equipment.
3. Put on disposable gloves.
4. Open the front of the card from an occult blood test collection kit. Obtain stool from a container with stool or the doctor's glove after a rectal examination using a wooden spatula, tongue depressor, or cotton-tipped applicator. The patient may also have placed stool in the card at home and returned one or more cards for testing in the office. If patients mail samples, they must use U.S. Postal Service approved mailing pouches, not ordinary envelopes.

Rationale: There are different ways to obtain stool for testing. Stool is a body excretion that must be treated with precautions to prevent transmission of microorganisms.

5. Apply a thin layer to the paper in the first box within the card. Using stool from a different part of the sample, apply a thin layer to the paper in the second box.
Rationale: The test requires a thin layer of stool for the chemicals to penetrate. For greater accuracy stool from two different areas of the sample is tested.

6. Wait 3 to 5 minutes before developing. Cards can be stored up to 14 days. They should not be directly exposed to heat.
Rationale: The stool must interact with the paper, which is impregnated with guaiac, a substance that will react with hemoglobin in blood, if present.

7. Open the back of the test card and drop two drops of the developer solution on the two boxes to which stool was applied.
Rationale: The developer is a solution containing hydrogen peroxide, which will cause the test paper to turn blue in the presence of hemoglobin.

8. Read the results as directed by the manufacturer. If any trace of blue appears on the paper of either box, read the results as positive.
Rationale: Different test kits may have different development times. In general the test should be read after between 30 seconds and 2 minutes have passed. After that the color of the paper may change.

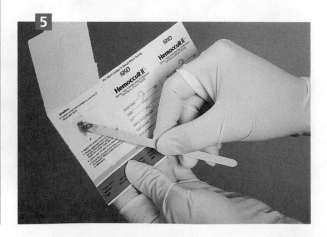

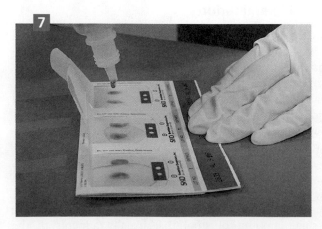

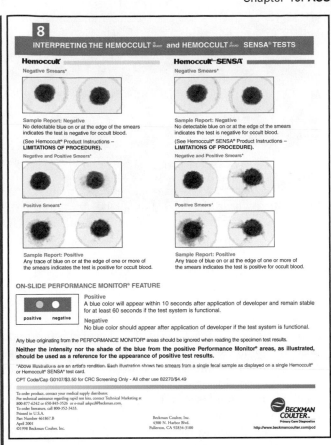

8

INTERPRETING THE HEMOCCULT ® BRAND **and HEMOCCULT** ® BRAND **SENSA** ® **TESTS**

9. While wearing disposable gloves, discard test card, applicator, and remainder of stool specimen in a biohazard waste container.
10. Clean contaminated surfaces with 10% household bleach solution and allow to air-dry.
11. Remove gloves and wash hands.
12. Record results in the medical record. If you are testing specimens obtained by the patient at home, record the date the specimens were collected.
    Rationale: The medical record provides an ongoing record of procedures performed and care given to the patient.

Charting Example	
Date	
10/25/XX	Stool specimens returned by patient tested for occult blood.
	Specimen 1 collected 10/19/XX: negative; specimen 2 collected 10/21/XX: negative; specimen 3 collected 10/22/XX: negative. ———
	——————————— P. Dean, RMA

Interpreting the Hemoccult Test. (Courtesy of Beckman Coulter, Palo Alto, CA.)

(Photographs from Bonewit-West K: *Clinical Procedures for Medical Assistants,* 5th ed. Philadelphia: W.B. Saunders, 2000.)

The medical assistant has four roles in the proctosigmoidoscopy:

1. patient instruction
2. assistance during rigid sigmoidoscopy
3. assistance during flexible sigmoidoscopy
4. care of the flexible sigmoidoscope.

Patient Instruction. When setting an appointment for a patient to have a sigmoidoscopy, the medical assistant often discusses the instructions with the patient. The colon must be thoroughly cleaned so the doctor can clearly see the colon walls and mucosa. Instructions for doing this are specific, and the medical assistant may need to take extra time with patients who have never been through the procedure before, especially patients who may be frightened because the sigmoidoscopy is a follow-up exam after other symptoms have appeared.

The patient may be advised to eat a light lunch the day before the exam, have a liquid supper, and drink only water after 9:00 PM until after the test is completed. The day before the test, the patient also takes a laxative (a medication that causes the colon to eliminate stool) such as citrate of magnesia, castor oil, or bisacodyl (trade name Dulcolax) tablets, all of which can be purchased without a prescription.

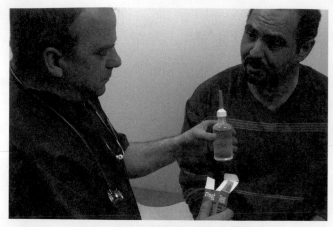

> **Figure 16–28** The medical assistant expains the use of a Fleet enema to a patient.

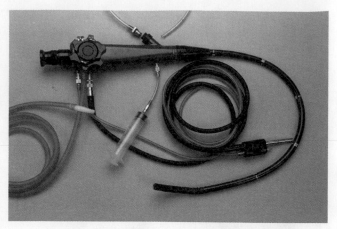

> **Figure 16–30** Flexible sigmoidoscope.

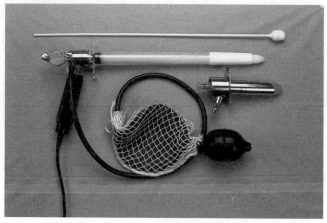

> **Figure 16–29** Rigid sigmoidoscope with insufflator and swab.

On the morning of the test, the patient needs to administer one or two Fleet enemas before coming to the office. An enema is a substance introduced into the rectum to cause emptying of the rectum and lower colon. Although there are various types of enemas, Fleet enemas are fairly well tolerated because they use only a small amount of fluid. The patient is instructed to hold the enema fluid in the rectum until the urge to defecate (pass stool) becomes strong. In Figure 16–28, the medical assistant explains the use of the Fleet enema to a patient.

Rigid Sigmoidoscopy. Some offices still use a plastic or metal sigmoidoscope about 10″ long, which is passed into the rectum with an obturator. The patient must be in the knee-chest position or kneeling on the step of a table that can be tilted to lower the head and raise the buttocks. The handle of the sigmoidoscope contains a light source, and a swab or biopsy forceps can be passed through the sigmoidoscope. The equipment for a sigmoidoscopy using a rigid sigmoidoscope is shown in Figure 16–29.

Flexible Sigmoidoscopy. The flexible sigmoidoscope, shown in Figure 16–30, has largely replaced the rigid sigmoidoscope for three main reasons.

1. It is much more comfortable for the patient.
2. It can be passed higher into the colon because it is flexible.
3. It can be hooked up to a monitor for excellent visualization.

Using a flexible sigmoidoscope, it is still possible to biopsy small lesions on the colon wall or obtain a culture. During the procedure, air is pumped into the colon for better visualization. This may stimulate abdominal cramping. Suction may be used to remove mucus, blood, or small amounts of stool. The patient is usually in Sims' position during flexible sigmoidoscopy. Procedure 16–7 describes assisting with a flexible sigmoidoscopy.

Flexible Sigmoidoscope Care. The flexible sigmoidoscope must be cleaned with soap and water (wearing protective equipment to avoid splashes), then sterilized using chemical sterilization. Each tube in the sigmoidoscope must be filled with chemical disinfectant, using a large syringe. Then the entire sigmoidoscope sits in disinfectant solution for several hours until it is sterilized. Many offices buy a special container that fits the sigmoidoscope and holds sterilizing solution. The sigmoidoscope is rinsed with sterile water to remove the disinfectant before use.

PROCEDURE 16–7

Assisting with Flexible Sigmoidoscopy

Performance Objective: The student will set up for flexible sigmoidoscopy and assist the doctor with the examination.

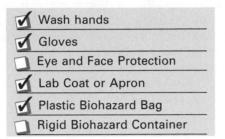

☑ Wash hands
☑ Gloves
☐ Eye and Face Protection
☑ Lab Coat or Apron
☑ Plastic Biohazard Bag
☐ Rigid Biohazard Container

Supplies and Equipment: flexible sigmoidoscope with light source, insufflator, video monitor, suction machine, suction catheter, gloves, drape, patient gown, water-resistant lab coat for doctor, water-soluble lubricant, 12″ sponge sticks, biopsy forceps (sterile), specimen container with preservative solution, gauze sponges, tissues.

Procedure Steps

1. Wash hands.
2. Assemble supplies and equipment. Hook up the sigmoidoscope to the light source, insufflator, and monitor. Prepare the suction equipment and test. Place a generous amount of lubricant on a gauze square.
3. Identify patient.
4. Explain procedure to patient.
5. Have the patient empty his or her bladder before the procedure. Collect a urine specimen if needed.
   Rationale: This examination is most comfortable for the patient if the bladder is empty.
6. Tell patient to undress from the waist down and put on a gown with the opening in the back.
7. Position the patient in Sims' position. Some offices have a special table for this examination. The patient kneels on the table, which is tilted when the examination begins so that the patient is supported in a knee-chest position. Place a drape over the patient's buttocks until the examination begins.
   Rationale: The examination requires access to the patient's rectum. The drape prevents unnecessary exposure.

8. The doctor puts on a fluid-resistant lab coat or gown, and both the doctor and medical assistant put on disposable gloves.
9. When the doctor is ready to begin the examination, remove the drape to expose the anal area.
   Rationale: This keeps the patient warm and keeps exposure to a minimum.
10. Instruct the patient to breathe deeply through the mouth. You may instruct the patient to bear down slightly (as if trying to pass gas) when the sigmoidoscope is first introduced.
    Rationale: Deep breathing and bearing down help relax the anal sphincter and may relieve discomfort.
11. Assist the doctor as needed during the examination. This may include:
    - Placing lubricant on the doctor's gloves or the sigmoidoscope
    - Plugging in or adjusting lights or equipment
    - Handing supplies to the doctor
    - Opening the specimen container and holding it to receive a specimen
    - Turning on the suction machine if it is needed.
    Rationale: The doctor advances the sigmoidoscope along the colon, observing the wall of the colon. During the examination, a specimen or biopsy of any suspicious area may be taken and mucus or small amounts of stool may be removed from the colon by suction.
12. Offer emotional support and encouragement to the patient.
    Rationale: The exam may be somewhat uncomfortable, and the patient appreciates gestures of support.
13. When the examination is completed, offer tissues to the patient.
    Rationale: The patient may wish to remove excess lubricant and/or stool from the anal area.
14. Remove gloves and assist the patient to sit up. Instruct the patient to remain sitting until any dizziness or light-headedness has passed.
    Rationale: The patient may be dizzy or light-headed after this exam.
15. Instruct the patient to dress, and provide pri-

Procedure continued on following page

PROCEDURE 16–7 (continued)

vacy unless the patient needs assistance. Give any follow-up instructions.

Rationale: Patients prefer to dress in privacy. The medical assistant assesses the patient's need for assistance in dressing.

16. Fill out the correct lab slip for each specimen, including where the specimen was obtained. Fasten each lab slip to the correct specimen. Place specimen(s) in a plastic biohazard bag for transport.

Rationale: Any specimens sent to the lab must be accompanied by lab slips with complete information.

17. Put on disposable gloves and discard paper gown, drape, and used supplies in biohazard container. Place cloth gown or drape in laundry bag.

18. Discard used table paper and clean examination table with 10:1 household bleach solution. Allow to air-dry.

19. Clean used equipment with soap and water and place in soaking solution until ready to sterilize. Do not soak the light attachment—clean it with alcohol swabs.

20. Rinse equipment and place in container with sterilizing solution. Use sterile syringes to push sterilizing solution into the interior chambers of the sigmoidoscope as directed by the manufacturer.

21. Remove gloves and wash hands.

STUDENT STUDY PLAN

To reinforce your understanding of the material in this chapter . . .

Complete *Complete* the **Review & Recall** questions below.

Discuss *Discuss* the situation in **If You Were the Medical Assistant** with your classmates and answer the questions.

Answer *Answer* the **Critical Thinking Questions** below and discuss with your classmates.

Visit *Visit* **Web sites** suggested below and search for additional Web sites using **Keywords for Internet Searches.**

Complete *Complete* the exercises in chapter 16 of the **Student Mastery Manual.**

Practice *Practice* Positioning the Patient Activities in the Clinical Skills section on the **CD-ROM.**

REVIEW & RECALL

1. List and describe methods used to perform the physical examination.

2. Identify the nine parts of the physical examination.

3. Identify the instruments and/or supplies needed by the doctor to perform each part of the physical examination.

4. Describe how the medical assistant prepares the patient for the physical examination.

5. Describe how six common positions are used for different parts of the physical examination.

6. Describe the role of the medical assistant when a woman is having a Pap test and pelvic examination.

7. Identify diagnostic tests used for screening distance vision, color vision, and hearing in the medical office.

8. Describe three methods for examining the anus, rectum, and/or sigmoid colon that may be used in the medical office.

IF YOU WERE THE MEDICAL ASSISTANT

When a female patient has a Pap test and pelvic examination, the medical assistant must ask additional questions in order to fill out the cytology requisition. Additional equipment must also be prepared.

1. What information must be obtained to fill out the form completely?
2. What equipment must be prepared for the Pap test and pelvic examination?

3. What position is usually used for this examination?
4. Describe how the medical assistant prepares the examination table and instructs the patient to assume the correct position for this examination.

CRITICAL THINKING QUESTIONS

1. Identify at least three circumstances when a Pap test might need to be delayed to avoid inaccurate results. How would the medical assistant explain this to a patient?
2. Discuss with your classmates the advantages and disadvantages of performing screening tests such as vision testing, hearing testing, Pap test, testing stool for occult blood, and proctosigmoidoscopy routinely as part of the physical examination.
3. Find out what diagnostic tests are recommended as routine for the following age groups: children, adolescents, young men, young women, men over age 40, women over age 40, men over age 60, and women over age 60. Why are the recommendations different?
4. Write down the instructions you would give a patient to collect, prepare, and return three cards to be tested for occult blood.
5. Obtain the instructions given to a patient who is going to have a sigmoidoscopy at a medical office or health facility in your area. Compare the instructions with those obtained by your classmates. Discuss any differences. Why do you think different facilities may have a different preparation for this test?

EXPLORE THE WEB

INTERNET WEB SITES

Pap test
www.cancernet.nci.nih.gov

sigmoidoscopy
www.sigmoidoscopy.com

sigmoidoscopy instructions
www.niddk.nih.gov/health/digest/pubs/diagtest/sigmo.htm

KEYWORDS FOR INTERNET SEARCHES

GYN exam
  occult blood
  patient physical
    examination
  Pap (smear) test

pelvic exam
proctosigmoidoscopy
rectal exam
sigmoidoscopy

ANSWERS TO ON THE JOB

1. The exam room should contain a lamp, otoscope with various sizes of disposable ear specula, ophthalmoscope, and sphygmomanometer. Sandra should prepare the following: tongue blade, tape measure, tuning fork, examination gloves, lubricant, and percussion hammer. Dr. Lopez will usually have his own stethoscope. Sandra may also need to prepare a penlight (if Dr. Lopez prefers it to the light on the otoscope), a head mirror, and a laryngeal mirror. She should have tissues available for after the exam.

2. Sandra should give Mr. Hilton a gown and drape and tell Mr. Hilton to undress completely, including his underwear. When Mr. Hilton has put on the gown, he should sit on the end of the exam table. He may or may not choose to place the drape over his knees.

3. Usually Sandra will not be present for the physical exam of a male patient because the patient will be more comfortable if he is alone with Dr. Lopez. Once the equipment is prepared Dr. Lopez will be able to carry out the exam without assistance.

Assisting with Surgical Procedures

Instructional Objectives

After completing this chapter, you will be able to do the following:

1. Describe the medical assistant's responsibilities during a minor surgical procedure.
2. List guidelines that should be observed during a sterile procedure to maintain surgical asepsis.
3. Identify and explain the use and care of instruments commonly used for minor office surgery.
4. Discuss the preparation of the patient for minor surgical procedures.
5. Discuss the techniques and principles of surgical handwashing, sterile gloving, and handling sterile supplies.
6. Explain the difference between a closed and open wound.
7. List and explain the three types of wound healing.
8. Describe the two different types of sutures (absorbable and nonabsorbable), and give examples of uses for each.
9. Explain the purpose of the procedures for incision and drainage, colposcopy, laceration repair, and suture removal.
10. List guidelines for applying a bandage.
11. Identify the common types of bandages used in the medical office.
12. Describe post-surgical patient care, including the procedures and principles for the application of sterile and nonsterile dressings.

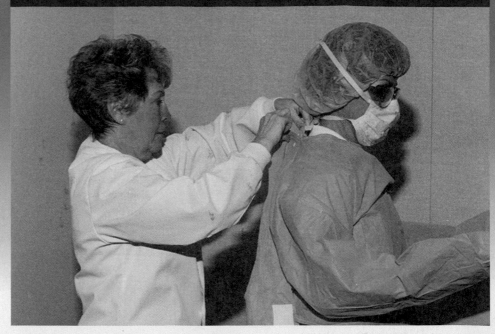

(From Kinn ME, Woods M: *The Medical Assistant, Administrative and Clinical,* 8th ed. Philadelphia: W.B. Saunders, 1999)

Performance Objectives

After completing this chapter, you will be able to do the following:

1. Perform surgical aseptic handwashing (Procedure 17–1).
2. Apply and remove sterile gloves using correct technique (Procedure 17–2).
3. Open a sterile barrier field using correct technique (Procedure 17–3).
4. Open a sterile surgical pack using correct technique (Procedure 17–4).
5. Add sterile solution to a sterile field (Procedure 17–5).
6. Prepare the skin for minor surgery (Procedure 17–6).
7. Prepare patients for and assist with minor surgery (Procedure 17–7).
8. Apply a tubular gauze bandage (Procedure 17–8).
9. Change a sterile dressing using correct technique (Procedure 17–9).
10. Remove sutures (Procedure 17–10).

VOCABULARY

abscess (p. 365)
approximated (p. 372)
bandage (p. 373)
biopsy (p. 364)
curette (p. 351)
cyst (p. 368)
debridement (p. 379)
dressing (p. 373)
excision (p. 365)

fenestrated (p. 353)
forceps, ring-handle (p. 346)
forceps, spring-handle
   (p. 346)
granulation (p. 372)
hemostasis (p. 347)
incision (p. 349)
informed consent (p. 359)
laceration (p. 368)

lesion (p. 365)
ligate (p. 347)
Mayo stand (p. 353)
primary intention (p. 372)
probe (p. 350)
proliferation (p. 372)
remodeling (p. 372)
retractor (p. 349)

scalpel (p. 349)
secondary intention (p. 372)
slough (p. 370)
sound (p. 350)
suture (p. 352)
swaged (p. 353)
tertiary intention (p. 372)

ABBREVIATIONS

I & D (p. 368)

need to know highlited yellow stuff

As a medical assistant in a doctor's office, you may be asked to assist with minor surgical procedures. In the past, most surgery, even minor surgery, was done in a hospital. Today, however, this surgery is increasingly being done in a doctor's office on an outpatient basis.

During these procedures, you may have a number of responsibilities, including preparing the sterile field, preparing the patient, and assisting the doctor during the surgery by controlling bleeding, passing instruments to the doctor, and assisting during skin closing.

SURGICAL ASEPSIS

As was stated in chapter 13, the reason for maintaining surgical asepsis is to keep harmful organisms from entering the body during a surgical procedure. Surgical procedures will be conducted with sterilized equipment and will occur within a sterile field, maintained by sterile drapes.

Surgical aseptic techniques are used whenever the doctor is going to penetrate below the skin or enter a sterile body cavity. A surgical incision causes a break in the skin where microorganisms could enter the body.

Surgical asepsis keeps harmful microorganisms and spores from entering the surgical incision.

TREATMENT OF THE SKIN

Skin cannot be sterilized. Yet harmful microorganisms live on the skin. To get the skin as free of pathogens as possible, the patient's skin around the surgical incision will be treated with an antiseptic such as Betadine.

The doctor and medical assistant will scrub their hands using surgical aseptic handwashing technique, as shown in Procedure 17–1. They will wear sterile gloves when touching sterile instruments and carrying out the surgical procedure, to prevent the skin on their hands from touching anything sterile. Procedure 17–2 shows how to put on sterile gloves.

PRINCIPLES OF SURGICAL ASEPSIS

To maintain sterility, it is imperative that a set of rules be followed. These rules are designed to assure that no harmful microorganisms are present where the surgery is taking place. Because harmful microorganisms cannot be seen, it should be assumed that they are present unless sterility is achieved by following the rules of surgical asepsis.

The following eight rules should be followed at all times:

1. Only use sterile objects to touch other sterile objects. Once a sterile object has been touched with an object that is not sterile, the formerly sterile object is no longer sterile.

2. Only areas in your direct line of vision are sterile. If you cannot see it, you must assume it is not sterile. Always keep the sterile field in your vision. If you must leave the area, back away from the sterile field so you do not contaminate it by accident.

3. Only the area above waist level is sterile. The draping around the sterile field that falls below the table level is not sterile. If you lower your hands below waist level, they are no longer sterile. Anything that falls to the floor, obviously, is no longer sterile. In addition, the outside 1″ of the sterile field on all sides is to be considered

nonsterile; sterile items should always be placed in the middle of the sterile field.

4. Avoid passing nonsterile objects over the sterile field. In fact, do not reach over the sterile field at all, if possible. Bring sterile instruments, dressings, and sponges into the sterile field; once used, do not return them to the sterile field.

5. When pouring sterile liquids, do not pour directly onto the sterile field. The area below the field is not sterile, and a wet surface can wick up harmful microorganisms. Pour the liquid into a bowl or onto a dressing on a waterproof wrapper. Do not let the edge of the bottle touch the sterile item (bowl or dressing) that you are pouring into.

PROCEDURE 17–1

Surgical Aseptic Handwash

Performance Objective: The student will be able to perform a surgical aseptic handwash using correct technique.

Supplies and Equipment: Sink with foot or arm control for water and antimicrobial soap, sterile towels, disposable hand and nail brush.

Procedure Steps

1. Remove all jewelry, and place for safekeeping. *Rationale:* A surgical handwash usually precedes donning of sterile gloves. Jewelry can puncture gloves and should not be worn during a sterile procedure.

2. Open package of sterile towels. *Rationale:* After hands have been washed, you may not touch anything that is not sterile.

3 Using foot controls, regulate water to a comfortable warm temperature and rinse hands and forearms, holding them upright at or above waist level. *Rationale:* Rinsing provides the removal of surface microorganisms before the application of

antimicrobial soap. Soap will lather best in warm water. The fingertips are held upright to encourage the flow of contaminants away from the hands.

4 Clean under and around nails with brush or wooden orange stick. Apply adequate soap, scrub one hand and forearm, and then the other, fingertips up, with brush, using friction for at least 3 minutes. Often a disposable brush containing Betadine (povidone-iodine) is used for the surgical handwash. Lather and scrub without touching faucet or sink. *Rationale:* Friction applied to the skin surface will loosen microorganisms for removal. Betadine acts as an antiseptic. The sink area is more contaminated than the hands so care must be taken not to touch while performing the remainder of this procedure; if you do touch sink, you should start over again.

5 Discard brush. Rinse hands and forearms thoroughly, holding hands and arms up. *Rationale:* Soap must be completely removed because microorganisms may shelter under soap residue.

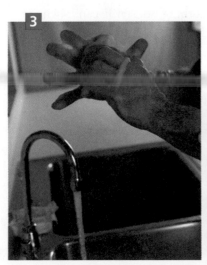
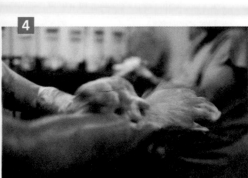
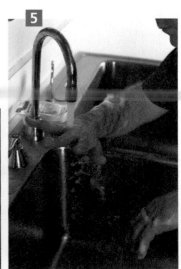

Procedure continued on following page

PROCEDURE 17–1 (continued)

6 If using foot or elbow controls, turn off water; otherwise leave water running for someone else to turn off. Hold hands above waist. *Rationale:* Once hands are clean you may not touch any part of the sink with them.

7. Pick up the sterile towel without touching the package and dry one hand from hand to arm. Use a new towel for the second arm. Drop each towel (rather than putting it down) after use to avoid contaminating hands. *Rationale:* The hands are considered cleaner than the arms.

8. Apply sterile gloves as described in Procedure 17–2. *Rationale:* The hands cannot be made sterile, but after making them as clean as possible, that level of cleanliness can be maintained by applying sterile gloves.

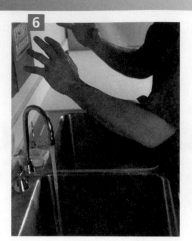

PROCEDURE 17–2

Sterile Gloving

Performance Objective: The student will be able to put on sterile gloves using sterile technique.

Supplies and Equipment: Pair of sterile gloves in appropriate size (ranges from size 5 to 10).

Procedure Steps

1. Remove all jewelry, place for safekeeping, and perform a medically aseptic handwash. *Rationale:* Sterile gloves can be punctured by jewelry. Hands must be clean before performing any procedure.

2. Place package of sterile gloves on clutter-free, flat surface that is waist level.

Rationale: Anything placed below the waist is outside one's peripheral vision and compromises maintenance of sterility.

3. Open package, being careful not to touch the sterile inner packaging. *Rationale:* Hands are not sterile.

4 Grasp the edge of the inner packaging and pull the paper open to expose both sterile gloves inside, touching only the edges of package to keep the area a sterile field for donning gloves. *Rationale:* Nothing nonsterile can touch the sterile gloves without making them nonsterile.

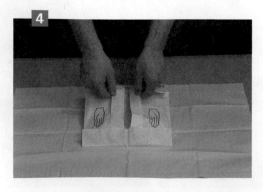

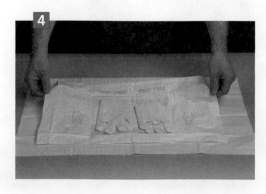

5 With the fingers and thumb of one ungloved hand (usually the nondominant hand is gloved first), pick up the glove for the other hand by grasping the inside of the glove and lifting the glove completely off the paper.

Rationale: The inside of the glove is not sterile, because it touches your skin. It does not matter which hand you glove first, but make sure that when you touch the sterile glove you are touching only the inside area that will be against your skin when you pull it on. To maintain sterility, prevent the fingers of the glove from falling back against the paper package.

6 Pull the glove on without touching the outside of the glove.

Rationale: The outside of the glove is considered sterile.

7 Using the gloved hand, pick up the second glove by placing the gloved fingers between the folded cuff and the fingers of the second glove and lifting the glove completely off the paper.

Rationale: The outside of the glove, including between the cuff and the fingers (as the gloves are folded in the package), is considered sterile, and may be touched by the sterile glove that you are already wearing.

8 Slide the second hand into the glove, being careful not to let the gloved hand touch the skin of the hand you are gloving. Pull the cuff away from your arm as you slide your hand into the glove to prevent accidental contact between the fingers of the sterile glove and the skin of your arm.

Rationale: Sterile items may only touch sterile items.

9 Hold both gloved hands above the waist. You may adjust the fingers, but do not touch anything that is not sterile.

Rationale: After sterile gloves have been put on, hands must remain above the waist to be considered sterile.

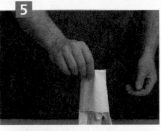

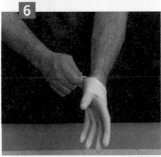

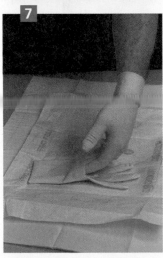

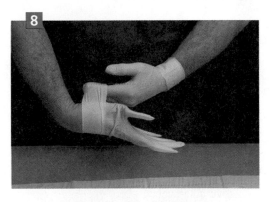

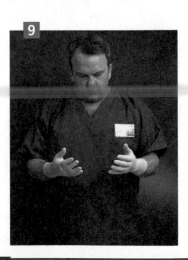

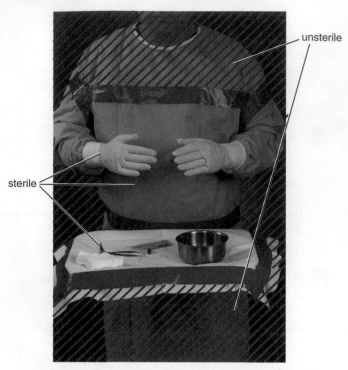

> **Figure 17–1** When wearing a sterile gown and gloves for a procedure, the sterile areas include the lower sleeves, gloves, front of gown, and the sterile field except for the outer inch and any part that hangs below the table.

6. Do not sneeze, cough, or talk above the sterile field. Microorganisms from the respiratory system can contaminate the sterile field and the objects on it.

7. Cover the sterile field with a sterile towel if it will not be under direct observation by anyone for even a moment.

8. When wearing a sterile gown to perform a procedure, the sterile areas are defined as follows, and as shown in Figure 17–1: Above the waist, front of gown, gloves, and the sterile field except the outer inch and any part that hangs below the table. Always hold hands above your waist if wearing sterile gloves; hold sterile instruments above your waist.

INSTRUMENTS AND SUPPLIES USED IN OFFICE SURGERY

Various instruments and supplies may be necessary for office-based surgery.

Instruments

Surgical instruments are metal, plastic, or rubber tools used in surgery for cutting, scraping, holding or

grasping, pulling back (retracting), or suturing (stitching). These include a number of different types of forceps, scissors, scalpels and blades, retractors, probes and sounds, and curets.

Many surgical instruments are named either for the activity for which they are used or for the individual(s) who designed the instrument.

Forceps

A **forceps** is a tool used for grasping, pulling, compressing, or holding tissue (skin and muscle) or other instruments and supplies during surgery. Forceps are held either with two fingerholes (**ring-handle forceps**) or with the thumb and forefinger (**spring-handle for-**

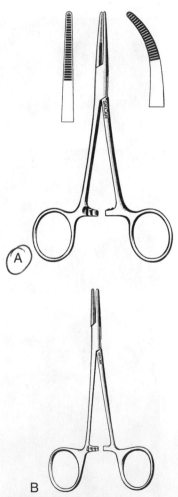

> **Figure 17–2** (A) Kelly hemostatic forceps. (B) Halsted mosquito hemostats. Kelly hemostatic forceps have longer, and thicker jaws than Halsted mosquito hemostats; Kelly hemostatic forceps may have straight or curved blades. (Courtesy of Sklar Instruments, West Chester, PA)

ceps). The tips of the forceps, called the jaws, can be blunt, sharp, or toothed.

Many forceps have three or more ratchetlike stops just below the ring handles, allowing the forceps to be locked in one of many positions to provide continuous pressure on the jaws.

Forceps come in a number of varieties, to serve a number of particular purposes, including:

Hemostatic forceps, such as Kelly forceps or mosquito forceps, are seen in Figure 17–2. Hemostats have slender jaws so they can tightly grasp blood vessels to achieve **hemostasis** (control of bleeding). Mosquito forceps, which have shorter and more delicate jaws, are used to grasp small blood vessels. Hemostats may have smooth or partially serrated jaws but do not have teeth. During surgery, blood vessels are first clamped, then **ligated** (tied off so they do not bleed).

Needle holders, such as the one seen in Figure 17–3, are designed to hold the suturing needle while taking stitches. Needle holders come in a number of different lengths, have short and strong jaws that may be serrated, or may have a groove in the middle.

Sponge forceps, such as the Foerster sponge forceps or the Bozeman forceps, shown in Figure 17–4, are

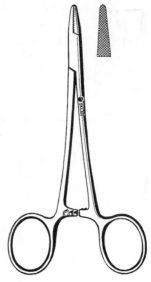

➢ **Figure 17–3** Baumgartner needle holder. (Courtesy of Sklar Instruments, West Chester, PA)

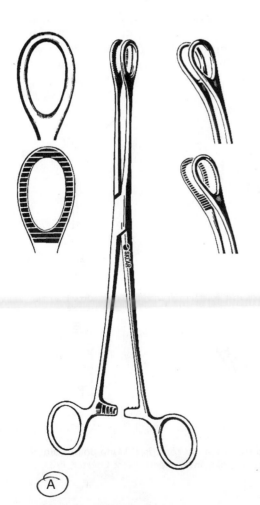

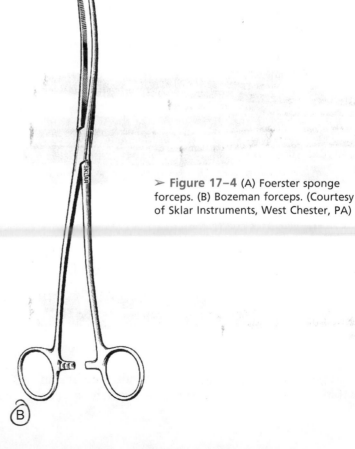

➢ **Figure 17–4** (A) Foerster sponge forceps. (B) Bozeman forceps. (Courtesy of Sklar Instruments, West Chester, PA)

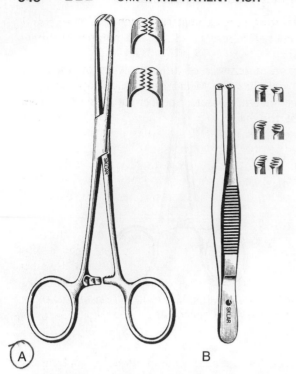

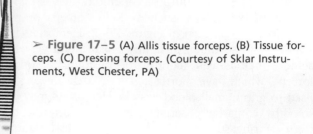

> **Figure 17–5** (A) Allis tissue forceps. (B) Tissue forceps. (C) Dressing forceps. (Courtesy of Sklar Instruments, West Chester, PA)

used to hold sterile squares of gauze, called sponges, which are used to clean away blood during surgery. Sterile sponge forceps can also be used to transfer sterile items without wearing gloves.

Tissue and dressing forceps, shown in Figure 17–5, are used to grasp tissue after the surgical incision has been made or to pick up gauze squares or dressings. If these forceps are the kind that are grasped with the thumb and forefinger, they are sometimes called thumb forceps. Allis tissue forceps come in many different lengths and jaw widths. Because the teeth are not sharp, it is less traumatic to tissue than many other forceps. Toothed tissue forceps have more of a pincer grip, and plain-tip dressing forceps are used mainly to grasp dressing or gauze sponges.

Splinter forceps are used to remove foreign bodies from wounds, and ear forceps are used to remove foreign bodies from the ear. Splinter forceps (Figure 17–6) may also be used to place packing in a wound. Splinter forceps have a number of different designs; they have a very sharp tip for retrieving small foreign objects. Ear forceps have a serrated tip and are manufactured in different lengths.

Tenaculum forceps have curved, sharp points. They are used for grasping tissue during surgery. If used within a body cavity, they have blades as long as shown in Figure 17–7. Towel clamps, such as the Backhaus towel clamp, are used to hold drapes in place during surgery. They look like tenaculum forceps but have shorter curved blades. They are also shown in Figure 17–7.

Biopsy forceps have a long rod with a cutting instrument at the end. They can pass through an endo-scope and take a piece of tissue for microscopic examination.

Scissors

Scissors are made up of two cutting surfaces, held together and pivoting on a pin. They are ring-handled (two fingerholes). Scissor blades can be sharp or blunt, depending on what they are used for. In surgery, scissors are used both for cutting tissue (skin and muscle)

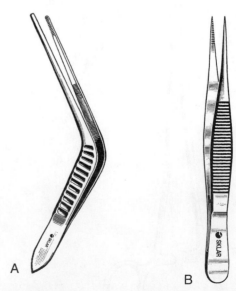

> **Figure 17–6** (A) Wilde ear forceps. (B) Fine point splinter forceps. (Courtesy of Sklar Instruments, West Chester, PA)

and for cutting surgical materials such as dressing and suture material. Figure 17–8 shows a number of different scissors.

There are a number of different types of operating scissors, including the Metzenbaum and Mayo scissors, which are straight scissors. Spencer suture scissors have a straight top blade and a hooked bottom blade that slides under sutures in the skin to cut them for removal. Lister bandage scissors are angled and have a blunt tip on the bottom blade to slide under the bandage, with a sharp straight top blade. The blunt tip prevents injury to the skin underneath the bandage.

Scalpels and Blades

A **scalpel** is a surgical knife. It has a straight handle and a sharp cutting blade, the style of which differs depending on the procedure performed. Some scalpels are completely disposable; others have reusable handles into which disposable blades are fit. Disposable scalpels with blades that can be retracted after use improve safety.

A straight or pointed blade is used for making an initial surgical **incision** (a cut made with a knife or scalpel) or for incision and drainage. For excising (removing) tissue, a curved blade is used. Figure 17–9 shows various kinds of scalpels and blades.

Retractors

A **retractor** is a surgical instrument used to hold open a flap of tissue so the doctor can view the area

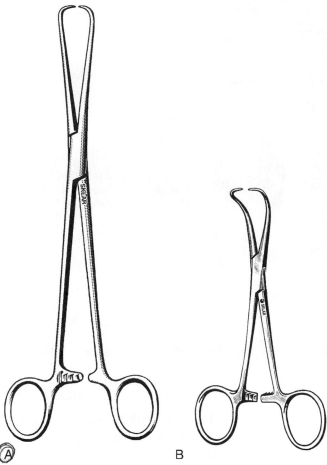

➤ **Figure 17–7** (A) Tenaculum forceps. (B) Backhaus towel clamp. (Courtesy of Sklar Instruments, West Chester, PA)

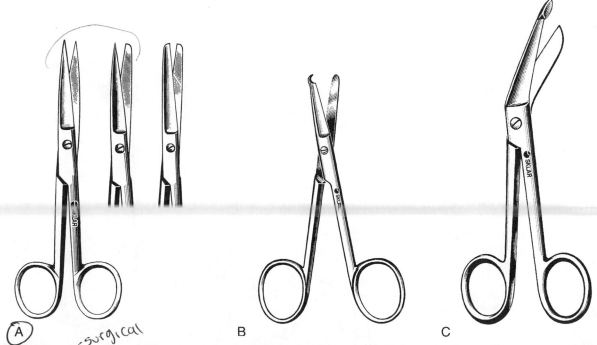

➤ **Figure 17–8** (A) Operating scissors. Operating scissors may have straight or curved blades with sharp or blunt tips. (B) Spencer stitch scissors. Scissors with a curved hook are often used to remove sutures. (C) Lister bandage scissors. Scissors with one long, blunt blade at an angle to the handles are often used to remove dressings. (Courtesy of Sklar Instruments, West Chester, PA)

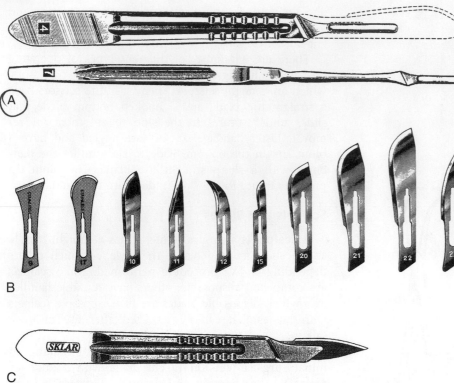

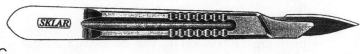

A

B

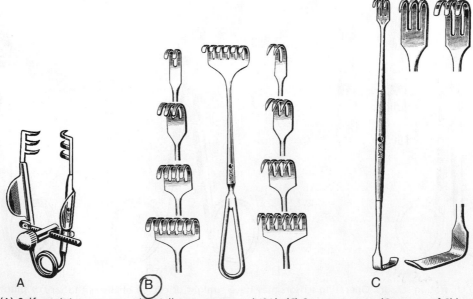

C

> **Figure 17–9** (A) Scalpel handles. (B) Scalpel blades. (C) Disposable scalpel. (Courtesy of Sklar Instruments, West Chester, PA)

underneath. Retractors may have smooth or toothed tips; toothed retractors may be sharp or blunt. Retractors may be held in place by an assistant or may be screwed in place and self-holding. Figure 17–10 shows a number of different retractors. Retractors used in the hospital for abdominal or chest surgery are much larger than those used for office surgery.

Some retractors have fingers or "rakes" for the tip; others are flat. Some have ring handles; others have a simple bar handle. The Senn retractor has a rake tip on one end and a blunt tip on the other end.

Probes and Sounds

Probes and **sounds** are instruments used by doctors to feel around inside an incision or measure the depth of a cavity before proceeding. They show the angle and depth of a wound and can show foreign bodies in the

A

(B)

C

> **Figure 17–10** (A) Self-retaining retractor. (B) Volkman retractor (USA). (C) Senn retractor. (Courtesy of Sklar Instruments, West Chester, PA)

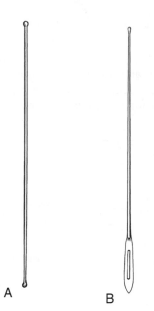

➤ **Figure 17–11** (A) Double-ended probe. (B) Probe with eye. (Courtesy of Sklar Instruments, West Chester, PA)

wound. Probes and sounds are shown in Figure 17–11.

Curettes

A **curette** is an instrument used to scrape. Uterine curettes are used to scrape away fetal tissue from the uterus. Ear curettes are used to remove earwax for better viewing of the tympanic membrane (ear drum). Curettes are shown in Figure 17–12.

Biopsy forceps are long, thin instruments with a blade at the end for cutting. When they enter a body cavity, the blade is closed; the blade can be released to obtain a specimen. The shape depends on where they are intended to be used. Biopsy forceps are shown in Figure 17–13.

Care of Instruments

Surgical instruments are delicate and require extensive care when using, cleaning, and storing, to avoid both injury to the user and damage to the instrument.

Many surgical instruments used today are disposable (especially scalpels). Scalpel blades, suture material, surgical needles, and gloves are always discarded after use; blades and needles in the rigid biohazard (sharps) container, gloves in a biohazard bag. Disposable scalpels should also go in the sharps container. Needles and syringes used for injection of local anesthetic are also usually discarded in the sharps container. Suture material, because it usually comes attached to the suturing needle, also goes into the rigid sharps container.

Reusable instruments are more durable and are made of better materials than disposables. Reusable in-

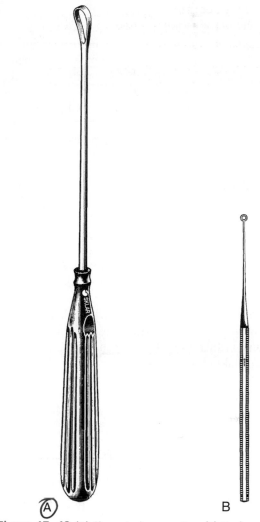

➤ **Figure 17–12** (A) Sims uterine curettes. (B) Buck ear curette. (Courtesy of Sklar Instruments, West Chester, PA)

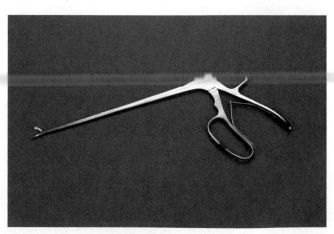

➤ **Figure 17–13** Biopsy forceps.

struments must be sanitized (cleaned), wrapped, and sterilized, using the following steps:

1. Immediately after they are used, instruments should be soaked in a room-temperature, neutral pH solution to prevent blood and other biological material from drying. A plastic basin should be used to prevent instrument edges and tips from being damaged.

2. After the procedure is over, the medical assistant needs to clean and sterilize the equipment. To clean, always wear protective equipment (apron, mask, eye protection, and heavy-duty rubber gloves.)

3. Carefully separate sharp instruments from other instruments that might have been soaking together. This reduces the likelihood of being cut by a sharp instrument every time you reach into the soak basin and reduces the likelihood that sharp instruments will be damaged. Also remove instruments that contain rubber (which can decompose if left in soaking solution too long) and plastic (which can discolor and lose its strength from soaking too long).

4. Wash each instrument thoroughly, checking to make sure it is in good working order. A soft bristle brush can be used to clean the ratchets, hinges, and serrated edges.

5. Dry each instrument thoroughly to avoid water spotting (even "stainless steel" will develop water stains). Separate instruments by the type of material used (stainless steel, chrome plate). Do not stack instruments on top of each other. Instruments with ratchets should be left with ratchets open.

6. Prepare instruments for sterilization, using the sterilization procedures discussed in chapter 13.

Supplies

To perform minor surgery, the doctor will need a number of supplies, including gauze in many forms, solutions to clean the skin, local anesthetic, suture material, dressings and bandages, and surgical drapes.

Gauze Squares (Sponges)

Prepackaged squares of gauze are called sponges. They are most commonly found in 2″ × 2″, 3″ × 3″, and 4″ × 4″ sizes. Sponges come in sterile packs of two or in nonsterile packs of 100 (which are much less expensive). A medical assistant can sterilize the number needed for a procedure or for a day, in a canister or a pack.

Sponges are either plain gauze or can have a cotton or rayon pad for extra absorbency and softer feel. Sponges are used to clean wounds, to prepare skin for surgery, and for padding, dressing, and covering wounds.

Sometimes a wound needs to remain open to drain. For this purpose, sterile wicking is used. This wick is a length of narrow sterile gauze, that comes in a bottle. The desired amount can be drawn from the bottle using sterile forceps and cut with a sterile scissors. It can be used for nasal packing or as a drainage wick in an open wound.

Solutions

A number of different solutions are used in minor office surgery.

Sterile water is used to dilute medications; sterile saline is used to irrigate and clean out wounds.

Liquid soap such as Hibiclens or Betadine scrub is used by the staff to scrub before surgery and to wash the patient's skin before applying an antiseptic.

Betadine (povidone-iodine) is usually used as an antiseptic to prepare (paint) the skin before surgery. It is a more effective disinfectant than isopropyl alcohol, which was often used in the past. Isopropyl alcohol is still used to prepare the skin before an injection, such as an injection of local anesthetic. Hydrogen peroxide is also not effective to prepare the skin for surgery but can be used after surgery for cleaning around the surgical incision.

Anesthetics

Many surgical procedures require a local anesthetic such as Novocaine or Xylocaine (lidocaine). The medical assistant should obtain the type and strength the doctor desires, and place it to the side of the sterile field.

Xylocaine is available in 0.5, 1.0, 1.5, and 2.0 percent solutions, with or without epinephrine. Epinephrine causes vasoconstriction (narrowing of the blood vessels), which prolongs the anesthetic effect. If the local anesthetic contains epinephrine, the area where it is used will become very pale.

Not all procedures require an injected anesthetic. A topical (surface) anesthetic spray can be used. The most frequently used is ethyl chloride spray, which freezes the skin and allows for simple piercing or lancing. An anesthetic cream such as EMLA cream can be applied for minor procedures. Procedures being done under topical anesthetic must be done quickly, because the anesthetic effect lasts a shorter time than the minutes or hours that an injected local anesthetic lasts.

Suture Material

Surgical stitches used to close a surgical incision or repair a laceration are called **sutures.** They hold the edges of the incision or wound together until healing occurs. Doctors have preferences about the type and size of sutures they use. The assistant opens the outside of the suture material package and either drops the inner pack on the sterile field or allows the doctor to remove the sterile inner pack with his or her sterile gloves.

Sutures are either absorbable or nonabsorbable.

Absorbable sutures are made from an organic material and are used for deep tissue layers. They are rarely used in the medical office.

Nonabsorbable sutures are made from silk, nylon, Tevdek, or another material and must be removed after the wound has partially healed. Sutures are normally removed after 6 to 10 days.

Adhesive mock sutures (Steri-Strips and other brands) are sometimes used when only a small amount of tension needs to be applied to the edges of an incision or laceration. They are applied close together along the incision or laceration and are allowed to fall off on their own over time (usually less than 1 week).

Suture material comes in a number of different diameters, ranging from 3, the thickest, to 000000 (called 6-O), the finest. Fine suture material is usually used in an office.

Needles

Most commonly, the doctor uses a **swaged** needle, that is, fused to the suture material. The more the needle is curved, the easier it is for the doctor to dip in and out of the skin. So-called "atraumatic" needles cause the least damage to skin as they are passed through.

The doctor holds the needle with a needle holder, never with a gloved hand, to avoid accidental injury.

Suturing needles are very sharp. After use, they must be immediately disposed of in a rigid biohazard (sharps) container, because they have been exposed to body tissues.

Dressings

A dressing is applied to the wound or incision site after it is closed. Dressings are usually made of sterile gauze and must be handled with care so they do not become contaminated. A dressing must be large enough to cover the entire wound or incision area. Topical ointment is often applied to the wound or incision site before the dressing is applied, to prevent infection.

Some types of dressing have a special surface that prevents it from adhering to the wound, such as Telfa.

Bandages

A bandage is a nonsterile material that is applied over the dressing to hold the dressing in place. Bandages also provide padding to the wound or incision site, and can even be used to immobilize the area. A bandage can be made from gauze. Premade tubular-gauze bandages are often used to cover fingers, toes, arms, or legs. Elastic bandages can also be used. Some bandages are impregnated with zinc oxide or another chemical and promote healing as well as providing pressure.

Tape

Tape is often used to fasten a bandage or to hold a dressing in place. There are several types of tape:

Stronger tapes such as waterproof tape are used to support a wound or joint. Cloth adhesive tape is strong, but can cause allergic reactions. Surgical tape is often made of paper or clear material. Paper tape is less likely to cause irritation, but for areas where movement is necessary, clear or elastic tape may be used.

Drapes

Surgical drapes are used to frame the surgical site. In most offices, disposable paper drapes have replaced linen towels, which must be sterilized in an autoclave.

After the surgical site has been framed by paper drapes, a clear incisional drape is placed over the surgical site. This drape has an adhesive back, which holds it in place against the colored drapes below. Many incisional drapes are **fenestrated**, meaning that they have an opening that should be fit right over where the incision will be made. This way, there is no need to cut through the clear drape.

PREPARING THE STERILE FIELD

The sterile field is the area on which sterile instruments and supplies will sit, awaiting the doctor's use. A sterile field can be formed from a square or rectangular piece of sterile cloth or paper The sterile field is set up either on a countertop or on a **Mayo stand**, a small table with wheels designed to hold a doctor's necessary instruments and supplies.

Some offices that do their own sterilization rather than purchasing disposables package all the items necessary for the most common surgical procedures within a single surgical pack. Disposable surgical packs are also available for common procedures, although they may not contain exactly the type or size items a particular doctor prefers.

Setting Up a Sterile Field

Whether the pack is made from autoclaved cloth drapes or prepackaged paper, the outside is considered to be nonsterile, whereas the inside and any inner packaging is sterile. Before opening the pack, check the expiration date. Items beyond their expiration date are no longer sterile. Autoclaved packs are sterile for 30

PROCEDURE 17–3

Opening a Sterile Barrier Field

Performance Objective: The student will be able to drape a Mayo stand or a tray with a sterile drape or cloth to create a sterile field.

Supplies and Equipment: Unopened package containing a sterile cloth or paper drape in package such as a sterile barrier field, Mayo stand.

Procedure Steps

1. Wash hands.
2. Place the package containing the sterile drape on flat surface near the Mayo stand or tray.
   Rationale: Sterile drapes are usually made of cloth or disposable paper. They may be plain or plastic backed. A paper drape with a plastic back is preferred for use as a sterile field because small splashes of fluid cannot penetrate to the surface beneath and allow microorganisms to penetrate into the sterile field.
3. Open package without touching the drape. Although the entire drape is sterile, usually if one side is blue, the blue side is placed toward the Mayo stand.
   Rationale: If the drape has a plastic backing, it may be the blue side. The outer inch of a sterile drape is not considered sterile.

4. Pick the drape up as you move away from the table and allow it to unfold without touching anything.
   Rationale: To avoid contaminating the drape.
5. Grasp the other corner of the long edge and lay the drape over the Mayo stand in one motion without waving it around or moving the drape once it has touched the stand.
   Rationale: To avoid contaminating the drape. The excess drape that hangs over the edge of the Mayo stand will not be considered sterile.
6. Add sterile items to the sterile field. Do not turn your back on the sterile field without covering it with a sterile towel or drape. Do not touch any item on the sterile field unless wearing sterile gloves or using sterile transfer forceps.
   Rationale: Only items that are in your direct line of vision can be considered to remain sterile unless they are covered by a sterile drape.

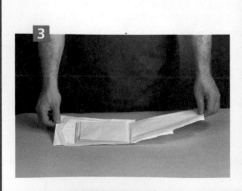

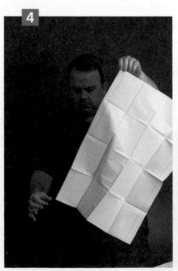

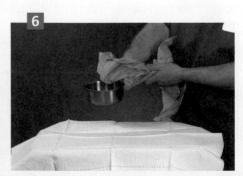

days after they have been sterilized; prepackaged items have a longer shelf life.

Take the package containing the sterile towel or drape and hold it so the top flap of the package opens away from you. Open the package on a flat surface (either the countertop or Mayo stand), handling only the outside of the wrapper so that you do not reach across the package. **Do not reach across the sterile field or across the sterile contents of a pack.**

Pick up the sterile towel by the corner and allow it to fall open without touching anything such as your uniform or the edge of the table. Hold the sterile towel by the top corners and allow it to fall onto the Mayo stand or counter. Practice until you can drop it accurately, because you should not move it from its original position. **The outside 1″ to 2″ of the field and any part that drapes down below the Mayo stand or table are not considered sterile.**

Sometimes, the outside wrapper of a large surgical pack is used to form the sterile field. In this case, the medical assistant only touches the outside corners of the wrapper, pulling each edge all the way open from each side to form the sterile field.

Procedure 17–3 takes you through opening a sterile barrier field, and Procedure 17–4 shows how to open a sterile surgical pack.

PROCEDURE 17–4

Opening a Sterile Surgical Pack

Performance Objective: The student will be able to open a sterile pack using the inside of the pack as a sterile field.

Supplies and Equipment: Sterile pack (wrapped in two layers of wrap) containing sterile instrument(s) or supplies, package containing sterile gloves or sterile transfer forceps, Mayo stand.

Procedure Steps

1. Wash hands.
2. Place a paper or cloth pack (wrapped in two layers of wrap) on the Mayo stand, which has been adjusted to be waist level or higher. Check pack to be sure that it has been sterilized within 1 month. Check tape to be sure that it has changed color during sterilization.

Rationale: If two layers of wrap have been used, the entire inner wrap will be sterile to create a sterile field. Packs wrapped in cloth or paper remain sterile for 1 month after sterilization. Black stripes on the tape of the pack indicate that the pack has been sterilized.

3. Remove tape that is holding the pack closed. Grasping the top flap by the corner, pull first flap away from the body.
Rationale: The outer one inch of the sterile field will not be considered sterile.

4. Touching only the corners pull out one side flap and then the other, leaving the last flap to open toward the body.
Rationale: Maintaining sterile technique while opening and exposing the contents of the package requires a routine whereby the last flap is

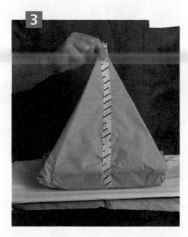

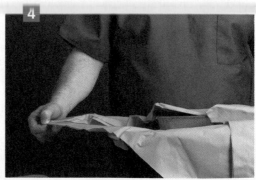

Procedure continued on following page

PROCEDURE 17–4 *(continued)*

opened toward the body last to avoid reaching over the pack.

5 Touching only the corners, pull the final flap toward you. Be sure each corner is fully extended and does not fall back toward the inside of the sterile field.

Rationale: Once you have touched a corner, it may not touch any part of the sterile field.

6. Lay a package of sterile transfer forceps (such as sponge forceps) on a table beside the Mayo stand and open the package. Touching only the handles of the forceps, you may move sterile items within the pack. You may also apply sterile gloves and use them to move items.

Rationale: Only sterile objects can touch sterile objects.

7. Arrange items on the sterile field as desired using sterile transfer forceps or sterile gloves leaving the outer inch of the field clear of objects.

Rationale: It may be necessary to arrange objects within the pack and you must have sterile

gloves or sterile forceps to touch the contents of the pack without contaminating them. The outer inch and any part of the field that hangs over the table is not considered sterile.

8. Cover with sterile drape if the sterile field is not going to be used immediately.

Rationale: If the sterile field is not in your direct field of vision it will not be considered sterile unless it has been covered with a sterile drape.

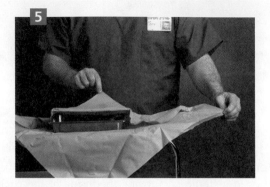

Opening Sterile Packages and Adding to the Sterile Field

Commercial sterile packages come in peel-apart packaging. To open these packages, peel back the edges of the wrapper while holding it and drop the contents gently onto the sterile field, as shown in Figure 17–14, in which suture material is being dropped onto the sterile field.

Open wrapped, autoclaved packages by holding the package so the first fold opens away from your body. If you hold the package in your hand, grab each flap of the wrapper as you open it, then gently drop the sterile item onto the sterile field. The item should not touch against the outside of the wrapper, as shown in Figure 17–15.

Adding Sterile Solution to a Sterile Field

To pour sterile solutions into a sterile basin on a sterile field, remove the cap and place it face up on a clean surface. Or hold it in your nondominant hand, with the inside of the cup facing downward. Pour the solution into the sterile container while holding the bottle approximately 6″ above the container. Replace the cap without touching the inside of the bottle or cap. This is detailed in Procedure 17–5.

Dry Sterile Transfer Forceps

In the past, transfer forceps were sterilized, then stored in a container of disinfectant. It is difficult to be sure that the forceps remain truly sterile if this method is used.

If a medical assistant wants to move a sterile object without putting on sterile gloves, it is more reliable to

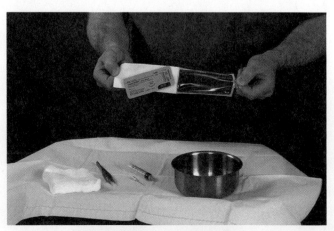

➤ **Figure 17–14** Adding suture material from sterile pack to sterile field (sterile bowl, instruments, and gauze squares already on field).

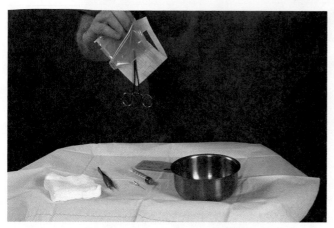

> **Figure 17–15** Holding package to drop sterile instrument onto sterile field.

open a sterile package of sponge forceps each time they are needed. The jaws of the forceps are considered sterile, but the handles are not because the medical assistant touches them.

To store these forceps temporarily, the medical assistant can open a tall sterile container beside the sterile field without touching the rim or the inside of the container. The forceps can be stored in this container during the procedure. After the procedure, the sponge forceps must be resterilized in a peel-apart package before being used for another sterile procedure.

The container used for temporary storage must be resterilized or discarded. Figure 17–16 shows a medical assistant taking sterile sponge forceps from a package to use as sterile transfer forceps.

PROCEDURE 17–5

Adding Sterile Solution to the Sterile Field

Performance Objective: The student will be able to pour a sterile solution into a container on a sterile field using sterile technique.

Supplies and Equipment: Bottle containing sterile solution, sterile field with a sterile container already placed.

Procedure Steps

1. Wash hands.
2. Obtain bottle of sterile solution and place it close at hand before setting up the sterile field.
   Rationale: Once the sterile field is set up, you must keep it in your direct vision at all times.
3. Read label of sterile solution three times to ensure what is to be poured is correct; check expiration date at this time as well.
   Rationale: To be sure that you have the correct solution and that its sterility and potency are assured.
4. Place label of the bottle toward the palm of your hand. Open the bottle and place the cap on the counter with the inside of the cap up. Pour off a small amount of solution into the sink to clean the lip of the bottle. Place the bottle near the place where you will set up the sterile field. Do not replace the cap.

Rationale: The solution label must be protected if bottle will be reused. Placing label in palm will allow any spillage to drain away from label. Care must be taken not to contaminate the cap if it will be replaced.
5. Set up the sterile field. Arrange items on the field using the steps of Procedure 17–4.
   Rationale: Sterile solution is usually poured into a sterile container on the sterile field last, after field is completely set up, to avoid spilling solution while arranging items on the field.
6. Approach field holding the open bottle with the label toward your hand and pour desired amount into the sterile container on the field, holding the bottle 2″ to 6″ above the container

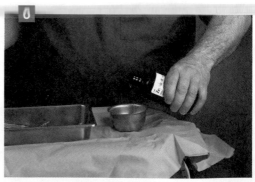

Procedure continued on following page

PROCEDURE 17–5 *(continued)*

without touching it. Avoid any splashes or spillage.

Rationale: The solution bottle is not sterile so it should not touch the sterile container or anything on the field. Pour at a comfortable height, 6″ or lower, that will not allow for splashing. If not using a barrier drape, wetness will contaminate the field because microorganisms from the surface below can penetrate a

wet drape. If the sterile field becomes wet, it will need to be set up again.

7. Replace cap on solution bottle. Drape field if not using immediately. Return the bottle to storage or discard if empty.

Rationale: If a sterile field is not going to be used immediately, then it should be covered with a sterile drape until used to protect items from contamination.

Figure 17–17 shows the use of sponge forceps to move a sterile bowl from inside a tray to another location on the sterile field.

Covering the Sterile Field with a Sterile Towel

Any time you must step away from the sterile field and it will be out of view, you must cover it with another sterile towel to make sure it does not become contaminated. The sterile towel is opened in the same way as the barrier field, held by the corners, and dropped over the sterile field. This is shown in Figure 17–18.

PREPARING THE PATIENT FOR SURGERY

For the doctor to work most effectively and efficiently, the medical assistant often does much of the preparation for a surgical procedure. This includes instructing the patient about what he or she needs to do

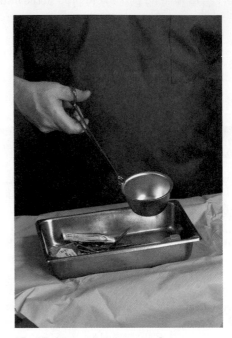

➤ **Figure 17–17** Using sterile sponge forceps to move a sterile bowl from a tray to another area on the sterile field.

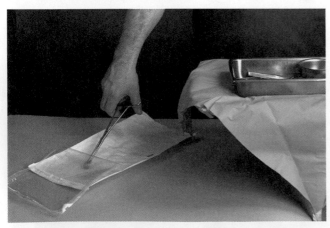

➤ **Figure 17–16** Taking sterile sponge forceps from package to use as sterile transfer forceps.

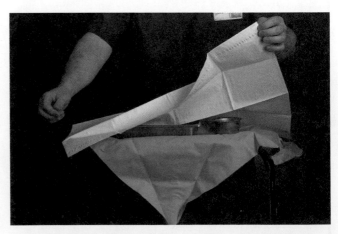

➤ **Figure 17–18** Placing sterile towel over sterile field.

for the procedure, helping the patient to get into a comfortable position for the procedure, and sometimes preparing the skin around the surgical site. The medical assistant also has the patient sign the consent form, giving the patient's **informed consent** to perform the procedure.

Preoperative Instructions

If the procedure is done on a scheduled basis, as opposed to an urgent basis, the medical assistant can be helpful in preparing the patient. Depending on the patient's circumstances and the type of procedure that will be performed, the patient may be asked to adjust diet or discontinue medications, such as anticoagulants. Other times, the patient may be prescribed antibiotics before surgery.

Diet modification may include restricting the amount or types of food or liquid in the 24 hours before surgery.

If the procedure is planned, the medical assistant can also help the patient understand what will be needed in the postoperative period, so those supplies can be purchased before the surgery. The patient may also need to make adjustments to his or her work and social schedule for a time before and after the procedure.

Whether the surgical procedure will take place in the office, in a day-surgery center, or in a hospital, the patient should usually have someone drive him or her to the procedure and home again. The patient may also need to have presurgical diagnostic tests performed, such as X-rays and blood tests. The medical assistant can help the patient arrange these at a convenient facility that is covered by the patient's insurance.

Using Procedure Manual or Procedure Cards

The office should have a set of procedure cards, or a three-ring binder that serves as a procedure manual. Either on a card or on a separate page in the manual is listed each procedure that is commonly done by any doctor in the office. (This means that if there are five doctors in the office who all do repair of lacerations, there will be up to five cards or sheets, one for each doctor.)

A separate card or page for each doctor is necessary because each doctor may have different preferences in the way he or she works. This may include whether the doctor is left- or right-handed; whether the doctor likes to sit or stand (which will have an impact on the height of the procedure table and Mayo stand); and what types of forceps, scalpel blades, suture material, and other instruments the particular doctor likes to use.

Each of the cards for that procedure contains information such as preoperative instructions; skin prep in-structions, including shaving and what prep solution to use; what personal protective equipment is to be used during the procedure; the equipment, supplies, and set-up necessary; and postoperative instructions.

Figure 17–19 shows the information contained on a procedure card for minor surgery.

Obtaining Informed Consent

Whether the surgical procedure is done on an emergency basis or as an elective procedure, the patient must sign an informed consent form, meaning that he or she has been instructed about the procedure, including what will be done and possible complications. (Parents or adult guardians sign for children, and adults who are not legally competent to sign must have another individual such as a conservator or the person who holds the medical power of attorney sign.) A consent form must be signed before the patient receives any medication that could affect his or her mental function, such as a tranquilizer or a narcotic.

Doctor Instructs Patient

It is the doctor's responsibility to instruct the patient about the procedure. The doctor tells the patients what steps will occur during the surgery and answers the patient's questions.

Medical Assistant Obtains Signature and Witnesses

The medical assistant gives the forms to the patient and shows the patient that the form says what the doctor has said verbally, then asks the patient to sign. The medical assistant then witnesses the signature with his or her own signature. Issues of informed consent will also be discussed in the chapter on legal liability issues.

If the procedure is performed on a date after the consent is given, the medical assistant may be asked to sign again or initial the form stating that the form is the one that was signed by the patient earlier. If the patient has additional questions about the procedure when signing the consent form, these should be referred back to the doctor. Although the consent form validates that the patient has been instructed, the patient must understand what he or she has signed.

Figure 17–20 shows a surgical consent form, and Figure 17–21 shows a doctor dressed for surgery, discussing the case with a medical assistant before the surgical handwash.

Positioning the Patient

A patient may have to sit or lie in an unnatural position for the duration of a surgical procedure.

Procedure Card for Minor Surgery

Supplies and Equipment:

For the doctor: Open sterile gown, sterile gloves, sterile towel. The doctor will put on surgical cap, shoe covers and mask before washing hands.

Sterile Pack: Assemble needed equipment such as surgical scissors, scalpel, hemostats, sterile bowls, etc.

Other Supplies: Betadine swab sticks, Xylocaine 1%, 3 ml syringe with 25G 5/8" needle attached, sterile 0.9% saline solution, Betadine solution, alcohol wipes, 1 inch cloth tape, fenestrated drape, bottle containing Formalin for specimens (if needed), sterile swabs for culture, sterile sponge forceps.

Patient position: Position the patient as indicated for the specific procedure.

Prepare sterile field: Open sterile pack on Mayo stand. Use sterile sponge forceps to arrange. Pour solutions into sterile bowls if needed. Add 3 mL syringe with needle for local anesthetic. Add suture material if needed. Add any other instruments requested by the physician if not included in the sterile pack.

Assist the doctor
- Tie gown, adjust mask if needed.
- Clean stopper and hold Xylocaine bottle upside down with label facing the doctor who will draw up the local anesthetic.
- Open Betadine swabsticks without touching ends of swabs and hold for the doctor to remove.
- Open package holding fenestrated drape and hold for the doctor to remove.
- If a specimen is to be sent to the lab, open bottle containing Formalin for the doctor to add specimen or hold culture transport medium for the doctor to insert swab for culture.

➤ **Figure 17–19** Sample procedure card for assisting with surgery.

Whenever possible, the medical assistant should help the patient into that position a couple of minutes before the procedure will begin and help the patient discover the most comfortable position that still affords the doctor the necessary access to the surgical site. Using pillows to prop an arm, leg, shoulder, or hip can often make the position more comfortable.

The medical assistant may also need to help the patient remove clothing to the extent necessary. Blankets can be used to keep a patient warm until it is time to drape the patient for the surgery and to keep other parts of the body warm during the surgery.

Preparing the Skin

The area of the body where the surgery will take place needs to be as free of bacteria and other pathogens as possible. It is never possible to completely sterilize the skin, but it is possible to keep almost all harmful organisms away from the surgical site. Skin should first be washed; then, if necessary, shaved; then rinsed and dried. Finally, an antiseptic containing iodine is "painted" on the skin around the area where the surgery will take place.

Gloves should always be worn when preparing the skin.

Washing

First the skin is washed with an antiseptic soap such as Hibiclens or Betadine scrub. The soap is applied with sterile 4" × 4" sponges, starting at the wound or site where the incision will be made and working outward in small tight circles.

If the procedure is planned, the patient may be instructed to wash with antiseptic soap for a number of days before the surgery. Figure 17–22 shows a medical assistant preparing a patient's arm before surgery.

Shaving, Rinsing, Drying

Again, work from the wound or incision site outward. Hold the skin taut to avoid nicks. At the same time, as much as possible, shave in the direction of the hair growth pattern, to try to avoid nicks.

After shaving, scrub the area again, then rinse with sterile water, and dry with sterile 4" × 4" sponges.

CONSENT FOR SURGERY

Date _2/15/00_

Time _10:30 AM_

I authorize the performance of the following procedure(s) _Incision and Drainage (L) axilla_
_____ on _Katherine McDonald_
to be performed by_Howard Lawler_____, MD.

The following have been explained to me by Dr._Howard Lawler_____

    1. Nature of the procedure: _Incision and Drainage_____

    2. Reason(s) for procedure: _inflamed cyst 5mm × 5mm (L) axilla_

    3. Possible risks: _fever, infection, drainage_____

    4. Possible complications: _infection with drainage, scar in left axilla_

I understand that no warranty or guarantee of the effectiveness of the surgery can be made.

I have been informed of possible alternative treatments including _oral antibiotics_ alone
_____ and of the likely consequences of receiving no treatment, and I
freely consent to this procedure.

I hereby authorize the above named surgeon and his/her assistants to provide additional
services including administering anesthesia and/or medication, performing needed diagnostic tests including but not limited to radiology, and any other additional service deemed
necessary for my well-being. I consent to have removed tissue examined by a pathologist
who may then dispose of the tissue as he/she sees fit.

Signed____*Katherine McDonald*____   Relationship to Patient _self_____
      (Patient/Parent/Guardian)

Witness *Kathy Anderson CMA*

> **Figure 17–20** Completed surgical consent form.

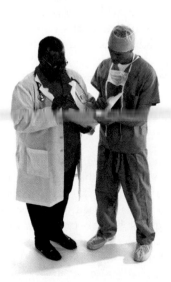

> **Figure 17–21** The doctor dresses in scrubs with a surgical cap and mask before the surgical handwash.

ON THE JOB INFORMED CONSENT

Kathy Anderson has been asked by Dr. Lawler to obtain informed consent from Katherine McDonald for an incision and drainage of an inflamed cyst in the patient's left axilla. Kathy enters the treatment room with the prepared consent form (as shown in Figure 17–21).

QUESTIONS
1. What should Kathy say to the patient?
2. Why is the consent form obtained?
3. Assuming that the patient appears to understand the procedure and has read the consent form carefully, both the patient and Kathy sign the form. What does Kathy's signature attest to?
4. What should Kathy do if each of the following situations occurs?
   a. The patient says, "I'm so glad he doesn't have to cut it out and all I need is an injection of antibiotics."
   b. The patient says: "I can't read this without my glasses, but I don't suppose it matters. You just want my signature."
   c. The patient says, "Dr. Lawler promised me that this will heal easily without a scar."

Applying Antiseptic

Pour antiseptic (Betadine [povidone-iodine]) into a sterile bowl, using the steps in Procedure 17–5. Either the medical assistant or the doctor will then paint the area around the wound or surgical site with the antiseptic, using sterile 4″ × 4″ sponges or sterile swabs and allow the antiseptic to air-dry. Procedure 17–6 discusses preparing the skin for minor surgery.

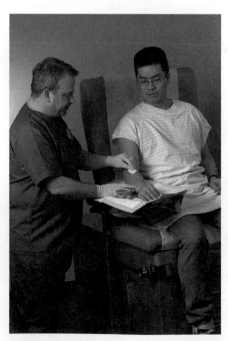

➤ **Figure 17–22** The medical assistant washes the patient's arm as part of the preparation for minor surgery.

Before beginning the procedure, the doctor performs a surgical handwash, as discussed earlier in the chapter. With hands held above the waist, the doctor dries his or her hands with a sterile towel and puts on a sterile gown and sterile gloves. The medical assistant ties the gown (the back is not considered sterile) and also ties the surgeon's mask.

Draping

The surgical site is framed with sterile surgical draping. This is usually done after the doctor puts on surgical gloves so that the drape remains sterile. A fenestrated drape (one that has an opening for the surgical incision) is placed over the area with the wound or where the incision will be made. Often, a piece of adhesive plastic is placed over or around the incision, or four drapes are laid out to form a rectangle and held in place with towel clamps. Figure 17–23 shows the patient prepared and draped for surgery.

Assisting the Doctor to Draw Local Anesthetic

When the doctor is ready to begin the procedure, the medical assistant wipes the rubber stopper of the anesthetic bottle with an alcohol swab and holds the bottle upside down, with the label facing the doctor so the doctor can make sure it is the proper solution. Wearing sterile gloves, the doctor picks up a sterile syringe and inserts a sterile needle into the bottle and draws up the solution. Normally, the doctor requires a

PROCEDURE 17-6

Preparing the Skin for Minor Surgery

Performance Objective: The student will be able to prep the skin for a minor surgery procedure.

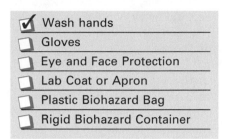

☑ Wash hands
☐ Gloves
☐ Eye and Face Protection
☐ Lab Coat or Apron
☐ Plastic Biohazard Bag
☐ Rigid Biohazard Container

Supplies and Equipment: Antiseptic soap solution, gauze sponges, sterile gloves, razor, sterile basin, underpad with plastic backing; if area is to be rinsed, an additional sterile basin and sterile solution such as sterile water or sterile saline.

Procedure Steps

1. Wash hands.
2. Assemble equipment.
3. Identify patient.
4. Check with patient and chart for any allergies to solutions to be used such as Betadine, or shellfish allergy.
   Rationale: Whenever a medication or chemical is used on the skin or internally, the patient should be questioned regarding allergy. Iodine allergy may be demonstrated by allergy to shellfish.

5. Explain procedure and prep to patient.
   Rationale: By talking with the patient while setting up for minor surgery, you will be able to answer questions and reaffirm consent for procedure.
6. Open sterile basin(s) and pour solution(s), open razor for surgical prep, open gauze sponges, and place underpad under area to be cleaned.
   Rationale: All items must be assembled and opened before putting on sterile gloves or gloves will become contaminated. An underpad will absorb water during the procedure.
7. Put on sterile gloves.
   Rationale: Even though skin cannot be sterilized, it is cleaned thoroughly using sterile procedure to avoid introducing any microorganisms.
8. Apply antiseptic soap with gauze sponges, beginning at operative site and moving outward. Use a circular motion from center outward. Continue scrubbing for 2 to 5 minutes to ensure a thoroughly cleaned area. Do not break the skin down with too much friction, though.
   Rationale: Soap cleans the skin and moistens the skin and hair before shaving. As in any procedure, the goal is to move from the cleanest area outward to the least clean area. Circular motion will dislodge organisms from skin crevices better than an up-and-down motion.

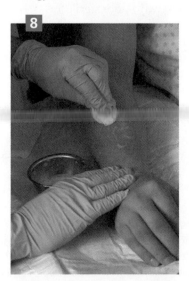

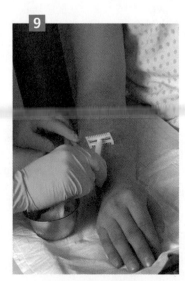

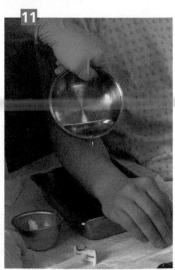

Procedure continued on following page

PROCEDURE 17-6 *(continued)*

9 Hold skin taut and shave hair in the direction of hair growth, if applicable. Scrub skin surface a second time after shaving or at least twice if the area does not require shaving.
Rationale: Hair holds microorganisms and should be removed before an invasive procedure. However, care should be taken to avoid cutting or nicking patient with razor, which could then lead to an infection.

10. If the doctor plans to clean the area again, wipe dry and cover area with a sterile towel if doctor is not ready to begin procedure.
Rationale: Area must stay as free from contamination as possible until procedure is performed.

11 If the doctor wishes the area to be rinsed, apply sterile solution from a separate sterile bowl using sterile gauze sponges. Dry with gauze sponges or sterile towel and cover with a sterile towel.
Rationale: Soap residue may harbor microorganisms.

12. Dry with gauze sponges or sterile towel and cover with a sterile towel.

13. Remove sterile gloves and discard; replace soiled and/or wet underpad with clean underpad for patient comfort.

14. Wash hands.
Note: Some doctors may choose to clean the operative site immediately before they incise. Have supplies available to be prepared should this need arise. Have extra sterile gloves on hand because the doctor will wish to change gloves after cleaning the site.

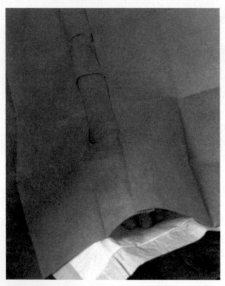

➤ **Figure 17-23** A patient prepared for arm surgery after Betadine has been applied to the incision area and a sterile fenestrated drape has been placed.

3-cc (cubic centimeter) syringe and a 5/8″, 25G (gauge) needle to infiltrate the skin surrounding the surgical site.

ASSISTING WITH MINOR SURGICAL PROCEDURES

Once a sterile field has been established and the surgical equipment and supplies are laid out on the sterile field, and once the patient is prepped and draped, surgery can begin. Depending on the complexity of the procedure and time it will take, the medical assistant will have different responsibilities.

Responsibilities During Surgery

The medical assistant can play an active part in assisting the doctor in more complex and time-consuming procedures or can play a more passive role in less complex, less time-consuming surgeries. The medical assistant may need to be sterile or may be able to remain nonsterile during a surgical procedure, depending on the type of help the doctor needs.

Medical Assistant Nonsterile. If the medical assistant is nonsterile, he or she may not touch any of the items on the sterile field. The following can be done by the medical assistant who is nonsterile:

1. Tie the back of the surgeon's sterile gown (The back of the gown is nonsterile.)
2. Obtain additional supplies and put them in the sterile field, using Procedure 17-4
3. Reassure the patient, speaking to him or her and being emotionally supportive
4. Adjust the light for the doctor
5. Adjust the doctor's mask, face shield, and/or protective glasses, and wipe sweat off the doctor's face as necessary
6. Hold a container with formalin to receive any specimen for **biopsy**. (A biopsy is an examination of tissue under a microscope to determine if cancerous cells are present.)

Medical Assistant Sterile. The medical assistant who is sterile for a surgical procedure may be gloved only for simple procedures, or may be gloved and gowned for more complex procedures. A medical assistant who is sterile may:

1. Hand instruments to the doctor
2. Hold a retractor
3. Suction or sponge blood from the surgical field, using a sterile suction catheter tip or sterile gauze sponges.

Control of Bleeding

During office surgery, it is often necessary to control bleeding. There are five ways to do this.

Tourniquet for extremities. For bleeding on the arm or leg, a cuff-type tourniquet placed above the operative site can slow the blood flowing down the artery to the site and reduce or stop bleeding. A cuff similar to a blood pressure cuff is often used for this purpose.

Electrocautery. In this process, a handheld wand is heated by electric current from a power source using wall current or a battery-powered unit. The tool is used to remove small growths. As the growth is being essentially burned off, blood vessels are sealed off to minimize bleeding.

Suction. Suction is used to remove blood from the surgical area so the doctor can better view the place he or she is working. Suction does not actually stop or lessen bleeding; it only lessens the amount of blood in the surgical area. The suction catheter must be sterile.

Sponge forceps and sponge. Again, sponging blood only removes it from the surgical area; it does not lessen the amount coming from blood vessels into the surgical area.

Clamp and tie. In this process, blood vessels that are cut during surgery are first clamped shut, then the end is tied off. This does reduce the amount of blood flowing into the surgical area. In the office, this technique is only used for blood vessels that bleed profusely (often called "bleeders" or "pumpers"). Hemostats for this purpose are often included in surgical packs.

Assisting During Skin Closure

After the surgical procedure is complete, the skin must be sutured to reclose it. If the doctor asks the medical assistant to assist, and he or she has not previously been sterile, the assistant must perform a surgical scrub, then glove before proceeding.

The three skin closing materials are sutures, staples, and adhesive sutures (Steri-Strips). Staples are not usually used to close wounds or surgical incisions in the medical office but can be removed there.

If assisting with suturing, the medical assistant needs to open a sterile suture pack and add the inner package to the sterile field. When the sterile package is opened and the suture material and needle revealed, the medical assistant wearing sterile gloves may clamp the needle with a needle holder on the upper one-third of the needle (the third of the needle closest to the suture).

Clamping too close to the end can damage the point; clamping too close to the suture material can cause the suture to detach from the needle.

After the needle is clamped, the medical assistant hands it to the doctor handle first. After the suture is complete, the assistant cuts the suture close to the stitch. Alternatively, the doctor may open the package of sutures, suture, and cut without assistance.

Adhesive stitches are used to close small wounds or to support a surgical incision after sutures have been removed. They are applied parallel to the wound at intervals of 1/4" to 1/2".

Figure 17–24 shows different types of skin closure: Steri-Strips, continuous, and interrupted sutures. In continuous suturing, the suture material is passed continuously through the wound without being cut and tied. In interrupted suturing, each stitch is separately cut and tied. The doctor may cut the sutures or the medical assistant, wearing sterile gloves, may cut them. Interrupted sutures are the most common type of suture used in the medical office.

Procedure 17–7 discusses assisting with minor surgery.

SURGICAL PROCEDURES AND METHODS

Following are brief discussions of some of the minor surgical procedures that may be performed in an office setting.

Excision of a Lesion

Excision means cutting out. A **lesion** is an irregularity on the skin, such as a mole or a skin tag. Lesions are usually "dry," meaning they do not contain fluid that must be drained.

Figure 17–25 shows the procedure card for excision of a lesion. Any small skin lesion is usually sent to a pathology laboratory for examination. When the doctor removes the lesion, the medical assistant removes the top from a small bottle containing formalin, a preservative, and holds the bottle for the doctor to drop the specimen in. After the surgery, the bottle is labeled and sent with a cytology request to the lab.

Incision and Drainage

Whereas a dry lesion is simply excised (cut out), an abscess or a cyst must often be incised (cut into) and drained. Abscesses are then allowed to heal. In many cases the cyst sac is removed, with or without drainage.

An **abscess** is a localized collection of pus, with inflammation of the surrounding tissue. An abscess is

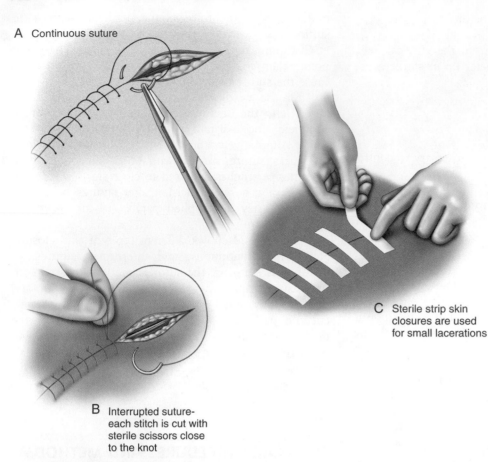

A Continuous suture

B Interrupted suture—
each stitch is cut with
sterile scissors close
to the knot

C Sterile strip skin
closures are used
for small lacerations

➤ **Figure 17–24** Types of skin closure.

PROCEDURE 17–7

Assisting with Minor Surgery

Performance Objective: The student will be able to assist in a minor surgery procedure.

- ☑ Wash Hands
- ☑ Gloves
- ☑ Eye and Face Protection
- ☑ Lab Coat or Apron
- ☑ Plastic Biohazard Bag
- ☑ Rigid Biohazard Container

Supplies and Equipment:

For the sterile field: a package containing a sterile barrier field and sterile packages containing instruments and supplies needed for the procedure (such as scalpel with blade, scissors, hemostats, thumb forceps, bowl/basin containing sterile cleansing solution, gauze squares, suture material, needle holder, etc.) and a sterile syringe with needle for the local anesthetic.

To prepare the doctor: sterile towels (for the doctor to dry hands), sterile gloves, and a sterile gown.

Additional supplies needed near the surgical table: local anesthetic that doctor can draw up, specimen container with formalin, one or more open packages containing sterile drapes, dressing/bandage material, biohazard waste container for cleanup, laboratory requests and labels for all specimens that may be sent for pathology (if applicable), and additional packages of sterile gloves in the correct size for both the doctor and the medical assistant.

Procedure Steps

1. Wash hands.
2. Identify patient and explain procedure.
3. Be sure that consent form has been signed or obtain patient's signature.

Rationale: Patients must give informed consent to all procedures. The patient's signature is obtained on a consent form for surgery and most invasive procedures.

4. Assemble equipment. Adjust Mayo stand for instrument tray setup and have available another stand or countertop for additional supplies.

   Rationale: Mayo stand should be positioned at doctor's waist level or higher to prevent contamination of sterile field.

5. Position patient on an examination or treatment table so that the surgical site is accessible to the doctor. Prepare the skin following the steps of Procedure 17–6 as directed by the doctor.

   Rationale: The patient's skin must be as clean as possible and free of hair before surgery begins. The doctor may choose to clean the skin as part of the surgical procedure. If so, additional sterile gloves will be needed.

6. Set up the sterile field following steps of Procedure 17–1 and/or 17–2. Add any needed items to the sterile field. Pour antiseptic solution into sterile bowl or basin if included in tray. Maintain sterile technique throughout setup. Cover the sterile field.

   Rationale: The sterile field should be covered if you cannot keep it in direct vision to avoid accidental contamination.

7. Set up next to surgical field additional wrapped sterile items and solutions that may be needed during procedure.

   Rationale: Items may become contaminated, or additional instruments or supplies may be needed during the procedure.

8. Alert doctor that patient and equipment are ready for procedure to begin. Uncover field. Assist doctor in gowning and gloving if indicated.

   Rationale: Do not leave sterile field once you have set it up, if possible. The patient may contaminate field by looking under cover or touching any part of the inside of the tray. It is for this reason that a sterile field should not be set up until immediately ready for procedure to begin. Once the tray is uncovered, only sterile items may touch the sterile field. Additional packages of gloves are necessary should the medical assistant or doctor need to leave the field to obtain nonsterile packages such as more suture or gauze.

9. Assist the doctor as needed for the procedure, being certain to follow principles of surgical asepsis. Before donning sterile gloves, wipe the top of the bottle of local anesthetic with alcohol and hold the bottle for the doctor to draw it up. The doctor will apply antiseptic solution and inject the local anesthetic. (Alternatively, the local anesthetic may be drawn up before surgery if indicated by doctor. This should be done using sterile technique if the syringe is to be placed on the sterile field. Open vial, wipe top with alcohol, open syringe, apply sterile gloves, and withdraw solution with nonsterile vial sitting on counter. Then place the syringe and needle on the sterile field.)

   Rationale: The medical assistant must assist the doctor to prepare the local anesthetic and surgical site before putting on sterile gloves.

10. The doctor will apply a sterile fenestrated drape or several sterile drapes laid across each other to isolate the surgical site.

    Rationale: One or more drapes are placed to allow only the surgical site to be exposed during procedure and to provide a sterile area around the incision site.

11. While wearing sterile gloves, the medical assistant may pass or hand instruments to the doctor during the procedure. Hand doctor instruments in functional position (i.e., handles first). Assist with handing suture material in needle holder, if indicated.

    Rationale: Assisting includes helping doctor make procedure flow smoothly and quickly. Assuring sterility is sometimes easier with help from an assistant.

12. During the procedure the assistant will be responsible for comforting and attending to the needs of the patient as well as keeping the doctor comfortable.

    Rationale: Doctor should be alerted to any unusual patient discomfort during procedure. Observing verbal and nonverbal communication is very important.

13. The medical assistant may need to remove sterile gloves to open new supplies, to adjust a light, or to remove perspiration from the doctor's face. If necessary, the medical assist-

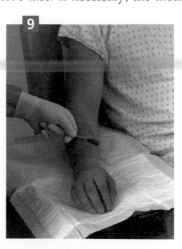

Procedure continued on following page

PROCEDURE 17-7 *(continued)*

ant puts on new sterile gloves for assisting with sterile parts of the procedure.
Rationale: The doctor cannot touch nonsterile objects without contaminating sterile gloves. Observing for signs of visible perspiration on the doctor's face will help keep him or her more comfortable during the procedure.

14. If tissue is removed, remove the lid from a specimen container and hold so that the doctor can drop the tissue specimen into it. Label any tissue specimen and complete the necessary requisition to send it to an outside laboratory for pathology/cytology.
Rationale: Tissue removed during any surgical procedure is commonly sent to a laboratory for analysis.

15. After inserting sutures (if needed) the doctor usually applies a dressing to the surgical area. The medical assistant prepares tape or other bandage material as directed and may finish applying the bandage.
Rationale: The dressing is sterile, but the tape or bandage that holds the dressing is not.

16. Be sure that the patient's condition is stable before he or she gets up. Check dressing for drainage.
Rationale: Even minor surgery can cause a patient to feel dizzy or faint. If a bleeding blood vessel was overlooked, the dressing may quickly become saturated with blood.

17. Give the patient instructions to care for the surgical site at home and instruct the patient when to return to the office for follow-up (if the doctor has not already done so).
Rationale: The patient must know how to care for the surgical site and when to return to the office to prevent complications from the surgery.

18. Using appropriate personal protective equipment, clean room, placing all disposable instruments and items contaminated with body fluids in a biohazard container. All sharps must be placed in a rigid biohazard container. Take precautions to avoid injury from needles or other sharps.
Rationale: Gloves, a fluid-resistant gown, and face protection are needed to avoid coming in contact with items contaminated with body fluids when cleaning room.

19. Use appropriate cleaning solutions to ready the room for next patient.
Rationale: Surfaces contaminated with blood or body fluids must be disinfected according to Occupational Safety and Health Administration guidelines.

20. Although the doctor will write or dictate a note about the surgery, the medical assistant may need to document that instructions were given to the patient on discharge and/or that a specimen was sent to the laboratory.

---

formed by the body's normal immune system response to a local attack by a foreign body. The pathogens are walled off in a self-contained area and are not allowed to spread throughout the body. An abscess may be drained to relieve pain and pressure and to facilitate healing.

A **cyst** is caused by an oil duct in the body becoming clogged, which causes an accumulation of sebum (oil) in the surrounding gland under the skin. Cysts that become infected or inflamed must be removed; noninflamed cysts are often also removed because they are ugly or are located in an area of the body that makes them uncomfortable.

Cysts are surrounded by a membrane and should be completely excised, because they tend to recur if they are not. However, sometimes it is necessary to incise and drain so the cyst sac does not explode during excision.

Incision and drainage **(I&D)** means cutting into the affected area to allow the collection of pus or sebum to drain out of the abscess or cyst in a controlled manner. Sometimes the material is cultured or sent for micro-

scopic examination, and the patient may be treated with oral antibiotics or antibiotic cream.

After an abscess is incised and drained, it is not sutured. A small abscess that the doctor is able to completely drain will normally close and heal by itself over a short time. A larger abscess may need to be left open for a period of time, with a wick inserted, to allow fluid deep in the affected area to drain out. This promotes healing from the inside out; if the skin closes before all of the fluid is out, the abscess will re-form. Usually, the patient receives an antibiotic to assist in wound healing.

If a cyst is incised and drained to prevent exploding during removal, it is usually removed after it is drained.

Figure 17–26 shows a procedure card for an incision and drainage.

Suturing

In addition to closing surgical incisions using sutures, suturing is also done to close accidental **lacera-**

Procedure Card for Surgical Excision - Dr. Hughes

Supplies and Equipment:

For the doctor: Open sterile gown, sterile gloves size 7, sterile towel. The doctor will put on surgical cap, shoe covers and mask before washing hands.

Sterile Pack: 2 hemostats, curved operating scissors (S/S), straight operating scissors (B/B), 4X4 gauze squares, tissue forceps, dressing forceps.

Other Supplies: Scalpel, 1 package 4-0 silk suture with attached reverse cutting needle FS-2, Betadine swab sticks, Xylocaine 1%, 3 ml syringe with 25G 5/8" needle attached, alcohol wipes, 1 inch cloth tape, fenestrated drape, bottle containing Formalin for specimens, sterile sponge forceps.

Patient position: Place the patient in a position so that the lesion is facing up.

Patient preparation: Wearing sterile gloves, wash, shave and rinse area at least 5 inches larger than area to be excised. Dry with sterile towel and cover area with sterile towel for Dr. Hughes to paint with Betadine.

Prepare sterile field: Open sterile pack on Mayo stqand. Add suture, disposable scalpel. Use sterile sponge forceps to arrange if needed. Add 3 mL syringe with needle for local anesthetic.

Assist the doctor
- Tie gown, adjust mask if needed.
- Clean stopper and hold Xylocaine bottle upside down for the doctor to draw up the local anesthetic.
- Open Betadine swabsticks without touching ends of swabs and hold for the doctor to remove.
- Open package holding fenestrated drape and hold for the doctor to remove.
- When the doctor removes a specimen, open bottle containing Formalin for the doctor to add it without touching inside of lid or bottle.
- Place lid on bottle. After procedure is done, label and fill out lab slip.
- Prepare tape for dressing and secure dressing as directed.

➢ **Figure 17–25** Procedure card for surgical excision.

---

tions (cuts). A surgical incision is straight, but an accidental laceration is often jagged and often not the same depth throughout.

Suturing a laceration helps facilitate healing. It also minimizes scarring and decreases the likelihood of infection.

Indications

A laceration should be sutured for one of four reasons:

1. It is gaping, meaning that the edges of the wound are far apart from one another rather than close together.
2. It is bleeding, and the bleeding cannot be controlled.
3. It is located on the face or neck, or in a part of the body where natural twisting and bending will open the wound.
4. It extends deep into underlying tissue.

Wound Cleaning

Before suturing, a laceration must be meticulously cleaned. Cleaning should be done in a similar manner to preparing for surgery, using antiseptic soap and working away from the laceration. In addition, the laceration itself should be irrigated (washed out) with sterile water. If the laceration has been caused by glass, wood, or rock, it may also need to be probed to make sure no particles of material are inside the wound before it is sutured closed.

Procedure 31–11 in chapter 31 on emergency treatment discusses cleaning of minor wounds.

The setup for suturing a wound is similar to that for a surgical excision, depending on the doctor's preference for instruments and suture material. Nonabsorbable sutures are usually used in the smallest size the doctor judges will keep the edges of the laceration firmly approximated (held together). Although the doctor usually cuts the stitches, the medical assistant may be asked to put on sterile gloves and assist.

Procedure Card for Incision and Drainage - Dr. Lawler

Supplies and Equipment:

For Dr. Lawler: Open sterile gown, sterile gloves size 8, sterile towel. Dr. Lawler will put on surgical cap, shoe covers and mask before washing hands.

Sterile I & D pack: 2 small bowls, 2 hemostats, curved operating scissors (S/S), straight operating scissors (B/B), 4X4 gauze squares, 2X2 gauze squares.

Other Supplies: Betadine swab sticks, Xylocaine 1%, 3 ml syringe with 25G 5/8" needle attached, 5 ml syringe without needle, sterile 0.9% saline solution, Betadine solution, alcohol wipe, bottle of packing strip, 1 inch cloth tape, fenestrated drape, bottle containing Formalin for specimens (if needed), sterile sponge forceps.

Patient position: Area to be incised up. Mayo stand beside patient. Plastic bag for used supplies beside patient.

Prepare sterile field: Open sterile I & D pack on Mayo stand. Use sterile sponge forceps to arrange as shown. Pour Betadine in one bowl and normal saline in the other bowl. Add 3 ml syringe with needle and 5 ml syringe to sterile field.

Assist Dr. Lawler:
- Tie gown, adjust mask if needed.
- Clean stopper and hold Xylocaine bottle upside down for Dr. Lawler to draw up the local anesthetic.
- Open Betadine swabsticks without touching ends of swabs and hold for Dr. Lawler to remove.
- Open package holding fenestrated drape and hold for Dr. Lawler to remove.
- Open bottle containing packing strip and hold for Dr. Lawler to remove packing.
- If a specimen is to be sent to the lab, open bottle containing Formalin for Dr. Lawler to add specimen.
- Place lid on bottle after procedure is done, label and fill out lab slip.
- Prepare tape for dressing and secure dressing as directed.

➤ Figure 17–26 Procedure card for incision and drainage.

Electrocautery

Electrocautery is the use of electricity to heat or burn tissue. It controls bleeding by coagulating blood vessels as the tissue is burned.

The doctor uses a handheld device with a blunt or sharp tip that applies electric current to the tissue. The power source may be a battery or a foot pedal connected to a power supply. With some devices, a grounding pad is placed under the patient's skin to complete the electric circuit.

As with any electrical device, care must be taken and all cables and connections must be inspected for frayed wires before use. Disposable tips or cautery devices should never be reused.

Because the electric current poses a fire risk, alcohol, flammable anesthetics such as ethyl chloride, and oxygen should not be used when the cautery device is being used.

After cauterization, the affected tissue necroses, meaning it dies and **sloughs** (separates from healthy tissue). It is then replaced by new, healthy tissue. Patients should be warned that the sloughing tissue may have an unpleasant odor for the first week or so. The patient may be instructed to wear a dressing, depending on the size and location of the cauterized area.

Cryosurgery

Cryosurgery is use of cold to destroy tissue. On the skin, liquid nitrogen is frequently used. It is kept in a pressurized tank and is applied to the skin directly from a probe or a cotton swab. Liquid nitrogen is used to destroy warts and other benign skin lesions.

After the application, the outer skin layers necrose and slough in the same way as after electrocauterization. The surrounding area may become inflamed, and the patient may experience local discomfort for a few days. If a blister develops, the patient should not disturb it. Usually, patients wear a dressing, and the doctor may also instruct the patient to apply an antibiotic ointment.

Cryosurgery is also used to treat chronic cervicitis by freezing the cervix. When the cells of the cervix are frozen, they slough and are replaced by new tissue that may not be subject to the same inflammation. For this procedure, the patient is placed in the lithotomy position. The doctor uses a vaginal speculum to view the cervix. The cryosurgery device probe is inserted into the vagina and used to bathe the cervix in the coolant liquid, usually liquid nitrogen, nitrous oxide, or carbon dioxide.

The patient may experience a cramping sensation similar to that of a menstrual period during this procedure. After the procedure, the patient wears a sanitary napkin to absorb the discharge, which continues for several days.

Again, the patient should be warned that the sloughing tissue has an unpleasant odor for the first week or so. The patient should also be instructed not to have intercourse for about 4 weeks so the area can heal. In addition, the doctor may prescribe douches or vaginal medication.

The medical assistant should follow the manufacturer's instructions for proper storage of the chemicals used in cryosurgery and should not allow any of the liquid nitrogen to come into contact with any skin or other surface other than the area intended for surgery.

Laser Surgery

Lasers are frequently used in office-based surgical procedures of the eye, ear, and nose. In hospitals, they are used in more complex surgery. The word laser is actually an acronym that has, over time, become a word. It is made up of the first letters of the words *light amplification by stimulated emission of radiation.*

In practical terms, a laser produces a highly concentrated light that is capable of destroying tissue. It is used both to coagulate blood vessels and to remove small bits of tissue without damaging the surrounding tissue. Lasers were first used in eye surgery on the retina, but now are used for surgery on many parts of the body.

When used on the skin, the laser causes tissue destruction that resembles a burn or may cause the entire outer layer of the skin to be lost, depending on the type of laser and the duration of exposure. All person-

nel in the room with the laser (and the patient as well) must wear goggles to prevent eye damage from the laser's intense light.

Warning signs need to be posted on the door when the laser is in use, to prevent a person entering the room without goggles. In addition, the laser can cause burns and pose a fire hazard.

Whenever laser surgery is being performed, the sterile field should include a basin of sterile saline, with a sterile syringe, in case tissue or equipment needs to be cooled urgently.

A medical assistant can only assist in laser surgery if he or she has undergone specific training on the type of laser being used, as well as on the specific accessories being used in the surgery, and on safety precautions for the patient, doctor, and assistant.

Microsurgery

Microsurgery is surgery using tiny instruments and is performed while the doctor views the surgical area under a microscope or wears magnifying glasses.

Magnifying Glasses

Magnifying glasses, called surgical loupes, as shown in Figure 17–27, are worn by the doctor. These both enlarge the image of the surgical site and improve the doctor's ability to visualize the surgical site.

Microscope

A surgical microscope is not like a tabletop microscope seen in a laboratory. A surgical microscope has a light source and lenses, and is hooked up to a camera or video recorder and a television monitor, for viewing. Lenses and cords must be inspected carefully before each usage and must be stored carefully.

POSTOPERATIVE CARE

Wounds are classified as either intentional or accidental, either open or closed. Closed wounds are bruises and hematomas, in which the skin is not broken but the underlying tissue is traumatized.

Postoperative wounds are, by definition, open wounds. Lacerations are accidental open wounds, and surgical incisions are intentional open wounds.

Wound Healing

All wounds must go through a process of healing. Suturing a wound does not equal healing a wound. Suturing is only a way to draw the edges of a wound together to promote healing. The healing process is biological and occurs over time. Figure 17–28 shows different types of wounds.

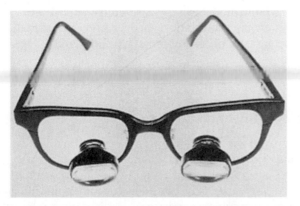

➤ **Figure 17–27** Surgical Loupes. (From Meeker MH, Rothrock JC, *Alexander's Care of the Patient in Surgery,* 11th ed. St. Louis: Mosby 1999.)

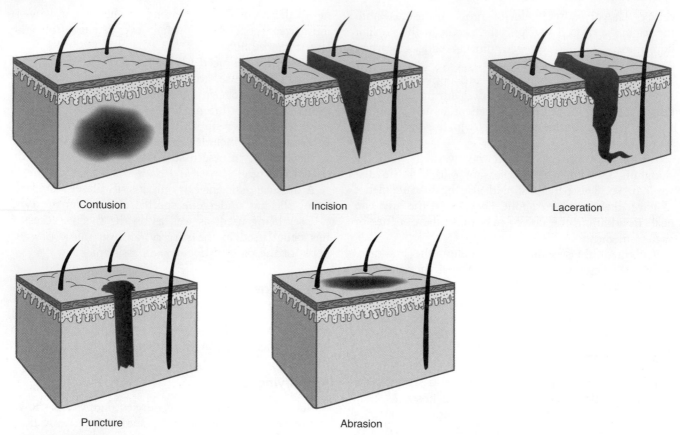

Contusion

Incision

Laceration

Puncture

Abrasion

➤ **Figure 17–28** Types of wounds. (From Bonewit-West K. *Clinical Procedures for Medical Assistants,* 5th ed. Philadelphia: W.B. Saunders, 2000.)

Wound healing takes place in three phases.

The first phase, called the inflammatory response, lasts for 3 or 4 days. Over the first day, blood vessels contract to control bleeding. Blood platelets come together to form a kind of glue that begins binding the wound. Finally, fibrin is released in the wound, which collects red blood cells into a clot, which becomes a scab. White blood cells arrive to clean up bacteria and tissue debris. Finally, the edges of the wound begin to pull together under the scab.

The second phase, called **proliferation,** lasts another 5 to 20 days. Cells continue to form, and the tissue continues to contract under the scab and pulls the edges together. Clean and shallow wounds usually completely heal by the end of this phase.

Deeper or more jagged wounds completely heal during a third phase, called **remodeling.** When it is necessary for the tissue to remodel, a thick fibrous protein substance called collagen forms into what is commonly called scar tissue. Scar tissue is stronger than skin but lacks a blood supply and elasticity.

Wounds can also be classified by the way they heal; this classification is known as healing by primary intention or secondary intention. Figure 17–29 shows different kinds of wound healing.

Primary Intention

A wound that heals by **primary intention** is one where the wound edges are **approximated,** meaning that the skin opening comes together in a near-perfect fit, with minimal scarring.

Secondary Intention

A wound that heals by **secondary intention** is one that heals by **granulation,** or filling in with granulated tissue instead of the original type of tissue, from the bottom up.

Tertiary Intention

Delayed primary intention or **tertiary intention** means keeping a large wound that may become infected open until the wound is clean. It is then sutured. The edges may not be completely approximated, and some granulation occurs.

Greater scar formation occurs in wounds that heal by secondary and delayed primary intention.

Dressings and Bandages

After a surgical incision or laceration is closed, it usually must be covered for at least a short time, to protect the wound from contamination while it goes through the first phase of healing. This is done by placing a dressing immediately over the wound and a bandage over the dressing.

Dressing and Bandage Material

A **dressing** is a sterile covering that goes immediately over a closed surgical incision or laceration. A sterile gauze sponge, sometimes lubricated with antibiotic ointment, or a nonadhesive dressing such as Telfa, should be used. A wick used to keep an incised infection open is also considered dressing material.

A dressing needs to be kept in place using bandage material. A **bandage** also helps to provide even pressure and support to the area around the wound.

A bandage can be made out of tape, gauze, cloth, or elastic. Very small wounds are covered by a bandage that combines gauze and tape (such as Band-Aids). Small surgical wounds are often secured by tape, which holds the dressing in place and provides some support for the incision.

If a large area on an extremity needs to be covered, or if the skin is delicate, the bandage may be held in place with conforming gauze bandage that encircles the limb over the dressing(s). Tape is applied to the gauze to hold it in place. Elastic bandages can provide pressure to reduce postoperative bleeding and/or swelling. These are secured with tape or metal clips.

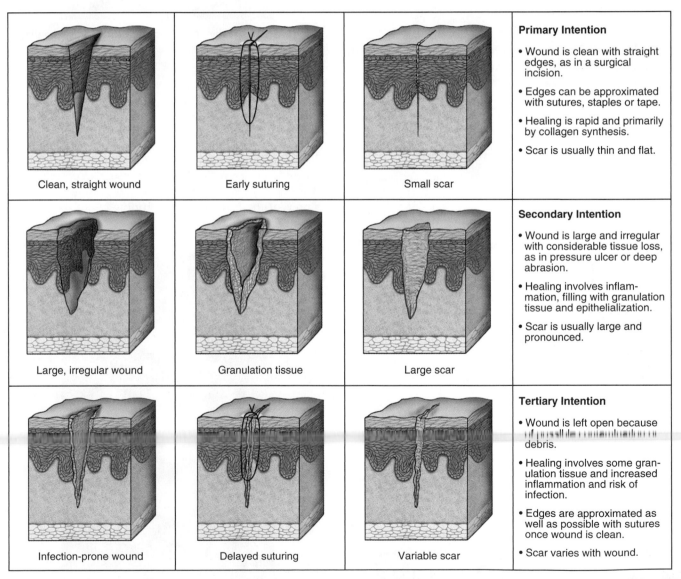

Primary Intention

- Wound is clean with straight edges, as in a surgical incision.
- Edges can be approximated with sutures, staples or tape.
- Healing is rapid and primarily by collagen synthesis.
- Scar is usually thin and flat.

Clean, straight wound / Early suturing / Small scar

Secondary Intention

- Wound is large and irregular with considerable tissue loss, as in pressure ulcer or deep abrasion.
- Healing involves inflammation, filling with granulation tissue and epithelialization.
- Scar is usually large and pronounced.

Large, irregular wound / Granulation tissue / Large scar

Tertiary Intention

- Wound is left open because of possible contamination or debris.
- Healing involves some granulation tissue and increased inflammation and risk of infection.
- Edges are approximated as well as possible with sutures once wound is clean.
- Scar varies with wound.

Infection-prone wound / Delayed suturing / Variable scar

> **Figure 17–29** Wound healing by primary, secondary and delayed primary (tertiary) intention. (From Monahan FD, Neighbors M. *Medical-Surgical Nursing: Foundations for Clinical Practice,* 2nd ed. Philadelphia: W.B. Saunders, 1998.)

Applying a Sterile Dressing

The doctor usually applies the dressing after surgery, but a medical assistant may apply or change a sterile dressing.

A number of dressings may be necessary to provide adequate coverage to the affected area and to absorb drainage. Place each sterile dressing carefully on the wound; do not drag them across the skin to get them into the proper position. The sterile package for each pair of dressings should be opened and used as a sterile field.

A bandage should completely cover the sterile dressing and extend at least 1″ beyond each border of the dressing.

Sterile gloves are used to apply a sterile dressing. Once the wound is covered with a sterile dressing, it is no longer necessary to wear sterile gloves.

Taping a Dressing

Enough tape should be used to secure the bandage and dressing. However, too much tape can make it difficult for the patient to move the affected area.

Gloves do not need to be worn when taping a dressing and bandages.

Principles of Bandaging

Bandages should be snug but comfortable. They should be fastened securely enough so that they do not fall off or come apart during normal activity.

The affected area should be bandaged in its normal position. Skin surfaces should not touch each other underneath bandaging, to keep the skin from adhering and forming scar tissue.

Bandages should be applied starting at the distal part of the body and ending at the proximal part (ankle toward knee, wrist toward elbow, and so on). Distal and proximal are measured in reference to the attachment of the arm or leg to the shoulder or hip. Closer to the shoulder or hip is proximal, farther is distal.

There are two reasons for this. First, a bandage wrapped from a smaller place toward a larger place stays more secure. Second, bandages wrapped from distal to proximal assist in venous blood return to the heart.

Bandage Turns

The following bandage turns are commonly used:

Circular:	Used to anchor a bandage.
Spiral:	Used to hold a bandage in place on the arm or leg.
Spiral Reverse:	Provides more support than the plain spiral.

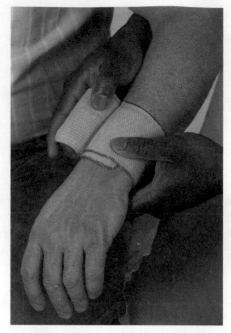

> **Figure 17–30** A circular bandage turn anchors a bandage.

Recurrent:	Used on the fingers, head, and the stump of an amputation.
Figure-of-Eight:	Used across a joint that bends, such as an ankle or hand.

Bandage turns may be combined; for example, an above-the-knee amputation may use a recurrent turn on the upper leg and a figure-of-eight around the waist to prevent the bandage from slipping off.

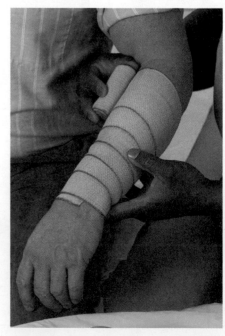

> **Figure 17–31** The spiral turn is used to wrap the arm or leg.

The circular and spiral or spiral-reverse turns are used to wrap the straight part of an arm or leg. Begin by wrapping the bandage straight around the extremity to anchor the bandage and prevent slipping. Figure 17–30 shows the circular bandage turn.

To use a spiral bandage turn, after one complete turn over the beginning of the bandage, begin to wrap the extremity at an angle, keeping the bandage smooth, as shown in Figure 17–31. Either wrap until the bandage is finished, or cut the bandage at the desired end and secure with clips or tape, as shown in Figure 17–32.

The spiral-turn can be done either by spiraling first up, then down on the extremity, as shown in Figure 17–33, or by using the thumb to fold the bandage on each turn so that it changes direction, as shown in Figure 17–34. The spiral-reverse provides more support because more bandage is used.

The figure-of-eight turn begins with a circular turn to anchor the bandage, then progresses around a joint

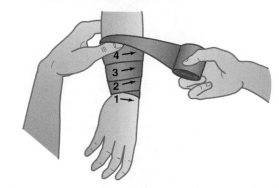

➤ **Figure 17–34** Spiral reverse turn made by folding the bandage. (From Bonewit-West K. *Clinical Procedures for Medical Assistants,* 5th ed. Philadelphia: W.B. Saunders, 2000.)

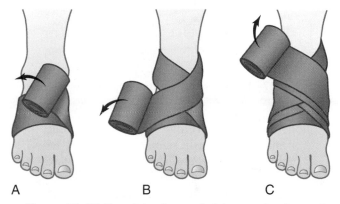

A   B   C

➤ **Figure 17–35** Use of the figure-of-eight turn for the ankle. (From Bonewit-West, K. *Clinical Procedures for Medical Assistants,* 5th ed. Philadelphia: W.B. Saunders, 2000.)

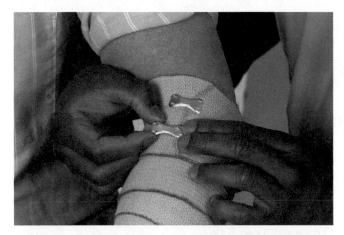

➤ **Figure 17–32** Clips or tape are used to secure the bandage.

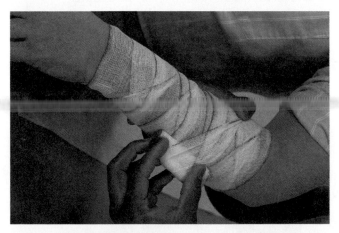

➤ **Figure 17–33** In the spiral reverse turn, the direction of the spiral changes each time the bandage is brought around the limb.

such as an ankle, knee, or wrist. Figure 17–35 illustrates the use of the figure-of-eight bandage turn.

The recurrent turn is used to cover the end of an extremity, an amputation, or to cover the head. The bandage is laid over the part in back and forth layers and is anchored with circular turns. It is sometimes prevented from slipping by figure-of-eight turns around the wrist for a finger bandage or the waist for an above-the-knee amputation. This bandage turn is shown in Figure 17–36.

Tubular Gauze Bandages

Tubular gauze is supplied in varying widths to be applied to fingers, toes, arms, or legs. Metal or plastic is loaded with enough gauze to complete the bandage. Several layers of gauze are applied using this applicator, as described in detail in Procedure 17–8.

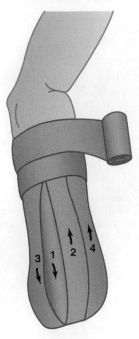

> **Figure 17–36** Recurrent turn used for a below-the-knee amputee. (From Bonewit-West K. *Clinical Procedures for Medical Assistants,* 5th ed. Philadelphia: W.B. Saunders, 2000.)

Montgomery Straps for Abdominal Dressing

Montgomery straps are used for draining abdominal wounds that will need frequent dressing changes. Montgomery straps avoid tissue breakdown that can occur when adhesive tape is changed frequently. The device is made of a pair of nonadhesive tape straps that run across the abdomen. They tie across thick absorbent dressings. The dressings can be changed as often as necessary, but the Montgomery straps are only changed when they become extremely soiled.

Changing a Sterile Dressing

Sterile dressings are changed maintaining surgical asepsis and wearing gloves.

First the old dressing is removed. Tape is pulled toward the incision. Bandages that encircle limbs may be cut off using bandage scissors. The bandage and dressing should not be cut near the incision site (i.e., if the incision is on the underside of the arm, the bandage should be cut away on the top of the arm).

If the dressing is sticking to the wound because of dried blood or wound exudate, it can be soaked with

---

PROCEDURE 17–8

Applying a Tubular Gauze Bandage

Performance Objective: The student will be able to apply a tubular gauze bandage.

✓	Wash hands
☐	Gloves
☐	Eye and Face Protection
☐	Lab Coat or Apron
☐	Plastic Biohazard Bag
☐	Rigid Biohazard Container

Supplies and Equipment: Seamless tubular gauze bandage and applicator.

Procedure Steps

1. Wash hands.
2. Identify patient and explain procedure.
   Rationale: The patient will be more comfortable and cooperative if he or she knows what to expect.

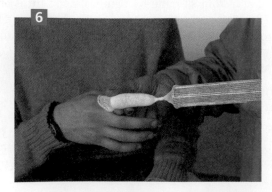

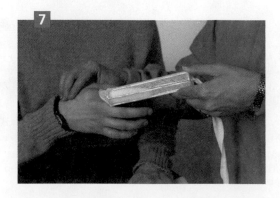

3. Assemble the applicator and seamless tubular gauze bandage. The applicator (made of stainless steel or plastic) should be somewhat larger than the extremity to be bandaged. The tubular gauze should be the correct size for the applicator.
   Rationale: The applicator must move freely over the extremity and bandage as it is applied. The bandage fits snugly but should not be too tight (because it can interfere with circulation) or too loose (because it will shift or fall off).

4. Cut a length of gauze 6 to 10 times longer than the extremity to be bandaged. Load applicator by stretching the gauze over it and feeding the length of gauze onto the applicator.
   Rationale: Several layers of gauze will be applied to form the bandage.

5. Place applicator over extremity to be bandaged. Pull the first part of the tubular gauze from the applicator and hold with your fingers to begin the bandage. Pull the applicator away from the end you are holding until the entire extremity is covered with a layer of gauze and the applicator is 1″ to 2″ beyond the end of the extremity.
   Rationale: If you do not hold the beginning of the bandage, it may not remain in place to cover the entire extremity.

6 Rotate the applicator one full turn to anchor the bandage.
   Rationale: The rotation of the bandage anchors the distal end before you apply another layer of gauze.

7 Move the applicator toward the extremity, adding a layer of gauze to the bandage. When the applicator reaches the proximal end of the extremity, rotate one full turn to anchor the bandage.
   Rationale: Unless the bandage is anchored, the gauze will not remain in place.

8 Continue adding layers with a full turn at each proximal and distal end until the bandage has reached the desired thickness. Finish the last layer at the proximal end. For a finger, you may wish to cut the final 8″ to 10″ of gauze into two sections to form strings that you can use to tie around the hand to secure the bandage.
   Rationale: Most appendages are bandaged several times to give proper support. Twisting gauze as the applicator is removed will cover the fingertip and help to hold bandage on securely.

9. Document procedure in the patient's medical record. Instruct the patient when and how to remove or change the bandage and when to return to the office for follow-up.

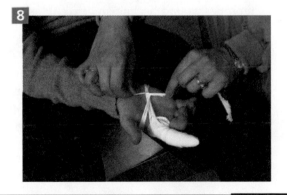

8

Charting Example	
Date	
6/7/XX	10:00 AM Tube gauze applied to right index finger to protect 1″ laceration.
	———————————— D. Cabot, RMA

sterile water or saline solution to loosen it. A dressing should not be pulled off, unless specified by the doctor. If soaking does not remove it, the doctor should be consulted.

After the wound is uncovered, the gloves used during this part of the process should be discarded.

The doctor needs to examine the wound to determine the degree of healing before exudate or drainage is cleaned. If the doctor wants a culture of the drainage, this needs to be done before the wound is cleaned.

After the doctor has checked the wound and it has been cultured, if necessary, the medical assistant puts on new sterile gloves and cleans the wound or incision with antiseptic solution or sterile saline solution. Working from the middle and using a new gauze sponge or sterile swab for each motion, the medical assistant cleans the wound from the center to the edge. When the wound or incision is dry, a new dressing is applied and held in place with tape or a bandage. This is discussed in detail in Procedure 17–9.

PROCEDURE 17–9

Changing a Sterile Dressing

Performance Objective: The student will be able to change a sterile dressing maintaining aseptic technique.

- ☑ Wash hands
- ☑ Gloves
- ☐ Eye and Face Protection
- ☑ Lab Coat or Apron
- ☑ Plastic Biohazard Bag
- ☐ Rigid Biohazard Container

Supplies and Equipment: Sterile dressing change kit that includes antiseptic solution, gauze sponges and thumb forceps or antiseptic swabs, sterile gloves, small plastic bag, tape, and sterile dressing. Additional supplies to have on hand: Nonsterile gloves, wound culture swab, tape, and other bandage material.

Procedure Steps

1. Wash hands.
2. Identify and position patient for dressing change. Explain procedure.
3. Assemble supplies.
4. Open disposable sterile kit. Remove plastic bag (which should be on top) for use outside of sterile field. If desired, tape bag to table for easy disposal of contaminated dressing change supplies.
   Rationale: The inside of the kit is sterile, but the plastic bag will be used to hold the contaminated dressing before the sterile part of the procedure.

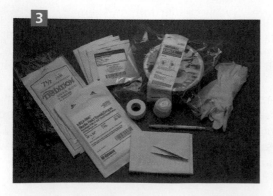

5. Put on nonsterile gloves. Loosen tape on dressing. Remove dressing and place in small plastic bag. If the dressing is stuck to the wound, use a small amount of sterile water or hydrogen peroxide to loosen it. Remove dressing without resistance.
   Rationale: The old dressing must be removed before the sterile part of the procedure. Nonsterile gloves protect you from contact with the wound.
6. Assess the wound for signs of infection such as redness, swelling (edema), crusts, streaks around wound, discharge or excessive buildup of wound material. If these are found, culture the wound using a sterile swab by running the swab along the length of the wound and then placing it in a culture transfer tube. Squeeze the tube to release the transfer medium.
   Rationale: If signs and symptoms of a wound infection are present, the wound should be cultured to identify the infecting microorganism.
7. If any signs and symptoms of infection or improper wound healing are present, ask the doctor to observe the wound before re-dressing.
   Rationale: The doctor must observe the wound before it is covered by a new dressing.
8. Remove nonsterile gloves and place in plastic bag with the old dressing. Wash hands. Apply sterile gloves.

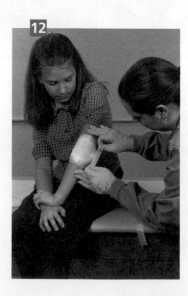

Rationale: Always wash hands after removing nonsterile gloves and before beginning any other procedure.

9. Set up sterile supplies, which may include opening and laying out a sterile towel, pouring sterile solution into a container within the tray, or opening a package of presaturated sterile swabs.

    Rationale: The contents of the tray are sterile and you are wearing sterile gloves, so you may touch all contents, but you must prevent all contents of the tray from touching nonsterile objects.

10. Clean wound using antiseptic solution with gauze and thumb forceps or swabs, being gentle so as not to irritate wound. Clean from the center of the wound to the edge using a new swab or gauze square each time you return to the center. Drop each used gauze square or swab into the plastic bag.

    Rationale: Avoid bringing potential contamination from the edge of the wound back to the center area.

11. When all exudate is removed from the wound, place sterile dressing material to completely cover the wound.

    Rationale: The wound must be covered with a sterile dressing to prevent introducing microorganisms into the area.

12. Secure new dressing either with strips of tape or a bandage secured by tape or clips depending on the size and location of the wound.

    Rationale: Large wounds, especially on or near joints, are usually secured with a conforming gauze bandage to facilitate movement. The doctor may prefer an elastic bandage to reduce swelling. For small wounds, it is usually sufficient to tape the dressing to the skin.

13. Remove gloves and place in plastic bag. Dispose of all contaminated items in plastic bag. Place plastic bag in biohazard container.

    Rationale: Items used in the procedure are considered contaminated with body fluids.

14. Wash hands.

15. Document observation and dressing change procedure in patient record.

Charting Example	
Date	
9/11/XX	9:30 AM Elbow dressing changed. Wound dry and appears to be healing well. Cleaned site and reapplied sterile dressing. _____ S. Dellarosa, RMA

Wet-to-Dry Dressings

Dead tissue must be removed for proper healing to take place (an activity called **debridement**). One way to do this is with a wet-to-dry dressing.

A dressing is applied wet and is pressed against the wound surface, where it dries. When the dressing is changed, the old dressing must be removed quickly. This pulls dead tissue away from the wound.

Suture or Staple Removal

Suture or staple removal is done wearing gloves, using sterile gloves and instruments. Suture-removal packs are prepackaged kits that contain a small thumb forceps and a scissors for cutting the sutures.

The forceps is used to gently lift the suture by the tail of the knot closest to the skin. The scissors is then used to cut the suture, and the suture is gently pulled out using the forceps.

After the sutures are removed, the incision should be cleaned with an antiseptic solution and patted dry. A dressing is usually not needed, but one may be applied to prevent clothing from rubbing the incision line.

Staples are removed using a prepackaged sterile staple remover. The staple remover is gently slipped under the staple; when the handle is pressed, the staple compresses in the center and can be gently lifted out.

Again, when the staples are all removed, clean the incision and pat dry. Either sutures or staples should be counted and compared to the number inserted, to be sure that all have been removed. A forgotten suture may cause infection due to tissue irritation. This is discussed in more detail in Procedure 17–10.

Cleaning the Surgical Area

After the surgical procedure is completed and the patient has left the treatment room, it must be cleaned. If one assistant has helped the patient (a circulating assistant) and another has assisted the doctor (a "scrub" assistant), the scrub assistant should clean up the materials before removing his or her gloves. If only one

ON THE JOB: POSTOPERATIVE INSTRUCTION

After Dr. Lawler has finished removing the inflamed cyst from Katherine McDonald's left axilla, he applies a dressing and asks Kathy Anderson to secure the dressing with tape. Dr. Lawler writes the following orders:

- Rest in bed or chair with at least two pillows overnight, then activity as tolerated.
- Change dressing after 48 hours to large adhesive bandage. Discard gauze packing when it falls out.
- Notify office for excessive drainage, yellow or green drainage, T > 101°F.
- No shower for 1 week; don't get area wet until healed.
- Notify office by telephone of condition in 1 week.

He has given her a prescription for pain medication that she can take every 4 hours to reduce discomfort.

 Make a sheet of take-home instructions for this patient with sections for elevation of the surgical area, care of the dressing, problems to report, activity, and follow-up.

PROCEDURE 17–10

Suture Removal

Performance Objective: The student will be able to remove sutures from a well-healed incision.

☑ Wash hands
☑ Gloves
☐ Eye and Face Protection
☐ Lab Coat or Apron
☑ Plastic Biohazard Bag
☑ Rigid Biohazard Container

Supplies and Equipment: Sterile suture-removal kit that includes thumb forceps, suture scissors, and gauze. Other needed supplies include antiseptic solution or antiseptic swabs, biohazard waste container, and gloves.

Procedure Steps

1. Wash hands.
2. Identify patient and explain procedure. Check the medical record for the number of sutures inserted. Position patient so that incision is easily accessible.
   Rationale: All sutures must be removed to prevent infection of a retained suture.

3. Assemble equipment. Open kit without touching contents. Pour solution into a sterile or open package of antiseptic swabs.
   Rationale: To clean the area around the sutures.
4. Put on gloves. Clean area around sutures to dislodge any exudate built up on suture material.
   Rationale: Removal of crusty exudate around sutures makes suture removal less painful for the patient. If the incision is completely healed the medical assistant does not need to wear sterile gloves.

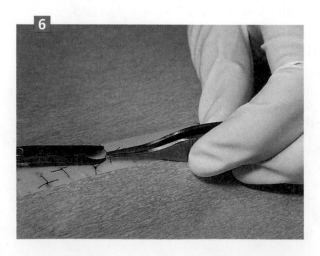

5. Using thumb forceps, gently find one knot of suture and lift upward.
   Rationale: Gentle upward traction creates a space to insert scissors.

6. Slip scissor notch under knot and clip.
   Rationale: The hook on the suture scissors allows the scissors to slide under the knot easily.

7. Using thumb forceps, pull stitch straight upward so that the entire suture slips out of the incision.
   Rationale: It is important to remove the suture intact. Any retained suture material can become infected.

8. Lay the sutures on a gauze square as they are removed. Count when finished.

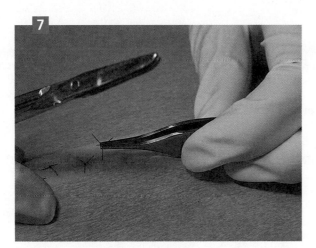

(Photographs from Chester GA: *Modern Medical Assisting.* Philadelphia: W.B. Saunders, 1998.)

Rationale: To be sure the same number of sutures have been removed as were inserted.

9. If any additional exudate or crusts are present, clean the wound again with more solution and dry. The wound may be supported with skin closure strips (such as Steri-Strips). You may also apply a dry dressing if the wound is in an area that can be rubbed or abraded by clothing.
   Rationale: The wound may be tender, but it should be completely healed if you have removed sutures.

10. Remove gloves and discard gloves, sutures, gauze, and disposable instruments used in the procedure in a biohazard waste container. Disposable forceps and scissors are sharps and must be discarded in a rigid biohazard waste container.

11. Instruct the patient that the wound should be protected while it remains tender. Skin closure strips remain in place until they fall off.

12. Document the procedure in the patient's medical record and give instructions for further care of the wound.

Charting Example	
Date	
9/11/XX	10:50 AM (7) seven sutures removed from well-healed incision. Steri-Strips applied. Written instructions given to pt.
	S. Williams, CMA

assistant has helped with the procedure, he or she should assist the patient back to the waiting area; then he or she needs to reglove to clean up.

Disposable materials need to be placed in the proper waste container. Blades, needles, and disposable scalpels, staple removers, or suture-removal kits need to go in the rigid biohazard sharps container.

Disposable drapes, gowns, masks, and other soft materials go into the biohazard bag. Linens that will be washed and sterilized go into the biohazard linen container.

After all the materials have been cleaned up, the room should be checked for blood spills and other contamination, and cleaned if necessary. Contaminated gloves should then be removed and put in the biohazard waste container.

After washing hands, the medical assistant then needs to put on clean gloves to sanitize and disinfect the room, as discussed in chapter 13.

Any specimens that need to be sent to a laboratory must be processed.

DOCUMENTATION

The medical assistant must fill out laboratory forms for any specimens and record details of any procedure in the medical record. These include dressing changes, wound cleaning, patient instructions, bandaging, and suture removal.

You should describe the location and the appearance of the wound or incision for each visit. Specific examples of documentation are given in the procedures throughout this chapter.

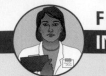

FOCUS ON
INSTRUCTION

After a surgical procedure is completed and the wound is dressed and bandaged, or after a wound is re-dressed and rebandaged, the medical assistant needs to give the patient instructions about wound care.

ELEVATE WHEN POSSIBLE

Whenever possible, the part of the body that has undergone trauma (either accidental or surgical) should be elevated. This helps reduce swelling.

CHECK DRAINAGE

Wounds drain to varying degrees. The medical assistant needs to explain to the patient approximately how much drainage to expect (how soiled the bandage is expected to become before it is changed). The patient should be instructed to call the office if drainage is excessive, if it turns yellow or green, if drainage increases, and if the oral temperature rises above 101°F.

RETURN VISIT FOR FIRST DRESSING CHANGE

A patient who has a wound that is expected to drain and that will need re-dressing is always asked to come to the office for the first dressing change. This allows the doctor to look at the wound to see that healing is progressing well. It also gives the medical assistant an opportunity to teach the patient how to re-dress the wound at a time when the patient is under less stress than immediately after he or she has undergone the surgery.

SUBSEQUENT DRESSING CHANGES

Sometimes the doctor will want the patient to come in to the office for subsequent dressing changes. This is usually because a problem has developed, such as infection or pulling apart of the wound edges.

If the patient is expected to do sterile dressing changes at home, the patient or a family member must be taught how to do this and must be given a list of supplies to purchase.

WOUND CARE

The patient must understand how to care for the surgical incision or wound. This includes keeping it dry, applying topical medications ordered by the doctor, knowing whether to cover with a dressing or expose the incision to air, and knowing when to return to the office for suture removal. Adhesive skin closures usually stay in place until they fall off and are not replaced.

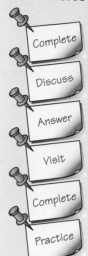

STUDENT STUDY PLAN

To reinforce your understanding of the material in this chapter . . .

Complete *Complete* the **Review & Recall** questions below.

Discuss *Discuss* the situation in **If You Were the Medical Assistant** with your classmates and answer the questions.

Answer *Answer* the **Critical Thinking Questions** below and discuss with your classmates.

Visit *Visit* **Web sites** suggested below and search for additional Web sites using **Keywords for Internet Searches.**

Complete *Complete* the exercises in chapter 17 of the **Student Mastery Manual.**

Practice *Practice* Surgical Assisting activities in the Clinical Skills section of the **CD-ROM.**

 REVIEW & RECALL

1. List the eight rules of surgical asepsis.
2. Describe several types of forceps and scissors that may be used for surgical procedures.
3. Identify how the following types of instruments are used: retractors, probes, sounds, scalpels, curettes.
4. How should the medical assistant prepare reusable instruments for sterilization?
5. List supplies commonly used for surgical procedures and wound care.
6. Describe how a medical assistant sets up a sterile field.
7. Describe the correct method to add sterile solution or a packaged instrument to a sterile field.
8. What types of information are contained in the procedure manual or on procedure cards for different surgical procedures?
9. List the steps necessary to prepare the patient for a surgical procedure.
10. Describe how the patient's skin is prepared for surgery.
11. How does the medical assistant assist the surgeon during surgery and skin closure and removal of sutures or staples?
12. Identify several reasons why the doctor may suture a laceration.
13. Compare laser surgery and cryosurgery to conventional surgery.
14. Describe the process of wound healing.
15. Compare and contrast a dressing and a bandage.

 IF YOU WERE THE MEDICAL ASSISTANT

Today Dr. Hughes, one of the doctors at Blackburn Primary Care Associates, is going to remove a small skin lesion from the upper outer aspect of the left leg of Jacqueline Tamar, a 28-year-old woman.

1. What will you discuss with the patient before the procedure? Does Ms. Tamar have to complete any paperwork?
2. What position would allow Dr. Hughes to have easy access to the lesion?
3. What sterile instruments and supplies will you need to put on the sterile field for this type of surgery?
4. Describe what needs to be done to the patient's leg before Dr. Hughes can make the incision.
5. What will happen to the tissue that is removed during the surgery?
6. What supplies will Dr. Hughes need to place a dressing and bandage over the surgical site after the surgery?
7. Describe in general the instructions that you should give Ms. Tamar before she goes home after the surgery.

CRITICAL THINKING QUESTIONS

1. What should the medical assistant do if he or she notices that the doctor has touched a nonsterile object while wearing sterile gloves?

2. Prepare a procedure card for removing sutures or staples.

3. Discuss the medical assistant's role in obtaining informed consent for surgery. Can you think of any difficult situations that could arise?

4. Discuss how the medical assistant decides the best method to keep a dressing in place. What factors influence this decision?

5. What instructions would you give a patient who is supposed to perform a sterile dressing change on a family member's wound at home?

 EXPLORE THE WEB

INTERNET WEB SITES

The American College of Surgeons
http://www.facs.org

CDC Hospital infection program
http://www.cdc.gov/ncidod/hip/Sterile/sterile.htm

KEYWORDS FOR INTERNET SEARCHES

asepsis
      bandaging
      dressing change
      office surgery
      sterile technique
      suture removal
      suture techniques

 ANSWERS TO ON THE JOB: INFORMED CONSENT

1. Kathy might say, "Mrs. McDonald, I need to have you sign a consent form for our records indicating that you understand the procedure that Dr. Lawler is about to perform. Did you understand his explanation completely?"

2. The consent form provides a permanent record that the patient was instructed about the procedure, the possible risks and complications of the procedure, and alternative methods of treatment.

3. Kathy's signature is a statement that she is a witness; that is, that she observed the patient, Katherine McDonald, sign the form on the date and at the time indicated.

4. a. This statement by the patient indicates that she doesn't understand what the doctor is going to do. Kathy should ask the doctor to explain the procedure again before obtaining the patient's signature.

   b. Kathy should remind the patient that it is unwise to sign things without reading them, then help the patient to find her glasses and read the form before allowing the patient to sign. If the patient does not have her glasses with her, Kathy should read the complete form to the patient before obtaining the signature.

   c. Before having the patient sign the form, Kathy should tell Dr. Lawler what the patient just said so that he can explain the possible results of the procedure to her again. When Kathy hears that the patient believes the doctor has promised that there will be no adverse effects, she must take steps to have the doctor correct the patient's mistaken belief. The consent form clearly states that the doctor does not make any promises about the outcome of the surgery, but if a court case arises later, what the patient believed carries more weight than what the consent form states.

ANSWERS TO ON THE JOB: POSTOPERATIVE INSTRUCTIONS

Patient: Mrs. Katherine McDonald
Incision and Drainage and removal of inflamed cyst, left axilla

Elevation of the Surgical Area: *Rest in bed and sleep for first night on at least two pillows to keep left armpit and shoulder somewhat elevated.*

Care of Dressing: *Keep dressing in place for 48 hours, then remove and replace with a large adhesive bandage. Packing (gauze strip) in the wound will fall out, probably when the surgical dressing is removed, and can be discarded.*

Activity: *Do not shower or get wet for 7 days; return to normal activity when you feel able to.*

Call the office: *If drainage seeps through the dressing, if you notice any yellow or greenish drainage, or if your temperature is higher than 101°F.*

Follow-up: *Call the office to report on your condition in 1 week.*

Chapter 18

Taking Electrocardiograms

Instructional Objectives

After completing this chapter, you will be able to do the following:

1. Define and spell the vocabulary words for this chapter.
2. Correlate the normal configuration of a single complex of the EKG tracing to the electrical activity of the heart.
3. Describe the purpose and procedure of the 12-lead EKG.
4. Identify and describe the different complexes and intervals of the normal EKG.
5. Describe lead placement for the 12-lead EKG.
6. Describe which part of the heart is measured by each of the 12 leads of the EKG.
7. Compare and contrast single-channel and three-channel EKG machines.
8. Discuss the role of the electrocardiograph, electrodes, electrolytes, and paper in obtaining the EKG tracing.
9. Identify three types of artifact, and describe measures to reduce or eliminate them.
10. Describe how to mount a single-channel EKG tracing.
11. Identify life-threatening arrhythmias.
12. Discuss lead placement for the Holter monitor.
13. Describe patient instructions given to a patient wearing a Holter monitor.
14. Identify reasons a doctor might order a cardiac stress test.
15. Compare the procedure for the cardiac stress test to the 12-lead EKG.
16. Identify potential adverse effects of the cardiac stress test.

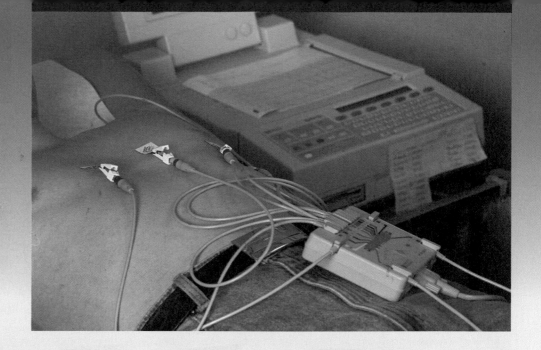

- Perform electrocardiograms
- Prepare patients for and assist with procedures and treatments
- Practice within the scope of education, training, and personal capabilities

- Document appropriately
- Instruct and demonstrate the use of patient care equipment
- Instruct individuals according to their needs

Performance Objectives

After completing this chapter, you will be able to do the following:

1. Perform a 12-lead electrocardiogram (Procedure 18–1).
2. Apply a Holter monitor and instruct a patient in its use (Procedure 18–2).

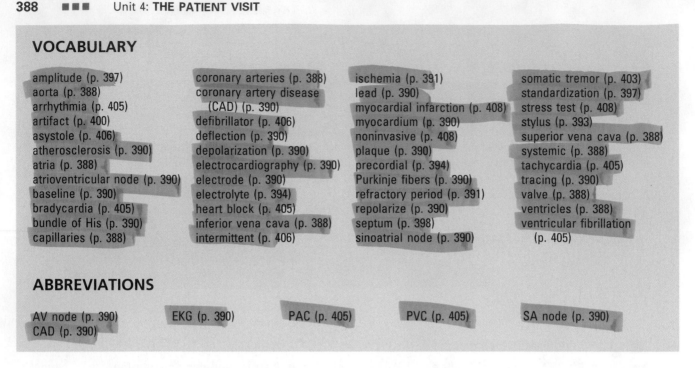

VOCABULARY

amplitude (p. 397)
aorta (p. 388)
arrhythmia (p. 405)
artifact (p. 400)
asystole (p. 406)
atherosclerosis (p. 390)
atria (p. 388)
atrioventricular node (p. 390)
baseline (p. 390)
bradycardia (p. 405)
bundle of His (p. 390)
capillaries (p. 388)

coronary arteries (p. 388)
coronary artery disease
   (CAD) (p. 390)
defibrillator (p. 406)
deflection (p. 390)
depolarization (p. 390)
electrocardiography (p. 390)
electrode (p. 390)
electrolyte (p. 394)
heart block (p. 405)
inferior vena cava (p. 388)
intermittent (p. 406)

ischemia (p. 391)
lead (p. 390)
myocardial infarction (p. 408)
myocardium (p. 390)
noninvasive (p. 408)
plaque (p. 390)
precordial (p. 394)
Purkinje fibers (p. 390)
refractory period (p. 391)
repolarize (p. 390)
septum (p. 398)
sinoatrial node (p. 390)

somatic tremor (p. 403)
standardization (p. 397)
stress test (p. 408)
stylus (p. 393)
superior vena cava (p. 388)
systemic (p. 388)
tachycardia (p. 405)
tracing (p. 390)
valve (p. 388)
ventricles (p. 388)
ventricular fibrillation
   (p. 405)

ABBREVIATIONS

AV node (p. 390)   EKG (p. 390)   PAC (p. 405)   PVC (p. 405)   SA node (p. 390)
CAD (p. 390)

THE HEART'S STRUCTURE AND FUNCTION

The cardiovascular system is made up of the heart, blood vessels, and blood. This system serves to transport oxygenated blood and nutrients to all of the body's organs and to transport carbon dioxide and wastes back from the organs for elimination.

A triangular-shaped organ, the heart is located in the central portion of the chest between the lungs, in a cavity between the lungs called the mediastinum. Its tip, or apex, extends to the left and rests on the diaphragm, which separates the thoracic cavity from the abdomen.

The heart is essentially two pumps, sitting side by side, separated by a partition, or wall, called the **septum.** It is divided into four cavities, or chambers. The two upper chambers are called **atria** (singular, atrium), and the two lower chambers are called **ventricles.** There is a membranous structure—a **valve**—at the bottom of each chamber, which keeps blood flowing in only one direction.

When the heart contracts, blood from the right lower chamber (right ventricle) is pumped through the pulmonic valve and the right and left pulmonary arteries to the lungs, where it passes through successively smaller arteries (arterioles) to the network of pulmonary **capillaries.** These are microscopic blood vessels whose walls are so thin that oxygen, carbon dioxide, glucose, and other substances can pass by osmosis between the circulatory system and the tissues. The blood leaving the lung carries oxygen. It is pumped through small veins (venules) that consolidate into larger veins

until it is delivered back to the left atrium of the heart through the right and left pulmonary veins.

When the atria contract, blood in the left side of the heart passes through the mitral (bicuspid) valve into the left ventricle. When the ventricles contract, the blood passes through the aortic valve into the **aorta,** the largest artery in the body. The arteries that supply blood to the heart itself branch from the aorta almost immediately. These are called the **coronary arteries;** if they become narrowed or blocked, the heart cannot receive adequate oxygen to function properly.

Blood is carried to all parts of the body through branching arteries and arterioles to capillaries, where it deposits oxygen and picks up carbon dioxide. It returns to the heart through veins that join to larger veins, which empty into either the **inferior vena cava** (coming from the lower part of the body) or the **superior vena cava** (coming from the upper part of the body) to enter the right atrium, pass through the tricuspid valve, and enter the right ventricle.

Each time the heart beats, blood is pumped through the heart and out to both the pulmonary and **systemic** (pertaining to the whole body) circulation. Figure 18–1 shows the anatomy and physiology of the heart and blood flow.

Any condition that affects the structure or function of the cardiovascular system may interfere with the body's ability to meet oxygen demands, either in a localized area or throughout the body.

Disturbances in the heart, such as an abnormal cardiac rhythm, decreased strength of heart contraction, abnormal blood flow through the heart, or decreased

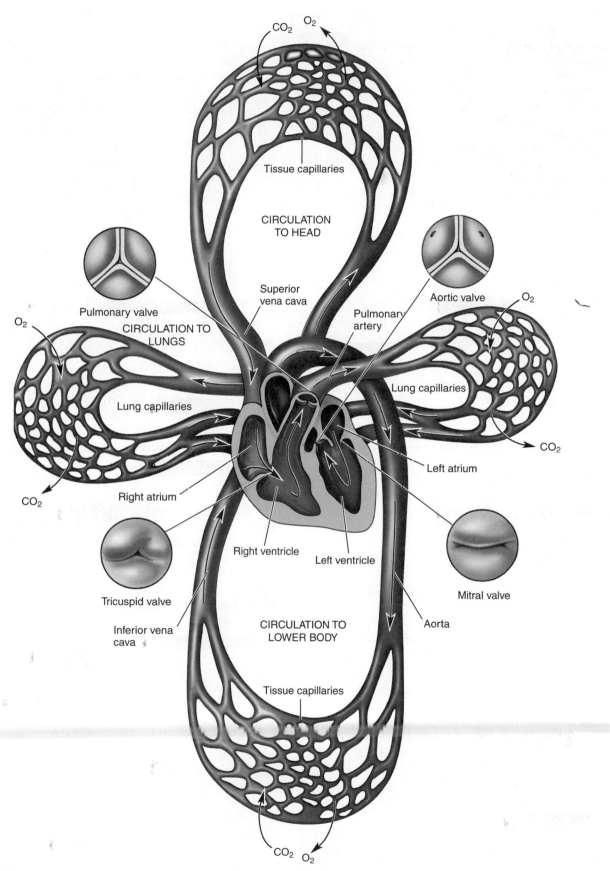

➣ **Figure 18–1** The heart and blood flow.

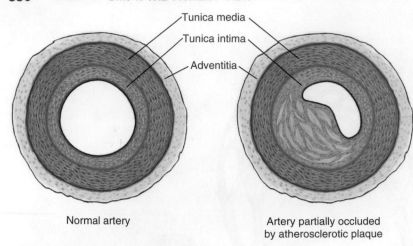

Tunica media
Tunica intima
Adventitia

Normal artery

Artery partially occluded
by atherosclerotic plaque

➤ **Figure 18–2** The normal artery compared to an artery partially blocked by atherosclerosis. (From Monahan FD, Neighbors M: *Medical Surgical Nursing: Foundations for Clinical Practice*, 2nd ed. Philadelphia: W.B. Saunders, 1998.)

blood flow to the **myocardium** (heart muscle), may be present. Blood flow through any large or small blood vessels may be impaired due to blockage or injury.

One common cause of blockage is **atherosclerosis**, a condition in which deposits of cholesterol and lipids occur along the walls of arteries and arterioles, resulting in decreased flexibility of the blood vessel and blocking part or all of the blood flow through that vessel. This is shown in Figure 18–2. Depending on the location and extent of atherosclerotic **plaques** (patches or deposits), the patient may experience different signs and symptoms. When plaques are located in the coronary arteries, the condition is called **coronary artery disease (CAD)**, a common cause of cardiac problems because narrowing of these arteries decreases the blood supply to the myocardium.

THE HEART'S CONDUCTION SYSTEM

Conduction of an electrical impulse through the heart works in the following way. The pumping action of the heart is regulated by electrical activity of cells in the myocardium. The electrical impulses follow a specific pathway through the heart. The heart rate is usually regular, but may speed up or slow down in response to the needs of the body's cells.

The **sinoatrial node (SA node)** is located on the right atrial wall just below the entrance to the vena cava. The cells in this area spontaneously depolarize together at a regular rate to begin the electrical impulse that starts the heartbeat.

Depolarization is a sudden change in the electrical charge of the cells, which allows an electrical impulse to begin to flow from one area to another. The SA node, which begins each heartbeat, is called the pacemaker. The depolarization wave spreads across both atria, causing them to contract.

The **atrioventricular node (AV node)** is located in the inferior portion of the septum (wall) between the two atria. The impulse is delayed for about 0.1 second (one-tenth of one second), to allow the atria to finish contracting. Then the impulse is passed into the bundle of His.

The **bundle of His** is a group of specialized cardiac muscle fibers, which divides into right and left bundle branches, down the walls of the septum between the ventricles. The electrical impulse follows this pathway into the **Purkinje fibers**, nerve pathways that penetrate into both ventricles. When the impulse reaches the ventricles, they contract together.

Each of the ventricles **repolarizes**, meaning that the cells of the myocardium become able to contract again. Then the SA node initiates another impulse.

Figure 18–3 shows the heart's conduction system.

ELECTROCARDIOGRAPHY

Electrocardiography is the recording of the electrical activity of a patient's heart. **Electrodes**, metal plates or metallic-coated paper tabs that conduct electricity, are placed at specific locations on the patient's skin and attached to the electrocardiograph (**EKG**) machine with wires.

The EKG machine records the electrical activity from various combinations of electrodes. The combinations are called **leads**. The standard 12-lead electrocardiogram allows a doctor to visualize the electrical activity of all parts of the heart and draw conclusions about how effectively the heart is pumping.

The pattern that shows up on the EKG paper from the various leads is called a **tracing**. The tracing is printed on special EKG graph paper. Each **deflection**, or movement on the tracing away from the **baseline**, is assigned a letter for purposes of discussing the tracing.

The baseline is the flat line that signifies no electrical activity.

The patterns that appear on a normal EKG tracing are described as waves, complexes, and intervals. A wave is a simple pattern, with one wavelike top. A complex is a series of usually sharper tops. An interval is the distance between one deflection and another.

EKG paper moves through the machine at a specific rate. This allows the distances between the different patterns to be measured precisely. It is known how long these intervals should be in a healthy patient. The amount of time it actually takes for the electrical impulses to move through the heart—and therefore for the patterns to show up on the tracing—gives information about how the electrical impulse is moving through the heart.

The P wave represents contraction of the atria. It is normally an upright round contour. The QRS complex represents contraction of the ventricles. The T wave represents the repolarization of the ventricles (repolarization of the atria occurs while the ventricles are contracting and is not visible on the EKG tracing).

The PR interval is the time from the beginning of the P wave to the middle of the QRS complex; if this is too long, it means that impulses are being blocked or delayed at the AV node, and the ventricles are not contracting quickly enough.

The QT interval is the time from the beginning of the QRS complex to the end of the T wave; this represents the time for ventricular depolarization and repolarization.

The ST segment may also be measured. This represents the refractory period, the time when the ventricles cannot contract again until depolarization is complete. Normally, the ST segment is on the baseline because there is no electrical activity. Elevation of the ST segment above the baseline may indicate myocardial ischemia, a lack of oxygen to the myocardium. Figure 18–4 shows how cardiac activity is related to the EKG tracing.

Equipment Necessary to Take the EKG

Four pieces of equipment are necessary to take an EKG:

1. The electrocardiograph machine
2. EKG paper
3. Electrolyte cream or liquid
4. Electrodes.

The electrocardiograph itself is a simple machine that receives electrical impulses from the heart through wires attached to the skin with electrodes and translates it into a tracing.

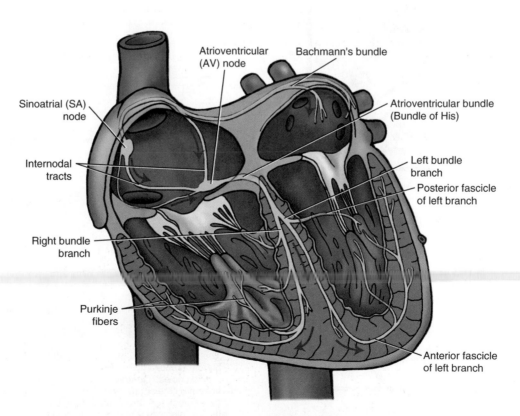

> **Figure 18–3** Conduction system of the heart. (From Monahan FD, Neighbors M: *Medical Surgical Nursing: Foundations for Clinical Practice*, 2nd ed. Philadelphia: W.B. Saunders, 1998.)

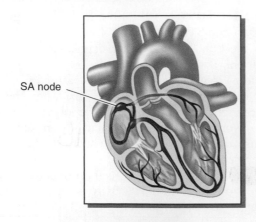

SA node

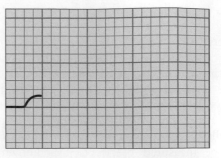

Impulse is initiated in the SA node and spreads throughout the atria. Upon completion of the P wave the right and left atria have begun to contract.

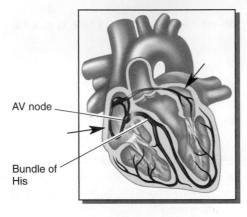

AV node

Bundle of His

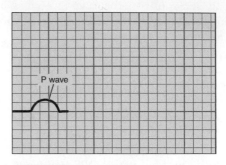

P wave

A short delay at the AV node (seen as an isoelectric or undeflected line) allows the atria to finish contracting. The impulse travels through the AV node and activates the bundle of His.

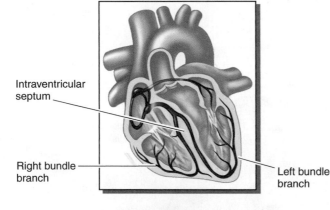

Intraventricular septum

Right bundle branch

Left bundle branch

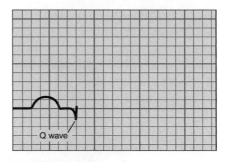

Q wave

Activation of the septum between the ventricles produces a small Q wave.

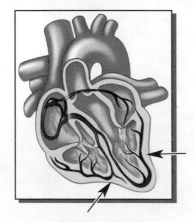

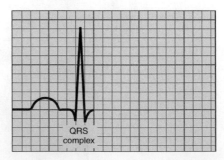

QRS complex

The impulse travels quickly along the right and left bundle branch into the Purkinje fibers in the wall of the ventricles. Contraction of the ventricles is represented by the sharp spike of the QRS complex. While the ventricles contract, the atria repolarize (return to their original state and become able to contract again.)

➤ **Figure 18–4** Cardiac activity related to the EKG tracing.

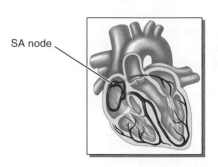

SA node

There is no electrical activity for a short period as represented by the isoelectric ST segment. Repolarization of the ventricles produces the T wave.

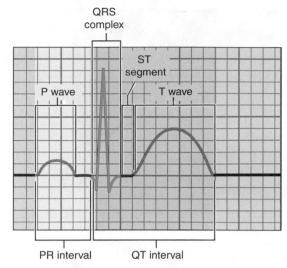

QRS complex

ST segment

P wave

T wave

PR interval

QT interval

> **Figure 18–4** (*Continued*)

EKG machines that produce a paper tracing either print a tracing based on one lead at a time or on multiple leads. The most common EKG in use today is the so-called three-channel EKG, which creates three parallel tracings—three leads at a time of the 12 possible leads. Figure 18–5 shows various EKG machines.

Modern technology has created paperless EKGs. The tracing is shown on a monitor and stored as a data file on a computer. EKGs can also be transmitted in real time over telephone lines to be read immediately at another location or stored on computer.

EKG tracings are made on graph paper that moves through the machine at 25 millimeters per second. The paper is black (or blue) underneath, with a white coating over the undersurface, which has a printed grid on it. Older machines have a piece of pointed metal called a stylus that moves to the right or left of the baseline, depending on the electrical current from the heart. The stylus is made hot enough by the electrical current running through it to melt the white coating, exposing the underlying black paper. This line of black is the tracing.

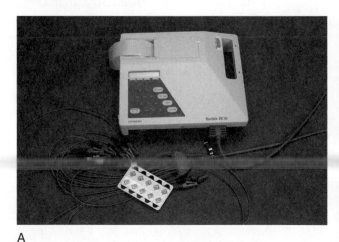

A

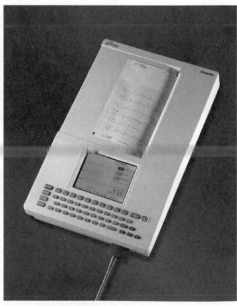

B

> **Figure 18–5** (A) Single-channel electrocardiograph machine. (B) Three-channel electrocardiograph machine. (Courtesy of Spacelabs Medical, Inc., Deerfield, WI)

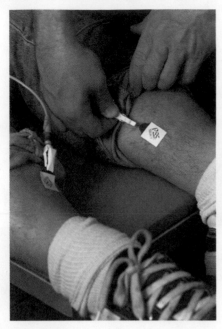

➢ **Figure 18–6** Applying leads with tab electrodes.

Skin is a poor conductor of electricity, so electrolyte cream or solution is used between the electrodes and the skin. An electrolyte is a substance that transmits electricity. The electrolyte either comes in a tube and is squeezed on before the metal electrode is put in place or is already on the adhesive electrode tab.

Electrodes are the actual devices that pick up the electrical current from the heart. Early EKG machines used metal plates held on by straps for the arms and legs, and metal suction cups for the chest lead. Most EKG machines today use disposable adhesive tab electrodes. Figure 18–6 shows a medical assistant applying electrodes.

Lead Placement

Placement of the electrodes on the body allows the transmission of electrical impulses to be recorded from different angles. Each angle is called a lead. Twelve leads are used to show a three-dimensional image of the impulse wave. Lead placement is extremely important. If the leads are not placed in the proper position, the EKG tracing or computer reading will be inaccurate.

Limb electrodes are placed on both arms and both legs, with the wires running toward the heart. The wires are color-coded: white for the right arm, which is abbreviated as RA; green for the right leg (RL); black for the left arm (LA); and red for the left leg (LL).

Limb electrodes must be positioned away from bony areas. Usually tab electrodes are placed just above the ankles on the legs and on the fleshy part of the upper arms (metal electrodes may be attached to the lower arms). The right leg electrode serves as a ground to reduce interference. It keeps the average voltage of the patient the same as that of the EKG machine.

Standard leads are also called bipolar leads, because they record electrical activity between two electrodes, one negative and one positive. Lead I records activity from the right arm to the left arm (RA to LA); lead II from the right arm to the left leg (RA to LL); and lead III from the left arm to the left leg (LA to LL). The standard leads are seen in Figure 18–7 with color coding as used on EKG machines.

Augmented leads use the same electrodes as the standard leads, only in different combinations. They are considered unipolar because they comprise one positive electrode recording the electrical potential of that point, with reference to the two negative electrodes. The machine augments (increases) the voltage at that point, so the tracing becomes bigger and easier to see, but the tracing of an augmented lead is usually smaller than the standard leads.

In this system, lead aVR measures potential at the right arm, lead aVL measures potential at the left arm, and lead aVF measures the potential at the left leg. Augmented leads are seen in Figure 18–8, color-coded like the standard leads.

Precordial (in front of the heart) leads are placed on the chest to view the activity of the heart in the horizontal plane. These must be placed in the spaces between the ribs in the correct position. Some machines use only one chest electrode, which must be moved; newer machines have all six attached at once.

- V_1 is placed in the 4th intercostal space just to the right of the sternum.
- V_2 is placed in the 4th intercostal space just to the left of the sternum.
- V_3 is placed directly between V2 and V4.
- V_4 is placed in the 5th intercostal space, at the midclavicular line.
- V_5 is placed in the 5th intercostal space, at the anterior axillary line.
- V_6 is placed in the 5th intercostal space, at the midaxillary line.

Precordial leads are shown in Figure 18–9.

Lead Coding

Manual lead coding is done by moving a dial for each lead and pressing a button to mark the place where the tracing stops being from one lead and begins being from the next lead. Short and long marks are made at the beginning of each new lead tracing to designate which lead is being used. Newer machines switch and mark leads automatically.

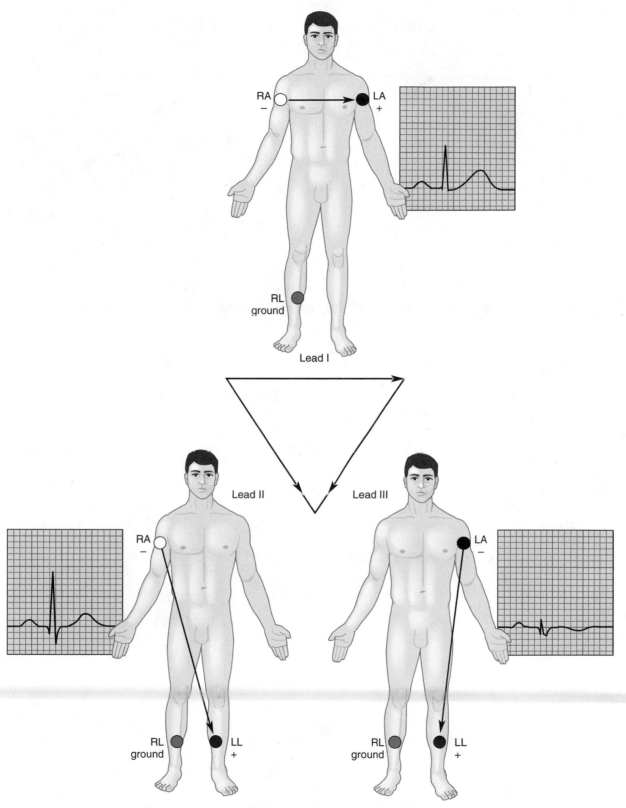

➤ **Figure 18–7** Standard (bipolar) leads with color coding as used on the EKG wires.

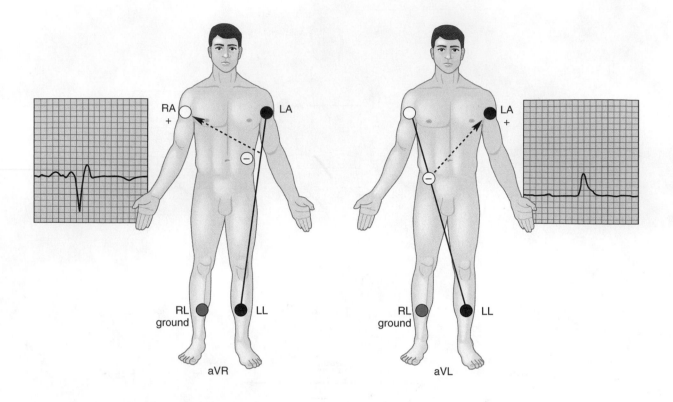

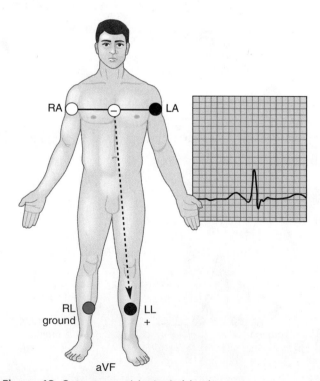

➤ **Figure 18–8** Augmented (unipolar) leads.

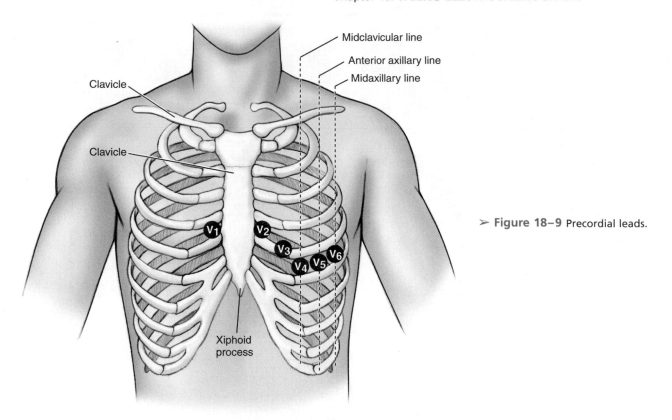

➤ **Figure 18–9** Precordial leads.

Standard leads are coded using one, two, or three dots. Augmented leads are coded using one, two, or three dashes. Precordial leads are coded with a dash, followed by one to six dots. See the box showing standard marking codes for leads.

Standardization

Standardization refers to the action of making sure the machine is working correctly and that the tracing is being done using one of three standard **amplitudes**, or amounts of current going through the machine. On older machines, each time the medical assistant changes leads, he or she must press a button to restandardize the machine; newer machines standardize automatically.

One millivolt (mV) of electrical activity deflects the stylus exactly 10 millimeters (10 mm). Each small box on the EKG graph paper equals 1 mm, so a 10-mm deflection equals 10 small boxes. Each time the machine is restandardized, a mark is placed on the tracing showing that the machines deflects 10 mm for 1 mV. Figure 18–10 shows normal standardization and amplitude alterations.

If the patient's EKG complexes are very large so the tracing is wider than the paper, the amplitude may be halved to get a half-size tracing that stays on the paper. This means that the standardization mark will only be 5 mm (half standardization). If the tracing of the augmented leads is very small and difficult to read, the amplitude may be doubled, creating a double-size trac-

ing that is easier to read. In this case, the standardization mark is 20 mm (2X standardization).

If the heart is beating very rapidly, the paper can be adjusted to pass through the machine at 50 mm per second instead of 25 mm per second. This creates

The Standard Marking Codes

	ELECTRODES CONNECTED	MARKING CODE
Standard or Bipolar Limb Leads		
Lead I	LL & RA	·
Lead II	LL & RA	··
Lead III	LL & LA	···
Augmented Unipolar Limb Leads		
aVR	RA & (LA-LL)	—
aVL	LA & (RA-LL)	— —
aVF	LL & (RA-LL)	— — —
Chest or Precordial Leads		
V	C & (LA-RA-LL)	V_1 — ·
		V_2 — ··
		V_3 — ···
		V_4 — ····
		V_5 — ·····
		V_6 — ·····'

(Courtesy of Spacelabs Medical, Inc., Deerfield, WI.)

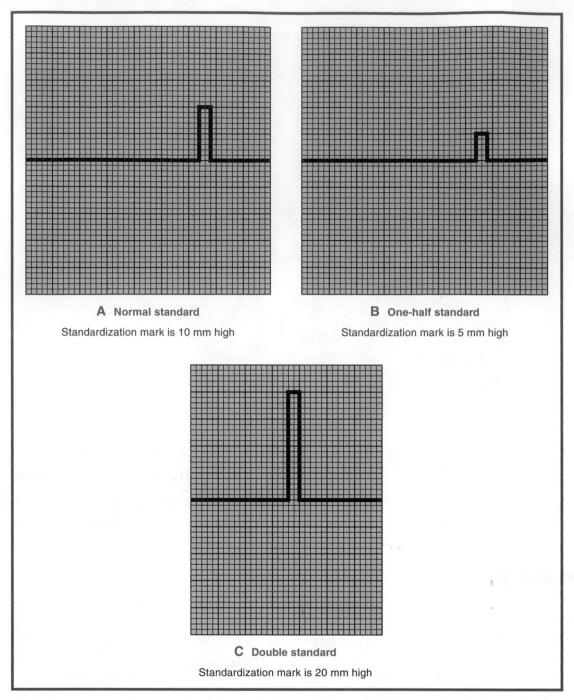

A Normal standard

Standardization mark is 10 mm high

B One-half standard

Standardization mark is 5 mm high

C Double standard

Standardization mark is 20 mm high

➤ **Figure 18–10** Normal standardization and amplitude alterations. (From Kinn ME, Woods M: *The Medical Assistant: Administrative and Clinical*, 8th ed. Philadelphia: W.B. Saunders, 1999.)

more space between complexes so they can be seen better. The change should be noted on the tracing.

When the doctor or EKG technician reading the tracing sees the different standardization marks, he or she knows that the amplitude of the lead in question has been altered.

At the end of the tracing, the machine should always be returned to the normal standardization of 10 mm.

EKG paper is normally set to pass through the machine at 25 mm/second. This means that each small square represents 0.04 second, and each large square represents 0.2 second. This permits calculation of the duration of each wave, segment, or interval. Figure 18–11 shows a representation of time and voltage on EKG paper.

In the normal EKG, each wave, segment, or interval should be within specific parameters for time, although

Voltage
Time
= 1 mm
= 5 mm
= 10 mm
or 1 mV
= .04 sec
= .08 sec
= .12 sec
= .16 sec
= .20 sec
= 1 sec

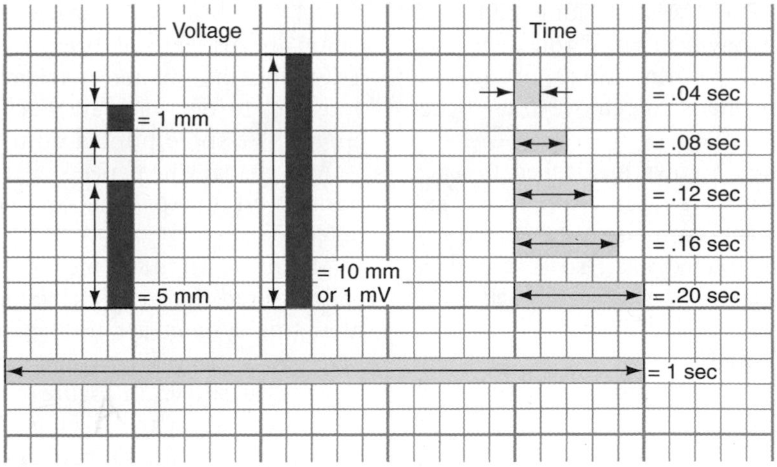

➢ **Figure 18–11** Representation of time and voltage on EKG paper. (From Chester GA: *Modern Medical Assisting*. Philadelphia: W.B. Saunders 1998.)

the size of the deflection varies from lead to lead. Figure 18–12 shows a normal lead II EKG complex.

Performing the EKG

Preparing the Machine

Both the machine and the patient must be prepared to take an EKG tracing. The machine is plugged into a grounded outlet and turned on to warm up. No sources of metal that might interfere with the reading should be in contact with the patient; he or she must not be in direct contact with anything metal except the electrodes.

Check to make sure the machine is set up correctly.

Instructing the Patient

The medical assistant should always ask if a patient has had an EKG taken before. If not, it should be explained that the machine will make a tracing of the electrical activity of the heart. The patient needs to lie still, without talking, for the short time it takes to perform the test. This explanation should be given to any patient who the medical assistant feels may be anxious about the test, even if the patient has had a prior EKG (this includes many teenagers, adults with mental retardation or mental illness, and some elderly patients).

Patient Preparation and Position

The patient needs to be instructed to remove clothing above the waist. Women must also remove their bras, because they can interfere with lead placement as well as the tracing.

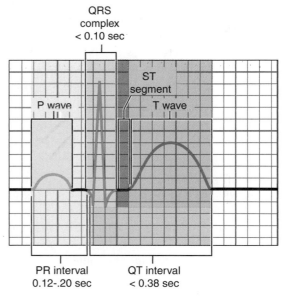

QRS
complex
< 0.10 sec
ST
segment
P wave
T wave
PR interval
0.12-.20 sec
QT interval
< 0.38 sec
P wave = atrial depolarization + contraction
PR interval (0.12-0.2 seconds) (beginning of P wave to beginning of QRS complex)
Q wave = beginning of ventricular depolarization
QRS complex (less than 0.10 seconds) = ventricular depolarization and contraction
ST segment = flat line occurring between depolarization and repolarization of the ventricles; should be isoelectric (on baseline)
T wave = ventricular repolarization
QT interval (less than 0.38 seconds)

➢ **Figure 18–12** Normal Lead II EKG complex.

Men and women who are wearing long pants are also instructed to remove any socks and roll their pant legs up. Women who are wearing skirts or dresses, along with tights or hose, need to remove their tights or hose.

Women should be given a gown and asked to leave it open in the front. Women's chests should be exposed as little as possible, but when the tracing is made, the gown must be pulled back so that it does not touch any of the electrodes, because this will cause interference.

The patient lies comfortably in a supine position. The head may be elevated slightly using a pillow. Legs should not be touching each other, and arms should be at the patient's sides. The patient needs to remain warm and the extremities need to be supported. Discomfort or cold may cause muscle movement and result in **artifact,** a change in the EKG tracing that has not been made by the heart's electrical activity.

To apply the electrodes, the skin must be clean and dry. If oily, sweaty, or slick with lotion, the skin should be rubbed with an alcohol wipe and allowed to dry before the electrodes are placed.

Arm electrodes are placed on the upper arm with the tab facing down. Leg electrodes are placed above the ankle with the tab facing up. Chest electrodes are placed with the tab facing down. If the chest or extremities are hairy, try to press the hair and separate it so tabs adhere to the skin. If they keep falling off, it may be necessary to shave a small area to apply the leads.

Taking the Tracing

The tracing takes a few minutes to run. If using an older, manual lead-change machine, the medical assistant should change leads, standardize, and mark the new lead about every 5″ to 6″ of paper that moves past the stylus. If using a newer machine, the medical assistant presses the AUTO button and the machine standardizes and changes leads automatically.

Procedure 18–1 describes performing a 12-lead EKG in more detail.

Mounting and Recording Information

If you are using a single-channel machine, when the paper tracing is complete, write the patient's name and the date on the strip and carefully roll it until it can be mounted. When using a 3-channel machine, you may be asked to enter the patient name before running the EKG; the patient's name will then be printed with the tracing. Or you may have to enter the information manually after the tracing is complete.

The patient's name and the date should be entered immediately. Before the patient is released, you also need to record the patient ID number, the name of the doctor, any history of cardiac problems, and any medication the patient has been taking that might affect an EKG. This information is recorded either on the mount you plan to use for a single-channel tracing or on the appropriate space printed on the three-channel tracing.

Any changes in paper speed, amplitude, and special position of the patient or electrodes should also be noted.

Mounting an EKG means preparing it to be read, and is used for single-channel EKGs. A number of mounting systems are used. Usually, the section of the EKG from each lead is cut and applied to a sticky backing, as shown in Figure 18–13. If any arrhythmias have occurred in the tracing, they should be included in the mounted sections, and the medical assistant should run a rhythm strip for 10 to 30 seconds to see if additional arrhythmias occur.

Single-channel tracings should be labeled with the patient's name immediately after being taken, in case mounting is delayed. Three-channel EKGs come out of the machine as a complete tracing and do not need to be mounted.

Troubleshooting Problems

You may need to make adjustments and rerun a tracing if problems occur.

Artifact, caused by unwanted movement of the stylus, interferes with interpretation of the EKG. Artifact is usually caused by one of four occurrences:

1. AC interference
2. wandering baseline
3. somatic tremor
4. baseline interruption.

Alternating current (AC) is the standard electrical current that comes from a wall socket. AC interference usually shows up as a series of regular peaks of spiked lines. To avoid AC interference, always use a grounded (3-prong) plug, don't use the EKG near x-ray equipment, and don't place the patient on a metal table. Lead wires should always be straight and not crossed. It may even be necessary to move the patient table away from the wall. Most machines also come with an additional ground wire, which can reduce AC interference. Figure 18–14 shows AC interference.

Wandering baseline occurs when the baseline is not level. This can be caused by electrodes applied too tight or too loose, or by tension on an electrode so it is pulling away from a patient's skin. Too little electrolyte, a dirty electrode, or skin cream or lotion in the area where the electrode is placed may be present. To avoid wandering baseline, keep electrodes clean and be sure the patient's skin is clean and free of lotion. It may be necessary to shave the skin where the electrodes will be placed. Figure 18–15 shows wandering baseline.

PROCEDURE 18–1

Taking Electrocardiograms

Performance Objective: The student will be able to perform a 12-lead electrocardiogram.

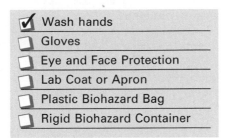

- ☑ Wash hands
- ☐ Gloves
- ☐ Eye and Face Protection
- ☐ Lab Coat or Apron
- ☐ Plastic Biohazard Bag
- ☐ Rigid Biohazard Container

Supplies and Equipment: Electrocardiograph (EKG) machine with paper and patient cable, disposable tab electrodes or metal limb electrodes with straps, suction cup chest electrodes and electrolyte pads, cream or liquid, alcohol prep pads, tissues, exam table, and gown/cape for patient to disrobe.

Procedure Steps

1. Wash hands.
2. Identify patient and ask him or her to remove clothing from the waist up and put on gown or cape with the opening in the front. Women should remove stockings; socks should be pushed down to ankles.
   Rationale: The chest leads will be placed directly on the skin of the left and right side of chest so disrobing is necessary for testing. Nylon is not a good conductor of electric

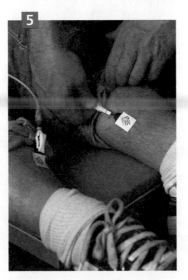

impulses so leads should be placed directly on the skin surface.

3. Place patient in a supine position for EKG.
4. Assemble and prepare equipment and explain the procedure to patient. Turn on electrocardiograph.
   Rationale: Understanding the procedure for performing the EKG will put the patient at ease. It will increase cooperation if the patient understands why he or she should not talk or move during the procedure. Older machines need to warm up to heat up the stylus.
5. Place the limb lead electrodes on nonbony areas, usually just above the ankles (pointing up) and on the fleshy part of the upper arms (pointing down). The electrodes may vary depending on the equipment. Metal plates that fasten with rubber straps may be used. Position an electrolyte pad on the extremity, place the metal pad over it, and fasten the rubber strap so that it is tight but not uncomfortable for the patient. If disposable tab electrodes are used, remove the paper backing and press the tab firmly into position with the tab pointing upward on the legs and downward on the arms.
   Rationale: There must be good contact between the skin and the electrode to transmit impulses to the EKG machine. An electrolyte pad improves conduction from the skin to the metal type electrode. The disposable tab electrode already contains an electrolyte layer. Metal electrodes must be held securely; if they are too loose or if they constrict the extremity, artifact may occur in the tracing.
6. If the tab electrode does not adhere completely, wipe the skin with an alcohol pad and allow to dry, then apply a new electrode.
   Rationale: Alcohol will remove skin oils and improve the ability of the tab electrode to adhere to the skin.
7. Place chest leads using specific designated intercostal spaces. Count each intercostal space on the left and right of chest. If tab electrodes are used, remove backing without handling electrodes and press each electrode firmly into place with the tab pointing down. On a male patient, press chest hair down and to the side before applying electrode. If the electrode does not adhere, shave a small area and apply a

Procedure continued on following page

PROCEDURE 17–6 *(continued)*

electrode. If Welch suction cup electrodes are used, apply a small amount of electrode cream or liquid where each electrode will be placed. Squeeze the rubber bulb of the electrode and place above the electrolyte cream. This creates suction to hold the electrode in place.
Rationale: Correct lead placement will help determine the accuracy of the EKG. Good contact between the electrode and the skin is necessary to conduct the electrical impulses. The electrolyte cream is necessary to transmit the impulse from the skin to the Welch suction cup electrodes.

8 Attach all electrode wires from EKG machine to tabs (or electrode plates and suction cups). Follow color coding and/or electrode marking on wires to be sure each is attached to the correct electrode.
Rationale: Each wire is color-coded and marked with abbreviations, which show which wire goes with which extremity or chest placement.

9. Enter any patient data your practice requires for identification purposes. Make any needed adjustments to the machine.
Rationale: Many EKG machines print data such as the patient name and clinic number directly on the EKG tracing.

10. Instruct the patient not to talk and to lie still. Press AUTO for automatic, and the machine will perform the EKG tracing. The machine performs standardization automatically and makes the tracing. The three-channel machine creates a tracing on a letter-size piece of paper. The single-channel machine prints each lead successively on a long strip of EKG paper.

Rationale: Standardization is needed to determine the voltage setting and whether the machine is calibrated correctly.

11. Before disconnecting lead wires, check the EKG tracing for artifacts, loose leads, and low voltage. If any are found, troubleshoot the problem and repeat the tracing.
Rationale: It can save time by reviewing the tracing before removing electrodes in case it is necessary to repeat the tracing.

12. Disconnect electrodes and assist patient in clean-up as needed.

13. Wash hands.

14. If not printed by the electrocardiograph, fill in information, including patient name, date, age, doctor, cardiac symptoms, cardiac medications, or other information requested. Record that the EKG was taken in the patient's medical record. If necessary, mount the EKG and give the completed EKG to the doctor.

Charting Example	
Date	
7/15/XX	2:00 PM 12-lead electrocardiogram taken without problems.
	K. Anderson, CMA

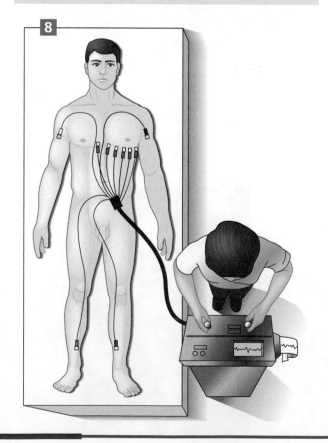

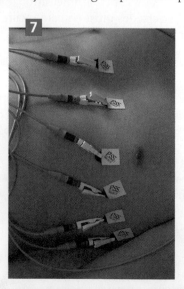

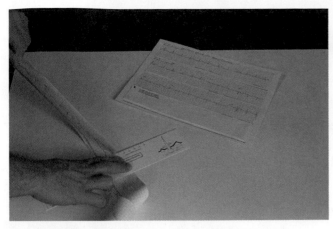

➤ Figure 18–13 Mounting single-channel EKG.

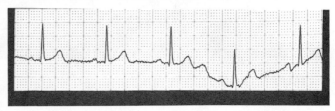

➤ **Figure 18–15** Wandering baseline. (From Chester, GA: *Modern Medical Assisting*. Philadelphia: W.B. Saunders, 1998.)

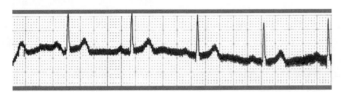

➤ **Figure 18–14** AC interference. (From Chester GA: *Modern Medical Assisting*. Philadelphia: W.B. Saunders, 1998.)

The electrode wires can be prevented from pulling on the electrode by taping the wire to the skin about 1″ to 2″ below the alligator clip.

Somatic tremor is an unnatural baseline deflection caused by muscle tension or talking. A somatic tremor may occur when the patient is tense, uncomfortable, or cold, or has a physical problem that causes tremors, such as Parkinson's disease. Somatic tremor can be prevented by making the patient comfortable, helping the patient to relax, and making sure the patient is warm enough. Figure 18–16 shows somatic tremor. The patient may also place the palms down flat on the examination table, under his or her buttocks, to alleviate somatic tremor.

Baseline interruption occurs when the patient moves around or when there is a break in the connection, usually due to a lead that comes loose from an electrode. If some leads show interrupted baseline and some show no problem, look for a loose connection.

Special Situations

Sometimes electrodes cannot be placed in the usual positions, and the medical assistant must make adaptations. These should be noted for the person interpreting the EKG.

Bandages, Casts, or Amputations

The electrode must be placed on the skin. If bandages or casts are on an arm or leg, or if the lower part of the extremity is missing, place the electrode higher on the limb, as near to the preferred site as possible but not directly on a bony prominence. Place the electrode symmetrically on the other limb.

Large Breasts or Obesity

It may be difficult to palpate intercostal spaces in a patient with large breasts or an obese patient. Place chest leads by eye to the best of your ability.

Lesions, Wounds, or Healing Incisions on the Chest

Do not place leads over open lesions, sutures, staples, or very recently healed areas on the chest. If you

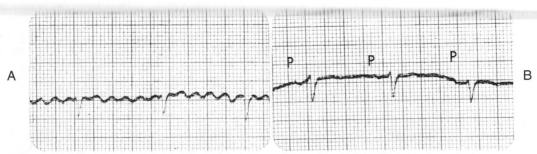

➤ **Figure 18–16** Somatic tremor. (A) Wavy baseline due to muscle tremor. (B) Same pattern without the artifact showing normal P waves. (From Goldberger A, Goldberger E: *Clinical Electrocardiography: A Simplified Approach*, 4th ed. St. Louis: Mosby, 1990.)

ON THE JOB

CHARACTERS: Robert Winthrop, 58-year-old male, patient of Dr. Lopez; Kathy Anderson, medical assistant

SCENE: In the examination room.

SITUATION: Kathy is taking an EKG using a single-channel machine. The machine is set up to run at 25 mm/second, switch leads, mark, and standardize automatically. While taking the tracing, Kathy notices that in the lead marked — . . . the stylus has wandered from the top to the bottom of the paper, forming spiky lines all over the tracing, as shown below. All other leads appear normal. Noticing Kathy's frown, Mr. Winthrop asks anxiously, "Is there something wrong with my heart?"

QUESTIONS

1. How should Kathy answer Mr. Winthrop?
2. Which lead should Kathy look at first?
3. What is most likely wrong? How does Kathy know?
4. Which leads would appear abnormal if the electrode on the left arm was not connected to the machine?
5. What should Kathy do before running another tracing?
6. Does Kathy have to report this problem to the doctor? Why or why not?

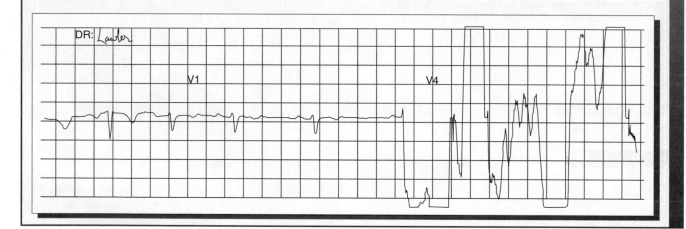

cannot position the electrodes near the preferred site, ask for guidance from the doctor.

Respiratory Problems

If a patient cannot tolerate a flat position, note how high the head is elevated. If the patient is using intercostal muscles to breathe, artifact may be seen in the chest leads. Repositioning the precordial leads may help, or you may need to ask for guidance from the doctor.

Caring for the EKG Equipment

After the EKG is complete and you have checked the tracing to make sure it is clear, remove the lead wires from the electrodes, then remove the electrodes from the patient. Discard disposable electrodes and other disposables items, and arrange the wires neatly over or beside the machine before returning it to storage.

If metal and bulb electrodes have been used, clean the patient's chest with a moist paper towel to remove the electrode cream or gel, and dry with a second paper towel. The metal electrodes, bulb electrodes, and rubber straps should be washed regularly with soap and water, and dried carefully. They must air-dry completely before they are used again.

Lotion or gel must be removed from the inside of bulb electrodes each time they are used; a cotton-tipped applicator is helpful to do this. Do not use metal polish or steel wool on the metal electrodes, because it can cause artifact.

EKG Interpretation

After the medical assistant has made the EKG tracing and mounted it, if necessary, it is given to the doctor for interpretation. Many modern machines print an interpretation, but the doctor still needs to make his or her own evaluation.

Common Arrhythmias

A number of abnormalities of heart rate or heart rhythm, collectively known as arrhythmias, can be seen immediately on the EKG tracing. If the medical assistant notices any of these distinctive patterns, he or she should alert the doctor as soon as possible.

Normal heart rate is between 60 and 100 beats per minute. Below 60 beats per minute is known as **bradycardia,** and more than 100 beats per minute is known as **tachycardia.** A medical assistant should recognize these conditions if they occur while taking the EKG.

A premature contraction, either a premature atrial contraction **(PAC)** or a premature ventricular contraction **(PVC),** is not usually abnormal, but either is considered serious if it occurs more than six to eight times per minute.

A PAC is characterized by a cardiac cycle that begins before the next cycle is due and contains an abnormally shaped P wave. PACs are often seen in healthy people who smoke and drink a lot of caffeinated beverages. The occurrence of multiple PACs can be a sign of later cardiac problems.

A PVC occurs early in the cycle and is characterized by lack of a P wave, an abnormal T wave, and a wide QRS complex, all followed by a pause before the next cycle. PVCs are usually seen in individuals with hypertension (high blood pressure), CAD, and lung disease. However, they can occur in healthy people from tobacco, alcohol, medications that contain epinephrine, and even anxiety.

A comparison of PAC and PVC is shown in Figure 18–17.

Serious or Life-Threatening Arrhythmias

The medical assistant should recognize the seriousness of life-threatening arrhythmias and obtain immediate help. These include third-degree heart block, ventricular tachycardia, and **ventricular fibrillation,** also called v-fib, an erratic heart rhythm that doesn't allow

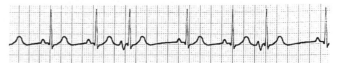
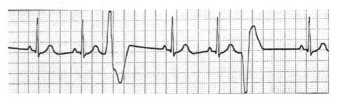

> **Figure 18–17** (A) Premature atrial contractions appear as an early beats with abnormal P waves. (B) Premature ventricular contractions show widened QRS complexes. (From Chester GA: *Modern Medical Assisting*. Philadelphia: W.B. Saunders, 1998.)

for sufficient blood to be pumped through the body. If a PVC occurs during repolarization of the ventricles, it may throw the heart into ventricular fibrillation.

If an individual undergoing an EKG shows a potentially dangerous arrhythmia, the medical assistant should obtain help to assess the seriousness of the problem before allowing the patient to get up or walk, even from the laboratory to the doctor's office (a reason why many doctors perform EKGs in an examination room rather than in the lab).

Heart block is a term used for conditions in which the electrical impulse is delayed or blocked at the AV node. When all impulses are blocked (complete, or third-degree, heart block) the ventricles contract in a regular rhythm, but the rate is usually very slow (20 to 60 beats per minute). The patient usually complains of weakness and fainting spells.

A patient with this condition should be kept lying down and will usually be transferred to the hospital for insertion of a pacemaker. On the EKG, QRS complexes occur without any relationship to P waves. The QRS complexes may appear relatively normal, or they may be widened (like PVCs), depending on which cells of the ventricles are initiating the contraction. This is shown in Figure 18–18.

Ventricular tachycardia (V tach) is an abnormal sequence of three or more PVCs. Short runs of ventricular tachycardia may not be serious. But if the condition

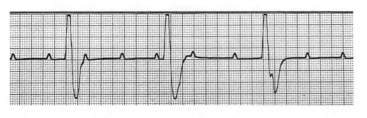

> **Figure 18–18** Third-degree (complete) heart block. (From Chester GA: *Modern Medical Assisting*. Philadelphia: W.B. Saunders, 1998.)

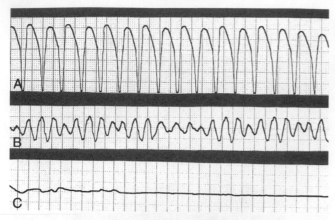

> **Figure 18–19** Life-threatening arrhythmias. (A) Ventricular tachycardia. (B) Ventricular fibrillation. (C) Asystole. (From Chester GA: *Modern Medical Assisting*. Philadelphia: W.B. Saunders, 1998.)

lasts longer than 30 seconds, the rapid heart rate (100 to 200 beats per minute) decreases the efficiency of the vascular system; the blood pressure falls rapidly; inadequate oxygen is carried to the brain, heart, and other tissues; and the person becomes unconscious.

With continued lack of oxygen, the heart rhythm usually turns into ventricular fibrillation. The heart's cells no longer contract together, and the complexes become irregular and gradually diminish in size until **asystole** (lack of heartbeat) occurs. This is shown in Figure 18–19.

If ventricular tachycardia or ventricular fibrillation are noticed during an EKG, continue to run a rhythm strip and get help immediately. If the patient becomes unconscious, the doctor may ask the medical assistant to call an ambulance and prepare equipment necessary for resuscitation.

If the office has a crash cart or emergency box, it should be brought to the area. The doctor or paramedic may administer medication and use a **defibrillator,** a machine that sends electric current through the patient's chest to depolarize the entire heart so that the SA node can reestablish a heartbeat. A defibrillator shown in Figure 18–20.

HOLTER MONITOR

If a patient has **intermittent** (not continuous, but rather coming and going) symptoms of arrhythmia, the doctor may order a Holter monitor test. A Holter monitor is an ambulatory EKG machine that can take a 24-hour reading of heart rate and rhythm while the patient engages in a normal day's activities. The results of this continuous EKG are recorded on either magnetic or computer tape, and stored on a recorder that the patient wears over the shoulder or on the belt.

The leads are round adhesive pads that come with electrolyte already applied. The lead wires attach to a snap on each of these disposable adhesive pads. After preparing the skin by shaving it and cleaning it with alcohol, leads are placed in the following way:

V_1 is placed in the 3rd intercostal space, 2″ to 3″ right of the sternum.

V_2 is placed in the 3rd intercostal space, 2″ to 3″ left of the sternum.

V_3 is placed in the 5th intercostal space on the left, next to the sternum.

V_4 is placed in the 6th intercostal space, on the right, in front of the axilla.

V_5 is placed in the 6th intercostal space, on the left, in front of the axilla.

The electrodes are taped and must be left in place for 24 hours. The patient needs to be instructed not to shower or bathe during that time, not to use an electric blanket, and not to touch the electrodes. The patient is instructed to briefly press the "event" button when he or she is experiencing any kind of symptom.

Most important, the patient needs to keep a detailed diary of activities, symptoms, and emotions. By cross-checking the time when activities, symptoms, and emotions are recorded by the patient against the real-time EKG results from the Holter monitor, the doctor can try to determine causal relationships between particular activities or emotions and various symptoms such as fatigue and chest pain.

The patient needs to record the times at which he or she eats, lies down to sleep, has a bowel movement,

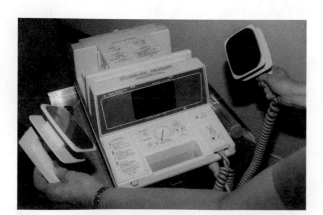

> **Figure 18–20** Cardiac defibrillator with paddles prepared for use. (From Kinn ME, Woods M: *The Medical Assistant: Administrative and Clinical*, 8th ed. Philadelphia: W.B. Saunders, 1999.)

PROCEDURE 18–2

Applying a Holter Monitor

Performance Objective: The student will be able to apply a Holter monitor for 24-hour Holter monitoring.

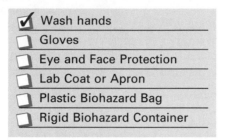

☑ Wash hands
☐ Gloves
☐ Eye and Face Protection
☐ Lab Coat or Apron
☐ Plastic Biohazard Bag
☐ Rigid Biohazard Container

Supplies and Equipment: Holter monitor, replacement battery, magnetic/computer tape, patient diary, razor, alcohol swabs, disposable round electrodes with snap fastener, skin-sensitive adhesive tape, carrying case with belt/shoulder strap.

Procedure Steps

1. Assemble and prepare equipment by removing previously used battery from monitor and replacing with a new one. Insert a blank magnetic/computer tape into monitor.
   Rationale: So that a malfunction will not occur, always replace battery and tape for each patient.
2. Identify patient and ask him or her to remove clothing from waist up.
3. Wash hands.

4. Explain procedure to patient.
5. With patient in sitting position, identify lead locations on chest wall. Prepare the skin by using an alcohol swab to rub the areas where the electrodes will be placed until reddened. If hairy, the area should be shaved. Let area dry.
   Rationale: The skin surface should be slightly abraded to allow for better adherence of electrodes and better conduction of impulses and to allow for easier removal when test is completed.
6. Place round electrodes with snap fastener in each area prepared by attaching adhesive backing to skin surface firmly.
   Rationale: The wires of the Holter monitor snap on to the electrodes. Round electrodes are larger and adhere better for the 24-hour test.
7. Attach lead wires to all electrodes.
8. Connect to patient cable.
9. Secure electrodes with adhesive, skin-sensitive tape.
10. The monitor may be plugged into an EKG machine to test for baseline tracing. Place electrode/patient cable so that it comes out at waist level, below the shirt. Tape patient cable to patient's chest.
    Rationale: Patient cable should not pull on electrode lead wires.
11. Place recorder in case and attach to belt or shoulder strap.

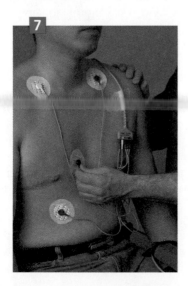

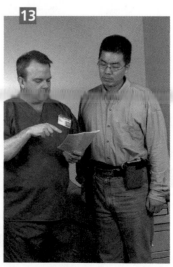

Procedure continued on following page

PROCEDURE 17–6 *(continued)*

12. Plug cable into Holter monitor and make sure the recorder is recording.
    Rationale: The connection into the monitor will begin the recording process. Making sure this is working correctly lets the medical assistant know that the entire monitor, battery, tape, and electrodes are working correctly before the patient leaves the office.
13. Provide the patient with verbal and written instructions on use of monitor, diary information to be kept, and when to return to have the unit removed.
14. Wash hands.
15. Document in patient record.

Charting Example	
Date	
7/15/XX	2:30 PM Holter monitor applied.
	Patient instructed to leave monitor
	in place for 24 hours, to record all
	activity and cardiac symptoms in
	patient diary, not to shower or allow
	unit to get wet, and to return on
	7/16/XX for removal of unit. ————
	K. Anderson, CMA

takes medication, goes up or down stairs, smokes, engages in physical exercise, or engages in sexual activity.

A day after the Holter monitor is fitted, the patient returns to have it removed. The tape is then sent to be analyzed.

Procedure 18–2 describes applying a Holter monitor.

Cardiac Event Monitoring

For patients with infrequent symptoms, cardiac event monitoring may be more useful than a Holter monitor. The patient uses an event recorder when symptoms occur to make a recording of cardiac activity.

Some recorders require two disposable electrodes. Others only require the patient to place the recorder on the chest above the heart. The patient records symptoms by pressing a button on the recorder and transmits the recording via telephone to a monitoring center after the event.

If the recording shows a serious arrhythmia, the monitoring center contacts the doctor and prompts the patient to seek immediate treatment. The patient must be instructed how and when to use the event recorder, how to transmit the recording to the monitoring center, and how to erase the recorder's memory for future recording.

Stress Testing

A **stress test** (sometimes called an exercise tolerance EKG) is performed on a patient who has symptoms such as chest pain or fatigue but shows no abnormalities on a resting EKG. A stress test is usually performed by a cardiologist. It is a **noninvasive** test, meaning it does not penetrate a body cavity.

Equipment used in a stress test, shown in Figure 18–21, includes a treadmill, stationary bicycle, or other device for exercise; a cardiac monitor; and a blood pressure cuff and stethoscope. A doctor is present during the stress test. A continuous EKG readout is taken, and blood pressure is monitored closely.

Although the stress test is noninvasive, the patient must sign a consent form, because the test can induce a **myocardial infarction** (heart attack) or stroke in a patient with underlying CAD.

During exercise, the heart must work harder to pump oxygenated blood throughout the body. The myocardium also needs more oxygen. When one or more coronary arteries are blocked or narrowed, the patient may experience pain and/or fatigue, which may also show up on an EKG taken while exercising as ST-segment elevation or other EKG changes. Emergency equipment and medications must be available when a stress test is performed.

The procedure for the stress test is simple. The patient is asked to come to the test wearing comfortable clothing and walking or jogging shoes. At the testing site, the patient is attached to a cardiac monitor, using chest electrodes like those used for a Holter monitor.

After proper stretching, the patient climbs on the exercise equipment and begins exercising. Gradually the exercise is made more demanding. On a treadmill, the speed, incline of the treadmill, or both, may be increased. On a bicycle, the tension is increased. The cardiologist actively monitors the real-time EKG readout and the blood pressure. The patient is also instructed to tell the doctor if he or she is feeling any symptoms.

If the patient experiences pain, excess fatigue, or shortness of breath, the doctor will end the test. If the patient is able to exercise comfortably to a sufficient degree of difficulty, the doctor eventually will end the test. Monitoring continues through the cool down until the heart rate returns to normal. The patient should rest, refrain from caffeine and other stimulants, not take a hot bath or shower, and avoid extreme temperature changes for a few hours after the test.

After the stress test, the doctor may wish to obtain a nuclear medicine scan of the heart (a thallium scan). This requires the stress test to be done at a facility that has a nuclear medicine department so the scan can be done as soon as the test ends.

REMOTE EKG

Pilots who fly commercial airplanes must have an annual physical—pilots over age 40 must have physicals every 6 months—and an annual electrocardiogram, to maintain their licensing with the Federal Aviation Administration (FAA).

Each year, the FAA office of aeromedical affairs receives over 80,000 EKGs, which must be examined to determine if any pilot has underlying heart problems that should keep him or her out of the cockpit of a commercial airplane.

Until the mid-1990s, the majority of those EKGs came to the FAA as paper tracings mailed in by pilots' doctors, who are known as aeromedical examiners and are licensed by the FAA to perform pilot physicals. These tracings then had to be manually read by an EKG technician. If an EKG looked suspicious, a cardiologist had to look at the tracing. This process often took weeks.

If the doctor wanted the pilot to have another EKG, the pilot's doctor would have to be notified, and the doctor would then notify the pilot to come in for another EKG.

For 20 years, the FAA has worked to build a system of remote EKGs. Today the technology is in place so that all pilot EKGs are sent immediately as they are taken, via telephone modem hookup from the aeromedical examiner's office to the FAA computer in Oklahoma City.

If an artifact is being transmitted, the computer can immediately alert a technician, who can telephone the doctor and ask that the EKG be retaken before the patient leaves the office. Using a sophisticated computer program, the EKGs receive a cursory screening for abnormalities. If one is detected, the tracing can be viewed immediately by a cardiologist, who can speak with the aeromedical examiner and even the pilot while he or she is still at the doctor's office.

Utilizing the most modern EKG equipment, as well as high-speed computers and sophisticated software, the FAA is working to make sure pilots are healthy and that air travel on American commercial airlines is as safe as possible.

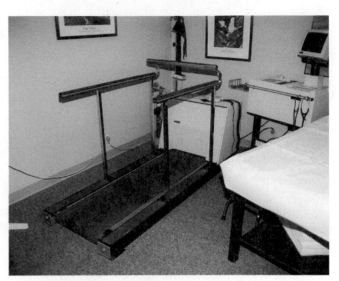

A

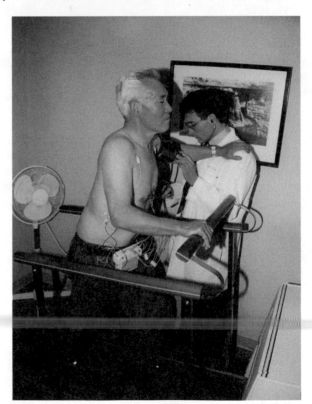

B

➢ **Figure 18–21** Cardiac stress testing. (A) Treadmill prepared for stress testing. (B) Doctor monitoring patient during stress testing. (From Kinn ME, Woods M: *The Medical Assistant: Administrative and Clinical*, 8th ed. Philadelphia: W.B. Saunders, 1999.)

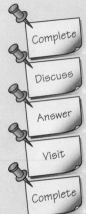

STUDENT STUDY PLAN

To reinforce your understanding of the material in this part of the chapter . . .

Complete the **Review & Recall** questions.

Discuss the situation in **If You Were the Medical Assistant** with your classmates, and answer the questions.

Answer the **Critical Thinking Questions,** and discuss them with your classmates.

Visit **Web sites** listed below and search for additional Web sites using the **Keywords for Internet Searches**.

Complete the exercises in chapter 18 of the **Student Mastery Manual.**

 ## REVIEW & RECALL

1. Describe the heart's conduction system.

2. What do each of the following parts of the EKG tracing represent in terms of heart activity: P wave, PR interval, QRS complex, QT interval, ST segment, T wave?

3. Where are the leads placed on the chest for a 12-lead electrocardiogram? For a Holter monitor?

4. What instructions should you give a patient before taking an EKG?

5. Define the term *arrhythmia*. Name several common arrhythmias. Which arrhythmias are considered life-threatening and why?

 ## IF YOU WERE THE MEDICAL ASSISTANT

Dr. Hughes has ordered a 24-hour Holter monitor test after a normal 12-lead EKG done in the office. The patient is Daniel Goldman, a 64-year-old man who presented with complaints of episodes of chest palpitations, mild chest pressure, and shortness of breath that last 10 to 20 minutes and occur almost every night.

1. How would you explain the test to Mr. Goldman?

2. Why is a more extensive skin preparation used before applying the leads for a Holter monitor than is used for a 12-lead electrocardiogram? What will you do before you apply the electrodes? Why is tape applied over the electrodes?

3. Where would you apply the six leads?

4. What instructions do you have to give to Mr. Goldman before he leaves the office?

5. When Mr. Goldman returns to the office tomorrow, what will you do?

CRITICAL THINKING QUESTIONS

1. What steps should the medical assistant carry out if the EKG tracing shows small jagged lines instead of a clear tracing?

2. How can you determine the heart rate from the EKG tracing? How can you determine if the heartbeat is regular?

3. What physical problems might prevent you from applying the EKG leads in their normal positions? What problems might interfere with obtaining a smooth tracing? What could you do to respond to these problems?

EXPLORE THE WEB

INTERNET WEB SITES

American Heart Association
www.americanheart.org

American College of Cardiology
www.acc.org

Education sites for cardiovascular diseases and procedures
www.med-edu.com
www.medhelp.org

Patient teaching: cardiac procedures
www.cardioassoc.com/patient_pgs/patientres.asp/

KEYWORDS FOR INTERNET SEARCHES

cardiac testing
  Holter monitor

ANSWERS TO ON THE JOB

1. Kathy should tell Mr. Winthrop that there seems to be a problem with one of the leads, so she is not obtaining a good tracing for Dr. Lopez to interpret.

2. Kathy should look at the chest lead V_4.

3. Because the tracing is clear, except for this particular lead, the most likely problem is that lead V_4 is not firmly attached to the skin. Kathy knows this because none of the other leads is affected.

4. If the electrode on the left arm was loose or not connected to the matching lead (lead I), lead III and the augmented leads (aVR, aVL, aVF) would be affected. The tracing from lead II and the precordial leads would appear normal.

5. Before running another tracing, Kathy should replace lead V_4. She should clean the skin at that area with alcohol and allow it to dry. She may also need to shave a small area so that the lead will adhere. And she could also apply tape to the wire 1″ or 2″ below the electrode.

6. Kathy does not need to report this to Dr. Lopez. She is responsible to correct a problem with the equipment and obtain a clear tracing.

Chapter 19

Assisting with Diagnostic Procedures

Chapter Topics

Overview of Diagnostic Procedures

Respiratory System
Diagnosis of Diseases and Conditions of the Respiratory System
Spirometry
Sputum Specimen
Pulse Oximetry and Blood Gases

Genitourinary System
Urinary Catheterization
Diagnosis of Diseases and Conditions of the Reproductive System
Colposcopy
Loop Electrosurgical Excision Procedure and Cryosurgery
Prostate-Specific Antigen Test

Sperm Count and Sperm Washing

Neurologic System
Diagnosis of Diseases and Conditions of the Neurologic System
Neurologic Examination
Lumbar Puncture

Instructional Objectives

After completing this chapter, you will be able to do the following:

1. Define and spell the vocabulary words for this chapter.
2. Explain the role of the medical assistant related to diagnostic testing.
3. Describe how blood levels of oxygen and carbon dioxide can be measured.
4. Discuss the role of the medical assistant during spirometry.
5. Identify appropriate precautions when obtaining a sputum specimen.
6. Describe the procedure for obtaining a sputum specimen.
7. Discuss the purpose and procedure for urinary catheterization.
8. Describe the role of the medical assistant when colposcopy is performed as an office procedure.
9. Discuss the importance of testing males over age 50 for prostate-specific antigen (PSA).
10. Describe the importance of a sperm count in the diagnosis of infertility.
11. Correlate the procedure for sperm washing to artificial insemination procedures.
12. Compare the neurologic examination to the general physical examination.
13. Describe the medical assistant's role in the neurologic examination.
14. Describe how the medical assistant assists with a lumbar puncture.

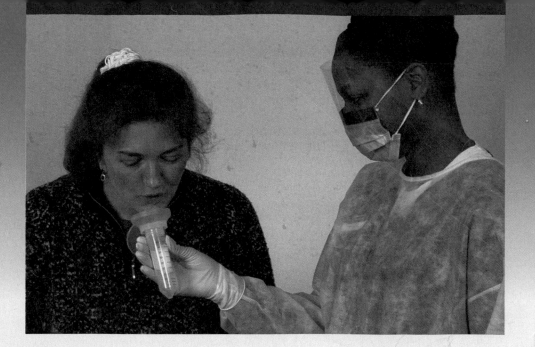

CMA/RMA CERTIFICATION
Content and Competencies

- Perform respiratory testing
- Prepare patient for and assist with routine and specialty examinations
- Prepare patients for and assist with procedures, treatments, and minor office surgery

- Instruct patients according to their needs
- Document appropriately

Performance Objectives

After completing this chapter, you will be able to do the following:

1. Perform spirometry (Procedure 19–1).
2. Obtain a sputum specimen (Procedure 19–2).
3. Perform urinary catheterization on a female patient (Procedure 19–3).
4. Perform sperm washing (Procedure 19–4).
5. Assist with a neurologic exam (Procedure 19–5).
6. Assist with a lumbar puncture (Procedure 19–6).

VOCABULARY

calculi (p. 424)	expiratory reserve volume (p. 417)	intracervical insemination (p. 429)	spirometry (p. 414)
catheter (p. 422)			sputum (p. 417)
catheterization (p. 424)	forced expiratory volume at 1 second (p. 417)	intrauterine insemination (p. 429)	subclinical (p. 425)
clonus (p. 431)		malignant (p. 415)	tidal volume (p. 417)
cryosurgery (p. 428)	forced vital capacity (p. 417)	motility (p. 428)	vital capacity (p. 417)
cystoscopy (p. 428)		precancerous (p. 415)	
endocervical curettage (p. 428)	inspiratory reserve volume (p. 417)	prostate-specific antigen (p. 429)	
		residual volume (p. 417)	

ABBREVIATIONS

AFB (p. 420)	CSF (p. 431)	FVC (p. 417)	LP (p. 431)	STD (p. 424)
BPH (p. 428)	FEV_1 (p. 417)	LEEP (p. 428)	PSA (p. 428)	

During the course of a physical examination, the doctor performs a number of diagnostic tests. For many of these tests, the medical assistant is called upon to set up the equipment and either assist with the test or perform the test himself or herself.

The doctor may order additional tests to be done outside the office, often in the hospital or at an outside laboratory.

This chapter discusses the diagnostic tests and procedures performed in the doctor's office during the office visit and the medical assistant's role in those tests. Some of these tests involve direct testing; others involve collecting specimens.

The next chapter discusses methods for diagnostic imaging, which may be done in the office, in an outside lab, or at a hospital. Finally, collection of blood, urine, and culture specimens for laboratory tests and the tests themselves, are discussed in the following unit, on the physician office laboratory and laboratory tests.

OVERVIEW OF DIAGNOSTIC PROCEDURES

Many types of diagnostic procedures help in the diagnosis of disease or medical conditions. Blood, urine, and other body fluids can be tested to identify cells, chemicals, or the presence of microorganisms. Samples can be taken of secretions, or discharge, to test for the presence of microorganisms. Cell samples can be examined to determine if they are normal or abnormal.

Obtaining some specimens requires fairly complex procedures. Two examples are urinary catheterization to obtain urine and lumbar puncture to obtain cerebrospinal fluid. Those procedures are discussed in this chapter.

In addition, instruments can be inserted into body openings to view body cavities and obtain samples for analysis. Because most body cavities require special equipment and sometimes anesthesia, most of these procedures are done in special procedure rooms in hospitals or large clinics. Colposcopy (visual examination of the vagina) is a common office procedure and is discussed in this chapter. Sigmoidoscopy, often part of the physical examination, was discussed in chapter 16.

A variety of tests measure whether parts of the body function normally, such as the electrocardiogram, discussed in chapter 18, or **spirometry** (measurement of breathing), which is discussed in this chapter.

Images can be made of the body or its parts to observe the structure and function of various organs. Diagnostic imaging, a branch of medicine whose complexity and variety increased dramatically in the second half of the twentieth century, is discussed in chapter 20.

The accompanying box offers an overview of various types of diagnostic tests.

RESPIRATORY SYSTEM

The respiratory system includes the lungs and the trachea—the tube that carries air to and from the lungs. The respiratory system brings oxygen into the body and eliminates carbon dioxide. Oxygen is the main ingredient needed for cell metabolism. If carbon dioxide is not eliminated, the body's acid-base balance changes, becoming more acid; this can eventually lead to a condition known as acidosis.

Diagnosis of Diseases and Conditions of the Respiratory System

The respiratory system is vulnerable to attack by microorganisms, which can be present in microscopic droplets in the air or are passed by direct contact

Overview of Types of Diagnostic Tests

BLOOD TESTS AND TESTS OF URINE AND OTHER BODY FLUIDS OR SECRETIONS

Blood gases—measurements of the amount of oxygen and carbon dioxide in a sample of arterial blood.

Chemistry analysis—tests of blood, urine, spinal fluid, or other body fluids to determine the presence or amount of specific chemicals (such as glucose, sodium, and blood urea nitrogen).

Coagulation studies—various tests of blood to determine whether specific clotting factors are present and effective and the time it takes for the blood to clot.

Culture and sensitivity—technique to grow microorganisms from samples of blood, secretions, or other body fluids using special materials and conditions (culture). The sensitivity test uses small disks impregnated with different antibiotics on the culture plate to determine which medications may be effective in killing the microorganisms or preventing them from growing.

Hematology—analysis of venous or capillary blood to determine the number and appearance of the various types of blood cells in the sample.

Serology—uses the antigen–antibody reaction to test blood serum, plasma, whole blood, or urine to determine past or present infections or the presence of certain hormones, such as those found only in pregnancy. Serologic techniques are also used to determine blood type and test blood for compatibility before transfusions.

Urinalysis—a physical, chemical, and microscopic examination of urine, which can provide information about the bladder, kidneys, and metabolic processes. The urine specimen may be obtained by having the patient void or by catheterizing the patient.

DIAGNOSTIC IMAGING

Diagnostic radiology—use of x-ray to form a diagnostic image. Continuous x-ray imaging is called fluoroscopy. Creation of a series of cross-sectional images is called tomography. When these images are linked by computer, the tests are called computed tomography scans (CT scans).

Magnetic resonance imaging—use of magnetic fields in combination with radio waves and computer technology to create cross-sectional views of tissue.

Nuclear medicine imaging—a process of diagnostic imaging using radioactive material injected into or swallowed by the patient and followed by a scan of various body parts to detect uptake of the radioactive material by body tissues.

Ultrasound (diagnostic medical sonography)—use of ultrasound (inaudible high-frequency sound waves) to form a diagnostic image. Ultrasonic waves directed toward the body form echos whose varying densities give information about underlying structures.

TESTS TO DETERMINE FUNCTION OF BODY ORGANS

Electrodiagnostic tests—methods to create a visual record of electrical activity of selected body tissues, especially the heart, brain, and muscles.

Pulmonary function tests—measurements of lung capacity and breathing, such as spirometry.

PROCEDURES TO VIEW BODY CAVITIES AND OBTAIN AND EXAMINE TISSUE SAMPLES

Biopsy—excision of a small piece of tissue for microscopic examination.

Cytology—cells are examined under the microscope, usually to determine if they are normal, **precancerous** (showing changes that may become malignant), or **malignant** (showing changes of cancer, which allow cells to grow without normal regulation).

Endoscopy—use of a flexible instrument to examine the inside of a body cavity. Modern endoscopes usually project images on a television screen. Tissue samples can usually be obtained for analysis during the procedure.

through respiratory secretions. Upper respiratory infections (URIs) affect mucous membranes of the nose, pharynx, and larynx, causing nasal stuffiness, sneezing, sore throat, fever, and headache.

The same viruses that cause URIs can also affect the lower respiratory system, causing inflammation of the bronchi, bronchioles, and alveoli. The increased mucus produced as part of the inflammatory reaction interferes with breathing and may collect in the alveoli, interfering with the exchange of oxygen and carbon dioxide. Symptoms of a lower respiratory infection may include fever, cough, shortness of breath,

■ ASTHMA

Asthma is a chronic disease in which lung function is compromised because of inflammation to the airway. Asthma can be caused by environmental factors and can be exacerbated by an upper respiratory viral illness, environmental conditions in which excessive dust is present, the presence of substances to which the individual is allergic, or even stress.

About 14 million Americans have asthma. Each year, asthma attacks account for over 500,000 visits to hospital emergency rooms and more than an equal number of visits to health centers, clinics, and doctors' offices. About 6,000 annual deaths in the United States are due to acute asthma attacks.

Asthma rates are higher in cities than in rural areas; in poor communities than middle- and upper-income communities; and in the Latino and African-American population than in Asian-American and white populations.

The goal of asthma treatment is to relieve chronic symptoms and manage the illness to reduce the possibility of an acute episode. A variety of new treatments are available, and research continues to improve the way older treatments are utilized. Management of asthma is a partnership between an individual who lives with the condition, his or her doctor, and often a medical assistant, nurse, or other patient educator.

Diagnosing asthma can be difficult. Many children will experience an episode of wheezing during a respiratory illness. It is only after such symptoms occur many times in conjunction with respiratory illness or after wheezing occurs in relation to exercise or spontaneously that a disagnosis of asthma is made.

In adults, cigarette smoking or working in a dusty or pollen-laden job (such as textile manufacturing, landscaping, and dry-wall installation) can lead to a misdiagnosis of chronic bronchitis, or even emphysema, before a proper diagnosis is made.

A detailed medical history, as well as a number of diagnostic tests, can be necessary to diagnose asthma. These tests include pulmonary function tests, as discussed in this chapter, or even a methacholine bronchial challenge test. Inhaling the chemical methacholine causes mild airway constriction in an individual with asthma.

The main medications used in asthma treatment are anti-inflammatory drugs, which both reduce the number of inflammatory cells in the airways and prevent blood vessels from leaking fluid into the airway tissue. Reducing inflammation helps reduce spontaneous spasms in airway muscles. Some asthma medications are taken by inhaler; others are taken as pills.

Corticosteroids can be either inhaled or taken as a pill. Inhaled corticosteroids are often used on a daily basis by individuals with moderate to severe asthma to reduce the incidence of severe acute attacks. Inhaled steriods have been shown to reduce the need for other medications.

Cromolyn sodium and nedocromil sodium are also inhaled; they are used daily by individuals with mild to moderate asthma.

Two other medications are used to moderate acute attacks and provide temporary symptomatic relief. These medications are known as bronchodilators.

Theophylline, the older of the two medications, is taken as a pill, often before bedtime to reduce nighttime symptoms.

$Beta_2$ adrenergic agonists are often prescribed for intermittent, mild asthma symptoms. These are administered through "puff" type plastic tubes that an individual can carry. They provide from 6 to 12 hours of acute relief (depending on the exact substance) from mild symptoms brought on by cold air or exercise. $Beta_2$ adrenergic agonists do not act against the underlying inflammation. Because they provide immediate relief, they can be overused; if the patient needs to use the substance on a daily basis, he or she should consult with a doctor about taking other medications used for long-term management.

In 1996, the first new asthma medication in 20 years—leukotriene receptor antagonists—became available. These substances block the action of leukotrienes, which are released by cells in the lungs during an asthma attack and cause inflammation to the lung tissue. Leukotriene receptor antagonists can be used for asthma that does not respond to more conventional treatment or in conjunction with other treatments for additional prevention of acute attacks.

rapid breathing, and sometimes painful breathing (dyspnea).

A second cause of respiratory diseases is related to structural changes caused by chronic inflammation. This inflammation may be related to hazardous substances inhaled into the lungs, such as cigarette smoke, dust, vapor, or toxic particles from various manufacturing processes (such as coal mining, sanding, or production of cotton thread or cloth). It may also be caused by chronic diseases such as asthma, allergies, or cystic fibrosis.

In response to chronic inflammation, production of thick mucus increases; this may overwhelm the normal cleansing mechanisms of the bronchial tree. This mucus may block the smaller bronchioles, trapping air in the alveoli, and eventually destroying their delicate membranes. The greater the extent of nonfunctioning lung tissue, the more respiratory problems the patient experiences, with symptoms including chronic cough, production of thick **sputum** (bronchial secretions and saliva coughed up from the lungs), and prolonged exhalation due to inelasticity of the alveoli.

As with any body system, abnormal growths called tumors or neoplasms can arise from the epithelial cells lining the nose, pharynx, larynx, and bronchial system. These tumors may be benign or malignant.

Lung cancer is the leading cause of death from cancer; its symptoms usually do not become severe until the disease is well established and the cancer has spread throughout the body.

Diagnosis of respiratory diseases focuses on identifying infectious agents, areas of infection, calcification (deposits of calcium used to wall off areas of inflammation), and tumors, and on monitoring decreases in blood oxygen levels and effective breathing.

Spirometry

Spirometry, a test of lung capacity, is one of a group of tests called pulmonary function tests. It measures how much air a patient can take in, and how forcefully and how fast he or she can blow it out. See the box on measurements of lung volumes.

In the doctor's office, spirometry is most frequently administered as part of a pre-employment physical or as part of the routine examination for a patient with a lung disease such as asthma, cystic fibrosis, or chronic obstructive pulmonary disease, which includes emphysema or chronic bronchitis.

The equipment used in spirometry, shown in Figure 19–1 consists of tubing and a disposable mouthpiece, the recording equipment, and usually a disposable noseclip. Old spirometry equipment consisted of paper, a circular drum, and a marking pen. Modern equipment contains a small computer that calculates the results of the test based on the patient's sex, age, and height. A report can usually be printed either from the spirometer itself or by connecting the spirometer to a

Measurements of Lung Volumes

Room air contains a combination of gases, including nitrogen (approximately 78%), oxygen (approximately 21%), carbon dioxide, water vapor, and traces of other gases. The air a person exhales contains a larger percentage of carbon dioxide. When breathing normally a person inhales and exhales about 500 milliliters of air with each breath (called the **tidal volume** or tidal air).

An individual with normal lungs can forcefully breathe in up to 3 liters of air after a normal breath (called the **inspiratory reserve volume**) and can forcefully breathe out about 1 liter of air after a normal exhale (called the **expiratory reserve volume**). The maximum amount of air that can be exhaled following a maximum inhalation is called the **vital capacity**. In addition, about 1 liter of air remains in the lungs at all times and cannot be forcibly exhaled or directly measured. This quantity is called the **residual volume.**

During spirometry, it is common to measure how much air a person can breathe against time. The person is instructed to breathe in as much air as possible and to blow the air out as rapidly and completely as possible. The total amount of air measured by the machine is corrected for temperature and barometric pressure and compared to predicted values based on age, height, and sex. The machine then prints a report identifying the total amount of air exhaled (**forced vital capacity,** or **FVC**), the amount of air exhaled in 1 second (**forced expiratory volume at 1 second,** or FEV_1), as well as other values.

Normally a person can expel at least 75% of his or her vital capacity within 1 second. If the ratio of the FEV_1 to the FVC is less than 75%, some obstruction to the flow of air is probably present, due to inflammation or constriction of the bronchioles. An individual who does not expend enough effort when performing the test is likely to demonstrate decreased values for all measurements.

printer. Figure 19–2 is an example of a printed spirometry report.

Patient preparation for spirometry is important. When the test is scheduled, the patient needs instruction on when to stop taking any medications (if necessary) and when to stop smoking (if the patient is a smoker); the patient may also be given other specific instructions, such as the need to remove dentures.

At the time of the test, the patient needs to be instructed closely. Proper posture is important to get an accurate reading; most spirometers require the pa-

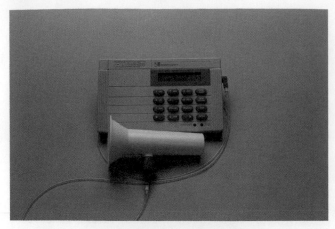

> **Figure 19–1** Spirometer.

bly refer the patient to a facility with larger, more sensitive equipment for additional testing. Patients with asthma often use a simple version of the spirometer called a peak flow meter to measure their breathing at home. The patient is instructed how to use the particular model he or she has been given, to perform the test at about the same time every day and, if he or she is

tient to be in a seated position, because the test can make some individuals light-headed, and standing could pose a danger. Legs should be uncrossed and both feet flat on the floor. The chin should be positioned slightly upward and the neck slightly outward.

The patient is told to relax, take a deep breath through the mouth then blow out, continuing to blow until the medical assistant instructs him or her to stop. Remind the patient to make a tight seal around the mouthpiece, keep the tongue from blocking the mouthpiece, and blow forcefully. If a paper mouthpiece is used, remind the patient not to bite down. A noseclip is often used to be sure all air passes into the mouthpiece.

During testing, continue to give encouragement to the patient to blow hard. Allow the patient to take at least three tries, with time in between attempts to recover. Follow instructions to save each attempt. Usually, the machine selects the best attempt to print.

Care of the equipment is important. Always dispose of the mouthpiece immediately and the noseclip as well if it is disposable. Change the external tubing, and discard or disinfect the old tubing using high-level disinfection techniques. If it is a water-seal unit, change the water regularly. Calibrate the equipment regularly and keep records of calibration; each model comes with directions for proper calibration.

If the computer does not automatically record the patient's name and date on the printed output, do so by hand. Document that the test was done. Place the results so the doctor can review them; the report can be inserted into the progress notes in sequence or placed in the section on diagnostic tests.

For more detail on performing spirometry, see Procedure 19–1.

Office spirometry is primarily a screening tool. If a patient's breathing is abnormal, the doctor will proba-

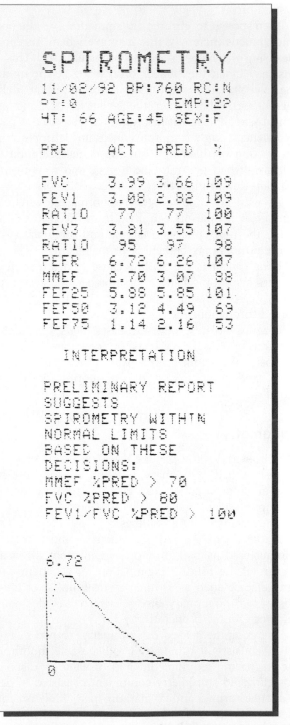

> **Figure 19–2** The spirometry report gives the values obtained and often offers a preliminary interpretation.

PROCEDURE 19-1

Performing Spirometry to Measure Lung Volume

Performance Objective: The student will be able to perform spirometry to measure lung volume.

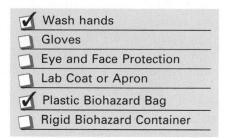

- ☑ Wash hands
- ☐ Gloves
- ☐ Eye and Face Protection
- ☐ Lab Coat or Apron
- ☑ Plastic Biohazard Bag
- ☐ Rigid Biohazard Container

Supplies and Equipment: Spirometer, disposable mouthpiece and plastic tubing, noseclip (depending on equipment), chair, biohazard bag.

Procedure Steps

1. Wash hands.
2. Identify patient, and explain procedure and purpose of test.
   Rationale: Patient needs to understand that he or she must inhale deeply and exhale as quickly and deeply as possible for the total volume of air expelled to be measured.
3. Assemble equipment and place new disposable mouthpiece and tubing on the spirometer.
   Rationale: To prevent transmission of infection, a new mouthpiece and tubing is used for each patient.
4. Place patient in chair, sitting straight.
   Rationale: The test is usually done with the patient seated to prevent faintness or dizziness. The patient should assume the position for which the machine was calibrated.
5. Enter information using the keypad according to the directions for the model of spirometer you are using.
   Rationale: Most spirometers request the patient's clinic number, height, weight, sex, and age to compare the actual values to expected values.
6. Apply noseclip if the machine you are using requires it. Instruct the patient to take a deep breath and blow out as rapidly and forcefully

as possible with lips around (not inside) the mouthpiece.
   Rationale: A noseclip may be used to be sure that no air is exhaled through the nose. The lips are placed around the mouthpiece to allow maximum exhalation.
7. Be sure the machine is recording while the patient blows out. Coach the patient and encourage him or her to blow rapidly and continue exhaling as much air as possible.
   Rationale: Coaching improves results.
8. Allow the patient to rest for a few minutes and repeat the test until three good efforts have been recorded or until the patient is too dizzy to continue.
   Rationale: The patient needs to rest to prevent dizziness and light-headedness from blowing off too much carbon dioxide.
9. Print results and label with the patient's name (if the machine does not do so).
10. Discard mouthpiece and tubing in a biohazard container. Disinfect the machine if necessary.
11. Wash hands.
12. Place the report in the patient's medical record and place in the designated area for the doctor to review. Note in the progress notes that a spirometry test was done and refer to the printed report.

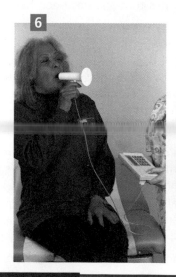

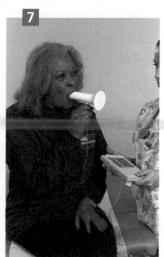

experiencing difficulty breathing, to record the results and sometimes to adjust his or her medication based on the results.

Sputum Specimen

A sputum sample may be necessary to diagnose tuberculosis, pneumonia, or other infectious disease of the lungs and lower respiratory tract.

Sputum can be collected in one of three ways: expectoration, suctioning, and bronchoscopy. Regardless of the method used, the medical assistant should wear gloves, mask, gown, and goggles or face shield when collecting a sputum specimen from a potentially infectious patient.

Expectoration is the coughing up of mucus from the lungs and throat. This is the least uncomfortable method for the patient and is used when the patient is able to produce sputum by coughing. If the expectoration method is to be used, the patient should be instructed to drink plenty of liquid the night before, not to brush his or her teeth or use mouthwash in the morning, and to give the specimen before eating. The patient is instructed to spit the specimen directly into the laboratory cup, or the medical assistant may use suction to collect the specimen from the back of the patient's throat.

When collecting a specimen using tracheal suction, a sterile catheter is passed through the patient's nose into the trachea. The suction machine pulls sputum out of the trachea. This method cannot be used if the patient has underlying heart disease or certain abnormalities of the trachea.

Bronchoscopy is a method of collecting specimens that involves placing a bronchoscope into the throat and the bronchus and removing secretions using a bronchial brush or aspirating the secretions directly into the bronchoscope tubing. A tissue sample is usually also obtained during the procedure. If bronchoscopy is to be used, the patient must fast for 6 hours before the procedure, because it is done under anesthesia.

The specimen is sent to a laboratory for culture and sensitivity, to determine the bacterium causing the infection. Figure 19–3 shows a completed laboratory requisition. These studies are usually available in 2 to 3 days. The doctor may also ask the lab to do a Gram stain or test for acid-fast bacillus (AFB) to determine if the patient has tuberculosis. Procedure 19–2 describes in detail how to obtain a sputum specimen.

Pulse Oximetry and Blood Gases

Pulse oximetry is a noninvasive test to determine the concentration of oxygen in the blood. Normal oxygen saturation is 97 to 99 percent. If the oxygen saturation drops below 94 percent, the doctor may order respiratory assistance such as oxygen. If oxygen concentration drops lower, more aggressive measures may be needed both to determine the cause of the decreased oxygenation and to provide appropriate therapy.

ON THE JOB

Sandra Morse, a medical assistant at Blackburn Primary Care Associates, has been asked by Dr. Hughes to perform a spirometry test on Mary Timmons. Mary, a 19-year-old woman with asthma, has told Dr. Hughes that she has been having increasingly frequent asthma attacks over the past 2 months.

Sandra: Dr. Hughes wants me to do a spirometry test today. Have you had one before?
Mary: I haven't had one for about a year, but before that I had them all the time.
Sandra: Then you remember that you are going to sit over here, take a deep breath, place your lips around the mouthpiece, and blow out into the mouthpiece as hard as you can.
Mary: This test always makes me dizzy. Why do I have blow as hard as I can?

QUESTIONS

1. Describe how asthma can interfere with a patient's ability to breathe and why it sometimes decreases the total amount of air that a patient's lungs can hold. You may need to do research to find the answer to this question.
2. Why is a patient usually seated for spirometry?
3. When Sandra begins the test, what should she tell Mary to do?
4. How can Sandra encourage Mary to produce her best effort?
5. How long should Sandra wait before asking Mary to repeat the test?
6. Why should Sandra give Mary at least three opportunities to repeat the test?

MICROBIOLOGY			GL 404	ST	BD	LAST NAME		FIRST NAME	

Form content:

MICROBIOLOGY — PLEASE PRINT • PRESS HARD

DRAWN BY | REMARKS: | DATE/TIME OF COLLECTION

ADDRESS

ROUTINE REQUEST

IF REQUEST IS OTHER THAN ROUTINE, PLACE STICKER WITH APPROPRIATE INSTRUCTIONS IN THIS SPACE

BIRTHDATE   AGE   SEX   CLASS

DATE | VERIFYING NURSE | DIAGNOSIS

PHYSICIAN   ROOM NO.   HOSP. NO.

DATE   PHONE

CIRCLE CODE NO. | **INDICATE** | SMEAR RESULT:

CULTURES | **SOURCE**

604 BLOOD — ☐ EYE
(600) (ROUTINE) — ☐ EAR
607 ANAEROBIC — ☐ CSF
620 URINE — ☐ NASOPHARYNX
606 CAMPYLO-BACTER — ☐ THROAT
618 AFB (SMEAR INCLUDED) — ☑ SPUTUM — CULTURE RESULT:
612 FUNGUS — ☐ URINE
616 GRAM STAIN — ☐ STOOL
(601) ANTIBIOTIC SENSITIVITY — ☐ CERVIX
— ☐ VAGINA
SCREENS — ☐ WOUND
625 BETA STREP — ☐ ASPIRATE
632 NEISSERIA — ☐ ABSCESS
INDICATE SITE:

TIME IN | TECHNOLOGIST | TIME CALLED OR TELETYPED | TIME OUT

MEDICAL RECORD

> **Figure 19–3** A sample laboratory requisition for a sputum specimen for culture and sensitivity. (From Zakus SM: *Clinical Procedures for Medical Assistants*, 3rd ed. St. Louis: Mosby, 1988.)

PROCEDURE 19–2

Collecting a Sputum Specimen

Performance Objective: The student will be able to instruct a patient on proper collection of a sputum specimen and assist in the collection if necessary.

☑ Wash hands
☑ Gloves
☑ Eye and Face Protection
☑ Lab Coat or Apron
☑ Plastic Biohazard Bag
☐ Rigid Biohazard Container

Supplies and Equipment: Sterile sputum specimen container, label and laboratory requisition, PPE (to include gloves, goggles, disposable gown and mask), plastic laboratory specimen bag, biohazard bag, tissues.

Procedure Steps

1. Wash hands.
2. Identify patient and explain procedure.
3. Assemble equipment. Label container with the patient's name, doctor's name, date, and clinic number.
4. Put on PPE, including gloves, goggles, disposable gown, and mask.
   Rationale: To protect the medical assistant from touching, inhaling airborne microorganisms, and/or contaminating the uniform.
5. Instruct patient on proper technique for collection; (1) Cough deeply. (2) Bring up secretions from lungs. (3) Expectorate directly into sterile container. Reinforce that the specimen must come from the lungs and not be brought down from the nose or cleared up from the throat.

Procedure continued on following page

PROCEDURE 19–2 *(continued)*

Rationale: Patient should be scheduled for specimen collection in the morning, preferably before breakfast, to prevent false-positive results from food or drink intake. Taking several deep breaths before coughing may help ability to cough up sputum and not produce

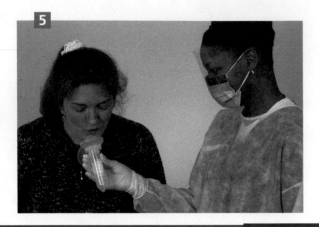

saliva instead. The specimen, which may be tested for specific bacteria such as M. tuberculosis, is placed in a sterile container to prevent contamination with other microorganisms.

6. After the specimen is collected, secure the lid tightly and place the specimen into the plastic laboratory specimen bag.
   Rationale: Specimens of body fluids are transported to the laboratory in securely closed plastic laboratory specimen bags to prevent contact with body fluids.
7. Complete lab request and place in plastic laboratory specimen bag. Close the bag securely.
8. Clean the area and dispose of soiled gloves, tissues, or other supplies in biohazard container.
9. Wash hands.
10. Document in patient record that the specimen was obtained and sent to the laboratory.

Many offices use an oximeter, a device that uses a photoelectric cell attached to a finger or earlobe to measure the oxygen saturation. If the oximeter is attached to a finger, the patient must remove any nail polish.

The device senses the amount of oxygenated and unoxygenated hemoglobin in the blood, calculates the percent of oxygen saturation, and displays the result within seconds. Figure 19–4 shows a pulse oximeter.

To determine if a person is experiencing a disturbance in acid-base balance, in addition to respiratory compromise, a sample of arterial blood can be tested (blood gas analysis). Low levels or excessive levels of carbon dioxide and bicarbonate (HCO_3) can alter the acidity of the blood, causing metabolic problems for the patient.

Blood gases are drawn from an artery. A medical assistant should never attempt to draw an arterial sample of blood without special training because of the possiblity of causing tissue damage or hemorrhage. The sample must be placed on ice and transported to the laboratory immediately for testing, as shown in Figure 19–5. For this reason, the patient is often sent to the facility that will test the blood to have the sample drawn.

GENITOURINARY SYSTEM

The urinary system is made up of three organs: the kidneys, the ureters, and the bladder. Urine travels from each kidney through each of the two ureters to

the bladder, where it is collected to be eliminated from the body. The bladder is considered a sterile cavity that normally does not contain microorganisms. Anatomy of the urinary system and examination of urine is discussed in detail in chapter 24, on urinalysis, as part of the section on the Physician Office Laboratory.

Sometimes it is important to obtain a sterile urine specimen or assist a person who cannot urinate by passing a sterile **catheter** (tube) through the urethra into the bladder. The urethra opens to the outside at

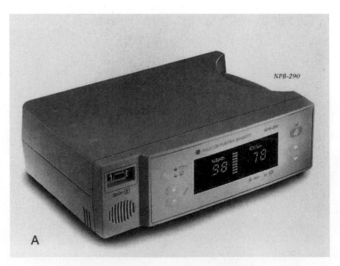

A

➤ Figure 19–4 (A) Pulse oximeter.

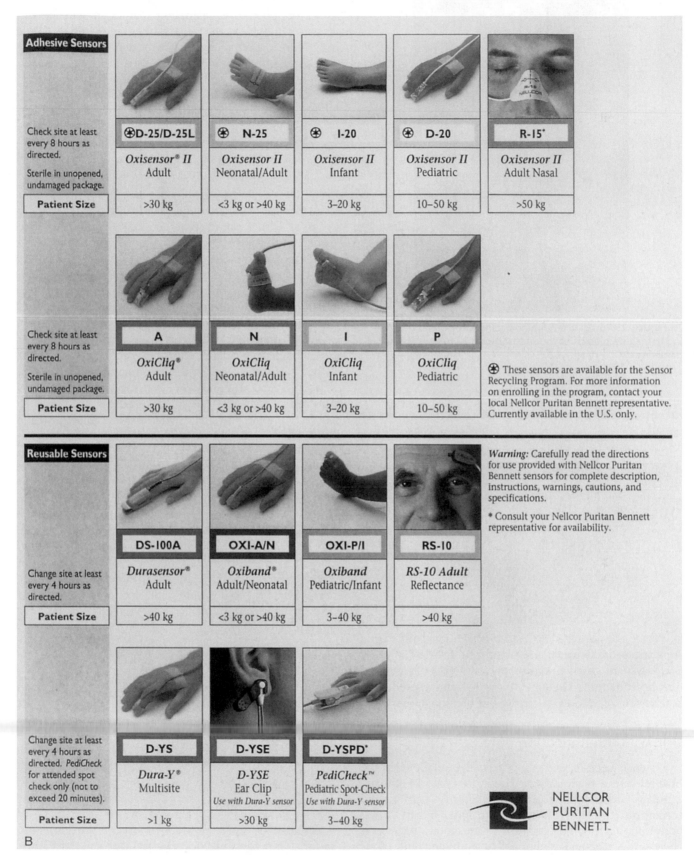

➤ **Figure 19–4** (B) Varied sites of placement of oximeter probe. (Reprinted by permission of Nellcor Puritan Bennett, Inc., Pleasanton, CA)

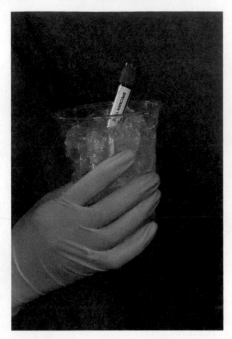

➤ **Figure 19–5** An arterial blood sample for blood gas testing should be placed on ice and transported to the laboratory immediately.

the tip of the penis in males and near the vagina in females.

Problems of the urinary system include:

- Infections, which are usually bacterial and are easily treated
- Kidney stones (**calculi**) are concretions composed of various substances that usually pass through the system but may cause severe pain during passage.
- Obstruction of the urine flow, which can be caused by inflammation of internal organs or prostate disease in men (discussed in detail later)
- Damage to kidney structures, caused by exposure to toxins or poor circulation.

When the kidneys do not function properly, toxic substances build up in the blood and can affect every body system, causing symptoms as diverse as congestive heart failure, swelling of the extremities (edema), severe itching, and even changes in mental status.

Urinary Catheterization

When it becomes necessary to collect urine from the bladder rather than allowing the individual to eliminate it on his or her own, a urinary catheter is used. **Catheterization** (use of a sterile tube to enter a part of the body) should not be used unless absolutely necessary, because of the possibility of introducing infectious agents into the urinary bladder.

The four reasons to use a catheter for urine elimination are:

1. To make sure a sterile urine specimen is obtained for laboratory evaluation. Although females can clean the genital area and urinate into a sterile cup (called a clean-catch midstream urine specimen), there is almost always some contamination from microorganisms in the genital area.
2. To relieve a urinary retention problem.
3. To allow a postoperative or incontinent patient to obtain bladder relief without having to use a bedpan or diapers.
4. To monitor urine production as an indicator of kidney function. Figure 19–6 shows various urinary catheters.

A medical assistant may either be asked to perform or assist with a catheterization. In catheterization, the catheter tube is inserted through the urethra into the bladder. Sterile technique needs to be maintained throughout the catheterization procedure. Introduction of any harmful microorganisms into the catheter can cause a bladder infection and/or invalidate any tests run on the urine specimen.

When removing urine for a specimen or to correct an immediate urinary retention problem, a straight catheter is used and immediately removed after the sample is taken. For females, the French catheter is most often used, size 14 to 20 for adults and size 8 to 10 for children. For males, the coudé catheter, which has a slight upturning on the end, is often used, because it more naturally fits the tract of the urethra up the penis to the bladder. The smaller the patient, the smaller the size of the catheter used.

If the catheter is to be left in place (after prostate surgery or bladder surgery or for a patient with serious medical problems), a Foley or other indwelling catheter is put in place. The indwelling catheter has a small balloon at the end that is blown up to keep it from sliding back out of the bladder into the urethra. Patients who have indwelling catheters for a long period of time may undergo dilation of the urethra and require progressively larger catheters.

Figure 19–7 shows the equipment and supplies needed to insert an indwelling catheter. Procedure 19–3 describes in detail urinary catheterization on a female patient. Catheterization of a male patient is usually done by a doctor, especially for a man over age 50 because of the possibility of causing trauma to the urethra if there is narrowing at the area of the prostate gland.

Diagnosis of Diseases and Conditions of the Reproductive System

Diseases of the reproductive organs are primarily bacterial and viral infections transmitted through sexual contact. These sexually transmitted diseases (**STDs**) include gonorrhea, syphilis, chlamydia, genital herpes, genital warts caused by human papillomavirus, and the

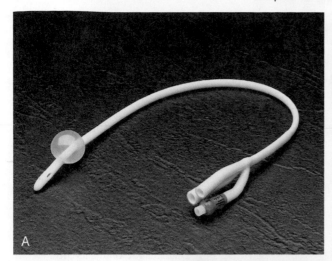

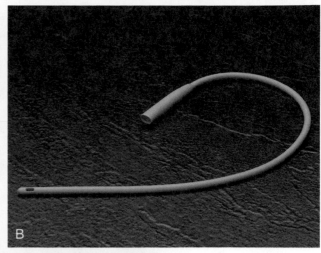

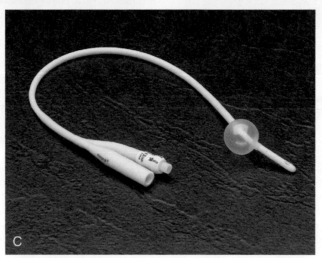

> **Figure 19–6** Urinary catheters come in various sizes and shapes. (Courtesy of Allegiance Healthcare Corporations, McGaw Park, IL)

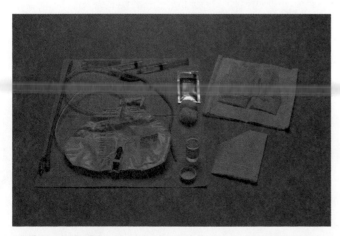

> **Figure 19–7** Equipment needed to insert an indwelling (Foley) catheter.

human immunodeficiency virus, which causes acquired immunodeficiency syndrome.

If a patient has an STD, you must conduct a thorough history of sexual contact and educate the patient about the need to notify all sexual partners about the disease. Some STDs that create clinical symptoms in men are **subclinical** (do not produce symptoms that are noticed by the patient) in women, and vice versa. STDs are usually diagnosed by culture and sensitivity tests of discharge from the vagina or penis, as discussed in chapter 26 on microbiology.

In women, other problems of the reproductive system include menstrual difficulties, such as excessive bleeding and an irregular cycle, and hormonal imbalances.

PROCEDURE 19–3

Performing Urinary Catheterization on a Female

Performance Objective: The student will be able to perform a urinary catheterization on a female patient.

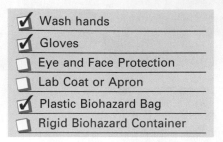

☑ Wash hands
☑ Gloves
☐ Eye and Face Protection
☐ Lab Coat or Apron
☑ Plastic Biohazard Bag
☐ Rigid Biohazard Container

Supplies and Equipment: Sterile, disposable urinary catheterization tray: straight catheter (No. 14 French), sterile drapes, lubricant, sterile gloves, cotton balls, sterile forceps, Betadine or cleansing solution, specimen container with label, biohazard bag.

Procedure Steps

1. Wash hands.
2. Assemble equipment.
3. Identify and explain procedure to patient. Verify allergies to such things as iodine or shellfish.
   Rationale: The most common cleansing solution is Betadine, which contains iodine. If a patient is allergic to Betadine, iodine, or shellfish, choose another antiseptic cleansing solution such as Zephiran (benzalkonium chloride).

4. Place patient in lithotomy or dorsal recumbent position. Pull out the table extension to provide a workspace or position a Mayo stand between the patient's legs.
   Rationale: Either of these positions permits proper access to the urinary meatus.
5. Drape patient to expose the genital area. Position light.
6. Open disposable sterile kit using aseptic technique. Remove drape and, holding by the corners, place on the table extension or Mayo stand to create a sterile field. Holding the fenestrated drape by the corners only, place it over the exposed genital area.
   Rationale: The outer edge of a sterile drape is not considered sterile and can be touched to place the drape.
7. Don sterile gloves and set up the rest of the kit: open Betadine and pour over cotton balls, open lubricant and lubricate approximately 2″ to 3″ of the catheter tip, and place container near the patient for draining urine.
   Rationale: All supplies must be ready for use before one hand becomes contaminated when cleaning urinary meatus.
8. Inform patient of beginning of procedure before touching her.
   Rationale: Patient compliance is essential in this procedure.
9. With nondominant hand, spread the labia as widely as possible to expose the urethra. Using the fingers to spread and then lift the labia will help to locate the urethral meatus.

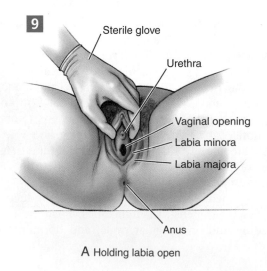

A Holding labia open

(labels: Sterile glove, Urethra, Vaginal opening, Labia minora, Labia majora, Anus)

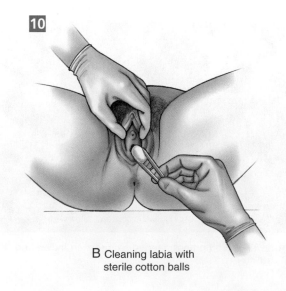

B Cleaning labia with sterile cotton balls

This can be difficult on some women. Once you have spread the labia, do not release your hand and let them fall back until the procedure is complete.

Rationale: You must locate the correct opening; the catheter will become contaminated if placed in the vagina or anus.

10. Pick up one cotton ball saturated with Betadine with the forceps and, using one motion, swipe downward on one side of the labia. Do the same with another cotton ball on the other side, using only a downward motion. Then lastly, down the middle. Discard the used cotton balls as you pick up another. Keep the labia open during this entire procedure. Should the labia be heavily contaminated with mucus, discharge, or blood, additional cotton balls may be necessary to repeat the entire three-step cleansing process. Most kits come with five or six cotton balls.

Rationale: Using only a downward motion will move all the contaminants one direction. The labia must be kept open once you begin to clean to prevent contamination from other parts of the genital area.

11. With dominant hand, pick up lubricated catheter and let patient know you are about to insert catheter.

12. Insert catheter into the urethral opening about 2″ to 3″ until urine begins to flow. Some resistance may be felt as the tip passes through the urinary sphincter. Should resistance be too great, do not attempt to continue. Notify the doctor of problem without alarming the patient.

Rationale: The urethra is normally about 2″ to 3″ long. Once the catheter reaches the bladder, urine will flow. If the urethra is narrowed, it may be difficult to insert the catheter.

13. Let some urine flow into the kit tray and then catch the sterile urine in the specimen collection container. When the specimen container is full, allow the remaining urine to flow into the kit tray.

Rationale: The initial urine flow may contain some Betadine or other contaminants.

14. When urine stops flowing, gently remove the catheter.

15. Secure top on container.

16. Remove and discard all supplies in a biohazard container.

17. Before removing gloves, clean patient and advise that the genital area may be stained yellow for a few days because of the use of Betadine.

18. Place specimen in a plastic laboratory specimen bag.

Rationale: Specimens of body fluids are transported to the laboratory in securely closed plastic laboratory specimen bags to prevent contact between medical and laboratory personnel and body fluids.

19. Complete lab request and place in plastic laboratory specimen bag. Close the bag securely.

20. Remove gloves and dispose of them in biohazard container.

21. Wash hands.

22. Document procedure in patient record, including color and amount of urine removed and the tests for which the specimen was sent.

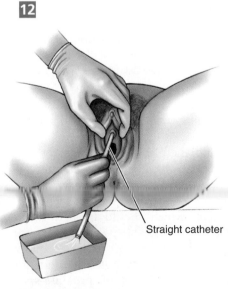

Straight catheter

C Collecting urine from straight catheter

Charting Example	
Date	
11/6/XX	10:15 AM Patient catheterized without difficulty for 240 cc clear yellow urine. Specimen sent to lab for urinalysis, culture, and sensitivity. ————————
	C. Johnson, RMA

In men, other problems of the reproductive system include impotence—the inability to achieve or maintain an erection.

In both men and women, many kinds of neoplasms of the reproductive system, both benign and malignant, may arise.

In men, testicular cancer is uncommon but can occur at any age; the incidence of prostate cancer increases drastically as a man ages. (Diseases of the prostate are discussed in detail later in the chapter.)

In women, ovarian cysts and fibroid tumors of the uterus are common benign conditions. Uterine and cervical cancers are extremely dangerous. Early detection is possibly by thorough examination, including a Pap smear for irregular cells. After an abnormal Pap test, additional tests are needed to locate and biopsy areas of the cervix that may have precancerous or cancerous cells. Some of the follow-up tests are done in the medical office.

Colposcopy

In colposcopy, the doctor uses a stereoscopic instrument called a colposcope to visualize the internal surfaces of the vagina and cervix. Colposcopy is normally performed after an abnormal Pap smear and is used to study collections of abnormal cells or to determine the best place from which to take biopsies. The patient signs a consent form because biopsies will be taken if abnormal areas are found. The procedure is done with the woman in the lithotomy position. Using a sterile speculum, the doctor examines the cervix through a colposcope, an instrument that magnifies the cervix so that tiny lesions can be visualized.

Before colposcopy the medical assistant needs to set up a sterile field containing a sterile vaginal speculum, normal saline, acetic acid (used to clean the cervix), Lugol's solution (used to stain the cervix so that abnormal cells show up white), long cotton-tipped applicators, cervical punch biopsy forceps, and any other instruments requested by the doctor. To the side of the sterile field sterile gloves, several specimen containers, laboratory request forms, a biohazard waste container, and a tray for used instruments should be set up.

If the doctor takes a biopsy specimen, the medical assistant removes the cover of the specimen container and allows the doctor to drop the specimen into it. A separate container is used for each specimen. Each container should be labeled with the date, patient's name, doctor's name, and location from which the specimen was taken. For the cervix, specimens are usually identified as if looking at a clock (e.g., cervical specimen 1 o'clock). A specimen may be obtained by **endocervical curettage** (scraping from within the cervical opening) and placed in a separate container.

Usually little or no bleeding results from colposcopy and cervical or vaginal biopsy. However, a chemical cauterizing agent such as Monsel's solution and sterile packing should be available.

Loop Electrosurgical Excision Procedure and Cryosurgery

Lesions that are larger than the biopsy punch may be removed in the office with an electrical loop that removes the lesion and cauterizes the site simultaneously. In the procedure, called a loop electrosurgical excision procedure **(LEEP)**, the cervix is frozen by applying liquid nitrogen, nitrous oxide, or carbon dioxide gas. This technique (called **cryosurgery**) can also be used alone as a treatment for chronic inflammation of the cervix. After application of the liquid gas, which is as cold as $-40°$ to $-80°C$, the outer cells of the cervix are destroyed. They will slough off and be replaced by new cervical tissue over a period of 4 to 6 weeks.

For a LEEP, a local anesthetic (Xylocaine [lidocaine]) is used. Cryosurgery is often done without anesthetic and may cause discomfort from cramping during and imediately after the procedure.

The patient should be instructed to use sanitary pads to collect the discharge over the next few weeks. Tampons should not be used, to avoid introducing microorganisms into the vagina. The patient usually returns for follow-up after 6 weeks.

Prostate-Specific Antigen Test

Older men commonly have a condition in which the prostate gland becomes enlarged and presses on the urethra, a condition called benign prostatic hypertrophy **(BPH)**. Symptoms of BPH are a reduced urine stream, difficulty urinating, and a feeling of urgency to urinate. If urine retention becomes an issue, part of the prostate can be removed through the urethra under **cystoscopy** (viewing the bladder through the urethra).

Malignant tumors of the prostate also occur with increasing frequency in older men. With the increasing sensitivity of testing technology, prostate cancer is rapidly becoming one of the most common cancers detected in men. Prostate cancer is often a slow-growing cancer, and there is some debate about proper treatment, especially in men diagnosed after age 70.

The most common test used to detect both benign and cancerous conditions of the prostate is a digital rectal exam, which should be performed on all men over age 40 as part of a complete physical examination. Beginning at age 50, it is recommended that as part of their annual physical, men undergo a blood test that measures the level of **prostate-specific antigen (PSA)** in the blood. This protein is usually elevated in men with prostate cancer. However, the PSA test does produce both false-negative and false-positive results, and an elevated PSA should be retested a few weeks later.

If PSA remains elevated, follow-up includes an ultrasound of the pelvis. However, a biopsy of the prostate is necessary to make a definitive diagnosis of prostate cancer.

Sperm Count and Sperm Washing

Counting and "washing" sperm are procedures usually carried out in an obstetrics practice that concentrates on infertility problems and artificial insemination. However, in the primary care setting, a drop of ejaculate may be viewed under a microscope to determine the approximate number of sperm and their **motility** (ability to move), both of which are issues in couples having problems conceiving.

If a couple is having severe difficulty conceiving, artificial insemination, usually with the male partner's sperm but sometimes with donor sperm, is an option that may be pursued.

Both **intracervical insemination,** in which sperm are placed in the cervical canal, and **intrauterine insemination,** in which sperm are placed directly into the uterus, are common office procedures.

If the sperm specimen is obtained from the male partner, he should be instructed to supply it in a sterile container. The specimen should be used or frozen within 30 minutes of being obtained. A frozen specimen, from the male partner or donor, should sit at room temperature for 10 to 15 minutes to liquefy.

Two to three cubic centimeters of semen are drawn up into a 3-cc syringe with an 18-gauge needle, and a drop of the specimen is analyzed under the microscope for number and motility of sperm. Five motile sperm in each microscope grid represents an adequate number of sperm in the specimen.

Intracervical insemination can be performed using an unwashed sperm specimen. But when the sperm count of an untreated specimen is low or the woman's cervical mucus does not support fertility, a sperm sample that has been separated from the semen may be introduced directly into the uterus, a process called intrauterine insemination.

By concentrating the sperm and decreasing the distance that sperm must travel, this method increases chance of fertilization. For this procedure, the sperm is separated from the seminal fluid, then suspended in a small amount of sterile fluid called sperm washing medium. The suspension is injected directly into the uterus through a sterile catheter inserted through the cervical opening. Procedure 19–4 discusses sperm washing in detail.

PROCEDURE 19-4

Performing Sperm Washing

Performance Objective: The student will be able to perform sperm washing techniques to prepare for intrauterine insemination.

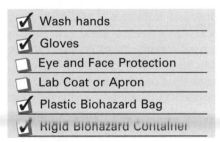

- ☑ Wash hands
- ☑ Gloves
- ☐ Eye and Face Protection
- ☐ Lab Coat or Apron
- ☑ Plastic Biohazard Bag
- ☑ Rigid Biohazard Container

Supplies and Equipment: 3-cc syringes with 18-gauge (18G) needles, microscope, slide marked with squares for counting sperm, centrifuge and tubes (2), incubator, intrauterine catheters, sperm sample in sterile container, sperm washing medium (modified HTF medium with human albumin 5.0 mg/ml), gloves, rigid biohazard container, biohazard bag.

Procedure Steps

1. Wash hands.
2. Using gloves, obtain sperm sample in sterile container within 30 minutes of washing. Allow to stand at room temperature for 10 to 15 minutes to liquefy. If it does not, draw through an 18G needle to thin out sample.
   Rationale: Sample must be liquid to draw up in syringe.
3. Draw 2 to 3 cc of sperm into sterile 3-cc syringe using sterile 18G needle. If sample is greater than 3 cc, use 3 cc for washing. If sample is less than 3 cc, use 2 cc or entire amount of sample for washing. If using frozen vials of donor sperm, use one or two vials, with two being ideal, to wash.
   Rationale: A needle with a large lumen must be used to avoid damaging cells.
4. Place one drop of the sample on a slide marked with boxes for counting sperm and view under the microscope for number of sperm and percent motility. There should be

Procedure continued on following page

PROCEDURE 19–4 *(continued)*

at least 5 sperm per square and the majority of the sperm should be moving forward.
Rationale: If the sample does not contain enough motile sperm, the likelihood of fertilization is decreased. The doctor should decide what to do about a sample with too few sperm or sperm with decreased motility.

5. Place sperm in a centrifuge tube and add sperm washing medium to sample in a 3:1 ratio.
Rationale: This provides the correct dilution of the sperm sample.

6. Gently invert tube three times to mix sample. Do not shake.
Rationale: As with any specimen of body fluid, cells can become damaged or destroyed by forceful handling.

7. Centrifuge specimen at 15,000 RPM for 7 minutes. If no pellet forms after 7 minutes, centrifuge for 2 to 3 additional minutes.
Rationale: After centrifuging, the sperm and other components of semen will clump together as a pellet.

8. Hold tube with pellet facing up. Discard supernatant (liquid in which the pellet is floating), being careful not to disturb pellet. There should be approximately 0.5 cc of supernatant remaining at the bottom of the centrifuge tube.
Rationale: The supernatant contains any impurities.

9. Carefully add 1 cc of fresh sperm washing medium to pellet, letting medium go down side of centrifuge tube, not directly onto pellet.
Rationale: If the fresh washing medium falls directly on the pellet, it may disturb it and disperse the sperm.

10. Allow sample to stand upright in 98.6° incubator for 40 to 50 minutes. During this time the sperm will begin swimming up from the pellet into the supernatant.
Rationale: The sperm will gradually become active at body temperature.

11. Draw up the supernatant into intrauterine catheter, which is attached to a 3-cc syringe. Be sure not to disturb the pellet at this time. If the client is not present at the end of the swim-up period, draw sample into a smaller tube and keep at body temperature.
Rationale: The supernatant contains the washed sperm without other components of semen.

12. Place one drop of the post-washed semen on a slide marked with boxes for counting sperm and view under the microscope for number of sperm and percent motility. There should be at least 5 sperm per square and the majority of the sperm should be moving forward.
Rationale: If the sample does not contain enough motile sperm, the likelihood of fertilization is decreased. The doctor should decide what to do about a sample with too few sperm or sperm with decreased motility.

13. Inform the doctor that the sample is now ready for intrauterine insertion. The doctor will continue the procedure and document.

14. Clean area and dispose of used needles and syringes in a rigid biohazard container. Dispose of other materials contaminated with body fluids in a biohazard container, including gloves after you remove them.

15. Wash hands.

NEUROLOGIC SYSTEM

The neurologic system comprises the brain, spinal cord, and nerves that run throughout the body, carrying sensation from the outside world to the brain for processing and from the brain to the muscles.

Involuntary body activities, such as breathing, circulation, and heart rate, are regulated by the autonomic nervous system, which has two major parts: the sympathetic nervous system and the parasympathetic nervous system. The sympathetic nervous system speeds up and heightens these actions and is responsible for the fight-or-flight response to emergency, which was discussed in chapter 6. The parasympathetic nervous system is responsible for everyday functions such as digestion and elimination and also balances the sympathetic nervous system to bring body systems back to normal function after an emergency is over.

Spinal nerves run out of the spinal cord, emerging through openings between vertebrae. These contain sensory fibers, which receive stimuli from the internal organs and skin, and motor fibers, which carry impulses from the brain to the muscles.

The cranial nerves arise from the bottom of the brain and carry sensory information to the brain from the head and neck region and motor impulses from the brain to specific parts of the head and neck.

Diagnosis of Diseases and Conditions of the Neurologic System

Because the nervous system affects all parts of the body, there are many manifestations of nervous system problems, which can be caused by trauma, infection, tumors, structural defects, or by interference with circulation or bleeding within the brain or spinal column.

Cerebrovascular disease is decreased blood flow to the brain, usually caused by atherosclerosis of the carotid arteries on either side of the neck that carry blood to the brain. The most common symptom of cerebrovascular disease is a cerebrovascular accident, commonly known as a stroke, which occurs when a blood vessel carrying blood in or to the brain either ruptures or becomes totally clogged off. Manifestations of a stroke depend on the region of the brain in which it occurs; they can include loss of speech, weakness or paralysis on one side of the body, or mental confusion.

A cerebral concussion occurs from a traumatic injury to the brain that results from an impact to the head. Concussion occurs frequently in body-contact athletics, such as football or boxing, but can also occur in such noncontact sports as soccer from an athlete heading a ball or baseball from an athlete diving on the ground to catch a ball or sliding into base and banging his or her head on the ground. Symptoms include nausea and vomiting, disturbed vision, and sensitivity to light.

Chronic neurologic diseases include multiple sclerosis and amyotrophic lateral sclerosis.

Multiple sclerosis (MS) is a chronic inflammation and deterioration of the myelin, the protective sheathing around the peripheral nerves. MS is not always progressive and is highly individual. Some people have one or a few periods of crisis, followed by long periods of remission, during which they may recover nearly all function. Other people deteriorate rapidly, becoming totally incapacitated.

MS is more common in women than in men. Onset usually occurs between ages 20 and 40. MS is considered an autoimmune disease, and there is a higher incidence in individuals who have other autoimmune conditions such as Crohn's disease, rheumatoid arthritis, or lupus than in the general population. Treatment is aimed at alleviating symptoms.

Amyotrophic lateral sclerosis, known as Lou Gehrig's disease after the baseball star who died of the disease in the 1940s, is a progressive, always fatal neurologic disease that causes muscle atrophy. It may start as localized muscle weakness, but within a few years the individual has trouble speaking, chewing, and even swallowing. Death usually occurs within 10 years of diagnosis.

Most neurologic diagnosis is conducted by specialists called neurologists. However, primary care doctors do carry out basic neurologic exams on their patients, in which the medical assistant is often asked to assist.

Neurologic Examination

A routine neurologic examination has four parts:

1. Test of mental status
2. Assessment of cranial nerves
3. Test of sensory and motor function
4. Assessment of reflexes.

The doctor may also choose to do or have done by others radiologic and/or electrical tests. A lumbar puncture may also be performed.

Parts of the Neurologic Exam

A test of mental status includes routine questions that help establish alertness, orientation, and the ability to focus. These include the current year, the name of the president of the United States, and counting forward by twos or some other number or backward from 100.

Each cranial nerve is tested individually, because poor function of one or more cranial nerves helps localize areas of pathology within the brain. Testing procedures are shown in Figure 19–8

Testing sensory function is performed by asking the patient to close his or her eyes, then using a brush or pin to gently press or prick the patient, and asking the patient to distinguish between the two sensations.

Motor function is tested in both the upper and lower extremities, looking for equal strength on both sides of the body in major muscle groups. Coordination and balance are tested by having a patient touch the examiner's finger, then his or her own nose, and also by having the patient walk so the examiner can assess the gait to see if there is any swaying, shuffling, or other gait abnormality.

Finally, assessing reflexes is done with a reflex hammer, testing the patella just below the knee, the biceps on the inner upper arm, the triceps on the outer upper arm, and the ankle or Achilles tendon behind the ankle. Reflex response is defined as none, diminished, normal, brisker than normal, or hyperactive (indicated by a repetitive muscle jerking called **clonus** which signals a neurologic problem).

The Medical Assistant's Role

The medical assistant may prepare the patient and equipment for the neurologic exam. During the examination, the medical assistant may hand equipment and supplies to the doctor, and support or assist the patient as needed. Procedure 19–5 describes assisting with the neurologic exam in detail.

Lumbar Puncture

A lumbar puncture (**LP**) is the insertion of a needle into the subarachnoid space at the level of the fourth or fifth lumbar vertebrae (L4 or L5), to remove cerebrospinal fluid (**CSF**). A lumbar puncture is performed to diagnose infection, inflammation, or bleeding problems in the brain.

The spinal cord itself ends at the level of the first or second lumbar vertebrae (L1 or L2). But the meninges,

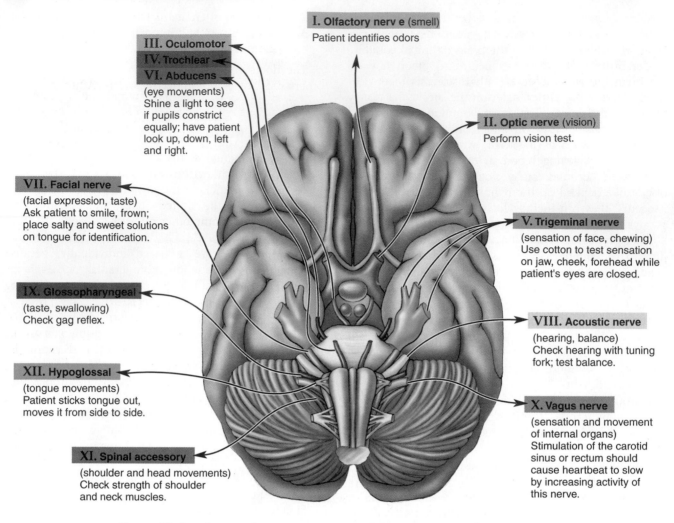

I. Olfactory nerv e (smell)
Patient identifies odors

III. Oculomotor
IV. Trochlear
VI. Abducens
(eye movements)
Shine a light to see
if pupils constrict
equally; have patient
look up, down, left
and right.

II. Optic nerve (vision)
Perform vision test.

VII. Facial nerve
(facial expression, taste)
Ask patient to smile, frown;
place salty and sweet solutions
on tongue for identification.

V. Trigeminal nerve
(sensation of face, chewing)
Use cotton to test sensation
on jaw, cheek, forehead while
patient's eyes are closed.

IX. Glossopharyngeal
(taste, swallowing)
Check gag reflex.

VIII. Acoustic nerve
(hearing, balance)
Check hearing with tuning
fork; test balance.

XII. Hypoglossal
(tongue movements)
Patient sticks tongue out,
moves it from side to side.

X. Vagus nerve
(sensation and movement
of internal organs)
Stimulation of the carotid
sinus or rectum should
cause heartbeat to slow
by increasing activity of
this nerve.

XI. Spinal accessory
(shoulder and head movements)
Check strength of shoulder
and neck muscles.

➢ **Figure 19–8** In the neurologic examination, the function of each cranial nerve is tested.

PROCEDURE 19–5

Assisting with the Neurologic Exam

Performance Objective: The student will be able to assist a doctor with a neurologic screening examination.

Supplies and Equipment: Percussion hammer, safety pin or neurologic pinwheel, cotton ball, tuning fork, tongue blade, flashlight, ophthalmoscope, hot and cold water, odorous substance for smell identification.

Procedure Steps

1. Wash hands.
2. Assemble equipment on tray. Cover.
3. Identify patient, and explain the purpose of the exam and what the doctor will be doing during examination.
   Rationale: Explanation improves patient co-operation.

☑ Wash hands
☐ Gloves
☐ Eye and Face Protection
☐ Lab Coat or Apron
☑ Plastic Biohazard Bag
☐ Rigid Biohazard Container

4. Perform a mental status examination during history taking. Pay particular attention to orientation, memory, coherence and understanding of questioning, awareness, overall behavior, and mood.

   Rationale: Mental status examination is the first part of the neurologic exam.

5. Perform a visual acuity test if applicable.

   Rationale: Assessment of the function of the optic nerve (the second cranial nerve) may be evaluated by a visual acuity test.

6. Assist doctor as needed during exam. This may include handing items to the doctor to test smell (test tube containing ammonia or other odiferous substance), simple touch (cotton ball), interpretation of sensation (safety pin or neurologic pinwheel), vibration and hearing (tuning fork), and/or temperature sensation (test tubes containing hot and cold water).

   Rationale: The neurologic examination tests all twelve cranial nerves, motor ability, and various types of sensation in all extremities.

7. Assist patient as needed during exam.

8. Clean room and equipment after the exam.

9. Wash hands.

10. Document findings in patient record as directed by doctor or as noted during history taking.

the covering of the brain and spinal cord, continue down the spinal canal, covering the roots of the lumbar and sacral spinal nerves. A needle inserted into the lower back, below the end of the spinal cord, cannot accidentally puncture it, which makes the lower back a relatively safe site from which to remove CSF for diagnostic testing, to introduce contrast medium for X-rays of the spinal cord (myelogram), or to introduce medications for spinal anesthesia. Figure 19–9 shows the lower spine and meninges.

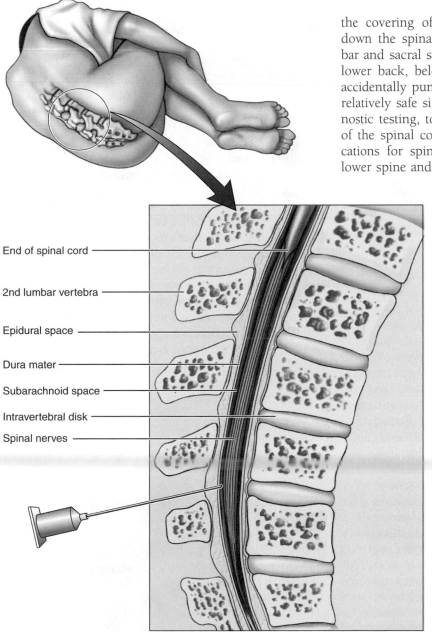

End of spinal cord

2nd lumbar vertebra

Epidural space

Dura mater

Subarachnoid space

Intravertebral disk

Spinal nerves

➢ **Figure 19–9** In a lumbar puncture, the patient's spine is flexed so that the needle can penetrate to the subarachnoid space between the vertebrae at L4 or L5.

Lumbar punctures are more often performed in outpatient clinics or day-surgery centers than in an office setting, because the patient must lie flat for 6 to 12 hours after the procedure to avoid irritation to the brain covering, which can result in a severe headache. If the procedure is performed in the medical office, the medical assistant may help the patient to get into and maintain one of the uncomfortable positions that must be used to perform the LP, either the side-lying, curled position or a supported, forward-bending sitting position. These positions help increase the space between the vertebrae so the needle can be introduced.

Talking to the patient and encouraging slow, deep breathing and other relaxation techniques is a primary role for the medical assistant during the lumbar procedure. The medical assistant is also vital to postprocedure recovery, because the patient may require intravenous fluids and pain medication to alleviate the severe headache sometimes experienced.

Procedure 19–6 describes the steps to an LP in detail.

PROCEDURE 19–6

Assisting with Lumbar Puncture

Performance Objective: The student will be able to assist with a lumbar puncture.

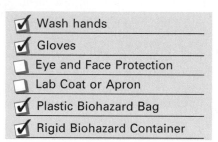

☑ Wash hands
☑ Gloves
☐ Eye and Face Protection
☐ Lab Coat or Apron
☑ Plastic Biohazard Bag
☑ Rigid Biohazard Container

Supplies and Equipment: Local anesthetic (lidocaine 1% to 2%), disposable sterile lumbar puncture tray (includes: povidone iodine swab sticks or other antiseptic, 3-cc syringe with 25-gauge (25G), 5/8″ needle, specimen vials [3 or 4] with tops, 3 1/2″ spinal needle with stylet [a slender metal rod that fits within the needle], sterile gloves, drape, stopcock, and manometer, exam light, labels for specimen vials, plastic laboratory specimen bag, lab requisition, biohazard bag, and rigid biohazard container.

Procedure Steps

1. Wash hands.
2. Identify patient and explain procedure. Verify signed consent form. Verify that the patient has an empty bladder.
   Rationale: Patient will be placed in a position with knees drawn up to chest for procedure, so bladder and bowels should be emptied before beginning procedure.

3. Assemble equipment and instruct the patient to remove clothing and put on a gown with the opening in the back. Place a Mayo stand or other clear surface to hold the lumbar puncture tray.
   Rationale: The back must be visible and accessible to perform the procedure.
4. Position patient on the side with knees drawn up to abdomen, grasping knees and flexing chin on chest. Place an absorbent pad under the patient's buttocks. Cover with a drape until the doctor is ready to begin the procedure.
   Rationale: Help the patient understand that this position allows for easier insertion into the proper space because this position widens the space between the lumbar vertebrae. The patient in the illustration is clothed to illustrate the position without embarrassment.
5. Reassure the patient while the doctor opens the tray, and prepares for the procedure. Re-

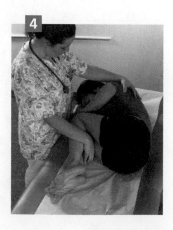

move the unsterile drape so that the doctor can clean the area with the povidone swab sticks and place the fenestrated drape.
Rationale: Because a sterile body cavity will be penetrated, the area is prepared as if for surgery and sterile technique is maintained by the doctor.

6. The doctor will put on sterile gloves. Clean the stopper of the vial of local anesthetic with an alcohol swab, invert the bottle, and hold for the doctor to draw up.
Rationale: The doctor must maintain sterile technique from this point until the procedure is finished.

7. Inform the patient that the doctor will inject a local anesthetic to minimize discomfort during the actual procedure.

8. Assist patient to maintain position by grabbing the knees while the doctor performs the actual lumbar puncture. Remind the patient to breathe normally, and not to hold the breath or talk while the needle is being inserted.
Rationale: The insertion of the spinal needle into the subarachnoid space and verification of placement requires the vertebrae to be separated as much as possible. Motion by the patient might prevent proper placement of the needle.

9. Encourage the patient to maintain the position while the doctor attaches the stopcock and manometer, measures the pressure of the spinal fluid, and collects specimens.
Rationale: Motion by the patient might dislodge the needle.

10. When the doctor directs, assist the patient to straighten legs and apply Band-Aid to site. Assist the patient to rest in a prone position for 2 to 3 hours.
Rationale: Resting in a prone position may help prevent a spinal headache by minimizing leakage of cerebrospinal fluid from the puncture site.

11. Fill out laboratory requisition and labels. Put on nonsterile gloves and apply labels to the specimen tubes, place tubes and requisition into a plastic laboratory specimen bag, and close bag securely.
Rationale: Specimen containers may have body fluids on the outside of the container.

12. Clean up area and dispose of used supplies. Be sure that the needle and syringe used for the local anesthetic and the spinal needle and stylet have been placed in a rigid biohazard container. Remove gloves and place in biohazard container.

13. Wash hands.

14. Document procedure in patient record. Note that specimens are being sent to the laboratory. Describe the patient's condition and instructions given to the patient.

Charting Example	
Date	
6/4/XX	11:00 AM Lumbar puncture performed by Dr. Hughes. 20 cc of CSF sent to lab. Patient instructed to remain prone for 2 hours in exam room. Patient instructed to lie down for at least 12 hours at home and to notify the office if there is fluid leakage at the puncture site. Instructed by Dr. Hughes to take acetaminophen if headache develops. ———— ———— S. Williams, CMA

STUDENT STUDY PLAN

To reinforce your understanding of the material in this chapter . . .

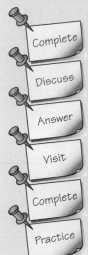

Complete the **Review & Recall** questions.

Discuss the situation in **If You Were the Medical Assistant** with your classmates, and answer the questions.

Answer the **Critical Thinking Questions** and discuss them with your classmates.

Visit **Web sites** listed below and search for additional web sites using the **Keywords for Internet Searches.**

Complete the exercises in chapter 19 of the **Student Mastery Manual.**

Practice spirometry testing activities in Case II (Raymond Johnson) on the **CD-ROM.**

 REVIEW & RECALL

1. Describe two ways that the level of oxygen in the blood can be measured.

2. Discuss how the amount of air a person can breathe in and out of the lungs can affect the levels of carbon dioxide and oxygen in the blood.

3. What personal protective equipment should the medical assistant use when collecting a sputum specimen?

4. What are four reasons for performing urinary catheterization? Describe the procedure.

5. Identify and describe three diagnostic procedures for identifying cancer of the reproductive system in males and females.

6. Describe the process for assessing that a semen specimen contains an adequate number of motile sperm and for preparing the sample for intrauterine insemination.

7. Describe the four parts of the neurologic exam. How does the medical assistant assist with the exam?

8. Describe the role of the medical assistant when assisting with a lumbar puncture.

 IF YOU WERE THE MEDICAL ASSISTANT

Both colposcopy and a lumbar puncture are sterile procedures. Describe how you would set up for each procedure, how you would prepare the patient, and what you might have to do to assist the doctor. Describe the care of each patient after the procedure. What kinds of specimens might be obtained, and what would you do with them?

CRITICAL THINKING QUESTIONS

1. Discuss the reasons that spirometric testing is repeated at least three times. What factors could result in test results that do not reflect the patient's actual breathing capacity?

2. Pulse oximetry has become a common diagnostic test in the medical office and in the hospital in the past 5 years. What makes this test so useful that doctors are willing to spend over $500 to buy the equipment to perform it?

3. Discuss why it is important to use good sterile technique when performing urinary catheterization.

4. Compare and contrast artificial insemination using intracervical and intrauterine methods. What are the advantages and disadvantages of each method?

5. When the doctor performs a lumbar puncture, blood may appear in the cerebrospinal fluid. Do research to find out why it is important to know whether the blood entered the fluid during the procedure itself or was already present.

EXPLORE THE WEB

INTERNET WEB SITES

American Cancer Society
www.cancer.org

American Lung Association
www.lungusa.org

Prostate Cancer Research Institute
www.prostate-cancer.org

Fertility treatment resource
www.fertilitext.org

American Society for Colposcopy and Cervical Pathology
www.asccp.org

National Institute of Allergy & Infectious Diseases
www.niaid.nih.gov

Virtual Hospital
www.vh.org

KEYWORDS FOR INTERNET SEARCHES

asthma
    colposcopy
    lumbar puncture
    pulmonary medicine
    pulse oximetry
    urinary catheterization

ANSWERS TO ON THE JOB

1. When a person has asthma, certain trigger factors (including exposure to allergens, changes in temperature, and exercise) cause the airways to constrict. During severe attacks the person has extreme difficulty breathing; during milder attacks the person wheezes and becomes short of breath. Treatment of asthma focuses on avoiding allergens and using medication to dilate the bronchioles and decrease the inflammatory response. Many individuals return to normal breathing between attacks, but the airways of other individuals remain somewhat constricted and inflamed, leading to chronic bronchitis.

2. Although the lungs can hold more air when a person is standing, the forceful blowing required for spirometry can make a person dizzy or light-headed. For safety reasons, most spirometers are calibrated to measure lung volumes of a person in the sitting position.

3. Sandra should tell Mary to take as deep a breath as possible, place her lips around the mouthpiece, and blow the breath out as quickly and as forcefully as possible.

4. When Mary starts to blow out, Sandra can tell her to blow as fast as possible and encourage her to keep blowing. Between attempts, Sandra can tell Mary that she is doing a great job but may be able to do even better on the next try.

5. Sandra should give Mary time to catch her breath and resume normal breathing before repeating the test.

6. The goal is to obtain the best possible results for the patients. Most patients improve their performance after the first attempt because they understand more clearly what the test is trying to achieve. Performance tends to decline after three attempts because the patient may become fatigued.

Chapter 20

Diagnostic Imaging

Instructional Objectives

After completing this chapter, you will be able to do the following:

1. Define and spell the vocabulary words for this chapter.

2. Explain the role of the medical assistant related to diagnostic imaging.

3. Describe safety precautions when x-rays are used.

4. Describe the use of various diagnostic imaging modalities, including x-rays, CT scan, nuclear medicine, MRI, PET, and ultrasound.

5. Describe the responsibility of the medical assistant when preparing a patient for x-ray studies of the gastrointestinal tract.

6. Explain the role of the medical assistant in diagnostic procedures of the urinary tract and male reproductive system.

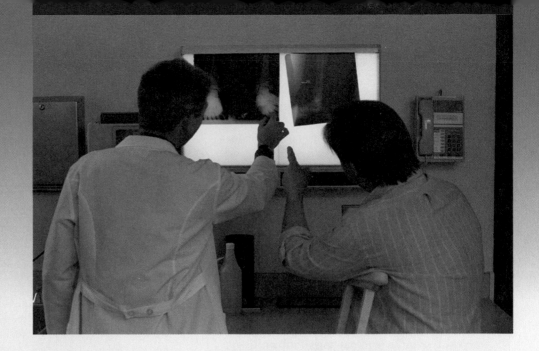

- Prepare patients for examinations, procedures, and treatments
- Assist with examinations, procedures, and treatments

- Practice within the scope of education, training, and personal capabilities
- Document accurately
- Instruct individuals according to their needs

VOCABULARY

aneurysm (p. 447)
angiography (p. 447)
anteroposterior projection
  (p. 441)
arteriogram (p. 447)
contrast medium (p. 441)
dosimetry (p. 442)
fluoroscope (p. 441)

fluoroscopy (p. 441)
intravenous pyelogram
  (p. 446)
lateral projection (p. 441)
magnetic resonance imaging
  (p. 449)
mammography (p. 446)
oblique projection (p. 441)

positron emission tomography
  (p. 449)
posteroanterior projection
  (p. 441)
radiograph (p. 440)
radiologist (p. 440)
single-photon emission computed
  tomography (p. 449)

tomograph (p. 448)
transducer (p. 449)
ultrasound (p. 449)
venogram (p. 447)

ABBREVIATIONS

AP (p. 441)
CAT (p. 448)

CT (p. 448)
IVP (p. 446)

KUB (p. 441)
lat (p. 441)

MRI (p. 449)
NPO (p. 445)

PA (p. 441)
PET (p. 449)

SPECT (p. 449)

DIAGNOSTIC RADIOLOGY

Diagnostic radiology allows a radiologist (a doctor who specializes in interpreting diagnostic radiology studies) to obtain a view of internal structures and organs.

The discovery of the x-ray in the late 19th century by Wilhelm Roentgen (1845–1923) changed medicine possibly more than any other scientific discovery; for the first time structures within the body could be visualized by noninvasive techniques.

Internists, pediatricians, and family practice doctors do not always have their own x-ray equipment and send patients in need of x-ray studies to radiology offices or hospital emergency rooms. However, x-ray facilities are usually found in larger clinics, as well as in the offices of some specialists such as orthopedic surgeons, podiatrists, and chiropractors. Also, in rural practices where the nearest hospital may be an hour or more away, there is usually at least a mobile x-ray machine used to take x-rays in the case of injuries, so patients do not have to go to the hospital emergency room.

Radiographs and X-ray Equipment

X-rays cannot be seen, felt, tasted, or smelled. They are high-energy electromagnetic impulses that travel at the speed of light. X-rays penetrate soft tissue easily and bone less easily. Figure 20–1 shows x-ray equipment. An x-ray, or radiograph, is produced by projecting x-rays from the machine's tube through the body and onto photographic film placed behind the body. When the film is processed, an x-ray image becomes visible, such as the one seen in Figure 20–2.

Because x-rays are absorbed by bone more than soft tissue, the bones show up as white images on the film.

Where the x-rays pass through the body, they strike the film, causing it to turn dark gray or black. Breaks or fractures in the bone can be seen clearly.

Depending on the part of the body to be examined, the x-ray technician helps the patient into a particular position, and adjusts the machine to direct the x-rays at a particular part of the body. Usually at least two images are made, at 90-degree angles to one another. The patient may be lying down or standing. The doctor specifies the path of the x-rays through the body.

Among the most common terms dealing with x-ray studies are:

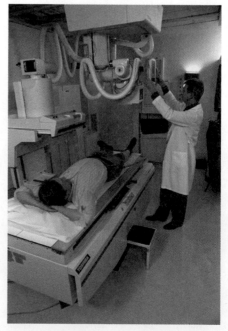

➤ **Figure 20–1** X-ray equipment.

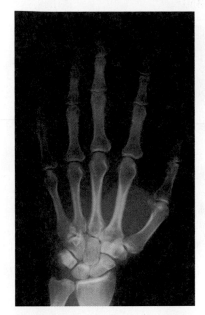

> ➤ **Figure 20–2** In an x-ray film of the hand the bones appear white. There appear to be spaces between the bones because the cartilage that cushions the ends of the bones does not absorb x-rays and therefore appears dark.

anteroposterior (AP) projection—The x-ray beam passes through the patient from front to back before striking the film.

posteroanterior (PA) projection—The x-ray beam passes through the patient from back to front before striking the film.

lateral (lat) projection—The x-ray beam passes through the patient from one side to the other before striking the film. The doctor may specify which side is positioned next to the film (e.g., for a right lateral projection, the right side is positioned next to the film).

oblique projection—The x-ray beam passes through the patient at an angle to the body part being studied. The doctor may specify which side of the body is close to the film and whether the x-ray beam should pass from front to back or back to front.

X-ray studies of particular organs are usually done with the patient in a standard position. For a chest x-ray the patient usually stands, whereas for an abdominal x-ray, also called a **KUB** (kidneys, ureters, bladder), the patient lies in the supine position. The standard position is used unless the doctor specifies something different on the x-ray requisition. The patient's right or left side is labeled on the x-ray using letters made of lead, which are placed between the patient and the film. Figure 20–3 shows a number of common positions used for x-rays.

Contrast Media and Fluoroscopy

Internal organs of the gastrointestinal (GI) tract and urinary tract show up in less detail than do bones. To produce more sharply focused x-ray films of internal organs, it is necessary to use a **contrast medium,** a substance that absorbs x-rays and highlights a specific organ.

For GI studies, the most common contrast medium is barium, an inert element the body does not absorb. Barium is introduced into the gastrointestinal tract either by having the patient drink liquid barium (for x-ray studies of the esophagus, stomach, and small intestine) or by administering an enema (for x-ray studies of the colon). Barium should never be given to a patient who may have a perforation of any GI organ; if barium enters the abdomen, it will not be absorbed and must be removed surgically.

Another common contrast medium is iodine, which may be taken by mouth several hours before the test, as for gallbladder studies, or injected either before or during the test. When iodine is used as a contrast medium, the patient should be questioned regarding allergy to iodine or shellfish (a food source high in iodine) before the test because some people may experience severe allergic reactions.

Because it is often important to observe the organs in motion, contrast media studies are usually done under continuous low-dose x-ray called **fluoroscopy,** using a special x-ray machine called a **fluoroscope.**

The patient is placed between the x-ray tube and screen, as with a conventional x-ray. However, in addition to simply taking moment-in-time static x-ray films, the radiologist uses a fluoroscope to view a real-time image of internal organs in motion. The radiologist can watch on a television screen and use a still camera to take moment-in-time x-ray films at certain points to highlight aspects of the patient's system.

Protection from Hazards of Radiation

Radiation is a general term for energy emitted into space in all directions. Ionizing radiation is the type of energy produced when atoms change from one form to another and emit rays, or particles, from the nucleus.

Substances that emit radiant energy because their atoms are constantly changing are called radioactive. Normally, this energy travels out from the source in all directions. Because radiation cannot pass through lead, this substance is used in the x-ray tube to contain the radiation at all times unless an image is being produced and to direct the x-ray beam during the imaging process. The room containing the x-ray machine contains lead within the walls and windows, to prevent radiation from leaking into the rest of the building.

Both the person performing the x-ray procedure and the patient need to have protection against excessive radiation or radiation reaching parts of the body to

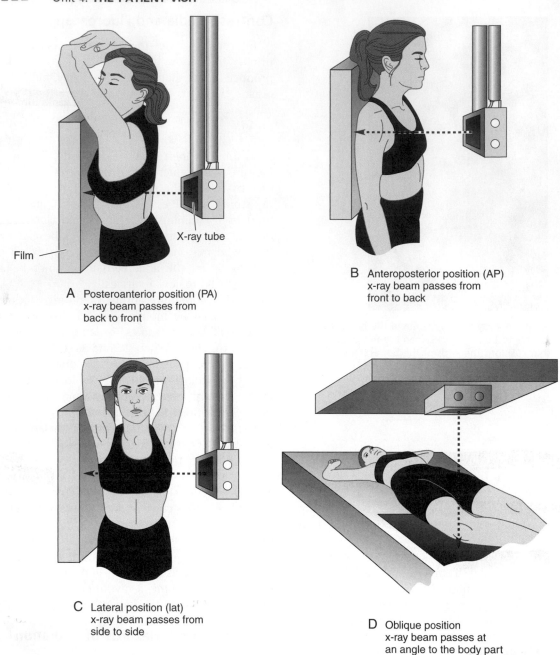

A Posteroanterior position (PA)
x-ray beam passes from
back to front

Film

X-ray tube

B Anteroposterior position (AP)
x-ray beam passes from
front to back

C Lateral position (lat)
x-ray beam passes from
side to side

D Oblique position
x-ray beam passes at
an angle to the body part

➤ **Figure 20–3** Positions used for x-ray studies.

which it is a danger, such as the reproductive organs and the thyroid.

Figure 20–4 shows some of the protective equipment the radiology technician or medical assistant wears; this includes gloves, a lead apron that reaches below the waist to protect the internal organs of the trunk and the reproductive organs of both women and men, goggles, and a leaded neck protector to shield the thyroid.

The x-ray technician or medical assistant takes additional precautions against excessive radiation exposure.

He or she stays as far away from the x-rays as possible, stepping out of the room or behind a lead-lined barrier while the x-ray machine is actually taking the image; ensuring proper working conditions of the machine to make sure it is not throwing off excess radiation; and, if a child is to have an x-ray, asking a parent to wear a lead apron and hold a young child still rather than doing it himself or herself.

X-ray technicians who work taking x-rays all day also practice **dosimetry**, the monitoring of the area and/or their own body to see how much radiation they

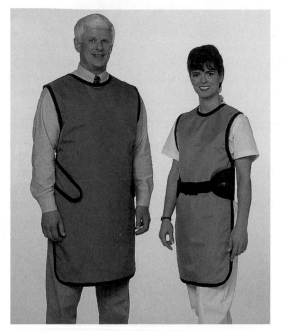

> Figure 20–4 Protective apron for x-ray treatment. (Courtesy of Bar Ray Products, Littlestown, PA)

have been cumulatively exposed to over a period of time. A piece of x-ray film is placed in a holder and either left in the x-ray room (area monitoring) or worn by the personnel taking x-rays (individual monitoring). Every month, the film is replaced and the sample from the holder is sent for processing to determine the amount of radiation it was exposed to. Records are kept to be sure that radiation emitted by the equipment remains below a hazardous level. Figure 20–5 shows a personal dosimeter.

Patients are also provided with a lead shield that protects the reproductive organs if the x-ray is of the trunk and a full-trunk apron if the x-ray is of an arm or leg. Patients should be exposed to the minimum amount of x-ray radiation possible consistent with a complete diagnostic evaluation.

Radiation during pregnancy is not considered safe and is used with extreme caution. Routine x-ray studies are not done for a patient who is or could be pregnant. All women of childbearing age should schedule x-ray studies during the first 10 days of the beginning of the menstrual period, if possible, and they should be asked each time an x-ray study is done whether there is any possibility of pregnancy. X-rays are most dangerous to the developing fetus during the first 6 weeks of gestation, the time when the woman is least likely to know that she is pregnant. Miscarriage or birth defects could be caused by the radiation.

Processing and Storage of X-ray Films

Most x-rays today are processed in automated processing equipment to ensure standard quality, which has greatly reduced the degree of human error. The patient is usually asked to wait until the exposures have been developed before dressing in case one or more x-ray films needs to be repeated, but modern processing methods have reduced the number of poor exposures.

The film used for x-rays must be stored in a cool, dry place where it is protected from moisture and light. Usually it remains in a sealed package until used. The cassettes used to hold film when x-rays are taken must be loaded with film in a darkroom.

X-ray films must be stored in a cool, dry environment. Sleeves of different sizes are used to store them. Medical assistants are often responsible for proper record keeping and filing of x-ray films. Sometimes all of a patient's x-ray films—or at least all studies of the same part of the body—are stored in a single sleeve, because comparison to previous films is often an essential part of the process of diagnosis.

The x-ray films themselves belong to the facility that produces them, but x-ray reports are sent to the referring doctor. X-ray films are also sometimes loaned to the patient for visits to a consulting doctor; patients can usually receive copies of original x-ray films by paying a fee to cover the costs of duplication.

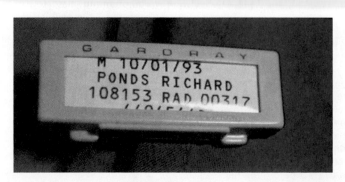

> Figure 20–5 A personal dosimeter worn to measure exposure to radiation. (From Zakus SM: *Clinical Procedures for Medical Assistants,* 3rd ed. St. Louis: Mosby, 1988.)

X-ray Studies of the Gastrointestinal System

The GI system is made up of a series of hollow tubelike muscles running from the mouth to the anus, as well as ancillary organs. The GI system's main purpose is to digest food, absorb nutrients from the food, and eliminate the nonnutritive and undigestible food elements as solid waste. Each of the GI tract's components—the mouth, esophagus, small intestine, large intestine (colon), rectum, and anus—is made up of the same sort of smooth muscular tissue and is governed by the autonomic nervous system, which gives it the ability to move slowly in some locations and more rapidly in other locations through an automatic muscle contraction known as peristalsis.

The three accessory organs to the GI system are the liver, the pancreas, and the gallbladder. The liver produces bile, which assists in breaking down fats. The pancreas produces many of the enzymes that break down the other food components—carbohydrates and protein. The gallbladder stores bile that is helpful but not necessary to break down a normally fatty meal.

Preparing Patients for Diagnostic X-ray Studies

X-ray studies of the gastrointestinal system are done in a hospital or sophisticated radiology center, under fluoroscopy. A radiologist performs the test with the help of a radiological technologist.

The radiologist observes the patient under continuous x-ray, decides when to expose images for a permanent record, interprets the findings, and sends a report to the patient's primary care doctor or gastroenterologist.

Because the tests are often scheduled from the doctor's office, the medical assistant must be able to instruct the patient in the proper preparation for the test. The office usually obtains preparation instructions from the x-ray department to give to the patient when the examination is scheduled. Chapter 32 gives specific information about instructing patients for diagnostic tests. See Table 20–1 for a summary of x-ray studies of the GI tract.

Upper GI Series (Barium Swallow)

Patients with problems of the upper GI tract, such as difficulty swallowing, epigastric pain, and continuous heartburn, and patients with known Crohn's disease suffering from more right lower quadrant pain than usual are often scheduled for an upper GI series, also known as a barium swallow.

Barium sulfate is used as the contrast medium for this test and is swallowed in a thick drink, usually

Table 20–1	X-ray Examinations of the Gastrointestinal Tract			
Test	**Purpose**	**Preparation**	**Instructions**
Upper GI series (barium swallow), sometimes with small-bowel follow-through	To visualize the esophagus, stomach, duodenum, and sometimes the small intestine. The patient swallows a flavored drink containing barium.	■ Light evening meal the day before the test ■ NPO after midnight	■ Schedule after barium enema or cholecystogram ■ Increased fluids and possibly milk of magnesia after the test to help evacuate barium
Barium enema (lower GI)	To visualize the colon by introducing barium through the rectum. The patient retains the enema while placed into various positions for x-rays. Air may be pumped into the colon.	■ Clear liquid diet the day before the test with regular fluids ■ Laxative(s) to empty the GI tract the evening before the test ■ NPO after midnight ■ Enema(s) to empty the lower colon and rectum the morning of the test	■ Increased fluids and possibly milk of magnesia after the test to help evacuate barium
Cholecystogram	To visualize the gallbladder and gallstones, if present	■ Fat-free evening meal the day before the test ■ Take all tablets prescribed by doctor the night before the test with 8 oz of water ■ NPO after taking the tablets, which contain contrast medium ■ Sometimes instructed to use laxative(s) and/or enemas to empty the GI tract before the test	■ Preparation may have to be repeated if the gallbladder cannot be seen ■ After initial films are finished, may be instructed to eat a fatty meal and return for additional X-rays
Intravenous cholangiogram	To visualize the gallbladder and biliary ducts after administration of intravenous contrast medium	■ NPO after midnight ■ Sometimes instructed to use laxative(s) and/or enemas to empty the GI tract before the test	■ Test may take several hours

flavored to make it more palatable. The individual must be **NPO** (no food or liquid taken by mouth) the night before the test so there is nothing in the stomach during the test.

After this test (and any other test using barium) the individual is instructed to increase fluid intake, and may be told to use a mild laxative, such as 2 table-spoons of milk of magnesia, to be sure that the barium passes through the digestive tract. Barium may turn the stool a whitish color for a few days until it is expelled. The test usually takes about 30 minutes, but it may take longer if the small intestines are also being examined, because the barium must flow all the way through the small intestine.

Barium Enema

The second barium study used for GI diagnosis is the barium enema, used to visualize the lower GI tract (the large intestine and lower portion of the small intestine). The colon may be examined directly by sigmoidoscopy and/or colonoscopy, as discussed in chapter 16. However, an x-ray study is often used because it can visualize the entire colon.

For the barium enema, also called a lower GI study, barium is delivered via an enema tube placed in the rectum. While the patient holds the enema in, he or she is placed into various positions to fill the colon. Air may also be pumped in to expand the large intestine and give the radiologist a better view of any constrictions or growths.

A barium enema is one of the most effective screening tests for early-stage colon cancer. Figure 20–6 shows results of a barium enema x-ray study.

Gallbladder Studies

The gallbladder stores bile, a fluid produced by the liver, which contains bilirubin, bile salts, and lipids. After a fatty meal, the gallbladder contracts, ejecting bile into the small intestine, where it helps break down fats for digestion.

Inflammation of the gallbladder is often caused by gallstones, which form when the bile salts precipitate out of solution, becoming hard, solid masses. An indi-

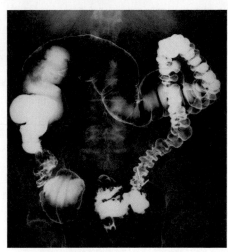

➤ **Figure 20–6** In the barium enema the entire colon shows up white because of the barium.

vidual with inflammation of the gallbladder usually experiences pain in the upper right part of the abdomen, which may radiate to the right back and shoulder blade. The doctor usually orders a cholecystogram, or ultrasound of the gallbladder, to evaluate this type of pain. Contrast material for the cholecystogram contains iodine and is taken by mouth the night before the test. Additional studies can be done of the bile ducts using an iodine contrast medium injected intravenously or directly into the bile ducts.

X-ray Studies of the Urinary System

The urinary system is made up of the kidneys, the ureters, and the bladder. The kidneys excrete urea, a waste product, from the body. Urine is formed when these wastes are mixed in some of the water that collects in the kidneys. Kidneys also help to maintain the acid-base balance in the body's fluids.

Urine travels from each kidney through each of the two ureters to the bladder, where it is collected to be eliminated from the body. The structure and function of the urinary system is discussed in detail in chapter 24.

ON THE JOB

Kathy Anderson, a medical assistant for Blackburn Primary Care Associates, has been asked to schedule a barium enema for Angela White, a 45-year-old female patient of Dr. Lawler. She calls the radiology department of Memorial Hospital and schedules the exam, but she cannot find the information sheet about the examination to give to Mrs. White. The receptionist tells her that another medical assistant gave the last one to a patient yesterday. What should Kathy do and why?

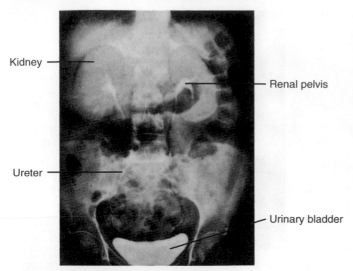

Kidney

Renal pelvis

Ureter

Urinary bladder

➤ **Figure 20–7** Intravenous pyelogram (IVP). (From Thibodeau GA, Patton KT: *The Human Body in Health and Disease.* St. Louis: Mosby, 1992.)

Several types of X-ray studies are used to give information about the urinary system. The most common is an **intravenous pyelogram (IVP),** which shows the kidneys, ureters, and bladder, using a contrast medium that has been administered to the patient by injection. Figure 20–7 shows an intravenous pyelogram.

To visualize the urinary system clearly, the examiner must be sure that the GI tract is empty. The medical assistant must therefore provide the patient with bowel preparation instructions similar to those for a barium enema. The patient must be NPO after midnight but

may be able to have a liquid breakfast if the test is scheduled for the late morning (depending on the particular procedures used by the radiology department conducting the test).

Iodine is usually used as the contrast medium for this test. The patient must be questioned about allergy to iodine or shellfish. In addition, the patient should be told that he or she may experience a flushing sensation or a metallic taste in the mouth after the injection. The contrast medium may also be introduced directly into the bladder through a catheter inserted into the bladder through the urethra. This test is called a retrograde pyelogram and requires the same preparation as the IVP. Because of the possibility of introducing infection into the bladder, this test is usually only used for patients known to have decreased kidney function.

Mammography

Mammography is a specialized form of X-ray study used to detect abnormal masses in the female breast tissue. Equipment is used to compress the breast tissue to a more uniform thickness to aid in diagnostic imaging. Mammography is a highly effective tool in early detection of breast cancer, making it possible to visualize collections of abnormal cells far earlier than they can be felt in manual examination by a doctor or in manual self-examination.

It is recommended that women have a baseline mammogram at age 40, a biannual mammogram from

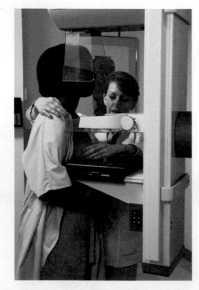

➤ **Figure 20–8** During a mammogram, each breast is compressed and flattened while an x-ray image is made.

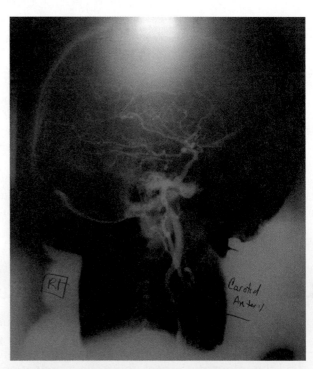

➤ **Figure 20–9** Cerebral angiogram. (From Kinn ME, Woods M: *The Medical Assistant: Administrative and Clinical,* 8th ed. Philadelphia: W.B. Saunders, 1999.)

ages 40 to 50, and an annual mammogram after age 50.

The examination is done by radiologic technologists who are certified in mammography to ensure high-quality studies that will show any abnormalities of the breasts. The patient should be told not to wear any deodorant or powder on the day of the test, because they may contain small amounts of metal that interfere with the x-ray. Although the test is somewhat uncomfortable, women should be reminded of the greatly improved prognosis for breast cancer when lesions are discovered before metastasis. Figure 20–8 shows a woman having a mammogram.

Angiography

Angiography uses iodine as a contrast medium to study whether abnormalities or narrowing of blood vessels are present in various parts of the body. When the contrast medium is injected into an artery, the test may be called an **arteriogram;** when injected into a vein the test may be called a **venogram**.

To introduce the contrast medium, a catheter is inserted into the blood vessel. During this type of test, a blood clot can be dislodged, causing a stroke or heart attack. The patient is usually given medication to reduce pain and promote relaxation. But because serious complications can occur, he or she must remain awake so that the patient's level of pain and mental status can be evaluated.

The patient needs to receive instruction and sign a consent form before any angiogram because this is considered an invasive procedure. Two common sites for angiography are the brain and the heart. Figure 20–9 shows a cerebral angiogram, used to identify the blood vessels flowing to the brain. These studies may show tumors, **aneurysms** (enlarged arteries due to weakness in the artery wall), shifts of the midline, and other abnormalities.

FOCUS ON
PROFESSIONALISM

WHO CAN TAKE X-RAYS?

In 1981, Congress adopted the Consumer-Patient Radiation Health and Safety Act, which directs states to develop minimum standards for state certification and licensure of personnel who perform radiologic procedures. State legislation was supposed to set minimum requirements for training and proficiency to achieve certification.

However, the act had no enforcement mechanism, and by the year 2000 only 35 states had created legislation to limit the performance of diagnostic radiology to certified/licensed radiographers. Even fewer states had passed specific legislation regarding the performance of therapeutic radiation and nuclear medicine imaging. Medical assistants had formerly performed many radiologic procedures and continue to do so in those states without specific legislation requiring certification/licensure.

In 1999, an organization, The Alliance for Quality Medical Imaging and Radiation Therapy, made up of 10 organizations that represent more than 200,000 professionals in the fields of radiography, nuclear medicine, magnetic resonance, radiation therapy, medical dosimetry, and other specialty areas, began lobbying Congress to pass legislation strengthening the Consumer-Patient Radiation Health and Safety Act of 1981. The organization wants federal standards for education and proficiency, and to add enforcement mechanisms to the 1981 act.

The group is hoping to use grass-roots activism by professionals and patients to move Congress to act, taking as its model the 1992 approval of the Mammography Quality Standards Act, the first time the federal government had ever established uniform standards for a radiologic procedure and identified minimum qualifications for those who perform and interpret radiologic diagnostic tests. This occurred in response to efforts of breast cancer survivors, women's groups, doctors, mammographers, and professional organizations, who generated thousands of letters and telephone calls in support of legislation.

If the Alliance for Quality Imaging and Radiation Therapy is successful in its efforts, it will be an important example of a situation in which action by other professional groups has limited the legal range of responsibility for medical assistants (and incidentally limited the ability of a doctor to delegate certain tasks). There are many ramifications, as offices with x-ray equipment are required to hire licensed radiographers in those states that have passed legislation; those offices may expand the duties of the radiographer to include those formerly performed by a medical assistant.

In most states medical assistants would be well advised to copy the behavior of other professional groups and organize to promote specific legislation that names medical assistants and would allow certified or registered medical assistants to carry out all tasks for which they have been trained.

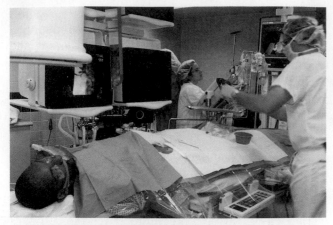

> Figure 20–10 A patient being prepared for an angiogram. (From Leahy JM, Kizilay PE: *Foundations of Nursing Practice: A Nursing Process Approach.* Philadelphia: W.B. Saunders, 1998.)

To study the coronary arteries, which supply blood to the heart, a catheter is inserted into an artery (usually the femoral artery) and advanced under fluoroscopy into the aorta where it arises from the left ventricle. The contrast medium is injected through the catheter, and x-ray films are taken to show if there are any blockages in the coronary arteries. Figure 20–10 shows a patient being prepared for an angiogram.

Bone Density Studies

Osteoporosis, or demineralization of the bones, is a common problem of women after menopause, individuals who have been on long-term steroid therapy, and those who have been immobilized for long periods. Special x-ray studies may be done to detect loss of bone density using two low-dose x-ray beams that pass through the body to a detector placed under the body.

Patients at risk for osteoporosis receive bone density studies because medications can be prescribed to increase the body's absorption of calcium, thus preventing further bone loss and possible pathologic fractures due to fragile bones. The bones tested are usually those of the pelvis; there is no special preparation for the test.

Computed Tomography

Tomography is a specialized radiologic technique used to produce multiple images in selected planes of tissue. Using a computer, machines can create cross-sectional images of both bone and soft-tissue structures within the body. The test is usually called a CT (computed tomography) scan, or sometimes a CAT (computed axial tomography) scan.

By moving the x-ray tube and the film's position in relation to one another over time, the CT scanner creates a radiographic exposure that blurs out all of the structures except those directly in the focal plane. In this way, the radiologist is able to focus attention on only the small area he or she wishes to scan. Contrast

media may be injected during CT scans to improve visualization of certain structures. Figure 20–11 shows a patient in position to enter the CT scanner. The patient must remain still during the test to provide a clear image.

The medical assistant should instruct a patient who will undergo a CT scan in which contrast media is expected to be used to remain NPO for 4 hours. He or she should also instruct the patient to remove metal jewelry before the test. As with other x-ray studies, a pregnant patient should normally not be scheduled for a CT scan.

DIAGNOSTIC IMAGING

In the past 25 years, diagnostic imaging has expanded to include producing images of body parts using ultrasound, radioactive isotopes, or one of the newer technologies such as CT, magnetic resonance imaging (MRI), or positron emission tomography (PET). Different tests may be preferred for different organs or systems, because of the nature of the images that can be produced.

Nuclear Medicine

Nuclear medicine is the medical specialty that uses radioactive materials (other than x-rays) for both diagnosis and treatment.

For testing, small amounts of radioactive substances called radionuclides are either ingested by the patient or injected into the patient's bloodstream. These radioactive isotopes are absorbed by the tissues of the patient's body. Depending on the area to be scanned, different isotopes are used.

After an interval that depends on the area to be visualized, the patient is placed under a large gamma camera, which is sensitive to radiation. The camera,

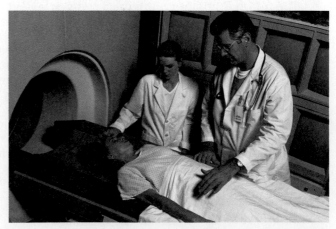

> Figure 20–11 The patient is positioned on a table that moves into the CT scanner.

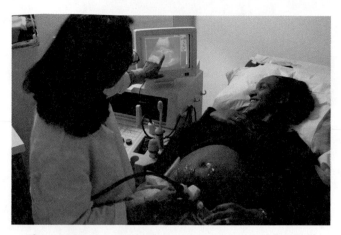

> **Figure 20–12** During a fetal ultrasound, the tecnician moves a transducer across the patient's abdomen, and the image appears on a television monitor.

which is connected to a computer, records an image of the radiation in the organs being studied. As the radioactive compound travels through the patient's body, the radiation is detected by the camera and is translated into light, which in turn exposes film. The substances used lose their radioactivity within hours, and there are usually no adverse effects to the patient.

The film is called a scan. Doctors who specialize in nuclear medicine interpret the scan, which is useful in evaluating the cause of many health problems. Scans are often used to diagnose problems in the brain, the thyroid, the liver, the lung, the gallbladder, or in a bone. They are used as follow-up studies for potential problems of the breast, the prostate, and the heart

One of the most common scans is the thyroid scan, used to diagnose abnormalities of the thyroid gland in the neck. Because the thyroid gland uses iodine to produce thyroid hormones, patients must discontinue vitamin pills containing iodine at least 2 weeks before the study. Also, a thyroid scan should not be scheduled until at least 3 weeks after any x-ray studies using

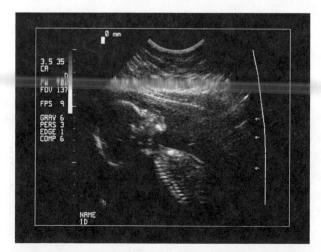

> **Figure 20–13** The head and spine of the fetus is clearly visible in a photograph made during the ultrasound.

iodine as a contrast medium. A patient who takes thyroid medication should be advised by the doctor if it is necessary to stop the medication for a certain time before the test.

Most nuclear medicine scans require no preparation, but some do require the patient to be fasting. When scheduling a test for a patient, the medical assistant should be sure to determine if the patient should be fasting and for how long before the test.

Positron Emission Tomography (PET) and Single-Photon Emission Computed Tomography (SPECT)

Two specialized types of nuclear medicine scans use computers to produce sectional images: positron emission tomography (PET) scan and single-photon emission computed tomography (SPECT) scan. These techniques produce images in colors that vary depending on how much of the radioactive material different cells absorb. In general, active cells show more intense colors than inactive cells. These tests are useful for studying cellular activity and for evaluating the effectiveness of circulation to specific areas of the body.

Diagnostic Medical Sonography

Diagnostic medical sonography (also called ultrasound) uses high-frequency sound waves to create real-time or still images of soft tissue and internal organs. The sound waves are emitted by an instrument called a transducer, which is pressed against the skin over the area being examined.

Sound waves bounce off the body's organs, back to the handset, where they are translated into a visual display on a screen. Because this modality is not known to be harmful to cells, sonography is commonly used in prenatal care. Many obstetricians and midwives routinely schedule an ultrasound exam around or before the fourth month of pregnancy to determine the fetus' size, head circumference, and position; sometimes the fetus' gender can also be determined. Figure 20–12 shows a technician performing fetal ultrasound. The image is shown in Figure 20–13.

Ultrasound exams are also used to examine heart function, gallbladder and other abdominal problems, and pelvic structures.

Most ultrasounds do not require specific patient preparation, but for the fetal ultrasound, the patient must have a full bladder to push the uterus up in the abdomen for easier visualization. The patient is instructed to drink several glasses of water in the hour before the test.

Magnetic Resonance Imaging

Magnetic resonance imaging (MRI) utilizes magnetic fields, in combination with radio waves and sophisticated computer technology, to create cross-sec-

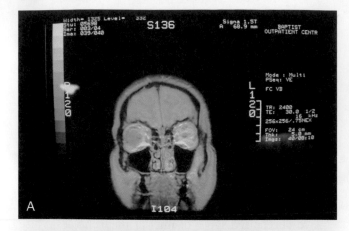

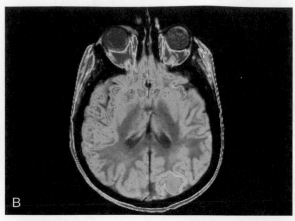

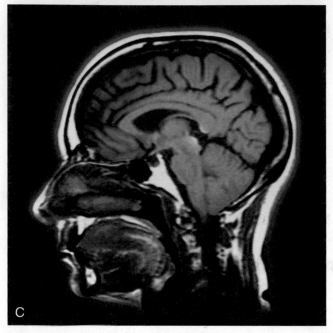

➢ **Figure 20–14** Images of the head. (A) CT scan. (B) color-enhanced cerebral scan. (C) MRI.

tional views of soft tissue. MRI is especially good at imaging tumors and masses on soft tissue, including many kinds of cancers. It is also used to diagnose joint problems.

Because MRI uses powerful magnets, it cannot be used on people with pacemakers or prosthetics that include metal parts. Unlike with an x-ray or CAT scan, the patient is completely enclosed in the MRI machine, and some people get anxious and claustrophobic. Because of this, a mild sedative is usually given before the exam. Newer machines allow more open space and are more comfortable for patients.

Figure 20–14 compares images of the head created by CT scan, color-enhanced cerebral scan, and MRI.

STUDENT STUDY PLAN

To reinforce your understanding of the material in this chapter . . .

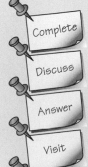

Complete *Complete* the **Review & Recall** questions.

Discuss *Discuss* the situation in **If You Were the Medical Assistant** with your classmates, and answer the questions.

Answer *Answer* the **Critical Thinking Questions,** and discuss them with your classmates.

Visit *Visit* **Web sites** listed below and search for additional web sites using **Keywords for Internet Searches.**

Complete *Complete* the exercises in chapter 20 of the **Student Mastery Manual.**

REVIEW & RECALL

1. Identify protective measures taken to prevent excessive radiation exposure to patients and health care personnel when diagnostic x-ray films are being taken.

2. Describe how barium and iodine are used in x-ray studies. What is their purpose? How do they affect the x-ray image?

3. Identify the kind of energy used for each of the following types of diagnostic tests: CT scan; MRI, diagnostic medical sonography, nuclear medicine, and PET scan. Which of these tests is considered safe to be performed during pregnancy?

4. Describe the role of the medical assistant related to x-ray and other diagnostic imaging tests.

5. Describe three common x-ray studies of the GI tract and the patient preparation for them.

IF YOU WERE THE MEDICAL ASSISTANT

What are some possible situations in which you might be able to help with the x-ray study even if you are not allowed to take x-rays in your state? If you are asked to assist with diagnostic x-ray studies by holding a patient, what instructions might you give to the patient? What equipment would you wear to protect yourself? Why might you wear more protective equipment than the patient?

CRITICAL THINKING QUESTIONS

1. What information should a medical assistant give a patient who is concerned about getting too much radiation from diagnostic x-ray studies?

2. If a medical office has x-ray equipment, summarize the safety precautions needed for the protection of patients and staff.

3. Assuming that a medical assistant has helped patients schedule each of the following diagnostic tests: CT scan of the head, ultrasound of the pancreas, thyroid scan, and MRI, what would be an appropriate explanation of each?

4. Constipation is common after x-ray studies of the GI tract. What can patients do to help prevent it?

5. Find information about kidney problems that may be diagnosed by intravenous pyelogram (IVP) and correlate to the x-ray findings.

EXPLORE THE WEB

WEB SITES

American Society of Radiologic Technicians
http://www.asrt.org

Virtual Hospital
http://www.vh.org

Patient information on x-ray tests and MRI
http://www.vh.org/Patients/IHB/DiagnosticRad.html

KEYWORDS FOR INTERNET SEARCHES

barium enema
bone density
diagnostic sonography
intravenous pyelogram
magnetic resonance imaging
mammogram

medical imaging
pulmonary medicine
radiology
ultrasound
x-ray

ANSWERS TO ON THE JOB

1. If Mrs. White does not receive the instructions to prepare for the barium enema, it is unlikely that the test can be performed as scheduled because of the presence of stool in the GI tract. Kathy should ask the radiology department to fax her a copy of the instructions to give to Mrs. White.

2. If Mrs. White must leave the office immediately, Kathy should take her address to send the instructions to her and, if possible, make a follow-up telephone call to be sure she understands the directions. Before Mrs. White leaves the office, Kathy should at least explain that Mrs. White needs to eat a fat-free meal for lunch the day before the test, drink fluids during the afternoon and evening, and take the laxatives as directed on the instruction sheet. She can purchase the laxatives at a pharmacy.

3. When Kathy receives the instructions from the radiology department, she should make several copies so they will be available in the office for other patients. She should place a "Post-it" type sticky note on one of the last copies to remind everyone in the office to make more copies before giving out the last one.

451

Chapter 21

Assisting with Treatments

Instructional Objectives

After completing this chapter, you will be able to do the following:

1. Define and spell the vocabulary words for this chapter.
2. Apply principles of medical asepsis to eye and ear irrigation and instillation.
3. Describe the procedure for instructing a patient in the use of a metered-dose inhaler.
4. Explain the purpose and procedure for a treatment using a nebulizer.
5. List guidelines for protecting patient safety during thermal treatments.
6. Describe proper use of hot soaks and hot moist compresses.
7. Identify measures used to apply dry heat safely.
8. Differentiate between the physiologic effects of heat and cold.
9. Describe common injuries to bones and joints, their diagnosis, and treatment.
10. Explain the procedure for applying a cast safely.
11. Describe patient-teaching needs after a cast has been applied.
12. List four potential problems that might be experienced by a patient with a cast.
13. Explain why a sling is used.
14. Describe the procedure for removing a cast.
15. Define and describe five treatments used in physical medicine and rehabilitation.

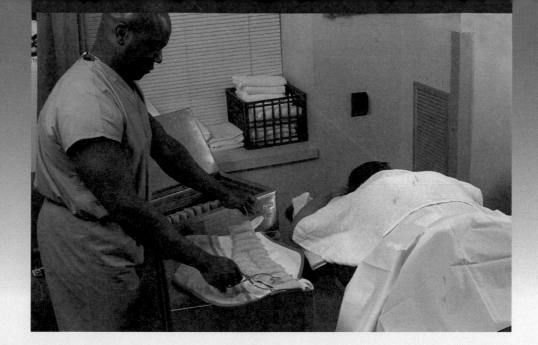

■ Prepare patient for and assist with procedures and treatments

■ Instruct individuals according to their needs

■ Instruct and demonstrate the use and care of patient equipment

■ Provide instruction for health maintenance and disease prevention

■ Document appropriately

Performance Objectives

After completing this chaper, you will be able to do the following:

1. Perform an eye irrigation (Procedure 21–1).
2. Instill eye medication (Procedure 21–2).
3. Perform an ear irrigation (Procedure 21–3).
4. Instill ear medication (Procedure 21–4).
5. Instruct a patient how to use a metered-dose inhaler correctly (Procedure 21–5).
6. Apply warm moist compresses (Procedure 21–6).
7. Apply an ice pack (Procedure 21–7).
8. Assist the doctor to apply a cast (Procedure 21–8).
9. Apply a sling using a triangular bandage (Procedure 21–9).

VOCABULARY

aerosol (p. 462)	cryotherapy (p. 465)	luxation (p. 471)	strain (p. 471)
atrophy (p. 478)	dislocation (p. 471)	nebulizer (p. 462)	subluxation (p. 471)
canthus (p. 454)	fracture (p. 471)	open reduction (p. 473)	thermotherapy (p. 465)
cast (p. 473)	hypertonic (p. 454)	pinna (p. 457)	traction (p. 473)
cerumen (p. 457)	hypotonic (p. 454)	reduction (p. 473)	vasoconstriction (p. 465)
closed reduction (p. 473)	irrigation (p. 454)	splint (p. 473)	vasodilation (p. 465)
compress (p. 465)	isotonic (p. 454)	sprain (p. 471)	

ABBREVIATIONS

DC (p. 480)   MDI (p. 462)   POP cast (p. 472)   RICE (p. 472)   TENS (p. 481)   UV (p. 480)
DO (p. 480)   ORIF (p. 473)

A medical assistant may be asked to assist with or perform independently one of a host of treatments. These treatments are prescribed by the primary care provider based on the patient diagnosis. They are often billed separately from the office visit. Sometimes, the doctor will not even see the patient if the patient is coming into the office for a follow-up treatment.

IRRIGATIONS

An **irrigation** is the application of a large amount of fluid to an area for the purpose of removing foreign material, cleaning the area, removing a harmful substance or, less commonly, applying medication.

Uses

Irrigation is used for any number of purposes. It may be to flush a burn or to clean a wound before medication is applied or the wound is sutured. Irrigation is also used to remove irritating chemicals from the skin or eyes or to flush a surgical field. Irrigation is also used to clean the lumen of a catheter.

Principles

The solution used in irrigation must be nonirritating; it must also be sterile if it enters a sterile body cavity or area. When sterile solution is used, it is applied from a sterile syringe or sterile applicator. Normal saline solution is often used because it is **isotonic** to body tissue, meaning that it has the same concentration of electrolytes as body tissue, so that the fluid and electrolyte balance of body tissue is not disrupted.

Figure 21–1 shows the effects of irrigating solutions of different concentrations. **Hypertonic** (more concentrated than body tissues) and **hypotonic** (less concentrated than body tissues) solutions are occasionally used depending on the desired effect.

There must be a way to collect, drain, or absorb the fluid so the patient does not get wet and the used fluid, which may contain harmful microorganisms, does not contaminate clean surfaces. Appropriate personal protective equipment should be worn to prevent contact with body fluids and splashes of solution.

Eye Irrigation

Eye irrigation is usually performed to remove a foreign object from the eye or to flush the eye of harmful chemicals. The procedure is described in detail in Procedure 21–1. It is important to position the patient properly and for comfort, either lying or sitting; place a basin and towel in the appropriate place to keep the patient dry; and always irrigate from the inner to the outer **canthus** (corner of the eye) to reduce the possibility of cross-contamination with the other eye.

Eye Instillation

To instill medication in the eye, have the patient sit with the eye looking up. Verify that you have the correct medication or drops, as ordered by the doctor. (The process to use in verifying medication orders is described in detail in chapter 22.)

Gently pull down the patient's lower eyelid, using a sterile gauze pad. Always wear gloves during eye instillation.

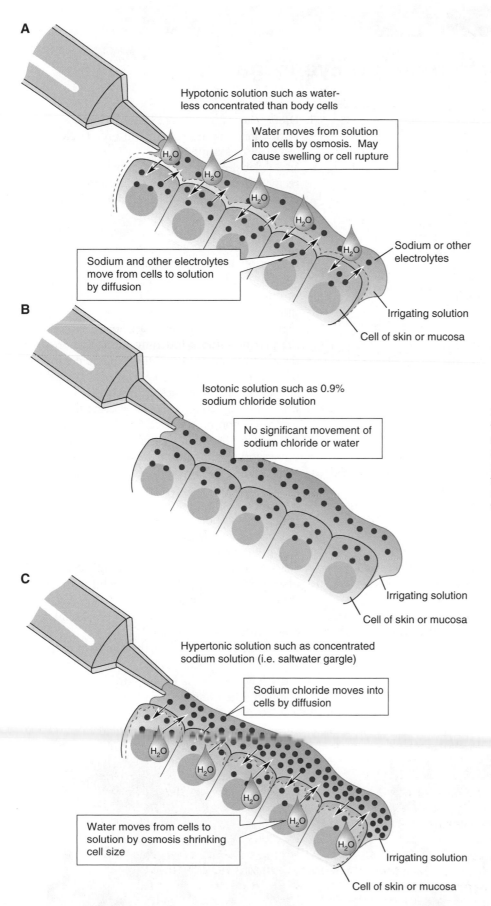

A

Hypotonic solution such as water-less concentrated than body cells

Water moves from solution into cells by osmosis. May cause swelling or cell rupture

Sodium and other electrolytes move from cells to solution by diffusion

Sodium or other electrolytes

Irrigating solution

Cell of skin or mucosa

B

Isotonic solution such as 0.9% sodium chloride solution

No significant movement of sodium chloride or water

Irrigating solution

Cell of skin or mucosa

C

Hypertonic solution such as concentrated sodium solution (i.e. saltwater gargle)

Sodium chloride moves into cells by diffusion

Water moves from cells to solution by osmosis shrinking cell size

Irrigating solution

Cell of skin or mucosa

➤ **Figure 21–1** Irrigating with solutions of different concentrations produces different effects on body cells. (A) Hypotonic solutions allow fluid to move into the cells. (B) Isotonic solutions do not result in water movement. (C) Hypertonic solutions pull water out of the cells.

PROCEDURE 21–1

Performing an Eye Irrigation

Performance Objective:
The student will be able to cleanse an eye to remove a foreign object or flush a harmful chemical.

☑	Wash hands
☑	Gloves
☐	Eye and Face Protection
☐	Lab Coat or Apron
☑	Plastic Biohazard Bag
☐	Rigid Biohazard Container

Supplies and Equipment:
Sterile irrigation solution and sterile container for solution or commercially prepared bottled solution, sterile syringe (bulb or 10-cc syringe), kidney-shaped basin, sterile gauze or cotton balls, draping towel, gloves, biohazard waste container.

Procedure Steps

1. Wash hands.
2. Identify patient. Explain procedure to patient.
3 Assemble equipment.
4. Position patient in supine position with head turned toward affected side. Place a draping towel under the patient's head to catch any drips.
   Rationale: Turning the head will help the solution drain away from the unaffected side. This will prevent cross-contamination. Irrigating solution and any exudate from the eye will flow across the affected eye and be collected in the kidney-shaped basin.

5. Drape patient, covering neck and chest area.
   Rationale: Draping patient will protect clothing from becoming wet.
6. Check label on sterile solution bottle for correctly ordered medication and expiration date. Solution should be body temperature.
   Rationale: The label on solution should be checked three times for accuracy. The solution must be used before the expiration date. A solution at body temperature will be most comfortable for the patient. Excessively cold or hot solutions could damage the sensitive tissue of the eye.
7. Open the sterile container and place beside the patient without touching the inside of the bowl. Pour sterile solution into the container without touching the rim of the sterile container. Open the package of the sterile syringe or bulb syringe and place beside the irrigating solution on the inside of the wrapper.
   Rationale: The solution, the container holding it, and the tip and inside of the irrigating syringe must remain sterile to avoid introducing microorganisms into the patient's eye.
8. If you are using a bottle of prepared eye irrigating solution, remove the cap.
9. Put on disposable gloves.
10. Ask the patient to look up and fix his or her gaze on an object. Hold the patient's eye open by pulling on the lower eyelid with the thumb of your nondominant hand to expose the conjunctiva and holding the top eyelid open with your forefinger.
    Rationale: Having the patient stare at a particular place will help hold the eye still. The eye must stay open to be exposed to the irrigating solution. The nondominant hand is used to

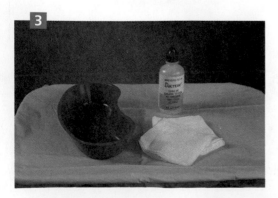

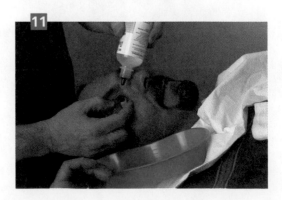

hold the eye so that the syringe can be manipulated with the dominant hand.

11 Fill the syringe with irrigating solution and irrigate the affected eye with solution from the inner canthus (corner) to outer canthus of the eye. The solution should fall onto the conjunctiva rather than the cornea. The tip of the syringe should remain about 1″ above the eye and should never touch the eye. *Rationale:* It is important to prevent cross-contamination by flowing solution from the inside to the outside corner and not allowing

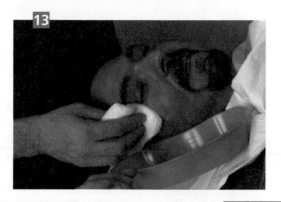

the solution to flow over to the unaffected eye. The procedure will be more comfortable for the patient if solution does not fall directly on the cornea. If the syringe touches the eye, it could damage the cornea.

12. Continue irrigation as ordered by doctor. You may need to refill the syringe several times.

13 Dry the eyelid and eyelashes with sterile gauze or cotton balls after the irrigation.

14. Discard waste in biohazard container.

15. Remove gloves and wash hands.

16. Document the procedure, including the type and amount of solution used for irrigation, in the patient's medical record.

Charting Example	
Date	
2/5/XX	2:15 PM Left eye irrigated with 250 mL normal saline. Pt tolerated procedure well.
	———————— P. Dean, RMA

For drops, hold the dropper about 1/2″ above the conjunctival sac and release the appropriate number of drops into the sac. Then have the patient gently close the eye and slowly roll the eye around to disperse the medication. Any medication left in the dropper must then be discarded.

When using ointment, discard the first bead without touching the top of the ointment tube. Then place a thin line across the inside of the lower eyelid, moving from the inner canthus to the outer canthus. Twist the tube gently to get the last bit of ointment to release from the tip; do not touch the tip of the ointment tube to the eye.

Procedure 21–2 describes eye instillation in greater detail.

Ear Irrigation

Ear irrigation is usually performed to remove excess cerumen from the ear canal so the doctor can better visualize the tympanic membrane (eardrum). **Cerumen** is the substance secreted by the sebaceous glands of the ear, commonly known as earwax. Cerumen can build up and harden in the ear canal. Figure 21–2 shows impacted cerumen in the ear canal, causing hearing problems and dizziness.

Solution is injected into the ear canal gently, with the patient's head tilted slightly toward the affected ear,

to allow solution and loosened cerumen to run out. An ear basin, towel, and plastic drape keep the patient's clothing from getting wet or soiled. Irrigation may be necessary if the doctor cannot visualize the tympanic membrane or if the patient complains of pain in the ear canal or difficulty hearing. Before the actual irrigation, it may be necessary first to insert warm oil eardrops or eardrops containing carbamide peroxide to help soften and loosen any hard, encrusted cerumen.

It is important when irrigating the ear that the **pinna,** or ear flap, be held correctly to straighten the canal as much as possible so solution can reach the built-up cerumen. For adults and children older than age 3, the pinna should be gently pulled back and up. For infants and toddlers younger than age 3, the pinna should be very gently pulled straight back.

Procedure 21–3 describes ear irrigation in more detail.

Ear Instillation

To instill ear medication, have the patient sit with the affected ear tipped up. Verify that you have the correct medication or drops, as ordered by the doctor (see chapter 22). For adults, pull the pinna of the ear up and back; for children, pull it straight back. Be careful when putting the dropper into the patient's ear not to touch the skin; let the drop flow along the ear canal.

After ear medication has been instilled, the patient

should sit or lie for a short time, with the affected ear up, to allow the medication to move throughout the ear canal. If the medication needs to be retained for a long period, gently place a cotton ball in the external ear canal.

Procedure 21–4 describes in more detail how to instill ear medication.

Nasal Irrigation

Nasal irrigation is occasionally used to remove a foreign object from the nose or to relieve inflammation and assist in drainage. Saline nasal spray is sprayed into each nostril or, less commonly, solution at body temperature is injected into the nasal passage using a

---

PROCEDURE 21–2

Instilling Eye Medication

Performance Objective: The student will be able to instill medication into the eye as ordered by doctor.

☑	Wash hands
☑	Gloves
☐	Eye and Face Protection
☐	Lab Coat or Apron
☑	Plastic Biohazard Bag
☐	Rigid Biohazard Container

Supplies and Equipment: Nonsterile gloves, eyedrops or tube of eye ointment, gauze pads, biohazard waste container.

Procedure Steps:

1. Obtain chart with doctor's medication order.

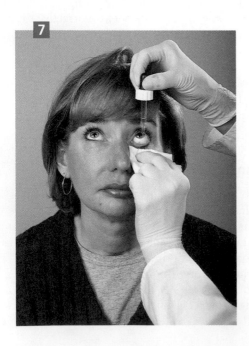

2. Calculate dosage if necessary. Recheck dosage with chart. Assemble medication and supplies to administer. Check the label three times to ensure accuracy. The three label checks should be first, when removing from cabinet, compare label to order; second, before removing cap or withdrawing medication into dropper; and third, before instilling medication into the eye. Check to be sure the medication has not expired.
   Rationale: The label is checked three times to ensure that the correct medication is being administered. Medications should be used before the expiration date to ensure potency.

3. Identify patient and explain procedure.

4. Place patient in sitting or supine position.

5. Wash hands and put on gloves.

6. Ask the patient to look up and, using a 2x2 gauze pad with your nondominant hand, gently pull the lower eyelid downward to expose the conjunctiva.

7. Place the ordered number of drops into the center of the lower conjunctiva, being careful not to touch the dropper tip to the eye. If the medication is an ointment, discard the first bead of ointment and squeeze a line of ointment onto the conjunctiva from inner to outer canthus (corner).
   Rationale: Prevent contamination by holding the dropper bottle or tip of dropper away from the eye and eyelashes. There is also a danger of corneal damage should the dropper scratch the eye surface.

8. Ask the patient to close his or her eye and roll the eyeball to distribute medication evenly.

9. Blot excess with another gauze pad, moving from inner to outer corner.

10. Assess patient for any adverse reactions.

11. Remove gloves and discard with waste in biohazard container. Wash hands.

12. Provide verbal and written instructions should the patient be required to continue treatment at home.
13. Document exact administration and instructions in patient record. Use the following abbreviations:

> OU—both eyes
> OS—left eye
> OD—right eye
> gt—drop
> gtt—drops.

Charting Example	
Date	
4/8/XX	9:35 AM Isopto-Tears gtt ii instilled OU. Pt. instructed to continue use at home to prevent excessive dryness of eyes.
	P. Dean, RMA

*Figure from Bonewit-West K: *Clinical Procedures for Medical Assistants*, 5th ed. Philadelphia: WB Saunders, 2000.

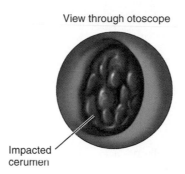

View through otoscope

Impacted cerumen

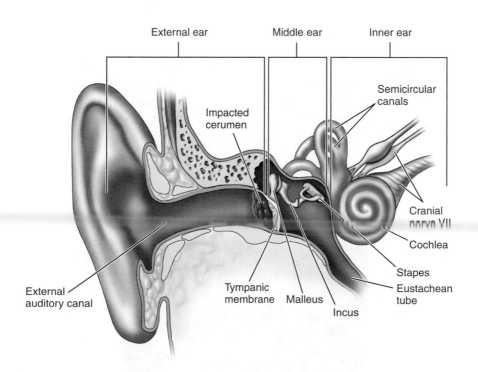

External ear | Middle ear | Inner ear

Semicircular canals

Impacted cerumen

Cranial nerve VII

Cochlea

Stapes

Eustachean tube

External auditory canal

Tympanic membrane | Malleus

Incus

➤ **Figure 21–2** Cerumen can become impacted in the external auditory canal.

PROCEDURE 21–3

Performing an Ear Irrigation

Performance Objective: The student will be able to irrigate the ear to remove foreign matter.

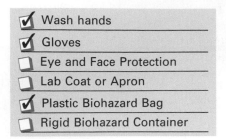

- ☑ Wash hands
- ☑ Gloves
- ☐ Eye and Face Protection
- ☐ Lab Coat or Apron
- ☑ Plastic Biohazard Bag
- ☐ Rigid Biohazard Container

Supplies and Equipment: Irrigating solution, container for irrigating solution, syringe (bulb or 10-cc syringe), ear basin for returned solution, plastic drape, gauze or cotton balls, gloves, biohazard waste container.

Procedure Steps

1. Wash hands.
2. Identify patient. Explain procedure to patient.
   Rationale: A feeling of dizziness may be felt during procedure and should be reported by patient if this happens. Too much dizziness may cause nausea and vomiting.
3. Assemble equipment.
4. Position patient in supine position with head turned toward affected ear.
   Rationale: Turning the head will help the solution drain into the basin. Patient may be placed in a sitting position if easier to administer.

5. Apply plastic drape under the ear and covering the patient's shoulder. Place the ear basin under the ear to catch the fluid after irrigation.
   Rationale: Draping the patient and using the ear basin will protect clothing from becoming wet.
6. Check label on solution bottle to be sure it is the solution ordered by the doctor and has not expired. Solution should be at body temperature.
   Rationale: Verify the label three times for accuracy. Expiration date needs to be current. Solution at body temperature will be more comfortable for the patient.
7. Pour solution into a container and fill the ear syringe or bulb syringe with solution. Place filled syringe and basin at tableside.
8. Place gauze squares or cotton balls for use if needed to catch drips.
9. Put on gloves and grasp the ear. Straighten the adult auditory canal by pulling back and up on the pinna (fleshy part of the ear). If irrigating a child's ear, pull straight back.
   Rationale: If the auditory canal has been straightened, the fluid can easily flow to loosen cerumen.
10. Irrigate by gently inserting tip of bulb or syringe into affected ear canal, being careful not to go too deep. Direct the solution upward at a minimally forceful rate.

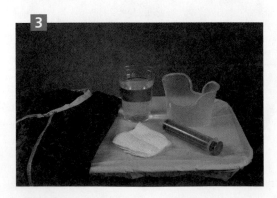

3

Rationale: Avoid injury to tympanic membrane and allow solution to drain out into basin. Cerumen or foreign matter will be dislodged and rinsed into basin.

11. Continue irrigation as ordered by doctor. Usually the syringe is refilled and the ear is irrigated several times.

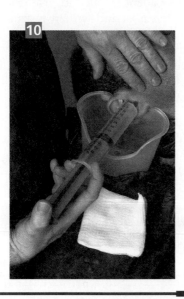

Rationale: More cerumen may be removed when the ear is irrigated several times.

12. Dry the ear with sterile gauze or cotton balls after the irrigation.
13. Remove gloves and discard waste in biohazard container.
14. Wash hands.
15. Document in patient record. Estimate whether a small, moderate, or large amount of cerumen was removed.

Charting Example

Date	
9/27/XX	4:15 PM Left ear irrigated with 500 mL normal saline. Mod. amt. of brown cerumen returned. Pt. complained of discomfort during procedure but was without complaints after the procedure.
	P. Dean, RMA

PROCEDURE 21–4

Instilling Ear Medication

Performance Objective: The student will be able to instill drops into the ear as ordered by doctor.

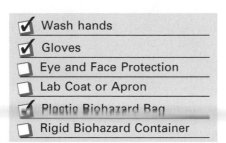

- ☑ Wash hands
- ☑ Gloves
- ☐ Eye and Face Protection
- ☐ Lab Coat or Apron
- ☑ Plastic Biohazard Bag
- ☐ Rigid Biohazard Container

Supplies and Equipment: Eardrops in self-dropper bottle or separate sterile ear dropper, gauze pads, gloves, biohazard waste container.

Procedure Steps

1. Obtain chart with doctor's medication order.

2. Calculate dosage if necessary. Recheck dosage with chart.
3. Assemble medication and supplies to administer. Obtain bottle of otic drops and check expiration date and label three times to assure accuracy. The three label checks should be first, when removing from cabinet compare label to order; second, before removing cap or withdrawing medication into dropper; and third, before instilling drops into the ear. *Rationale:* The label is checked three times to ensure accuracy. Expired medications may have lost potency and should not be used.
4. Identify patient and explain procedure.
5. Place patient in sitting or supine position with affected ear tilted up.
Rationale: This will help medication flow into affected ear more evenly.
6. Wash hands and put on gloves.
7. Using the nondominant hand, gently pull the pinna (fleshy part of the ear) up and back

Procedure continued on following page

PROCEDURE 21–4 *(continued)*

(for an adult) or straight back (for a child).
Rationale: If the ear canal is straight, the drop(s) can easily flow into the ear.

8 Place the ordered number of drops into the ear and have the patient hold the position for about 5 minutes to allow medication to fully enter ear canal. Do not insert the tip of the dropper into the ear.
Rationale: Inserting the dropper into ear canal could cause injury.

9. Blot excess, if necessary, being careful not to

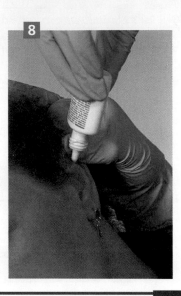

absorb medication. A moistened cotton ball may be placed in canal if ordered by the doctor to help hold medication in place.

10. Remove gloves and discard with waste in biohazard container.

11. Assess patient for any adverse reactions.

12. Provide verbal and written instructions should the patient be required to continue treatment at home.

13. Document exact administration and instructions in patient record. Use the following abbreviations:

> AD—right ear
> AS—left ear
> AU—both ears
> gt—drop
> gtt—drops

Charting Example	
Date	
6/14/XX	2:45 PM Otocort otic sol. gtt ii instilled AU. Instillation demonstrated for the patient's mother, who was instructed to continue use at home as directed by Dr. Lopez. ————
	———————— P. Dean, RMA

bulb syringe. The patient should try to let the solution drain out and avoid blowing his or her nose for 5 minutes after the procedure, so solution is not moved into the sinuses.

INHALATION TREATMENTS

Inhalation treatments are used to introduce moisture and/or medication directly into the lungs. The patient breathes in a mist containing very fine droplets of water and/or medication. In the lungs, the liquid acts to loosen secretions; the medication directly affects lung tissue, usually causing the bronchi to dilate so that breathing is more efficient.

Metered-dose Inhalers

Metered-dose inhalers **(MDI)** are used for administering medications for asthma treatment, as well as some anti-inflammatory medications. The patient uses a mouthpiece to inhale medication that has been vaporized deeply into the lungs. A plastic chamber may be

used to extend the inhaler to facilitate breathing in as much of the medication as possible. Procedure 21–5 discusses instructing a patient in how to use an MDI.

Nebulizers

Nebulizers are devices that deliver fluid as wet mist **(aerosol).** The patient either uses a mouthpiece or a mask to breath in the vapor, which is produced by a machine called a compressor. Sterile solutions are used in nebulizers, because the tiny particles enter the tracheobronchial tree.

Portable nebulizers are often used by people with asthma for short treatments. This compressor is fairly small and usually contains a rechargeable battery. Nebulizers with a larger compressor and the ability to hold large volumes of fluid are needed for continuous production of mist, for example, if a patient has a tracheostomy.

Medication can be added into the holder. If a mouthpiece is used, the medical assistant should have the patient brush his or her teeth and rinse afterward, to prevent soreness.

Figure 21–3 shows a nebulizer.

PROCEDURE 21-5

Instructing a Patient to Use a Metered-Dose Inhaler

Performance Objective: The student will be able to instruct a patient on using a metered-dose inhaler to deliver aerosol medication.

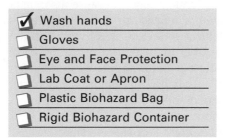

☑ Wash hands
☐ Gloves
☐ Eye and Face Protection
☐ Lab Coat or Apron
☐ Plastic Biohazard Bag
☐ Rigid Biohazard Container

Supplies and Equipment: Placebo inhaler with mouthpiece and extended delivery chamber/spacer.

Procedure Steps

1. Wash hands.
2. Identify patient.
3. Open inhaler packaging and demonstrate use to patient. Point out parts, such as medication canister, plastic holder, plastic spacer (extender). Explain that the spacer (if recommended by the doctor) helps more of the medication to enter the lungs.

4. Instruct the patient to place the medication canister into the plastic holder and shake. If the spacer is used, fit the plastic holder into the spacer and shake both the spacer and the plastic holder containing the medication canister up and down.
   Rationale: Shaking mixes the medication evenly in the liquid.

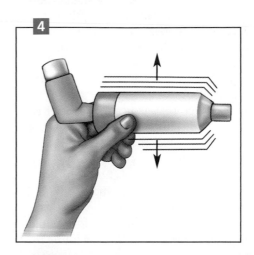

5. Instruct the patient remove the cap from the mouthpiece of the plastic holder or spacer.
6. Instruct the patient to sit in an upright position and place lips around the mouthpiece of the plastic holder or spacer.

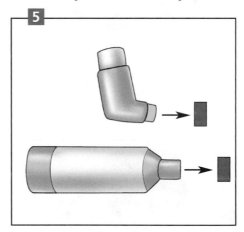

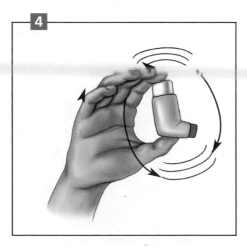

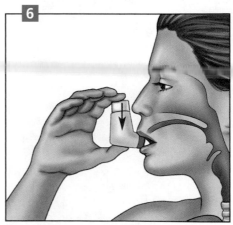

Procedure continued on following page

PROCEDURE 21–5 *(continued)*

Rationale: An upright position and tight seal allows as much medication as possible to reach the lungs.

7 Instruct the patient to press the medication canister down while taking a deep breath and inhaling. If a spacer is used, the patient will not need to coordinate inhaling as closely with release of the medication. If a spacer is used, instruct the patient to inhale slowly but deeply.
Rationale: When the medication canister is depressed, medication is released. The more medication is inhaled, the more effective the medication will be.

8. Instruct the patient to hold the breath for 3 to 5 seconds, exhale slowly, and repeat as ordered by the doctor.
Rationale: It takes a few seconds for the medication to be absorbed by the cells lining the airways.

9. Have the patient return the demonstration on his or her own plastic holder or spacer.
Rationale: A return demonstration allows you to evaluate the effectiveness of teaching.

10. Explain common patient reactions to many inhaled medications. Reinforce that the patient should remain seated and not drive or use machinery when taking medication such as this until breathing has stabilized and all unusual sensations have passed.
Rationale: An increase in heart rate and nervousness are common occurrences the patient may experience after a metered-dose medication is administered. Patients should be reassured that these are normal reactions. The medication may also cause insomnia or difficulty falling asleep. If this is a problem, the patient should discuss it with the doctor.

11 Instruct the patient to rinse the plastic holder with tap water and allow to dry. When the holder is dry, the medication canister is reinserted and the cap is reapplied to keep the mouthpiece clean.
Rationale: This cleans the holder and prevents sticky buildup.

12. Wash hands.

13. Document instructions in patient record. Provide written instructions as well as verbal.

Charting Example	
Date	
11/18/XX	9:45 AM Patient instructed in use of metered-dose inhaler. Able to return demonstration accurately. Able to verbalize common side effects and information to report to report to the doctor. ——————— ——————— S. Williams, CMA

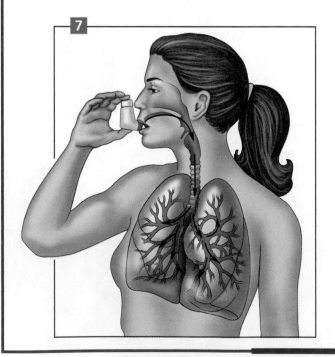

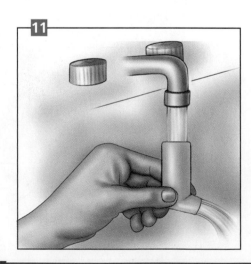

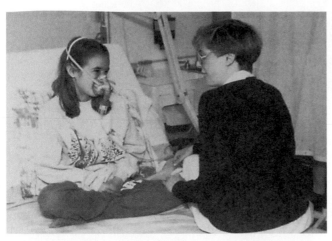

➤ **Figure 21–3** A nebulizer is often used to keep airways from drying out and to deliver medication directly to bronchioles. (From Betz CL, Hunsberger MM, Wright S: *Family Centered Nursing Care of Children,* 2nd ed. Philadelphia: W.B. Saunders, 1994.)

THERMAL TREATMENTS

Both heat and cold are useful in treating certain conditions. Heat or cold can be applied in either a moist or a dry manner. Moist heat or moist cold penetrate deeper and last longer than dry treatments.

Thermal treatments are often used by physical therapists, in which case the medical assistant's role will most often be to complete the referral from the doctor's office to the physical therapist. Thermal treatments may also be given in the office. The medical assistant may also instruct the patient in how to use thermal treatments at home.

Treatment with heat, sometimes called **thermotherapy,** promotes **vasodilation,** the opening of blood vessels, which sends more blood to the affected area. Heat treatments, whether moist or dry, should never be more than 110° F; above that temperature, tissue begins to break down.

Heat is used to relax muscle spasms or loosen muscles in preparation for range-of-motion exercises, relieve pain from strained muscles or joint stiffness due to injury or arthritis, promote drainage from an infection, or relieve localized congestion, such as in the sinuses. Heat should not be used immediately after an injury, because it promotes the inflammatory process and tends to increase swelling.

Treatment with cold, sometimes called **cryotherapy,** promotes **vasoconstriction,** the closing of blood vessels, which brings less blood to the affected area. Cold slows the inflammatory process and thus helps prevent swelling immediately after an injury.

Table 21–1 shows the various thermal treatments available.

Moist Heat

Moist heat feels moist against the skin. Treatment with moist heat can consist of either a soak in warm water or the application of moist **compresses,** material that has been soaked in warm water and is placed on the affected area.

A soak can be as simple as soaking an infected finger or toe in a basin of warm water and Epsom salts in an effort to drain the infection. If salts are added to the soaking solution, the hypertonic solution tends to pull fluid from the tissue and reduce swelling, as shown in Figure 21–4. A soak may also involve instructing a patient with a bad back on how to most comfortably get into and out of a warm bath or administering a whirlpool treatment at a physical therapist's office before beginning range-of-motion or strengthening exercises to warm the muscles and improve the blood flow. A whirlpool bath has an electrical motor

Table 21–1	**Effects of Heat and Cold Application**	
Heat Application Causes	**Tissue Response**	**Therapeutic Result**
Vasodilation	Increased blood flow	Increased nutrients at site
		Faster removal of wastes
	More white blood cells to area	Phagocytosis
Muscle relaxation	Reduced muscle spasm	Decreased pain
Increased metabolism	Local warmth	Faster tissue repair
Cold Application Causes	**Tissue Response**	**Therapeutic Result**
Vasoconstriction	Decreased blood flow	Prevention of swelling
		Reduced inflammation
Numbness of nerve endings	Local anesthesia	Reduced pain
Reduced metabolism	Decreased oxygen needs	Reduced pain
Increased blood viscosity	Promotion of blood clotting	Prevention of swelling

---

Precautions to Prevent Injury from Thermal Treatments

- Do not use heat in the first 24 hours of acute inflammatory process (after injury) or on burned skin.
- Assess the patient's ability to respond to the sensation of burning or excessive cold. Infants, the elderly, and patients with paralysis are more easily burned than others.
- Instruct the patient to report changes in sensations, or discomfort, immediately.
- Never leave a patient alone who cannot feel if a hot pack is too warm or too cold, or who is paralyzed, or too confused to remove the pack if it becomes uncomfortable.

- Use caution in using heat with a pregnant woman. Heat can cause uterine contractions.
- Always wrap hot or cold appliances with cloth before applying to skin.
- Determine the correct temperature for treatment, and use a timer to control duration of exposure.
- Because metal is a good conductor of heat, have the patient remove all jewelry before any heat application.

---

that agitates the water, creating a gentle massaging action on the affected area.

Hot moist compresses are used to soak a small area; they are often used to soak an infected area or developing boil or cyst on the arm, trunk, face, or neck. They can be made at home from a clean washcloth, soaked in water below 110° F, then squeezed out. If possible, plastic should be put over the compress to help retain heat.

In the office, they are usually made with gauze sponges and solution. If applied to an open lesion, sterile supplies and solution should be used. Commercially made hot moist compresses are also available.

They are made of canvas and contain a silicon gel that retains heat over time. They are heated by immersing them in hot water. Procedure 21–6 details how to apply a hot moist compress.

To test temperature, the water should feel warm but not too hot to immerse the wrist or elbow comfortably (the hands are usually less sensitive to heat). Patients who are directed to use hot moist compresses at home must be warned to avoid water that is too hot, because burns can easily occur.

Moist heat can be applied to a larger area using a commercial hot pack, which is kept warm in a container of hot water. The pack contains a gel that retains heat. To apply this type of pad, the medical assistant removes the pad from the hot water using metal tongs, wraps the pack in a towel or commercial holder, and applies the pack. The doctor determines the area to receive heat and the duration of the treatment. The use of commercial hot packs is shown in Figures 21–5 and 21–6.

One other kind of moist heat is called a paraffin bath. This treatment is often used for patients with longstanding joint disease such as rheumatoid arthritis. The paraffin bath is made of a mixture of seven parts paraffin to one part mineral oil, heated to its boiling point, 127° F. The joint is bathed in the paraffin mixture, either by dipping (for a hand or foot) or by coating (for instance, for a knee or elbow). The paraffin is left on for about 30 minutes, then peeled off. The outside of the coating is hard and quickly cools to room temperature, but the inside retains warmth for a long time. The skin underneath should be warm and smooth, and the effects of the deep heat in the joints should last 3 to 4 hours.

Dry Heat

Dry heat is used mostly to reduce discomfort in joints and muscles. The two most frequently used

➤ **Figure 21–4** A patient may soak an infected finger or toe in warm water.

PROCEDURE 21–6

Applying Warm Moist Compresses

Performance Objective: The student will be able to apply heat therapy in the form of a warm moist compress.

☑	Wash hands
☑	Gloves
☐	Eye and Face Protection
☐	Lab Coat or Apron
☑	Plastic Biohazard Bag
☐	Rigid Biohazard Container

Supplies and Equipment: 4″ × 4″ gauze pads, gloves, basin, thermometer, warm water, biohazard waste container.

Procedure Steps

1. Wash hands.
2. Identify patient.
3. Explain therapy to patient and reason for applying compress.
   Rationale: Moist heat penetrates the skin better than dry heat, helps to improve vascular circulation, and promotes relaxation and mobility.
4. Place an absorbent pad with a plastic backing under the area to be treated. Pour warm water into basin.
5. Measure water temperature to read not over 125°F for adults and 115°F for children or elderly. If no thermometer is available, water that feels comfortably warm on the medical assistant's forearm or elbow is the correct temperature.
   Rationale: The water should be warm to promote vasodilation, but excessively hot water can cause skin irritation or burns. The hands should not be used to test water temperature because temperatures higher than 125°F may not feel excessively hot.
6. Put on gloves.
7. Immerse gauze in water. Squeeze to remove excess water.
   Rationale: This prevents dripping and softening of the patient's skin.
8. Apply compress to area as ordered by doctor and leave in place for the time specified.
   Rationale: Heat therapy is usually not applied for longer than 15 minutes at one time. After that time vasodilation has occurred. Moist packs may cause skin softening or irritation if left in place for a longer period.
9. Remove gloves and discard with used sponges in biohazard bag.
10. Document therapy in patient record. Provide written instructions if the patient is to continue therapy at home.

Charting Example	
Date	
2/16/XX	1:30 PM Warm moist compresses applied to patient's elbow for 15 minutes. Patient instructed to continue application at home b.i.d. ——— ——————— S. Dellarosa, RMA

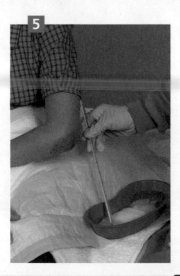

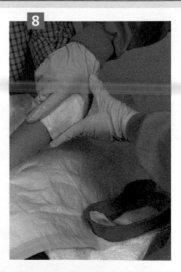

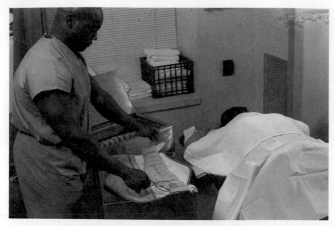

> **Figure 21–5** Commercial hot packs are heated in warm water and retain heat well because they contain gel.

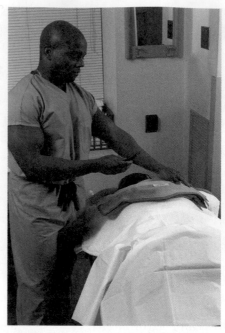

> **Figure 21–6** A towel is used to protect the patient's skin when a commercial hot pack is applied.

methods of dry heat are a heating pad and disposable chemical hot packs. Figure 21–7 shows disposable hot and cold packs.

Heating pads are small plastic pouches with radiant-heat coils inside. Most come with a fabric cover, so the heated plastic surface never touches the skin. Newer model heating pads often have an automatic thermostat that allows temperature to be adjusted much more precisely than older models, which have low, medium, and high heat settings. Some heating pads have water circulating through tubing within a waterproof pad.

An individual should be instructed to use the heating pad at low or medium heat, never on high, for a prescribed period (usually 20 to 30 minutes at a time), never to lie directly on the heating pad, because heat can build up and lead to burns even if the plastic pad is covered with fabric, and never to fall asleep while using a heating pad.

Disposable hot packs have a chemical gel in them that retains heat for up to 60 minutes. They are usually used for 20 to 30 minutes at a time, because they retain maximum heat for this period. Some disposable packs are activated by squeezing the pack to start a chemical reaction. They can be used only once. Another type of gel pack can be heated in a microwave oven for several uses. Instruct the patient to inspect such a pack for leaks before each use. If a leak develops during use, remove the pack as soon as the leak is noticed. If any of the pack's contents have touched the skin, flush with water and follow any other directions on the pack.

A hot-water bottle can also be used to deliver dry heat. A hot-water bottle is never used in the doctor's office, because it can leak and cause burns.

If used, the water temperature inside the bottle should not be over 125° F for adults, and 115° F for children or the elderly. If a patient wants to use a hot-water bottle, he or she should be instructed to fill the bottle one-half or two-thirds full, then expel the excess

air before putting the stopper in. The bottle should always be covered with a towel or flannel cover.

Cold

Cold compresses and ice packs are used to control swelling and bleeding after an injury or surgery.

Cold compresses are made from gauze sponges or washcloths and are used on small areas on the face or head. Over time, the cold will numb the pain, but the first one or two compresses will probably hurt, so they should be applied gently. Prepare the patient by explaining what he or she should expect. Compresses should be changed every 3 minutes, and the total treatment should last about 20 minutes.

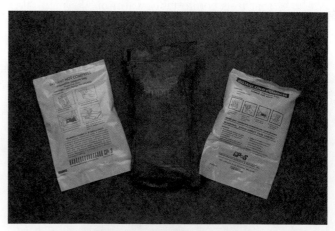

> **Figure 21–7** Commercial hot packs (red) and cold packs (white with blue letters). Twisting the pack to break the inner lining activates a chemical reaction.

Dry cold can be applied using an ice pack. Ice packs can be made from real ice, or a commercial chemical cold pack can be used. To make an ice pack, put ice cubes or crushed ice into a disposable latex glove and tie the glove off (a patient at home can use a zip-top plastic bag or a commercial ice bag). Crushed ice has the advantage of being easily molded around body contours. The bag should be wrapped in a towel to protect the skin from excessive cold and to prevent water from getting on and possibly irritating the skin.

Various kinds of commercial cold packs are available. One is the pack used to keep food cold in lunch boxes and coolers, which consists of a hard plastic case with a chemical in it that can be refrozen in the freezer an unlimited number of times. Because the container is rigid, these do not work as well for injuries as the reusable gel-filled cold packs. These should always be used with a towel to prevent applying excessive cold to the tissue. For acute injury, disposable chemical cold

packs are often used. When they are banged with the heel of the hand and the inner pouch holding the chemical bursts, they become flexible cold packs that stay cold for 30 to 60 minutes. They are discarded after one use.

Procedure 21–7 explains how to apply an ice pack.

CASTS, SPLINTS, AND SLINGS

Casts, splints, and slings are used to provide different levels of immobilization for limbs after an injury to the bone, the joint, or the muscle. The medical assistant generally assists in applying a cast or forming a splint. The medical assistant may apply a commercial splint or sling. In addition, the medical assistant is often responsible for educating the patient about how to care for the cast or splint and how to put the sling

---

PROCEDURE 21–7

Applying an Ice Pack

Performance Objective: The student will be able to perform a cold therapy treatment using an ice pack.

☑	Wash hands
☐	Gloves
☐	Eye and Face Protection
☐	Lab Coat or Apron
☐	Plastic Biohazard Bag
☐	Rigid Biohazard Container

Supplies and Equipment: Commercially prepared ice pack or ice bag and ice, cloth to cover bag/pack.

Procedure Steps

1. Wash hands.
2. Identify patient.
3. Explain therapy to patient and reason for applying pack.
   Rationale: Cold will relieve swelling, pain, and tenderness and can reduce body temperature.
4. Place ice cubes in a disposable glove or ice bag and secure, remove reusable ice pack from the freezer, or apply enough pressure to a commercially prepared cold pack intended for

one-time use to activate chemicals that will cause the bag to become cold.

5. Cover pack with cloth to protect skin surface.
   Rationale: A layer of cloth between the ice pack and the skin is necessary to prevent the skin from excessive cold, which can cause skin damage.
6. Apply pack to area and for the length of time ordered by doctor.
   Rationale: Cold therapy may be applied for 20 to 45 minutes. Leaving it on skin longer will have opposite effect of intended treatment.
7. Document therapy in patient record. Provide written instructions if the patient is to continue therapy at home.

Charting Example	
Date	
9/15/XX	3:20 PM Ice pack applied to patient's back at the midthoracic area for 20 minutes. Pt. instructed to purchase reusable ice pack and given written instructions to continue using ice packs at home q.i.d. ——— ——— S. Williams, CMA

Table 21–2	**Types of Fractures**

Spiral

Greenstick

Twisting or rotating of the bone during fracture causes a coiled fracture line

Bending the bone with or without a partial break; may splinter along the fracture line, as seen with a fresh or "green" stick; seen in children

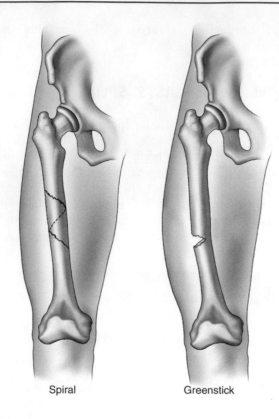

Spiral   Greenstick

Transverse

Oblique

Comminuted

A break in the bone across the axis of the bone

A break in the bone that slants diagonally

A break in the bone resulting in several fragments; usually caused by direct force

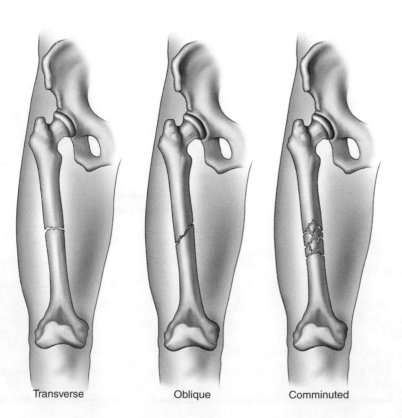

Transverse   Oblique   Comminuted

Depressed

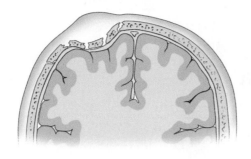

Depressed

A break in a flat bone, such as one of the skull bones, with bone ends forced down into the tissue below the main part of the bone

Longitudinal

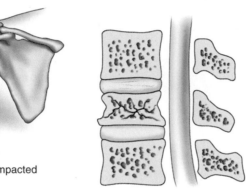

Longitudinal

A break in the bone that runs the length of the bone

Impacted

Compression

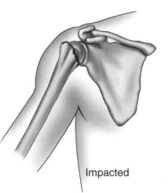

Impacted

A break in the bone in which one bone end is forced into the other; occurs when force is applied from the end of the arm or leg

A break in the bone caused by strong force to both ends; often seen in the bones of the spine

Compression

on each morning. The medical assistant must emphasize that following the doctor's orders to rest the injured extremity can avoid excessive swelling and facilitate healing.

Joint and Bone Injuries

A **strain** is an injury to a muscle and the tendons that support it that is caused by overstretching.

A **sprain** is an injury to a joint capsule and the ligaments that support the joint when the joint has been twisted beyond normal limits.

A **dislocation** occurs when a bone is displaced from the articular surface of the joint. A dislocation is sometimes called a **luxation,** and a partial dislocation is called a **subluxation.** Dislocation, especially of the

shoulder, is a common athletic injury. Dislocation also frequently occurs in the weakened shoulder of a stroke victim. Children frequently suffer a subluxation of the elbow as the result of being pulled along by a parent or other caretaker, an injury termed nursemaid's elbow.

A **fracture** is a break in the bone (Table 21–2). Fractures are characterized as either simple (also called a closed fracture, meaning that the two ends of the broken bone do not penetrate the skin) or compound (also called an open fracture, meaning that the ends of the broken bones cause a break in the skin). A fracture can occur in the middle of a bone or at a joint, where it is accompanied by dislocation. Some types of fractures, especially those that involve the wrist or ankle, must be surgically set before a cast can be applied.

Figure 21–8 shows various joint and bone injuries.

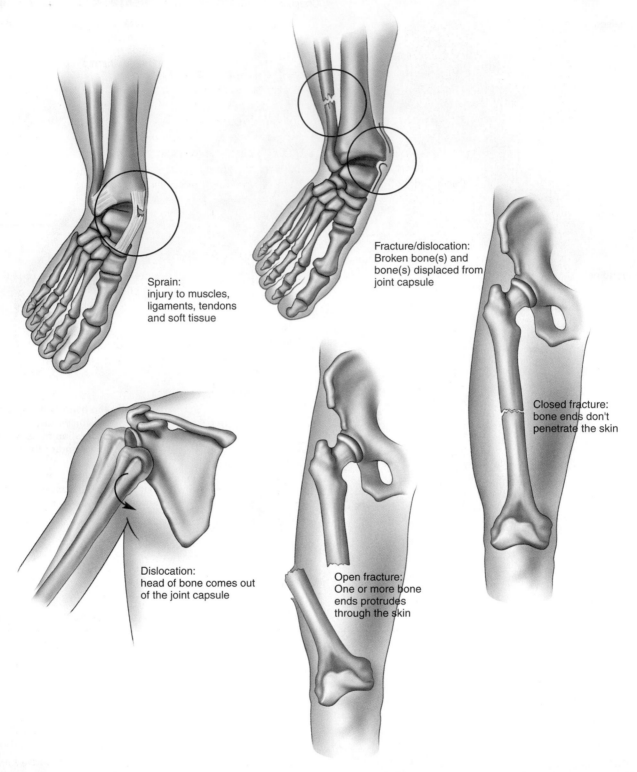

Sprain:
injury to muscles,
ligaments, tendons
and soft tissue

Fracture/dislocation:
Broken bone(s) and
bone(s) displaced from
joint capsule

Closed fracture:
bone ends don't
penetrate the skin

Dislocation:
head of bone comes out
of the joint capsule

Open fracture:
One or more bone
ends protrudes
through the skin

➤ **Figure 21–8** Various types of bone and joint injuries.

It is often difficult to differentiate between a sprain and a more serious injury. Diagnostic imaging is often used to determine the extent of the injury. X-ray films are taken from several angles to determine if a fracture has occurred. If no fracture is shown on the x-ray film, sometimes an MRI (magnetic resonance image) is taken to determine the degree of injury to the muscles, ligaments, tendons, or the soft tissue, especially if the injury is to a joint. An MRI scan is illustrated in chapter 20.

Treatment

Treatment of sprains and strains is generally described by the acronym **RICE:** rest, ice, compression, and elevation. Ice packs are used to decrease swelling.

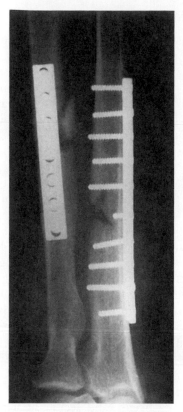

> **Figure 21–9** A severe fracture may require surgery to insert plates, screws, rods, or other hardware to hold the fracture in place. The comminuted fracture of the radius and ulna show up as dark lines on the bones. The hardware, which absorbs X-rays, shows up white. (From Mettler, FA: *Essentials of Radiology.* Philadelphia: W.B. Saunders, 1996.)

For fractures, the treatment is usually immobilization for a time in a cast or splint. For some fractures, reduction is necessary. Reduction can either be closed or open. A **closed reduction** is the term for "setting" the fracture, or placing the bones into alignment without surgically opening the skin over the fracture. An **open reduction** is the term for alignment of the bones after a surgical opening is made at the fracture site. During surgery, screws, plates, nails, or other hardware may be needed to hold the bones in place so that the fracture will heal, as shown in Figure 21–9. This type of surgery—open reduction with internal fixation (**ORIF**) is often necessary for complicated fractures of wrists or ankles.

Assisting in Applying a Cast or Splint

A fracture of a bone in a limb will almost always be immobilized by using a **cast,** a solid material molded to the extremity. Fractures to bones in the trunk do not always require a cast. Rib fractures may be protected by taping and extra padding during athletic activity, and collarbones will sometimes be immobilized by use of a clavicle strap that holds the shoulder back while healing takes place.

Some fractures require **traction**—using a weight to pull on bone ends. Traction can be built into a cast using metal rods and pins placed into the bones during surgery. Traction can also be applied by using weights applied to an apparatus over a patient's bed.

This type of traction requires the patient to be immobilized for 1 to 6 months and is avoided if possible because prolonged immobility predisposes a person to respiratory and circulatory problems and results in severe muscle wasting.

Casts and **splints,** molds that partially encircle a part, can be made in a number of different ways, from a number of different materials.

Before and during transport, a splint should be applied to a suspected fracture to prevent further injury. (This is discussed in more detail in chapter 31 on emergency care.) In addition to traditional plaster-molded casts, many casts today are molded from synthetic material, usually fiberglass. There are also commercially produced rigid appliances for the leg and ankle called walkers, which provide compression and support.

Casts wrap the entire limb and are not removable; splints can be removed. They can be custom molded using either plaster or fiberglass casting material or can be commercially produced. Custom-molded splints are held on with bandages; commercially made splints are secured by Velcro or straps.

Casts on the arm or leg can be long or short. A short arm cast runs from below the elbow to the mid-palm, whereas a long arm cast runs from the axilla to the mid-palm, with the elbow usually at a 90-degree angle. A short leg cast runs from below the knee to the

Immediately after the injury occurs, the pain may not be significant, but the injured person will later show sudden discomfort, immediately stopping activity and taking weight off an injured leg or foot, or not using an injured arm or wrist. Compression can be provided by an elastic bandage (Ace bandage); this supports the injury and prevents swelling. The bandage should not be too tight. It should feel comfortable, and the skin beyond the bandage should be pink or normal color, not pale or purple.

Elevation means that the affected joint should be placed above the level of the heart if possible, to enhance venous drainage and reducing swelling.

Treatment for dislocation is first to get the joint back into its proper alignment, a process called **reduction.** This is done in a medical facility after x-ray studies have established the exact position of the dislocated bones. Medication to decrease muscle spasms facilitates reduction. After reduction, the joint may be immobilized for a time to limit the amount of swelling that occurs with normal use. The patient may be taught appropriate exercises to strengthen the joint in an effort to prevent a recurrence.

toes, with the foot in a natural position. A long leg cast runs from the upper thigh to the toes, with the knee usually slightly flexed and the foot in a natural position.

Either a short or long leg cast can be designed as a walking cast; a walking cast is built to be strong enough to support the weight of the body and often has a rubber walking heel on it. The patient is instructed by the doctor when partial and/or full weight can be put on the leg. A cast boot may also be used over the cast to provide support when walking, as seen in Figure 21–10.

Body casts cover the trunk, and semi-body casts (spica casts) cover part of the trunk as well as one or two extremities. These are rarely applied in an office setting, because supporting the patient during application may require a special table and/or equipment.

A custom-molded cast is applied after the limb has been covered in a soft, knitted, tubular fabric called stockinette and further in soft roller padding, which is sometimes referred to as sheet wadding. Extra knitted fabric is rolled above and below where the cast lines will be, to keep the cast material away from the skin. It is usually folded over the outside of the cast and secured during the casting process.

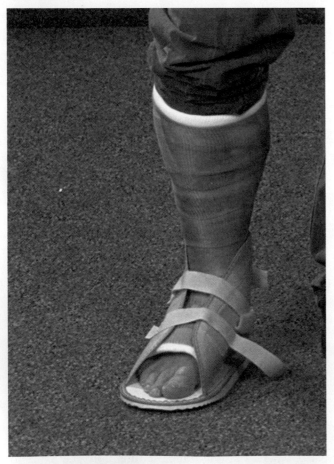

➣ **Figure 21–10** A canvas cast boot with a rigid sole is held in place by Velcro straps to support the right short leg cast when the patient places weight on it.

Plaster of Paris (POP) Casts

Plaster casting comes in rolls of material in various widths. The rolls are dry, with calcium sulfate crystals impregnating the material. When the material is dipped into warm water, the calcium sulfate undergoes a chemical reaction that turns it into a pastelike substance. The casting material is rolled around the injured extremity, smoothed, and shaped. The paste hardens to a rigid cast over time. The chemical reaction causes heat to be generated, which some patients find uncomfortable for 30 minutes or so. It takes about 72 hours (3 days) for a plaster cast to fully cure and harden.

The doctor applies the wet casting material to the limb, working from distal to proximal. The medical assistant is usually responsible for preparing the casting material rolls. Each roll must be submerged in water until no more bubbles appear around the roll. Then it is pressed—not wrung out—until it is wet but not dripping. Utility gloves are worn to keep the casting material from damaging hands.

When the cast is fully rolled out onto the limb, the doctor trims the edges with a plaster knife, then folds the knitted fabric back over the ends of the cast to form cuffs at each end, and secures it with additional plaster rolls. Any excess casting material must then be gently cleaned off the patient's exposed skin.

Patients with leg casts are given crutches to use, either until the cast is taken off or, if it is a walking cast, until the cast cures, at which point the patient may use a cane or no assistance at all. Patients with arm casts often have the arm placed in a sling to relieve the shoulder muscles of the extra weight of the cast.

Water used to moisten rolls of plaster must only be discarded in a sink equipped with a trap for plaster particles. If discarded in an ordinary drain, the plaster will harden and block the drain.

Fiberglass Casts

Fiberglass casting material also comes as rolls in airtight pouches. When opened, they are applied in the same manner as plaster casting, but the polyurethane additive in the fiberglass resin hardens in minutes after exposure to air to create a rigid cast that is more durable than plaster. Figure 21–11 shows supplies needed for applying a cast.

A plaster cast decomposes and becomes musty when wet—making bathing a chore—but fiberglass casts, once set, are relatively waterproof. They must, however, be thoroughly dried to prevent skin lesions from occurring. Patients can shower with a fiberglass cast simply by covering it with a plastic bag.

If a cast becomes wet, the patient should check with the office. Depending on the doctor's preferences, the patient may be instructed to dry the cast using a hair dryer on low to medium heat.

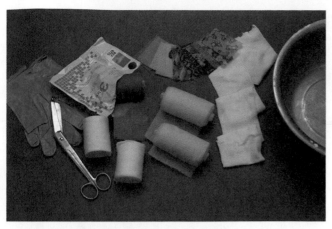

➤ Figure 21–11 Supplies needed to apply a fiberglass cast.

Procedure 21–8 describes assisting with applying a cast.

Splints

Sometimes a support must only be worn when actively using the limb. In this case, the patient may be fit with a custom-made or commercial rigid splint. A custom-made splint is made in much the same way as a cast. After stockinette and sheet wadding are applied to the extremity, casting material is applied lengthwise and shaped to support part of the limb. The stockinette and wadding are removed from the limb and the edges are finished into the splint with an additional layer of casting material. The splint is held in place by

---

PROCEDURE 21–8

Assisting with Cast Application

Performance Objective: The student will be able to assist with applying a fiberglass cast.

☑	Wash hands
☑	Gloves
☐	Eye and Face Protection
☐	Lab Coat or Apron
☐	Plastic Biohazard Bag
☐	Rigid Biohazard Container

Supplies and Equipment: Rolls of fiberglass casting material, stockinette, sheet wadding and/or spongy padding, tape, water, basin, bandage, scissors, gloves, stand to support foot (for lower extremity).

Procedure Steps

1. Wash hands.
2. Identify patient.
3. Explain procedure for applying cast and answer any questions before application.
   Rationale: Knowing what to expect will reassure patient about the procedure. Questions regarding injury should be directed to the doctor.
4. Assemble equipment.
5. Seat patient comfortably, as directed by the

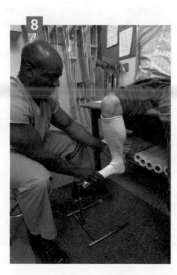

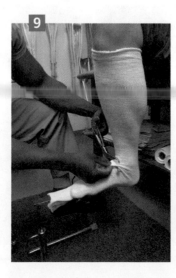

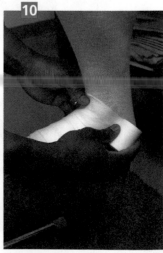

Procedure continued on following page

PROCEDURE 21-8 *(continued)*

doctor. If applying a cast to the lower extremity, the toes may be supported by a stand.
Rationale: The amount of flexion of the ankle can be controlled by supporting the toes so that the patient can more easily maintain the desired position without fatigue.

6. Clean area that cast will cover. Note any objective signs and ask for subjective symptoms to chart at end of procedure.
Rationale: The condition of the area under the cast must be noted before the cast is applied. This will be compared to site when cast is removed. Clean with mild soap solution or as directed. Dry thoroughly.

7. Cut stockinette to fit area cast will cover.

8. Apply stockinette smoothly to the area that the cast will cover. Leave 1″ to 2″ of excess stockinette above and below the cast area to finish the cast.

9. Excess stockinette may be cut away where wrinkles form as, for example, at the front of the ankle.
Rationale: Stockinette must lie smooth and cannot be too bulky or wrinkle, as this may cause a pressure wound.

10. Apply sheet wadding along the length of the cast using a spiral bandage turn. Extra padding may be used over bony prominences such as the bones of the elbow or ankle.
Rationale: Padding the cast helps reduce pressure against bony prominences that could cause skin breakdown.

11. Put on gloves.

12. With lukewarm water in basin, wet fiberglass tape.
Rationale: Immersing the roll of fiberglass

tape in water begins the chemical reaction that will cause the cast to harden. The cast can be shaped while wet and will harden in the shape that is formed.

13. Assist as directed to apply the inner layer of fiberglass tape (shown in the photograph as beige). Roll 1″ to 2″ of stockinette over the inner layer of the cast to form a smooth edge when the outer layer is applied.

14. Assist as directed to open and apply outer layer of fiberglass tape (shown in the photograph as blue).

15. Assist to shape cast as directed. All contours must be smooth.
Rationale: If flat or dented areas develop on the cast, they may cause pressure on the skin below.

16. Discard water and excess materials. Remove gloves.

17. Reassure patient and review cast care verbally and by providing written instructions.

18. Document observations and procedure in patient record.

Charting Example	
Date	
4/5/XX	2:22 PM Assisted with application of short leg cast to right leg. Skin under cast intact. Swelling of right ankle noted before cast applied. Pt. given standard written instructions and able to summarize in own words. ———————— K. Doyle, CMA

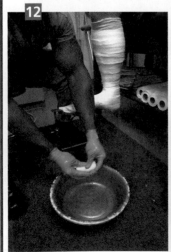
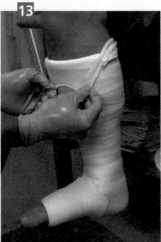
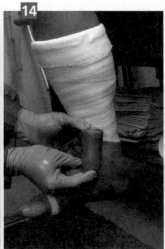
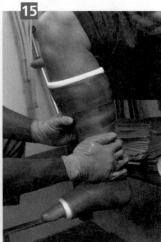

a compressing bandage, but can be removed for showers and sleeping, as specified by the doctor.

If a patient cannot bear weight on a lower-extremity cast, he or she is measured for crutches. See chapter 32 for a complete discussion of teaching a patient to use crutches.

Potential Problems with Casts

A number of potential problems can arise for a patient who is wearing a cast.

Excessive swelling under the cast can cause nerve damage after a cast is applied. The patient should always be instructed to wiggle fingers or toes frequently over the first 24 hours to improve circulation. If the patient cannot move the fingers or toes freely, if they are bluish or white, or if they are numb to the touch, the patient should call the doctor.

Bleeding from a wound under the cast can also be a problem. Any discoloration of the surface of the cast should be circled and observed for increase in size. If the size increases, the patient should report it to the doctor; this is a sign that a wound is continuing to bleed under the cast.

A third problem is a possible infection under the cast. This can be at the site of an open wound or can be caused by the patient poking a sharp instrument down the cast to scratch an itchy spot under the cast. A bad smell or drainage from under the cast should be reported to the doctor.

Finally, deterioration of the cast can be a problem. Until a plaster cast dries, it can crumble if it gets wet or is subjected to excess pressure. A plastic bag should be used to cover the cast while showering with a fiberglass cast, and the patient must be careful not to get a plaster cast wet at all.

Applying a Sling

The reason for using a sling is to keep the hand and wrist elevated to reduce swelling, promote healing, decrease movement, or immobilize a broken collarbone and, when an arm cast has been applied, to reduce pressure on the shoulder muscles caused by the weight of the cast. Commercially made slings are available, many of which have foam padding inside to maintain the arm in a particular angle. These slings buckle or belt at the shoulder.

A sling can also be made from a large piece of cloth, folded into a triangle and knotted at the shoulder. Figure 21–12 shows various types of commercial slings, and Procedure 21–9 explains how to apply a triangular cloth sling.

Cast Removal

A cast is removed after the bone has healed. Usually this takes about 6 to 8 weeks for a simple fracture. Usually, an x-ray film is taken to determine if a bone has healed sufficiently for the cast to be removed. The medical assistant may be responsible for removing a cast or for assisting a doctor in its removal.

Cast removal is accomplished using two instruments, a cast cutter, shown in Figure 21–13, and a cast spreader, shown in Figure 21–14.

The cast cutter is a saw that does not actually cut but vibrates rapidly, slicing through the cast material. Because it does not actually cut, it does not cut into the skin underneath the cast. The medical assistant needs to assure the patient that although he or she will hear a loud noise and feel vibration and some heat from the cast cutter, it will not cut the skin.

Cast Care Instructions

1. Keep the cast uncovered for the first 24 hours to dry thoroughly. Don't allow the plaster cast to rest on a hard surface until it has thoroughly cured (24 to 48 hours), because it can become flattened.
2. Elevate the limb in the cast above the level of the heart as much as possible during the first 24 hours after the cast has been applied. Support it using pillows.
3. Use ice packs around the cast for the first 24 hours, as instructed by the doctor, to reduce swelling.
4. Wiggle fingers or toes frequently to improve circulation. Report any absence of movement, any numbness, or abnormally pale or bluish color.
5. Use a plastic bag over the cast while showering. This is more important for plaster than for fiberglass, but even fiberglass casts should be covered.
6. Note any discoloration of the cast, which may indicate bleeding under the cast. Use a pen to circle discoloration and report if discolored area enlarges over time.
7. Do not insert any object under the cast to scratch, because it can cause skin irritation and infection.
8. Do not seal the cast with paint or varnish. This prevents air from circulating and can cause skin breakdown.
9. Report extreme pain or tightness of the cast, numbness, swelling, or tingling of fingers or toes. Also report any drainage, sharp edges on the cast, or a broken or damaged cast.

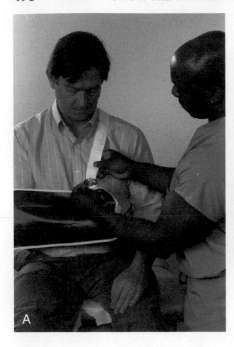
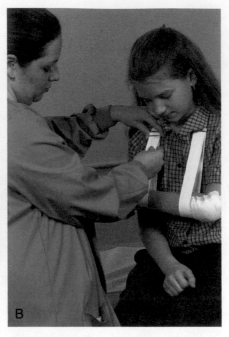

➢ **Figure 21–12** (A) Commercial sling that supports the entire forearm. (B) A sample sling consisting of two loops.

The cast is cut lengthwise along both sides until it is essentially cut in two halves. Then the cast spreader is used to split the cast apart. The padding is cut with large bandage scissors and the two pieces are removed.

Under the cast, the skin is usually pale, dry, sensitive to temperature, and tender to the touch. Depending how long the cast has been on, there may be significant muscle **atrophy** (wasting) under the cast. Skin tone returns to normal relatively quickly, within a few days in most cases. Cream or lotion is used to alleviate the dryness. Over a short time, normal sensation returns.

The doctor may prescribe exercises to strengthen weakened muscles and restore joint mobility. The patient should be encouraged to follow the doctor's instructions in this regard. And, if necessary, physical therapy is used to improve muscle tone and mobility of the extremity.

PROCEDURE 21–9

Applying a Sling Using a Triangular Bandage

Performance Objective: The student will be able to apply a sling using a triangular bandage.

- ☑ Wash hands
- ☐ Gloves
- ☐ Eye and Face Protection
- ☐ Lab Coat or Apron
- ☐ Plastic Biohazard Bag
- ☐ Rigid Biohazard Container

Supplies and Equipment: Large square cloth or muslin bandage material.

Procedure Steps

1. Wash hands.
2. Identify patient.
3. Explain procedure for applying sling.
4. Assemble equipment.
5. Seat patient comfortably as directed by doctor.
6. Fold cloth/muslin material in triangle.
7. Support arm while placing triangular material on chest. Place half of the material under arm on chest and let the other half hang below arm.
8. While continuing to support arm, bring up bottom half of triangle and tie knot on

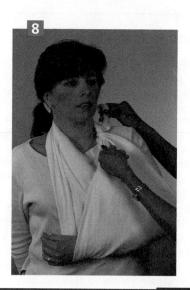

shoulder. Sling should draw arm up slightly as it supports but should not misalign shoulder or wrist placement. The wrist should also be supported, but the hand does not have to be covered by the sling.

Rationale: The sling should support the arm in a functional position with the hand elevated if possible to reduce swelling. The knot should be to one side or over the spine to avoid pressure on the cervical vertebrae.

9. Check for patient comfort and support.
10. Wash hands.
11. Document sling application in patient record.

ON THE JOB

John Daley is a middle-aged, mentally retarded patient who comes to Blackburn Primary Care Associates with a fracture of the right radius. He is accompanied by his brother.

Dr. Hughes applies a short arm cast and gives instructions that John should stay home from his job packing groceries at the local supermarket for 2 days. Although you give John's brother, with whom John lives, complete written and verbal instructions regarding cast care, you need to give John instructions as well.

QUESTIONS

1. What is your goal in giving John instructions for taking care of his cast?
2. How will you adapt your instructions to John's level of comprehension?
3. Why does John need to wear a sling in addition to the cast? What is important when applying the sling each morning?
4. Identify three "do's" and three "don'ts" for John to focus on. Draw simple pictures to illustrate each.

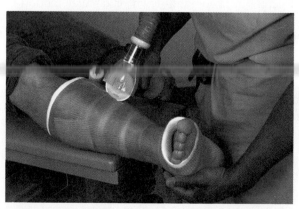

➤ **Figure 21–13** The cast cutter makes a separation in the cast without cutting through the wadding underneath.

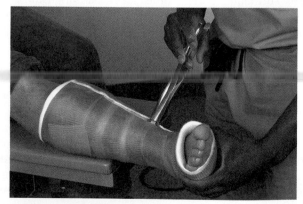

➤ **Figure 21–14** The cast spreader is used to increase the space between the two sections of the cast so that the wadding and stockinette can be cut with scissors.

Physical Medicine, Rehabilitation, and Related Disciplines

Physical Medicine and Rehabilitation. Medical specialty that focuses on restoring function and well-being of patients following injury and disease.

Occupational Therapist. A health care practitioner who evaluates the self-care, work, and play skills of an individual and plans activities to restore, develop, and maintain daily tasks. The occupational therapist may supervise an occupational therapist assistant.

Osteopathy. A medical system that emphasizes the relationship between the musculoskeletal system and organ function as a basis for healthy functioning. The first college of osteopathic medicine was established in Missouri in 1882 by Andrew Taylor Still.

Osteopath (DO). Doctor of Osteopathy; a graduate of an accredited college of osteopathy. In all states, osteopaths are licensed as physicians and able to practice all medical and surgical specialties.

Chiropractic. A system that relies primarily on manipulation of spinal vertebrae to improve body function and comfort.

Chiropractor (DC). A doctor of chiropractic; a licensed practitioner who manipulates the spinal vertebrae and spinal column as a means of restoring health and function of the body. Chiropractors are licensed and their role is limited by state law.

Massage Therapist. Receives training in the use of massage to improve circulation, improve well-being, and induce relaxation.

OTHER PHYSICAL THERAPY TREATMENTS

There are a number of other treatments used in physical medicine and rehabilitation. The doctor in general practice or family medicine may order these treatments in the office, or may refer the patient to a specialist or a physical therapist. Medical assistants may perform these treatments in various settings.

These treatments include:
Ultraviolet (UV) light
Ultrasound
Electric stimulation
Traction
Massage.

Ultraviolet Light

Ultraviolet (**UV**) light refers to the rays beyond the violet end of the light spectrum, invisible to the naked eye. Ultraviolet rays are generated by the sun, as well as by sun lamps and tanning tables. Although ultraviolet rays generate no heat, they do cause changes in the skin (tanning or burning), kill bacteria, and activate formation of vitamin D.

Doctors use the bacteria-killing quality of ultraviolet light rays to treat skin diseases such as acne and psoriasis, and they use the vitamin D formation qualities to promote wound healing.

The angle at which the light hits the skin, as well as the duration of the exposure, are the critical factors in treatment. Treatment is usually for a period of seconds or minutes at the most. The patient's ability to tolerate ultraviolet treatment is determined by testing different length exposure on small patches of skin on the arm and seeing the effect the next day. Redness is acceptable, but burning is not.

Both the patient and the light source operator must wear ultraviolet-blocking goggles, and portions of skin that are not being treated should be covered during treatment. Treatment is usually administered every other day. The length of the exposure must be timed exactly for patient safety, and the patient should never be left unattended while receiving a treatment.

Ultrasound

Ultrasound uses acoustic vibrations beyond human hearing to stimulate tissue. Therapeutic ultrasound works on the same principle as diagnostic ultrasound, producing acoustic vibration of the soft tissue. But whereas diagnostic ultrasound uses the sound signal after it bounces off tissue to visualize an image on a monitor, therapeutic ultrasound uses the vibration, as well as the heat produced by the vibration, to relax muscle tissue or increase elasticity of tendons and ligaments.

The ultrasound applicator (transducer) is about 2″ in diameter. The operator moves the applicator slowly and gently in an up-and-down or circular motion over the skin surface of the area being treated. Because air does not conduct ultrasound, a special gel is used to conduct the ultrasound onto the skin. The applicator must stay in motion all the time, because the intensity of diagnostic ultrasound being used can cause internal burns or tissue damage in the deep tissues being treated if left stationary.

Figure 21–15 shows an ultrasound treatment.

Electrical Stimulation

In electrical stimulation, electrodes are applied to the skin and a small amount of electric current is sent to the patient. The current passes from one electrode to the other through the skin.

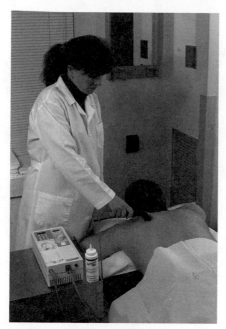

➢ **Figure 21–15** Treatment with an ultrasound machine.

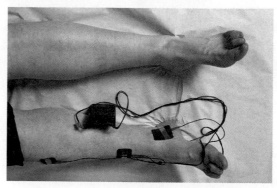

➢ **Figure 21–16** Transcutaneous electrical nerve stimulation (TENS) unit being used on a patient's leg. (From Leahy J, Kizilay P: *Foundations of Nursing Practice.* Philadelphia: W.B. Saunders, 1998.)

The procedure should tingle but not hurt, and the amount of current is regulated by the patient reaction. Electrical stimulation is used to stimulate muscles and joints. It may be used to hasten wound healing, or to reduce pain impulses by overloading neurons with stimulation that is less unpleasant than pain.

A transcutaneous electrical nerve stimulator (**TENS**) unit may be used in the office, or a patient may obtain his or her own unit with a prescription. Figure 21–16 shows a TENS unit. The medical assistant applies the TENS electrodes to the areas as directed and times the treatment.

Traction

Traction is a procedure in which a patient is pulled into a particular position by means of weights, pulleys, and harnesses to correct a musculoskeletal problem. It is most frequently used to:

maintain a proper position over a period of time, for instance in a complex fracture, or a dislocated joint, which must be held stationary for a period of time to promote healing
achieve relief of a compressed vertebral joint
decrease lower back spasm; or
prevent or correct a deformity.

Various types of traction are used in hospitals. Traction may also be built into a cast by means of metal rods attached to the cast and the bones of the patient's skull or extremities.

In the office setting, traction is used most frequently in chiropractors' offices; chiropractors use cervical traction to place tension on the cervical vertebrae and improve the cervical curve. The patient is placed in traction for a limited time, usually 5 to 15 minutes. The treatment may be preceded or followed by application of heat or cold.

Massage

Massage is possibly the original form of physical therapy and is still a regularly utilized piece of the physical therapy regimen. It is a systematic pressure applied to bare skin by rubbing, kneading, stroking, or rolling.

Massage is used to reduce tension, relieve pain, and relax muscles. It is also used to help restore range of motion and function to an injured or diseased area. To obtain the best results, both the patient and practitioner should be in a comfortable, relaxed position. The practitioner's hands should be warm, and he or she should work without straining.

Massage also helps the healing process, by removing blood and waste products from injured tissue and allowing fresh blood to flow to the injured area. A massage is illustrated in Figure 21–17.

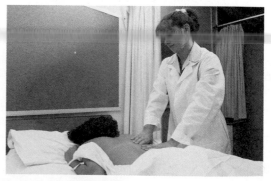

➢ **Figure 21–17** Massage helps relax muscles and relieve pain. (From Leahy J, Kizilay P: *Foundations of Nursing Practice.* Philadelphia: W.B. Saunders, 1998.)

STUDENT STUDY PLAN

To reinforce your understanding of the material in this chapter . . .

Complete the **Review & Recall** questions.

Discuss the situation in **If You Were The Medical Assistant** with your class-mates, and answer the questions.

Answer the **Critical Thinking Questions** and discuss them with your classmates.

Visit the **Web sites** suggested, and search for additional web sites using **Key-words for Internet Searches.**

Complete the exercises in chapter 21 of the **Student Mastery Manual.**

REVIEW & RECALL

1. Describe the measures used to prevent infection during eye irrigations and eye instillations.
2. What instructions should be given to a patient about use of a metered-dose inhaler?
3. Describe how a nebulizer moves medication to the patient's airways.
4. List characteristics of treatments with heat and cold. Identify situations when each modality is used.
5. Differentiate between the use of moist heat and dry heat.
6. List and define five types of bone and joint injuries.
7. How are specific bone and joint injuries usually diagnosed?
8. Describe how a cast is applied and removed.
9. Identify four specific problems with a cast that should be reported promptly to the medical office.
10. Explain why a patient is instructed to elevate an extremity with an injury to bone, joint, or other tissues. Describe specific ways to elevate an arm and a leg.
11. Define the following treatments, and identify what each might be used for: ultraviolet light, ultra-sound, electrical stimulation, traction, and massage.

IF YOU WERE THE MEDICAL ASSISTANT

You have been asked to perform an ear irrigation for Ann Lister, a 12-year-old girl who has never experienced this procedure before. After assembling the equipment, you enter the examination room to begin the procedure.

1. What explanation do you give to Ann about what you are going to do and why the doctor has asked you to do it?
2. How do you position Ann, and what equipment do you set up before you begin the procedure?
3. Just before you begin to introduce the irrigating so-lution, you have to prepare Ann for a sensation that most people find unpleasant. Discuss what it feels like to have your ears irrigated with your classmates or with a friend who has undergone the procedure. How should you describe it for Ann?
4. What should you do if Ann jerks her head away during the procedure, before any cerumen has been removed, so that irrigating solution and your irrigat-ing syringe spill on the floor? Identify your actions in order of importance.

CRITICAL THINKING QUESTIONS

1. Discuss why metered-dose inhalers and nebulizers are an important part of asthma treatment. Consider what could happen if a patient or a patient's family member does not understand how to use them properly.

2. Both heat and cold must be used carefully to avoid skin and tissue damage. Identify several types of patients who are more susceptible to burns or to damage due to cold, and describe ways to prevent tissue injuries to those patients.

3. Compare the guidelines for using heat and cold given in this chapter with beliefs and practices you have experienced before. Identify situations in which you may have seen a person use heat when cold might be more appropriate, or vice versa. What explanation might you use to persuade a person to use cold instead of heat for an acute injury?

4. Describe how you would instruct a patient to apply an elastic bandage (Ace bandage) to a sprained ankle and to determine if it is too tight or too loose. What bandage turn would be most appropriate? Discuss the problems that could arise if the bandage is too tight or not tight enough.

EXPLORE THE WEB

INTERNET WEB SITES
National Rehabilitation Information Center (NRIC)
www.naric.com

KEYWORDS FOR INTERNET SEARCHES

casts	heat treatments	nebulizer	physical therapy
crutch walking	ice packs	occupational therapy	traction

ANSWERS TO ON THE JOB

1. Because it is impossible for John's brother to supervise him from minute to minute, it is important for John to understand what he should and should not do with his cast. Even if he needs frequent reminders, he is more likely to comply if he understands what is important, such as keeping the cast dry or keeping the arm elevated.

2. Focus on instructions for daily care with John. His brother will be responsible for understanding signs and symptoms to report to the doctor. Use short sentences and simple terms to give explanations John can understand. Repeat them as needed.

3. John needs to wear a sling to keep his right forearm elevated with his hands above the elbow and, if possible, above the heart. This helps prevent venous congestion and swelling in the hand. The sling should fit comfortably, and the straps should not press on the bones of his cervical spine. His fingers should be visible beyond the end of the sling.

4. DO'S
Keep cast elevated above heart level.
Wear sling when walking to keep arm elevated.
Wear a plastic bag over the cast for showering.
DON'TS
Let the arm hang down.
Get the cast wet.
Poke anything under the cast.

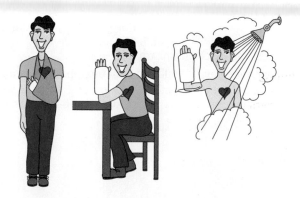

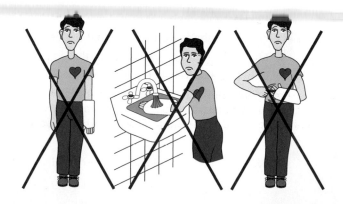

Chapter 22

Preparing and Administering Medications

PART I

Instructional Objectives

After completing this chapter, you will be able to do the following:

1. Define and spell the vocabulary words for this chapter.
2. List five sources of drugs.
3. Differentiate between chemical, generic, and trade names for medications.
4. Differentiate between prescribing, dispensing, and administering a medication.
5. Identify government agencies that regulate medications in the United States.
6. Define and give examples of nonprescription, prescription, and controlled drugs.
7. List the five schedules of controlled substances and regulations for prescription and storage of medication on each schedule.
8. Describe each part of a prescription.
9. Discuss measures to store and dispose of drugs correctly.
10. List four methods to classify medications.
11. Describe the processes that affect the action of a drug in the body.
12. Define forms of medication that can be used for various routes of administration.
13. Use and translate abbreviations commonly used in pharmacology, including the metric, apothecaries', and household systems of measurement.
14. Identify factors affecting medication dosage.
15. Calculate accurate medication doses for adults and children using the apothecaries' and metric systems.
16. Identify principles of safe preparation and administration of medications.

17. List the parts of a needle and syringe, and identify those parts that must remain sterile.
18. Differentiate between subcutaneous, intradermal, and intramuscular injections in terms of appropriate sites, angle of injection, and reasons each route is used.
19. Discuss methods to prevent needle-stick injuries.
20. Identify precautions and their rationales when administering medications.

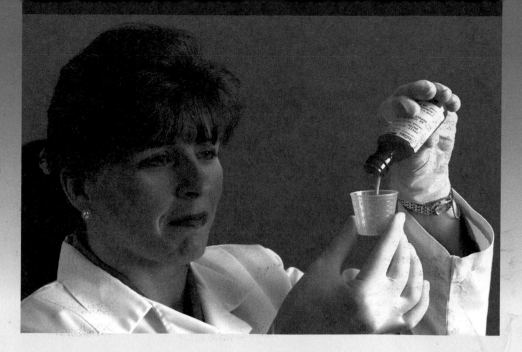

CMA/RMA CERTIFICATION
Content and Competencies

- Apply principles of aseptic technique and infection control
- Prepare and administer medications and immunizations
- Maintain medication and immunization records
- Maintain and dispose of regulated substances in compliance with government guidelines

- Document accurately
- Comply with established risk management and safety procedures
- Maintain awareness of federal and state health care legislation and regulations

Performance Objectives

After completing this chapter, you will be able to do the following:

1. Prepare and administer oral medications (Procedure 22–1).
2. Prepare an injectable medication from an ampule (Procedure 22–2).
3. Prepare an injectable medication from a vial (Procedure 22–3).
4. Reconstitute a powdered medication to prepare an injectable medication (Procedure 22–4).
5. Administer a subcutaneous injection (Procedure 22–5).
6. Select an appropriate site for an intramuscular injection (Procedure 22–6).
7. Administer an intramuscular injection (Procedure 22–7).
8. Administer a Z-track injection (Procedure 22–8).
9. Administer an intradermal injection (Procedure 22–9).
10. Administer a tine or Mantoux test (Procedure 22–10).

VOCABULARY

addiction (p. 488)	diluent (p. 523)	ointment (p. 499)	synergism (p. 497)
administer (p. 488)	dispense (p. 487)	parenteral (p. 502)	syrup (p. 501)
allergy (p. 497)	dorsogluteal (p. 528)	percentage (p. 507)	systemic (p. 494)
ampule (p. 518)	drug (p. 486)	pharmacodynamics (p. 495)	tablet (p. 501)
anaphylaxis (p. 497)	drug abuse (p. 488)	pharmacokinetics (p. 495)	teratogenic (p. 497)
antagonism (p. 497)	elixir (p. 501)	pharmacology (p. 486)	time-release (p. 501)
antidote (p. 497)	enteric coated (p. 501)	potentiation (p. 497)	tolerance (p. 496)
bevel (p. 518)	gauge (p. 518)	prescribe (p. 487)	topical (p. 494)
buccal (p. 501)	generic name (p. 487)	prescription (p. 489)	transdermal (p. 500)
caplet (p. 501)	idiosyncratic (p. 497)	proportion (p. 507)	urticaria (p. 497)
capsule (p. 501)	installation (p. 501)	ratio (p. 507)	vastus lateralis (p. 529)
contraindicated (p. 497)	liniment (p. 499)	solution (p. 501)	ventrogluteal (p. 529)
controlled substance (p. 488)	lumen (p. 518)	sublingual (p. 501)	vial (p. 518)
cross-sensitivity (p. 497)	meniscus (p. 514)	suppository (p. 501)	wheal (p. 540)
deltoid (p. 528)	nomogram (p. 509)	suspension (p. 501)	

ABBREVIATIONS

BSA (p. 496)   DEA (p. 488)   FDA (p. 487)   OTC (p. 490)   USP/NF (p. 497)   VO (p. 511)
cc (p. 504)

PART I

BASICS OF PHARMACOLOGY

Pharmacology is the study of the sources, uses, and means of action of pharmaceuticals (**drugs**). Pharmacologists study the potentially helpful effects of the various chemical components of animal, mineral, plant, synthetic, or genetically engineered substances. Pharmacology also involves the scientific study to determine active ingredients and to verify that chemicals do have the desired effect and do not have dangerous side effects.

Sources of Drugs

Throughout history, people have derived medicinal compounds (drugs) from natural sources, especially plants. Today, the majority of drugs are derived from chemical compounds synthesized in the laboratory. However, many of those chemical compounds have their origins in the chemicals found in natural substances. In the 21st century, scientists are finding it increasingly possible to genetically engineer substances that occur naturally in humans or other animals.

One example of a drug produced from an animal is insulin. An individual whose pancreas does not produce enough insulin cannot use glucose effectively for the body's energy needs (a condition known as diabetes mellitus). Insulin from the pancreas of animals such as cattle or pigs has long been used for injections for diabetic patients.

Minerals such as salt (sodium chloride), iron, calcium, and potassium are all necessary for good health. For people whose bodies do not absorb enough of these, supplement tablets provide concentrated doses. Even the mineral gold has been used to treat rheumatoid arthritis.

Plants provide a multitude of both medical and mind-altering substances. Many Americans use "natural" plant remedies such as garlic, ginkgo biloba, ginger, and chamomile. Individuals from Asian, South American, and Caribbean cultures often supplement Western medical treatment with herbal or plant-based treatments such as ginseng, Ma huang (which contains ephedrine), Dong quai, or Kava Kava. Even the Western medical list has its share of plant-based medications in it. Digitalis comes from the foxglove plant and quinine from cinchona bark.

Legal mind-altering drugs such as nicotine, found in tobacco (which has sedative and vasoconstrictive properties), and the stimulant caffeine, found in coffee, tea, chocolate, and cola, are the most common. Alcohol, a sedative, comes from the natural fermentation process of various grains such as rye, barley, corn, and potatoes, as well as grapes.

Many illegal mind-altering drugs also are plant based. Heroin, a sedative-hypnotic, comes from the opium poppy; cocaine, a stimulant, from coca leaf (a shrub called *Erythroxylon coca*) and marijuana, a sedative, from the hemp plant (*Cannabis sativa*). These plant compounds have some medicinal properties.

When refined, heroin becomes morphine, which is used to relieve severe pain. Cocaine was used medicinally in the early part of the 20th century as a local anesthetic. And the argument continues today over medicinal uses of marijuana, which has been shown in some experiments to reduce the intraocular pressure of glaucoma, as well as the nausea caused by some cancer treatments.

Chemically synthesized compounds have replaced some of these natural substances. For instance, many people take vitamin C tablets instead of drinking citrus fruit juice. Multivitamins contain many of the minerals people do not get enough of, either because of their diet or because these minerals are found in small quantities in food.

Genetic engineering is also used to produce synthetic analogs of some substances. For instance, the genetically engineered product Humulin has replaced most bovine or porcine insulin for diabetics because it does not contain the variations in chemical structure that have often caused allergic reactions to bovine insulin.

Drug Names

Any manufactured drug (not a naturally occurring substance) has three types of names. The first is the chemical name. This describes the chemical compound. The second name is called the **generic name.** This name is assigned by the United States Adopted Name Council and is given to the company that discovers the chemical compound. The third name is the trade name, or brand name. This name is applied for by any company that manufactures the compound, approved by the U.S. Food and Drug Administration (FDA), and registered with the U.S. patent office.

The trade name is always capitalized and usually identified with the symbol for being patented; a generic name may be spelled lower case.

When a new chemical compound is discovered, a patent is applied for. When the patent is approved, the company that owns the patent has 17 years during which to conduct all safety and effectiveness research, manufacture, and market the drug under the trade name it has chosen. After the 17-year patent life has expired, any company can manufacture the compound under a different brand name, or sometimes under no brand name at all, as "generic" drugs. Any company that manufactures a generic of a formerly patented brand-name drug must match the chemical composition and must manufacture to the same FDA standards.

For instance, a particular drug has the chemical name: 4-dimethylamino-1, 4, 4a, 5, 5a, 6, 11, 121-octahydro-3, 6, 10, 12, 12-a-pentahydroxy-6-methyl-1, 11-dioxo2-naphthacenecarboxamide.

The generic name for this drug is tetracycline, a broad-spectrum antibiotic.

No company has held a patent on tetracycline for a number of years. Tetracycline is thus considered an "off-patent" drug and has been manufactured by a number of companies under the brand names Achromycin, Panmycin, Robitet, Sumycin, Tetracyn, Topicycline, and other names.

Many times, a doctor will specify in a prescription that a brand-name drug be used. But for tetracycline, all of the brands are manufactured to the same degree of purity, strength, and chemical composition. What varies are substances used to shape the pill or capsule, called binders. There may also be slight variation in the medication's inactive chemical structures.

Brand-name medications are usually more expensive than their generic counterparts. A doctor can order a specific brand name and stipulate that no generic form can be substituted. In most states, the pharmacist can substitute a generic unless the doctor indicates that no substitutions are allowed. Doctors have had to learn about reimbursement procedures of many health maintenance organizations (HMOs); although a doctor can always order any medication, in some HMO plans the patient must either pay a larger co-payment for brand-name drugs than for generics or must pay the actual difference in cost between the generic and the brand name. In the case of "new" drugs, for which there are not yet any generic substitutes, the higher co-payment rule usually applies.

Laws Regulating Medications and Controlled Substances

Three activities take place in the medical office regarding medication. For each of these—prescribing, dispensing, and administering—federal and/or state laws and regulations come into play.

To **prescribe** a drug is to determine that an individual should take a drug as treatment for a specific illness or condition. Prescribing is a responsibility of a licensed professional. In some states, only an M.D., D.O., D.M.D. (dentist), D.D.S. (dental surgeon), or D.P.M. (podiatrist) can prescribe. In other states, advanced-practice nurses (nurse practitioners) and physician's assistants are legally allowed to prescribe.

A medical assistant cannot prescribe and should not tell a patient or a friend what medications to take to treat a particular condition. A medical assistant should not authorize pharmacy refills without written direction from a doctor.

If the doctor has established written guidelines for a patient, a medical assistant may review those with the patient. For example, the office may have written instructions for pregnant patients that state that the pregnant patient may take acetaminophen for headaches.

To **dispense** a drug means to give a patient a supply of a medication to take later. This is primarily a job of a pharmacist working from a prescription written by a licensed health care provider. A doctor can dispense medication, usually in small amounts. This is usually done by giving a patient one or two one-day dose samples provided by drug companies. If instructed by a doctor, a medical assistant may also give samples, but always as an agent of the doctor. A medical assistant should never dispense samples independently.

To **administer** a drug is to give one dose of a medication as directed by a licensed practitioner who can prescribe. State laws vary, but some states permit medical assistants to administer medication as directed by a doctor. A medical assistant is responsible for knowing the law in the state in which he or she is working.

A medical assistant should never administer medication unless there is a doctor in the office and able to respond to any problem that might arise. When a doctor delegates administration of a medication, the medical assistant is acting as an agent of the doctor. At the same time, however, the medical assistant is responsible for his or her own actions.

A medical assistant must always follow proper procedures for administering medication. These procedures will be discussed in detail later in this chapter. In general, a medical assistant cannot give medication as an agent of a nurse practitioner or a physician's assistant.

The FDA, part of the Department of Health and Human Services, regulates which drugs can be sold in the United States. The FDA is also responsible for regulating and enforcing standards of purity for drug manufacture, labeling, and interstate transport of drugs.

Before a new drug can be sold, it must be approved by the FDA. This requires animal trials, as well as a series of clinical trials in humans. The first human trials are conducted on a small number of healthy patients to judge the safety of the compound. Then a series of studies on larger groups of people with the condition to be treated are conducted to determine how effective the compound is at various doses.

All preparations of a drug need to conform to standards of quality, purity, and strength. If drug safety is questioned during clinical trials or after the drug is on the market, the FDA may order the drug removed from the market. An example of this was the removal in 1997 of the diet drug fenfluramine. The "fen" in phen-fen was found to cause serious heart-valve problems.

Controlled Substances

The Controlled Substances Act of 1970 regulates the prescription, dispensing, and administering of controlled substances. A **controlled substance** is a drug that has a potential for addiction and abuse, and is therefore subject to additional legal restrictions. **Addiction** is a need to continue using a substance due to

physiological or psychological dependence. **Drug abuse** is the continued desire for and willful misuse of a substance that is not medically indicated.

The Drug Enforcement Agency **(DEA)** enforces the Controlled Substances Act. Doctors who prescribe controlled substances must register with the DEA and renew their registration every 2 years. Appendix A contains the address, phone, and Web site for the DEA. Table 22–1 shows the five schedules of controlled substances. The DEA constantly updates these schedules and mails them to doctors on its mailing list. Schedule I controlled substances have the highest potential for abuse and currently have no accepted medical use in the United States, whereas Schedule V controlled substances have the lowest potential for abuse.

Federal law requires that controlled substances be stored away from other medications, in a secure, double-locked box or drawer—a box or drawer with an outer lock or key and an inner compartment that also has a lock or key. A doctor may not legally obtain Schedule I controlled substances, unless participating in an authorized experiment. Schedule II controlled substances are ordered from a manufacturer or a distributor using the Federal Triplicate Order Form DEA 222. Schedule III through V controlled substances do not require the special triplicate form; however, they do require that invoices and packing slips be kept for 2 years.

If controlled substances are kept in a medical office, an inventory sheet must be maintained. The controlled substance stock must be counted daily and verified by a second person. The two people must sign the inventory sheet. Every 2 years, a record of daily inventory of controlled substances must be submitted to the DEA. If controlled substances need to be wasted or destroyed, two witnesses must sign the inventory sheet. If any controlled substances are stolen, local police must be alerted immediately.

Prescribing, dispensing, and/or administering controlled substances also requires documentation. States vary on what paperwork is necessary; some require a triplicate form for Schedule II prescriptions, while others do not. Any doctor copies from controlled substance triplicate forms should be kept in a secure, fireproof safe or other storage. If controlled substances are administered or dispensed only rarely, records can be kept in the patients' records and made available to DEA investigation.

The doctor's DEA registration number should not be preprinted on prescription forms. Some doctors write their DEA number on any prescription for a controlled substance; others do not and the pharmacy independently gets the DEA number after the prescription has been delivered by the patient.

A medical assistant must know the legal requirements regarding controlled substances that have been set by the DEA and the state in which he or she works. A medical assistant will often be responsible for

Table 22–1	**Controlled Substances**		
Schedule	Description	Legal Restrictions	Examples
Schedule I	No accepted medical use High potential for addiction and/or abuse	May only be used in certain controlled research experiments	Heroin, marijuana, lysergic acid diethylamide (LSD), mescaline, peyote
Schedule II	High potential for addiction and/or abuse Narcotics; stimulants such as cocaine and amphetamines; depressants in the barbiturate group	Can only be prescribed by doctor who has received a license from the Drug Enforcement Administration (DEA number) Requires a handwritten prescription with DEA number; prescription cannot be refilled. A special prescription form is used in many states.	Morphine, injectable codeine, secobarbital (Seconal), meperidine, methadone, methylphenidate (Ritalin); Percodan (oxycodone/aspirin); Percocet (oxycodone/acetaminophen)
Schedule III	Potential for dependence but lesser potential for abuse Combination drugs may contain small amounts of narotics or amphetamine-like substances	Requires handwritten prescription; up to five refills in 6 months as written on the original prescription	Codeine in combination with non-narcotic drugs (such as acetaminophen with codeine); anabolic steroids, hydrocodone and butabarbital compounds in combination with non-narcotic drugs
Schedule IV	Minor tranquilizers and sleep-inducing medications with less potential for abuse	Up to five refills in 6 months Prescription requires doctor signature but refills may be authorized by telephone.	Chlordiazepoxide (Librium), diazepam (Valium), phenobarbital, flurazepam (Dalmane), chloral hydrate, propoxyphene (Darvon)
Schedule V	Miscellaneous mixtures containing limited amounts of narcotic drugs; cough syrups containing codeine Less potential for abuse	Prescriptions and refills are the same as Schedule IV	Diphenoxylate (Lomotil); various cold and cough syrups such as brompheniramine and guaifenesin in preparations that contain codeine

flagging the doctor's DEA registration renewal date, as well as for providing security and inventory record keeping of all controlled substances. A medical assistant may also be responsible for properly disposing of expired controlled substances and keeping records.

Prescriptions

Federal law also identifies drugs that require a prescription. A **prescription** is an order from a doctor or other licensed health care provider to a pharmacist to dispense a supply of medication. Individual states have different regulations within a set of federal guidelines. The medical assistant must know the laws of the state in which he or she works.

Eight pieces of information are found on a prescription, in addition to the doctor's address and telephone number:

1. Date: A prescription must be filled within 6 months of the date.
2. Patient name and address: A prescription can only be filled for the person named.
3. Superscription: The abbreviation Rx, which

means "take thou." This is usually preprinted on the prescription pad.
4. Inscription: The name of the drug, its desired form, and strength.
5. Subscription: The amount of the drug the pharmacist is to dispense. This is written either as a number of pills, suppositories, and so on, or an amount of liquid medication.
6. Signature: Sig. means "write on label." This is the instructions to be written for the patient, such as how often to take the medication, what conditions to take it for, and other special instructions.
7. Refills: Controlled substances can usually be refilled for up to 6 months, other drugs for up to 1 year. The number of refills is indicated by a number, the abbreviation NR (no refills), or the abbreviation PRN. The pharmacy will only refill a prescription at the time interval that indicates the patient is taking the medication as directed (i.e., 30 pills at a time each month for a once-a-day prescription).
8. Provider's signature.

The doctor may also write on the prescription whether a generic substitute may be provided. Different

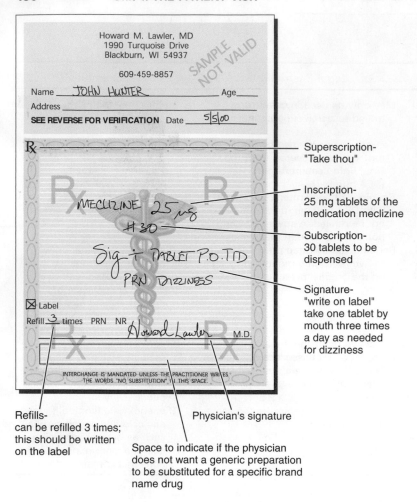

Howard M. Lawler, MD
1990 Turquoise Drive
Blackburn, WI 54937

SAMPLE NOT VALID

609-459-8857

Name _JOHN HUNTER_____ Age____

Address _____

SEE REVERSE FOR VERIFICATION Date __5|5|00__

℞

MECLIZINE 25 mg

30

Sig – 1 TABLET P.O. TID

PRN DIZZINESS

☒ Label

Refill _3_ times   PRN   NR

Howard Lawler M.D.

INTERCHANGE IS MANDATED UNLESS THE PRACTITIONER WRITES
THE WORDS "NO SUBSTITUTION" IN THIS SPACE.

Superscription–
"Take thou"

Inscription–
25 mg tablets of the
medication meclizine

Subscription–
30 tablets to be
dispensed

Signature–
"write on label"
take one tablet by
mouth three times
a day as needed
for dizziness

Refills–
can be refilled 3 times;
this should be written
on the label

Physician's signature

Space to indicate if the physician
does not want a generic preparation
to be substituted for a specific brand
name drug

➤ **Figure 22–1** Parts of a prescription; many prescription pads are white, but colored forms are more difficult to copy or alter.

states have different laws regarding whether a generic may be substituted for a brand-name drug.

Figure 22–1 shows the parts of a sample prescription.

In most states, a doctor or a member of the office staff may telephone a prescription for any drug except a Schedule II controlled substance to a pharmacy. When a medical assistant calls in a prescription, he or she must have the doctor's order and give the pharmacist or pharmacy technician all of the necessary information about the patient's name, the drug name, the desired form and strength, the amount to dispense, instructions to the patient, refills if applicable, and if a generic substitution is proper.

Prescription pads should always be stored in a secure location to avoid theft. The doctor usually keeps one in his or her pocket when seeing patients. If the doctor wears a white coat and the office uses a laundry service, whoever sends coats to be laundered must check the pockets and remove any prescription pads.

All prescriptions should be documented in the medical record. The doctor documents when he or she writes a prescription during the patient visit. The medical assistant may document in the progress note when calling a prescription to the pharmacy if the doctor has written the order on a telephone message slip. (It is good practice to keep the message slip with the patient's record.)

Table 22–2 shows the most commonly prescribed drugs in 1999.

Over-the-Counter Drugs

Nonprescription drugs, called over-the-counter **(OTC)** medications, are considered safe enough to be used without a doctor's advice and prescription. When obtaining the list of medications a patient is taking as part of the medical history, a medical assistant should always ask about which OTC medications the patient

Table 22—2	**Most Common Prescriptions (New and Refill) Dispensed in 1999**	

Rank	Brand Name (Manufacturer)	Generic Name
1	Premarin (Wyeth-Ayerst)	Conjugated estrogens
*2	Synthroid (Knoll)	Levothyroxine
3	Lipitor (Parke-Davis)	Atorvastatin
4	Prilosec (Astra)	Omeprazole
*5	Hydrocodone w/APAP** (Watson)	Hydrocodone w/APAP**
6	Albuterol (Warrick)	Albuterol
7	Norvasc (Pfizer)	Amlodipine
8	Claritin (Schering)	Loratadine
*9	Trimox (Apothecon)	Amoxicillin
10	Prozac (Lilly)	Fluoxetine
11	Zoloft (Pfizer)	Sertraline
12	Glucophage (B-M Squibb)	Metformin
13	Lanoxin (Glaxo Wellcome)	Digoxin
14	Prempro (Wyeth-Ayerst)	Conjugated estrogens/medroxyprogesterone
15	Paxil (SK Beecham)	Paroxetine
16	Zithromax Z-Pack (Pfizer)	Azithromycin
17	Zestril (Zeneca)	Lisinopril
18	Zocor (Merck)	Simvastatin
19	Prevacid (Tap Pharm)	Lansoprazole
*20	Augmentin (SK Beecham)	Amoxicillin/clavulanate
21	Celebrex (Searle)	Celecoxib
*22	Hydrocodone w/APAP** (Mallinckrot)	Hydrocodone w/APAP**
23	Coumadin (Dupont)	Warfarin
24	Vasotec (Merck)	Enalapril
*25	Amoxicillin (Teva Pharm)	Amoxicillin
26	Furosemide (Mylan)	Furosemide
*27	Levoxyl (Jones Medical Ind)	Levothyroxine
28	Cipro (Bayer Pharm)	Ciprofloxacin
29	Cephalexin (Teva Pharm)	Cephalexin
30	K-Dur (Key Pharm)	Potassium chloride
31	Prednisone (Schein)	Prednisone
32	Pravachol (B-M Squibb)	Pravastatin
*33	Amoxil (SK Beecham)	Amoxicillin
34	Trimethoprim/sulfa (Teva Pharm)	Trimethaprim/sulfamethoxazole
35	Biaxin (Abbott)	Clarithromycin
36	Ortho Tri-Cyclen (Ortho Pharm)	Norgestimate/ethinyl estradiol
37	Acetaminophen/codeine (Teva Pharm)	Acetaminophen/codeine
38	Atenolol (Geneva)	Atenolol
39	Zyrtec (Pfizer)	Cetirizine
40	Ambien (Searle)	Zolpidem
*41	Propoxyphene N/APAP** (Mylan)	Propoxyphene N/APAP**
*42	Propoxyphene N/APAP** (Teva Pharm)	Propoxyphene N/APAP**
43	Alprazolam (Greenstone)	Alprazolam
44	Ultram (McNeil)	Tramadol
45	Accupril (Parke-Davis)	Quinapril
46	Prinivil (Merck)	Lisinopril
47	Cardizem CD (Hoech Mar R)	Diltiazem
48	Glucotrol XL (Pfizer)	Glipizide
49	Allegra (Hoech Mar R)	Fexofenadine
50	Toprol-XL (Astra)	Metoprolol

* Note that some popular drugs are prescribed in more than one strength or by specific brand name(s) as well as by generic name.
** APAP is an abbreviation for acetaminophen.
From www.rxlist.com/top 200.htm

takes regularly. OTC medications can have adverse interactions with prescription drugs.

For example, a patient taking the prescription drug Coumadin, an anticoagulant, may be advised not to take aspirin or ginkgo biloba, both of which have side effects like the prescription anticoagulant.

Storage and Disposal of Medications

Medication, including samples, as well as prescription pads, should always be stored away from patients. They should never be stored in examination or treatment rooms but in a central secure cabinet. Medications should be stored in a cool place and protected from light (they should be stored in opaque bottles). Some medications need refrigeration; if they do, it will be written on the label. External medications such as creams, lotions, eye drops, and eardrops should be stored separate from internal medications, in order to avoid accidental ingestion of the external medications.

When disposing of expired medications, take care to prevent accidental ingestion by patients. Review expiration dates on medication regularly and discard outdated medication. Also discard any medication that has become discolored, any medications without labels, and any tablets that have dropped or been touched. Any medication that has been prepared but for some reason was not given should also be discarded.

Liquids should be discarded down the drain. Powders should be mixed with water, then discarded down the drain. Pills should be flushed down the toilet. For controlled substances, expired medication should be sent back to the pharmacy or distributor. Any that has been spilled or excess medication in a prefilled syringe must be wasted. Two people must witness such disposal and document it.

Syringes should be disposed of in rigid biohazard containers (sharps containers) that have been constructed to prevent retrieval. Never cut needles to prevent needle-stick injury. Never recap a syringe. Biohazard containers in exam rooms must be bolted to the wall with a lock mechanism to prevent removal of the box or individual syringes.

All prescriptions need to be recorded in the patient record. Before issuing a new prescription, most doctors require the patient to visit the office. If a patient is taking a medication that can be easily abused, most doctors require more frequent visits. The biggest clue

---

IDENTIFYING AND PREVENTING DRUG ABUSE

Drug abuse is one of the most underreported and undertreated diseases. Any drug can be abused. Drug abuse is overuse of a drug or use of a drug for the wrong purpose. Abuse can be one-time use that is excessive or it can be chronic use.

Research is increasingly pointing to the likelihood of a genetic predisposition to drug abuse. And more is being learned about the relationship between drug abuse and brain chemistry.

For instance, most people can take a powerful painkiller such as Percocet or Demerol and be relieved of acute pain. When the effect of the drug wears off, assuming the pain has gone away, those people have no need for another dose of the painkiller.

Other people, however, have a psychological or physiologic need to take painkilling medication. They engage in constant drug-seeking activity to get the pleasurable "high" or relief from unpleasant feelings that comes from a "hit" of Percocet or Demerol. If they cannot acquire prescription pain medication, they may fulfill their need with legal drugs such as alcohol, caffeine, or nicotine; abuse prescription drugs; or turn to street drugs such as cocaine, heroin, or marijuana, among others.

Prescription drugs that are commonly abused are those that have a significant effect on the central nervous system, either as central nervous system depressants/sedatives, such as Valium or barbiturates, or as stimulants, such as Dexedrine or Ritalin.

Some of the tip-offs that a patient is abusing prescription drugs include:

1. A new patient complaining of severe pain, insomnia, or severe agitation
2. An established patient who calls for refills more frequently than prescribed, especially with lots of excuses for "losing" medication or lots of "new problems" that cause anxiety and stress
3. A pharmacist who calls with questions about a prescription or a patient.

Clues that a patient is using street drugs include:

1. In a teenage patient, behavior changes, poor grades, new "undesirable" friends, and/or withdrawal from formerly enjoyable social activities
2. Stuffy nose, constant sniffing, or visible damage to nasal mucosa from cocaine use
3. Complaints of severe pain requiring an injection (more

commonly seen in hospital emergency rooms, because most offices don't keep narcotics)

4. Jumpiness, sweating, and needle marks.

If you believe a patient is either using street drugs or abusing prescription drugs, encourage the patient to discuss the use/abuse with the doctor.

Tell any patient wishing for a telephone refill of any drug that can be abused that the patient must be seen in the office before any refill can be issued. Refer any pharmacy questions to the doctor, with the patient's chart. Record *all* refills in the patient record. Keep needles, syringes, and prescription pads out of exam rooms.

If a patient has a drug problem, support and understanding are essential. Encourage the patient to have an honest, open discussion with the doctor about options for treating the drug problem. Offer referrals to treatment programs.

Perhaps more difficult than dealing with a patient with a drug problem is dealing with a colleague, or even a supervisor or doctor in the office, who has a drug (or alcohol) problem. It is not considered "cool" to "squeal" or "rat" on a coworker or to "blow the whistle" on someone higher in the organization.

There is a long tradition of loyalty to one's own social group, be it family, coworkers, or larger social units. Doctors especially have stuck together, regarding their loyalty to each other as an integral part of their profession.

Fortunately, the current mindset is to put the public welfare above personal loyalty, even in issues where there are not clear legal guidelines. Each medical assistant needs to establish his or her own process for deciding how to make difficult choices when loyalties conflict.

If a law is being broken, a medical assistant's duty is obvious. If a medical assistant becomes aware that a coworker's illegal actions threaten the patients or the medical practice, she or he has an obligation to report that knowledge to the person's

supervisor or even to regulatory, licensing, or criminal justice authorities. Any such report should be based on sufficient evidence to be sure that the report is justified. This applies to supervisors and doctors as well.

For example, if there is evidence that a coworker is stealing prescription pads from the office, the medical assistant must report it.

When no law is being broken, or when the medical assistant has suspicions but no firm evidence, it may be more difficult to decide what to do.

For example, it is not illegal to drink alcohol, even to excess. But it is considered unprofessional to perform any medical procedure requiring physical coordination or mental acuity (essentially to practice medicine) while under the influence of alcohol.

When a suspicion arises that a coworker, supervisor, or doctor is impaired by his or her use or abuse of alcohol or prescription drugs, the medical assistant should consider:

1. The frequency and degree of impairment
2. The amount of evidence
3. The potential harm to patients and, less urgently, to the practice's reputation.

Possible interventions include discussing the problem with the individual who is suspected to be abusing drugs or alcohol, discussing the problem with a colleague, discussing the problem with the person's supervisor and, in the case of a licensed professional, making a report to the state licensing agency. Substance abuse is often accompanied by a tendency to dismiss or downplay the problem and a willingness to make promises that will not be kept.

Unless patient care is directly threatened, the medical assistant should give the person a reasonable opportunity to correct his or her behavior in the office setting, while being aware that the impaired person may not be in control of his or her behavior because of the addiction.

that a patient is abusing a prescription medication is frequent telephone calls with excuses for needing "emergency" refills, such as:

medication was lost
medication was left at someone's house
medication fell in the toilet.

Other clues are a call from a patient who hasn't been seen recently requesting a prescription for a controlled substance, a reluctance to make an appointment, and calls from a number of pharmacies confirming the amount and the drug prescribed for a single patient. If you suspect that a patient is abusing pre-

scription drugs, street drugs or alcohol, do not confront the patient yourself; rather, refer the matter to the patient's primary practitioner.

Classification of Drugs

There are a number of different ways of classifying drugs. The most frequently used classification systems are: 1) the extent of the drug's effect; 2) the desired action; how the drug works; 3) the body system affected; and 4) the chemical structure.

The extent of the effect describes whether the drug acts locally or throughout the body. A drug that has a

Table 22-3	Classification of Medications by Therapeutic Effect	
Group	Therapeutic Effect	Example(s)
Analgesic	Relieves pain	
narcotic analgesic	relieves moderate to severe pain	morphine, codeine
non-narcotic analgesic	relieves mild to moderate pain	acetaminophen, ibuprofen
Anesthetic	Produces loss of sensation	Xylocaine, Novocain
Antacid	Decreases gastric acidity	Maalox, calcium carbonate
Antianginal	Decreases angina pectoris by dilating arterioles	nitroglycerin
Antiarrhythmic	Decreases abnormal heartbeats	lidocaine
Anticoagulant	Delays blood clotting	heparin, Coumadin
Anticonvulsant	Prevents seizures	phenytoin, phenobarbital
Antidepressant	Reduces depression	Prozac
Antidiabetic (hypoglycemic)	Reduces serum glucose	insulin
Antihypertensive	Prevents high blood pressure	atenolol
Anti-infective	Prevents growth of microorganisms	penicillin, tetracycline
Anti-inflammatory	Prevents or decreases inflammation	
steroidal	mimics anti-inflammatory action of hormones	cortisone, prednisolone
nonsteroidal	relieves inflammation by inhibiting prostaglandin synthesis	ibuprofen
Antineoplastic	Reduces growth of tumors	methotrexate
Antipyretic	Reduces fever	acetaminophen, ibuprofen
Antitussive	Suppresses cough reflex	dextromethorphan, codeine
Antiulcer	Prevents ulcers	cimetidine, ranitidine
Bronchodilator	Dilates bronchioles	albuterol, epinephrine
Cardiotonic	Increases force of cardiac contraction	digoxin
Diuretic	Increases urine output	furosemide, hydrochlorothiazide
Expectorant	Makes oral secretions more liquid	guaifenesin
Hematinic	Promotes formation of blood cells	ferrous sulfate
Hormone	Decreases serum glucose	insulin
Laxative	Promotes bowel movements	milk of magnesia, magnesium citrate
Sedative/ hypnotic	Reduces anxiety; in larger doses causes sleep	phenobarbital
Skeletal muscle relaxant	Reduces spasm of skeletal muscles	methocarbamol
Thrombolytic	Reduces size of blood clots	alteplase

topical effect acts in the areas where it is applied, as for example, eyedrops and antibiotic skin cream. A drug that works by remote action targets a specific organ or tissue. An example would be a diuretic, which targets cells of the kidney to prevent water reabsorption. A **systemic** drug has effects on cells throughout the body and can be taken by mouth or by an injection. An example would be ibuprofen or another analgesic.

Desired action is a common classification system that identifies the effect for which the drug is given. Examples of desired action are analgesia (pain relief) and mood elevation (antidepressant). Table 22–3 shows common drug groups classified by their desired effect.

How a drug works, or physiologic action, is a classification system that identifies groups of medications that affect similar types of tissues or receptors. Examples include anticholinergics, which interfere with the parasympathetic nervous system; beta-adrenergic blocking agents, which block certain cells (beta cells) of the sympathetic nervous system; or calcium channel blockers, which prevent calcium from being transported into cardiac muscles and other smooth muscle. Table 22–4 shows common drug groups classified by physiologic action.

Another way of grouping medications is through identification of the body system that the drug is given to affect, such as the cardiovascular system or the musculoskeletal system.

Finally it is possible to classify drugs is by chemical structure. Hormones, alcohols, and minerals are examples of a chemical class of drugs; a more specific group is cardiac glycosides, substances affecting the heart that can be chemically broken down into a sugar and another substance. These are active chemical ingredients of digitalis preparations.

Action of Drugs in the Body

There are five stages of a medication's action in the body:

1. absorption
2. distribution

3. effects on cells and tissues (sometimes called the action)
4. metabolism (sometimes called biotransformation)
5. excretion.

The study of how a specific drug undergoes these five stages is called **pharmacokinetics.**

Absorption

Absorption refers to how a drug is broken down and absorbed into the body's circulating fluids. How the drug is administered plays a large part in how quickly it is absorbed. Even drugs used for a local effect have some systemic effects.

For drugs taken orally, it is possible for a drug manufacturer to put the active ingredients inside a transport substance that breaks down in a specific region of the gastrointestinal system. This allows the medication to either be released over a specific time or to target specific areas of the body more effectively.

Examples of time-release medications are certain cold preparations, in which some of the medication dissolves quickly and other parts have a coating that delays digestion and absorption. Some drugs break down in the small intestine to treat small-bowel disease (mesalamine [Asacol]); others break down in the large intestine to treat disease in the colon (sulfasalazine [Azulfidine]).

Distribution

Distribution refers to the way a medication is transported from where it enters the body to various parts of the body, especially the area on which it is supposed to have a therapeutic effect.

One of the most important issues is how much of a particular drug crosses the blood-brain barrier, the barrier between the brain's tissue and the capillaries that carry blood through the brain. For a medication to relieve pain and discomfort, it must cross the blood-brain barrier in sufficient amounts for the brain to process fewer pain signals from the body.

Many medications can also cross the barrier from a woman to a fetus, which is why it is so important for a pregnant woman to speak with her doctor before taking any OTC medication as well as prescription medication. Many medications that are harmless to an adult or even a child are dangerous to a developing fetus.

Action

Effects on cells and tissues, or drug action, refers to how the medication actually causes a physiologic change. The study of these actions is called **pharmacodynamics.**

Every drug causes some kind of cellular change, either temporary or permanent. Drugs called agonists bind to particular cells and produce a functional change in that cell's behavior. Other drugs, called an-

Table 22–4	Classification of Medications by Physiologic Action	
Group	Therapeutic Effect	Example(s)
Anticholinergic	Blocks the effects of acetylcholine	atropine
Antihistamine	Blocks the effect of histamine; results in decreased nasal stuffiness and suppression of itching or other allergic response	diphenhydramine
Beta-adrenergic blocking agent	Blocks effects of epinephrine and norepinephrine at β-adrenergic receptor; results in decreased blood pressure	propranolol
Antacid	Decreases gastric acidity	Maalox, calcium carbonate
Calcium channel blocker	Causes vasodilation, resulting in decreased blood pressure and less severe angina pectoris	diltiazem
Cholinergic	Prolongs the action of acetylcholine; used in the treatment of myasthenia gravis	pyridostigmine
Histamine (H_2) antagonist	Inhibits gastric secretions; used in the treatment of ulcers and gastric hyperacidity	cimetidine
Immunosuppressants	Inhibits lymphocytes; used to prevent rejection of transplants	cyclosporine
Neuromuscular blocking agent	Inhibits transmission of nerve impulses; used when an endotracheal tube is placed in the trachea and while a patient is on a ventilator	succinylcholine
Vasodilator	Causes dilation of blood vessels; used in the treatment of angina pectoris	nitroglycerin
Vasopressor	Causes constriction of blood vessels; used in the treatment of shock	dopamine

tagonists, bind to particular cells and block a sequence of biochemical events from happening. Depending on what the cells normally do, an agonist or antagonist can either stimulate (enhance) or depress (reduce) the cell's normal function.

Still other drugs act by changing the way a particular enzyme functions, thus preventing the enzyme from interacting with cells the way it usually does. Other drugs alter the biochemical process within certain cells or affect the cell membrane. Such a change in a cell membrane changes the membrane's permeability, the ability of ions to cross the membrane. Some drugs act not by changing the cellular function of body cells but of the cells of an invading microorganism.

Metabolism

Metabolism of a drug refers to the process by which the drug is broken down into harmless chemical by-products. Most of this metabolism takes place in the liver. Once a medication is metabolized by the liver, it is transported to the kidneys, where it is diluted in the water the body is going to eliminate.

Excretion

Excretion refers to the process of eliminating the drug's byproducts from the body. Most excretion of drug metabolites (byproducts) occurs in urine, which is formed in the kidneys, stored in the bladder, and then eliminated. This is why urine is used as the quickest, easiest, and least costly way to screen for illegal drug use by employers, schools, and drug-treatment programs. Different metabolites remain in the body for different amounts of time, and several random urine samples may be necessary to establish a pattern of abuse.

Factors Influencing Drug Action

Six factors influence how a drug acts in any particular person.

The first factor is the amount of medication given. In general, the more medication given, the greater the effect.

The second factor is the individual's age. Elderly people often have a slower metabolism, so drugs take longer to clear the body in them. Because of this it is important to monitor the patient for the cumulative effect of medication over time. On the other hand, children often react to medication quickly. Both the young and the old are especially sensitive to drugs that affect the central nervous system.

The third factor is a person's size. This can be a combination of body surface area (BSA) and body weight. In general, the larger the person, the larger the dose needs to be to have a therapeutic effect. However,

individuals vary. If an adult medication is used for a child, the dosage must be calculated carefully to take the child's body weight into consideration. A child has a greater proportion of body surface area to body weight than an adult.

The fourth factor is the person's gender. In general, men and women respond to drugs differently. There are two major reasons for this. One is the differences in levels of particular hormones. The second is the difference in the ratio of muscle to fat in men's and women's body compositions. Women's musculature has less blood supply than that of men; therefore, intramuscular injections remain in women's tissue longer than in men's tissue.

The fifth factor is pathological processes that might be present in a particular person. Absorption, distribution, metabolism, or excretion may be affected in a person with underlying disease. For example, in a person with liver disease, the period when the drug is being metabolized will be longer, so the period of action will be prolonged. A person with kidney disease may have difficulty excreting all of the medication's metabolites. A person with vascular disease will not distribute medication as effectively as a healthy person.

The final factor is tolerance, the tendency of some drugs to require a greater amount of time to achieve the same result. Over a period of time, the body may become tolerant to a particular drug, meaning that its effectiveness will be reduced. In the case of tolerance, a larger dose may be required to produce the same effect, or it may be necessary to change to a different medication.

Additional Effects of Drugs

Four types of drug effects may occur in addition to the drug's therapeutic action. These are side effects, allergy, drug interaction, and teratogenic effects.

Side Effects

Side effects are effects other than those the drug is given for. Most drug side effects are mild, such as gastrointestinal upset, dry mouth, drowsiness, or headache. When side effects are more serious they are sometimes called adverse effects and can prevent continued use. Some drugs can interfere with or damage vital organs such as the kidneys, liver, bone marrow, or heart.

An adverse effect that causes death is called a significant adverse effect. Sometimes a drug is approved for use by the FDA even though there have been a significant number of adverse effects during the drug's study period. This usually occurs because the drug treats a previously untreatable condition or significantly improves treatment of a condition that many suffer from. Many of these drugs must continue to undergo safety studies in large populations after approval, and adverse effects must be reported to the drug manufacturer, which then informs the FDA in periodic reports.

Allergy

Allergy is a specific untoward effect due to stimulation of the allergic response by some ingredient in the drug. It may also be called hypersensitivity to the drug. A mild allergic reaction is rash or **urticaria** (hives). A severe allergic reaction can lead to **anaphylaxis,** a generalized hypersensitivity reaction that causes severe respiratory distress and circulatory system failure. If a patient is known to have a particular drug allergy, this is always noted in the chart and on the medical record cover in red.

Because related drugs may cause allergic reactions, they are given with extreme caution to patients who have had a reaction to one of them. The ability of related drugs to cause reactions is called **cross-sensitivity.** Patients with severe allergies are recommended to wear medical alert identification bracelets. When a patient responds to a medication in an unexpected way, it is sometimes called an **idiosyncratic** effect.

Drug Interactions

A drug interaction is what happens when a patient takes two or more drugs together. There are three desirable drug interactions, referred to as potentiation, synergism, and antagonism.

Potentiation describes a situation in which one drug's action either prolongs or multiplies the effect of a second drug. For example, acetaminophen is often combined with narcotics to increase pain relief without increasing the amount of narcotic, as in Tylenol #3 (acetaminophen with codeine) or Percocet (acetaminophen with oxycodone).

Synergism describes a situation in which two drugs work to enhance each other. For example, before surgery patients are often given a combination of medication to decrease anxiety and to reduce oral secretions.

Finally, **antagonism** describes a situation in which one drug reduces the effect of another. A drug that antagonizes another can be given as an **antidote** for an overdose of the first medication. For example, vitamin K reduces the effect of Coumadin (warfarin), an anticoagulant.

Teratogenic Effects

The final kind of undesired effect is a **teratogenic** effect, one that may prevent a fetus from developing normally. A drug that has teratogenic side effects is **contraindicated** (meaning it should not be used) for a pregnant woman. It is extremely important for a woman who is pregnant or trying to become pregnant to inform a doctor about this before accepting any prescription.

The FDA has established five categories that describe safety levels for pregnant women:

- Category A medications present no risk to the fetus in the first trimester and no apparent risk in the second or third trimesters.
- Category B medications have shown no risk to the fetus in human tests, although there may have been risks identified in animal studies.
- Category C medications have insufficient data in studies on pregnant women to say whether there may be risks to the fetus, although risks were clearly shown in animal studies. The clinical benefits must be weighed carefully against potential risks.
- Category D medications have been shown in clinical investigations and/or postmarketing studies to pose risks to a fetus. Any possible clinical benefits of using the drug must be determined in relation to the clear risks the drug poses.
- Category X medications have been clearly documented to pose risks to a fetus, and these risks outweigh any clinical benefits of using the medication.

Sources of Information

There are many important sources that can and should be used to learn more about drugs.

The *United States Pharmacopeia/National Formulary* **(USP/NF)** is the official list of standardized drugs in the United States. It is published every 5 years. *New Drugs,* which updates the USP/NF, is published each year by the Council on Pharmacy of the American Medical Association.

The *Physicians' Desk Reference* (PDR) is published annually and is widely used by doctors and other health professionals. The PDR has three different indexes, which all cross-reference drugs. There is a Manufacturers' Index, which lists each manufacturer and its product line; a Brand and Generic Name Index; and a Product Category Index. It also has a Product Identification Guide, which has color photos of all the different drugs available. The PDR also contains product information, including side effects, and diagnostic product information.

A host of drug guides, as well as pharmacology textbooks, are published, many targeted to specific populations.

Package inserts are especially useful. These come with all prescription medications and contain detailed information about the specific product. Most pharmacies also provide information sheets for patients with all prescriptions.

The Internet is increasingly becoming a good source of information about medications. A number of Web sites, listed at the end of the chapter, provide good information.

FOCUS ON
INSTRUCTION

LEARNING ABOUT MEDICATIONS

Before administering a medication, always be familiar with the drug. Remember, the person administering the drug is responsible for giving the medication safely.

Make drug cards like the ones shown below to learn about drug groups and individual medications. A drug card should have the following information on it:

1. The name of the medication, both generic and trade (trade names are brands of the drug). Remember, the generic name is lower case, and any trade name is capitalized.

2. Whether the generic is commonly used or the branded drug is always used.

3. The classification or group.

4. Related medications.

5. Use: What the drug is used for.

6. Action: How the drug works in the body.

7. Common side effects.

8. Usual route and dose.

9. Contraindications, cautions, and warnings: Conditions in which the drug might be dangerous or require special monitoring. Include whether it may be used by pregnant women, as well as any special information about use in children or the elderly.

10. Patient teaching needs.

Front of card:

ATENOLOL (generic)
Brand Name: Tenormin

Related medications
acebutolol, bexolol, bisprolol, esmolol, metarpolol

Group
antihypertensive, antiangianal, antiarrythmic

Use
hypertension

Action
beta-adrenergic blocking agent. Works primarily on beta adrenergic receptors of the heart and arteries.

Common Side Effects
fatigue, weakness, dizziness, impotence

Severe Side Effects
bradycardia, congestive heart failure, pulmonary edema

Back of card:

Patient Teaching Needs

Instruct to take exactly as directed; do not skip or double up on missed doses; take a missed dose up to eight hours before the next dose.

Teach patient/family to take pulse and/or blood pressure if directed by the doctor. Make position changes slowly because may cause orthostatic hypotension when patient sits up.

Notify doctor if slow pulse, difficulty breathing, severe dizziness or fainting.

Contraindications

uncompensates congestive heart failure, pulmonary edema, cardiogenic shock, heart block

Caution

renal impairment, hepatic impairment, diabetes mellitus, thyrotoxicosis, history of severe allergic reactions

Pregnancy and Children

safety not established

MEDICATION FORMS, MEASUREMENTS, AND DOSAGE CALCULATIONS

Before medication can be administered, it must be prepared. Preparing medication for administration is a series of activities that takes concentration and precision. Sometimes doses need to be calculated.

Common Abbreviations

Several abbreviations are commonly used when prescribing, ordering, and administering medications. Table 22–5 shows common abbreviations used for ordering and administering medications.

The Medication Label

The medication label is the source of information about the medication that is being prepared. The label contains 10 pieces of important information:

1. Trade (brand) name
2. Generic name
3. Dosage strength in a given amount of medication; for instance, 250 mg per tablet; 80 mg/½ tsp; or 25 mg/mL
4. Total contents (number of pills, volume of liquid)
5. Usual adult dose and how often the dose is given

6. Form in which the drug is supplied (such as capsules, tablets, liquid)
7. List of all active and inactive ingredients
8. Expiration date; lot or batch code
9. Storage instructions
10. Manufacturer's name.

Figure 22–2 shows the information on a medication label.

Routes of Medication Administration

The form of the drug often determines the method by which it will be administered. There are 11 methods by which a drug may be administered: topical, transdermal, buccal, rectal, inhalation, instillation, sublingual, oral, parenteral, implanted, or pump.

Topical Medications

Topical medications include creams, lotions, sprays, **ointments** (semisolid), or **liniments** (emulsions). A cream has active ingredients that disappear when they are rubbed into the skin. Lotions are often used on dry, cracked skin. The active ingredients in ointments are suspended in a base such as petrolatum or lanolin. They can protect skin for a long time. Liniments are similar to lotion, but with a higher proportion of oil and stronger active ingredients.

Table 22–5	**Common Abbreviations Used for Ordering and Administering Medications**						

ac	before meals	IM	intramuscular	pm, PM	afternoon
ad lib	as desired	IU	international units	prn, PRN	as needed
AM; am	morning	IV	intravenous	pt	patient or pint
amp	ampule	kg	kilogram	q	every
amt	amount	L	liter	qd	every day
aq	aqueous	lb	pound	q 2 h	every 2 hours
AD	left ear	m, min, ℳ	minim	qid	four times a day
AS	right ear	mcg, μg	microgram	qs	quantity sufficient
AU	both ears	mEq	milliequivalent	Rx	take, prescribe
bid	twice a day	mg	milligram	s̄	without
c̄	with	mL	milliliter	SC, subq, S/Q	subcutaneous
cap	capsule	NaCl	sodium chloride	Sig	directions to patient
DC, disc, d/c	discontinue	NKA	no known allergies	sl, SL	sublingual
dr, ʒ	dram	noc, noct	night	sol	solution
DW	distilled water	npo, NPO	nothing by mouth	ss, s̄s̄	half
elix	elixir	NS	normal saline	stat, STAT	immediately
et	and	OD	right eye	supp	suppository
ext	extract	ophth	ophthalmic	T, Tbsp	tablespoon
fl	fluid	os	mouth	t, tsp	teaspoon
g	gram	OS	left eye	tab	tablet
gr	grain	OU	both eyes	tid	three times a day
gt(t)	drop(s)	oz, ʒ	ounce	tinc, tinct	tincture
h, hr	hour	p̄	after	ung	ointment
hs, HS	hour of sleep	pc	after meals	U	units
ID	intradermal	po, PO	by mouth		

Transdermal Medications

A **transdermal** medication is one that is placed on a patch that sits on the skin. The medication is absorbed slowly and consistently from the patch through the skin. A transdermal patch usually administers medication for 3 days. Some patients with angina (chest pain) use a nitroglycerin patch. Replacement estrogen for postmenopausal women is also sometimes administered via a patch. Nicotine patches are often used by people trying to stop smoking cigarettes; each successive patch has slightly less nicotine, giving the body a chance to gradually get used to a nicotine-free state and reducing cravings. Nicotine patches are also under study as a treatment for ulcerative colitis.

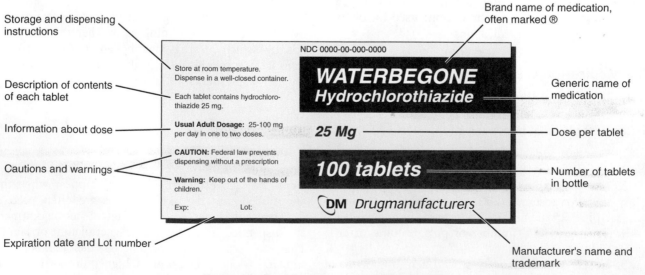

➤ **Figure 22–2** Information on a medication label.

Buccal and Sublingual Medications

Buccal administration means placing the medication, in the form of a lozenge, between the cheek and gum so the medication can be absorbed through the vascular oral mucosa.

Sublingual medication is administered as a tablet, which is placed under the tongue and dissolves, allowing medicine to enter the system through the oral mucosal membrane. Nitroglycerin tablets for relief of angina are often given this way, because they are rapidly absorbed.

More often, medication held in the mouth is used for topical relief of a sore throat rather than for its systemic effect.

Rectal and Vaginal Medications

Medications can be administered rectally either in the form of an ointment, a liquid administered as an enema, or a **suppository.** A suppository is medication in a glycerin or cocoa-butter base that melts at body temperature, releasing the medication. Rectal suppositories are often given to patients who are vomiting and cannot keep down pills or oral liquids, to patients who are not allowed to take anything by mouth, or to promote a bowel movement.

Medication can be administered vaginally either as an ointment or a suppository.

Inhalation

Inhalation refers to medications that are inhaled either as a spray, a gas, or an aerosol vapor. Inhalation is usually targeted at local results, although general anesthesia or oxygen can be administered by this route. Inhalation can take place through the nose or through the mouth, through a mask or a nebulizer. A common example is medication used for asthma, which expands the breathing passages.

Instillation

Instillation refers to drops used in the eyes, nose, or ears.

Oral Medications

Oral solid medication can be administered as a tablet, a capsule, or a caplet, which are all referred to as "pills." A **tablet** is a disk of compressed medication. A **capsule** is an oblong gelatin sheath that contains powdered medication. A **caplet** is a capsule in the shape of a tablet.

Figure 22–3 shows various types of oral solid medications. Some of these medications are **time-release** capsules that contain many tiny doses inside, which dissolve over different time periods depending on the material that makes up the minicapsule. Others are **enteric coated**, meaning coated with a material that does not break down until they are in the intestine, so they do not upset the stomach. Aspirin and ibuprofen can be purchased in enteric-coated tablets. Figure 22–4 shows a cross-section of an enteric-coated tablet.

Oral liquids come either as a solution, a syrup, a suspension, or an elixir. Liquid preparations taken orally are rapidly absorbed in the stomach and small intestine.

A **solution** is a preparation in which the medication is completely dissolved in liquid, usually water. A **syrup** is a concentrated solution containing sugar or a sugar substitute. A **suspension** is an insoluble medication, contained in a liquid, such as milk of magnesia or liquid antacid. Suspensions need to be shaken before administering to get the liquid and medication to mix. An **elixir** is a sweetened preparation; originally, elixirs were dissolved in alcohol. Because many elixirs are intended for use by children, such as ibuprofen or acetaminophen elixir, they are now produced without alcohol.

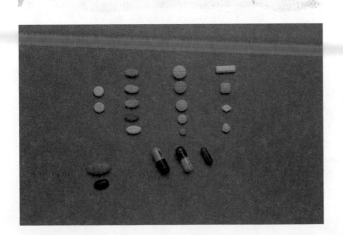

➤ **Figure 22–3** Oral solid medication can be in the form of tablets or capsules.

Parenteral Medications

When medication is given by injection, the route is termed **parenteral** (literally, beyond the intestine). Injections can be given into body tissue or directly into a vein.

Parenteral liquids are sterile preparations that are either solutions or oil-based preparations. Depo-Provera (medroxyprogesterone) is an oil-based contraceptive injected under the skin that lasts for 3 months.

Implants

Implantable medications are surgically placed below the skin, where they continue to release a constant dose of medication over a long period of time. Norplant (levonorgestrel) is a contraceptive implanted in six cylinders under the skin of the upper arm.

Pumps

Finally, medication can be administered via a pump to provide continuous flow of the medication. The pump is becoming an increasingly popular way of administering a constant dose of insulin to diabetic patients who engage in competitive athletics such as golf and bicycling, do not want to have to constantly monitor their sugar, and do not want the volatility of blood sugar that normally occurs with injected insulin.

Systems of Measurement Used in Pharmacology

A doctor orders an amount of medication to be administered based on the patient's age and gender, weight, size, and any other important factors such as underlying disease that will change drug metabolism. The medical assistant often has to calculate a dose from the supply on hand. To do this properly, he or she must know three different measurement systems—the metric, the apothecaries', and the household, as well as how to do conversions from one system to another.

The Metric System

The metric system is the most common system of measurement used in pharmacology. It was developed in France in the late 1800s. The metric system is easy to use, because all units of measure are based on multiples of ten.

The basic unit of length is a meter, which is a little longer than a yard. For volume, the basic unit is a liter, which is a little more than a quart. For weight, the basic unit of measure is a gram. A gram is very small; it takes nearly 500 grams to equal 1 pound. Words for larger and smaller units are formed by adding prefixes. All units of length end in -meter; all units of volume end in -liter; and all units of weight end in -gram. Figure 22–5 shows the basic units of measurement in the metric system, with abbreviations used to indicate larger and smaller amounts.

Prefixes. In the metric system, Latin prefixes are used for amounts smaller than the basic unit, and Greek prefixes for amounts larger than the basic unit.

Three prefixes are commonly used in medicine for units smaller than the basic unit, and one prefix is in common use for units larger than the basic unit. These are shown in Table 22–6.

The three prefixes for smaller units are:

1. milli, which equals one thousandth (0.001), and is used in describing units of length or weight. For example, 1000 milligrams equals 1 gram.
2. centi, which equals one hundredth (0.01), and is used in describing units of length. For example, 100 centimeters equals 1 meter.
3. micro, which equals one millionth (0.000001), and is used for describing units of weight. For example, 1000 micrograms equals 1 milligram, or 1,000,000 micrograms equals 1 gram.

The prefix for larger units is kilo, which means one thousand (1000), and is used for describing units of weight. For example, 1000 grams equals 1 kilogram.

Metric Abbreviations. Standard abbreviations for metric units use the first letter(s) of the prefix, if there is one, and the first letter of the unit of measure. The lower case is used, except in the case of L for liter, which is capitalized to avoid confusion with the number 1. The abbreviation for micro is either mc, or the Greek symbol μ ("mu"). Metric abbreviations are:

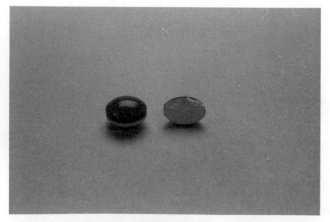

➤ **Figure 22–4** In cross-section the thick outer covering of enteric-coated medication is visible.

Basic unit of weight: gram (g)

A candle used on a birthday cake weighs about one gram. We could also say that the candle wieghs 1,000,000 µg or 1,000 mg or 0.001kg.

Conversion equations for weight:

    1,000 µg (micrograms) = 1 mg (milligram)
    1000 mg (milligrams) = 1 g (gram)
    1000 g (grams) = 1 kg (kilogram)

Basic unit of volume: liter (L)

A quart of milk contains a little less than a liter. We could say that the carton contains approximately 1000 mL.

Conversion equation for volume:

    1000mL (milliliters) = 1 L (liter)

Basic unit of distance: meter (m)

A yard is slightly less than a meter. A centimeter is slightly less than a half inch.

Conversion equation for distance:

    1 cc (cubic centimeter) = 1 mL (milliliter)

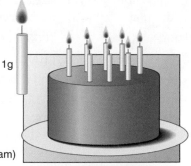
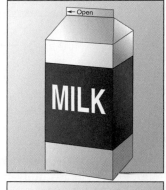
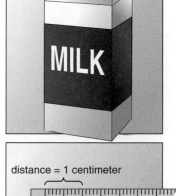

1g

← Open

MILK

distance = 1 centimeter

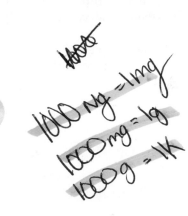

➤ **Figure 22–5** Basic units of the metric system.

---

g = gram
kg = kilogram
mg = milligram
mcg = microgram
m = meter
cm = centimeter
mm = millimeter
L = liter
mL = milliliter

Metric Notation. Standard notation for the metric system uses Arabic numbers, followed by the abbreviation for the units. Partial units are written as decimals. For instance:

    2.6 cm = two and six tenths centimeters

    0.012 g = twelve thousandths of a gram

    25.05 L = twenty-five and five hundredths liters

    64.2 mcg = sixty-four and two tenths micrograms

Table 22–6	**Prefixes Used in the Metric System**						
	Latin Prefixes			No prefix		Greek prefixes	
micro-	milli-	deci-		**none**	deka-	hecto-	kilo-
0.000001	0.001	0.1		**1**	10	100	1,000
millionth	thousandth	tenth		**one**	ten	hundred	thousand

When the metric system was established, units of volume and weight were linked to the meter, the unit of length. One milliliter (0.001 L) is defined as the volume of water contained in a cube that measures 1 centimeter on each side. The weight of this volume of water is defined as 1 gram. Figure 22–6 shows the relationship between length, volume, and weight in the metric system.

Because the volume of a cubic centimeter is 1 mL, health professionals use the terms milliliter and cubic centimeter (**cc**) interchangeably.

Conversions Within the Metric System. Sometimes it is necessary to convert measurements within the metric system. If the doctor orders a medication dose in grams, for example, but the label on the medication bottle is written in milligrams, the medical assistant will need to convert from grams to milligrams to calculate how much of the medication to give.

You remember from arithmetic that any number divided by itself equals one. Therefore, if you write 1000 mcg/1 mg, you have written 1 in another form. To convert within the metric system, simply multiply the number you want to convert by the conversion equation (shown below), expressed as a fraction with the units you want to convert to in the numerator.

Metric System Conversion Equations

Weight	Volume
1000 mcg = 1 mg	1000 mL = 1 L
1000 mg = 1 g	1 mL = 1 cc
1000 g = 1 kg	

Conversion Example 1. Conversion from smaller units to larger units.

To convert milligrams to grams, multiply the number of milligrams by 1 g/1000 mg, because there are 1000 milligrams in 1 gram.

How many grams are there in 400 mg?

$$400 \text{ mg} \times \frac{1 \text{ g}}{1000 \text{ mg}} = \frac{400 \text{ mg} \times 1 \text{ g}}{1000 \text{ mg}} = \frac{4 \text{ g}}{10} = 0.4 \text{ g}$$

Remember that all numbers in the metric system are expressed as decimals. The units you are converting from cancel out, and you are left with only the units you are converting to.

Because the metric system is based on decimals, converting from smaller units to larger units can be done simply by moving the decimal point to the left. When you want to divide by 1000, as in this case, move the decimal point three places to the left, one place for each 0.

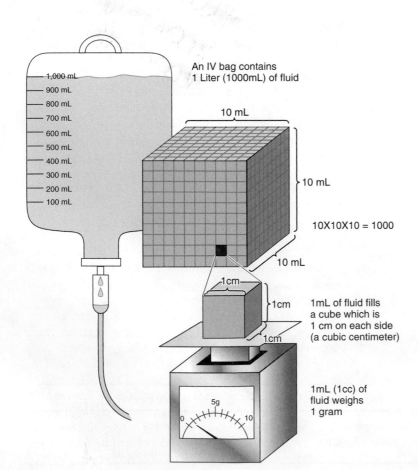

> **Figure 22–6** The relationship between length, volume, and weight in the metric system.

$$400 \text{ mg} = 400 = 0.4 \text{ g}$$

Remember that if there is no decimal point, it is assumed to follow the number. **When a decimal is smaller than one, in scientific notation, you must put a zero before the decimal point. This helps prevent overlooking the decimal point.**

Conversion Example 2. Conversion from larger units to smaller units.

To convert liters to milliliters, multiply the number of liters by 1000 mL/1 L because there are 1000 milliliters in 1 liter.

How many milliliters are there in 0.976 L?

$$0.976 \text{ L} \times \frac{1000 \text{ mL}}{1 \text{ L}} = \frac{0.976 \text{ L} \times 1000 \text{ mL}}{1 \text{ L}} = \frac{976 \text{ mL}}{1}$$
$$= 976 \text{ mL}$$

Converting from larger units to smaller units can also be done by moving the decimal point to the right. When you want to multiply by 1000, as in this case, move the decimal point three places to the right.

$$0.976 \text{ L} = 0.976. = 976 \text{ mL}$$

Apothecaries' and Household Systems

The oldest system of measurement is the apothecaries' system. The word apothecary comes from the Greek and means the one who runs a store. Original apothecary measurements were based on the size or volume of items found in nature. The apothecaries' system was used for hundreds of years in England and the United States, and is still used in some situations.

Apothecaries' Measurements. Originally, in apothecary measurement of weight (known as apothecaries' weights) 1 grain equaled the weight of a plump grain of wheat. Today, the weight of 1 grain has been standardized at 65 milligrams. Twenty grains equals 1 scruple; 3 scruples equals 1 dram; and 8 drams equals 1 ounce. Therefore, 480 grains equals 1 ounce.

Originally, in apothecary measurement of volume, a minim was equal to 1 drop of water. Today, it is standardized at 0.06 milliliters. Sixty minims equals 1 fluidram, and 8 fluidrams equals 1 fluidounce. Sixteen fluidounces equals 1 pint; 2 pints equal 1 quart; and 4 quarts equal 1 gallon.

Abbreviations for apothecaries' measures are:

gr = grain
oz or ℥ = ounce
m, min, or ♏ = minim
fl oz or fl ℥ = fluidounce

Household Measures. Ounces and pounds, fluidounces, pints, quarts, and gallons are used in household measuring as well. Household measures are those in general use for cooking and are often used for liquid medication. Household measures used in pharmacology are:

gt = drop
gtt = drops
t or tsp = teaspoon
T or Tbsp = tablespoon
oz = 2 tablespoons
C = cup (8 ounces)

Liquid medication doses may be expressed as drops (for eye or ear medication), teaspoons, or tablespoons. Bottles for medication are manufactured using fluidounces, and doctors must specify the size of a bottle on any prescription. Because it is obvious on a prescription that a bottle holding liquid is intended, many doctors use the abbreviation for ounces instead of fluidounces.

Notation using the apothecaries' system. The most common notation for the apothecaries' system uses Roman numerals for numbers up to 15 or 16. Arabic numbers are used for fractions, except ½, for which the abbreviation ss̄ is commonly used. Decimals should not be used. The unit being described is written before the numeral. This helps avoid confusion with the metric system.

For example, two grains would be written as gr II or gr ii; one sixtieth of a grain would be written as gr 1/60; four fluidounces would be expressed as fl oz IV or fl oz iv. Doctors use this notation for many prescriptions. For example, one tablet will be tab I or tab i; two drops would be gtt II or gtt ii.

Because the apothecaries' system is older and less precise than the metric system, there is little standardization of notation. You may see Roman numerals written in either lower or upper case or, when handwritten, a combination form with both lines and dots. Arabic numbers are sometimes used with the units before or after the numerals.

It is important not to be confused between the apothecaries' and metric system. The most likely confusion will be caused by the similarity between g for grams and gr for grains. Because 1 grain equals 60 milligrams, a serious error could occur. Most doctors are careful to write gr I for 1 grain and 1 g for 1 gram. But if you are confused or a pharmacist calls with a question, always ask the doctor for clarification.

Conversion Between the Metric and Apothecaries' Systems. You will probably not need to convert from apothecaries' to metric measures often, but it is important to know the basic principles involved. First you need to know a conversion equation. The following are the most useful equations of approximate equivalents between the apothecaries' and household system and the metric system. These equivalents are not exact because the apothecaries' system is not exact. Some manufacturers will use standardized measurements for the apothecaries' system, and others will use nonstandardized conversion equations; therefore, the numbers you see on manufacturers' bottles may not agree exactly with these calculations. See Table 22–7, the conversion tables for the apothecaries', household, and metric systems.

For volume:

$$1 \text{ teaspoon} = 5 \text{mL (cc)}$$
$$1 \text{ tablespoon} = 15 \text{ mL (cc)}$$
$$1 \text{ fluidounce} = 30 \text{ mL (cc)}$$

For weight:

$$1 \text{ grain} = 60 \text{ mg}$$
$$15 \text{ grains} = 1 \text{ g}$$

To set up the conversion equation, multiply the number you want to convert by the conversion factor, expressed as a fraction. Put the units you want to convert to in the numerator.

For instance, if you want to convert 15 teaspoons to its equivalent in milliliters, you multiply $15 \times 5 \text{ mL}/1$ tsp (numerator/denominator). $15 \times 5/1 = 75/1 = 75$.

Table 22–7	Conversion Tables for Apothecaries', Household, and Metric Measurements

Apothecaries' / Metric Units of Weight

Apothecaries'	Metric
gr 1/60 (one sixtieth of a grain)	1 mg
gr 1/30	2 mg
gr 1/20	3 mg
gr 1/15	4 mg
gr 1/10	6 mg
gr 1/6	10 mg
gr 1/4	15 mg
gr 1/2	30 mg
gr i (one grain)	60 mg
gr v (five grains)	300 mg
gr x (ten grains)	600 mg
gr 15	1000 mg
dr i (60 grains = 1 dram)	4 g

**For easier calculation a gram is commonly considered to be 60 milligrams instead of 65 milligrams in conversion tables. This means that a 5-grain tablet of aspirin or acetaminophen actually contains 325 milligrams of medication.

Household (Avoirdupois)/Metric Units of Weight

Household	Metric
1 oz (one ounce)	30 g
1 lb (one pound = 16 ounces)	454 g
2.2 lb	1 kg

Apothecaries'/Household/Metric Units of Volume

Apothecaries'	Household	Metric
min i (one minim)	gt i (one drop)	0.06 mL
min xv (15 minims)	tsp ss (1/2 teaspoon)	
min 16		1 mL (1 cc)
fl dr i (one fluidram)	tsp i (one teaspoon)	5 mL (5 cc)
fl oz i (one fluidounce)	Tbsp ii (3 tsp = 1 Tbsp)	30 mL (30 cc)
fl oz iv		120 mL (120 cc)
fl oz viii	1 cup	
fl oz 16	1 pint	500 mL (500 cc)

**The conversion equivalents used for liquid measurement are also approximate for ease in calculation.

To convert back the other way, from 15 mL to its equivalent in teaspoons, multiply 15 × 1 tsp/5 mL. 15 × 1/5 = 15/5 = 3.

To convert 1000 mL into fluid ounces, multiply 1000 × 1 fl oz/30 mL, or 1000 × 1/30 = 1000/30 = 333.3 fl oz.

Other Units

Certain medications, such as penicillin, insulin, and heparin, are measured in international units. For instance, the normal adult dose of penicillin G is 200,000 to 800,000 units. The volume necessary to provide a medication measured in units will vary, because the strength of each batch varies depending on the manufacturer, the conditions under which it was manufactured, and the method by which the medication was obtained. For instance, synthetic insulin (Humulin) will have a different strength than insulin from a pig.

Calculating Dosages Correctly

Like conversions from one system of measurement to another, dosage calculations are based on mathematical principles. A **ratio** is a relationship between two numbers that can be expressed in one of three ways:

1. two numbers separated by a colon and expressed as "first number" to "second number" (i.e. 1:4, or 1 to 4).
2. two numbers written as a fraction (i.e. ¼, or one fourth).
3. the relationship of the two numbers per hundred, also called a **percentage**.

A percentage is obtained by dividing the second number of the ratio (the denominator of the fraction) into 100 and multiplying by the first number (i.e., 100 divided by 4 = 25, therefore 4 is 25 percent of 100).

When you have two equal ratios, it is called a **proportion**. For example, 1:4 = 25:100 are proportional ratios.

When calculating medication doses, one of the elements of the proportion is unknown. Solving an equation to determine the value of the unknown element is done by cross-multiplying, then solving for the unknown using the following steps:

Step 1. Set up the proportion.

$$\frac{5}{20} = \frac{1}{X}$$

Step 2. Cross-multiply (multiply the numerator of the first fraction times the denominator of the second fraction, and vice versa).

$$5 \times X = 20 \times 1$$
$$5X = 20$$

Step 3. Solve for X by dividing both sides of the equation by a number that will leave X alone on one side of the equation (in this case, divide by the number 5). Remember, you can always divide both sides of an equation by the same number.

$$\frac{5X}{5} = \frac{20}{5}$$
$$X = 4$$

Calculating a Dose of Solid Medication

Any medication calculation can be expressed as a proportion, where the unknown (X) is the amount to give. The relationship between the weight of a medication in a given amount (such as a tablet, capsule, or liquid) is proportional to the desired weight in an unknown quantity of tablets, capsules, or liquid.

$$\frac{\text{medication ordered (by weight)}}{X} = \frac{\text{amount on hand (by weight)}}{\text{per tablet, capsule, tsp., mL, etc.}}$$

X equals the desired number of tablets, capsules, teaspoons, and so on of the medication to be given.

In the case of tablets or capsules, it is customary to convert the proportion to a formula that makes the process of calculation easier, namely:

Number of tablets (capsules) to give

$$= \frac{\text{dose ordered}}{\text{dose per tablet (capsule)}}$$

Example. The doctor orders 750 milligrams of an antibiotic, ciprofloxacin (Cipro). The label of the bottle in the office says 250 milligrams per tablet. Using the formula, calculate the number of tablets to give.

$$\frac{\text{dose ordered}}{\text{dose per tablet}} = \frac{750 \text{ mg}}{250 \text{ mg/tab}} = 3 \text{ tablets}$$

(Note, cancel the units out when doing the division, so it becomes

$$\frac{750}{250}$$

Remember, to solve a fraction always divide the bottom number into the top number.

Example. The doctor has written an order to give Zoloft (sertraline) 50 mg. The medication label of the bottle in the office says that each tablet contains 100 mg. Calculate as follows.

$$\frac{\text{dose ordered}}{\text{dose per tablet}} = \frac{50 \text{ mg}}{100 \text{ mg/tab}} = \frac{1}{2} \text{ tablet}$$

To be sure that you set up your formula correctly, always look at your answer and compare to the original order. If the order is larger than the amount of medication in each tablet, your answer should be more than one tablet. If the order is smaller than the amount per tablet, your answer should be a fraction of one tablet.

If the dose ordered is not expressed in the same units as the dose on hand, before setting up the calculation, it is necessary to convert the dose ordered into the same units as those on the medication label.

Example. The doctor has written an order to give lithium carbonate 0.6 g. The medication label says lithium carbonate capsules, 300 mg per capsule.

Step 1. Express 0.6 g in milligrams.

There are two ways to do this, by the formula, or by moving the decimal point.

Formula method: $0.6 \text{ g} \times \dfrac{1000 \text{ mg}}{1 \text{ g}} = 600 \text{ mg}$

Decimal point method: $0.600. \text{ g} = 600 \text{ mg}$

Step 2. Using the answer to step 1, solve a ratio of the dose ordered to the dose on hand (dose per capsule).

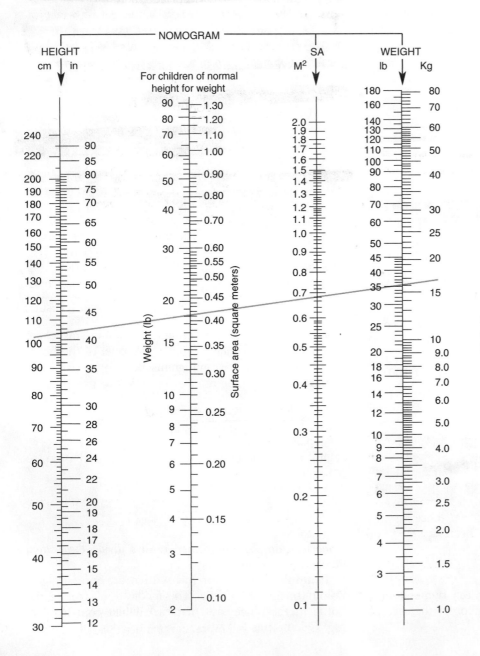

➤ **Figure 22–7** A diagonal line connecting a child's height and weight allows calculation of body surface area.

$$\frac{\text{dose ordered}}{\text{dose per capsule}} = \frac{600 \text{ mg}}{300 \text{ mg/cap}} = 2 \text{ capsules}$$

Calculating a Dose of Liquid Medication

When the liquid medication is expressed in a unit of one (such as per one teaspoon or per one milliliter) the calculation is done in the same way as for oral solid medication.

Example. The doctor has written an order to give atropine sulfate 0.6 mg by injection. The medication label says atropine sulfate 0.4 mg per mL. Calculate the dose as follows:

$$\frac{\text{dose ordered}}{\text{dose per mL}} = \frac{0.6 \text{ mg}}{0.4 \text{ mg/mL}} = 1.5 \text{ mL}$$

When an amount of medication is in liquid units other than one, it is necessary to do a more complex calculation. The first method is to calculate in two steps, by first finding the amount of medication in one unit, then calculating the number of units. It is also possible to use a formula that allows you to calculate the correct dose in one step.

Example. The doctor has written an order to give erythromycin oral suspension 250 mg. The label on the bottle says that there are 125 mg per 5 mL.

Two-step method.

Step 1. Calculate the number of milligrams in 1 milliliter by dividing 5 into 125.

$$\frac{125 \text{ mg}}{5 \text{ mL}} = \frac{25 \text{ mg}}{1 \text{ mL}}$$

Step 2. Using the number of milligrams per milliliter, calculate the desired dose.

$$\frac{\text{dose ordered}}{\text{dose per mL}} = \frac{250 \text{ mg}}{25 \text{ mg/mL}} = 10 \text{ mL}$$

One-step method. Use the following formula:

$$\frac{\text{dose ordered (weight)} \times \text{quantity (volume)}}{\text{dose on hand (weight)}}$$

$$= \text{amount to give}$$

The solution for this example is:

$$\frac{250 \text{ mg} \times 5 \text{ mL}}{125 \text{ mg}} = \frac{1250 \text{ mg}}{125 \text{ mg}} = 10 \text{ mL}$$

As with solid medication, the doctor may order medication in units that are different from those on the medication label. In this case, it is necessary first to convert to the units on the label.

Example. The doctor has written an order to give medroxyprogesterone 1 g intramuscularly. The medication label says that each milliliter contains 400 mg/mL.

Step 1. Convert 1 g to 1000 mg.

Step 2. Calculate the dose.

$$\frac{1000 \text{ mg}}{400 \text{ mg/mL}} = 2.5 \text{ mL}$$

Sometimes liquid medication is ordered by volume instead of by weight. This is the case with most immunizations. If the doctor orders tetanus toxoid 0.5 mL, the amount to give is already stated and no calculation is needed.

Calculating Pediatric Doses

Calculating the appropriate dose of medication for a child involves using either the body weight method or the BSA method. Figure 22–7 shows a nomogram chart for calculating BSA, which is determined by drawing a straight line from the child's weight to his or her height and finding the place where the line intersects the BSA column. A **nomogram** is a chart that shows the relationship between three variables.

The dose is then calculated as the child's BSA, expressed in square meters, over 1.7 square meters, times the adult dose. The equation looks like this:

$$\text{Child dose} = \frac{\text{BSA(m}^2)}{1.7(\text{m}^2)} \times \text{Adult dose}$$

Body weight is the method usually performed, because it is a straightforward calculation. The BSA calculation is more cumbersome.

For medication calculations, body weight is expressed in kilograms. One kilogram equals 2.2 pounds. A doctor will order medication for a child as milligrams per kilogram of body weight. Sometimes the dose will be divided into portions at different times of day. For instance, if a doctor wants a 75-pound child to have 10 milligrams per kilogram, divided equally into a morning and evening dose, the calculation is as follows:

Step 1. Calculate the number of kilograms in 75 pounds.

$$75 \text{ pounds} = X \text{ kilograms}$$
$$75/2.2 = 34 \text{ kilograms}$$

Step 2. Calculate the number of milligrams to give each day.

$$34 \text{ kilograms} \times 10 \text{ milligrams per kilogram}$$
$$= X \text{ milligrams}$$
$$34 \times 10 = 340 \text{ milligrams per day}$$

Step 3. Calculate the number of milligrams to give in each dose.

$$340 \text{ milligrams divided by two doses}$$
$$= X \text{ milligrams per dose}$$
$$340/2 = 170 \text{ milligrams per dose}$$

STUDENT STUDY PLAN: PART I

To reinforce your understanding of the material in Part I of this chapter . . .

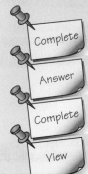

Complete the **Review & Recall** questions.

Answer the **Critical Thinking Questions** and discuss them with your classmates.

Complete the exercises for Part I in chapter 22 of the **Student Mastery Manual.**

View Part Two of the **Medications** videotape: "Evaluating Medication" and "The Follow-up."

 ## REVIEW & RECALL

1. Describe five sources from which medications are derived.

2. How do you know the difference between the trade name and the generic name of a medication?

3. Differentiate between prescribing a medication, administering a medication, and dispensing a medication; then identify which activities a medical assistant is legally allowed to perform.

4. Describe the five schedules of controlled substances.

5. What information must be included on a prescription?

6. How should medications be stored in the medical office?

7. Identify four ways of classifying medications.

8. Define the following terms as they apply to medications: absorption, distribution, action, metabolism, and excretion.

9. Define the term "side effect" and identify some common side effects of medication.

10. List several references for obtaining information about specific drugs.

11. Identify eleven methods by which medications can be given.

12. List the basic measures of volume, distance, and weight in the metric and apothecaries' systems of measurement.

 ## CRITICAL THINKING QUESTIONS

1. Discuss with your classmates several reasons why different doses of medication may be ordered for different people.

2. Patients often believe that it is not important to include vitamins, OTC medications, or herbal preparations when they list what medictions they take regularly. Is this a valid perception or not? Justify your thinking.

3. Because science and medicine use the metric system for most measurements, should the United States seriously consider going metric? Do research to identify several reasons for and against this idea.

4. If the same medication is given by different routes, it may be given in a different dosage, and it may have different effects. Discuss with your classmates why this happens and the implications it might have for a medical assistant.

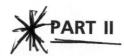

PART II

PRINCIPLES OF ADMINISTERING MEDICATIONS

The Medication Order

The doctor is responsible for identifying the medication, the dose, and the route of administration (the way the medication gets into the patient's body) for each individual patient.

In the case of a prescription (described earlier in this chapter) the doctor directs a pharmacist to dispense a supply of a medication to the patient. A single order is an order to administer one dose of a medication; this is usually done during the patient visit. A stat order is an order to give the medication immediately. A written order is an order written by the doctor on the patient's medical record.

A verbal order (VO) is an order expressed in words but not written. In the case of a verbal order, the person who is responsible for giving the patient the medication should repeat the order back to the provider, clarify any questions, and then write the order in the medical record exactly as he or she understood it for the provider to countersign at a later time.

A routine or standing order refers to medication administered to a patient who regularly comes to the office to receive a medication. An example of this might be vitamin B_{12} administered by intramuscular injection monthly. In this case, the injection may be given each month based on an order written within the past 12 months. A standing order may also be part of a protocol that describes actions to be taken in a specific situation rather than with a particular patient.

Preparing Medication

Medication preparation is a delicate task. Whoever prepares medication for administration is responsible for making sure that the right patient receives the right dose of the right medication at the right time, by the right route. These are known as "The Five Rights." The accompanying box describes these five rights in more detail.

The first thing to do before preparing medication is to be mindful of keeping aseptic technique. This means washing hands, working in a clean area, and not touching the medication surface area. For medications that will penetrate below the skin, sterile technique should be maintained at all times.

Make sure you have adequate knowledge of the drug you are preparing. This means looking up the drug in an appropriate reference, knowing how the drug works, and knowing what to instruct the patient about the drug.

To avoid giving a drug to a patient with a known allergy, check the patient's medical record. Drug allergies should be noted on the cover of the chart, usually on a red label. Because injections tend to cause more severe reactions in an allergic patient, it is good practice to ask the patient about medication allergies before giving parenteral medication.

The work space should be clean, quiet, well-lighted, and have adequate space. Follow the five rights closely. Be sure you have a valid order, either written by the doctor or one you have written after taking a verbal order from the doctor. You may work from the patient's medical record or, in some facilities, you may be expected to transcribe the order onto a medication card. The card is used to administer the medication, and after the medication has been given and documented, the card is thrown away (Figure 22–8).

Make sure to do any calculations necessary to prepare the correct dose. Have a colleague double-check your calculations if you are not sure.

Before pouring or drawing up any medication, check the expiration date, and discard any expired medication. Check medication for any discoloration, odor, or change in consistency. Discard any medication that is questionable.

Check the label of any medication against the medication order three times: when you remove the medication from storage, before you pour or draw up the medication, and when you replace it in the medication cabinet or drawer. Read the label thoroughly each time. Follow the proper procedural steps for the type of medication you are preparing. Never return a medication to the bottle. Throw away any dropped or spilled medication.

Measure exactly. There should be no bubbles in liquid medication. Once a medication is prepared, do not leave it unattended. Only give medication you have personally prepared.

Exam Room #	2
Patient Name:	McAllister, Keith
Drug:	Rocephin
Dose:	250 mg
Route:	IM
Date & Time:	6/9/00 – 10AM

➤ **Figure 22–8** A sample medication card that may be used in some facilities (instead of the medical record) to give medication. The card is destroyed after the medication has been given and documented.

Part 2 *#1*

The "Five Rights" of Correct Medication Administration

Right drug Prepare the medication from the written order in the patient's medical record. In hospitals, drugs are prepared from transcribed medication orders. Check the label of the bottle or package containing the drug against the medication order to be sure that they are the same. The label should be checked three times: when the bottle is removed from the medication drawer or cabinet, when the medication is removed from the bottle, and when the medication is returned to storage.

Right dose The drug is prescribed to achieve a specific effect. Giving too little medication may be ineffective; giving too much may cause harm to the patient. If a calculation is necessary, calculate the dose accurately before preparing the medication and work from your written calculation. If you have questions, ask another staff member to verify your calculation. Measure liquid medications accurately.

Right patient Always verify that medication is being given to the correct patient. To do this in an ambulatory care setting, take the patient's medical record with the medication to the patient. Ask the patient to state his or her name and verify it from the page of the medical record that contains the written medication order. In a hospital setting, the patient's name can be verified from the identification bracelet and checked against the written medication administration record.

Right time In the doctor's office the time of day is usually less important than the interval between doses, as for example, when giving a series of hepatitis B immunizations or DPT immunizations. Verify that the correct amount of time has passed since the last dose of the medication and refer any questions to the doctor.

Right route The medication must be given by the correct route to have the desired effect and, in the case of some injections, to prevent tissue injury. When giving injections, choose a needle length that will deposit the medication into the desired tissue based on the size of the patient and angle of administration. If you have questions, clarify the order with the doctor.

Administering Medication

Administering medication is one of the most important activities a medical assistant performs. It is tremendously important when administering medication to follow the 13 principles of safe medication administration:

1. Never give medication without a valid order from a doctor or other licensed practitioner.
2. Bring the medication, the medical record, or a prepared medication card and any other necessary supplies, to the patient—in one trip if possible so the patient is not left in an examination room alone with medication.
3. Identify the patient before giving the medication, to be sure that the correct patient is receiving the correct medication.
4. Always check for medication allergies by asking the patient before giving medication.
5. Administer medication by the route ordered by the practitioner.
6. Observe the patient taking oral medication; do not leave the patient to take medication alone.
7. Wear gloves if there is any possibility of coming into contact with body fluids.
8. When giving an injection, massage the injection site after administration to facilitate absorption. The exceptions to this are injections of heparin, as well as intradermal injections. *Not on all meds.*
9. For an injection, select an appropriate site for the type, amount, and route of medication to avoid nerve, tissue, and/or blood vessel damage.
10. Never break, recap, or bend a used needle.
11. Dispose of the used needle and syringe in a rigid biohazard container as quickly as possible.
12. Never leave a biohazard container that contains used needles in the exam room unless it is attached to the wall and is tamperproof. Figure 22–9 shows a wall-mounted rigid biohazard container.
13. Document all medications you give immediately after administration.

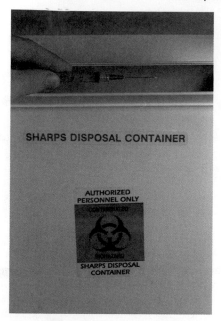

➤ **Figure 22–9** Exam rooms usually contain rigid biohazard container attached to the wall for disposal of sharps.

Documentation

Once a medication has been given, it should be documented immediately in the patient's medical record, including the following information: date, time given, name of the medication, amount (exactly as ordered by the doctor), and route. The signature of the person who gave the medication must accompany the documentation. In addition, if an injection was given, the route and site should be documented, in case a problem occurs.

Medications may be documented in the progress notes or on a special medication flow sheet. Medication flow sheets are used when patients receive the same medication over a period of time, especially in an inpatient setting such as a hospital or nursing home. They may also be used in a doctor's office for immunizations or other medications that the patient receives on a regular basis.

Never document a medication before giving it. If a patient refuses a medication for which there is a written medication order, tell the doctor and write a note describing the patient's reason for refusal, with the statement that the doctor has been notified.

Adverse Reactions to Medication

Any patient can have an adverse reaction to a medication, even a patient with no known medication allergies or someone who has had the medication before with no reaction. Adverse reactions can range from mild to severe.

Mild reactions usually occur after a patient has left the office; more severe reactions usually occur immediately and are more often associated with injections than with oral medication.

Reactions to oral medications usually include a rash and/or gastrointestinal upset. Usually, the patient calls the office to inform the doctor of the side effect. A medical assistant should take a message for the doctor. If the patient is troubled by the reaction, instruct him or her to wait for the doctor to call back before taking any more of the medication. Also take the number of the pharmacy the patient uses, in case the doctor wishes to change the medication and call in a new prescription.

To deal with the possibility of an immediate, severe reaction to an injection, a patient should always be instructed to stay at the doctor's office for about 15 minutes after having an injection.

Early signs of a reaction may be urticaria (hives), redness, and itching at the injection site. This can progress to more serious problems, including anaphylaxis, a swelling of the trachea, which leaves the patient unable to breath (anaphylaxis is described in detail in chapter 31, Emergency Care).

If a reaction occurs, have the patient lie down to prevent injury if he or she loses consciousness and to improve circulation. Take the patient's pulse and blood pressure. Monitor the patient's breathing.

In a severe reaction, the pulse will be rapid and weak, the blood pressure will be low, and the patient may have difficulty breathing.

Do not leave the patient alone. Call for help and ask whoever responds to get the doctor immediately. Also have the person get the emergency box or crash cart in case it is needed.

After a reaction, document the patient's symptoms and any treatment given in the patient's medical record. Also, fill out an incident report describing the problems the patient experienced and the response of all office personnel involved. Fill it out as completely as possible and file according to the office's procedures for reporting. (Incident reports are not normally filed in the patient's medical record.)

Medication Errors

Procedures for preparing and administering medications may seem cumbersome. But they are designed in such a way as to check and recheck that the right medication is being given to the right patient, at the right time, in the right dose, and by the right route. This prevents most medication errors from occurring.

But somehow medication errors do continue to occur. After all, people are only human, and all of us make mistakes. The most important thing to remember if you should make a medication error is to report it as soon as it is noticed and to monitor the patient to see if he or she has any adverse reaction to the medication. Whether the right medication was given to the wrong patient or the wrong medication to the right patient, a prompt response usually prevents any serious consequences.

Fortunately, most medication errors do not actually harm the patient. For example, if an immunization or usual dose of medication is given to the wrong patient, it will rarely harm the patient who receives it.

It is also important to make sure that the error is rectified by giving the right medication to the intended patient.

Medication errors must be documented in the medical record and signed by the person who made the error. Charting must include the date and time, the nature of the error, signs and symptoms experienced by the patient who was given the incorrect medication, and the patient's response to any treatment given.

In addition, an incident report should be filled out with as complete information as possible and should be reviewed by the office's head of risk management, so he or she can see if there are any system problems that can be addressed through better procedures or training to make sure similar errors do not happen in the future.

ORAL MEDICATIONS

The oral route is the most common route of medication administration, yet it is the route most rarely used in the office setting itself. That is because the doctor usually writes a prescription, which the patient has filled at the pharmacy. The patient then self-administers most oral medication.

Medication taken orally is absorbed through the lining of the gastrointestinal tract, where it is broken down. Oral medication is usually taken in the form of tablets or capsules. Oral liquid medication is available for children and for adults who have difficulty swallowing pills.

Preparing Solid Medication

To prepare solid medication, you need a plastic or paper medication cup. Be sure to check the label three times, as described above. Pour the medication into the bottle cap until the correct number of pills is in the cap. Then pour the pills into the medication cup.

You can pour medication back into the bottle from the bottle cap, but not from the medication cup. If any medication drops during the transfer or is not used after it is in the medication cup, it must be discarded.

If needed, scored tablets may be divided along the indentation in the pill surface. Use a paper towel or a plastic pill splitter to avoid touching the tablet. Cap-

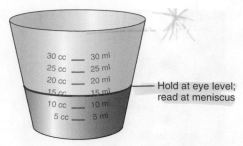

> **Figure 22–10** A medication cup containing 15 cc of medicine.

sules cannot be divided accurately. Enteric-coated medication cannot be divided or crushed.

Preparing Oral Liquid Medication

To prepare oral liquid medication, you need a plastic medication cup or plastic dropper with lines for medication doses.

Shake the medication well, especially if it is a suspension. Hold the bottle with the label toward your palm to keep the label clean. Hold the cup at eye level. The correct dose is read at the **meniscus**, the lowest point of the curved surface of the liquid in the cup.

You cannot pour unused medication back into the bottle. If you pour too much, discard the excess carefully. Add more medication if you discard too much. Figure 22–10 shows a medication cup with the exact dose (15 cc) measured at the meniscus.

Administering Oral Medication

Remember when administering oral medications that the inside of the bottle is considered sterile and cannot be touched. Liquid medication should be poured into a medicine cup with measurements on the side. Any overage must be discarded rather than poured back into the bottle. Solid oral medications should be poured into the cap, then transferred to a medicine cup. Pills can be poured back into the bottle from the cap but not from the medicine cup.

The patient should be given a cup of water either to wash down the pills or help get the taste of the liquid out of the mouth and keep the liquid from remaining on teeth.

Water should not be given with medications that are administered for local effects, such as cough medicine or antacids, or with sublingual or buccal medications that are dissolved under the tongue or between the gum and the cheek. Procedure 22–1 describes in detail the steps in administering oral medication.

PROCEDURE 22–1

Administering Oral Medications

Performance Objective: The student will be able to prepare and administer oral medications in tablet and liquid form following a doctor's order.

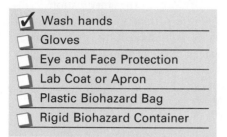

☑ Wash hands
☐ Gloves
☐ Eye and Face Protection
☐ Lab Coat or Apron
☐ Plastic Biohazard Bag
☐ Rigid Biohazard Container

Supplies and Equipment: Medication ordered by the doctor, medicine cup, cup of water, written medication order.

Procedure Steps

1. Obtain chart with doctor's medication order.
2. Calculate dosage if necessary so that you can give the **right dose** of the medication. Verify that it is the **right time** to administer the medication. Verify that giving the medication orally is the **right route**.
3. Wash hands.
4. Assemble medication and supplies to prepare and administer the medication.
5. Check the label of the medication as you remove it from the cabinet where it is stored to be sure that it is the same medication as ordered by the doctor in the patient's medical record.

Rationale: The label of the bottle of medication is checked three times to be sure that it is the **right medication.** This is the first check.

6. Check expiration date.
Rationale: Expired medication may have lost its potency or have undesired effects and should not be used.

7. Shake liquid medication, especially if directed to "Shake well" on the label.
Rationale: Many liquid medications consist of solid particles of medication suspended in a liquid vehicle. The medication tends to sink to the bottom during storage and requires shaking to redistribute evenly.

8. Check the medication label as you remove the cap to be sure that it is the same medication as ordered by the doctor in the patient's medical record. If preparing oral solid medication, use the cap to pour the medication. If preparing oral liquid medication, place the cap on the counter with the inside facing up.
Rationale: The label of the bottle of medication is checked three times to be sure that it is the **right medication.** This is the second check. The inside of the cap of the medication bottle must not touch the counter or any other object.

9a. For oral solid medication: Pour the correct number of tablets (as identified in your drug calculation) into the cap of the medication bottle and from the cap into the medication cup. Do not touch the medication with your hands. Do not touch the inside of the bottle cap or the inside of the medication cup.

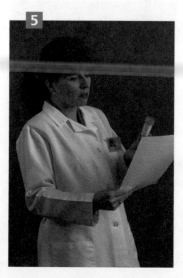

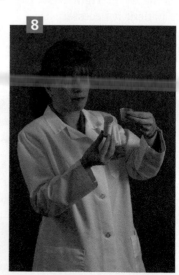

Procedure continued on following page

Rationale: The inside of the bottle is considered part of the bottle and if you pour extra tablets into the cap, you can return them to the bottle. Solid medication cannot be returned to the original bottle after it has been poured into a medication cup or has been dropped on the floor.

9b For oral liquid medication: Place your thumbnail at the level of the correct amount of medication to pour into the medication cup. Holding the label of the medication bottle against your palm, pour out the medication at eye level to the level marked by your thumbnail. The liquid may appear higher at the sides than in the middle of the cup. Read the correct dose at the meniscus (lowest level). Discard any excess in the sink.
Rationale: Read the dose at eye level for accuracy. Place the label against your palm to avoid staining the label if any medication drips accidentally. Wipe up any spills with a tissue. Once liquid medication has been poured out of a bottle, it cannot be poured back into the bottle.

10 Place the medication cup on the counter and recap the medication bottle. As you place the cap on the bottle and return it to storage, read the medication label to verify that it is the correct medication as ordered by the doctor in the patient's medical record.
Rationale: The label of the bottle of medication is checked three times to be sure that it is the **right medication.** This is the third check.

11. Take the medication and the medical record to the patient. Using the medical record, identify patient.
Rationale: Using the medical record allows you to be sure that you are going to give the medication to the **right** patient.

12. Assess patient if necessary.
Rationale: Vital signs may need to be checked before administering medication, even if the patient comes for a medication visit only. Should the patient exhibit any signs of illness, it may be necessary to check with the doctor before administering.

13. Seat patient in chair for comfort. Explain purpose of medication administration.
Rationale: Explaining that the doctor has ordered a particular medication will verify that the patient understands and is expecting administration of that medication.

14. Give the patient the medication. If the medication is in solid form, give it with a glass of water. If it is a liquid, you may give it with water if the patient desires, unless the medication label says otherwise.

15. Assess patient for any adverse reactions.

16. Wash hands.

17. Document the date, time, name of the medication, dose given, and route of administration. The abbreviation po (by mouth) is used by both the doctor and the medical assistant for oral medication. The dose given is documented as ordered by the doctor. An order written in milligrams is documented in milligrams regardless of the number of tablets or amount of liquid medication used, e.g. ibuprofen 800 mg. An order for a medication containing a combination of ingredients that specifies a number of tablets or amount of liquid is documented in the same form it was ordered, e.g. Maalox 30 cc.

Charting Example	
Date	
6/13/XX	12:30 PM Acetaminophen elixir 160 mg given po.
	K. Anderson, CMA

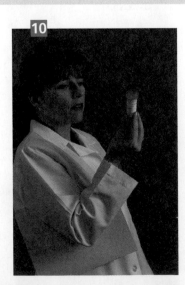

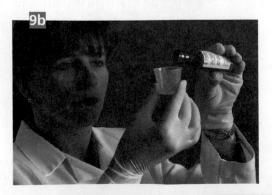

OTHER NONPARENTERAL MEDICATIONS

It is relatively rare that topical, rectal, or transdermal medication will be administered in the office. Eye and ear instillation are more common and were discussed in Chapter 21.

Topical Medication

When administering topical medication such as a cream or ointment containing medication, always use a tongue blade or large cotton swab to apply the medication. Wash your hands first, then wash the affected area, both to remove any dirt and any leftover medication. If the skin on the area is broken, use surgical asepsis, including sterile gloves; if the skin is intact, use medical asepsis. If the area is going to be bandaged, apply the medication to the bandage.

Rectal Medication

When a patient is vomiting, medication may be given by rectal suppository, to be absorbed through the tiny blood vessels of the rectum. Some suppositories also induce bowel movements.

When administering a rectal suppository, either you or the patient needs to insert the suppository above the anal sphincter so it will not be eliminated immediately. Suppositories are usually stored in the refrigerator to keep them firm for easier insertion. A water-soluble lubricant may also be used to ease insertion but not a petroleum-based lubricant. Always wear gloves when administering a rectal suppository. Figure 22–11 shows proper insertion of a rectal suppository above the anal sphincter.

Transdermal Medication

When administering a transdermal patch, try to rotate placement of the patch on the body. The most common places used are the upper arms, chest, and back. Gently wash the area where the new patch will be placed and clip any hair close (do not shave the area).

Before putting on a new patch, always remove any old patch. Be careful not to touch the inside surface of the patch, where the medication is located, so you do not absorb any medication. Discard the old patch by folding the sticky sides together.

Apply a new patch to the area you have prepared. Grasp only the adhesive, not the inside part with the medication. Beginning at the inside, firmly press down the adhesive-backed patch. Paper tape may be used to further hold the edges if they do not stick on their own.

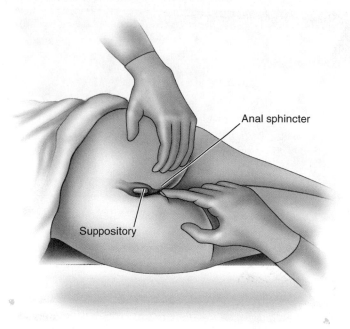

> **Figure 22–11** Proper position of a rectal suppository above the anal sphincter.

Anal sphincter

Suppository

PARENTERAL MEDICATIONS

There are a number of advantages to administering a medication by the parenteral route (via an injection). For systemic medications, the medication can get into the bloodstream faster because it bypasses the gastrointestinal tract. In addition to this more rapid response, absorption in the GI tract is often incomplete, so the parenteral route allows for a more accurate medication dosage to be administered.

Also, some medications, such as insulin, are made inactive by digestive enzymes. And in some cases, the patient is not allowed to take anything by mouth, so medication must be administered parenterally.

Finally, parenteral administration allows for targeting a medication to a specific place. The best examples of this are local anesthetics, intended only to numb the affected area so the doctor can work there without causing the patient discomfort, and injections into a particular joint or even into the spinal canal.

The physician or licensed practitioner must specify if the injection should be given intradermally, subcutaneously, intramuscularly, or intravenously.

Preparing Parenteral Medication

To prepare parenteral medication, you need a syringe and the medication, which comes either in an ampule, a vial, or a prepackaged single-dose syringe. Ampules are single-dose; vials may be single-dose or multi-dose.

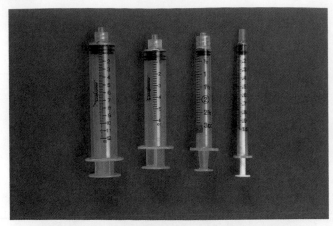

> **Figure 22–12** Various sizes of syringes: (from left) 12 cc syringe, 6 cc syringe, 3 cc syringe, and tuberculin (1 cc) syringe.

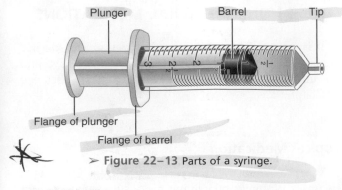

> **Figure 22–13** Parts of a syringe.

An **ampule** is a small glass flask with a glass top that breaks off when appropriate pressure is applied. Before opening, tap the top of the ampule to settle all medication out of the top. Then wipe the neck with an alcohol swab. Finally, tap or twist the ampule top so that it breaks apart at the weak spot on the neck. You may also use a file to weaken the glass at the neck before breaking the ampule. You can then insert a syringe needle into the ampule to draw out the medication.

A **vial** is a small glass bottle, with a rubber stopper at the top, through which a needle is inserted to draw out a dose of medication. Before inserting a needle to withdraw medication, the rubber stopper must be cleaned with alcohol. When using a multi-use vial, you need to be extremely careful not to allow the vial to become contaminated. Once you have removed the needle from the vial, discard any excess medication by squirting it into a sink. Do not return it to the vial.

There are many different types of syringes, but they all have the same parts. These include the barrel, which holds the medication and has the markings; the plunger, the movable part that pushes medication out through the needle; the flange, the protracted rim of the barrel used for gripping when pushing the plunger; and the tip, the part at the end of the barrel where the needle is placed. The inside of the barrel, as well as the plunger, and the tip of the syringe must all remain sterile during administration of medication. Figure 22–12 shows four types of syringes; Figure 22–13 shows the different parts of a syringe.

Some syringes come prefilled with a single dose of medication. Some prefilled syringes come as part of a cartridge injection system. The cartridge is attached to each prefilled syringe.

Needles have two size variables, length and diameter of the opening, or **lumen** (called the **gauge**). Different lengths are used for injections at different sites, and different gauges are used depending on the thickness of the medication and length of the needle. A longer needle must also be thicker to prevent bending or breaking. As with syringes, all needles have the same basic parts. These are the point, the sharp end that penetrates the skin; the **bevel**, the slanted edge just behind the point, where the medication emerges from the needle; the shaft, through which the medication flows; the hub, which mounts on the syringe; and the hilt, where the shaft attaches to the hub. Figure 22–14 shows various needles; Figure 22–15 shows the parts of a needle.

A number of variables go into selecting the proper needle and syringe to use to give an injection. These include the type and amount of medicine being given, the consistency or thickness of the medication, the size of the patient, and the type of injection. These variables effect both the length and gauge of the needle you select.

Intradermal injections (between layers of skin) require only a short needle, ⅜″. Subcutaneous injections (under all of the skin layers) require a needle that is ½″ or ⅝″. An intramuscular injection (into the muscle) requires the longest needle. Depending on which mus-

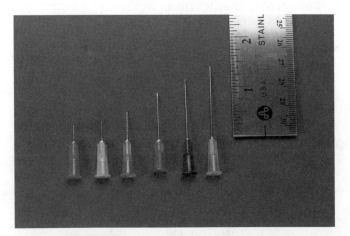

> **Figure 22–14** Various sizes and lengths of needles; the color of the hub identifies the gauge (diameter) of the needle for a particular manufacturer.

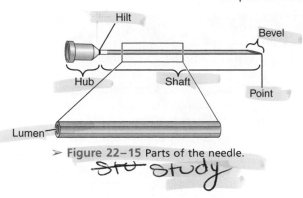

> Figure 22–15 Parts of the needle.

Stu Study (handwritten)

cle mass is being injected and how much fat you need to get through before you get to muscle, a needle anywhere from 1″ to 3″ should be used.

With regard to the gauge, the narrower (or finer) the gauge the smaller the opening inside the needle through which medication passes. Finer gauge needles hurt less, but they can generally penetrate less tissue without bending. When describing needle gauge, the higher the number the finer the gauge.

The finest gauge needles are 27-gauge (G) and 28 G, which are used for intradermal injections, when you only want to place a small amount of medication under the top layers of skin. Needles of 25 G or 26 G are generally used for subcutaneous injections. Wider-gauge needles—20 G to 24 G—are used for deeper, intramuscular injections. Needles of less than 20 gauge are used for venipunctures and other procedures in which deeper tissues must be penetrated.

Different techniques are used to draw medication from an ampule and a vial.

After breaking the top off the ampule, you should hold it sideways to upside down, with the syringe at eye level or slightly above, and draw out the correct amount of medication by pulling back the plunger. As long as only the shaft of the needle enters the ampule, hydrostatic pressure keeps the liquid from draining out, even if the ampule is inverted. No air is injected into an ampule because doing so would force the medication to run out over the side.

Procedure 22–2 describes the correct method of drawing medication from an ampule.

(handwritten notes: Smaller the # the bigger the needle; glass ampules; Tb test - 1ml; 27 G 1/2; DRAW w w/needle w/needle only on new)

PROCEDURE 22–2

Drawing Up Medication from an Ampule

Performance Objective: The student will be able to prepare an injectable medication from an ampule.

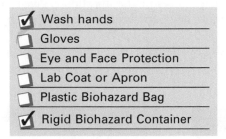

☑	Wash hands
☐	Gloves
☐	Eye and Face Protection
☐	Lab Coat or Apron
☐	Plastic Biohazard Bag
☑	Rigid Biohazard Container

Supplies and Equipment: Syringe with needle, ampule of medication, alcohol swab, gauze, rigid biohazard container.

Procedure Steps

1. Obtain chart with doctor's medication order.
2. Calculate dosage if necessary so that you can draw up the **right dose** of the medication. Verify that it is the **right time** to administer the medication.

3. Wash hands.
4. Assemble medication and supplies to prepare the medication.
5. Check the label of the ampule as you remove it from the cabinet where it is stored to be sure that it is the same medication as ordered by the doctor in the patient's medical record.
   Rationale: The label of the bottle of medication is checked three times to be sure that it is the **right medication.** This is the first check.
6. Check expiration date.
   Rationale: Expired medication may have lost its potency or have undesired effects and should not be used.
7. Tap the top of the ampule until all medication falls from the neck into the bottom part of the ampule.
   Rationale: If medication is caught in the neck or top of the ampule, the amount of medication remaining in the ampule may not be sufficient for you to draw up.
8. Check the label of the ampule to be sure

Procedure continued on following page

PROCEDURE 22-2 *(continued)*

that it is the same medication as ordered by the doctor in the patient's medical record.
Rationale: The label of the bottle of medication is checked three times to be sure that it is the **right medication.** This is the second check.

9 Wipe neck of the ampule with alcohol swab. Wrap a gauze square around the neck of the ampule.
Rationale: The sterile needle wil pass through the neck once the top has been removed so disinfection of the neck of the ampule is necessary.

10 Holding the top and bottom of the ampule with fingers protected by the gauze square, push the top away from yourself, breaking the top completely off. Discard the upper part of the ampule in a rigid biohazard container.
Rationale: Safety is practiced by breaking glass away from self to prevent any possible injury from glass fragments. The upper part of the ampule has a sharp edge that could tear a plastic bag.

11. Place the opened ampule on a flat surface.
12. Open syringe with needle attached, remove needle cover, and insert needle into the ampule. Do not touch anything with the tip of the needle or the shaft of the needle except the solution in the ampule.
Rationale: Safety is practiced by inserting needle into ampule on flat surface and not holding ampule in your hand when inserting the needle to avoid needle-stick injuries.
13. Withdraw ordered amount of medication by pulling back on the plunger of the syringe. You may withdraw the medication with the ampule standing on a flat surface or you may

invert the ampule and withdraw the medication.
Rationale: Ampules are made of special glass that will not allow contents to escape if they are turned upside down.

14. Draw up enough medication from the ampule for the dose ordered by the doctor. Withdraw the needle from the ampule and, with the needle pointing upward, tap the syringe until all bubbles rise toward the needle. Push the plunger toward the syringe to expel the air. If there is excess medication, holding the syringe over the sink, push the plunger to the desired dose, expelling excess medication.
Rationale: Air bubbles take up space in the syringe and prevent an accurate measurement of the dose of medication. When drawing up medication from an ampule, it is better to draw up more medication than needed and measure the dose after expelling any air than to keep putting the needle in and out of the ampule.

15. Recap the needle using a method to avoid needle sticks. If the needle becomes contaminated or if a filter needle was used, change the needle before administering the injection.
Rationale: The needle guard keeps the needle sterile until you give the injection. When drawing up medication from an ampule, a filter needle is sometimes used to filter any minute particles of glass and prevent them from entering the syringe. The needle must be changed before the injection is given to remove any particles that were filtered by the needle.

16. Check the label of the ampule to be sure that it is the same medication as ordered by

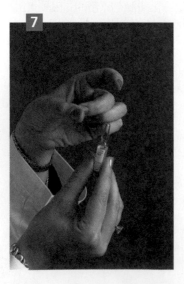

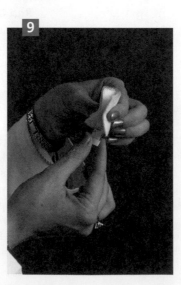

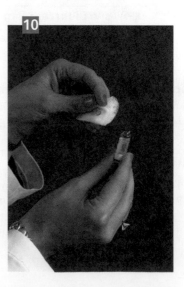

the doctor in the patient's medical record.
Rationale: The label of the bottle of medication is checked 3 times to be sure that it is the right medication. This is the third check.

17. Discard the ampule in a rigid biohazard container.

Rationale: This provides safe disposal of both the glass ampule and any unused medication.

18. Wash hands.

A vial is also held sideways to upside down, with the syringe at eye level, to draw medication from it. Vials are vacuum sealed. To be able to draw the medication easily, you must insert air into the vial to fill the space that will be left empty when the medication is drawn. To do this, pull the syringe back to the mark to which you will draw the medication. Then put the needle in the vial and push down, injecting the air in

the syringe into the vial. Then, invert the vial and pull the plunger back to the correct mark, drawing the correct amount of medication into the syringe.

The tip of the needle should be above the fluid line when injecting air (to avoid producing bubbles) and in the fluid when withdrawing medication.

Procedure 22–3 describes how to draw up medication from a vial.

check lable @ least 3 times

PROCEDURE 22–3

Drawing Up Medication from a Vial

Performance Objective: The student will be able to prepare an injectable medication using a medication vial.

☑	Wash hands
☐	Gloves
☐	Eye and Face Protection
☐	Lab Coat or Apron
☐	Plastic Biohazard Bag
☑	Rigid Biohazard Container

Supplies and Equipment: Syringe with needle, vial of medication, alcohol pads, rigid biohazard container.

Procedure Steps

1. Obtain chart with doctor's medication order.
2. Calculate dosage if necessary so that you can draw up the **right dose** of the medication. Verify that it is the **right time** to administer the medication.
3. Wash hands.
4. Assemble medication and supplies to prepare the medication.
5. Check the label of the vial as you remove it from the cabinet where it is stored to be sure

that it is the same medication as ordered by the doctor in the patient's medical record.
Rationale: The label of the bottle of medication is checked three times to be sure that it is the **right medication.** This is the first check.

6. Check expiration date.
Rationale: Expired medication may have lost its potency or have undesired effects and should not be used.

7. Wipe off vial top with alcohol swab.
Rationale: The sterile needle will pass

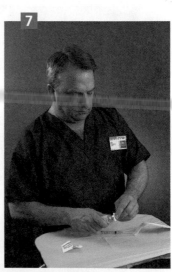

Procedure continued on following page

PROCEDURE 22–3 *(continued)*

through the rubber stopper so disinfection of top is necessary.

8. Check the label of the vial to be sure that it is the same medication as ordered by the doctor in the patient's medical record.
Rationale: The label of the bottle of medication is checked three times to be sure that it is the **right medication.** This is the second check.

9. Open the syringe and draw up air into the syringe equal to the amount of medication to be removed from the vial.
Rationale: If air is not injected into a multiple-dose vial to replace fluid that is removed, a vacuum will be created that will make it difficult to withdraw subsequent doses of medication.

10 Place the vial on a flat surface, remove needle cover by pulling it straight away from the needle, and insert needle into vial without holding the vial in your hand until the tip of the needle has safely entered the rubber stopper. Do not touch any part of the needle with your fingers.
Rationale: Accidental needle sticks can be avoided by practicing procedures to keep your hands away from all possible contact with an unsheathed needle. The needle is sterile and can only touch the rubber diaphragm of the vial that has been cleaned with alcohol.

11 Inject air above the fluid line to avoid bubbles. Invert the vial so that the tip of the needle is now below the fluid line and, hold-

ing the vial in your nondominant hand, pull back on the plunger of the syringe. Withdraw the correct amount of medication. Be sure that the tip of the needle is below the fluid line.
Rationale: You will need to bring vial up to eye level to withdraw the exact dose ordered.

12 If air bubbles appear in the syringe, tap the syringe to allow the bubbles to rise to the top. Holding the syringe in a vertical position, push the air through the needle and withdraw more medication if needed for the correct dose.
Rationale: Air bubbles can displace a volume of medication causing an incorrect dosage, especially if the bubbles are large.

13. Withdraw the needle from the vial and recap the needle using a method to avoid needle sticks. If the needle becomes contaminated change the needle to administer the injection. Discard the contaminated needle in a rigid biohazard container.
Rationale: The needle guard keeps the needle sterile until you give the injection.

14. Check the label of the vial as you return it to storage to be sure that it is the same medication ordered by the doctor in the patient's medical record.
Rationale: The label of the bottle of medication is checked three times to be sure that it is the **right medication.** This is the third check.

15. Wash hands.

.1 -air before putinto actual ↓ (handwritten)

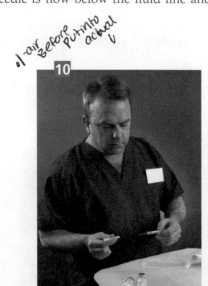

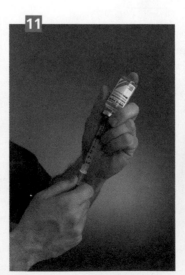

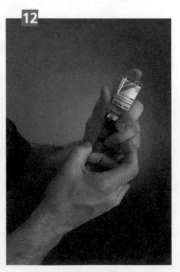

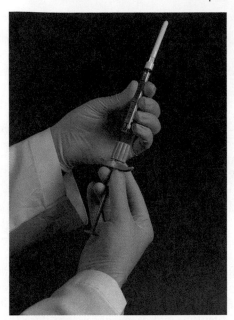

➤ **Figure 22–16** Loading a Tubex syringe: placing the cartridge in.

Increasingly, medications are coming in prefilled cartridges, which are loaded into a cartridge holder. Figure 22–16 shows the proper way to place a prefilled cartridge into a holder; Figure 22–17 shows how to tighten the handle.

After use, the entire cartridge is removed from the holder and discarded in a rigid biohazard container. The holder can be used again.

Some parenteral medications come in powdered form in single- or multi-dose vials. In this case, the medication must be reconstituted before it can be administered as an injection. Usually sterile water or sa-

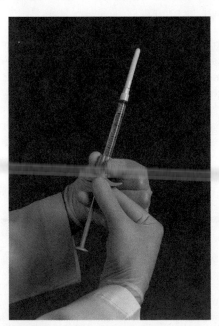

➤ **Figure 22–17** Loading a Tubex syringe: tightening the handle.

line is used as the **diluent**—the liquid used to dilute a powder. They are mixed with the powder to turn it into a liquid. A few powdered medications come with their own special diluent.

To reconstitute a powdered medication, follow the package directions to identify the correct amount and type of diluent (usually sterile water for injection or sterile 0.9 percent sodium chloride solution, also called normal saline). Draw up the correct amount of diluent from the multi-use vial. Then gently inject the diluent into the vial containing the powder. Injecting it directly into the powder can cause bubbles. After removing the needle, roll the vial from side to side and upside down, gently mixing the powder and the diluent, so as not to cause bubbles. Be sure that all the powder has dissolved before using the medication.

When a powdered drug is reconstituted, notations must be made on the vial's label about the date the medication was reconstituted, the diluent used, and the person who did the reconstitution. Procedure 22–4 describes in more detail how to reconstitute a powdered medication.

It may be necessary to calculate the dose of a reconstituted medication. The package instructions give instructions about the concentration after a specific amount of diluent has been added. Remember, after the powdered medication dissolves, there may be a greater volume of liquid than was added.

You need to take a number of special precautions when administering medication parenterally. You need to avoid major muscles and nerves, because these can be damaged by injections. You need to avoid blood vessels, unless the injection is intended to be intravenous.

Sterile technique must always be used, because the needle is going to penetrate the skin. Finally, always have the patient stay for 10 to 15 minutes after administering an injection, because any allergic reaction the patient is going to have will probably occur rapidly and may be intense.

Documentation of medication administration must be accurate. In the patient's chart, record the name of the medication; the exact dose ordered by the practitioner; the route and site of administration; and the time and date the injection was given. If there are any problems, these must also be documented thoroughly. Figure 22–18 shows the types of injections and angle of administration.

Subcutaneous Injections

Subcutaneous injections are given into the layer of fatty tissue below the skin. Injections are given by this route because the medication is something that would irritate the muscle, or is one that does not need to be absorbed rapidly. The subcutaneous route is used for insulin, heparin, and for the vaccination against mea-

PROCEDURE 22-4

Reconstituting a Powdered Medicine

Performance Objective: The student will be able to prepare an injectable medication by reconstituting the powdered form to a liquid using a diluent.

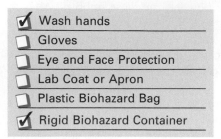

- ☑ Wash hands
- ☐ Gloves
- ☐ Eye and Face Protection
- ☐ Lab Coat or Apron
- ☐ Plastic Biohazard Bag
- ☑ Rigid Biohazard Container

Supplies and Equipment: Syringe with needle, vial of powdered medication, vial of diluent as specified on the label of the powdered medication, alcohol pads, rigid biohazard container.

Procedure Steps

1. Read the label of the powdered medication to identify the amount and type of diluent (liquid used to dilute) to add and the resulting concentration of the powdered medication.
   Rationale: Powdered medications are diluted either with sterile water, sterile saline for injection, or a diluent supplied by the manufacturer. You must use a solution that will dissolve the medication correctly as directed by the manufacturer.
2. Wash hands.
3. Assemble medication and supplies to prepare the medication.
4. Check expiration date of the powdered medication and the diluent.
   Rationale: Expired vials of medication may have lost their potency or sterility and should not be used.

5. Wipe off the top of the bottle of powdered medication and the bottle of diluent with an alcohol pad.
   Rationale: The sterile needle will pass through the rubber stopper of both bottles so disinfection of both tops is necessary.
6. Open the syringe and draw up air into the syringe equal to the amount of medication to be removed from the vial of diluent.
   Rationale: If air is not injected into a multiple-dose vial to replace fluid that is removed, a vacuum will be created that will make it difficult to withdraw subsequent doses of medication.
7. Inject the air into the bottle of diluent and withdraw the correct amount of diluent.
8. Inject diluent into the vial of powdered medication.
9. After removing the needle, roll the vial of medication between your hands until the medication is completely mixed.
   Rationale: Rolling the medication mixes the powder with the diluent without creating bubbles which can make it difficult to measure the dose accurately.
10. Label the bottle with the date, time, your initials, and the concentration of the reconstituted medication. Store as directed by the manufacturer.
    Rationale: Medication is usually manufactured in powdered form because it only remains stable for a short time when reconstituted. It may be stable for a longer time if refrigerated.
11. If you are not going to use the syringe to draw up the medication immediately or if you change the needle, dispose of used needle and/or syringe in a rigid biohazard container.
12. Wash hands.

---

sles, mumps, and rubella (MMR vaccination), usually given at age 15 months and again when the child enters middle school.

For a subcutaneous injection, select the appropriate site, pinch the skin gently, and inject at a 45-degree angle. Use a short, fine needle, ½" or ⅝" and 25G to

27G. An insulin syringe should be used for insulin injections, a 3-cc or tuberculin syringe for other subcutaneous injections.

Proper sites for a subcutaneous injection are those where there is a substantial layer of fatty tissue, such as the lateral aspect of the upper arm about 3" above the

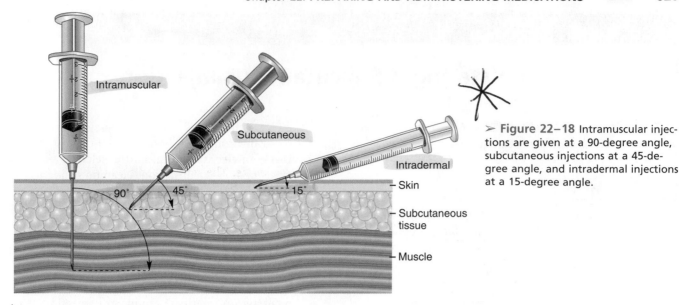

> **Figure 22–18** Intramuscular injections are given at a 90-degree angle, subcutaneous injections at a 45-degree angle, and intradermal injections at a 15-degree angle.

elbow, the abdomen, the top of the leg, and the back below the shoulder blades. Figure 22–19 shows subcutaneous injection sites.

Subcutaneous injections should be aspirated. This means that once the needle is in the tissue, the plunger should be gently pulled back to make sure the needle is not in a blood vessel. If it is, blood will enter the syringe. To avoid intravenous injection, which can alter the medication's intended action, the needle must be removed and the medication discarded. A new dose should be drawn up with a new needle and syringe.

After injection, massage the injection site to facilitate absorption and decrease discomfort. (This should not be done for injections of heparin, insulin, or medication given intradermally.)

If you are giving an insulin injection, it will often be part of a teaching session for a newly diagnosed diabetic or family of a diabetic. Education for the patient

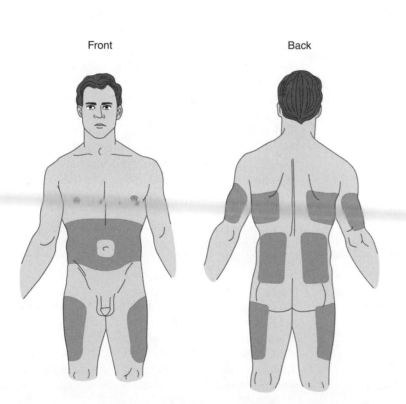

Front Back

> Figure 22–19 Subcutaneous injection sites.

PROCEDURE 22–5

Administering a Subcutaneous Injection

Performance Objective: The student will be able to administer a subcutaneous injection.

- ☑ Wash hands
- ☑ Gloves
- ☐ Eye and Face Protection
- ☐ Lab Coat or Apron
- ☐ Plastic Biohazard Bag
- ☑ Rigid Biohazard Container

Supplies and Equipment: Syringe and needle containing medication as ordered by the doctor, alcohol pad, gauze pad, gloves, bandage, biohazard container, medical record of the patient to receive the injection.

Procedure Steps

1. Wash hands.
2. Using the medical record, identify the patient, explain the procedure, and tell the patient the reason for the injection.
3. Ask the patient if he or she knows of any allergies to the medication.
4. Put on disposable gloves.
5. Select an injection site. The most common sites are the upper outer aspect of the arm, the top of the upper leg, or the abdomen.
   Rationale: A site with adequate subcutaneous tissue should be selected. Avoid injecting into moles, skin lesions, or blood vessels that can be seen through the skin.
6. Using an alcohol pad, clean the selected site by using a circular motion, cleaning inside to outside.
   Rationale: Move from the cleanest area to a less clean area without going back over any area already cleaned for best results.
7. Remove needle cover.
8. With thumb and first two fingers of your nondominant hand, form a skin fold by pinching up the tissue around the injection site.
   Rationale: Pinching up the skin lifts the subcutaneous tissue off the muscle and avoids accidental intramuscular injection.
9. Grasp the syringe between the thumb and first two fingers of your dominant hand with your palm up and, with one swift movement, insert the entire needle up to the hub at a 45-degree angle into the subcutaneous tissue.
   Rationale: The depth of the injection is determined by the choice of needle length. The 45-degree angle helps position the needle tip within the subcutaneous tissue. Inserting the needle with one swift movement reduces discomfort for the patient.
10. Without moving the needle in the tissue, aspirate: Pull back on the plunger slightly and observe to be sure that no blood enters the syringe. If blood appears, withdraw the needle, apply pressure to the site, and prepare a new injection.
    Rationale: Blood in the syringe means that the tip of the needle has penetrated a blood-vessel. If medication is injected, the route will be intravenous rather than subcutaneous, which could change the effect of the medication. A new syringe and medication will have to be prepared because blood contaminates the medication and may be irritating to the tissue if used.
11. If no blood appears when you aspirate, push in the plunger slowly and steadily until all medication has been administered.
    Rationale: Rapid injection may cause tissue damage and will not allow for proper absorption.
12. Withdraw needle swiftly at the same angle it was inserted.

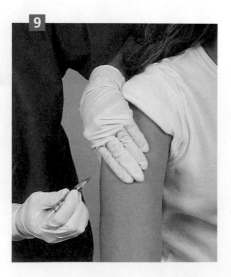

Rationale: Withdrawing the needle at the same angle reduces pressure on the tissue and minimizes discomfort.

13. Apply pressure to the site using a gauze pad or alcohol pad. Gently massage the injection site (except when injecting heparin or insulin, which should never be massaged.)
    Rationale: Pressure helps control bleeding, and massage facilitates absorption of the medication. Heparin is never massaged because it is an anticoagulant.

14. Place the syringe and needle in a rigid biohazard container without recapping the needle.
    Rationale: It is a standard precaution never to recap a needle that has been used to give an injection because of the potential to contract a blood-borne disease if a needle-stick injury were to occur. Disposing of used needles in a rigid biohazard container prevents injury.

15. Assess the injection site. Continue applying pressure if the injection site is still bleeding freely. Apply an adhesive bandage if bleeding has stopped.

Rationale: An adhesive bandage is reassuring to many patients. In addition, it may protect the patient's clothing if a small amount of bleeding or leakage of serous fluid occurs.

16. Remove gloves and discard.
17. Wash hands.
18. Ask the patient to remain in the office for 10 to 15 minutes in case a reaction occurs.
    Rationale: A severe medication reaction will usually begin within 10 to 15 minutes.
19. Document the medication, the dose as ordered by the doctor, the injection site, and any reaction that you observe in the patient's medical record.

Charting Example	
Date	
8/8/XX	11:13 AM Heparin 10,000 U SC given in the epigastric area of the abdomen. No bleeding or bruising noted at site. ———
	——— S. Williams, CMA

*Figure from Bonewit-West K. *Clinical Procedures for Medical Assistants,* 5th ed. Philadelphia: W.B. Saunders, 2000.

with diabetes will be discussed in detail in chapter 33.

Procedure 22–5 describes administering subcutaneous injections.

Intramuscular Injections

An intramuscular injection is one given directly into muscle tissue. Intramuscular injections are usually absorbed rapidly, but some oil-based preparations are long acting. These often contain the prefix "depo" in the name; a depot is a storage place.

When giving an intramuscular injection, select the appropriate site, spread the skin with your thumb and forefinger, and administer the injection at a 90-degree angle.

The needle must be both long enough and wide enough to penetrate to the middle of the muscle. The longer the needle, the thicker it must be to prevent bending. For infants, a $5/8''$, 25 G needle will penetrate to the middle of the muscle; for an adult the needle may need to be as long as $1\frac{1}{2}''$ and as heavy as 20 G.

A syringe must be chosen that is appropriate for the dosage. Different sites can absorb different amounts of medication. The site should be chosen for safety and for absorption of the particular amount and type of medication. If too much medication is injected into a small muscle, excessive tissue damage and/or poor absorption could result.

As with a subcutaneous injection, an intramuscular injection should be aspirated to make sure no blood vessel has been entered. When a medication is extremely irritating to subcutaneous tissue, the Z-track injection method should be used to minimize irritation. In the Z-track method, the skin at the injection site is pulled to the side before injection, displacing the layer of subcutaneous tissue. If the medication is irritating, the needle should be changed after the medication is drawn from the ampule or vial, so there is no medication on the needle to cause irritation to the subcutaneous layer while the needle is passing through to the muscle.

For most intramuscular injections, massaging the site after administration helps the medication be absorbed more quickly. However, the site should not be massaged after administering the iron supplement Imferon.

Choosing a Site for Intramuscular Injections

A number of different sites can be used to administer an intramuscular injection. The choice should be made both for patient comfort and for a site that can absorb the amount of medication being administered. Wherever you are going to inject, make sure you identify the anatomic area properly. Be sure you have prepared the injection using the proper needle length and gauge.

The **deltoid** muscle of the upper arm is the most common site for giving intramuscular injections in the office. The deltoid provides both maximum comfort and maximum modesty for the patient, and is what most patients expect when they think of an injection. An injection into the deltoid site usually leaves the deltoid muscle slightly sore for a day or two.

The deltoid is a rather small muscle. The most common volume for an injection in the deltoid is 0.5 mL. Although the stated maximum amount of medication that can be injected is 2.0 mL, more than 1.0 mL may be poorly absorbed and may cause pain by tearing muscle fibers. For an averaged sized adult, a 1″ 23 G to 25 G needle is used. A small adult or older child will require a shorter needle; for an obese adult a 1½″ needle may be required.

Infants and young children should not be given injections in the deltoid muscle. Figure 22–20 shows the deltoid site.

A proper deltoid injection is given about three fingers (1″ to 2″) below the acromion process of the scapula (shoulder blade), the triangular projection coming from the spine that forms the point of the shoulder. An injection should be given in the center of the deltoid, rather than the upper or lower portions. The brachial, axillary, and radial nerves cross the deltoid and must be avoided. The acromion process and the humerus must also be avoided, as well as major blood vessels.

The **dorsogluteal** site is traditionally used for deep intramuscular injections. The gluteus medius is a large muscle that lies over the curve of the ilium. An injection in this region must be given in the upper quadrant of the buttock to avoid the sciatic nerve and large blood vessels. This site can absorb a large amount of fluid. Up to 3 mL of fluid can be injected, and some resources say up to 5 mL.

To find the proper injection site, you need to mark both the posterior iliac spine and the greater trochanter of the femur. The area above and outside the imagi-

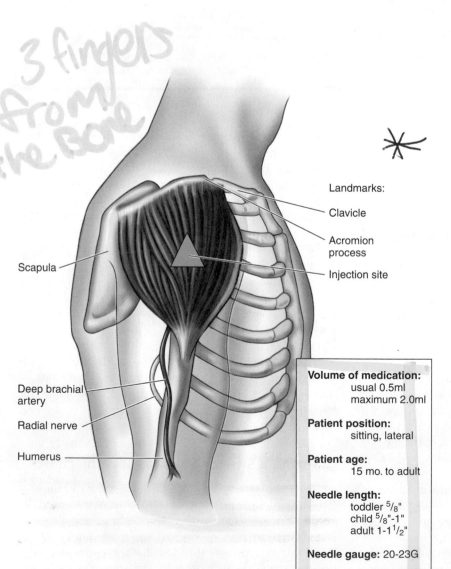

Landmarks:

Clavicle

Acromion process

Injection site

Scapula

Deep brachial artery

Radial nerve

Humerus

> **Figure 22–20** Deltoid injection site.

Volume of medication:
usual 0.5ml
maximum 2.0ml

Patient position:
sitting, lateral

Patient age:
15 mo. to adult

Needle length:
toddler 5/8″
child 5/8″-1″
adult 1-1½″

Needle gauge: 20-23G

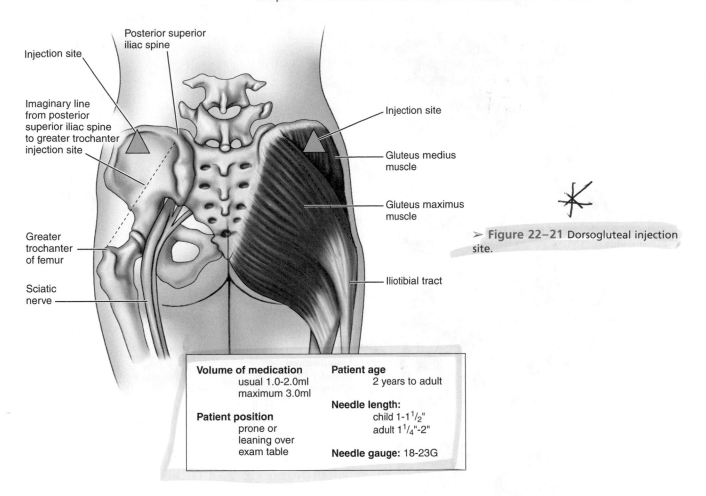

Posterior superior
iliac spine

Injection site

Imaginary line
from posterior
superior iliac spine
to greater trochanter
injection site

Greater
trochanter
of femur

Sciatic
nerve

Injection site

Gluteus medius
muscle

Gluteus maximus
muscle

Iliotibial tract

➤ **Figure 22–21** Dorsogluteal injection
site.

Volume of medication	Patient age
usual 1.0-2.0ml maximum 3.0ml	2 years to adult
	Needle length:
Patient position	child 1-1$^1/_2$"
prone or	adult 1$^1/_4$"-2"
leaning over exam table	**Needle gauge:** 18-23G

nary line between these two locations is appropriate for a dorsogluteal injection. Another way to find the correct site is to divide the buttock into four equal quadrants and inject into the upper outer quarter of the upper outer quadrant.

The gluteal muscles, using both the dorsogluteal and the ventrogluteal injection sites, are the least painful muscles for adults to receive an injection in. Also, the patient can not see the needle, which reduces anxiety and "psychic pain." However, they are not used as frequently as the arm.

The patient should lie on the examination table, in the prone position. This is not an appropriate injection site for an infant, because the muscle does not develop until after walking begins. Figure 22–21 shows the dorsogluteal site.

The **ventrogluteal** site is more to the side of the hip (gluteus minimus) than the dorsogluteal site. The ventrogluteal site is relatively free of nerves and blood vessels.

Although this is an excellent site and no more painful than the dorsogluteal site, it is not used extensively in the ambulatory care setting.

The ventrogluteal site can be used from infancy to adulthood. Figure 22–22 shows the ventrogluteal site.

To find the site, place the heel of the hand on the greater trochanter, using two fingers to point to the anterior superior iliac spine and the iliac crest. The area between the two fingers marks the injection site.

The **vastus lateralis** is the site used most often for intramuscular injections in infants and toddlers. It is the site of choice for infant immunizations because the muscles of the back and buttock are poorly developed. The site is located on the outside of the upper leg.

In an infant, an injection to this site is given with a $^5/_8$" 25 G or 26 G needle, and may be given at a 45- or 90-degree angle, depending on the size of the muscle and the amount of subcutaneous tissue over the muscle. The site is relatively large at birth and relatively free of nerves and blood vessels. The rectus femoris muscle, which runs down the front of the leg, may also be used for childhood immunizations. Figure 22–23 shows the vastus lateralis site in an infant.

The child must be restrained. He or she may sit on the parent's lap and be held closely, or may lie on the exam table, with office personnel immobilizing all extremities to prevent injury during the injection.

The vastus lateralis is rarely used for adults in an office setting. An injection to this site can be painful for an active person, especially if the person is athletic.

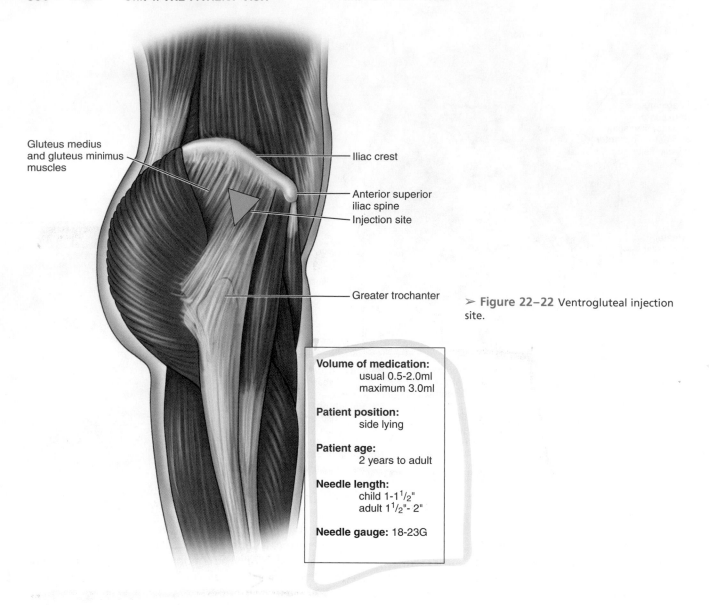

Gluteus medius and gluteus minimus muscles

Iliac crest

Anterior superior iliac spine

Injection site

Greater trochanter

➤ **Figure 22–22** Ventrogluteal injection site.

Volume of medication:
usual 0.5-2.0ml
maximum 3.0ml

Patient position:
side lying

Patient age:
2 years to adult

Needle length:
child 1-1$\frac{1}{2}$"
adult 1$\frac{1}{2}$"- 2"

Needle gauge: 18-23G

It can cause muscle soreness after the injection. The vastus lateralis is used more often in hospitals and nursing homes, for inactive or bedridden patients. Figure 22–24 shows the vastus lateralis site in an adult.

Procedure 22–6 describes how to select the proper site for an intramuscular injection.

Administering an Intramuscular Injection

After you have washed your hands, chosen the correct injection site, chosen the correct needle and syringe, and prepared the medication, it is time to perform the actual injection. Although gloves are not needed to prepare the injection, put them on before administering the injection. Instruct the patient to relax the muscles before injecting, to reduce discomfort.

There are eight principles for properly administering an injection.

1. Clean the site with alcohol, using a circular motion and friction. Let the site dry to prevent stinging.
2. Do not inject into any moles, skin discolorations, or obvious blood vessels.
3. Put the needle in quickly. Select the needle length to reach the appropriate area for the injection. Do not move the needle once it has been inserted.
4. Always aspirate before injecting the medication, to make sure you are not in a blood vessel.
5. If no blood enters when you aspirate, inject the medication slowly.
6. Withdraw the needle quickly.
7. Dispose of the needle immediately in a rigid biohazard container.
8. Immediately after the injection, apply pressure with a gauze pad until any bleeding stops.

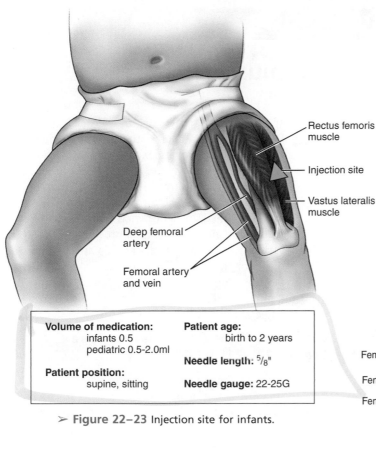

Volume of medication:
    infants 0.5
    pediatric 0.5-2.0ml

Patient position:
    supine, sitting

Patient age:
    birth to 2 years

Needle length: $^5/_8"$

Needle gauge: 22-25G

➢ **Figure 22–23** Injection site for infants.

Preventing Adverse Effects from Injections

A number of adverse effects can result from an injection. These include allergic reactions such as rash or nausea and vomiting. The most severe allergic reactions lead to anaphylactic shock, the sudden systemic reaction caused by massive histamine release, which causes low blood pressure and bronchoconstriction.

Other adverse effects include a sterile abscess at the injection site, an accidental intravenous administration of medication, bleeding from the injection site, infection of the site, nerve injury, or muscle contractures. Also, rarely, a needle breaks during an injection.

Some important measures can be taken to reduce the likelihood of an adverse effect occurring from the injection.

First, *never* give an injection unless there is a licensed practitioner in the office, in case a problem arises. If you need assistance because of a problem, interrupt whatever the practitioner is doing and make it clear that you need assistance immediately.

In addition to checking the chart for allergies, always ask the patient about allergies, especially if you are giving antibiotics. Always have the patient remain for 10 or 15 minutes after an injection to make sure there are no adverse reactions. A severe reaction will probably begin within this time.

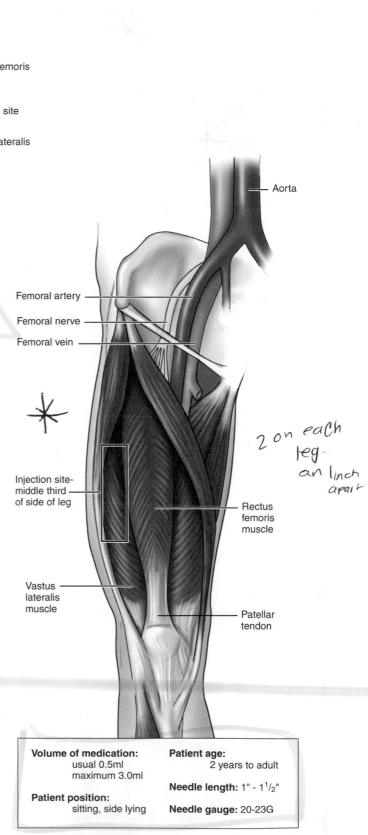

2 on each leg. an 1 inch apart

Volume of medication:
    usual 0.5ml
    maximum 3.0ml

Patient position:
    sitting, side lying

Patient age:
    2 years to adult

Needle length: 1" - $1^1/_2"$

Needle gauge: 20-23G

➢ **Figure 22–24** Vastus lateralis injection site (adults).

PROCEDURE 22-6

Selecting a Site for an Intramuscular Injection

Performance Objective: The student will be able to select appropriate sites for various intramuscular injections to a patient.

Supplies and Equipment: Manikin or student to locate the following injection sites: deltoid, ventrogluteal, dorsogluteal, vastus lateralis (in infants).

Procedure Steps:

Injection Site: *Deltoid* (see Figure 22–20)

1. Place patient in sitting, prone, supine, or lateral position.
2. Locate the deltoid injection site by placing hand on shoulder, palpating the acromian process of the scapula (sharp protrusion at the top of the shoulder), and dropping down to the middle of the muscle. The deltoid muscle can usually be visualized easily.
3. Precautions: Do not inject medication into the extreme upper and lower aspects of the deltoid or damage may be done to surrounding nerves and the humerus bone.
4. Needle gauge: 23 G to 25 G. Needle length: Toddler ⅝"; child ⅝" to 1"; adult 1" to 1½". Injection angle should be 90 degrees."

Injection site: *Ventrogluteal* (see Figure 22–22)

5. Place patient in supine or lateral position.
6. Locate the ventrogluteal site by palpating the greater trochanter, the anterior superior iliac

spine, and the bony ridge of the iliac crest.
7. Placing the palm against the greater trochanter, with the tip of index finger on the anterior superior iliac spine, spread the middle finger as far away from index finger as possible and locate the center of area for injection site. The injection will penetrate the gluteus medius or gluteus minimus muscle.
8. Precautions: Few dangers as this area is free of major nerves and vessels.
9. Needle gauge: 18 G to 23 G. Needle length: child 1" to 1½"; adult 1½" to 2". Injection angle should be 90 degrees.

Injection Site: *Dorsogluteal* (see Figure 22–21)

10. Place patient in prone position with appropriate draping of buttocks area.
11. Locate the dorsogluteal injection site by finding the posterior iliac spine and the greater trochanter of the femur. Draw an imaginary diagonal line between the two landmarks and locate the injection site above this line, about 2" below the iliac crest in the upper outer quadrant of the buttocks.
12. This site can also be located by visually dividing the buttock into four quadrants. The upper outer quadrant is then divided again into four quarters. The upper outer quarter of the upper outer quadrant is used for the injection.
13. Precautions: Caution should be used to keep this injection site well above the sciatic nerve, which runs down each side of the fatty portion of the buttocks. Nerve damage may occur if the sciatic nerve is accidentally injected. Do not use this site for infants because the gluteal muscles are small and

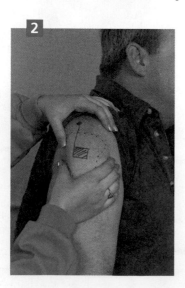

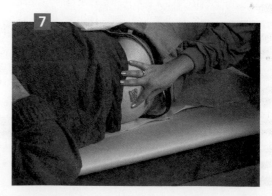

poorly developed until the child begins to walk.

14. Needle gauge: 18 G to 23 G. Needle length: child 1′ to 1½″; adult 1½″ to 2″. Injection angle should be 90 degrees.

Injection site: *Vastus Lateralis (Infant)* (see Figure 22–23)

15. Place child in supine or lateral position with parent holding child still.

16 Locate the vastus lateralis muscle below the greater trochanter of the femur and within the upper lateral quadrant of the thigh. You may divide the thigh in thirds down to the kneecap and give injection in the middle third area.

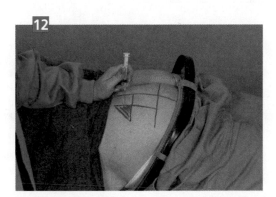

17. Precautions: Few dangers because this is a large muscle area. (This site is not usually used for ambulatory adults because it can cause discomfort.)

18. Needle gauge: 22 G to 25 G. Needle length: infant ⅝″. Injection angle can be 90 or 45 degrees, with the needle pointing toward the knee, depending on the size of the infant's muscle.

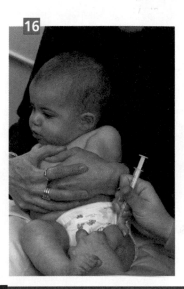

Remember to use the air-lock and Z-track methods when injecting irritating medications. The air-lock and Z-track methods are used to prevent medication from leaking back from the muscle mass into the subcutaneous tissue. After drawing the medication, change needles to prevent irritation going through the subcutaneous tissue to the muscle.

To create an air lock, after drawing up the medication, hold the syringe so medication does not run out and draw in 0.2 to 0.5 mL of air. When the syringe is held for injection, this air will rise above the medication and will follow the medication into the muscle to clear the entire injection track with air (Figure 22–25).

Before giving the injection using the Z-track method, draw the tissues to one side. Insert the needle, aspirate, and then inject and inject slowly. Wait 10 seconds. Then release the tissue. This causes the track where the needle entered through the subcutaneous tissue to move laterally, preventing any medication from flowing backward.

Figure 22–26 shows the Z-track technique. Procedure 22–7 describes administering an intramuscular injection, and Procedure 22–8 describes administering a Z-track injection.

Despite the best efforts of any health care professional, problems will occasionally occur during administration of an injection. These problems can run from a patient who refuses an injection to a patient having a violent allergic reaction.

If a patient refuses an injection or is not comfortable with you giving the injection, try to convince him or her that you are perfectly capable. If the patient insists, refer the matter to the doctor, but if you appear capable and professional, the patient should accept the injection from you.

If you aspirate blood, withdraw the needle, discard the medication, and draw up another dose for administration.

If the patient complains about severe pain or numbness while you are injecting a medication, stop inject-

Text continued on page 538

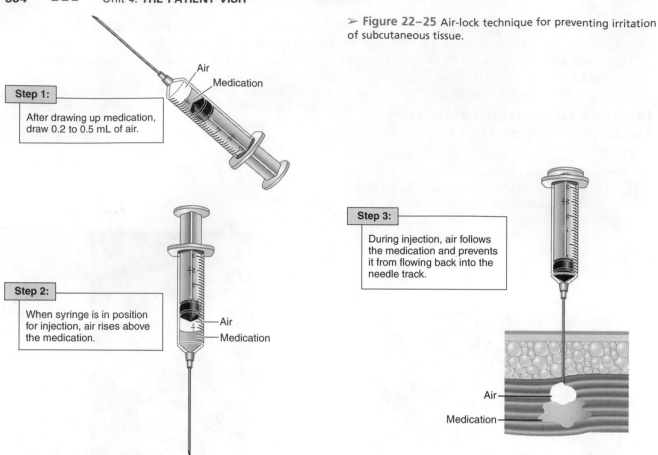

➢ **Figure 22–25** Air-lock technique for preventing irritation of subcutaneous tissue.

Step 1:

After drawing up medication, draw 0.2 to 0.5 mL of air.

Air
Medication

Step 2:

When syringe is in position for injection, air rises above the medication.

Air
Medication

Step 3:

During injection, air follows the medication and prevents it from flowing back into the needle track.

Air
Medication

➢ **Figure 22–26** Z-track injection technique prevents fluid from leaking into the subcutaneous tissue.

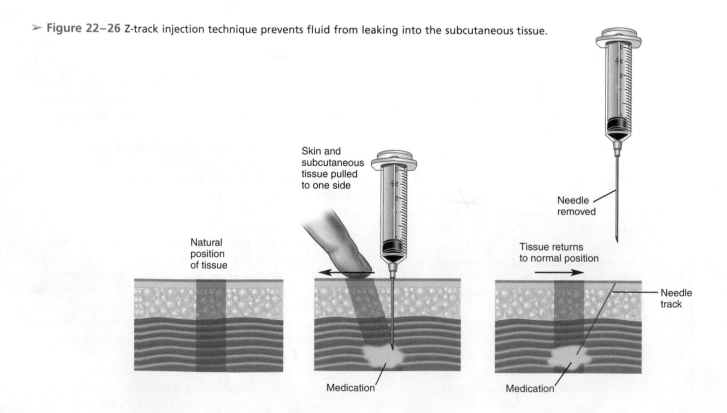

Skin and subcutaneous tissue pulled to one side

Natural position of tissue

Needle removed

Tissue returns to normal position

Needle track

Medication

Medication

Medication

PROCEDURE 22–7

Administering an Intramuscular Injection

Performance Objective: The student will be able to administer an intramuscular injection.

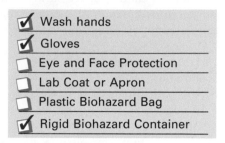

- ☑ Wash hands
- ☑ Gloves
- ☐ Eye and Face Protection
- ☐ Lab Coat or Apron
- ☐ Plastic Biohazard Bag
- ☑ Rigid Biohazard Container

Supplies and Equipment: Syringe and needle containing medication as ordered by the doctor, alcohol pad, gauze pad, gloves, adhesive bandage, rigid biohazard container, medical record of the patient to receive the injection.

Procedure Steps

1. Wash hands.
2. Using the medical record, identify the patient, explain the procedure, and tell the patient the reason for the injection.
3. Ask the patient if he or she knows of any allergies to the medication.
4. Put on disposable gloves.
5. Select an injection site as discussed in Procedure 22–6.
   Rationale: A site with a well-developed muscle should be selected. Avoid injecting into moles, skin lesions, or blood vessels that can be seen through the skin.
6. Using an alcohol pad, clean the selected site by using a circular motion, cleaning inside to outside.
   Rationale: Move from the cleanest area to a less clean area without going back over any area already cleaned for best results.
7. Remove needle cover.
8. With thumb and first two fingers of your nondominant hand, spread the skin around the injection site.
   Rationale: Spreading the skin compresses the subcutaneous tissue and allows the needle to penetrate the muscle.
9. Grasp the syringe between the thumb and first two fingers of your dominant hand with your palm up, and with one swift movement, insert the entire needle up to the hub at a 90-degree angle into the muscle.
   Rationale: The depth of the injection is determined by the choice of needle length. The 90-degree angle allows the needle tip to penetrate into the muscle. Inserting the needle with one swift movement reduces discomfort for the patient.
10. Without moving the needle in the tissue, aspirate: Pull back on the plunger slightly and observe to be sure that no blood enters the syringe. If blood appears, withdraw the needle, apply pressure to the site, and prepare a new injection.
    Rationale: Blood in the syringe means that

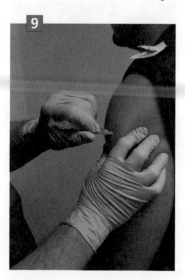

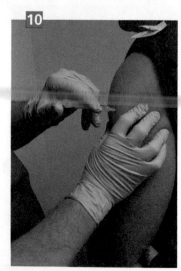

Procedure continued on following page

PROCEDURE 22-7 *(continued)*

the tip of the needle has penetrated a blood vessel. If medication is injected, the route will be intravenous rather than subcutaneous, which could change the effect of the medication. A new syringe and medication will have to be prepared because blood contaminates the medication and may be irritating to the tissue if used.

11. If no blood appears when you aspirate, push in the plunger slowly and steadily until all medication has been administered.
Rationale: Rapid injection may cause tissue damage and will not allow for proper absorption.

12. Withdraw needle swiftly at the same angle it was inserted.
Rationale: Withdrawing the needle at the same angle reduces pressure on the tissue and minimizes discomfort.

13. Apply pressure to the site using a gauze pad or alcohol pad. Gently massage the injection site (except when injecting heparin, which should never be massaged.)
Rationale: Pressure helps control bleeding and massage facilitates absorption of the medication.

14. Place the syringe and needle in a rigid biohazard container without recapping the needle.
Rationale: It is a standard precaution never to recap a needle that has been used to give an injection because of the potential of contracting a blood-borne disease if a needle-stick

injury were to occur. Disposing of used needles in a rigid biohazard container prevents injury.

15. Assess the injection site. Continue applying pressure if the injection site is still bleeding freely. Apply an adhesive bandage if bleeding has stopped.
Rationale: A bandage is reassuring to many patients. In addition, it may protect the patient's clothing if a small amount of bleeding or leakage of serous fluid occurs.

16. Remove gloves and discard.

17. Wash hands.

18. Ask the patient to remain in the office for 10 to 15 minutes in case a reaction occurs.
Rationale: A severe medication reaction will usually begin rapidly, usually beginning within 10 to 15 minutes.

19. Document the medication, the dose as ordered by the doctor, the injection site, and any reaction that you observe in the patient's medical record.

Charting Example	
Date	
9/17/XX	2:30 PM Solganol 25 mg given IM in ℞ buttock. No adverse reaction noted. Pt. released after 15 minutes of observation. ————— ————— S. Williams, CMA

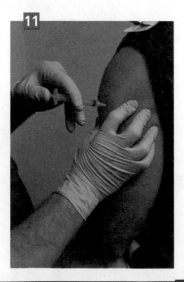

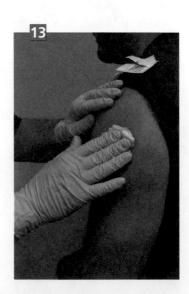

PROCEDURE 22–8

Administering a Z-Track Injection

Performance Objective: The student will be able to administer a Z-track injection to a patient.

- ☑ Wash hands
- ☑ Gloves
- ☐ Eye and Face Protection
- ☐ Lab Coat or Apron
- ☐ Plastic Biohazard Bag
- ☑ Rigid Biohazard Container

Supplies and Equipment: Syringe and needle containing medication as ordered by the doctor, alcohol pad, gauze pad, gloves, bandage, biohazard container, medical record of the patient to receive the injection.

Procedure Steps

1. Wash hands.
2. Using the medical record, identify the patient, explain the procedure, and tell the patient the reason for the injection.
3. Ask the patient if he or she knows of any allergies to the medication.
4. Put on disposable gloves.
5. Select the dorsogluteal injection site. Be sure that the needle was changed after drawing up the medication to prevent tissue irritation.
   Rationale: The dorsogluteal site is used when a medication is extremely irritating to the subcutaneous tissue so that the medication can be injected deep intramuscularly using the Z-track method. The needle is always changed before administration in case any drops of medication adhere to the outside of the needle used to draw up.
6. Using an alcohol pad, clean the site by using a circular motion, cleaning inside to outside.
   Rationale: Move from the cleanest area to a less clean area without going back over any area already cleaned for best results.
7. Remove needle cover. Before injecting, draw 0.2 to 0.5 mL of air into the syringe.
   Rationale: The air will rise to the top of the syringe when you administer the injection and follow the medication as you inject, forcing all medication through the subcutaneous tissue into the muscle.

8. With your fingers, pull the skin at the injection site to the left of its usual position about 2″ to 3″. Hold the tissue to the side while you inject and aspirate.
   Rationale: You want to move the subcutaneous tissue to the left of its normal position so that the needle track through the subcutaneous tissue does not connect to the needle track in the muscle tissue after the injection (see Figure 22–26).
9. Grasp the syringe between the thumb and first two fingers of your dominant hand with your palm up, and with one swift movement, insert the entire needle up to the hub at a 90-degree angle into the muscle.
   Rationale: The depth of the injection is determined by the choice of needle length. The 90-degree angle allows the needle tip to penetrate into the muscle. Inserting the needle with one swift movement reduces discomfort for the patient.
10. Without moving the needle in the tissue, aspirate: Pull back on the plunger slightly and observe to be sure that no blood enters the syringe. If blood appears, withdraw the needle, apply pressure to the site, and prepare a new injection.
    Rationale: Blood in the syringe means that the tip of the needle has penetrated a blood vessel. If medication is injected, the route will be intravenous rather than subcutaneous, which could change the effect of the medication. A new syringe and medication will have to be prepared as blood contaminates the medication and may be irritating to the tissue if used.
11. If no blood appears when you aspirate, push in the plunger slowly and steadily until all medication has been administered.
    Rationale: Rapid injection may cause tissue damage and will not allow for proper absorption.
12. Withdraw needle swiftly and release the tissue being held by your nondominant hand at the same time.
    Rationale: When you release your nondominant hand, the tissue returns to its original position.
13. Apply pressure to the site using a gauze pad or alcohol pad. Do not massage the injection site.

Procedure continued on following page

PROCEDURE 22–8 *(continued)*

Rationale: Pressure helps control bleeding, but you do not want the medication to be pushed back into the subcutaneous tissue before absorption.

14. Place the syringe and needle in a rigid biohazard container without recapping the needle.
Rationale: It is a standard precaution never to recap a needle that has been used to give an injection because of the potential of contracting a blood-borne disease if a needle-stick injury were to occur. Disposing of used needles in a rigid biohazard container prevents injury.

15. Assess the injection site. Continue applying pressure if the injection site is still bleeding freely. Apply a bandage if bleeding has stopped.

Rationale: A bandage is reassuring to many patients. In addition it may protect the patient's clothing if a small amount of bleeding or leakage of serous fluid occurs.

16. Remove gloves and discard.
17. Wash hands.
18. Ask the patient to remain in the office for 10 to 15 minutes in case a reaction occurs.
Rationale: A severe medication reaction will usually begin rapidly, within 10 to 15 minutes.

19. Document the medication, the dose as ordered by the doctor, the injection site, the Z-track method used for the injection, and any reaction that you observe in the patient's medical record.

---

ing. Before removing the needle, try to determine if the pain is radiating, which is a sign of nerve damage. If you think there is a chance you have hit a nerve, withdraw the needle, change needles, and inject at a new site. Document the patient's symptoms and report to the doctor.

Needle breaks are extremely rare, but if this happens, immediately call for help from a second person. Determine quickly if you can see the needle. If you can, pull the skin gently away and try to remove the needle with a hemostat or forceps. If you can not see the needle, mark the spot, keep the patient absolutely still, and apply a tourniquet on the arm or leg above the injection site to prevent the needle traveling in the bloodstream. Tell the doctor or other practitioner im-

mediately, call 911, and have the patient transported to the hospital for X-rays and surgical removal.

If the patient has a reaction to the injection, have the patient lie down and take his or her pulse and blood pressure immediately. If the pulse is strong and regular, reassure the patient and have him or her lie quietly. If the pulse is rapid and weak, the blood pressure low, and/or the patient is having trouble breathing, get the doctor or other practitioner and then get the emergency drug box. Be prepared to assist in administration of oxygen and/or epinephrine. (This will be discussed in greater detail in chapter 31.)

If any problem occurs, the doctor will discuss it with the patient. Following correct technique is the best way to prevent problems, but a rapid response

ON THE JOB

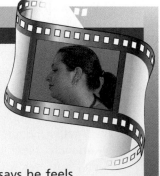

From Medications videotape: "The Reaction"

Stacy Dellarosa, a medical assistant at Blackburn Primary Care Associates, has given Lonnie Graham, a 42-year-old black male, an injection of Solu-Medrol, ordered by the doctor because Mr. Graham has a severe case of poison ivy. Immediately after receiving the injection, Mr. Graham complains of feeling dizzy. Stacy says loudly that she needs some help in the exam room.

QUESTIONS
1. What possibilities are probably going through Stacy's mind when Mr. Graham says he feels dizzy?
2. Why does Stacy ask for help immediately?
3. What should Stacy do next?
4. After a few minutes, Mr. Graham says the dizziness has gone away. His pulse is 80 and strong. His respirations are 16. His blood pressure is 118/72. Stacy has him rest in the office for another 15 minutes. How should she document the entire incident?

TUBERCULOSIS AND TUBERCULOSIS TESTING

Tuberculosis is a bacterial infection of the respiratory system, caused by *Mycobacterium tuberculosis*. Tuberculosis was one of the most feared diseases of the 19th and early 20th centuries. The disease thrived in the crowded, unsanitary conditions of Europe and the United States during the Industrial Revolution.

An individual with active tuberculosis can infect those in close contact by sneezing, coughing, speaking, or even singing. Tuberculosis is overwhelmingly a disease of the poor and those who live in close quarters, such as prisons and military barracks. For instance, it is estimated that up to 70 percent of men in Russian prisons have active tuberculosis. Although many die in prison, others are released after having little if any treatment and can infect the communities in which they live.

In one case, a former Russian prison inmate flew to the United States after release and infected 15 passengers on the flight.

Individuals with compromised immune systems are at especially high risk of acquiring tuberculosis.

Although tuberculosis is primarily a disease of the lungs, it can spread anywhere in the body. If untreated, the respiratory form causes death over a period of months or years; the systemic forms are more severe, especially in the young, old, and people with compromised immune systems.

With the advent of antibiotics in the middle of the 20th century, the World Health Organization and US Department of Health and Human Services expected that tuberculosis would eventually be wiped out in the industrialized world, then throughout the world.

Unfortunately, tuberculosis continues to be a public health problem, even in the United States, where there are 20,000 new cases diagnosed each year. Since the mid-1980s the incidence of tuberculosis has been rising, despite increased public health efforts. In addition, at times large groups of antibiotic-resistant tuberculosis cases have appeared.

Skin tests merely show if the body has produced antibodies to the tuberculin bacillus. The true diagnosis of tuberculosis comes from x-ray studies of the lungs that show calcified lesions. Symptoms are coughing (sometimes including bloody sputum), wheezing, and shortness of breath.

Treatment consists of at least 6 months of up to four different powerful antibiotics. Many people have side effects from the medication and are tempted to stop taking it when their respiratory symptoms become better. However, unless they finish the course of antibiotics, the tuberculosis has not been eradicated and another episode can occur, this time from a bacterium that has mutated and is now resistant to the antibiotics used the first time.

In the 1980s there was a major outbreak of drug-resistant tuberculosis in New York City, especially among intravenous drug abusers and people with AIDS. A program of aggressive intervention, with medical personnel who went to patients' homes and visually made sure the patient took the medication, helped end the outbreak.

A vaccine, BCG (bacillus Calmette-Guérin), is used in some African and Asian countries to prevent systemic tuberculosis and its complications in infants. This vaccine is not believed to be effective for the adult form of tuberculosis and is rarely used in the United States. It has the additional disadvantage that a person who has been immunized will always exhibit a positive reaction and possibly a severe reaction to a skin test for tuberculosis. Therefore, an individual who has been immunized and develops symptoms of possible tuberculosis must always be tested with chest x-rays.

Efforts continue to develop a more effective vaccine for this disease.

---

helps minimize damage from any problem that might occur. And thorough documentation provides the best evidence of care if legal questions arise after an incident.

Intradermal Injections

An allergy test or a test for exposure to tuberculosis is usually performed via an intradermal injection. Intradermal injections are given between layers of the skin. A small amount of material—an allergic extract in the case of an allergy test, and purified protein derivative (PPD), a cell protein from the tuberculosis bacillus in the case of a Mantoux tuberculosis test—is injected intradermally.

If the patient has an allergic reaction to an extract, the skin reaction will begin within 20 to 30 minutes. When a person has been exposed to the tuberculosis antigen, the antibody response will produce a reaction at the injection site in 48 to 72 hours.

When giving an intradermal injection, use a short, thin needle; from 3/8″ to ⅝″, and 25 G to 27 G. Insert just under the skin and almost parallel to the skin, at a 10- to 15-degree angle, with the bevel pointed up, as

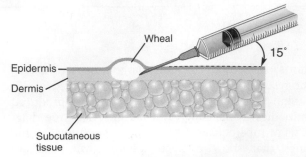

> **Figure 22–27** For an intradermal injection the needle is inserted, bevel up, between the epidermal and dermal skin layers. As the fluid is injected it forces the skin layers to separate, and a raised wheal appears.

seen in Figure 22–27. The needle should seem to be visible under the skin, so that the fluid can be injected between the skin layers to form a **wheal** (fluid-filled elevation of the skin).

Proper sites for an intradermal injection include the inner (anterior) forearm, the upper arm, the upper chest, or across the back. If giving a series of intradermal injections for allergy testing, the sites on the back will allow several substances to be tested. For a single-injection Mantoux test, the forearm is most often used. Figure 22–28 shows sites for intradermal injections.

Gloves must be worn while performing an intradermal injection. It is not necessary to aspirate an intradermal injection. Slowly inject the substance under the skin. When the fluid is injected, it forces the epidermis to separate from the dermis. The raised area is called a

wheal, or a bleb. If the needle penetrates too deeply, the wheal will not form, and there may not be a skin reaction. It is important to hold the syringe very steady, so all of the material will be deposited in a small area.

The needle should be removed at the same angle at which it was inserted. Do not apply pressure or massage the injection site. A small amount of capillary bleeding may occur. This may be gently wiped away with a gauze square, but do not apply a bandage to control bleeding, because this may put pressure on the wheal and force the fluid into deeper tissue layers.

Procedure 22–9 describes in detail how to perform an intradermal injection.

Before performing a Mantoux or tine test, make sure to ask the patient about previous positive tests (Mantoux or tine) and about any previous immunization to tuberculosis. Do not test a patient who has had a previous positive reaction, because each subsequent reaction tends to be increasingly severe. A chest x-ray is necessary to diagnose tuberculosis in such a patient.

The tuberculosis immunization (BCG) is seldom used in the United States, but immigrants from many Asian and African countries may have received it. These patients should never be given a Mantoux or tine test, because they will have a positive and often severe reaction. Notify the doctor, so that he or she can decide whether the patient needs further testing.

Procedure 22–10 describes in detail testing for tuberculosis using a Mantoux or tine test.

To test a patient for allergies, give a dose of a separate allergen in each space of a numbered grid,

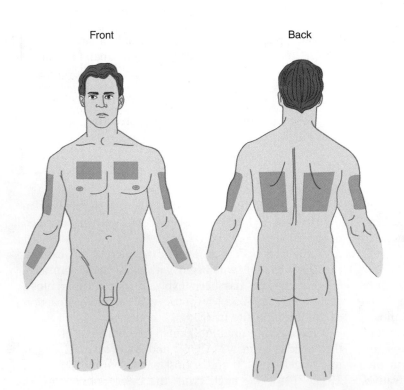

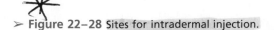

> **Figure 22–28** Sites for intradermal injection.

Administering an Intradermal Injection

Performance Objective: The student will be able to administer an intradermal injection.

- ☑ Wash hands
- ☑ Gloves
- ☐ Eye and Face Protection
- ☐ Lab Coat or Apron
- ☐ Plastic Biohazard Bag
- ☑ Rigid Biohazard Container

Supplies and Equipment: Syringe and needle containing medication as ordered by the doctor, alcohol pad, gauze pad, gloves, bandage, rigid biohazard container, medical record of the patient to receive the injection.

Procedure Steps

1. Wash hands.
2. Using the medical record, identify the patient, explain the procedure, and tell the patient the reason for the injection.
3. Ask the patient if he or she knows of any allergies to the medication. (Sometimes intradermal injections are used for allergy testing; in that case the medication is given in spite of possible allergies.)
4. Put on disposable gloves.
5. Select an injection site. The most common sites are the upper back or the inner aspect of the lower arm.
   Rationale: A site free from hair is usually used for an intradermal injection. Avoid injecting into moles, skin lesions, or blood vessels that can be seen through the skin.
6. Using an alcohol pad, clean the selected site using a circular motion, cleaning inside to outside. Allow to dry.
   Rationale: Move from the cleanest area to a less clean area without going back over any area already cleaned for best results.
7. Remove needle cover.
8. With thumb and index finger of your non-dominant hand, pull skin taut.
   Rationale: Stretching or pulling the skin taut will ease the needle insertion and cause it to be less noticeable.
9. Hold the syringe bevel up between the thumb and first two fingers of your dominant hand with your palm up, and insert needle at a 10 to 15-degree angle under the skin. **Do not aspirate.**
   Rationale: The needle is just under the skin surface so that many times you can see the needle color and tracking under the skin. This 10- to 15-degree angle with the bevel up allows the fluid to enter the tissue between the layers of the skin, forming a wheal.
10. Slowly inject the medication to form a bubble or wheal on the skin surface.
11. Withdraw needle slowly and gently, not to disturb the wheal.
12. Dab site with gauze but do not apply pressure or massage.
    Rationale: The medication must be absorbed slowly from the intradermal area and not pressed into deeper tissues or a reaction, if it occurs, may not be visible.
13. Dispose of supplies in biohazard container.
14. Assess patient and wound site. Instruct patient when the reaction, if any, will occur.
15. Document injection in the patient's medical record. Observe reaction, if any, and document after the appropriate interval.

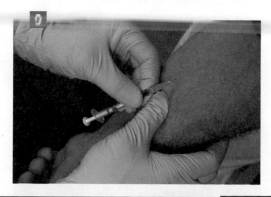

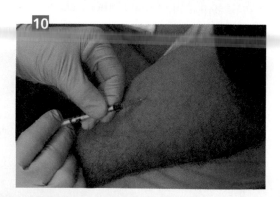

PROCEDURE 22–10

Administering a Tine or Mantoux Test

Performance Objective: The student will be able to perform a tine or Mantoux injection to test for tuberculosis.

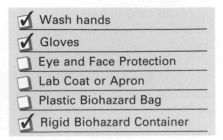

- ☑ Wash hands
- ☑ Gloves
- ☐ Eye and Face Protection
- ☐ Lab Coat or Apron
- ☐ Plastic Biohazard Bag
- ☑ Rigid Biohazard Container

Supplies and Equipment: Tuberculin/1-cc syringe with ⅜" to ½" needle containing PPD (Purified Protein Derivative); if performing a tine test: 4-prong multiple-puncture unit, gloves, alcohol swabs, 2" × 2" gauze pad, rigid biohazard container.

Procedure Steps

1. Wash hands.
2. Using the medical record, identify the patient, explain the procedure, and tell the patient the reason for the injection.
3. Ask the patient if he or she has ever had a reaction to a test for tuberculosis or has ever been immunized for tuberculosis. If the patient answers in the affirmative, consult with the doctor before proceeding.
   Rationale: Although immunizations for tuberculosis are not used in the United States, they are common in some countries. Once a person has been immunized or has had a skin reaction to a TB test, that person will always react to a skin test and other tests (such as a

chest x-ray) must be performed to identify if active tuberculosis is present. Skin reactions tend to increase in severity and be very uncomfortable for the patient.

4. Put on disposable gloves.
5. Select a site on the anterior aspect of the lower arm free from moles, lesions, or skin discolorations.
6. Using an alcohol pad, clean the selected site by using a circular motion, cleaning inside to outside.
   Rationale: Move from the cleanest area to a less clean area without going back over any area already cleaned for best results.
7. Remove needle cover or plastic protective cover of tine test.
8. With thumb and index finger of your nondominant hand, pull skin taut. You may want to hold the forearm with your nondominant hand under the patient's arm, pulling skin taut from underneath.
   Rationale: This will ensure that the needle or tines will enter skin with ease and be placed at the correct tissue depth.
9. If administering the tine test: press firmly into designated forearm area. Press, hold, and release to distribute medication that is on the prongs. If administering the Mantoux test, grasp the syringe bevel up between the thumb and first two fingers of your dominant hand with your palm up, and insert the needle at a 10- to 15-degree angle. Do not aspirate.
   Rationale: The depth of the injection is determined by the choice of needle length. Once the needle is at the tissue layer, do not move the needle while injecting the medication.
10. For the Mantoux test, inject the medication slowly to form a wheal.

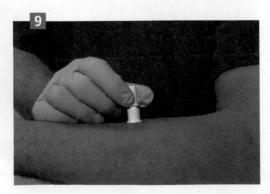

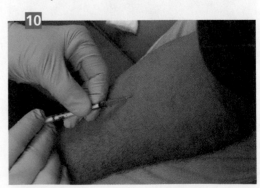

11. Withdraw needle and dab site, but do not massage or apply pressure.

12. Dispose of supplies in biohazard container.

13. Instruct the patient to return to have the test read in 48 to 72 hours. Alternatively, the patient may be instructed to observe the site in 48 to 72 hours and to call the office with a description of any reaction. Usually if a reaction occurs, the patient is instructed to come to the office so that trained personnel can measure the amount of induration (swelling).

14. Document the type of TB test, the location, and instructions given to the patient in the patient's medical record.

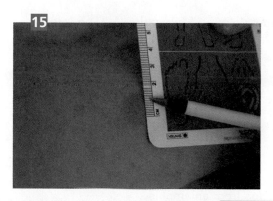

15 When the patient returns, observe the site of the TB test. Measure the diameter of induration (raised, hard, and reddened area) in millimeters and record. If redness is present without induration, the test is considered negative. Redness beyond the area that is hard and swollen is not measured. Notify the doctor of any positive results.

Charting Example	
Date	
12/04/XX	10:45 AM Mantoux test performed on ® forearm. Pt. instructed to return on 12/6/xx to have test read.
	———————— P. Dean, CMA
12/06/XX	3:20 PM Redness and induration noted at site of Mantoux test measuring 8 mm in diameter. Pt. states that he has never had a reaction in the past. Dr. Hughes notified. ————
	———————— P. Dean, CMA

usually on the patient's back, as shown in Figure 22–29. Instruct the patient to wait for 20 to 30 minutes, then read the results of each test.

Allergens may also be applied by a needle scratch to the skin (scratch test) or by taping a gauze square impregnated with the allergen (patch test) in each square of the grid.

For the Mantoux test, be sure to instruct the patient to return between 48 and 72 hours after the injection to have the test read. In some offices, the patient may be instructed to telephone if there is no reaction and only to return for redness, swelling, and/or itching at the injection site.

Be sure to document the injection site and the instructions given to the patient. The medical record may be placed on one side for documentation when the patient returns or telephones for follow-up.

Check for the reaction after the specified interval. Figure 22–30 shows reactions to intradermal injections.

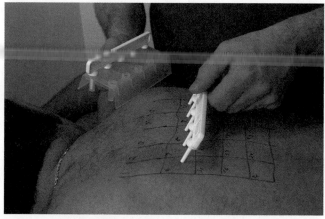

➤ **Figure 22–29** Sites marked for allergy testing on the patient's back.

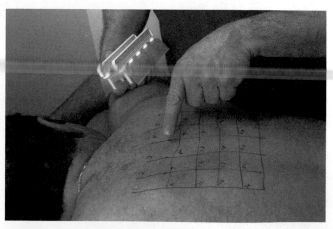

➤ **Figure 22–30** After 15 minutes, some of the allergens have caused the skin to redden.

STUDENT STUDY PLAN, PART II

To reinforce your understanding of the material in this chapter . . .

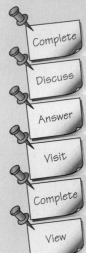

Complete the **Review & Recall** questions.

Discuss the situation in **If You Were the Medical Assistant** with your classmates and answer the questions.

Answer the **Critical Thinking Questions** and discuss them with your classmates.

Visit suggested Internet **Web sites** and search for additional Web sites using **Keywords for Internet Searches.**

Complete the exercises in chapter 22, Part II of the **Student Mastery Manual.**

View Part One of the **Medications** videotape: "Giving Medication," "The Injection," "The Reaction."

REVIEW & RECALL

1. When a doctor orders medication to be given to a patient in the office, what information must be given in the order?

2. Identify guidelines for preparing and administering medication.

3. What are measures a medical assistant should take to prevent medication errors? What should be documented if an error occurs?

4. Describe how to be sure the correct dose of liquid medication has been prepared.

5. What are the advantages to giving medication by injection?

6. Differentiate between the procedures for drawing up medication from a vial and drawing up medication from an ampule.

7. Describe the characteristics of a good site for intramuscular injections.

8. Describe how to locate the following injection sites: deltoid, ventrogluteal, dorsogluteal, and vastus lateralis.

9. Identify principles for proper administration of an intramuscular injection.

10. Why are intradermal injections used for TB and allergy testing?

IF YOU WERE THE MEDICAL ASSISTANT

Perform the following drug calculations. Prepare a medication card for each medication.

1. The medication order states: give Compazine 2.5 mg IM. The bottle is labeled Compazine (prochlorperazine) 5 mg/mL. How much would you draw up? What route would you use?

2. The medication order states: give atropine 0.6 mg SC. The bottle is labeled 400 mcg/mL. How much would you draw up? What route would you use?

3. The medication order states: give cefaclor oral suspension 500 mg po. The bottle is labeled 250 mg per 5 mL. How much would you pour? What route would you use?

4. The medication order states: give digoxin 0.25 mg po. The bottle is labeled 0.125 mg per tablet. How many tablets would you pour? What route would you use?

5. The medication order states: give Lasix (furosemide) 5 mg IM. The bottle is labeled 20 mg/2 mL. How much would you draw up? What route would you use?

CRITICAL THINKING QUESTIONS

1. Why is it important for the medical assistant to give injections only if there is a doctor present in the office? Discuss with your classmates what could happen if a medical assistant ignored this rule and gave an injection when he or she was alone in the office.

2. The medical assistant is instructed not to massage the site after administration of heparin, insulin, or an injection given using the Z-track method. Why are some injections massaged and others not?

3. Give reasons why larger and longer needles may be chosen for some injections when shorter and finer needles are chosen for others. Identify as many factors as you can that influence needle selection.

4. Research the law in your state related to giving injections. Are medical assistants allowed to give injections? If yes, under what circumstances? Write a short essay proposing specific legislation allowing certified or registered medical assistants to give injections. Include reasons in your essay.

EXPLORE THE WEB

INTERNET WEB SITES

Infomed
www.infomed.org

medication calculation exercises
www.utep.edu/nurs4710/tutorials

Medline drug information
www.nlm.nih.gov/medlineplus/druginformation.html

PCS Health Systems
www.druglist.com

Physicians' Desk Reference (PDR)
www.pdr.net

Rx list
www.rxlist.com

KEYWORDS FOR INTERNET SEARCHES

dosage calculations
    medications
    metric system
    prescription medications
    prescription drugs

ANSWERS TO ON THE JOB

1. Mr. Graham may be about to faint, or he may be having an allergic reaction to the injection.

2. If Mr. Graham is having a reaction, the speed at which it began indicates that it may be serious. Stacy wants to be sure she has assistance available because someone must stay with the patient at all times.

3. Stacy should have Mr. Graham lie down, and she should check his vital signs and blood pressure. If the problem is that he is about to faint, lying down will prevent injury and probably keep him from fainting by improving circulation to the brain. If the patient's vital signs are normal, he is probably not having a serious reaction. If he were going into ana-

phylactic shock, his pulse would be rapid and thready, and his blood pressure would be low. Mr. Graham's pulse is 80 and strong; his respirations are 16; and his blood pressure is 118/72.

4. Stacy should chart as follows: After receiving the injection, the patient complained of dizziness. He was placed in the supine position on the examination table. P:80 and strong. R:16. BP:118/72. Within a few minutes, pt stated that the dizziness had passed. Pt instructed to remain lying on the exam table for 15 minutes. After that time, pt was assisted to sit up, stated he felt fine, and left the office without further problems. (Signed: S. Dellarosa, RMA)

UNIT 5 The Laboratory and Laboratory Tests

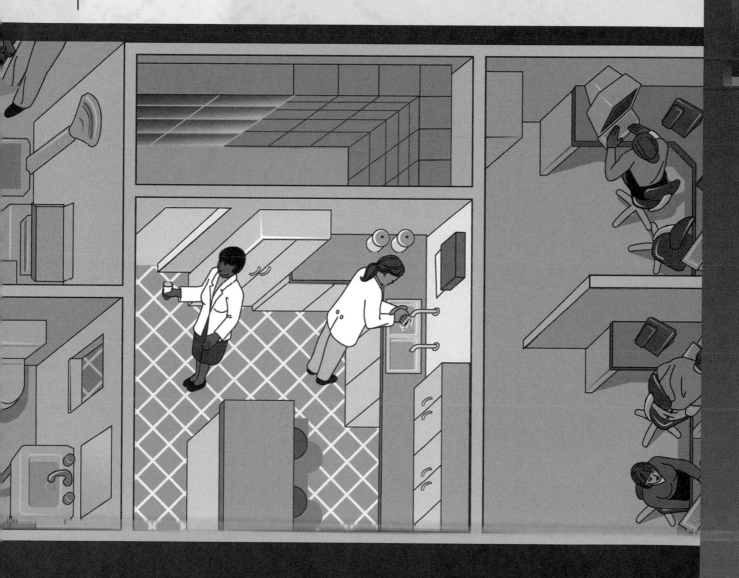

Chapter 23

The Physician's Office Laboratory

Instructional Objectives

After completing this chapter, you will be able to do the following:

1. Define and spell the vocabulary words for this chapter.
2. Differentiate among four different types of laboratories.
3. Describe how CLIA '88 and OSHA regulate types of laboratories and the activities performed in those laboratories.
4. Explain how quality control is used to maintain standards in a laboratory.
5. Describe the process for obtaining a certificate for a physician's office laboratory.
6. Identify measures to maintain safety within the laboratory.
7. List equipment and supplies used in the clinical laboratory.
8. Explain the proper use and maintenance of a microscope.
9. Describe a safe method for transferring fluid using a pipette.
10. Compare and contrast various methods for labeling and transporting laboratory specimens.

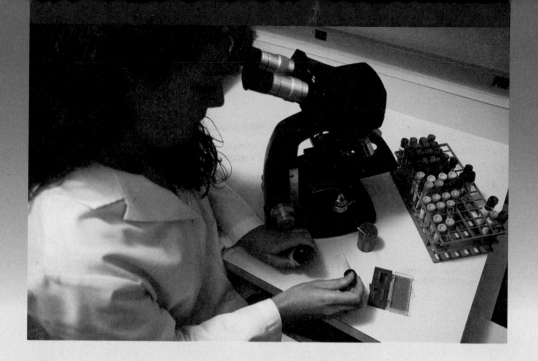

- Dispose of biohazardous materials
- Practice standard precautions
- Use methods of quality control
- Document appropriately
- Perform risk management procedures
- Perform routine maintenance of clinical equipment

Performance Objectives

After completing this chapter, you will be able to do the following:

1. Use a microscope to view slides (Procedure 23–1).

VOCABULARY

accuracy (p. 554)   hematology (p. 550)   pathologist (p. 551)   quality assurance (p. 554)
calibration (p. 555)   histology (p. 551)   pathology (p. 551)   quality control (p. 554)
centrifuge (p. 559)   objective (p. 560)   pipette (p. 564)   reference laboratory (p. 551)
control reagent (p. 554)   ocular (p. 560)   precision (p. 554)   urinalysis (p. 550)
fluorescence microscope (p. 561)   oil-immersion objective (p. 560)

ABBREVIATIONS

CLIA '88 (p. 552)   JCAHO (p. 554)   POL (p. 551)   QC (p. 554)   RPM (p. 559)   UV (p. 561)
HCFA (p. 553)   OSHA (p. 554)   QA (p. 554)

INTRODUCTION TO THE CLINICAL LABORATORY

Doctors use the results of laboratory tests to diagnose illness, as well as to manage chronic illnesses and assess patient well-being. Laboratory tests of blood, urine, and other specimens can confirm a diagnosis made through clinical assessment, detect symptoms of disease that do not appear in clinical examination, and distinguish between diseases that may present the same set of clinical symptoms.

The medical assistant has a number of responsibilities with regard to obtaining samples for laboratory analysis and may also be asked to perform some simple laboratory analysis on his or her own.

What Is a Clinical Laboratory?

Many doctors have a clinical laboratory in their office, in which various patient specimens are examined and analyzed. Large primary care practices, especially public health clinics and community health centers, have large laboratories that perform comprehensive tests. Most other doctors' offices have smaller labs that perform only the simplest tests, sending specimens to commercial laboratories for more complex testing.

Laboratory/Pathology Sections

There are nine specific sections in a laboratory:

1. Processing
2. Urinalysis
3. Hematology
4. Chemistry
5. Microbiology
6. Immunology/serology
7. Blood bank
8. Histology
9. Coagulation (which may be a separate section or may be included in hematology).

Processing

Most hospitals and department labs have a processing department to receive and disperse specimens after they have been collected from the patient. Processing includes order- and data-entry, generation of bar codes for specimen identification, and proper labeling of specimens. If a specimen has to be routed to more than one department, it is split and poured off in the processing department. A medical assistant could be employed as a processor in a hospital laboratory.

Urinalysis

The physical, chemical, and microscopic examination of urine is called **urinalysis.** Physical examination involves checking for color, transparency, and specific gravity. Chemical analysis measures the amount of glucose (sugar), red blood cells, ketones, bilirubin, protein, white blood cells, urobilinogen, and nitrites in the urine, as well as the urine's pH. Urine is examined under the microscope for evidence of red blood cells, white blood cells, bacteria, mucus, crystals, epithelial cells, and other cells. If bacteria are detected in a routine urinalysis, the microbiology department performs a culture to identify the specific bacteria present.

Hematology

Hematology is the study of blood; it includes the examination of blood cells. Red blood cells, white cells, and platelets are all counted. The size, shape, and maturity of these cells are examined. The hematology department may also test the ability of the various types of blood cells to carry out their proper function, such as clotting, or the lab may have a separate department to study blood coagulation.

Chemistry

The most frequently run tests by the chemistry section are the standard panels that analyze 12 to 20 components of blood, including the level of blood sugar, electrolytes (sodium, chloride, potassium, and bicarbonate), cholesterol, blood urea nitrogen, and several other substances. It is also possible to test for levels of alcohol, street drugs, or prescription medications. The chemistry department also conducts chemical analysis of other body fluids, such as urine, cerebrospinal fluid, joint fluid, and peritoneal fluid.

Microbiology

In the microbiology department, microorganisms that cause infection in blood, throat, urine, wound specimens, or other body fluids, such as urine and cerebrospinal fluid, are grown in the appropriate medium and identified. Microbiology includes bacteriology (study of bacteria), parasitology (study of parasitic microorganisms), virology (study of viruses), and mycology (study of fungi and yeasts). Identification is important in determining the appropriate treatment for any infection.

Immunology/Serology

Tests performed in the immunology department determine if antibodies are present against particular diseases, such as mononucleosis, rheumatoid arthritis, and various sexually transmitted diseases.

Blood Bank

This section, sometimes called immunohematology, is where blood typing and crossmatching are performed, and where donated units of blood are separated and stored for later use either by the individual or by others.

Histology

Histology is the microscopic study of tissues. In the clinical laboratory setting, histology examinations are usually of tissues removed in a biopsy procedure to determine if cancer or other disease is present. Many histology sections are part of hospital pathology departments. **Pathology** is the scientific analysis of the cause and effects of disease, which includes microscopic study of cells.

Coagulation

Coagulation tests are used to determine how rapidly or slowly a person's blood clots. Several tests evaluate the effectiveness of blood clotting. Patients who are taking anticoagulant medication have their blood tested frequently.

Types of Lab Personnel

There are four categories of laboratory personnel. The medical director for large laboratories must be a **pathologist,** a doctor who specializes in the study of disease processes. Two types of consultants are available for laboratories. The clinical consultant is available to consult on testing methods, quality assurance, and other such issues. The technical consultant is available to consult on equipment.

Finally, testing personnel perform the various tests and collect some of the necessary specimens. Other specimens are collected by other personnel, either at the lab or at doctors' offices that contract with the lab for testing services.

TYPES OF LABORATORIES

There are four types of laboratories:

1. Hospital-based laboratories
2. Reference laboratories
3. Clinical laboratories, including physician office laboratories **(POLs)**
4. Other laboratories.

Hospital-based Laboratories

Hospital laboratories handle most of the lab work for the hospital departments; hospitals may send specimens for highly specialized tests to a particular reference lab. Hospital-based labs can be housed in a government-run hospital, a university-based hospital, a private hospital, or a not-for-profit hospital.

Hospital laboratories also conduct tests on specimens for private doctors. This is especially true for pathology and microbiology specimens.

Reference Laboratories

Reference laboratories are large laboratories, either privately owned or run by universities or research centers, that handle more complex tests for many doctors and clinics in a geographic area.

MEDICAL LABORATORY PERSONNEL

Certified Medical Technologist. A certified medical technologist (MT) has a bachelor's degree, as well as 1 year of formal training in clinical laboratory matters, and has passed an examination given by one of several national certifying agencies. A medical technologist can perform tests in all areas and assume supervisory and consultant roles. Training programs must meet the standards set by the National Accrediting Agency for Clinical Laboratory Sciences (NAACLS).

Medical Laboratory Technician. A medical laboratory technician (MLT) has completed 1 year of college and 1 year of clinical training. MLTs are also eligible for certification from the same associations as MTs. An MLT performs laboratory tests but may not assume a supervisory role.

Clinical Laboratory Technician. A clinical laboratory technician (CLT) has completed a 1-year program, which includes schooling and clinical training. Many schools only offer the MLT program, so many CLTs received their certification years ago. CLTs perform most laboratory tests but may never assume a supervisory role.

Certification agencies for medical technologists and medical laboratory technicians are:

American Society of Clinical Pathologists (ASCP) certifies phlebotomy technicians, hisotechnologists, medical technologists, medical laboratory technicians, and other laboratory professionals.

American Medical Technologists (AMT) certifies both medical technologists and medical laboratory technicians.
National Certification Agency for Medical Laboratory Personnel.
International Society for Clinical Laboratory Technology.

Certified Medical Assistant (CMA) or Registered Medical Assistant (RMA). Certified and registered medical assistants have completed a 1 to 2-year training program and have passed a national certification examination that includes training in collecting specimens and basic laboratory tests. A CMA or RMA works under the supervision of a technically certified supervisor or consultant.

Certification agencies for medical assistants are:
American Association of Medical Assistants (AAMA)—CMA
American Medical Technologists (AMT)—RMA
California Certifying Board for Medical Assistants (CCBMA)

Phlebotomist or Laboratory Assistant. A phlebotomist or laboratory assistant has received training in the collection and preparation of laboratory specimens and works under the supervision of a technically certified supervisor. Phlebotomists are eligible for certification from the ASCP to use the title phlebotomy technician.

Clinical Laboratories

Clinical laboratories are present in a number of different settings. Many cities have clinical laboratories in their health departments. Nursing homes usually have laboratories to perform basic-level tests. POLs are the laboratories found in individual medical offices. The military runs a large number of clinical laboratories, located in the troop medical clinics on military bases.

Other Laboratories

There are also research laboratories, forensic laboratories, and veterinary medical laboratories. Some laboratories conduct pure research, although they do many of the same types of examinations as other laboratories.

Forensic laboratories conduct laboratory tests of samples taken from crime scenes. Veterinary laboratories conduct tests on samples from pets and/or farm or zoo animals similar to those conducted on samples taken from humans.

LEGISLATION REGULATING LABORATORIES

Clinical laboratories are regulated under the Clinical Laboratory Improvement Act of 1988, referred to as **CLIA '88.** CLIA '88 is federal legislation, developed by the Department of Health and Human Services (DHHS) to oversee the work of all clinical laboratories. The intention of the CLIA '88 legislation is to ensure the quality of laboratory testing by enforcing laboratory standards such as quality assurance and quality control.

Categorization of Laboratories by Level of Testing under CLIA '88

Laboratories are categorized according to the kinds of tests they perform. They fall into one of three categories:

Laboratories that conduct only low-complexity tests
Laboratories that conduct moderately complex tests, including subcategories of physician performed microscopy (PPM)
Laboratories that conduct highly complex tests.

CLIA Certification

Every laboratory must either be exempt from CLIA or possess one of the following five CLIA certificates:

Certificate of Waiver. This is issued by the Health Care Financing Administration (**HCFA**) of DHHS to labs that only perform low-complexity, or "waived," tests (i.e., tests that are exempt from many of CLIA's requirements). Table 23–1 summarizes the types of waived tests.

Registration Certificate. This enables a lab to perform moderate- to high-complexity testing, until the lab is determined to be in compliance through a survey conducted by HCFA or one of its agents.

Certificate of PPM Procedures. This certificate allows a doctor, mid-level practitioner, or dentist to perform only microscopy procedures and/or waived testing. Medical assistants perform waived tests and some moderate-complexity tests, in a lab with a certificate of compliance that is under the supervision of a medical laboratory technician or medical technologist.

Certificate of Compliance. This is issued to a lab after an inspection in which the lab is found to be in compliance with all applicable condition-level requirements. A medical assistant may prepare slides for microscopic examination by the doctor.

Certificate of Accreditation. This is issued when a lab is deemed to meet applicable CLIA requirements by an accredited organization approved by HCFA.

Table 23–1	CLIA-Waived Laboratory Tests
Category	**Type of Test**
Bacteriology	Tests for *Helicobacter pylori*
	Tests for *Streptococcus*, group A
Endocrinology	Tests for ovulation using visual color comparison
	Urine pregnancy tests using visual color comparison
General Chemistry	Approved tests for the following chemicals:
	Vaginal amines and pH
	Serum glucose using monitoring devices approved for home use
	Fecal occult blood
	Serum cholesterol and HDL cholesterol
	Gastric occult blood
	Glycosylated hemoglobin
General Immunology	Bladder tumor–associated antigen
	Helicobacter pylori antibodies
	Infectious mononucleosis antibodies
Hematology	Erythrocyte sedimentation rate, nonautomated
	Hematocrit
	Hemoglobin by copper sulfate, nonautomated
	Prothrombin time
	Spun microhematocrit
Toxicology	Saliva alcohol (ethanol) tests
	Tests for nicotine and/or metabolites
Urinalysis	Urine dipstick or tablet analytes, nonautomated, multiple tests
	Urine qualitative dipsticks; single test for bilirubin, blood, glucose, ketones, leukocytes, nitrites, protein, specific gravity, urobilinogen, or pH

These laboratory tests are considered simple, and many of them can also be performed by patients at home. A list of approved tests can be obtained from the Centers for Disease Control and Prevention (CDC) at http://www.phppo.cdc.gov/clia/waived.asp.

OSHA

The federal Occupational Safety and Health Administration **(OSHA)**, discussed in detail in chapter 6, is the federal agency that oversees the health and safety of employees who work in clinical laboratories, based on guidelines established by the Centers for Disease Control and Prevention (CDC).

JCAHO

The Joint Commission on Accreditation of Healthcare Organizations **(JCAHO)**, discussed in detail in chapter 11, is the organization that monitors quality assurance programs, personnel training, and quality improvement programs related to POLs.

QUALITY ASSURANCE, QUALITY CONTROL, AND CLINICAL STANDARDS

Just because a laboratory is approved under CLIA to perform a certain type of tests does not mean that results of those tests are always accurate or precise. **Accuracy** is a measure of how close a laboratory measurement is to the true value. **Precision** is a measure of the testing method's capability to reproduce results. A laboratory can produce results that are precise but not accurate, but if the results are accurate they must also be precise.

Quality assurance (QA) is a comprehensive set of policies and procedures utilized to assess the reproducibility of a test result. **Quality control (QC)** is a process to ensure the validity or accuracy of test results.

The focus of QA is to provide a series of procedures to ensure the quality of laboratory testing. These procedures include:

1. a system to identify specimens and report results accurately
2. personnel education and training
3. quality control
4. enrollment in a proficiency testing program.

Purpose of QA and QC

Every lab needs to establish a quality assurance, quality control, and clinical standards program to monitor its performance and improve in areas in which it determines it is deficient. QC monitors the proficiency of employees, as well as the precision of laboratory test kits and instrumentation, to assure the doctors who use the lab and the patients whose specimens are being tested that the results are accurate.

Types and Levels of QC

Quality control is a method of ensuring that all factors involved in the testing procedure are performing as expected. The factors assessed are the personnel, the manufactured test kits or reagents, instruments, and supplies used in the testing process. QC identifies human error in the procedure, problems with the reagents or chemicals in the test kits, or automated testing equipment that is not performing as expected.

Manufacturers prepare a sample of a tested substance with a known value, or a positive or negative outcome; this is known as a **control reagent**. Lab personnel run the control sample as if it were a patient's specimen, and results are compared with the expected values provided by the manufacturer of the control reagents.

For example, a positive control should yield a positive result, and a negative control should produce a

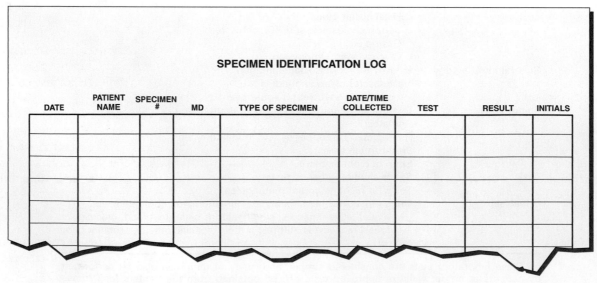

> Figure 23–1 Specimen identification log.

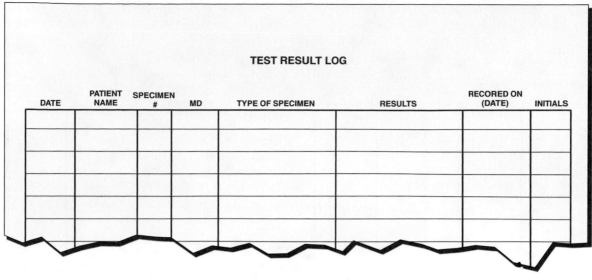

TEST RESULT LOG

DATE	PATIENT NAME	SPECIMEN #	MD	TYPE OF SPECIMEN	RESULTS	RECORED ON (DATE)	INITIALS

➤ **Figure 23–2** Test result log.

negative result. Some controls such as glucose controls have numerical values. The expected value is provided as a range. As long as the control falls within the range, the testing procedure can be used for patients.

If the test is run manually, human error can cause incorrect results. Another reason for a faulty result may be a problem with the chemicals or reagents being used. Chemicals and reagents should always be checked to see if they have expired or are otherwise bad. Reagents may get contaminated with bacterial growth from improper use, and if not refrigerated or exposed to light may appear more cloudy than usual.

A third reason for faulty results is a problem with the laboratory equipment. In situations where automated testing equipment is used, control samples are sometimes run along with the patient samples; other times the samples are run first and results checked to see if they are within the acceptable range.

Preventive maintenance of laboratory equipment is an integral factor of a QA program. Daily cleaning and replacement of faulty parts ensure equipment reliability. Maintenance schedules are provided by the manufacturer, and performance should be monitored.

Accurate record keeping is also an important part of laboratory quality control. The four key records are specimen identification, QC, test results, and instrument maintenance and history. Forms can be obtained from the National Committee for Clinical Laboratory Standards (NCCLS), which establishes the rules for safety, standards, and integrity of laboratory testing on human samples.

A sample of a specimen identification log is shown in Figure 23–1; a test result log is shown in Figure 23–2; a QC log is shown in Figure 23–3; and an instrument history and maintenance log is shown in Figure 23–4.

When QC Is Performed

QC tests should be performed on all instruments at the start of each day, before any patient tests are run. Results of QC tests are recorded in the QC log. For many pieces of automated testing equipment, QC tests are performed first thing in the morning, before running patient specimens, and at regular intervals throughout the day or after a certain number of tests have been run. Instruments should be cleaned daily, and preventive maintenance should be performed according to manufacturer's recommendation.

Calibration and Verification

Laboratory equipment is complex and sensitive and must be regularly calibrated to make sure it is producing accurate and precise results. **Calibration** is the testing and adjustment of test equipment to provide the known relationship between the measurement response and the substance value measured by the test.

Manufacturers provide a set of calibrations for every piece of equipment. The calibration procedure, which can be simple or complex, is outlined in a booklet provided by the manufacturer. Proper care and maintenance of laboratory equipment should be part of employee orientation.

Records must also be kept of the temperature of the incubator(s) and refrigerator/freezer. If their temperatures are too high or too low, these pieces of equipment must also be calibrated.

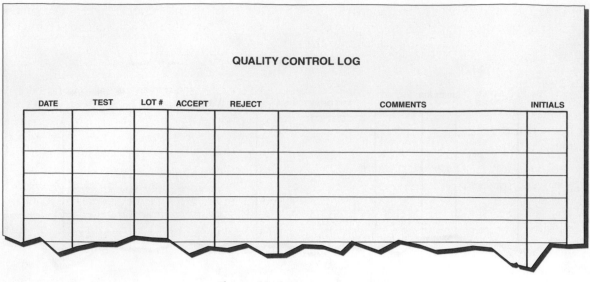

➤ Figure 23–3 Quality control log.

➤ Figure 23–4 Instrument history and maintenance record.

FILING FOR CERTIFICATION AS A PHYSICIAN'S OFFICE LABORATORY

Filing an Application and Paying Fees

To become certified as a POL, the office must file an application, be sure that the requirements for becoming certified are met, and pay the appropriate fees.

Obtaining a Certificate of Accreditation

As part of the accreditation process under CLIA, laboratories must submit to regular proficiency testing of laboratory personnel, as well as a physical inspection by an authorized agent of HCFA. In addition, OSHA or the CDC can, at any time, conduct an unannounced inspection of any laboratory facility.

CLIA requires proficiency testing for all procedures except waived tests. Proficiency testing is a form of QC, conducted by outsiders. Laboratories that perform moderate- and high-complexity tests must undergo proficiency testing three times a year.

Each time, an approved agency will ship the laboratory a set of specimens. These must be tested using the same procedures used for patient evaluation. The results are mailed to the agency conducting the proficiency testing.

During the physical inspection of the laboratory, the HCFA-authorized inspector will check to see that dozens of conditions are being met, which all fall into the following five categories:

1. Personnel
2. Patient test management
3. Quality control
4. Proficiency testing
5. Quality assurance.

LABORATORY SAFETY

Working safely is mostly a matter of common sense. The three major kinds of hazards in a medical laboratory are physical hazards, the most common of which is fire from alcohol lamps, burners, and electrical equipment, as well as spills and broken glass; chemical hazards, from caustic or volatile chemicals such as acids and alkalis, and fumes from chemicals; and biological hazards, from pathogenic microorganisms such as tuberculosis, HIV, and hepatitis B virus.

If an accident occurs, you must report it to your supervisor immediately. Laboratory safety records and incident reports must be maintained for any inspection by OSHA or by an agent of HCFA.

Follow Rules

The best way to make sure you and your colleagues are safe in the laboratory is to follow the rules of laboratory safety, which are highlighted in the accompanying box. Most laboratory accidents are caused by people who are skilled and believe because they are skilled they can take safety shortcuts. Laboratories are often busy, and supervisors, doctors, and patients are often anxious to receive lab results as quickly as possible. Despite these pressures, laboratory employees must consider their personal safety, and the safety of their colleagues, first.

Fire Extinguishers and Fire Blankets

Every laboratory should have a fire extinguisher by each door and easily accessible fire blankets. Employees should all know the location of fire extinguishers and fire blankets.

When using an open flame, a laboratory employee should have a fire blanket at hand and work carefully so that loose clothes—such as lab coat sleeves—do not catch fire.

Fire extinguishers can contain small fires, but they may not be effective against larger fires, and employees are not expected to totally extinguish any fire that breaks out. Fire extinguishers near doors can contain a fire long enough for laboratory employees to exit safely.

Fire blankets can be used either to smother a fire or to help put out a fire on a lab coat or other clothing.

Eyewash Station/Shower

Although standard precautions should be used at all time, sometimes caustic chemicals do get into the eyes, even under protective eyewear. For this reason, each laboratory has an eyewash station. If a caustic chemical gets in the eyes, the eyes should be thoroughly washed for 5 minutes.

If hazardous chemicals are used in the lab, there should be a shower in the lab area so employees who become exposed to the hazardous chemicals can completely wash off before leaving the lab, for their own safety and to prevent them contaminating other areas of the medical office.

Material Safety Data Sheets (MSDS) should be maintained for every hazardous chemical used in the lab, and all laboratory employees should be thoroughly briefed on these chemicals. An example of an MSDS was shown in chapter 6.

Spill Cleanup Kits

In addition to maintaining personal protection against hazardous and caustic chemicals and biohazards, the lab must also have spill cleanup kits available. All laboratory personnel need to know where they are and how to use them, as well as the regulations about cleaning up hazardous spills.

If a spill involving hazardous or caustic chemicals or biohazardous materials occurs, the office's designated safety officer must be notified immediately and must either personally clean up the spill or directly supervise the cleaning. The safety officer then fills out the required paperwork for OSHA and HCFA. Figure 23–5 shows a commercial acid spill cleanup kit.

Biohazard Waste Containers

Labs need to have both rigid biohazard (sharps) containers and biohazard waste bags in sufficient quantities and easily available to personnel working at any station where they might be necessary. Used or contaminated personal protective equipment, including gloves, masks, and disposable gowns or aprons, should be thrown away in biohazard bags. Lab coats and gowns or aprons should be placed in the hamper for laundry that is considered hazardous.

Disposal of Blood and Body Fluids

All laboratory specimens that contain blood or other body fluids or human tissue should be considered contaminated. If these are being sent to another lab, they should be packaged in a plastic biohazard transfer bag,

FOCUS ON
SAFETY

LABORATORY RULES

1. No eating, drinking, or smoking in the laboratory. Food and beverages can be contaminated or can contaminate laboratory specimens and reagents.

2. Never use a biohazard refrigerator for storing food or beverage.

3. Always wear a lab coat or apron in the lab area.

4. When entering or leaving the lab area, wash hands. Remove lab coat or apron when leaving the lab area.

5. Keep hair off shoulders or contained in a laboratory cap. No jewelry (plain wedding band is okay). Loose clothing, hair, and jewelry can be a fire hazard and can be contaminated by biological debris.

6. Follow standard precautions at all times.

7. Do not touch face, mouth, or eyes with hands, pens, or equipment from the lab area.

8. Avoid inhaling fumes of any chemicals used in the lab area.

9. Disinfect contaminated surfaces immediately, and disinfect all surfaces at the end of the day. Use a 10 percent bleach solution or other approved disinfectant.

10. Use proper procedure to clean up spills, as discussed in chapter 6.

11. Never use a mouth pipette to draw specimens.

12. If skin or eyes come in contact with chemicals, flush area with water for at least 5 minutes.

13. Label all chemicals and store them properly. Chemicals that can evaporate should be used in a well-ventilated area. Never store chemicals above eye level. Store flammable materials in a fireproof cabinet.

14. Keep an up-to-date safety manual with Material Safety Data Sheets (MSDS) in the laboratory. All personnel should be familiar with them.

15. Mark hot surfaces (unless obvious), and keep flammable items away from them.

---

inside a strong container with a secure lid. Surfaces where blood, body fluid, or tissue has splattered during testing should be decontaminated with a 10 percent solution of household bleach or other approved disinfectant. Equipment that has been contaminated with blood or body fluids should also be disinfected. Bulk blood or body fluids should be poured into a sanitary sewer.

CARING FOR LABORATORY EQUIPMENT AND SUPPLIES

Literally hundreds of different pieces of equipment and supplies may be used in a laboratory. Depending on the kinds of tests performed in the POL where you work, you may have to familiarize yourself with only a few pieces of equipment or dozens.

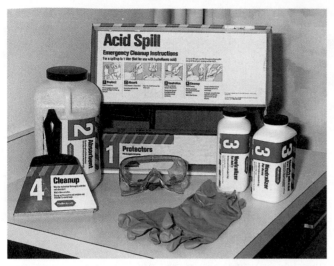

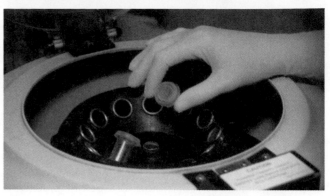

> **Figure 23–7** When placing tubes in the centrifuge, the medical assistant must always be sure they are balanced. (From Zakus SM: *Clinical Procedures for Medical Assistants*, 3rd ed. St. Louis: Mosby, 1995.)

> **Figure 23–5** Commercial acid spill cleanup kit. (From Stepp CA, Woods MA: *Laboratory Procedures for Medical Office Personnel*. Philadelphia: W.B. Saunders, 1998.)

Each piece of equipment comes with manufacturer's specifications about how it should be maintained and how often it should be professionally serviced. In addition, equipment must be cleaned each day and calibrated according to schedule, with records kept on proper forms or logs.

Types of Equipment and Supplies

The most common equipment found in POLs are cell counters, analyzers, centrifuges, refrigerators and freezers, incubators, various forms of glassware, microscopes, and test kits.

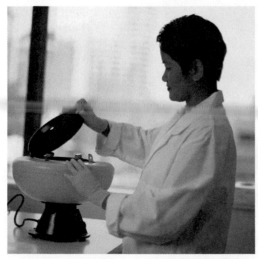

> **Figure 23–6** The cover of the centrifuge must be tightly closed before a sample of urine or blood is spun.

Simple cell counters most often found in doctor's offices are used to count the number of red blood cells, white blood cells, and platelets in a single patient sample. Some also measure the hemoglobin. Results are either printed out or appear on a display screen, depending on the machine being used.

Most chemistry analyzers found in medical office labs analyze one sample at a time. They often use strips onto which a blood or urine sample is placed for the machine to analyze.

Centrifuges are used to "spin down" a substance, using centrifugal force—a rapid rotation that separates the components of a liquid depending on their density. Centrifuges are used in every department in a medical laboratory. Figure 23–6 shows a centrifuge.

For instance, when blood is processed in a centrifuge, the heavy red blood cells sink to the bottom, white blood cells and platelets are in the middle (known as the buffy coat), and a liquid layer floats on top. If the sample is not allowed to clot, the top layer is called plasma; if a clot has formed, the top layer is called serum.

Centrifuges come in many different sizes, and all have variable speeds at which they spin, which are calculated in revolutions per minute (**RPMs**). Within the centrifuge, special rubber-cushioned cups hold the test tubes containing the blood or other samples. Any tube placed into the centrifuge must be counterbalanced; that is, a tube of the same design and weight must be placed in the space exactly opposite. Figure 23–7 shows a medical assistant placing tubes in a centrifuge.

Refrigerators and freezers are used to store samples, as well as chemical reagents and various testing kits. Food should never be stored in the laboratory's refrigerator, because of the possibility of cross-contamination.

Glassware includes beakers, flasks, graduated cylinders, test tubes, glass pipettes, and glass microscope slides.

Many laboratory tests are now conducted using individual, disposable kits; the two most common kits found in medical office labs are strep tests and pregnancy tests.

Routine Maintenance and Checks

Maintenance logs must be kept, and any unscheduled maintenance or repair must also be documented.

Microscopes

A microscope is an indispensable piece of equipment for every laboratory. There are many types of microscopes. Monocular microscopes have one eyepiece for viewing specimens; binocular microscopes have two eyepieces. Dual microscopes have two sets of eyepieces so two people can view the same specimen.

The eyepiece, or **ocular,** is attached to the barrel of the microscope, and magnifies the field by ten times

(10X). At the bottom of the barrel is the microscope's arm, which usually has three objectives attached. Each **objective** is a lens that magnifies the specimen by a different power of magnification.

The highest power of magnification is 100X, which is the **oil-immersion objective.** More light must be available to actually see this much magnification; hence, the lens is immersed in oil, which serves to prevent the scattering and loss of light that occurs when light waves pass through air.

When multiplied by the 10X magnification in the ocular, the microscope magnifies samples by 100X to 1000X.

Figure 23–8 shows the parts of a microscope.

When adjusting the microscope to increase or decrease the magnification, you should always rotate the nosepiece using the grip and not handle the objectives. The three different objectives are used for different kinds of lab work. The objective with the most magnification also has the narrowest field of view.

The most common microscope used in medical office labs is a binocular brightfield microscope. The brightfield microscope has a light source that passes

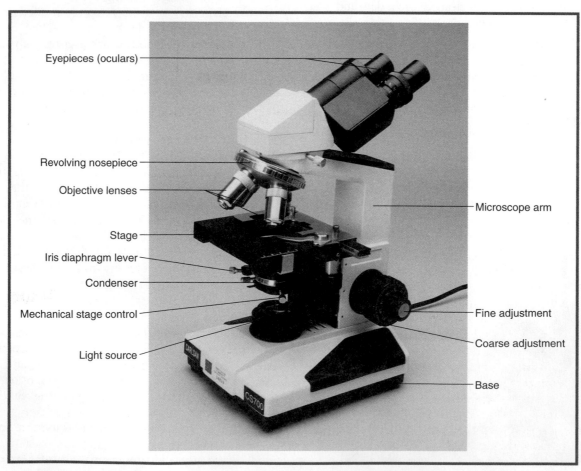

> **Figure 23–8** Parts of a microscope. (From Kinn ME, Woods M: *The Medical Assistant: Administrative and Clinical,* 8th ed. Philadelphia: W.B. Saunders, 1999.)

light through the specimen, then through both the objective and ocular lenses.

Other kinds of microscopes include the following:

The darkfield microscope, in which light comes from the side and the only light to come through the lenses is reflected off the specimen. Darkfield microscopy is often used to view very small bacteria.

The phase-contrast microscope, in which light is refracted at different wavelengths off the microorganisms and the medium they are in. This allows for better differentiation. This type of microscope is used to view living microorganisms.

The **fluorescence microscope,** which uses an ultraviolet (UV) light source that illuminates the object but does not pass through the objective lens. Dyes and pigments are used to assist the UV light, highlighting important aspects of the sample in question. This type of microscope is often used in immunology laboratories.

The electron microscope, which uses an electron beam instead of natural light and focuses using magnets instead of lenses. The image is viewed on a screen instead of through ocular lenses. Electron microscopy can be used to view very tiny viruses.

For best viewing when using a binocular microscope, keep both eyes open and do not squint. A microscope's lenses will correct for nearsightedness or

---

PROCEDURE 23–1

Using a Microscope

Performance Objective: The student will be able to use a microscope to view slides under all magnifications.

Supplies and Equipment: Compound light microscope with dust cover, immersion oil, lens paper, prepared microscope slides, lens cleaner.

Procedure Steps

1. Using both hands, one hand on the arm and one under the base, carry the microscope to the work area.
   Rationale: Dropping the microscope can result in permanent damage to the instrument.

2. Set the microscope on a secure flat surface and remove the dust cover.

3. Unwind the cord and plug the instrument into a grounded outlet. Place excess cord on the table.
   Rationale: Proper grounding of electrical instruments helps prevent unwanted electrical discharge. Dangling cords may cause accidents.

4. Clean the lenses and oculars of the microscope with lens cleaning solution and lens paper. Start with the oculars and the low-power lenses. Clean the oil-immersion objective (100X) last.

Rationale: Glass lenses are especially easy to scratch. Lens paper is designed to prevent scratching of lenses.

5. Turn on the light at the rheostat control, keeping light intensity at a low level.
   Rationale: Light will appear more intense on lower power objectives and may cause a temporary blinding effect. If no light appears when the light is turned on, the bulb or fuse may need to be replaced.

6. Place a prepared slide, coverslip up, or a prepared smear onto the center hole of the mechanical stage.
   Rationale: Light passes through the hole from the light source of the mechanical stage to allow viewing of objects.

7. Secure the slide with clips or slide holder to prevent slipping.

8. Swing the low-power or scan objective into place. You will feel and hear a click when the objective engages.
   Rationale: The lowest power objective has the longest working distance from the stage. Scratching of the objective is less likely to occur when the lower power is used for initial focus.

9. Adjust the width of the oculars until a single image appears. Adjust the iris diaphragm if more light is necessary.

Procedure continued on following page

PROCEDURE 23–1 *(continued)*

Rationale: Light should first be adjusted with the iris diaphragm, followed by the rheostat control.

10. Observe the slide with the naked eye while raising the stage using the coarse adjustment.
    Rationale: If you view the slide while raising the stage, you can avoid contact, which can cause the slide to crack or can scratch the objective.

11. Look into the oculars and begin to focus by lowering the stage with the coarse adjustment.
    Rationale: The coarse adjustment allows rapid focusing.

12. Bring the object into focus with the fine adjustment.
    Rationale: Fine adjustment allows more precise focusing.

13. Switch to the high-power (40X) objective lens. Use the fine adjustment to focus.
    Rationale: The longer lens is used after the object has been brought into focus with the low-power lens to avoid damaging the slide or the lens. Wet specimens are covered with a cover slip.

14. To observe an object on a prepared slide with the oil-immersion objective (100X), place a drop of immersion oil on the slide and click the oil-immersion objective into place.
    Rationale: A prepared slide can be viewed with greater magnification to reveal more detail.

15. Use the fine adjustment knob to bring the objective down until it touches the oil but not the slide.
    Rationale: The oil allows the light to be collected in the ocular rather than being dispersed. If the stage is lowered too rapidly, contact may occur between the ocular and the slide.

16. Adjust the light if necessary by opening the iris diaphragm.
    Rationale: You may need more light for higher magnification.

17. When finished, turn the oil-immersion objective to the side before removing the slide.
    Rationale: The objective or slide may be cracked or scratched if removed while under the oil-immersion objective.

18. Record or report results of identification as appropriate for specimen type.

19. Clean the slide and the oil-immersion objective with lens paper before storing the microscope.

20. Turn off the microscope and grasp the plug to remove. Do not pull on the cord.

21. Wrap the cord around the microscope and replace the dust cover before returning to storage.
    Rationale: The lenses will be easier to clean if accumulation of dust is prevented.

farsightedness, so it is only necessary to wear glasses when using a microscope if you have an astigmatism.

Procedure 23–1 describes using a microscope in detail.

Microscopes are delicate, precise, and expensive instruments. They must be taken care of, both when being used and when being stored. The objectives and ocular lenses must be cleaned carefully, especially the oil-immersion lens. Lens paper and gentle solutions should be used. Xylene and other harsh chemicals can damage the mounting cement. Paper towel or regular facial tissues can scratch the lens or leave particles.

A cotton swab moistened with mild lens cleaner can be used to clean especially difficult smudges or film. Swab gently, beginning at the middle of the lens and working toward the outside, using a clockwise motion.

The oil-immersion lens should always be cleaned immediately after it is used.

The microscope's body should be dusted regularly, using a soft cloth. When the microscope is not being used, it should be covered with a plastic dust cover and stored in a dry, clean, ventilated place.

LABELING AND TRANSPORTING SPECIMENS

To make sure that the correct specimen is taken from the correct patient, that the correct tests are undertaken on the correct specimen, and that the correct results are provided to the correct patient, meticulous attention to the paperwork that accompanies all laboratory tests is crucial.

Laboratory testing begins with a requisition for a particular procedure or test. All samples must be properly labeled with the patient's unique identifier. In-

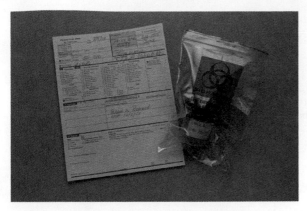

➤ **Figure 23–9** Laboratory requisition and specimen in plastic biohazard bag.

creasingly, a bar code system is being used for identification purposes. Finally, proper attention needs to be paid to transportation, in particular using appropriate containers and mailing packets.

Laboratory Requisition

If a doctor requests an outside lab to perform tests, a laboratory requisition needs to be sent either with the patient who is going to have a sample taken or with a sample that has been taken in the office. A laboratory requisition is shown in Figure 23–9.

Many labs have their own requisition forms. In other instances doctors use a generic requisition form, often one that is computer generated. Both preprinted and computer-generated requisitions list the most common laboratory tests in a logical order and have space for the doctor to write special requests.

The requisition must have the doctor's name and the practice's address written on it so the lab can return results appropriately, as well as the telephone number in case the lab has a question. It must also have the patient's name, address, telephone number, and Social Security number, as well as the patient's billing information if the bill is to be sent to the patient or to the patient's insurance company.

If the specimen has been taken in the office, information about the specimen must also be included: the time and date the specimen was taken, the source of the specimen, if the patient was fasting, the clinical diagnosis, medications the patient was taking at the time the specimen was taken, the tests being requested, and the urgency of the request.

Finally, the requisition must be signed by the doctor making the request.

Patient ID and Labeling Protocol

The medical assistant's role in the accuracy of laboratory test results is substantial, from obtaining the specimen to ensuring safety and making sure samples are properly identified and labeled.

The medical assistant is responsible for obtaining the specimen. The patient must be told if there are any requirements for advance preparation, such as fasting. Fasting involves abstaining from intake of any fluids or food for a specified period before collection of a specimen. Water is sometimes allowed during the fast. A typical fast lasts 8 to 12 hours, depending on the test to be performed.

Standard safety precautions must be followed during specimen collection to protect those involved in the procedure. Before collection, all supplies should be assembled and checked for quality. Needles should be checked for burrs or bending. Blood collection tubes must be inspected for cracks, chips, or other damage that occurs during shipping.

Proper identification of the patient is a crucial step in the collection process. In a doctor's office, you can usually confirm the patient's identification verbally. Ask the patient to tell you his or her name and to spell the last name to check and make sure it matches the lab slip.

Once the specimen is collected, using procedures explained in detail in other chapters, it is imperative to

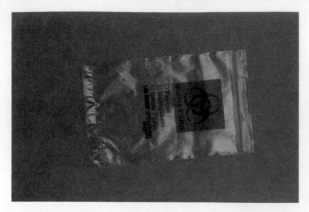

> **Figure 23–10** Plastic biohazard bag for transporting laboratory specimens.

label the container or tube with the patient's name, the date, the time of collection, your initials, and any other information required by the testing laboratory, such as the specimen source. Some facilities use a computer-generated label.

Ideally, testing occurs immediately on the specimens, because results are more accurate when specimens are fresh. Most tests are reliable on specimens taken within an hour, but this is not always possible. If a reference laboratory is involved, it has a protocol outlined for each specific test as to the proper way to handle, store, and transport the specimen.

If the specimen is blood, it may have to be centrifuged, and the serum or plasma separated into a separate container. Remember to properly label the transport container with the same information as on the original specimen. Refrigeration and sometimes freezing may be required to preserve the integrity of the constituents being tested.

Using a Pipette to Transfer Fluid

A **pipette** is a small glass or plastic vessel used to transfer fluid from one place to another. Pipettes are used to transfer specimens from collection containers such as urine sample cups onto glass slides, strips for chemical analysis, and test tubes.

When transferring liquid using a pipette, always keep the pipette vertical. Wear disposable gloves. Draw fluid up by putting pressure on the suction apparatus—do not use your mouth—until the top of the fluid is slightly above the calibration line for the desired amount. Put your finger over the top of the pipette to maintain suction.

Bring the pipette out of the vessel containing the fluid, wipe off the end with a tissue, and release a small amount until the desired amount of fluid is in

the pipette. Then, transfer the fluid. If a spill occurs, clean up and disinfect immediately.

Transporting Specimens

Specimens of body fluids must be transported in specially designed containers and mailing pouches. The documentation you fill out for the service that is delivering the samples must state clearly that the samples include body fluids or human tissue. Figure 23–10 shows a plastic biohazard bag for transporting specimens.

Bar Code System

Increasingly, laboratories are using bar code systems; each doctor's office that uses the lab is given a unique identifier and the patient is also given an identifier. These are entered into the office computer, and stickers with bar codes are printed. Stickers are put on the requisition form and on each of the samples.

When the samples and requisition form arrive at the lab, a bar-code reader is used to read the codes. Computerized analysis equipment can also read the bar codes; after each test is performed the results are transferred to the computer database and are collected into a report about each patient and a report packet for each doctor. This is then sent either by mail or fax, or is transferred within a computer network.

Lab Results

Lab results can arrive at the doctor's office either in the mail, via the fax, over the phone (if urgent) and followed up by mail, or by direct computer-to-computer transfer.

DEPARTMENT OF HEMATOLOGY
COMPLETE BLOOD COUNT

Date Time		09/03/99 3:46 PM		Reference Units
=>WBC		4.5		(3.8 - 10.2) THOU/CMM
=>RBC		4.34		(4.12 - 5.64) MIL/CMM
=>HGB		8.4		(11.6 - 15.8) G/DL
=>HCT		28.7 (A)	Lo	(35.9 - 46.8) %
		* * * * **PLEASE NOTE** * * * * CBC methodology and reference ranges have changed effective 8/12/99		
=>MCV		66.0	Lo	(84.4 - 101.2) FL
=>MCH		19.4	Lo	(26.6 - 35.0) PG
=>MCHC		29.4	Lo	(33.2 - 36.8) G/DL
=>RDW		17.5	Hi	(11.4 - 15.0) %
=>PLTCT		367	#	(140 - 390) THOU/CMM
=>MPV		6.6	Lo	(7 - 9) FL
=>PDW		46.9	Lo	(47 - 69) %
=>NEUTS		48.3		(45.9 - 84.5) %
=>LYMPH		35.5		(7.8 - 43.2) %
=>MONO		7.8		(2.3 - 8.7) %
=>EOS		2.4		(0.0 - 5.9) %
=>BASO		1.2	Hi	(0.0 - 1.1) %
=>ANISO		SLIGHT		
=>MICRO		MARKED		
=>HYPO		MARKED		

ROUTINE HEMATOLOGY

Date Time		09/03/99 3:46 PM		Reference Units
=>ESR	32		Hi	(0 - 20) MM/HR

HEMATOLOGY SENDOUTS

Date Time	09/03/99 3:46 PM	Reference Units

➢ **Figure 23–11** Sample hematology report.

Results of tests carried out in the medical office lab are usually handwritten, either directly into the patient's record or on a lab slip that is filed in the record.

Most results from commercial labs are machine generated, as shown in the sample hematology report in Figure 23–11.

The doctor reviews these results, and then they are filed in the patient's record. The medical assistant should never file lab results until after the doctor has initialed them, signifying that he or she has seen them.

When laboratory reports are sent directly from the lab's computer to the doctor's computer, they can be printed out at the doctor's office and placed for the doctor to read, or, if the office uses computerized medical records, simply transferred from the incoming lab report database to the patient's electronic record.

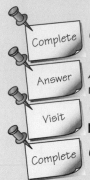

STUDENT STUDY PLAN

To reinforce your understanding of the material in this chapter . . .

Complete the **Review & Recall** questions.

Answer the **Critical Thinking Questions**, and discuss them with your classmates.

Visit **Web sites** suggested below, and search for additional Web sites using **Keywords for Internet Searches**.

Complete the exercises in chapter 23 of the **Student Mastery Manual**.

REVIEW & RECALL

1. Describe nine sections in a large medical laboratory.

2. Differentiate between hospital-based laboratories, reference laboratories, and clinical laboratories. Name two other types of laboratories.

3. Describe the categories of laboratories under CLIA 88.

4. What is the purpose of quality assurance and quality control?

5. Identify four types of records that must be kept as part of a quality control program.

6. What measures must be taken to be sure laboratory instruments are functioning correctly?

7. List 10 rules of laboratory safety.

8. What safety equipment should be present in a laboratory?

9. Describe how to use a microscope.

10. What information must accompany a laboratory specimen when it is transported to an outside lab?

CRITICAL THINKING QUESTIONS

1. What could happen if office personnel began storing their lunches in the laboratory refrigerator?

2. Why is it necessary to keep records of the temperature in the refrigerator, freezer, and laboratory incubator?

3. If you entered a laboratory and saw a spill on the laboratory table, what would you do? Why? Would your actions be different if someone told you exactly what the spill was? Why?

4. Discuss how a medical office can establish procedures to be sure all laboratory reports sent by computer are seen by a doctor before they are filed in the patients' medical records.

5. Do research to identify different types of fire extinguishers and their uses. What type of fire extinguisher would you recommend for a physician's office laboratory? Give reasons for your answer.

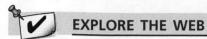

EXPLORE THE WEB

INTERNET WEB SITES

Types of lab tests under CLIA 88
www.phppo.cdc.gov/clia/default.asp

Virtual microscope
micro.magnet.fsu.edu

Health Care Financing Administration (HCFA)*
www.hcfa.gov

*Effective 6/2001, the name of this agency has been changed to the Centers for Medicare and Medicaid Services (CMMS). A new website address will probably be created.

KEYWORDS FOR INTERNET SEARCHES

medical laboratory
microscope
quality assurance
quality control
virtual microscope

Chapter 24

Urinalysis

Instructional Objectives

After completing this chapter, you will be able to do the following:

1. Define and spell the vocabulary words for this chapter.
2. Explain the role of each organ of the genitourinary system in forming urine.
3. Describe the normal function of the nephron.
4. Compare methods of obtaining urine specimens and the laboratory tests done on them.
5. Discuss quality-control methods for various types of urine tests.
6. Describe the proper technique for the physical examination of urine.
7. Correlate chemical abnormalities detected in the urine to abnormal physiologic conditions.
8. Describe the purpose and procedure of three tests done to confirm results of urine chemistry using a reagent strip.
9. Describe how urine is prepared for microscopic examination.
10. Identify normal and abnormal structures found during microscopic examination of urine.
11. Explain how physical, chemical, and microscopic urine tests should be documented.

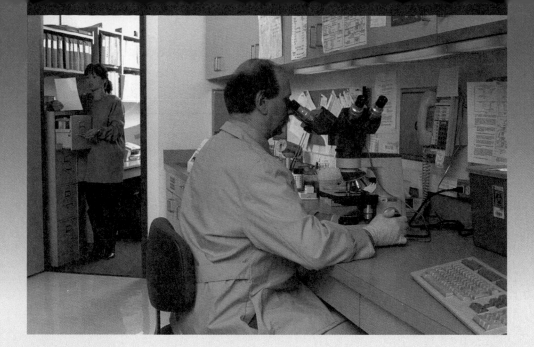

- Dispose of biohazardous materials.
- Practice standard precautions.
- Instruct patients in the collection of a clean-catch midstream urine specimen.
- Perform urinalysis.

- Use methods of quality control.
- Document appropriately.
- Instruct individuals according to their needs.
- Perform within legal and ethical boundaries.

Performance Objectives

After completing this chapter, you will be able to do the following:

1. Inform a patient of the correct procedure to collect a clean-catch midstream urine specimen (Procedure 24–1).

2. Inform a patient of the correct procedure to collect a 24-hour urine specimen (Procedure 24–2).

3. Measure the specific gravity of urine using a refractometer (Procedure 24–3).

4. Perform a urinalysis using the reagent strip method (Procedure 24–4).

5. Test urine for sugars using the Clinitest 5-drop method (Procedure 24–5).

6. Perform urine testing using the Acetest method (Procedure 24–6).

7. Perform urine testing using the Ictotest method (Procedure 24–7).

8. Prepare urine for microscopic examination (Procedure 24–8).

VOCABULARY

anions (p. 573)
bilirubin (p. 583)
Bowman's capsule (p. 572)
calyces (p. 571)
casts (p. 589)
cations (p. 573)
chain of custody (p. 576)
crystals (p. 592)
epithelial cells (p. 578)

filtration (p. 572)
glomerular filtrate (p. 572)
glomerulus (p. 572)
ketones (p. 583)
nephron (p. 571)
nitrites (p. 583)
oxidation (p. 581)
papilla (p. 571)

qualitative tests (p. 578)
quantitative tests (p. 581)
reagent strip (p. 581)
refractive index (p. 579)
refractometer (p. 579)
rugae (p. 570)
solute (p. 579)
specific gravity (p. 578)

turbid (p. 578)
urea (p. 573)
ureter (p. 570)
urethra (p. 571)
urinalysis (p. 570)
urinary meatus (p. 571)
urinometer (p. 579)
urobilinogen (p. 583)

ABBREVIATIONS

HPF (p. 589)   pH (p. 584)   SG (p. 578)   UTI (p. 571)

Perhaps the most common laboratory test performed in the physician's office laboratory is the urinalysis. The formation and excretion of urine is one of the most important of bodily functions; without the capacity to form and excrete urine, the human body would drown in its own waste materials. **Urinalysis**—the analysis of the physical, chemical, and microscopic composition of urine—is an efficient and effective way of determining how well the body is processing nutrients and excreting waste, and can be used to detect, confirm, or monitor a host of illnesses and chronic conditions.

FORMATION OF URINE

Urine is formed in the kidneys. As blood passes through each kidney, it is cleansed of impurities. These impurities are then mixed with water that is drawn out of the tissue by the kidneys. The waste-filled water—urine—is then excreted. An adult produces about 1.5 liters of urine each day, and excretes 1 to 2 liters per day, depending on the body's level of hydration.

The Urinary System

The urinary system is one of the body's most efficient homeostatic mechanisms. Our kidneys continually monitor and cleanse the bloodstream, processing about 180 liters (47 gallons) of blood per day, removing waste, and producing about 1.5 liters of urine to eliminate the waste. Normal adult kidneys can filter 1,000 to 1,200 milliliters of blood per minute. That means that one quarter of the body's total blood volume is cleaned every minute of the day.

The urinary system's primary function is regulation. A healthy urinary system serves to maintain the body's normal status in five main ways:

1. Disposing of toxic waste substances produced by chemical reactions within the body
2. Maintaining a constant blood pH (level of acidity) through the selective elimination or conservation of certain ions
3. Preventing loss of vital nutrients by reabsorption
4. Maintaining a constant blood pressure, through the regulation of water loss
5. Regulating other body systems through production of substances that stimulate blood cell production and regulate blood pressure.

Urinary System Anatomy

Anatomically, the urinary system, shown in Figure 24–1, is composed of two major organs—the two kidneys—and a few accessory organs. Each bean-shaped kidney is located retroperitoneal (in the rear of the abdominal cavity) in the upper lumbar region underneath the lower part of the ribcage. Because the liver is a large organ, the right kidney is slightly lower than the left kidney.

The urinary tract's accessory organs serve to transport, store, and eliminate urine. A long, cylindrical tube called a **ureter** is attached to each kidney to drain urine from the renal pelvis.

Urine produced in each kidney drains through a ureter into the bladder, a muscular, saclike structure that temporarily stores the urine until it is eliminated. The bladder's inner walls are composed of special, stretchy cells known as transitional epithelium. Layers of these unique cells form ridges called **rugae**, which allow the bladder to expand as it becomes filled with urine, much as a balloon fills with water. A normal adult bladder can hold 300 to 500 ml of urine, and more if necessary.

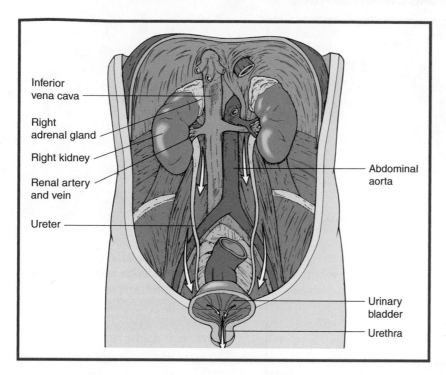

Inferior
vena cava

Right
adrenal gland

Right kidney

Renal artery
and vein

Ureter

Abdominal
aorta

Urinary
bladder

Urethra

➢ **Figure 24–1** The urinary system. (From Frazier M, Drzymkowski J, Doty S: *Essentials of Human Diseases and Conditions.* Philadelphia: W.B. Saunders, 1996.)

Urine is eliminated through the body through another tubelike structure, the **urethra.** A sphincter muscle located beneath the bladder can be controlled voluntarily to open or shut, allowing urine to leave the bladder. If urination is not initiated deliberately, involuntary reflex action causes the bladder to empty. Urine passes through the urethra and exits the body through the **urinary meatus,** the external opening.

The urinary structure differs somewhat in males and females.

Females have a much shorter urethra than males, only about 4 cm, which is separated from the female sexual organ, the vagina. The urinary meatus is located anterior to the vaginal opening and posterior to the clitoris. Due to the close proximity of the female urethra to both the vagina and the anus, and to its short length, females suffer from urinary tract infections **(UTIs)** 10 times as often as males.

In contrast, the adult male urethra averages 20 cm, and serves as the passageway for both urine and semen. The longer length of the male urethra makes it more difficult for bacteria to reach the bladder.

Kidney Anatomy

Because the kidneys use much of the body's total oxygen—about 23 percent at rest—a rich blood supply is needed for each kidney. Two renal arteries branch from the lower aorta of the heart, entering each kidney at the concave portion known as the renal hilum. These arteries supply the kidneys with oxygenated blood, which the kidneys filter of toxins, as well as nutrients. Deoxygenated, filtered blood exits the kid-

neys through the renal veins, which empty into the inferior vena cava.

Examination of a kidney reveals three major regions. The most superficial region is known as the renal cortex. The middle region, composed of several triangular areas, is called the renal medulla. The innermost region is the renal pelvis. The renal capsule, a thin, fibrous outer layer, covers each kidney.

A close look at these regions reveals important details about kidney function. The triangular structures located in the renal medulla are known as renal pyramids. Each pyramid is composed of a bundle containing thousands of tubular structures, which converge at the base of each pyramid to form a flowerlike structure called the **papilla.** Urine drains from the pyramids through very small holes in the papilla. Tubular extensions from the renal pelvis, called **calyces,** enclose each papilla. Urine collects in the smaller branches of the calyces, the minor calyces, then drains into the larger branches, the major calyces. All of the calyces in the kidney converge into a single renal pelvis. Urine exits the kidney through an opening from the renal pelvis to the ureter.

The Nephron

The **nephron,** shown in Figure 24–2, is the kidney's microscopic filtration unit. Each kidney contains over 1 million nephrons, located in the renal cortex and the medulla. The nephron contains two major parts, the renal corpuscle and the renal tubule. The renal corpuscle is the site of filtration; filtrate then

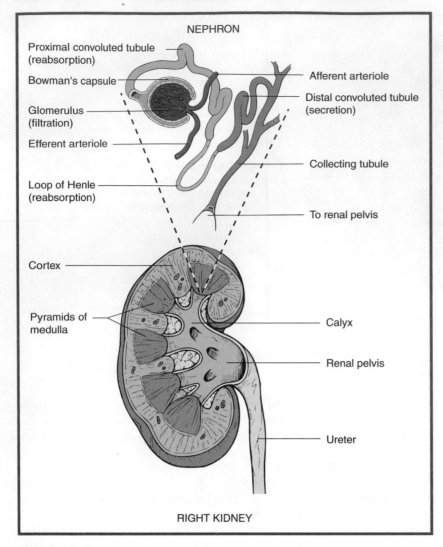

NEPHRON

Proximal convoluted tubule (reabsorption)

Bowman's capsule

Glomerulus (filtration)

Efferent arteriole

Loop of Henle (reabsorption)

Afferent arteriole

Distal convoluted tubule (secretion)

Collecting tubule

To renal pelvis

Cortex

Pyramids of medulla

Calyx

Renal pelvis

Ureter

RIGHT KIDNEY

➢ **Figure 24–2** The kidney and nephron. (From Frazier M, Drzymkowski J, Doty S: *Essentials of Human Diseases and Conditions.* Philadelphia: W.B. Saunders, 1996.)

passes through the renal tubule, where it undergoes various changes before becoming urine.

Filtration is the act of straining out large particles the body desires to keep, such as proteins.

The two major parts of the nephron can be further segmented into smaller structures, each playing a distinct role in urine formation. The renal corpuscle is composed of the **glomerulus,** a tuft of very small capillaries that filter blood, and the **Bowman's capsule**, a cuplike structure that surrounds the glomerulus and captures the filtrate produced from the blood.

After the renal artery enters the kidney, it branches into smaller and smaller arterioles. A single afferent arteriole enters each nephron, joining the glomerular capillary bed. Because the diameter of the glomerular capillaries is so much smaller than that of the afferent arteriole, a high pressure is created. This pressure forces liquid and small molecules out of the blood and into the space surrounding the glomerulus. This is known as **glomerular filtrate.**

Blood exits the glomerulus through the efferent arteriole, still oxygenated and newly filtered. The efferent

arteriole is continuous with the capillaries that surround the renal tubule. Oxygen and nutrients are exchanged for waste products from the cells of the nephron in these capillaries.

Glomerular filtrate contains almost everything that blood plasma contains, except for large molecules such as large proteins, and is very different from urine. This filtrate must undergo further changes and extreme concentration in the renal tubule, which is attached to Bowman's capsule, before it becomes the final urine product.

The renal tubule is divided into three distinct sections, each composed of different types of cells with different permeability characteristics, as shown in Figure 24–3.

In the first section, the proximal convoluted tubule, a process known as tubular reabsorption occurs, in which 65 percent of the filtrate's water, along with vital nutrients such as glucose, amino acids, sodium, calcium, and vitamins, are reabsorbed into the blood.

The second section, called the loop of Henle, is where another 15 percent of the filtrate's water is reabsorbed into the blood, but by a different process than that which occurs on the proximal convoluted tubule. More sodium, chloride, and potassium are redeposited into the blood.

In the third section, the distal convoluted tubule, tubular secretion, in which substances are transported from the blood to the renal tubule, occurs. Hormones such as antidiuretic hormone (produced by the pituitary gland) and aldosterone (produced by the adrenal gland) help regulate this process. Waste products and excess ions are eliminated from the blood in the distal convoluted tubule. Water may be reabsorbed or eliminated, depending on the person's current hydration status. Other substances such as urea, some hormones, and drug metabolites are also secreted into the distal convoluted tubule.

The renal tubule's final region is the collecting tubule. At this point, 99 percent of the original filtrate has been reabsorbed into the body, leaving the final urine product. Urine passes into the collecting tubule,

draining through the papilla, and combines with urine produced from all of the kidney's nephrons.

Composition of Urine

Normal urine is approximately 95 percent water and 5 percent solute, a combination of organic and inorganic molecules. One organic compound, a product of protein metabolism, is **urea.** Organic waste products also include nitrogenous (nitrogen-containing) waste such as ammonia. Creatinine and uric acid are two other examples of organic wastes found in normal urine. Creatinine is the metabolite—the breakdown product—of creatine, a product important in muscle metabolism.

Inorganic molecules are usually found in ionic form. Excess ions are eliminated from the body in urine. Positively charged ions are called **cations;** negatively charged ions are called **anions.** Ions such as sodium and chloride play an important role in electrolyte bal-

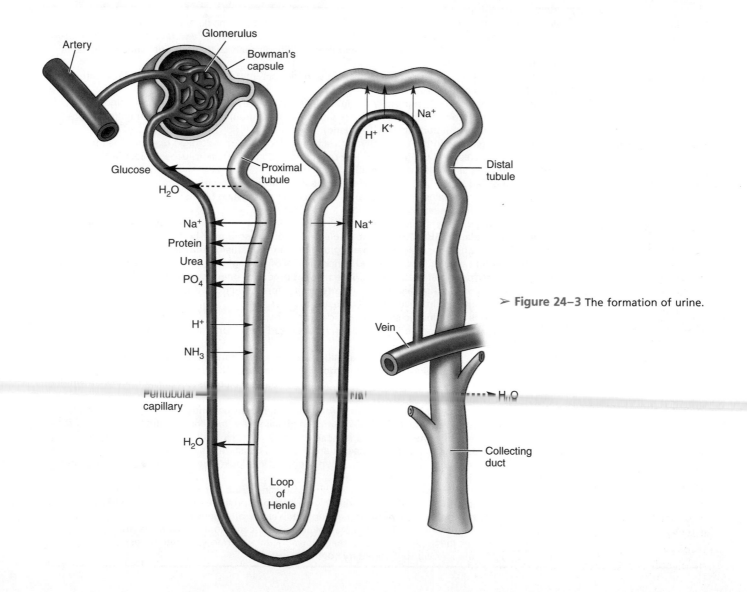

> **Figure 24–3** The formation of urine.

ance; the hydrogen ion maintains pH balance. Other ions, such as potassium, help regulate heart function. Calcium and magnesium are vital for healthy bones. It is essential for normal body functions that all of these ions be present in specific amounts. The kidneys eliminate excess ions while conserving ions that are needed.

Other substances that may be found in urine are hormones, enzymes, and drug metabolites. The presence of these substances is linked to the body's current status.

Urine is normally a sterile liquid, until it reaches the distal urethra, when it comes into contact with microorganisms and cells from the surrounding genital area. Special precautions can be taken when obtaining urine specimens to greatly reduce contamination.

Table 24–1 contains urinary-related terms.

OBTAINING A URINE SPECIMEN

To ensure the accuracy of test results, following proper technique for collecting urine specimens is crucial. Various testing methodologies require the use specific techniques of urine collection. The medical assistant needs to be familiar with several urine collection procedures and needs to be able to match the appropriate collection procedure with the particular tests ordered.

The following urine collection procedures are general guidelines. Each procedure gives an overview of the ordered urine tests, patient preparation, materials needed, and the suggested collection technique. The medical assistant should follow the guidelines required

Table 24–1	**Urinary-Related Terms**
Anuria	Failure to produce urine. Causes of anuria are severe dehydration, shock, and advanced renal disease.
Diuresis	Secretion and passage of large amounts of urine. Drugs such as caffeine and diuretics or large intake of fluids may induce this condition. Pathological conditions such as diabetes insipidus or diabetes mellitus may also induce diuresis.
Dysuria	Difficult or painful urination. Conditions such as urinary tract infections (UTIs), enlarged prostate, and genital infections can cause dysuria.
Enuresis	Inability to control urination, especially at night. Nocturnal enuresis is known as bedwetting.
Frequency	A condition in which the patient must urinate often. Increased fluid intake, bladder retention, pregnancy, and UTIs may induce urinary frequency.
Glucosuria, glycosuria	The presence of glucose in the urine. Glycosuria can be found in uncontrolled diabetes mellitus, gestational diabetes, and conditions of low renal threshold to glucose (glucose is lost in the urine at lower blood glucose levels than normal).
Hematuria	The presence of red blood cells (RBCs) in the urine. Hematuria can be found normally during the menstrual cycle in females. Pathological conditions that may cause blood in the urine are UTIs, kidney stones, renal disease, and trauma.
Hemoglobinuria	Hemoglobin may be present due to destruction of RBCs in hypotonic urine or destruction of large numbers of circulating RBCs. Hemoglobin released in the plasma may be filtered by the kidneys and found in urine. Conditions leading to hemoglobinuria are transfusion reactions, drug-induced hemolysis, and hemoglobinopathies, inherited abnormalities of hemoglobin such as sickle cell anemia.
Ketonuria	Ketones are a product of fat metabolism. When fat is burned for energy, as in starvation, decreased carbohydrate intake, and severe vomiting, ketones are formed and may appear in the urine. Ketonuria may also be present in uncontrolled diabetes mellitus.
Lipiduria	Found in conditions of nephrotic syndrome and poisonings.
Nocturia	Excessive voluntary urination during the night. A prolapsed uterus or bladder, pregnancy, and UTIs may induce nocturia.
Oliguria	Decreased output of urine; usually less than 400 mL in a 24-hour period on a consistent basis. The most common cause of oliguria is early to moderate stage renal disease.
Polyuria	Increased urine output; usually greater than 2000 mL per day on a consistent basis. Diabetes insipidus and diabetes mellitus are two causes of polyuria.
Proteinuria	Many forms of protein can be found in urine. Albumin, the most frequently detected protein in urine, is often associated with renal disease. Refer to the chemical and microscopic sections of this text for an in-depth description of proteinuria and its causes.
Pyuria	White blood cells that fight bacterial infections are the main constituents of pus. These white cells are more accurately known as neutrophils or polymorphonuclear leukocytes. Pyuria is most commonly associated with kidney and bladder infections.
Retention	The inability to empty the bladder. The kidneys are producing urine normally, but the bladder cannot be emptied. Bladder-neck obstruction caused by an enlarged prostate or cancer can cause retention.
Urgency	The immediate need to void; an overfilled bladder is one cause of urgency.
Urinary incontinence	The inability to retain urine in the bladder. Mental illness and conditions of paralysis may cause the loss of control over the sphincter muscle that allows voluntary urine elimination, resulting in reflex emptying of the bladder without voluntary control.

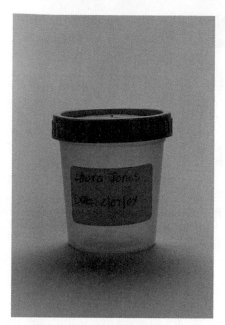

> **Figure 24–4** Urine specimen cup labeled with the patient's name.

by the testing facility when conducting any specimen collection.

In addition, proper labeling of urine specimens is critical to a quality assurance program. Each facility uses a unique patient identification system. Careful attention to specific labeling is important. Some of the more common specimen-identification methods use computerized bar code labels. Whether the specimen is labeled manually or by computer, the medical assistant should note the patient's name, date, and time of collection, and then initial the specimen.

Containers

Three different types of containers are used for collecting urine specimens. Urine cups for single samples can be either sterile (for culturing urine to see if bacteria grow) or nonsterile (for random specimens to conduct general urinalysis). Urine bottles for 24-hour collection are larger and may contain preservatives, such as boric acid or hydrochloric acid. Check the procedure manual to determine which preservative to add before giving the collection bottle to the patient. Figure 24–4 shows the most common type of urine collection container.

Routine or Random Specimen

Random urine specimens can be used for a variety of tests, including urine pregnancy confirmation tests and routine physical screening tests. Random specimens are not recommended when a UTI is suspected.

To collect a random urine sample, the patient should be instructed to void into the specimen cup, filling the cup with approximately 50 to 100 ml of urine. After the specimen is collected, the container must be tightly capped to avoid leaking. If the patient is unable to void, he or she should be instructed to drink water and try to eliminate later, perhaps after the physical examination.

Clean-Catch Midstream Specimen

Collection of clean-catch midstream urine is the method of choice for most health care providers. This type of specimen, if properly collected, provides an excellent sample for most urine tests. A clean-catch midstream specimen can be used for routine urinalysis, urine pregnancy testing, and microscopic examination, as well as for culture and sensitivity testing. It may be helpful to post instructions for clean-catch specimens in appropriate urine collection sites. Procedure 24–1 describes this urine collection method in detail.

First Morning Specimen

When concentration of a urine specimen is a factor, as in pregnancy testing, for example, the first morning sample is the specimen of choice. Formed elements and urine chemicals such as nitrites are best studied in the first morning specimen. Unless the patient is hospitalized, first morning specimens must often be collected by the patient at home. Label the specimen cup with the patient's name and give it to the patient with explicit instructions and any necessary supplies before the patient leaves the office.

The patient should be instructed to deliver the specimen as soon as possible, no more than 4 hours after the urine is collected. If the specimen cannot be transported immediately to the testing facility, it should be refrigerated.

24-Hour Urine Specimen

The 24-hour urine collection can be used for a number of tests. One of the most important factors affecting the specimen collection is determining the specific container in which the specimen will be collected. A laboratory test reference guide should be consulted whenever a 24-hour urine test is ordered. Some 24-hour procedures require the addition of a preservative into the container before the specimen is collected, other tests use no preservative but require that the specimen be refrigerated between voids.

If a preservative is added to the 24-hour specimen container, the container must be labeled as to the type and amount of preservative added. Most tests require that urine specimens be protected from light.

The test may also require that blood samples be drawn from the patient over the period of the urine collection. Patient information such as height, weight, sex, and age may be needed to calculate test results.

PROCEDURE 24-1

Collecting a Clean-Catch Midstream Urine Specimen

Performance Objective: The student can teach a patient the correct procedure to collect a clean-catch midstream urine specimen.

Supplies and Equipment: A sterile urine specimen kit, which should include at least two aseptic cleansing towels and a sterile specimen container.

Procedure Steps

1. Assemble supplies or prepackaged kit.
2. Identify patient.
3. Explain procedure to patient. Tell the patient that you are trying to collect a specimen of urine that is as pure as possible from the middle of the stream of urine.
4. Give the patient the kit or supplies and specific instructions.

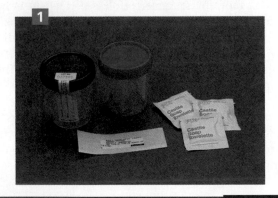

Collection procedure for females
- Wash hands before collecting the urine specimen.
- Loosen the lid of urine container without touching the inside.
- Spread the labia and clean the genital area from front to back using each cleansing towel only once.
- Continue to hold the labia apart and void a small amount into the toilet. Then void into the specimen cup until it is about half full and void any remaining urine into the toilet.
- Replace the cover without touching the inside of the cover or the specimen cup.
- Wash hands after collection is complete.

Collection procedure for males:
- Wash hands before collecting the urine specimen.
- Loosen the lid of urine container without touching the inside.
- Retract the foreskin of the penis (if uncircumcised) and clean the glans using each cleansing towel once.
- Holding the foreskin retracted, void a small amount into the toilet. Then void into the specimen cup until it is about half full and void any remaining urine into the toilet.
- Replace the cover without touching the inside of the cover or the specimen cup.
- Wash hands after collection is complete.

When the specimen is received, the medical assistant may be required to measure and record the volume of the 24-hour sample.

Other factors that must be taken into consideration are specific to the patient. If the patient is female or a physically impaired male, a special collection apparatus must be provided to collect the urine specimen. If a chemical preservative has been added to the collection container the patient should not void directly into the 24-hour collection container but into a collection cup that is then poured into the 24-hour container.

Although many variables affect the 24-hour urine collection, a general guideline may be followed. Again, follow any specific guidelines required by the laboratory in which the specimen will be tested. Procedure 24-2 discusses collecting a 24-hour specimen in detail.

Urine Specimen for Drug Screen

Sometimes a specimen is collected for a drug screen. A urine specimen may be taken after a traffic accident to see if the individual was driving under the influence of alcohol or illegal drugs; as a condition of employment either before being employed or at random times during employment; as part of a drug-treatment program such as methadone maintenance for heroin addiction; or even, in some states, as a condition of high school students being allowed to participate in after-school sports.

In urine specimen collection for drug screens, steps must be taken to preserve the chain of custody of the sample, so that the results cannot be disputed. **Chain of custody** is a legal term meaning that a record has been kept of each person who has been responsible for the sample.

PROCEDURE 24–2

Collecting a 24-Hour Urine Specimen

Performance Objective: The student can teach a patient the correct procedure to collect a 24-hour urine specimen.

Supplies and Equipment: Appropriate collection containers (2) for test ordered, preservative to be added to containers, urinal or toilet inserts for urine collection, a funnel for urine transfer to collection container.

Procedure Steps

1. Consult procedure manual to identify the type of container and amount and type of preservative to add.

2. Add preservative to the containers and label each with the type and amount of preservative.

3. Label containers with the patient's name and other identifying information required by the laboratory.

4. Inform the patient that the test requires all urine to be collected in a 24-hour period for testing.

5. Give the patient the containers and specific instructions both verbally and in writing.
   Rationale: The patient may have questions at home and may need to refer to written instructions.

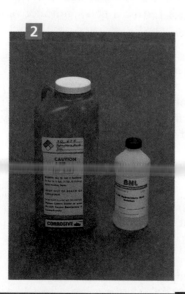

Collection procedure:

• Avoid alcoholic beverages, vitamins, and over-the-counter medications for at least 24 hours before and during specimen collection. Check with the doctor if you have questions about taking medication while the test is in progress.

• The container may contain a chemical to preserve the urine. Do not empty the bottle before starting the test. This chemical might burn your skin, so avoid all contact with it. Keep the container out of the reach of children.

• Keep the collection bottle in a cool place, preferably in the refrigerator.

• Collect the urine on a day that you will be able to collect all urine (each time you void) and bring it to the collection facility promptly when specimen collection is complete.

• It is best to begin this test in the morning. Do not collect the first specimen when you get up. Void the first time that day into the toilet and flush. Note the time and date of this void on the container.

• Collect all urine specimens for the next 24 hours. Collect the specimens in a urinal (males) or toilet insert (females) and pour into the collection bottle using a funnel. Make your final collection when you empty your bladder the first time the next morning (24 hours after the time you wrote on the container). You may need to set your alarm to be sure your last void occurs at the same time of day as you began the collection.

• Do not put anything except urine into the container (such as toilet paper, stool, tampons, etc.).

• Do not dip urine from the toilet bowl because that urine will be diluted with water.

• Call the office if you have questions or concerns. If you miss a void or if you spoil a void with stool, you will need to obtain a new bottle and begin the collection again.

• Return the specimen to the laboratory the morning the test is completed.

When the sample is obtained—either with the patient being observed, or wearing only a gown in the bathroom where clear water is not available (water in the toilet where drug screen samples will be provided should be colored)—the record is begun and initialed by the person who receives the specimen. A seal is placed over the specimen and initialed, so it would be obvious if the specimen were tampered with before testing. As the specimen is passed from person to person, each must inspect the seal and initial the "custody record." This close supervision of the specimen is necessary to ensure that results of drug tests truly represent substances found in the particular specimen.

When maintaining the chain of custody every individual who handles the specimen must physically hand it to the next person who will be responsible for it and sign a log that is maintained about the sample. Medical assistants do not test urine for drugs unless they have additional training, but they may obtain specimens and prepare them for transport.

PHYSICAL PROPERTIES OF URINE

Urine samples are tested for three sets of physical properties: color, clarity, and specific gravity. Abnormal results to any of these examinations can signal illness. Color and clarity are **qualitative tests** (i.e., they determine something about the composition of urine).

Determining Color and Clarity

Normal urine color intensifies with concentration. Urine color classification is based on subjective analysis, meaning the way it looks to the observer. Some laboratories provide a color chart for comparison, but experience and training provide the best judgment of urine color.

The four terms used to describe urine are colorless, straw, yellow, and amber. These colors are illustrated in Figure 24–5. Abnormal urine colors include brown, blue, green, red, pink, and orange, as described in the box "Abnormal Urine Color and Corresponding Conditions."

Fresh, normal urine is usually clear; urine may be cloudy due to illness, because it has been standing, or because it has been refrigerated. The terms used to

Abnormal Urine Color and Corresponding Conditions	
Urine color	**Condition**
Red or pink	Hemoglobin or blood
Green	Bile pigments
Yellow-brown	Bilirubin
Brown-black (standing)	Melanins (from melanoma)
Orange (with bubbles)	Hepatitis
Bright yellow	Carrots
Red-brown	Rhubarb
Red-orange	Pyridium (phenazopyridine)
Pronounced dark yellow	Multivitamins
Brown	Furadantin (nitrofurantoin)
Milky white	Pus or fat droplets
Colorless	Diabetes

Abnormal urine color may indicate a pathological condition. Some drugs and foods may also cause abnormal urine colors. Abnormal urine colors and conditions are as follows:

describe urine clarity are clear, slightly hazy, cloudy, and **turbid** (very cloudy).

Cloudiness in acidic urine is the result of amorphous urates, or phosphates. Cloudiness in a freshly voided urine specimen may be due to blood cells, bacteria, sperm, yeast, mucus, crystals, or **epithelial cells** (skin cells). Figure 24–6 shows turbid urine. Experience and training provide the best judgment of urine clarity.

Although urine odor is not reported on urinalysis test results, it can be a good indicator of disease. Some common aromas associated with urine, and their causes, are:

Ammonia—a UTI or stale urine
Sweet and/or fruity—acetone, possibly ketones due to diabetes
Putrid or foul—a UTI, bacterial growth, or white blood cell decomposition
"Mousy"—PKU (phenylketonuria)
Musty—asparagus
Alcohol, sweet—alcohol ingestion.

When performing urinalysis, the medical assistant should first observe the specimen and record the color and clarity using the terms given above.

Determining Specific Gravity

Specific gravity (SG) defines the concentration of dissolved particles in a specimen. It is expressed in relation to distilled water, which has a value of 1.000,

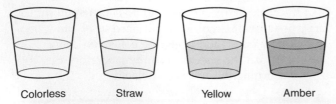

| Colorless | Straw | Yellow | Amber |

> **Figure 24–5** Different colors of normal urine. (From Stepp CA, Woods MA: *Laboratory Procedures for Medical Office Personnel.* Philadelphia: W.B. Saunders, 1998.)

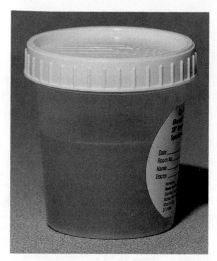

➢ **Figure 24–6** Turbid urine. (From Stepp CA, Woods MA: *Laboratory Procedures for Medical Office Personnel.* Philadephia: W.B. Saunders, 1998.)

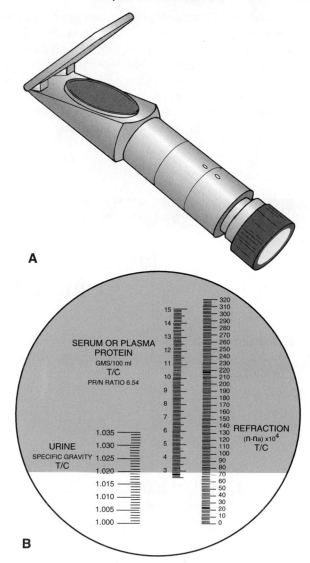

A

B

➢ **Figure 24–8** (A) Refractometer. (B) Refractometer scale as seen through the eyepiece. (From Stepp CA, Woods MA: *Laboratory Procedures for Medical Office Personnel.* Philadelphia: W.B. Saunders, 1998.)

as distilled water is free of **solutes,** substances that dissolve in a solution. The specific gravity of normal urine is between 1.005 and 1.030.

Several methods are used to measure specific gravity. One is to use a **urinometer,** a small glass tube that floats in a container of urine. The specific gravity is read at the meniscus (the bottom of the curve that is formed when the urine is contained in a narrow container).

Urinometers are calibrated and marked to read 1.000 at the meniscus for distilled water at room tem-

perature with a scale that reads up to about 1.040. Although urinometers are rarely used today, because they require at least 1.5 mL of urine and because the instrument is easily broken, they illustrate the principle of measuring specific gravity. The more highly concentrated the urine is, the higher the urinometer floats. The lower the concentration, the lower it floats. Figure 24–7 shows how to read a urinometer.

Another way to measure specific gravity is with a **refractometer,** an instrument that measures the refractive index of a solution. The **refractive index** is a comparison of the velocity of light in air with the velocity of light in a solution, such as urine. The velocity is dependent on the concentration of particles in the urine specimen. The angle at which light passes through the urine is measured and mathematically converts to specific gravity. Figure 24–8 shows a refrac-

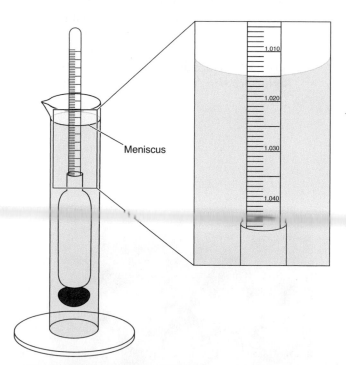

Meniscus

➢ **Figure 24–7** A urinometer is read at the meniscus. The specific gravity of the specimen in this illustration is 1.015.

tometer and an illustration of the scale seen through the eyepiece.

The refractometer only requires one or two drops of urine to generate a reading. The refractometer is also not affected by temperature; however, high concentrations of glucose and protein may falsely elevate the specific gravity readings. Procedure 24–3 discusses in detail measuring urine specific gravity using a refractometer.

The specific gravity of urine is significant because it is a measure of the ability of the kidneys to concentrate the toxins that must be excreted from the body. Urine specific gravity varies with the amount of fluid intake, as well as fluid loss through skin, bowel, and lungs. Increased specific gravity may be found in patients with severe dehydration, adrenal insufficiency, liver disease, diabetes mellitus, and congestive heart failure. Low specific gravity may be found in increased

---

PROCEDURE 24–3

Measuring Urine Specific Gravity Using a Refractometer

Performance Objective: The student will be able to measure the specific gravity of a urine specimen using a refractometer.

☑	Wash hands
☑	Gloves
☐	Eye and Face Protection
☑	Lab Coat or Apron
☑	Plastic Biohazard Bag
☐	Rigid Biohazard Container

Supplies and Equipment: Urine specimen, distilled water, disposable pipette, refractometer, lint-free tissues, distilled water, biohazard waste container.

Procedure Steps

1. Wash hands.
2. Assemble supplies and equipment. The urine should be at room temperature for an accurate reading.
3. Put on disposable gloves.
4. Make sure that the refractometer is clean and free of debris. Use a lint-free tissue to wipe the instrument if necessary, being careful not to scratch the lens.
5. Calibrate the refractometer daily using distilled water using the procedure below. The specific gravity of distilled water should read 1.000. If the boundary line does not fall on 1.000, use a screwdriver supplied by the manufacturer to adjust it.
   Rationale: Alterations in temperature can

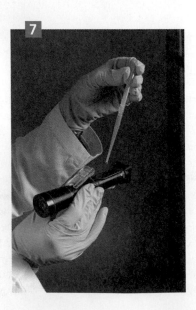

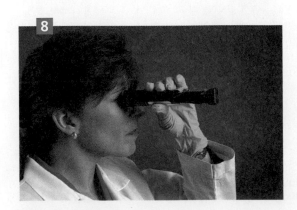

cause small changes in the readings of the refractometer.

6. Be sure that controls have been run for the day. Controls are run (with the same procedure as outlined below) using purchased urine controls with a known specific gravity. Record the values of the controls.
Rationale: Controls with known values are run daily to be sure that laboratory equipment is functioning correctly.

7 Using a disposable pipette, stir the urine to mix it and draw up urine from the urine specimen. Drop one to two drops of urine onto the chamber entrance of the refractometer. Allow the specimen to be drawn into the chamber by capillary action.
Rationale: The drop(s) of urine will spread across the chamber of the prism to create a reading.

8 Hold the refractometer to a light source. The specific gravity urine scale will be visible. Read the specific gravity from the urine scale at the boundary between the light area and the dark area.
Rationale: The reading is made by light reflected from the prism within the refractometer.

9. Clean the prism by dropping a few drops of distilled water on it and wiping with a lint-free tissue.

10. Discard the remainder of the urine specimen (unless needed for further testing) and used supplies in a biohazard waste container. Remove gloves and discard in the biohazard container.

11. Wash hands.

12. Document results, including date, time, and the specific gravity reading.

Charting Example	
Date	
8/2/XX	2:35 PM Urine SG 1.014 ————
	———————— C. Martin, CMA

fluid intake, as well as in individuals with chronic renal insufficiency, diabetes insipidus, and malignant hypertension. Specific gravity is also measured on some reagent strips.

CHEMICAL PROPERTIES OF URINE

Chemical analysis of urine can provide valuable insights into disease pathology. Many chemical tests are available; however, the urine dipstick is the most common testing method used in medical offices.

Reagent strips, better known as dipsticks, are strips that are impregnated with various chemicals or reagents that react to urine components. They are used to detect chemicals in urine. Most tests on the reagent strips are **quantitative tests** (i.e., they determine how much of a substance is present in the urine). Each test is based on a semi-quantitative color change that is easy to interpret. Urine dipsticks may be read manually or may be placed in an automated analyzer. Strips that perform from 1 to 10 individual chemical tests are available from different manufacturers. Figure 24–9 shows a semi-automated urine analyzer.

Quality Assurance/Quality Control

The expiration date and lot number of each urine reagent vial should be checked before use. Initial and date each newly opened bottle. Vials must remain tightly closed until testing is performed, and must be closed immediately after dipsticks are removed because light can affect the pads. Do not remove the desiccant (a substance that absorbs water) from vials. Vials should be stored according to the manufacturer's instructions.

To verify reagent strip performance, a quality-control program utilizing normal and high-abnormal urine external controls should be performed at the beginning of each laboratory shift, before any patient testing, when the vial lot number changes, or if reagent strips appear changed on some way.

Urine specimens should be analyzed as soon as possible after collection. If analysis is delayed, specimens should be protected from light and refrigerated. Specimens should be free of preservatives.

Urine Reagent Strip Test Reactions

Following are a number of reagent strip test reactions and the significance of each.

Blood

Reaction. Erythrocytes (red blood cells) and free hemoglobin from cells that have been broken down contain a chemical that catalyzes the oxidation of chemical compounds to produce a color change. **Oxidation** is a chemical reaction in which a compound unites with oxygen, forming a new compound.

Small, dotlike color changes on the reagent pads occur when only a few red blood cells are present.

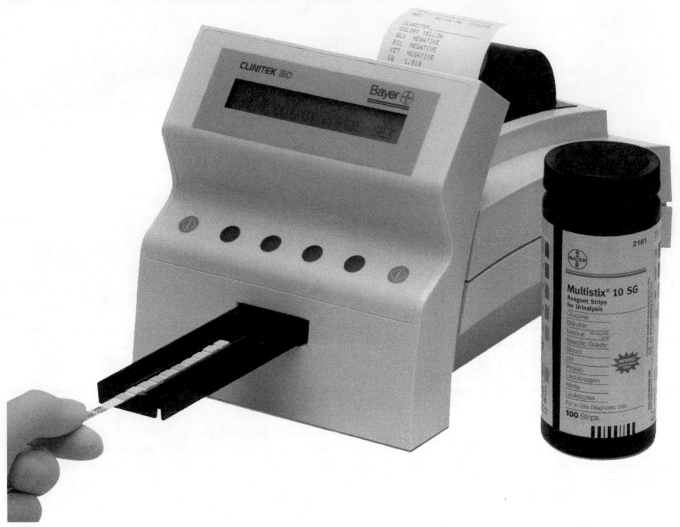

> **Figure 24–9** Clinitek 50 urine chemistry analyzer, a semi-automated instrument designed to read the reagent strip. (Courtesy Diagnostic Division, Bayer Corporation, Tarrytown, NY.)

Free hemoglobin or myoglobin may produce a color change to the entire test pad.

To confirm the presence of intact red blood cells when large amounts of blood are present, a microscopic examination must be performed.

Significance. Blood found in urine indicates bleeding into some part of the urinary tract. Blood in urine may be caused by trauma, UTIs, or renal disease. Free hemoglobin is due to destruction of red blood cells; the presence of free hemoglobin may be due to auto-immune disease, drug reaction, or a blood transfusion reaction.

False Positives. May be caused by menstrual blood, bleach or other oxidizing compounds, or peroxidase produced by microbes.

False Negatives. May be caused by formalin, excess nitrites, elevated specific gravity, or particular drugs such as captopril.

Leukocytes

Reaction. If white blood cells (WBCs) are present, a chemical reaction occurs that causes the pad to change from off-white to varying shades of purple.

Significance. The most common cause of elevated WBCs in urine is UTIs. Infection of the kidney, bladder, or urethra can introduce WBCs, or pus, into the urinary tract. Leukocyte esterase is only found in the WBCs known as granulocytes. Neutrophils, a type of granulocyte found commonly in bacterial reactions, produces leukocyte esterase in the greatest amounts. Other WBCs such as monocytes and lymphocytes will not produce a positive reaction. It is not normal to have enough WBCs in the urine to cause a positive leukocyte esterase reaction.

False Positives. May be caused by vaginal contaminants.

False Negatives. May be caused by drugs such as tetracycline, gentamycin, or cephalexin. Elevated glucose, high specific gravity, or oxalic acid can interfere with the chemical reaction, even if WBCs are present in the urine.

Nitrites

Reaction. In an acid pH, nitrite reacts with chemicals to produce pink color of varying intensity.

Significance. The presence of **nitrites** (compounds containing nitrogen) in fresh urine indicates bacterial growth.

Enteric bacteria are believed to establish themselves in the perineal and genital areas as a result of imperfect cleaning after bowel movements, sexual activity, or fecal incontinence. The closeness of the external anatomic surfaces of the intestinal and urinary tract in females, combined with the short urethra, may explain the increased incidence of UTIs in women versus men.

False Positives. May be caused by bacterial growth in an "old" urine specimen or a specimen placed in a container found around the house.

False Negatives. May be caused by urine that is abnormal in color.

Protein

Reaction. Colors range from yellow for negative to green or blue for positive.

Significance. Protein in the urine can be the first indication of renal disease. Small amounts of protein can be associated with physical or emotional stress, or the early stages of renal disease. Small to moderate amounts can indicate a UTI, kidney stones, or acute renal disorder. Large amounts are found in advanced renal disease such as nephrotic syndrome and chronic glomerulonephritis.

False Positives. May be caused by some drugs, as well as by contaminants such as bleach or alkaline urine with a high pH level.

False Negatives. May be caused by high salt levels in the urine. The reagents are more sensitive to albumins, so if other proteins, such as globulins, are present, the result may be falsely negative.

Glucose

Reaction. Reagent strips are specific for the presence of glucose. The color intensity is proportional to the glucose concentration.

Significance. The most common cause of glycosuria is diabetes mellitus. Rarely, a low renal threshold to glucose, associated with hypoglycemia or normal blood sugar levels, can cause a positive urine glucose.

False Positives. This test is specific for glucose, meaning no other compounds cause a positive result.

False Negatives. May be caused by an excess of ascorbic acid, elevated specific gravity, or a high level of ketones.

Ketones

Reaction. The presence of ketones produces a pink or purple color.

Significance. **Ketones** are the products of incomplete fatty acid metabolism and occur when glucose is limited. Elevated urine ketones may be found in conditions of starvation or when severe vomiting, diarrhea, or pregnancy are present. Ketoacidosis is a condition of prolonged elevated blood glucose in diabetes mellitus and may be associated with diabetic coma.

False Positives. May occur because of highly pigmented urine or certain dyes.

False Negatives. May occur if bacteria are present in the urine and the specimen is not tested immediately. Ketones are lost at room temperature and will dissipate if not kept in a closed container.

Bilirubin

Reaction. If bilirubin is present the pad turns tannish purple.

Significance. The presence of bilirubin in urine suggests liver disease such as infectious hepatitis, liver sclerosis, or obstructive jaundice. **Bilirubin** is a breakdown product of hemoglobin.

False Positives. May be caused by intensely colored urine or certain drugs.

False Negatives. May be caused by excess ascorbic acid and large amounts of nitrite. Light exposure will also decrease levels of bilirubin; urine samples should be protected from light if immediate analysis cannot be performed.

Urobilinogen

Reaction. If urobilinogen is present, the pad turns pink or red.

Significance. Normally, bilirubin is converted to **urobilinogen** by bacteria and excreted in the feces and urine. Elevated urobilinogen may occur in hepatitis and conditions involving excessive breakdown of red blood cells. Lower than expected values can be found in obstructive jaundice.

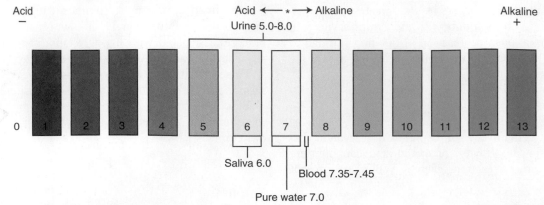

> **Figure 24–10** pH scale. (From Stepp CA, Woods MA: *Laboratory Procedures for Medical Office Personnel.* Philadelphia: W.B. Saunders, 1998.)

pH

Reaction. The colors range from orange through yellow and green to blue.

Significance. The acidity or alkalinity of urine is referred to as **pH,** or parts hydrogen. The average pH of normal urine is 6.0, or slightly acidic. The natural acidity of urine is an inhibitor to microbial growth. The pH of urine provides an indication of the kidneys' ability to maintain normal hydrogen ion concentration and may vary with an individual's diet. An acid urine may be seen with a diet high in meat protein; an alkaline urine may be produced by a diet high in certain fruits and vegetables.

Very alkaline urine, with a high pH, may indicate bacterial growth. Urine pH values ranging from 4.0 to 8.5 are represented by various colors on the reagent strip.

If runover of urine from another reagent strip occurs, a false color change can cause a misinterpretation of the pH test. Chemical additives or contaminants may also cause a false pH level.

Figure 24–10 shows the pH scale.

Specific Gravity

A test of specific gravity is included in many reagent strips. A refractometer may be used to confirm the reagent strip test.

False High Specific Gravity may be caused by glycosuria or proteinuria, because of the increased concentration.

False Low Specific Gravity is caused by highly alkaline urine.

PROCEDURE 24–4

Chemical Testing of Urine Using Reagent Strip Method

Performance Objective: The student will be able to perform a urinalysis using the reagent strip method.

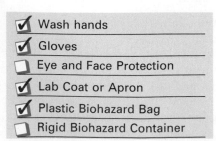

☑ Wash hands
☑ Gloves
☐ Eye and Face Protection
☑ Lab Coat or Apron
☑ Plastic Biohazard Bag
☐ Rigid Biohazard Container

Supplies and Equipment: Disposable gloves; vial of urine reagent dipsticks (e.g., Multistix 10 or Chemstix); clean, dry gauze pads; timer that measures seconds and minutes; fresh, well-mixed urine specimen, biohazard waste container.

Procedure Steps

1. Wash hands.
2. Assemble supplies and equipment.
3. Put on disposable gloves.
4. Be sure that controls have been run that day

for the bottle of reagent strips you will use.
Rationale: Running controls exposes the reagent strips to a solution whose values are known. If running controls produces unexpected results, discard the bottle of reagent strips.

5. Open a bottle of urine reagent strips and remove a reagent strip. Immediately close the vial.
Rationale: The vial is kept closed to prevent light and moisture from causing alteration in the unused reagent strips.

6 Quickly dip the urine strip into the urine sample, ensuring that the strip is completely immersed in the urine sample. Remove the strip and hold in a horizontal position so that urine does not run from one test pad to another.
Rationale: All test pads on the reagent strip must be saturated with urine. If chemicals from one test pad are carried onto another pad, the results may be inaccurate.

7. Blot the strip sideways onto clean gauze, being careful not to touch the reagent test pads onto the gauze.

Rationale: This helps remove excess urine and prevents runover.

8. Begin timing the procedure.

9. Read each urine chemical result at the appropriate time indicated by the reagent strip manufacturer.
Rationale: Each test takes a specific amount of time and must be read within time limits specified by the manufacturer for accuracy.

10 Match the color of each test pad on the strip to the color chart on the back of the reagent strip bottle. Make a mental note of each abnormal test.
Rationale: The results of each test are based on possible color changes.

11. Dispose of the reagent strip, used supplies, and the specimen (unless further tests are needed) in a biohazard waste container. Remove gloves and discard in the biohazard waste container.

12. Wash hands.

13. Record results in the patient's medical record. Note the date, time, brand name of reagent strips, color and clarity of the sample, and the results of each test.

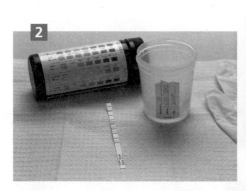

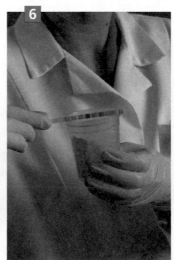

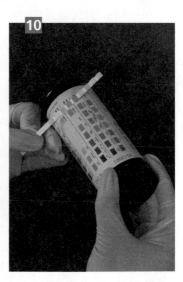

Procedure 24–4 describes in detail how to test urine using reagent strips. Machines are available to analyze reagent strips automatically. The strip is dipped in urine, held level, and inserted into the machine, eliminating the need to time the reading for each pad.

Confirmatory Testing

Other tests are available to confirm the results of the reagent strip tests. These are:

Clinitest (to determine the presence of other sugars besides glucose)
Acetest (ketones)
Ictotest (bilirubin).

Clinitest

Clinitest is the quantitative method used to determine the presence of sugars other than glucose. Be-

PROCEDURE 24-5

Urine Testing Using the Clinitest 5-Drop Method

Performance Objective: The student will be able to test urine for sugars using the Clinitest 5-drop method.

- ☑ Wash hands
- ☑ Gloves
- ☐ Eye and Face Protection
- ☑ Lab Coat or Apron
- ☑ Plastic Biohazard Bag
- ☐ Rigid Biohazard Container

Supplies and Equipment: Disposable gloves, a freshly voided urine specimen, a Clinitest kit that contains a thick glass test tube, dropper, and holding rack, bottle of Clinitest tablets, distilled water, clean pair of thumb forceps, timer that measures seconds and minutes, biohazard waste container.

Procedure Steps

1. Wash hands.
2. Assemble supplies and equipment. Place the test tube in the rack. Do not hold the test tube in your hands while performing this test. Do not place face close to the test tube during the reaction.
   Rationale: The test tube will become hot during the chemical reaction and the contents of the tube may bubble and even spill out.
3. Put on disposable gloves.
4. Using the dropper from the kit, place 5 drops of urine into test tube. Rinse dropper with distilled water.
   Rationale: The dropper is rinsed to remove urine before measuring water.
5. Add 10 drops of distilled water to test tube.
6. Using forceps to pick up Clinitest tablet, drop tablet into test tube. Do not handle tablet with hands.
   Rationale: Any water adhering to the gloves may start the chemical reaction and cause a burn.
7. The mixture will begin to boil and produce heat. Do not shake the test tube during boil-

ing or for 15 seconds after boiling has stopped.
   Rationale: Shaking the test tube could cause the contents to rise out of the tube. The test tube will become hot and should not be handled until the reaction has stopped.
8. At the end of the 15-second period, shake test tube gently to mix contents.
9. Compare color of liquid to the color chart provided by the manufacturer. Record the percent result that most closely matches the color chart. Ignore any color changes that occur after the 15-second time period.
   Rationale: The results are accurate after 15 seconds, but later changes may be inaccurate.
10. Discard contents of the test tube and rinse with water. Discard other supplies and urine specimen (if not needed for other tests) in a biohazard waste container. Remove gloves and discard in a biohazard waste container.
11. Wash hands.
12. Record date, time, and results in the patient's medical record.

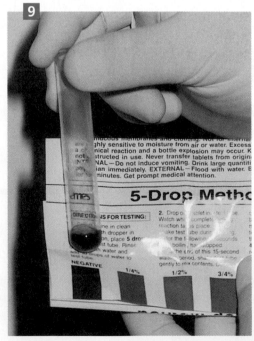

*Photograph from Stepp CA, Woods MA: *Laboratory Procedures for Medical Office Personnel.* Philadelphia: W.B. Saunders, 1988.

cause reagent dipsticks are specific for the presence of glucose only, Clinitest may be used to detect the presence of elevated amounts of other sugars, such as galactose, which is elevated in malabsorption; fructose; lactose; and pentoses. Non-sugar reducing substances, such as creatinine and uric acid, will also yield a positive Clinitest result.

Reaction and Interpretation. When the Clinitest tablet is placed in urine, a color change occurs, ranging from blue through green to orange, if sugar is present. A blue color is negative.

Interfering Substances. A number of drugs interfere with Clinitest when they appear in high concentrations. The presence of x-ray contrast media may produce false negatives. High levels of protein may extend reaction time.

QA/QC. To ensure test results, the Clinitest bottle should remain tightly capped and protected from light when not in use. Do not touch the contents with hands or allow moisture to enter the vial because the Clinitest tablets deteriorate rapidly with moisture or heat. A desiccant is provided to prevent moisture from contaminating tablets and should not be removed.

Check the expiration date, and initial and label a newly opened bottle. Store bottles according to manufacturer's instructions. Perform external urine tests using normal and high abnormal controls before patient testing.

Procedure 24–5 discusses using the Clinitest 5-drop method in detail.

Acetest

The Acetest is the confirmatory test for the presence of ketones. It is a semi-quantitative method used to determine ketones in urine, serum, plasma, and whole blood specimens.

Ketones are produced by fatty acid metabolism in conditions such as diabetes mellitus and starvation.

Reaction and Interpretation. If ketones are present in the urine, the color of the tablet will change. The color change becomes more intense as ketone concentration increases. A purple color indicates a positive result; no color change is a negative result.

QA/QC. Check the bottle for expiration date. Date and initial newly opened bottles. Acetest tablets must not come into contact with moisture. Recap the bottle immediately after tablets are removed. Do not store bottle in direct light. Tablets will darken when reagent reactivity has been altered.

Perform external urine tests using normal and high abnormal controls before patient testing.

Procedure 24–6 discusses in detail urine testing using the Acetest method.

PROCEDURE 24–6

Urine Testing Using Acetest Method

Performance Objective: The student will be able to perform urine testing using the Acetest method.

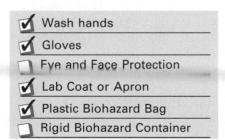

☑ Wash hands
☑ Gloves
☐ Eye and Face Protection
☑ Lab Coat or Apron
☑ Plastic Biohazard Bag
☐ Rigid Biohazard Container

Supplies and Equipment: Disposable gloves, a freshly voided urine specimen, a bottle of Acetest tablets, clean white test paper, clean pair of thumb forceps, dropper, timer that measures seconds and minutes, biohazard waste container.

Procedure Steps

1. Wash hands.
2. Assemble supplies and equipment. Place the clean white test paper on the table.
3. Put on disposable gloves.
4. Remove one tablet from the bottle using forceps and place on the test paper. Recap bottle immediately.
   Rationale: You should not touch the tablet with your hands to avoid chemical contamination. The vial is kept closed to prevent light or moisture from causing alteration in unused tablets.
5. Using the dropper, place one drop of urine directly on top of the tablet.
6. Compare the color of the tablet to the color chart provided by manufacturer at 30 seconds after application of specimen.

Procedure continued on following page

PROCEDURE 24-6 (continued)

Rationale: Color changes caused by ketones in the urine will have occured at 30 seconds after the drop of urine is applied to the tablet.

7. Discard tablet, test paper, and urine specimen (if not needed for further testing) in a biohaz-ard waste container. Remove gloves and dis-card in a biohazard waste container.

8. Wash hands.

9. Record date, time, and results in the patient's medical record.

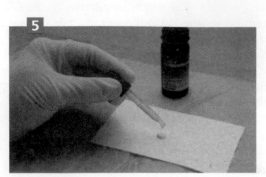
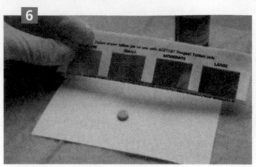

*Photographs from Zakus SM: *Clinical Procedures for Medical Assistants,* 4th ed. St. Louis: C.V. Mosby, 1995.

Ictotest

Ictotest is the confirmatory test for the presence of bilirubin in urine. Urine bilirubin is an important find-ing in evaluation of liver disease.

Reaction and Interpretation. A color change occurs if bilirubin is present. A blue to purple color is inter-preted as positive; no color change or a tan, pink, or red color is negative.

Interfering Substances. Large amounts of certain drugs may cause a false-positive reaction, and speci-mens exposed to light may exhibit decreased levels of bilirubin.

QA/QC. Do not store the bottle in direct sunlight. Keep the bottle and test pads free from moisture. Re-cap the bottle tightly when tablets are removed. Deteri-oration of tablets can be detected by tan to brown discoloration. Perform external urine tests using normal and high abnormal controls before patient testing.

Procedure 24-7 discusses in detail urine testing us-ing the Ictotest method.

Preparing a Urine Specimen for Microscopic Examination

A microscopic examination of urine may be re-quested as part of a urinalysis or may be required due to abnormal reagent chemical test results. Abnormal chemical test results that would initiate a microscopic exam include positive readings for blood, leukocyte esterase, protein, or nitrite.

A fresh urine specimen is the best sample for micro-scopic examination. Urine samples that are not to be analyzed immediately after collection should be pro-tected from light and refrigerated at 4° to 60° C for up to 8 hours before analysis.

Microscopic examination of urine is not a waived test under CLIA 88. It may be done by the doctor if the laboratory has a certificate of PPM procedures or in a laboratory that has a certificate of compliance. There-fore, many medical offices send this type of urinalysis to a larger laboratory, or a medical assistant may set up the slide for the doctor to examine.

QA/QC. Urine samples that are allowed to sit at room temperature and become stale undergo changes that can result in misinterpretation during the micro-scopic exam. Bacterial growth increases and cellular components degenerate. A salting out of minerals con-tained in urine occurs, making microscopic examina-tion difficult.

Urine centrifuge tubes must be filled with 12 ml of urine to provide a consistent interpretation of sediment elements. Tubes filled with less than 12 ml of urine should be noted on the patient report. After the centri-fuge is balanced, the urine is centrifuged for 5 minutes at 1500 RPM. To prepare the slide, the liquid portion of the urine is poured off and a drop of the remaining sediment is placed on a slide with a pipette for exami-nation under the microscope.

Procedure 24-8 discusses in detail preparing urine for microscopic examination.

Components of Urine Sediment

Components of urine sediment may be normal or abnormal, depending on the number or amount in the sample. Proper training is essential to identify and enu-merate urine sediment elements. Normally, a medical

PROCEDURE 24−7

Urine Testing Using Ictotest Method

Performance Objective: The student will be able to perform urine testing using the Ictotest procedure.

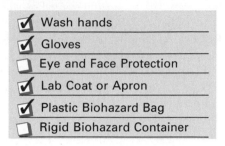

☑ Wash hands
☑ Gloves
☐ Eye and Face Protection
☑ Lab Coat or Apron
☑ Plastic Biohazard Bag
☐ Rigid Biohazard Container

Supplies and Equipment: Disposable gloves, a freshly voided urine specimen (or one that has been protected from light and is no more than 8 hours old), an Ictotest kit including tablets and test pads, distilled water, clean paper towel, clean pair of thumb forceps, dropper, timer that measures seconds and minutes, biohazard waste container.

Procedure Steps

1. Wash hands.
2. Assemble supplies and equipment. Place the clean white test paper on the table.
3. Put on disposable gloves.
4. Place a square of the absorbent test mat from the kit on a clean paper towel.
5. Using the dropper, drop 10 drops of urine onto the center of the test mat.
6. Remove one tablet from the bottle using forceps and place on the test paper. Recap bottle immediately.
   Rationale: You should not touch the tablet or the test mat with your hands to avoid chemical contamination. The vial is kept tightly closed to prevent light or moisture from causing alteration in unused tablets.
7. Place 1 drop of water onto the tablet.
8. Wait 5 seconds, and then place a second drop of water onto tablet, so that water runs off tablet and onto the mat.
9. Observe color of the mat around the tablet after 60 seconds. A blue to purple color is a positive result. A tan color, red, or pink is a negative result.
   Rationale: Color changes caused by bilirubin in the urine will have occurred at 60 seconds after the drop of urine is applied to the tablet.
10. Discard tablet, test mat, paper towel, and urine specimen (if not needed for further testing) in a biohazard waste container. Remove gloves and discard in a biohazard waste container.
11. Wash hands.
12. Record date, time, and results in the patient's medical record.

---

assistant is not qualified to report out microscopic results without additional training. The following information is given to help the medical assistant understand the types of elements seen in microscopic examination.

Components are divided into two classifications, organized and unorganized.

Organized

Organized components are red blood cells (RBCs), white blood cells (WBCs), epithelial cells, casts (hyaline, granular, cellular), bacteria, fungi, yeast, parasites, and spermatozoa, as shown in Figures 24−11 through 24−15.

Red Blood Cells. A large number of RBCs in the urine is known as hematuria and is indicative of trauma or renal disease. They may also appear in a specimen from a woman who is menstruating. Red blood cells appear under high magnification as pale, light-reflecting disks, with no nucleus. Red blood cells are counted by sight in a high-powered field (**HPF**) and reported as number per HPF. The normal value is 0 to 3/HPF.

White Blood Cells. More than 0.3 WBCs per HPF in urine indicates a UTI. White blood cells are larger than RBCs, and contain a nucleus. They are counted and reported in the same way as RBCs.

Epithelial Cells. Presence of a large number of renal epithelial cells indicates kidney disease.

Casts. Casts form when protein accumulates in the kidney tubules and is then deposited in the urine as it passes through the tubules. Presence of casts in urine

PROCEDURE 24–8

Preparing Urine for Microscopic Examination

Performance Objective: The student will prepare a urine specimen for microscopic examination.

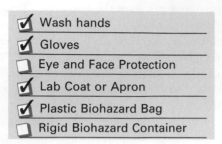

- ☑ Wash hands
- ☑ Gloves
- ☐ Eye and Face Protection
- ☑ Lab Coat or Apron
- ☑ Plastic Biohazard Bag
- ☐ Rigid Biohazard Container

Supplies and Equipment: Disposable gloves, at least 15 mL of fresh, well-mixed urine, plastic urine centrifuge tubes with caps (e.g., Kova tubes), disposable transfer pipette (e.g., Kova pipette), test tube rack, urine centrifuge, plain glass slides and cover slips or commercially available urine plastic slides, brightfield binocular compound microscope with 10X and 40X power objectives, biohazard waste container.

Procedure Steps

1. Wash hands.
2. Assemble supplies and equipment.
3. Put on disposable gloves.
4. Mix the urine specimen with the transfer pipette.
5. Place a centrifuge tube in the test tube rack and pour in 12 mL of urine.
6. Place a cap on the tube and place in the centrifuge.
7. Balance the centrifuge by placing another centrifuge tube filled with 12 mL of water directly opposite in the centrifuge.
   Rationale: The load in the centrifuge must be balanced for the machine to operate correctly.
8. Centrifuge at 1500 revolutions per minute (RPM) for 5 minutes.

Rationale: Spinning the urine specimen in the centrifuge forces heavier elements (sediment) to the bottom of the tube.

9. Remove urine tube from centrifuge. Do not shake tube.
10. Remove the cap from the tube and, using a plastic transfer pipette, remove the clear liquid (supernatant) from the top of the tube, leaving 0.5 to 1.0 mL of urine on top of the sediment. Discard supernatant.
    Rationale: The sediment is concentrated in a small amount of urine so that elements can be seen under the microscope.
11. Resuspend sediment by gently flicking the bottom of the urine tube. A urine stain may be added at this point (consult stain directions for use).
    Rationale: A urine stain such as Kova stain enhances the sediment for better visualization.
12. Draw up urine into the pipette and place one drop of urine mixture onto a glass slide. Add coverslip, being careful not to introduce bubbles. OR Place a drop of urine into commercial urine slide counting chamber.
13. Place slide onto the center of the microscope stage.
14. Prepare the microscope by turning on the light, closing the diaphragm, and keeping the rheostat at a low setting. Rotate the nosepiece until the low-power objective (10X) clicks into place. Use the coarse adjustment to bring the slide into coarse focus.
15. Inform the doctor or lab technician that the specimen is ready for examination.
16. After the doctor has completed the microscopic examination recap the centrifuge tube and discard with the slide and pipette in a biohazard waste container. Remove gloves and discard in a biohazard waste container.
17. Wash hands.

---

usually indicates kidney disease. Casts appear cylindrical, with either a round or a flat end. They take experience and expertise to recognize.

The most common cast is the hyaline cast, which may appear in normal urine and may not imply renal disease. Hyaline casts can simply signal fever, stress, or

that the individual has recently engaged in high-intensity exercise.

Cellular casts contain either RBCs, WBCs, or renal epithelial cells. Granular casts contain the remnants of disintegrated RBCs, WBCs, or epithelial cells and appear as granules. The presence of cellular inclusions

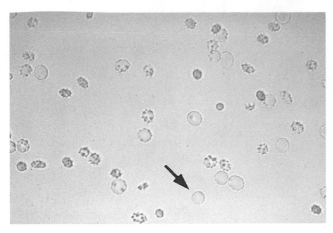

> ➣ **Figure 24–11** Red blood cells in urine. (From Stepp CA, Woods MA: *Laboratory Procedures for Medical Office Personnel.* Philadelphia: W.B. Saunders, 1998.)

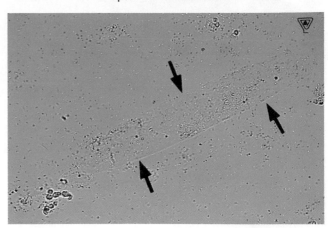

> ➣ **Figure 24–13** Hyaline casts in urine. (From Stepp CA, Woods MA: *Laboratory Procedures for Medical Office Personnel.* Philadelphia: W.B. Saunders, 1998.)

provides valuable information regarding the disease process. For example, red blood cell casts are indicative of glomerular disease.

Bacteria. Bacteria can appear round, rod-shaped, or amorphous, meaning without real shape. Bacteria in urine are reported as few, moderate, many, or loaded. An alternate reporting system designates the number of bacteria as 1+, 2+, or 3+.

Yeast. When present in large numbers, yeast cells, which are smaller than RBCs or WBCs, indicate a yeast infection in the urinary tract. Yeasts often appear to be "budding." If there is confusion between possible yeast and RBCs, a drop of dilute acetic acid added to the specimen will cause the RBCs to lyse while the yeast cells will not.

Parasites. Parasites present under a microscope with more motion than other organic cells. The most com-

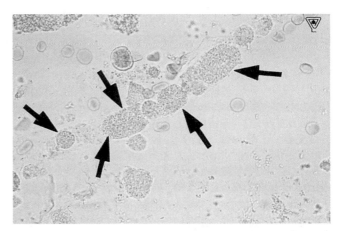

> ➣ **Figure 24–14** Granular casts in urine. (From Stepp CA, Woods MA: *Laboratory Procedures for Medical Office Personnel.* Philadelphia: W.B. Saunders, 1998.)

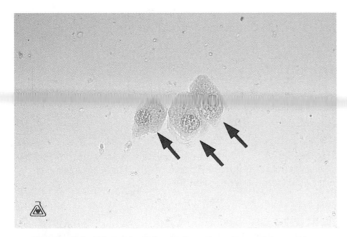

> ➣ **Figure 24–12** Epithelial cells in urine. (From Stepp CA, Woods MA: *Laboratory Procedures for Medical Office Personnel.* Philadelphia: W.B. Saunders, 1998.)

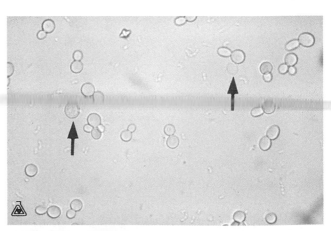

> ➣ **Figure 24–15** Fungus (yeast) in urine. (From Stepp CA, Woods MA: *Laboratory Procedures for Medical Office Personnel.* Philadelphia: W.B. Saunders, 1998.)

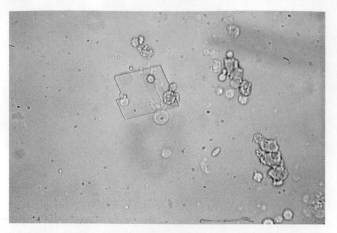

> **Figure 24–16** Cholesterol crystals in urine. (From Stepp CA, Woods MA: *Laboratory Procedures for Medical Office Personnel.* Philadelphia: W.B. Saunders, 1998.)

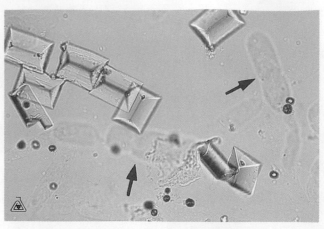

> **Figure 24–18** Triple phosphate crystals in urine. (From Stepp CA, Woods MA: *Laboratory Procedures for Medical Office Personnel.* Philadelphia: W.B. Saunders, 1998.)

mon parasite in the urinary tract is *Trichomonas vaginalis*, which can be recognized by its tail, or flagella. A doctor should always conduct a microscopic exam if parasites are suspected.

Spermatozoa. Sperm cells have oval bodies and long, thin tails. Sperm is only reported in male urine samples, unless specifically requested by a doctor for a female urine sample.

Unorganized

Unorganized components include **crystals** and other chemical elements with no regular shape, as shown in Figures 24–16 through 24–18.

Although crystals are large, they are mostly insignificant artifacts. A few, however, such as cystine, uric acid, and sulfa drug crystals, can be clues to disease.

Table 24–2 shows urine sediment elements.

Reporting Results

The most common components of the routine urinalysis a medical assistant is responsible for are the physical and chemical examinations. Most reference laboratories have a urinalysis report form similar in appearance to the one shown in Figure 24–19. The chemical components analyzed are reported out as negative, trace, small, or using plus signs (1+, 2+, 3+).

The key to quality urinalysis reporting is to be consistent. The laboratory should have a urinalysis procedure manual that indicates proper reporting techniques and terminology. If you are uncertain, ask your supervisor.

All laboratory reports must have documentation as to the date, time of completion, and initials of the technician who performed the test. Results must then be charted on the patient's chart, under the laboratory report section.

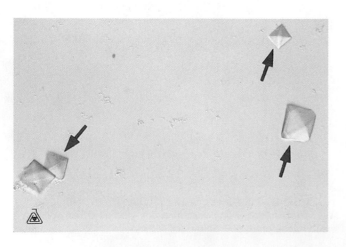

> **Figure 24–17** Calcium oxalate crystals in urine. (From Stepp CA, Woods MA: *Laboratory Procedures for Medical Office Personnel.* Philadelphia: W.B. Saunders, 1998.)

Table 24–2	**Components of Urine Sediment**

Cells: Type	Normal Values	Possible Reasons for Abnormal Increase
Red blood cells (RBCs)	0–3 cells per high power field	■ Trauma to the urinary tract ■ Menstruation (especially in a random specimen) ■ Kidney or bladder stones ■ Bleeding diseases and use of anticoagulants ■ Kidney diseases
White blood cells (WBCs)	0–3 cells per high power field	■ Urinary tract infection or infection of any part of the genitourinary system ■ Transplant rejection ■ Inflammation of the urethra or bladder
Epithelial cells	Squamous epithelial cells or transitional epithelial cells may be present in moderate amounts Renal epithelial cells may be present in small amounts	■ Vaginal contamination ■ Catheterization ■ Increased in kidney diseases

Casts: Type	Appearance	Possible Reasons
Hyaline casts	Colorless, transparent	■ Strenuous exercise ■ Kidney disease ■ Malignant hypertension
Cellular casts	RBCs, WBCs, epithelial cells seen in a hyaline matrix	■ Kidney disease ■ Collagen diseases ■ Vascular disease
Granular casts	Opaque granules seen in a matrix	■ Proteinuria ■ Acute or chronic renal disease
Other casts; include waxy casts, fatty casts, broad casts, and mixed casts	Seen as irregular or globular outlines, alone or in combination	■ Kidney disease ■ Fatty casts seen in some types of poisoning

Crystals: Type	Type of Urine	Possible Reasons
Amorphous urate Uric acid Calcium oxalate	Normal acid urine	■ Usually nonpathologic
Amorphous phosphate Triple phosphate Ammonium biurate Calcium phosphate Calcium carbonate	Normal alkaline urine	■ Usually nonpathologic
Tyrosine Leucine Cystine Hippuric acid Bilirubin Cholesterol Creatine	Abnormal urine	■ Liver disease ■ Liver disease ■ Cystinuria ■ Usually nonpathologic ■ Bilirubinuria ■ Bladder or kidney disease ■ Destruction of muscle tissue or ingestion of salicylates

URINALYSIS

Specimen Type: Urine-Clean Catch
Collected: 10/24/99

Pt. Number: 1127864
Physician: J. Hughes, MD

Test	Result	Reference Range
Color	YELLOW	
Character	HAZY	Clear
Specific Gravity	1.015	1.001 - 1.035
pH	6.0	4.6 - 8.0
Protein	++	NEG
Glucose	NEG	NEG
Ketone	NEG	NEG
Bilirubin	NEG	NEG
Blood	Trace	NEG
Nitrite	Positive	NEG
Leukocytes	Small	NEG

MICROSCOPIC URINALYSIS

RBC	None
WBC	10 - 20/hfp
Squamous Epithelial	10 - 15/hfp
Bacteria	1 +/hfp
Casts	None
Crystals	None

➤ **Figure 24–19** Laboratory report: urinalysis.

STUDENT STUDY PLAN

To reinforce your understanding of the material in this chapter . . .

Complete · *Complete* the **Review & Recall** questions.

Discuss · *Discuss* the situation in **If You Were the Medical Assistant** with your classmates, and answer the questions.

Answer · *Answer* the **Critical Thinking Questions,** and discuss them with your classmates.

Visit · *Visit* suggested **Web sites** and search for additional Web sites using the **Keywords for Internet Searches.**

Complete · *Complete* the exercises in chapter 24 of the **Student Mastery Manual.**

REVIEW & RECALL

1. Describe how urine is produced in the kidney.

2. Differentiate between a random urine specimen, a first morning urine specimen, a clean-catch midstream specimen, and a 24-hour urine specimen, in respect to how each is collected and the tests that might be performed on each.

3. What quality control methods are used when performing urinalysis?

4. Describe the three components of the physical examination of urine.

5. Describe 10 tests that may be part of a urinalysis using the reagent strip method, and correlate to reasons for possible abnormal findings.

6. Identify three additional urine tests that may be done to confirm the findings of the urinalysis using the reagent strip method.

7. What additional information may be obtained from a microscopic examination of urine?

8. What is the medical assistant's role related to the microscopic examination of urine?

9. Give several examples of organized and unorganized components of urine sediment.

10. Describe how to centrifuge urine to prepare for the microscopic examination.

 ## IF YOU WERE THE MEDICAL ASSISTANT

It is possible that some doctors' offices do not perform daily controls for urinalysis using the reagent strip method. What supplies are needed to perform controls? What arguments would you make to the clinical supervisor as reasons to begin a system of performing and documenting controls?

 ## CRITICAL THINKING QUESTIONS

1. Why does the composition of urine vary between different people and at different times in the same individual? Give at least five reasons.

2. Why might a doctor prefer to obtain a catheterized urine specimen from a female patient to diagnose kidney disease?

3. What can happen if the person performing the urinalysis using the reagent strip method does not read the tests at the specified time? What implications could this have for patient care?

4. Identify at least three different things that might indicate to you that a patient did not understand the instructions for obtaining a clean-catch midstream urine specimen.

 ## EXPLORE THE WEB

INTERNET WEB SITES

urinalysis tutorials
www.netwellness.org/healthtopics/labtesting/faq13.cfm
telpath2.med.utah.edu/WebPath/TUTORIAL/URINE/
URINE.html

virtual hospital-urinalysis for the physician office lab
www.vh.org/Providers/CME/CLIA/UrineAnalysis/Urine-
Analysis.html

picture gallery of substances in urine
www.insc.on.ca/lab/renal

KEYWORDS FOR INTERNET SEARCHES

CLIA
urinalysis
urine crystals

Chapter 25

Phlebotomy, Hematology, and Coagulation Studies

Instructional Objectives

After completing this chapter, you will be able to do the following:

1. Describe the composition of blood and how its elements are formed.
2. Identify the function of the circulatory system and each of the elements in blood.
3. Describe the equipment and supplies needed for venipuncture.
4. Describe the steps to prepare a patient for venipuncture.
5. Compare and contrast venipuncture using the evacuated tube, syringe, and butterfly methods.
6. Correlate additives in evacuated tubes to stopper color and use of tubes.
7. Discuss possible problems during and after venipuncture, and the appropriate measures to prevent or respond to them.
8. Identify two sites that can be used for capillary puncture.
9. List the tests included in a complete blood count.
10. Identify possible causes for an increased or decreased white blood cell count.
11. Describe how a blood smear is properly prepared.
12. Identify the characteristics of the five types of white blood cells that can be seen in a blood smear.
13. Correlate variations in red blood cell size and shape to pathologic conditions.
14. Identify the purpose of testing hemoglobin and microhematocrit.
15. Compare and contrast the Wintrobe and Westergren procedures for determining the erythrocyte sedimentation rate.
16. Discuss variations in erythrocyte sedimentation rate in health and various inflammatory processes.
17. Describe the purpose of coagulation studies.
18. Describe when the prothrombin time (PT) and partial thromboplastin time (PTT) are used for patients receiving anticoagulant therapy.

CMA/RMA CERTIFICATION
Content and Competencies

- Dispose of biohazardous materials.
- Practice standard precautions.
- Perform venipuncture.
- Perform capillary puncture.
- Perform hematology testing.
- Screen and follow up test results.
- Use methods of quality control.
- Document appropriately.
- Perform risk-management procedures.

Performance Objectives

After completing this chapter, you will be able to do the following:

1. Collect a venous blood specimen using the evacuated-tube method (Procedure 25–1).
2. Collect a venous blood specimen using the syringe method (Procedure 25–2).
3. Collect a venous blood specimen using the butterfly method (Procedure 25–3).
4. Collect a capillary blood specimen using a finger stick (Procedure 25–4).
5. Collect a capillary blood specimen using a heel stick (Procedure 25–5).
6. Collect a capillary blood specimen from an infant for PKU testing (Procedure 25–6).
7. Prepare a blood smear for a differential count (Procedure 25–7).
8. Test hemoglobin using a hemoglobinometer (Procedure 25–8).
9. Perform a microhematocrit test (Procedure 25–9).

VOCABULARY

agranulocyte (p. 599)
anemia (p. 599)
antecubital (p. 601)
basophil (p. 599)
capillary action (p. 623)
cell-mediated immunity (p. 600)
eosinophil (p. 599)
erythrocyte (p. 598)
evacuated tube (p. 601)

fibrinogen (p. 598)
fibrinolysis (p. 601)
granulocyte (p. 599)
hematoma (p. 616)
hematopoiesis (p. 599)
hemoglobin (p. 599)
hemolysis (p. 607)
hemostasis (p. 601)
humoral immunity (p. 601)

leukocyte (p. 598)
lymphocyte (p. 599)
microhematocrit (p. 631)
monocyte (p. 599)
neutrophil (p. 599)
phenylketonuria (p. 621)
phlebotomy (p. 601)
plasma (p. 598)
platelet (p. 601)

reticulocyte (p. 599)
sclerosed (p. 601)
serum (p. 603)
syncope (p. 613)
thrombocyte (p. 598)
thrombosis (p. 601)
tourniquet (p. 604)
venipuncture (p. 601)

ABBREVIATIONS

CBC (p. 599)
diff (p. 621)
ESR (p. 621)

Hb (p. 621)
Hct (p. 621)
MCH (p. 622)

MCHC (p. 623)
MCV (p. 622)
PKU (p. 621)

polys (p. 599)
PT (p. 634)

PTT (p. 634)
RBC (p. 598)

segs (p. 599)
WBC (p. 598)

REVIEW OF BLOOD

The average adult has 10 to 12 pints (about 6 liters) of blood in his or her body. Blood is transported throughout the body through the circulatory system. The heart pumps blood through the lungs, where it collects oxygen. Oxygenated blood is transported through arteries to the organs and tissues. Once oxygen is absorbed into these organs and tissues, deoxygenated blood is transported through veins to the kidneys, where harmful wastes are removed, then back to the heart, where the cycle begins again.

Composition

About 45 percent of blood is made up of formed elements, which consist of **erythrocytes** (red blood cells), **leukocytes** (white blood cells), and **thrombocytes** (platelets).

About 55 percent of blood—the liquid portion—is known as **plasma.** Plasma contains a substance called **fibrinogen.** When blood clots, the fibrinogen is transformed into fibrin, a sticky substance that traps all of the formed elements. While the fibrin and formed elements form the clot, the liquid that is left, called serum, is extracted from the clot.

Some laboratory tests are performed on blood that has been separated into the formed elements and serum. Over time, blood sitting in a test tube will clot on its own and separate out the serum. However, to facilitate testing, a centrifuge is used to separate the blood into the clot material and the serum. Other tests, in which the number, size, and shape of blood cells will be measured, must be performed on blood with

the plasma intact; in this case, an anticoagulant chemical must be added to the blood sample to keep the blood from clotting.

Function

Blood has a number of functions.

Blood brings oxygen and nutrients to all of the body's cells after it is pumped from the heart through the lungs. It also removes carbon dioxide and wastes from the cells after they have used the oxygen and nutrients. On its return trip from the cells to the heart, the blood passes through the kidneys so the carbon dioxide and wastes can be removed and formed into urine for excretion.

Erythrocytes (red blood cells, or **RBCs**) are the main transportation vehicles for this purpose. They are formed in the bone marrow. In a healthy individual, there are 4.5 to 5.5 million RBCs per cubic millimeter of blood. Red blood cells live for about 100 to 120 days, and after they die are removed from the body via the liver and spleen.

Blood also helps maintain a uniform body temperature and maintain the proper acid-base balance (pH level) for cells. Finally, it transports hormones, medication, and other chemicals throughout the body.

Leukocytes (white blood cells, or **WBCs**) are the body's main defense against dangerous microorganisms. They are formed in the bone marrow and the lymph system. There are many different types of WBCs, which fight against particular microorganisms. They live anywhere from 1 day to years. In a healthy individual, there are about 5,000 to 10,000 WBCs per cubic millimeter of blood. When they die, they are removed from the body via the bone marrow, liver, and spleen.

Thrombocytes (platelets) function to stop bleeding. They carry fibrinogen, which sets off the coagulation process. Platelets are also formed in the bone marrow and live for 9 to 12 days. In a healthy individual, there are approximately 250,000 to 450,000 platelets per cubic millimeter of blood. After platelets die, they are removed from the body via the spleen.

Blood Cell Formation

The formation of blood cells is called **hematopoiesis** and occurs mainly in red bone marrow. Other production sites for blood formation are lymph nodes, the spleen, the thymus gland, and the gastrointestinal tract.

Each type of blood cell has a slightly different formation process.

Stem cells form blast cells, which in turn become erythroblasts. These are the immediate precursors to RBCs. Myeloblasts, monoblasts, and lymphoblasts are all precursors to WBCs. Megakaryoblasts are the precursors to platelets. Figure 25–1 shows formation of blood cells.

Erythrocytes (Red Blood Cells)

Mature RBCs are anuclear, meaning they have no nucleus. They are pink-red disks, concave on each side, approximately 7 micrometers (μm) in diameter.

Red blood cells' function is to carry oxygen to tissue cells. Their color is attributed to **hemoglobin**, a protein that contains iron molecules. **Anemia,** a decreased ability of RBCs to carry oxygen, can result from either a decreased number of RBCs or abnormal size and shape.

Red blood cell formation is controlled by a hormone, erythropoietin, which is produced by the kidneys. When RBCs die, the iron is recycled, and the heme portion is eliminated by the liver in the form of bile.

Reticulocytes are young RBCs that contain fragments of RNA in their cytoplasm. An adult has a reticulocyte count of 0.5 percent to 1.5 percent; the normal range for infants and children is 0.5 percent to 5.0 percent. This measure helps determine if RBCs are being produced at a rate fast enough to retain the necessary number of RBCs in circulation.

Reticulocyte counts are useful in helping a doctor differentiate among various forms of anemia. Reticulocytosis, or an increase in the number of circulating reticulocytes, may be due to blood loss or an intrinsic anemia. Reticulocytopenia, or a decrease in the number of circulating reticulocytes, indicates a problem with the bone marrow's ability to produce RBCs.

Leukocytes (White Blood Cells)

There are two major types of WBCs: **granulocytes,** which contain granules in their cytoplasm, and **agranulocytes,** which do not contain granules in their cytoplasm.

The three different kinds of granulocytes are neutrophils, eosinophils, and basophils.

1. After staining, segmented **neutrophils** have pink granules in their cytoplasm and a multilobed nucleus (two to five lobes). An increase in neutrophils is associated with the body's defense working against a bacterial infection. The immature form of a neutrophil is called a band or stab. It has a horseshoe-shaped nucleus and is associated with severe stress and pyogenic infection. Neutrophils are the most numerous of the circulating WBCs in adults, and may be referred to as polymorphonuclear neutrophils (**polys**) or segmented neutrophils (**segs**).

   Toxic granulation occurs in severe infections and is noted when viewing the WBCs in the differential portion of the complete blood count (**CBC**). The granules appear enlarged and stain more distinctly.

2. After staining, **eosinophils** have large, red-orange refractive granules in their cytoplasm, and the nucleus may have two or three lobes. An increase in eosinophils is associated with defense against allergies or parasitic infection.

3. Afer staining, **basophils** have a multilobed nucleus (three or four) and large dark purple granules that contain histamine. An increase is associated with an allergic response. Basophils are the least numerous of the circulating WBCs.

The two different kinds of agranulocytes are lymphocytes and monocytes.

1. **Monocytes** are the largest WBCs, about 12 to 20 cm in diameter each. Their cytoplasm stains gray to blue-green, and they have a nucleus with brainlike convolutions that may have a horseshoe shape or appear as ground glass.

   An increase in monocytes is associated with rickettsial infections such as Rocky Mountain spotted fever, fungal infections, and some bacterial infections, such as brucellosis, tuberculosis, and typhoid fever. Some leukemias (cancer of the blood) also cause an increase in monocytes. Monocytes play a role in immunity.

2. The second most numerous WBCs in adults are lymphocytes. After staining, **lymphocytes** are scant blue to blue-gray cytoplasm with a large round nucleus. They are between 6 and 15 μm in diameter, with few or no purple-red granules.

   Viral infections and leukemia are common causes of lymphocytosis, or an increase in the

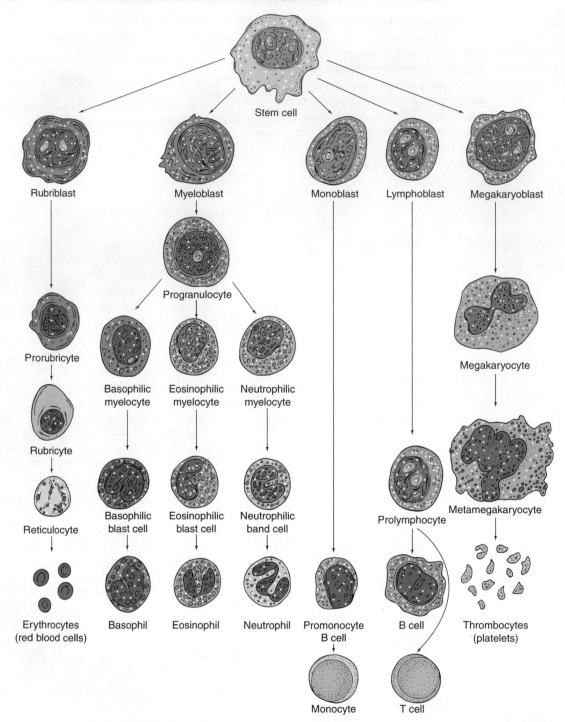

Stem cell

Rubriblast | Myeloblast | Monoblast | Lymphoblast | Megakaryoblast

Prorubricyte

Progranulocyte

Rubricyte

Basophilic myelocyte | Eosinophilic myelocyte | Neutrophilic myelocyte

Megakaryocyte

Reticulocyte

Basophilic blast cell | Eosinophilic blast cell | Neutrophilic band cell

Prolymphocyte | Metamegakaryocyte

Erythrocytes (red blood cells) | Basophil | Eosinophil | Neutrophil | Promonocyte B cell | B cell | Thrombocytes (platelets)

Monocyte | T cell

> **Figure 25–1** Development of blood cells. (From Frazier M, Drzymkowski J, Doty S: *Essentials of Human Diseases and Conditions.* Philadelphia: W.B. Saunders, 1996.)

number of circulating lymphocytes. Lymphocytes may become reactive, or atypical, in viral infections such as mononucleosis. Occasionally, an increase in lymphocytes is seen in a bacterial infection.

T-lymphocytes are influenced by the thymus, though they are produced in the secondary lym-

phoid tissues of the spleen, lymph nodes, and intestine-associated lymph tissue. T-lymphocytes are responsible for **cell-mediated immunity**, resistance to disease caused by cell actions. This type of immunity includes graft-versus-host reactions in transplant patients and delayed hypersensitivity reactions. About 80 to 90 percent of the circulating lymphocytes in the normal adult are T-lymphocytes.

B-lymphocytes are produced in the secondary lymphoid tissues and are responsible for **humoral immunity,** the production of antibodies.

Lymphocytes may become atypical with certain viral infections, such as mononucleosis, meaning that their cell shape appears less regular under the microscope, and the cytoplasm may contain deep blue edges. The untrained eye may confuse atypical lymphocytes with monocytes.

In acute lymphocytic leukemia and chronic lymphocytic leukemia, the number of circulating lymphocytes is increased dramatically, with a high percentage of lymphoblasts or immature lymphocytes present.

Thrombocytes (Platelets)

After staining, **platelets** are purple or gray fragments of cytoplasm, which originate from megakaryocytes in the bone marrow. Because platelets serve to form clots, platelet disorders or deficiencies (thrombocytopenia) can lead to hemorrhage. An increased number of platelets can lead to **thrombosis** (formation of a stationary clot that blocks a vein and keeps deoxygenated blood from returning to the heart). An embolus is a moving mass of blood, tissue, air, or fat in the bloodstream. If an embolus travels to the heart or lungs, it can be fatal.

Hemostasis is the process that stops bleeding. The mechanism of hemostasis is:

1. Vasoconstriction. Narrowing of blood vessels leads to a decrease in blood flow. Hormones and chemicals that cause vasoconstriction are released when damage to the vascular system occurs.
2. Platelets become sticky and adhere to the damaged blood vessel when the endothelium is exposed. This is called the formation of a "platelet plug." The complex process of blood clotting begins.
3. The platelets break down at the site of injury, releasing coagulation factors that stimulate the conversion of prothrombin to thrombin, which in turn stimulates the conversion of fibrinogen to fibrin, the substance that forms a mesh to trap RBCs and stop bleeding.

After a period of time, the fibrin clot is removed by the action of **fibrinolysis.** Plasminogen, an inactive circulating plasma protein, is converted into plasmin, which acts to dissolve the clot. Natural anticoagulants such as heparin and antithrombin III serve to prevent clot formation or at least regulate clotting activity.

A decrease in fibrinolytic proteins results in hypercoagulation diseases, which increase clot formation. A decrease in clotting factors results in bleeding diseases such as hemophilia, a sex-linked, hereditary disorder in which one of the coagulation factors, Factor VIII, is dysfunctional.

OBTAINING BLOOD SAMPLES BY VENIPUNCTURE

Venipuncture, also known as **phlebotomy,** is the removal of a sample of blood, usually from a superficial vein. The procedure is performed to obtain a blood sample for analysis, as a source for blood donation, or to remove blood from an individual with polycythemia vera, a condition in which an individual produces too many blood cells.

Venipuncture is a safe procedure for both the patient and the medical assistant if undertaken with proper care. Standard precautions should be used when performing a venipuncture. The medical assistant must make sure to make the patient as comfortable as possible, both by positioning him or her properly and by engaging in conversation to relieve any anxiety.

Collection Sites

A venipuncture is most frequently performed using the veins of the forearms and the inside of the elbow—the **antecubital** space—as shown in Figure 25–2.

Other sites that can be used are the back of the hand or back of the wrist. Sites on the ankle or lower leg can only be used if the patient has good blood flow to the lower extremities and with the permission of a supervisor or the doctor.

A suitable vein for venipuncture is large and easily accessible near the surface. Do not use a vein that is "rolling"—a vein that appears pronounced but moves easily from side to side when touched—or one that is **sclerosed** (hardened by repeated venipuncture "sticks"). Look for a vein that can be palpated but is better anchored in the tissue.

A venipuncture will be difficult if the individual is dehydrated, or has been taking certain medication such as steroids for a long period of time.

Methods

Blood may be drawn from a vein using one of two methods. Blood may be drawn directly into an **evacuated tube,** a glass or plastic tube sealed with a rubber stopper using a double-pointed needle. Or blood may be drawn using a needle and syringe.

In the evacuated-tube method, the vacuum inside the tube provides the pressure to pull blood out of the vein. In the syringe method, manual pressure on the plunger pulls blood from the vein.

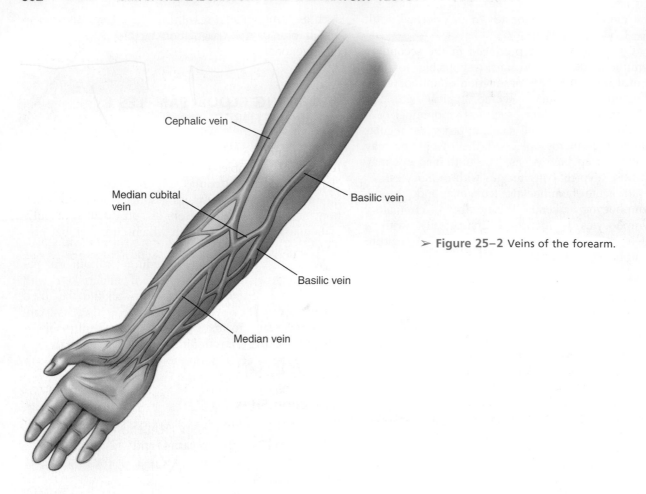

➢ **Figure 25–2** Veins of the forearm.

Equipment

Having the proper equipment and supplies at hand is one of the keys to being able to perform a fast and easy blood draw. The most common method of drawing blood is using evacuated tubes, and the equipment described here is necessary for an evacuated tube blood draw.

Figure 25–3 shows the parts of the evacuated-tube venipuncture system.

A double-pointed 20-gauge to 22-gauge needle, is screwed into a plastic holder. Remember, gauge is the diameter of the needle; the higher the gauge, the smaller the diameter and finer the needle. A needle for drawing blood must have a large enough opening to prevent damage to RBCs. Different needles are used for

a single sample or for multiple samples; a multiple-sample needle has a rubber sheath that fits over the end of the needle and penetrates the rubber stopper of the evacuated tube, so blood does not leak out while tubes are being changed. Figure 25–4 is a drawing of single-sample and multiple-sample needles.

The needle length is 1″ to 1½″. The 1″ needle may be less frightening to patients. The medical assistant should choose the needle length that is easiest to control, using a combination of personal preference and an evaluation of the stability of the vein. Figure 25–5 shows a number of different types of needles for drawing blood.

If it is not possible to perform an evacuated-tube blood draw, blood can be drawn using a needle and syringe. This technique will be described in detail a

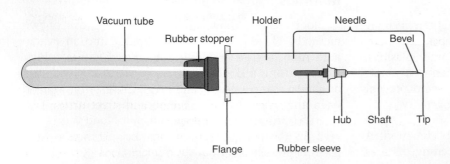

➢ **Figure 25–3** Parts of the evacuated-tube system for venipuncture.

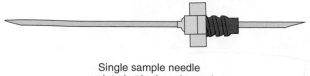

Single sample needle
pointed at both ends used
when only one tube is needed.

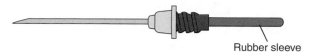

Rubber sleeve

Multiple sample needle -
short needle covered with rubber
sleeve to prevent escape of blood
when tubes are changed.

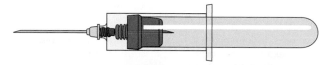

Multiple sample needle when penetrating
rubber stopper - rubber sleeve compressed
between hub and stopper.

➤ **Figure 25–4** Single sample and double sample needle; the rubber sleeve on the multiple sample needle prevents bleeding when the evacuated tubes are changed.

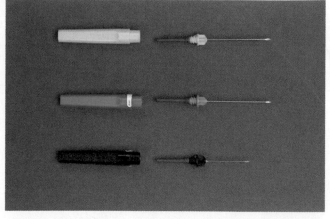

➤ **Figure 25–5** Needles for venipuncture may be single sample or multiple sample (shown), of various lengths and gauges.

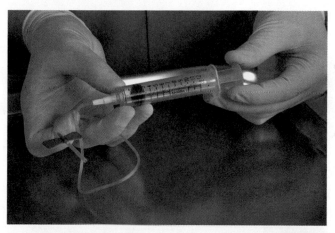

➤ **Figure 25–6** Butterfly needle connected to a syringe.

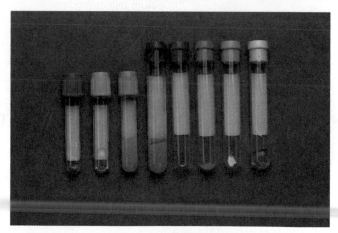

➤ **Figure 25–7** Evacuated tubes with different color stoppers.

little later in the chapter. For a needle and syringe draw, a luer-lock syringe and needle are used.

A winged infusion set (butterfly needle) can be used for a patient with small veins. It may be attached to a syringe, as shown in Figure 25–6, or it may be attached to a hub and needle that screws into a plastic holder for use with an evacuated-tube system.

When using the evacuated-tube method, a plastic holder holds the needle in place and supports the evacuated tube(s). Evacuated tubes are glass tubes that are sealed with a rubber stopper. They are called evacuated tubes because each one has had the air evacuated from the tube to create a vacuum. The vacuum in the tube draws blood into the tube. Each tube is filled with blood until the vacuum is exhausted.

Some tubes contain one or more additives, depending on the test that will be done on the sample. The stopper color identifies the additive in the tube. Different brands of evacuated tubes (called systems) have a different color coding. The medical assistant must learn and remember the color-coding for the particular system used in any office in which he or she works. Figure 25–7 shows a set of evacuated tubes.

Blood drawn by the syringe method is usually put into an evacuated tube for transport to the lab.

Tubes with no additives are used to allow a clot to form. These are used to perform tests on chemicals in the **serum** (the liquid portion of the blood after all of the cells and clotting elements have settled and formed a clot). These include blood chemistry analysis such as tests for the presence of glucose, cholesterol, electrolytes, therapeutic drugs, alcohol, and street drugs; hormone measures; and serology.

If blood analysis cannot be done immediately, a tube with a silica gel (called a serum separator tube, or

wed.

Table 25–1	Evacuated Tube Arranged in Correct Order of Draw		
Vacutainer Stopper Colors*	**Additives**	**Testing Purpose**	**Handling Instructions**
Yellow	Additive: Sodium polyanethole sulfonate (SPS)	Blood and body fluid cultures	Ensure sterility on collection.
Plain red	None	Serum testing, immunology, serology, blood bank, chemistry	Allow to clot at least 40 minutes, centrifuge; access to clot for blood bank testing.
Light blue	Sodium citrate (anticoagulant)	Coagulation testing utilizing plasma	Centrifuge immediately on collection; or separate plasma and refrigerate and test within 4 hours or freeze.
Green	Sodium/lithium heparin (anticoagulant)	Plasma; used for chemistry plasma testing or when patient on anticoagulant therapy	Centrifuge immediately and separate to analyze.
Lavender/purple	Ethylenediaminetetraacetic acid (EDTA) (anticoagulant)	Whole blood; hematology testing and manual erythrocyte sedimentation rate; malarial stains *CBC pregnancy*	Mix well; analyze within 4–8 hours of collection.
Red and black marble; ("tiger top")**	No additives but contains a gel serum separator	Serum; most chemistry analysis; ideal for most chemistry instrumentation	Allow to clot at least 40 min; centrifuge and analyze. No access to clot.
Gray	Potassium oxalate/sodium fluoride (anticoagulant)	Plasma; glucose determinations, esp. when delay in testing anticipated; alcohol levels	Centrifuge and separate to analyze.

YRBLTTG

*Stopper colors are based on Becton-Dickinson tubes.
**The manufacturer recommends treating this tube as one containing additives and using it in the order listed above, but some labs consider it a tube without additives and use it immediately after a plain red-capped tube.

you are bossy. lemvs to the Group

SST) is used. This tube must be centrifuged as soon as possible after clot formation. After centrifuging, the gel separates the serum from the cells. Separating the serum from the blood cells prevents the cells from altering the chemistry of the serum.

Tubes with additives are used to prevent blood from clotting. Each type of tube has a different colored stopper. Table 25–1 contains a list of evacuated tubes, stopper colors, and additives in each.

A few other supplies are necessary: a **tourniquet,** which is a strip of narrow rubber that is wrapped around the upper arm to dilate the veins in the lower arm by preventing venous return; gauze sponges, to cover the needle hole and help stop bleeding after the blood is drawn; alcohol or iodine prep pads, to clean the area before the blood is drawn; and bandages, to prevent bleeding from the venipuncture site.

The patient should be seated for this procedure, preferably at a drawing chair with an arm rest that can be rotated in front of the patient to prevent falls, as seen in Figure 25–8.

Order of Draw

The order of draw refers to the order in which tubes are filled when multiple tubes are collected for multiple blood studies. The following order is recommended to minimize problems if small amounts of additives from a previous tube get into tubes drawn later.

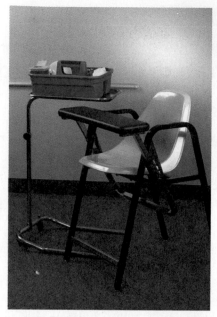

> **Figure 25-8** A chair used for phlebotomy. *R*

1. Sterile tubes for blood culture — *yellow*
2. Tubes without additives (red-capped tubes)
3. Tubes for coagulation studies (light-blue-capped tubes)

   (If only coagulation studies are ordered, a red-capped tube should be drawn first [and discarded] to prevent tissue thromboplastin from entering the light-blue-capped tube.)
4. Other tubes containing anticoagulants (green- and lavender-capped tubes)
5. SSTs—tubes that contain silica gel — *tiger top*
6. Other tubes with additives. *grey*

Evacuated-Tube Method

The evacuated-tube method is appropriate for medium and large veins. The best veins are the median cephalic or lateral basilic veins in the antecubital area. Do not use scarred, sclerosed, or injured veins, or veins in areas with a rash, bruise, tattoo, or other skin lesion, or an arteriovenous fistula for renal dialysis.

If a patient has had a mastectomy (removal of a breast), do not draw from the arm on the side of the removed breast. Do not draw from an edematous area (an area of swelling due to fluid collection). Do not draw from the arm in which an intravenous drip (IV) is in place. After two unsuccessful attempts another phlebotomist or the doctor should try to draw blood.

If a patient becomes faint, stop the procedure immediately. Call for assistance. Protecting the patient is the first responsibility. Be aware of exposed needles at all times.

The medical assistant must also be careful for his or her own safety. To avoid needle-stick injuries, the medical assistant should never recap a needle using the two-handed method and should use an available sharps container or one of the safety devices designed for blood drawing. These include holders that slide down to enclose a needle after use, needles that blunt while still in the vein, sharps containers that automatically remove the needle from the holder, and holders with buttons that release the needle.

Procedure 25–1 describes drawing blood using the evacuated-tube method in greater detail.

Causes of Failed Draw

A blood draw may fail for a number of reasons. The angle of the needle's entry into the vein may be too shallow, causing the needle to be above the vein or to only nick the top of the vein. The angle may be too deep and may puncture through the vein.

An absence of vacuum in the tube may cause the tube not to fill. If a tube does not fill, it is proper to assume a problem with the tube and replace the tube. If a second tube does not fill, it is appropriate to assume that the vein has been missed.

If a vein has been missed, slightly withdraw the needle and repeat at a steeper angle. Do not completely withdraw the needle from the skin, to avoid losing the vacuum in the evacuated tube. Avoid "digging"—moving the needle around in search of the vein.

If the tube does not fill but there is some blood in the tube, the vein may have collapsed. You need to find another vein and repeat the procedure using the syringe or butterfly method. If you must use the same arm, apply the tourniquet lower on the arm, so you do not precipitate bleeding from the vein that was just pierced.

Figure 25–9 gives a complete list of causes for failed blood draws.

Text continued on page 610

PROCEDURE 25-1

Drawing Blood Using the Evacuated-Tube Method

Performance Objective: The student will be able to collect a venous blood specimen using the evacuated-tube method.

- ☑ Wash hands
- ☑ Gloves
- ☒ Eye and Face Protection
- ☑ Lab Coat or Apron
- ☑ Plastic Biohazard Bag
- ☑ Rigid Biohazard Container

*Although eye and face protection is not routinely worn by phlebotomists, it is recommended, especially for students, because blood can spray from the puncture site.

Supplies and Equipment: Disposable gloves, alcohol pad, 2″ gauze squares, tourniquet, double-pointed needle (20G–22G, 1″–1½″) plastic holder, evacuated tubes appropriate for tests ordered, biohazard waste containers (rigid and bag), bandage.

Procedure Steps

1. Wash hands.
2. Review the lab slip or encounter form and choose appropriate collection tubes for ordered tests. Gather other supplies. Screw the posterior needle into the needle holder se-

curely and open the alcohol pad. You may place the first tube into the holder with the stopper just making contact with the needle. Do not push the stopper of the tube beyond the line on the holder.

Rationale: The tip of the needle should make contact with the stopper to hold the tube in place in the holder, but if pushed too far into the stopper, the tube may lose its vacuum and fail to fill.

3. Greet the patient. Explain the procedure and reassure the patient. Do not discuss test orders. Refer the patient to the doctor for patient test questions.

Rationale: The patient will be more cooperative if he or she understands how the blood will be drawn, although many patients are apprehensive. The doctor should provide explanations about the specific tests to be done by the lab.

4. Identify the patient by asking if he or she is the person named on the lab slip or encounter form.

Rationale: You must collect the correct blood specimens from the correct patient.

5. Review the requisition and question the patient about any required preparation; for example, if a fasting specimen is ordered, ask the patient when he or she last ate.

Rationale: If the correct preparation for a test was not done, the results may be inaccurate or misleading.

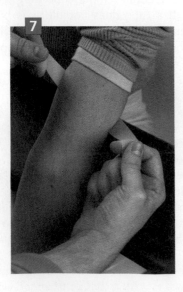

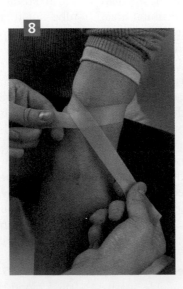

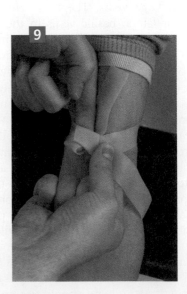

6. Visually assess the patient's veins; if veins appear moderate to large and in good condition, proceed with the collection procedure.

7 If veins are not visible, place a tourniquet on the patient, 3″ to 4″ above the bend in the elbow. Place the tourniquet behind the arm, holding an end with each hand.

8 Cross the ends of the tourniquet in front, putting tension on the tourniquet.
Rationale: The tourniquet should be tight enough to allow arterial blood to flow into the arm while preventing venous blood from returning to the heart. The arm may turn pink or red (but should not turn white).

9 Hold the place where the tourniquet ends cross with one hand and tuck the flap of one end under.
Rationale: One end is tucked under (instead of tied) so that the tourniquet can be released with one hand.

10. Assess vein status on both arms. Veins should feel spongy. You may ask the patient which veins have been used for this procedure in the past. **Do not leave the tourniquet on for more than 1 minute at a time.** (If you are unable to locate a large vein, consider using a butterfly needle, either attached to the evacuated tube or using the syringe method of drawing blood.) You may release the tourniquet and reapply after allowing a brief period for the circulation to be reestablished.
Rationale: Leaving the tourniquet on for more than a minute at a time may interfere with circulation to the arm and cause unnecessary discomfort for the patient. A medium size vein may be easier to penetrate with a butterfly needle. A small vein may collapse if the evacuated-tube system is used. When learn-

ing how to do venipuncture, do not reapply the tourniquet until after the puncture site has been cleaned. Once experienced, you will be able to palpate the vein, apply gloves, clean the site, and draw the blood within 1 minute.

11 Put on disposable gloves, reapply the tourniquet to the arm you have selected, and ask the patient to make a fist and to hold the arm straight. Palpate the site again to determine the location and direction of the vein.

12. Clean the site selected with an alcohol pad. Begin above the vein and clean in an outward concentric circle. If the pad appears excessively dirty, repeat with a second pad.
Rationale: It is important to clean outward to avoid bringing contamination from dirtier areas to areas that have already been cleaned.

13. Wipe the area you have cleaned with a gauze square. Do not blow on the area to dry it.
Rationale: If the alcohol is not dry, it can cause stinging at the puncture site. Furthermore, if any alcohol gets into the evacuated tube, it can cause **hemolysis** (rupture) of red blood cells.

14. Pick up the prepared holder with needle and tube attached. Remove the needle cover.

15 Holding the equipment in your dominant hand at a 15-degree angle with your thumb on top of the holder and your fingers curled under the holder, stabilize the vein with the thumb of your nondominant hand.
Rationale: This helps prevent the vein from rolling as the needle enters it.

16. Penetrate the vein just at the bend of the elbow to what you judge to be the middle in one rapid motion.
Rationale: In most patients the vein is close to the surface at the bend of the elbow. Intro-

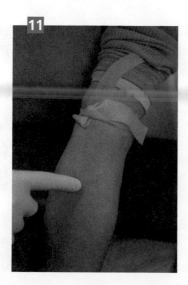

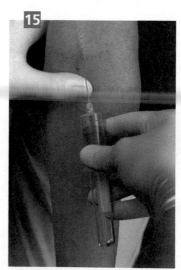

Procedure continued on following page

PROCEDURE 25–1 *(continued)*

ducing the needle too slowly can result in bleeding at the puncture site. This is upsetting for the patient and can interfere with your own concentration.

17 Allow the holder to rest on your fingers against the skin of the paitent's lower arm and do not move the holder or the needle. Using your nondominant hand, push the evacuated tube completely into the holder. If you have penetrated the vein, the tube will begin to fill.
Rationale: The vacuum within the tube pulls blood into the tube until the vacuum is exhausted.

18 Allow the tube to fill by vacuum action. When full withdraw the tube and, without moving the holder or needle, put on the next tube, following the correct order of draw.

19 When the last tube begins filling, release the tourniquet by pulling on the end that was tucked under.
Rationale: It is very important to release the tourniquet before withdrawing the needle to prevent excessive bleeding. Bleeding beneath the skin can cause bruising or a hematoma.

20. Remove the last tube from the holder.
Rationale: This prevents blood from leaking out of the needle.

21. Place a gauze square over the puncture site and remove the needle rapidly at the same angle it entered. Apply pressure to the puncture site after the needle has been removed.
Rationale: Removing at the same angle minimizes discomfort and prevents the needle from sticking up and possibly causing injury

to you. Pressure to the puncture site minimizes bleeding, but if pressure is applied before the needle is completely removed, it could be uncomfortable for the patient and you could accidently be stuck by the needle.

22. Ask the patient to apply pressure for 1 to 2 minutes (or longer if the patient takes anticoagulant medications). Do not allow the patient to bend his or her arm.
Rationale: Bending the arm may interfere with clot formation and cause bleeding under the skin.

23 Dispose of the needle in a rigid biohazard waste container. **Do not recap the needle.** If you are using a needle with a safety device, activate the device. If the holder is contaminated with blood, discard it.
Rationale: The needle should be disposed of as soon as possible after use to prevent the possiblity of a needle-stick injury.

24 While the patient is holding the gauze square, gently rotate any tubes with additives 8 to 10 times to mix the blood with the additive. Do not shake the tube.
Rationale: An additive such as an anticoagulant must be mixed with the blood to prevent the blood from clotting. Shaking the tube can cause hemolysis (rupture) of red blood cells.

25 Label the tubes with the date, time, patient's name, doctor's name, and your initials or apply preprinted labels.
Rationale: It is best to label tubes after they have been drawn. If tubes labeled before the draw and for some reason are not used, they might accidentally be used for another pa-

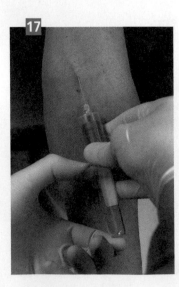

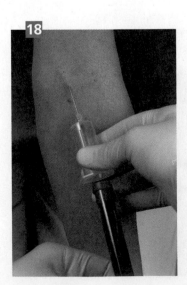

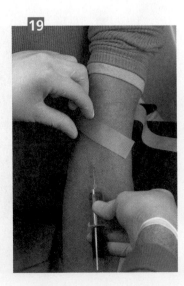

tient and not relabeled, causing results to be reported for the wrong patient.

26 Remove the gauze square from the puncture site to see if bleeding has stopped. If so, fold the gauze square into quarters, place over the puncture site, and apply a bandage to hold it in place. Instruct the patient to keep in place for 30 minutes. If the site is still bleeding, continue to apply pressure and check again in 2 to 5 minutes.

Rationale: The gauze square and bandage function as a pressure dressing to keep the puncture wound from bleeding until a secure clot has formed.

27. After the tubes have been labeled and mixed, place them in the appropriate area for testing or transfer with the appropriate requisitions. If preparing for transfer, place into plastic biohazard transfer bags.

28. Remove gloves and discard in a biohazard waste container.

29. Wash hands.

30. Document in the patient's medical record the date, time, lab tests for which blood was drawn, the arm blood was drawn from, and any adverse reaction of the patient.

Charting Example	
Date	
12/4/XX	2:30 PM Venous blood drawn from Ⓡ arm for SMA 12, Cardiac Panel and CBC with differential. Placed for pickup by Memorial Laboratory. ——————————— S. Morse, CMA

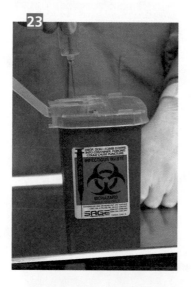

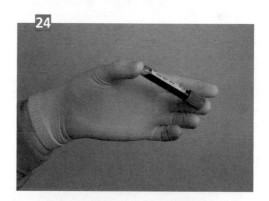

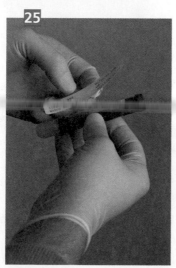

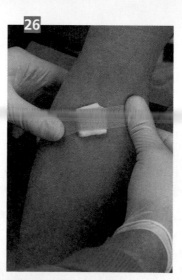

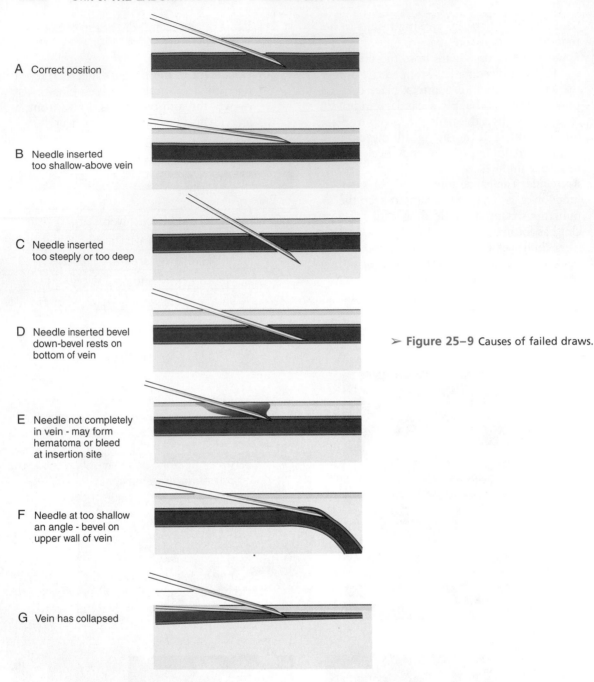

A Correct position

B Needle inserted
too shallow-above vein

C Needle inserted
too steeply or too deep

D Needle inserted bevel
down-bevel rests on
bottom of vein

E Needle not completely
in vein - may form
hematoma or bleed
at insertion site

F Needle at too shallow
an angle - bevel on
upper wall of vein

G Vein has collapsed

➤ **Figure 25–9** Causes of failed draws.

Syringe Method

The syringe method is appropriate for small and delicate veins. This method is rarely used by itself, although it may be used with a butterfly needle, as discussed in the next section. The syringe method should be used on the veins of the antecubital area. A 22G or 23G, 1″ to 1½″ needle should be used. Only about 10 mL of blood can be obtained using this method.

The blood must be transferred from the syringe to evacuated tubes before it clots. For safety, set up the tubes in a rack and do not hold them during transfer.

Tubes with additives are filled first, in the same order as for the evacuated-tube method, so anticoagulants can be mixed with the blood as soon as possible. Tubes without additives (red-capped tubes) are filled last in this method.

Procedure 25–2 describes drawing blood using the syringe method in greater detail.

Butterfly (Winged Infusion Set) Method

The butterfly method is appropriate when drawing blood from veins in the back of the hand or from small and delicate veins in the antecubital area. This

PROCEDURE 25–2

Drawing Blood Using the Syringe Method

Performance Objective: The student will be able to collect a venous blood specimen using the syringe method.

☑ Wash hands
☑ Gloves
[*] Eye and Face Protection
☑ Lab Coat or Apron
☑ Plastic Biohazard Bag
☑ Rigid Biohazard Container

*Although eye and face protection is not routinely worn by phlebotomists, it is recommended, especially for students, because blood can spray from the puncture site.

Supplies and Equipment: Disposable gloves, alcohol pad, 2″ gauze squares, tourniquet, 20G–22G needle, syringe large enough to contain blood for tests ordered, evacuated tubes appropriate for tests ordered, test tube rack, biohazard waste containers (rigid and bag), bandage.

Procedure Steps

1. Wash hands.
2. Review the lab slip or encounter form and choose appropriate collection tubes for ordered tests. Prepare the needle and syringe and open the alcohol pad.
3. Greet the patient. Explain the procedure and reassure the patient. Do not discuss test orders. Refer the patient to doctor for patient test questions.
   Rationale: The patient will be more cooperative if he or she understands how the blood will be drawn, although many patients are apprehensive. The doctor should provide explanations about the specific tests to be done by the lab.
4. Identify the patient by asking if he or she is the person named on the lab slip or encounter form.
   Rationale: You must collect the correct blood specimens from the correct patient.
5. Review the requisition and question the patient about any required preparation; for ex-

ample, if a fasting specimen is ordered, ask the patient when he or she last ate.
   Rationale: If the correct preparation for a test was not done, the results may be inaccurate or misleading.
6. Visually assess the patient's veins; if veins appear moderate to large and in good condition, proceed with the collection procedure.
7. If veins are not visible, place a tourniquet on the patient, 3″ to 4″ above the bend in the elbow, as described in Procedure 25–1, steps 7 through 10.
8. Assess vein status on both arms, apply disposable gloves and clean the selected site as described in Procedure 25–1, steps 10 through 14.
9. Remove the needle cover from the syringe.
10. Holding the syringe in your dominant hand at a 15-degree angle with your thumb on top of the holder and your fingers curled under the holder, stabilize the vein with the thumb of your nondominant hand.
    Rationale: This helps prevent the vein from rolling as the needle enters it.
11. Penetrate the vein at the bend of the elbow to what you judge to be the middle in one rapid motion.
    Rationale: In most patients the vein is close to the surface at the bend of the elbow. Introducing the needle too slowly can result in bleeding at the puncture site. This is upsetting for the patient and can interfere with your own concentration.
12. Pull back on the plunger of the syringe slowly until blood fills the syringe. Keep pulling slowly until you have obtained as much blood as is necessary for the tests ordered.
    Rationale: Pressure on the plunger pulls blood into the syringe. It is necessary to fill the syringe slowly to avoid collapsing the vein through too much sudden pressure.
13. When you have obtained the desired amount of blood, release the tourniquet by pulling on the end that was tucked under.
    Rationale: It is very important to release the tourniquet before withdrawing the needle to prevent excessive bleeding. Bleeding beneath the skin can cause bruising or a hematoma.

Procedure continued on following page

PROCEDURE 25-2 (continued)

14. Place a gauze square over the puncture site and remove the needle rapidly at the same angle it entered. Apply pressure to the puncture site after the needle has been removed. *Rationale:* Removing at the same angle minimizes discomfort and prevents the needle from sticking up and possibly causing injury to you. Pressure to the puncture site minimizes bleeding, but if pressure is applied before the needle is completely removed, it could be uncomfortable for the patient and you could accidentally be stuck by the needle.

15. Ask the patient to apply pressure for 1 to 2 minutes (or longer if the patient takes anticoagulant medications). Do not allow the patient to bend his or her arm. *Rationale:* Bending the arm many interfere with clot formation and cause bleeding under the skin.

16. Place the correct evacuated tube(s) in a test tube rack in the correct order of draw and transfer the blood by inserting the needle through the rubber stopper and allowing the vacuum to pull the blood into the tube. Do not hold the tube while inserting the needle. *Rationale:* Transferring the blood immediately allows you to avoid recapping the needle. In addition the blood must be transferred as soon as possible before it begins to clot in the syringe. The evacuated tube(s) should stand in a test tube rack to avoid needle-stick injuries. If transfer must be delayed by even a few minutes, place the needle cover on the table and maneuver the syringe so that the needle enters the needle cover without having your hands near it.

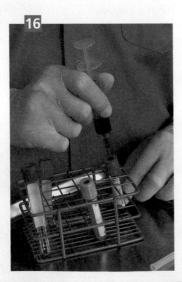

17. Dispose of the needle and syringe in a rigid biohazard waste container. **Do not recap the needle.** If you are using a needle with a safety device, activate the device. *Rationale:* The needle should be disposed of as soon as possible after use to prevent the possibility of a needle-stick injury.

18. While the patient is holding the gauze square, gently rotate any tubes with additives 8 to 10 times to mix the blood with the additive. Do not shake the tube. *Rationale:* An additive such as an anticoagulant must be mixed with the blood to prevent the blood from clotting. Shaking the tube can cause hemolysis (rupture) of red blood cells.

19. Label the tubes with the date, time, patient's name, doctor's name, and your initials or apply preprinted labels. *Rationale:* It is best to label tubes after they have been drawn. If tubes are labeled before the draw and for some reason are not used, they might accidentally be used for another patient and not relabeled, causing results to be reported for the wrong patient.

20. Remove the gauze square from the puncture site to see if bleeding has stopped. If so, fold the gauze square into quarters, place over the puncture site, and apply a bandage to hold it in place. Instruct the patient to keep in place for 30 minutes. If the site is still bleeding, continue to apply pressure and check again in 2 to 5 minutes. *Rationale:* The gauze square and bandage functions as a pressure dressing to keep the puncture wound from bleeding until a secure clot has formed.

21. After the tubes have been labeled and mixed, place them in the appropriate area for testing or transfer with the appropriate requisitions. If preparing for transfer, place into plastic biohazard transfer bags.

22. Remove gloves and discard in a biohazard waste container.

23. Wash hands.

24. Document in the patient's medical record the date, time, lab tests for which blood was drawn, the arm blood was drawn from, and any adverse reaction by the patient.

technique is often used to draw blood from children or the elderly.

A butterfly needle can either be attached directly to a syringe or to an adapter that screws into a plastic holder for use with evacuated tubes. This allows more tubes to be drawn.

Procedure 25–3 describes drawing blood using a butterfly in more detail.

Possible Problems During and After Venipuncture

The five most common problems that occur during or after venipuncture are:

fainting (**syncope**)
nausea
hematoma
continued bleeding
collapsed veins/failure to obtain a sample.

If any of these situations arise, the medical assistant's first responsibility is to the patient's safety. To respond appropriately to any of these situations, the medical assistant must remain calm.

If the patient becomes faint while sitting and having blood drawn, discontinue the venipuncture and have the patient place his or her head between the knees. Check and record the patient's pulse, respiration, and blood pressure. Continue to observe the patient. Obtain assistance by calling for help or using the office intercom. Do not leave the patient alone.

As soon as possible, place the patient in the supine position. If a patient informs you that he or she is likely to faint, always draw blood with the patient lying down.

If a patient becomes nauseated, place a cold cloth on his or her forehead. Give the patient a basin in case

PROCEDURE 25–3

Drawing Blood Using the Butterfly Method

Performance Objective: The student will be able to collect a venous blood specimen using the butterfly method.

☑	Wash hands
☑	Gloves
✳	Eye and Face Protection
☑	Lab Coat or Apron
☑	Plastic Biohazard Bag
☑	Rigid Biohazard Container

*Although eye and face protection is not routinely worn by phlebotomists, it is recommended, especially for students, because blood can spray from the puncture site.

Supplies and Equipment: Disposable gloves, alcohol pad, 2″ gauze squares, tourniquet, 21G to 23G winged-infusion set with a Luer adapter, plastic holder or syringe, evacuated tubes appropriate for tests ordered, test tube rack, biohazard waste containers (rigid and bag), bandage.

Procedure Steps

1. Wash hands.
2. Review the lab slip or encounter form and choose appropriate collection tubes for ordered tests. Gather other supplies.
3A. Prepare the winged-infusion set by attaching the end of the plastic tubing to the syringe.
OR

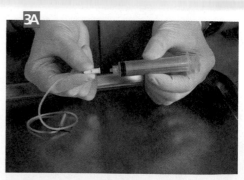

Procedure continued on following page

PROCEDURE 25–3 *(continued)*

3B Prepare the winged-infusion set by attaching the end of the plastic tubing to the Luer adapter and attached needle. If using the evacuated-tube method, screw the needle into a plastic holder and place the first tube loosely into the holder with the tip of the needle just making contact with the rubber stopper.

Rationale: The butterfly needle can be used with either a syringe or an evacuated-tube system. For small to medium veins, the evacuated-tube system works well. If veins are very small, the evacuated-tube method may pull blood so quickly that the veins collapse.

4. Greet the patient. Explain the procedure and reassure the patient. Do not discuss test orders. Refer the patient to doctor for patient test questions.

Rationale: The patient will be more cooperative if he or she understands how the blood will be drawn, although many patients are apprehensive. The doctor should provide explanations about the specific tests to be done by the lab.

5. Identify the patient by asking if he or she is the person named on the lab slip or encounter form.

Rationale: You must collect the correct blood specimens from the correct patient.

6. Review the requisition and question the patient about any required preparation; for example, if a fasting specimen is ordered, ask the patient when he or she last ate.

Rationale: If the correct preparation for a test was not done, the results may be inaccurate or misleading.

7. Assess the patient's veins on both arms. You may look for a small vein at the bend of the elbow by placing a tourniquet on the patient, 3″ to 4″ above the bend in the elbow. You may also look for a vein in the lower arm or hand by placing the tourniquet 2″ to 3″ below the elbow, in the middle of the arm, or 1″ to 2″ above the wrist.

Rationale: When using the butterfly needle method, a smaller vein may be used in the lower arm or hand.

Follow steps 7 through 13 in Procedure 25–1 to place the tourniquet, put on gloves, and clean the selected site with alcohol.

8. Pick up the prepared holder or syringe with butterfly needle and tubing attached. Remove the needle cover from the butterfly needle.

9 Hold the blue wings in your dominant hand with the needle at a 15-degree angle and enter the middle of the vein in one rapid motion. If you are afraid the vein will roll, stabilize the vein with the thumb of your nondominant hand.

Rationale: Introducing the needle too slowly can cause discomfort and result in bleeding at the puncture site. This is upsetting for the patient and can interfere with your own concentration.

10 Allow the needle to rest in the vein supported by the "wings." Rotate the needle if necessary until the needle rests flat. If you have penetrated the vein, blood will enter the tubing.

Rationale: The pressure of the blood in the veins forces a small amount of blood into the tubing.

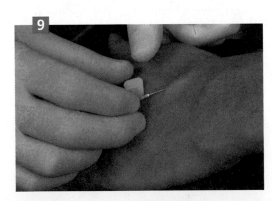

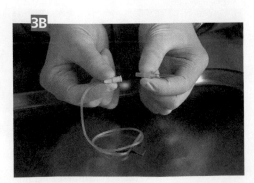

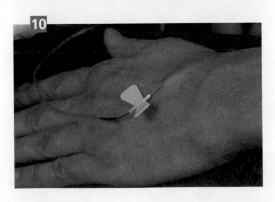

11A. If using the evacuated-tube method, push the first tube completely onto the needle and allow the tube to fill by vacuum action. When full, withdraw the tube and, without moving the holder or needle, put on the next tube, following the correct order of draw. OR

11B. If using the syringe method, slowly pull back on the plunger until the syringe has filled with the desired amount of blood.

12. When the last tube begins filling, or when you have drawn enough blood into the syringe, release the tourniquet by pulling on the end that was tucked under.
Rationale: It is very important to release the tourniquet before withdrawing the needle to prevent excessive bleeding. Bleeding beneath the skin can cause bruising or a hematoma.

13 Place a gauze square over the puncture site and remove the needle rapidly at the same angle it entered. Apply pressure to the puncture site after the needle has been removed.
Rationale: Removing at the same angle minimizes discomfort and prevents the needle from sticking up and possibly causing injury to you. Pressure to the puncture site minimizes bleeding, but if pressure is applied before the needle is completely removed, it could be uncomfortable for the patient and you could accidentally be stuck by the needle.

14. Ask the patient to apply pressure for 1 to 2 minutes (or longer if the patient takes anticoagulant medications). Do not allow the patient to bend his or her arm or wrist.
Rationale: Bending the arm or wrist may interfere with clot formation and cause bleeding under the skin.

15. Dispose of the winged-infusion needle and tubing in a rigid biohazard waste container. **Do not recap the needle.** If you drew blood in a syringe, attach a new needle to the syringe to keep the tip of the syringe sterile until you transfer the blood to the evacuated tubes.
Rationale: The needle should be disposed of

as soon as possible after use to prevent the possibility of a needle-stick injury.

16. If you drew blood in a syringe, place the correct evacuated tube(s) in a test tube rack in the correct order of draw and transfer the blood by inserting the needle through the rubber stopper and allowing the vacuum to pull the blood into the tube. Do not hold the tube while inserting the needle.
Rationale: The blood must be transferred as soon as possible before it begins to clot in the syringe. The evacuated tube(s) should stand in a test tube rack to avoid needle-stick injuries.

17. While the patient is applying pressure with the gauze square, gently rotate any tubes with additives 8 to 10 times to mix the blood with the additive. Do not shake the tubes.
Rationale: An additive such as an anticoagulant must be mixed with the blood to prevent the blood from clotting. Shaking the tube can cause hemolysis (rupture) of red blood cells.

18. Label the tubes with the date, time, patient's name, doctor's name, and your initials or apply preprinted labels.
Rationale: It is best to label tubes after they have been drawn or filled. If tubes are labeled before the draw and for some reason are not used, they might accidentally be used for another patient and not relabeled, causing results to be reported for the wrong patient.

19. Remove the gauze square from the puncture site to see if bleeding has stopped. If so, fold the gauze square into quarters, place over the puncture site, and apply a bandage to hold it in place. Instruct the patient to keep in place for 30 minutes. If the site is still bleeding, continue to apply pressure and check again in 2 to 5 minutes.
Rationale: The gauze square and bandage functions as a pressure dressing to keep the puncture wound from bleeding until a secure clot has formed.

20. After the tubes have been labeled and mixed, place them in the appropriate area for testing or transfer with the appropriate requisitions. If preparing for transfer, place into plastic biohazard transfer bags.

21. Remove gloves and discard in a biohazard waste container.

22. Wash hands.

23. Document in the patient's medical record the date, time, lab tests for which blood was drawn, the arm blood was drawn from, and any adverse reaction by the patient.

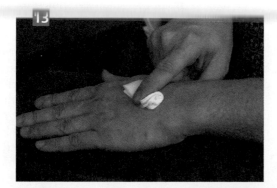

ON THE JOB

Craig Johnson, a medical assistant at Blackburn Primary Care Associates, has been asked to draw blood from Janine Sanders, a 40-year-old woman, to send to Memorial Hospital Laboratory for a chemistry screen (SMA-12) and a complete blood count. Craig has called Ms. Sanders into the phlebotomy area.

Craig: Hello, my name is Craig. I am going to draw your blood for some tests. Can you spell your last name for me? (He is writing on a lab slip.)
Ms. Sanders: S-A-N-D-E-R-S. You know, I don't do very well having my blood drawn.
Craig: And your first name is Janine.
Ms. Sanders: Yes. I get so nervous about this test. Maybe it's because I usually faint.

QUESTIONS

1. Did Craig identify the patient?
2. How should Craig respond to the information Ms. Sanders has just given him?
3. Craig notices that Ms. Sanders has veins that are clearly visible at the bend of the elbow. What venipuncture method should he use?
4. What tubes should Craig prepare for Ms. Sanders' blood? In what order should he draw them?
5. What must be done to the tube used to collect blood for the chemistry screen before it is sent to the lab? Why?

he or she vomits. Tell the patient to take slow, deep breaths. Obtain assistance, but do not leave the patient alone.

A **hematoma** is a large bruised area at the puncture site, caused by blood leaking into the tissue surrounding the vein. Hematomas can be very painful.

There are two common causes of hematoma. One is when the needle goes completely through the vein and the needle's bevel is only partially in the lumen (the open space) inside a vein. The other is when not enough pressure has been applied to the puncture site after the needle has been removed, allowing blood to seep into surrounding tissue.

If a hematoma forms, immediately stop the procedure. Apply firm pressure for 3 minutes, then apply an ice pack to the area. Notify the doctor and continue to observe the site to make sure bleeding stops. An incident report must be completed and placed in the patient file reporting any hematoma.

If bleeding continues and is difficult to control after blood has been drawn, apply pressure for a minimum of 3 to 5 minutes. Have the patient raise his or her arm straight above the head to decrease blood supply while applying pressure to the site. It may be helpful to apply an ice pack to the area to initiate vasoconstriction. If bleeding continues, call the doctor.

A patient may warn that he or she has veins that collapse. Either the person's veins are thin-walled or the lumen is very small in diameter. The evacuated-tube method of collection should not be performed on individuals with small veins.

A collapsed vein is a result of the force from the vacuum tube. The pressure causes the top of the vein to touch the bottom of the vein, impeding or stopping the flow of blood. If the patient's veins are small or do not feel resilient, use the butterfly method and either try to obtain the blood specimen using evacuated tubes with a smaller volume or with a syringe.

OBTAINING CAPILLARY BLOOD SPECIMENS

Capillaries are the small blood vessels that carry blood to and from the small arterioles to the tissues and return blood to the small venules. Usually, capillary specimens are obtained from a finger or from the heel of a foot, used when drawing newborn infants' blood. The earlobe is not a recommended capillary draw site, because blood flow is minimal and hemoglobin concentrations on blood drawn from the earlobe have been shown to be inaccurate. Capillary specimens may be taken on infants and children when small amounts of blood are needed or when it is difficult to perform venipuncture because of inaccessible or collapsed veins.

Any blood test can be performed with blood from a capillary specimen, but not enough blood is drawn for multiple tests or for repeating a test to confirm results.

Equipment and Supplies

To obtain a capillary blood specimen, the following equipment and supplies, shown in Figure 25–10, may be used:

A lancet, to pierce the skin
Blood collection device, such as microhematocrit tubes or a microtainer tube
Glass slides or strips of various types
Blood-diluting pipettes
Alcohol pads or alcohol and cotton balls, and gauze sponges
Sealing clay.

Manual lancets are single blades for making a small incision. Figure 25–11 shows disposable lancets for adults and a disposable automatic lancet used for an infant. The Autolet and pen-type lancets are examples of semi-automated capillary draw systems, which contain spring-loaded plastic holders. A disposable lancet is placed in a plastic holder, and the system's platform

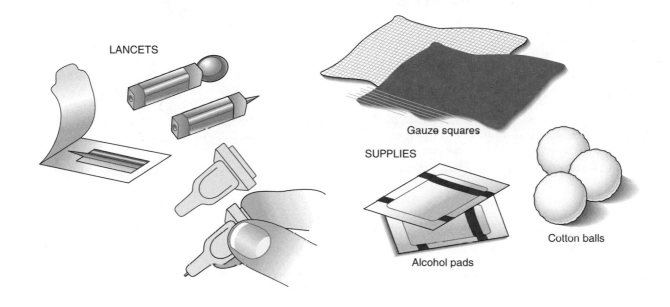

LANCETS

Gauze squares

SUPPLIES

Cotton balls

Alcohol pads

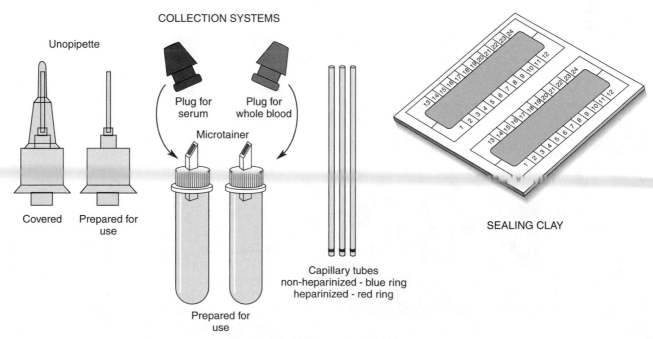

COLLECTION SYSTEMS

Unopipette

Covered   Prepared for use

Plug for serum   Plug for whole blood

Microtainer

Prepared for use

Capillary tubes
non-heparinized - blue ring
heparinized - red ring

SEALING CLAY

> **Figure 25–10** Capillary puncture supplies.

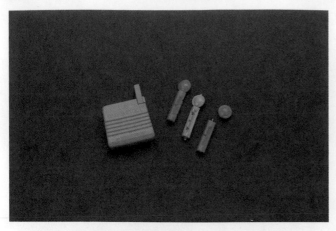

➤ **Figure 25–11** Disposable lancets: manual and automatic.

is placed on the patient's finger. A plunger is depressed, and the spring causes the lancet to puncture the skin. The advantage of such a system is that it standardizes the depth of puncture.

Microhematocrit or capillary tubes are either plastic or glass-coated with a plastic sheathing to minimize the risk of shattering. Capillary tubes can be either plain or heparinized to avoid blood clotting. They are closed by pressing one end in sealing clay.

Microcollection containers are small plastic tubes with removable, color-coded caps. The tip is shaped like a scoop, to direct the blood flow off the side and down the tube. The color of the cap indicates the type of additive, if any, in the tube. For instance, a lavender-colored top indicates there is EDTA in the tube, as in evacuated tubes.

Blood-diluting pipettes, called Unopettes, as shown in Figure 25–12, are used for conducting manual blood counts.

A test strip, test paper, or slide may be used if the test can be done using one drop of blood, such as tests for glucose, cholesterol, or prothrombin time.

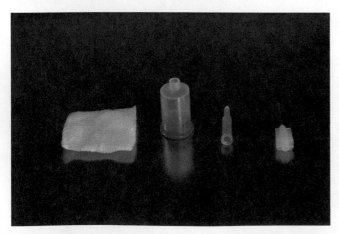

➤ **Figure 25–12** The Unopette system consists of a prefilled reservoir, pipette shield, and capillary pipette.

Finger Stick

Finger sticks are usually performed on the middle or ring finger of the nondominant hand; the index finger may be used if necessary. There is good capillary flow in this area and enough subcutaneous tissue to prevent accidental puncture of the bone (as might occur on the little finger). A finger stick should not puncture deeper than 3.1 mm on an adult, or 2.4 mm on an infant or child. Figure 25–13 shows preferred sites.

To prepare the site, the skin should be warm and dry. If the skin is cold, warm it up by gently rubbing it to increase blood flow or use a warm pack for 2 to 5 minutes. Use an alcohol prep pad or alcohol-soaked gauze sponge to clean the area, then either let the site air-dry or wipe it dry gently with a sterile gauze pad.

When the puncture is made, it must be deep enough for blood to flow freely. For test strips, the first drop should be wiped away, and a large, well-rounded drop allowed to form before applying the strip. Squeezing the finger may cause tissue damage, resulting in an inaccurate test result.

Gloves should be worn for the procedure; hands should be washed and a fresh pair of gloves put on between performing procedures.

Procedure 25–4 describes performing a finger stick in detail.

Heel Stick

Heel sticks are performed only on newborns and infants not yet walking, when the skin on the heel is still without calluses. The procedure should not be done on a part of the heel that is bruised. The procedure should not be done on the center of the foot, but rather on the outer portion of the heel. This prevents injury to the calcaneous bone and cartilage, which could cause osteomyelitis.

Site preparation is similar to that for a finger stick. Warm and clean the area, then dry it to prevent alcohol from hemolyzing the specimen. Always wash hands and change gloves between procedures.

Procedure 25–5 describes performing a heel stick in greater detail.

Some children will need to be restrained to obtain a blood sample from a heel or finger stick. For infants, a parent may hold the child in some kind of a back or chest "snuggly" apparatus, while the medical assistant holds the foot and performs the heel stick. Older children may have to have their arm gently but firmly held in place by a parent or another health care provider while a finger stick is performed.

To avoid injury, both to the child and the medical assistant, the medical assistant should consult with a doctor and/or the parent(s) before deciding what kind of restraint strategy to use with the child.

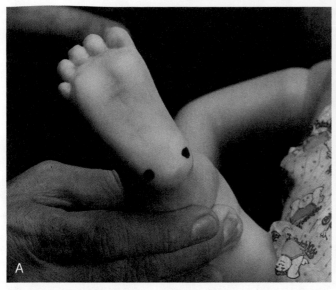
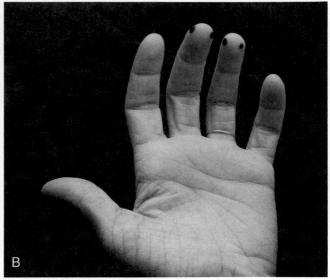

➤ **Figure 25–13** Capillary puncture sites. (From Kinn ME, Woods M: *The Medical Assistant: Administrative and Clinical,* 8th ed. Philadelphia: W.B. Saunders, 1999.)

PROCEDURE 25–4

Obtaining a Capillary Blood Specimen Using a Finger Stick

Performance Objective: The student will be able to collect a capillary blood specimen using a finger stick.

- ☑ Wash hands
- ☑ Gloves
- ☐ Eye and Face Protection
- ☑ Lab Coat or Apron
- ☑ Plastic Biohazard Bag
- ☑ Rigid Biohazard Container

Supplies and Equipment Disposable gloves, alcohol pads, sterile gauze, collecting device or test strip, disposable lancet, biohazard waste containers (rigid and bag).

Procedure Steps

1. Wash hands.
2. Assemble supplies and equipment. Open the alcohol pad and sterile gauze square.
3. Identify patient.
4. Explain procedure to patient or parent.

5. Clean the finger selected for puncture with alcohol and allow to air-dry.
   Rationale: Wet alcohol on the patient's finger may cause hemolysis of the blood specimen, in addition to causing stinging at the puncture site.
6. Put on disposable gloves.
7. Twist the small knob off a manual lancet or prepare an automatic lancet for use.
   Rationale: The needle is covered by a plastic knob to keep it sterile and safe until use.
8. Hold the finger in a downward position.
   Rationale: This position facilitates blood flow.
9. Without touching the area you have cleaned,

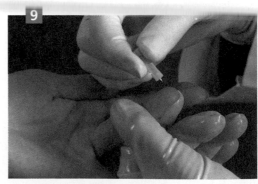

Procedure continued on following page

PROCEDURE 25–4 *(continued)*

make a puncture with the sterile lancet perpendicular to the fingerprint swirls on the lateral surface of the finger and 2 to 3 mm deep for an adult.
Rationale: The puncture must bleed freely.

10. Drop the lancet into a rigid biohazard waste container.
Rationale: The lancet has been contaminated with blood and must be discarded immediately to prevent possible transmission of blood-borne disease.

11 Allow blood to flow. Wipe away the first drop of blood.
Rationale: The first drop of blood contains tissue enzymes that could affect test results.

12 Collect the blood specimen in the desired microcollection device and seal if necessary, or apply a hanging drop of blood to a test strip.

13. When collection is complete, place sterile gauze over puncture site and apply pressure. When bleeding stops, apply a bandage.

14. Test specimens as appropriate. If specimens are to be transported to a lab for testing, label properly and package in plastic biohazard transfer bags.

15. Remove gloves and discard with the soiled gauze in a biohazard waste container.

16. Wash hands.

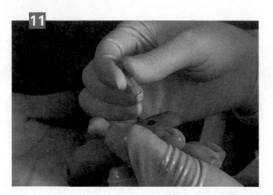

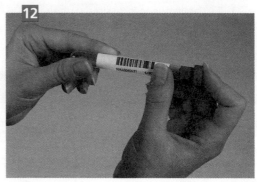

*Photograph from Bonewit-West K: *Clinical Procedures for Medical Assistants,* 4th ed. Philadelphia: W.B. Saunders, 1995.

PROCEDURE 25–5

Obtaining a Capillary Blood Specimen Using a Heel Stick

Performance Objective: The student will be able to collect a capillary blood specimen using a heel stick.

- ☑ Wash hands
- ☑ Gloves
- ☐ Eye and Face Protection
- ☑ Lab Coat or Apron
- ☑ Plastic Biohazard Bag
- ☑ Rigid Biohazard Container

Supplies and Equipment: Warm compress, disposable gloves, alcohol pads, sterile gauze, pediatric collection tubes or capillary tubes, sealing clay (for capillary tubes), disposable pediatric lancet, biohazard containers (rigid and bag).

Procedure Steps

1. Wash hands.
2. Assemble supplies and equipment. Open the alcohol pad and sterile gauze square.
3. Identify the infant.
4. Explain procedure to the infant's parents.
5. Warm the infant's heel with a compress for about 5 minutes.
Rationale: Warmth dilates the blood vessels in the capillaries of the heel.
6. Clean the heel selected for puncture with alcohol and allow to air-dry. Appropriate

sites include the lateral and medial aspects of the heel.

Rationale: Wet alcohol on the infant's heel may cause hemolysis of the blood specimen, in addition to causing stinging at the puncture site. The lateral and medial aspect of the heel contains an adequate capillary bed but will avoid damage to the calcaneus (heel bone).

7. Put on disposable gloves.
8. Prepare a pediatric lancet (which is usually shorter than a lancet designed for adults).
   Rationale: The lancet should not penetrate a greater distance than 2.4 mm for an infant.

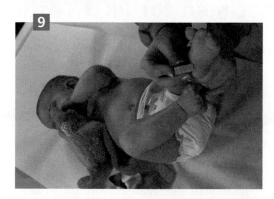

9. Grasp the infant's heel firmly. If using an automatic device, press the device firmly against the skin of the heel and activate it to cause a puncture.
10. Drop the lancet or device into a rigid biohazard waste container.
    Rationale: The lancet has been contaminated with blood and must be discarded immediately to prevent possible transmission of blood-borne disease.
11. Allow blood to flow. Wipe away the first drop of blood.
    Rationale: The first drop of blood contains tissue enzymes that could affect test results.
12. Collect the blood specimen in the desired microcollection device and seal if necessary.
13. When collection is complete, place sterile gauze over puncture site and apply pressure. When bleeding stops, apply a bandage.
14. Test specimens as appropriate. If specimens are to be transported to a lab for testing, label properly and package in plastic biohazard transfer bags.
15. Remove gloves and discard with the soiled gauze in a biohazard waste container.
16. Wash hands.

Heel Stick for Phenylketonuria

Phenylketonuria (PKU) is a metabolic condition in which an individual is missing the gene that codes for phenylalanine hydroxylase and is therefore unable to metabolize the amino acid phenylalanine. Phenylalanine is present in dairy and meat products. In normal individuals, it is converted into tyrosine.

When the enzyme is absent, phenylalanine accumulates in the blood of infants consuming either breast milk or formula. The child excretes phenylketones in its urine. If left untreated, a child with phenylketonuria develops mental retardation and other abnormalities. A special diet that eliminates phenylalanine can prevent the condition. PKU occurs in approximately 1 in 10,000 births.

Most states require PKU screening of infants. Formula-fed infants are usually tested before leaving the hospital. Because of shorter postnatal hospital stays (most women and infants go home about 48 hours after the delivery) the PKU test may need to be done at the child's 2-week office visit. Breast-fed infants have to wait 2 to 7 days to be tested, because the colostrum and the first breast milk do not contain phenylalanine.

Procedure 25–6 describes collecting a capillary specimen via a heel stick and preparing it for a PKU test.

HEMATOLOGIC TESTING

A number of tests are performed to examine blood elements in a sample of blood. Some of these are:

Complete blood count (CBC)
Differential cell count (**diff**)
Hemoglobin determination (**Hb**)
Microhematocrit (**Hct**)
Erythrocyte sedimentation rate (**ESR**)

Complete Blood Count

A CBC is minimally composed of five studies:

1. The WBC count, which is measured as the number of WBC (thousands) per cubic millimeter of blood (#wbc $\times 10^3$/mm^3).
2. The RBC count, measured as the number of

RBCs (millions) per cubic millimeter of blood ($\#rbc \times 10^6/mm^3$).

3. Hemoglobin measured in grams per deciliter of blood (g/dl).

4. Hematocrit measured as percent (%).

5. Platelet count (Plt), measured as the number of platelets in hundred thousands per cubic millimeter of blood ($\#platelets \times 10^5/mm^3$).

A CBC also includes the RBC indices (singular, index) of MCV, MCH, and MCHC. Indices are calculations that determine the size, content, and hemoglobin concentration of RBCs. They are useful in categorizing anemias.

MCV is the mean cell volume. It is the average size of RBCs and is calculated from the hematocrit and the RBC count. **MCH** is the mean cell hemoglobin. It is

PROCEDURE 25–6

Obtaining a Capillary Blood Specimen for PKU Testing

Performance Objective: The student will be able to collect a capillary blood specimen from an infant for PKU testing.

☑ Wash hands
☑ Gloves
☐ Eye and Face Protection
☑ Lab Coat or Apron
☑ Plastic Biohazard Bag
☑ Rigid Biohazard Container

Supplies and Equipment: Warm compress, disposable gloves, alcohol pads, sterile gauze, PKU test card and mailing envelope, disposable pediatric lancet, biohazard containers (rigid and bag).

Procedure Steps

1. Wash hands.
2. Assemble supplies and equipment. Open the alcohol pad and sterile gauze square.
3. Identify the infant.
4. Obtain information from the mother to complete the PKU test card.
5. Warm the infant's heel with a compress for about 5 minutes.
   Rationale: Warmth dilates the blood vessels in the capillaries of the heel.
6. Clean the heel selected for puncture with alcohol and allow to air-dry. Appropriate sites include the lateral and medial aspects of the heel.
   Rationale: Wet alcohol on the infant's heel may cause hemolysis of the blood specimen, in addition to causing stinging at the punc-

ture site. The lateral and medial aspect of the heel contains an adequate capillary bed but will avoid damage to the calcaneus (heel bone).

7. Put on disposable gloves.
8. Prepare a pediatric lancet (which is usually shorter than a lancet designed for adults).
   Rationale: The lancet should not penetrate a greater distance than 2.4 mm for an infant.
9. Grasp the infant's heel firmly. If using an automatic device, press the device firmly against the skin of the heel and activate it to cause a puncture.
10. Drop the lancet or device into a rigid biohazard waste container.
    Rationale: The lancet has been contaminated with blood and must be discarded immediately to prevent possible transmission of blood-borne disease.
11. Allow blood to flow. Wipe away the first drop of blood.
    Rationale: The first drop of blood contains tissue enzymes that could affect test results.
12. Apply the infant's heel to each circle of the PKU test card, holding the infant's heel

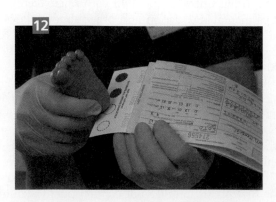

firmly but not squeezing. Each circle must be filled with blood so that blood can be seen on the reverse side of the card.

Rationale: The lab requires adequate blood to test. Squeezing the heel may cause increase in tissue enzymes, which can change the concentration of the blood.

13. When collection is complete, place sterile gauze over puncture site and apply pressure. When bleeding stops, apply a bandage.
14. Remove gloves and discard with the soiled gauze in a biohazard waste container.
15. Wash hands.
16. Allow the test card to dry for 2 hours at room temperature.
17. Document collection of the specimen in the infant's medical record.

18. Place the card in the mailing envelope and mail within 48 hours.

Rationale: The test must be completed in a timely manner for accuracy.

Charting Example	
Date	
1/30/XX	10:25 AM Capillary specimen for PKU obtained from medial aspect of ⓡ heel. Sent to Memorial Laboratory for testing. ——————————— ——————————— S. Williams, CMA

the content of hemoglobin in the average RBC and is calculated from the hemoglobin and RBC counts. **MCHC** is the mean cell hemoglobin concentration. It is the average concentration of hemoglobin in a given volume of RBCs and is calculated from the hemoglobin and the hematocrit.

Typically, all three indices are low in microcytic anemias, such as iron deficiency anemia, whereas the MCV and MCH are increased and the MCHC is normal or decreased in macrocytic anemias, such as folic acid anemia.

If the doctor requests a differential count, which identifies the number and type of WBCs, it is usually ordered as a CBC with differential on the requisition. A differential may be manual or automated.

For the manual differential, a blood smear is made, and after staining with Wright's stain, a technologist counts 100 WBCs, categorizes them, and reports them out as a percentage. The morphology of the RBCs, WBCs, and platelets are also noted in the differential. In an automated differential, a machine reports out the percentages.

Red cell and white cell morphology can also be examined. Red cells are examined to determine the cells' size, shape, and color, and whether there is a nucleus or remnant of a nucleus present. If RBCs are abnormal, their oxygen-carrying capacity can be harmed. White cells are examined to determine the cytoplasmic shape, as well as the condition of cells' nuclei (plural of nucleus).

Red and white cells can be counted either manually or using an automated system. Most physicians' office laboratories (POLs) that do their own cell counts use automatic cell counters. Manual cell counts are not usually performed by medical assistants, but medical assistants should understand the principles of manual counting.

Because both RBCs and WBCs are heavily concentrated in blood, it is necessary to dilute a precisely measured amount of blood with a precisely measured amount of diluting fluid to count cells. Manual cell counts can be performed with blood-diluting pipettes and diluting fluids, or using premeasured and prefilled blood-diluting pipettes called Unopettes. A counting chamber called a hemocytometer, a coverslip for the hemocytometer, and a microscope complete the equipment necessary to perform the manual count.

In the Unopette system, a precisely measured amount of blood is introduced into the Unopette. This blood can be taken directly from a capillary puncture or can be collected during a venipuncture in an EDTA anticoagulant tube, then transferred to the Unopette capillary tube later. Like the microhematocrit, blood rises in the tube by **capillary action,** which is the movement of fluid because of surface tension. After the blood is in the Unopette, it is rotated gently to mix it thoroughly with the diluting solution, then allowed to stand for 10 minutes. For WBC counts, Unopettes come prepared to produce a 1:20 or 1:100 dilution. For RBC counts Unopettes come prepared to produce a 1:200 ratio. Figure 25–14 describes how to fill a Unopette.

After the blood is diluted it is placed in a hemocytometer, a heavy glass slide for counting blood cells. When viewed from the top, the hemocytometer has two raised platforms, three depressions, and a series of ruled lines etched in the glass. Another piece of thin glass, a coverslip, is placed over the ruled portion of the hemocytometer. The coverslip controls the depth of the fluid on the slide, as seen in Figure 25–15.

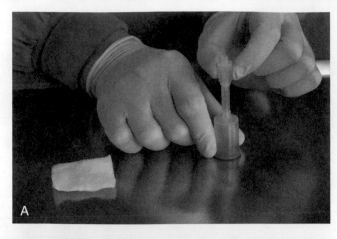

A

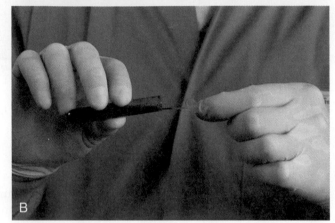

B

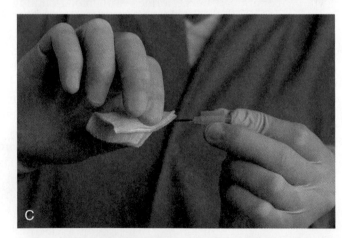

C

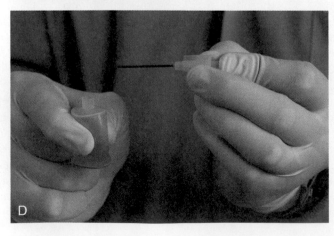

D

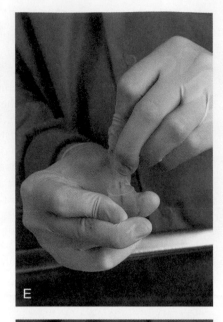

E

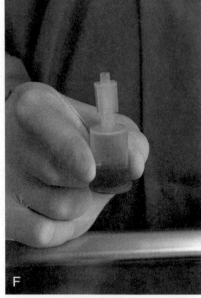

F

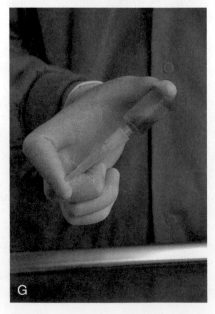

G

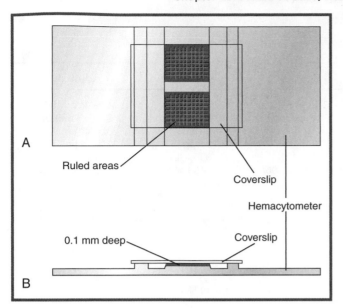

➤ **Figure 25–15** Hemocytometer. top (A) and side (B) views. The blood sample should fill the shaded area. (From Kinn ME, Woods M: *The Medical Assistant: Administrative and Clinical,* 8th ed. Philadelphia, W.B. Saunders, 1999.)

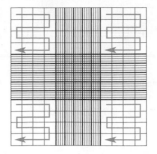
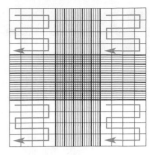

➤ **Figure 25–16** White blood cells are counted under the microscope in the pattern shown in the outer four squares of each section of the hemocytometer.

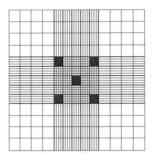
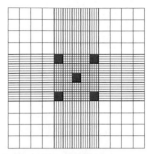

➤ **Figure 25–17** Red blood cells are counted under the microscope in five of the 25 center squares of each section of the hemocytometer.

The area under the coverslip is ruled to create two counting areas. In each of the four corners is an area 3 millimeters by 3 millimeters, divided into nine squares of 1 square millimeter each. These four areas are used for counting WBCs, as seen in Figure 25–16. In the center of the hemocytometer is another area 3 mm by 3 mm. This area, however, is divided into 25 tiny squares, each a little more than $\frac{1}{3}$ square mm. The four tiny squares in the corners and the one in the center, are used for counting RBCs, as seen in Figure 25–17.

Then, using a microscope, the cells in each of the four WBC counting boxes in the corners of the hemocytometer and the five tiny RBC counting squares within the RBC counting box in the center can be counted. The average number of RBCs in five areas is multiplied by 10,000 to obtain the total RBC count per mm^3. The average number of WBCs in four areas is multiplied by 50 to obtain the total WBC count per mm^3.

Most POLs use automated cell counters, as shown in Figure 25–18. With most automated counters, the blood is diluted using a fluid that conducts electricity. As the diluted blood moves through the counting chamber in the machine, each passing cell interrupts the flow of electricity, and the number of interruptions is counted. Other counters use a laser beam to spot the cells as they pass by.

Table 25–2 shows the reference ranges for complete blood counts.

➤ **Figure 25–14 (A)** Choose the correct Unopipette for the type of blood cells you want to count. Working on a flat surface, use the pipette shield to puncture a hole in the pre-filled reservoir. **(B)** Fill the pipette with blood from an evacuated tube containing EDTA-anticoagulated and well-mixed blood, or fill the pipette with blood from a finger or heel stick. The pipette will fill by capillary action to the end of the capillary tube. **(C)** Wipe the excess from the outside of the capillary tube without losing any of the sample from inside. **(D)** Hold finger over top end to keep blood sample from leaking out of the capillary tube. **(E)** Squeeze reservoir to remove some air, but do not squeeze out any liquid. Insert capillary tube into reservoir. Remove finger from top end and blood will drain into the reservoir. **(F)** Squeeze reservoir two or three times. This will rinse blood from the capillary tube. **(G)** Place pipette shield on reservoir and invert to mix the diluted blood.

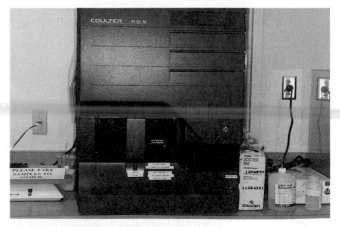

➤ **Figure 25–18** Automated cell analyzer for a physician's office laboratory. (From Stepp CA, Woods MA: *Laboratory Procedures for Medical Personnel,* Philadelphia, W.B. Saunders, 1998.)

Table 25–2	Reference Ranges for Complete Blood Count and Differential				
	Neonates	Infants to 6 Months	Children	Adult Men	Adult Women
WBC	9–30 × 1000/mm³	6–16 × 1000/mm³	5–12 × 1000/mm³	4.5–11 × 1000/mm³	4.5–11 × 1000/mm³
RBC	4.8–7.0 million/mm³	3.8–5.5 million/mm³	4.5–4.8 million/mm³	4.6–6.2 million/mm³	2.4–5.4 million/mm³
MCV	96–108 μm			82–98 μm	82–98 μm
MCH	32–24 pg			26–34 pg	26–34 pg
MCHC	31–33 g/dL			31–33 g/dL	31–33 g/dL
Platelets	140–300 × 1000/mm³	200–475 × 1000/mm³	150–450 × 1000/mm³	150–400 × 1000/mm³	150–400 × 1000/mm³
Differential					
Neutrophils				50–60%	50–60%
Bands				0–3 %	0–3 %
Eosinophils				1–3 %	1–3 %
Basophils				0–3 %	0–3 %
Monocytes				4–9 %	4–9 %
Lymphocytes				25–40 %	25–40%

Differential Cell Count

A differential cell count is performed for the purpose of counting the different kinds of WBCs and checking the ratio of platelets to white cells, as well as to study the morphology of WBCs and RBCs. Abnormalities in cell morphology can be a sign of an underlying disease.

The test is performed by first preparing a peripheral blood smear (using capillary or venous blood), then staining the smear, and finally identifying the normal blood cells on the smear.

The smear is prepared by using one glass slide as a blade to spread a small sample of blood across another slide that will then be used for viewing. Procedure 25–7 describes preparing a blood smear in detail.

Blood smears are stained using a polychromatic stain that contains methyl blue and eosin. The most common stain used is Wright's stain. Under Wright's stain, each different type of cell shows up in a different color.

Red blood cells appear pale red or pink. White blood cells will stain according to their various charac-

PROCEDURE 25–7

Preparing a Peripheral Blood Smear

Performance Objective: The student will be able to prepare a blood smear for a differential count.

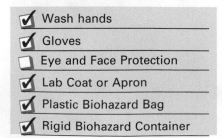

☑ Wash hands
☑ Gloves
☐ Eye and Face Protection
☑ Lab Coat or Apron
☑ Plastic Biohazard Bag
☑ Rigid Biohazard Container

Supplies and Equipment: Disposable gloves, alcohol pads, sterile gauze, glass slides with a frosted end, disposable lancet, biohazard waste containers (rigid and bag).

Procedure Steps

1. Wash hands.
2. Assemble supplies and equipment. Label at least two slides with the patient's name and date in pencil.
3. Identify patient.
4. Explain procedure to patient.
5. Perform finger stick following Steps 5 through 11 of Procedure 25–4. Be sure to wear disposable gloves and dispose of the lancet in a rigid biohazard container immediately after use.

6 After wiping away the first drop of blood, allow a second drop to form. With the patient's finger facing down, touch the drop (but not the patient's finger) to the slide about ¼″ from the frosted end.

Rationale: The drop of blood should remain in place and not spread out as it would if the patient's finger touched the slide.

(Note: It is also possible to obtain a drop of blood from a venipuncture needle immediately after venipuncture or from a lavender-capped tube of blood collected within 2 hours using a capillary tube.)

7. Hold another slide at a 30- to 35-degree angle. Bring edge of spreader slide into blood drop and let blood spread.

8. With a smooth gliding motion, spread blood about three quarters across slide. A nice feathered edge is the desired effect.

Rationale: The smear should be even without ridges or bubbles and should cover the entire slide for about 1½″.

9. Repeat to prepare a second slide if required by the lab.

10. Allow slides to air-dry.

11. Remove gloves and discard in biohazard container.

12. Wash hands.

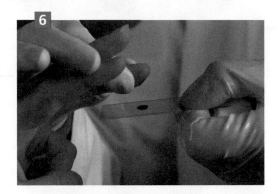

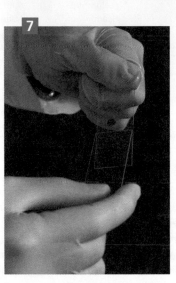

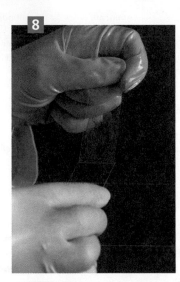

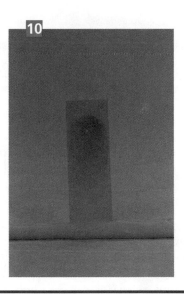

teristics. Basophil granules will appear dark blue. Eosinophilic granules will appear red-orange. Neutrophilic granules will appear colorless or light pink. Nuclei stain dark blue. The cytoplasm of monocytes will appear gray-blue. Lymphocytes will have sky blue cytoplasm and dark-blue nuclei. Platelets will stain gray to purple.

Stain can be applied in either a two-step or three-step method.

In the two-step method, methylene blue, eosin, and a fixative (methanol) are combined in a single solution and placed on the dried smear. After being allowed to stand for 1 to 3 minutes, a buffer is added to the stain.

Although the three-step stain has an extra step, it takes less time, under 1 minute. First, the slide with the dried smear is dipped in a fixative, then into two separate staining solutions. The slide is dipped into each of the three solutions five times, and allowed to drip off for a few seconds between dips. At the end of the five dips in each solution, excess is dabbed off the end of the slide with a paper towel.

After staining, the smear is examined under the oil-immersion objective of the lab microscope (the highest magnification power). The slide should be examined near the feathered end of the slide, where the smear is the thinnest and the cells are barely touching each other.

Under the microscope, it is possible to differentiate the three types of normal blood cells—RBCs, WBCs, and platelets—as well as the different kinds of WBCs

Table 25–3	Characteristics of Leukocytes

	Granulocytes				Agranulocytes	
	Neutrophil Segmented (mature)	Neutrophil Band (immature)	Eosinophil	Basophil	Lymphocyte	Monocyte
Cell size	10–15 μm	10–15 μm	10–15 μm	10–15 μm	6–15 μm	12–20 μm
Nucleus shape	2–5 lobes connected by threadlike filaments	Band or U-shaped	Bilobed or band	Slightly segmented, granular, or band	Round or oval	Round, indented, or superimposed lobes
Nucleus structure	Coarse	Coarse	Coarse	Obscured by granules	Smudged, lumpy, or clumped	Brainlike convolusions or folded
Cytoplasm amount	Abundant	Abundant	Abundant	Abundant	Scant	Abundant
Cytoplasm color	Colorless to light pink	Colorless to light pink	Colorless to light pink	Colorless to light pink	Sky blue to dark blue	Dull gray to blue-gray
Cytoplasm inclusions	Many tiny tan, pink, or red-purple granules	Many tiny tan, pink with increased red-purple granules	Large rounder oval red to red-orange granules	Large, coarse blue-black granules	None to few round red-purple granules	Ground glass appearance, fine red-purple granules, rare blue granules

(From Stepp CA, Woods MA: *Laboratory Procedures for Medical Office Personnel.* Philadelphia, W.B. Saunders, 1998.)

described earlier in the chapter. It is also possible to evaluate cell size, characteristics of each cell's nucleus, and various characteristics of each cell's cytoplasm. Various forms of WBCs are shown in Table 25–3.

A manual differential WBC count can be performed in a laboratory that is certified under CLIA to perform tests of moderate complexity, although a medical assistant would not usually perform this test. The count is performing by counting 100 white cells and classifying them according to what kind of cells they are, then determining the ratio of the various kinds of WBCs.

First, it is necessary to find an area on the smear where the cells are barely touching and not overlapping. This is usually done on a low power of magnification. Then the area is focused under the oil-immersion objective. To count the WBCs, it is necessary to move through the field of vision in a certain pattern so cells are not counted twice.

After doing the differential WBC count, red cell morphology is studied. Normally, all RBCs are the same size and shape and are filled with hemoglobin. Different RBC abnormalities are shown in Figure 25–19.

Stained RBCs may be paler than they should be, which signals a lack of hemoglobin, a condition known as being hypochromic. Although normal RBCs are round or slightly oval, they can be crescent-, sickle-, or target-shaped; a significant variation in the shape of RBCs is known as poikilocytosis. Finally, the condition in which the RBCs are of differing sizes is called anisocytosis.

Any RBC abnormality is reported.

Hemoglobin Determination

Hemoglobin is a protein molecule present in normal RBCs. Hemoglobin, which gives RBCs their color, makes up about 85 percent of the dry weight of RBCs. Each hemoglobin molecule is made up of four globin chains, each of which has a heme group attached.

Hemoglobin's key function is to transport oxygen to tissue and organ cells as blood circulates. Hemoglobin carries approximately 95 percent of all oxygen from the lungs to cells and returns approximately 25 percent of carbon dioxide back to the lungs to be removed.

A number of diseases are associated with abnormal hemoglobin. The degree of pink stain taken on by each RBC gives a rough indication as to the amount of hemoglobin in the cell. In a normal RBC, the center stains slightly lighter than the periphery, due to the cell's biconcave shape. When the hemoglobin level decreases, the central pale area becomes larger and paler. This condition is referred to as hypochromia.

Another disease of abnormal hemoglobin is sickle-cell anemia. In sickle-cell anemia, hemoglobin S molecules have undergone change that alters the structure of the RBCs. Instead of being rounded, the RBCs are sickle shaped, which makes it difficult for the cells to pass through capillary beds, causing a traffic jam of RBCs in some capillary spaces. This loss of blood flow to tissue causes the pain and other symptoms associated with a sickle-cell crisis.

Hemoglobin volumes may be determined in various ways. Many POLs use a hemoglobinometer, an instrument into which a slide containing a drop of blood is placed. The instrument has a scale that measures hemoglobin volume. When the instrument is then held up to the light, it is clear where on the scale the hemoglobin volume falls.

Procedure 25–8 discusses in detail how to determine hemoglobin using a hemoglobinometer.

The hand-held reflectance photometer reads a reagent test strip containing blood from a finger stick to determine hemoglobin. The HemoSite test or HemoCue

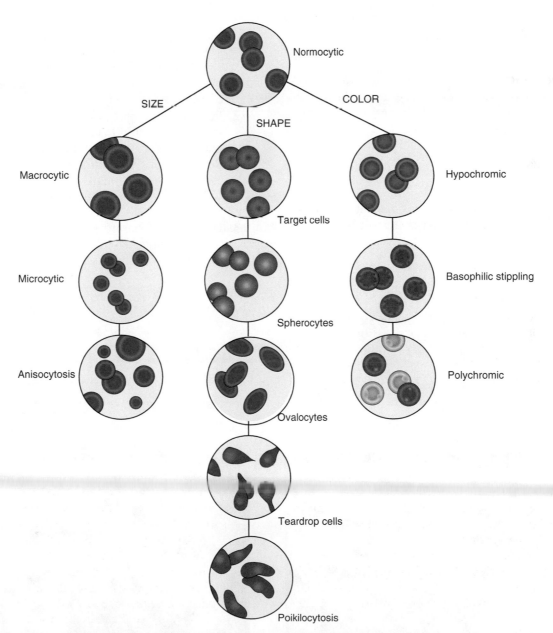

➤ **Figure 25–19** Abnormal red blood cells. (From Stepp CA, Woods MA: *Laboratory Procedures for Medical Office Personnel.* Philadelphia: W.B. Saunders, 1998.)

PROCEDURE 25–8

Testing Hemoglobin Using a Hemoglobinometer

Performance Objective: The student will be able to test hemoglobin using a hemoglobinometer.

- ☑ Wash hands
- ☑ Gloves
- ☐ Eye and Face Protection
- ☑ Lab Coat or Apron
- ☑ Plastic Biohazard Bag
- ☑ Rigid Biohazard Container

Supplies and Equipment: Disposable gloves, alcohol pads, sterile gauze, disposable lancet, hemoglobinometer, reagent applicators, biohazard waste containers (rigid and bag).

Procedure Steps

1. Wash hands.
2. Assemble supplies and equipment. Prepare the hemoglobinometer by removing the chamber and opening it so that the chamber slide is visible.
3. Identify patient.
4. Explain procedure to patient.
5. Put on disposable gloves.
6. Perform finger stick following Steps 5 through 11 of Procedure 25–4. Be sure to dispose of the lancet in a rigid biohazard container immediately after use.
7. After wiping away the first drop of blood, allow a second drop to form. With the patient's finger facing down, touch the drop (but not the patient's finger) to the chamber slide.
   Rationale: Contact with the patient's finger may alter results.
8. Using a reagent stick, stir the drop of blood to hemolyze the red blood cells. This will take about 45 seconds.
9. Close the chamber slide and insert into the hemoglobinometer.
10. Holding the device horizontally at eye level, turn on the light.
11. As you look through the eyepiece, you will see a split green field. Move the slide on the right side of the instrument until both sides of the split field appear to be the same shade of green.
12. Read the scale on the side of the instrument that will identify the hemoglobin reading in grams per deciliter (100 mL) of blood.
    Reference ranges: Adult males: 13.5–18.0 g/dL
                            Adult females: 12.0–16.0 g/dL
13. Dispose of biohazard waste and clean the hemoglobinometer chamber and work area.
14. Remove gloves and discard in hazardous waste container.
15. Wash hands.
16. Record the test results in the patient's medical record.

Charting Example	
Date	
4/18/XX	8:30 AM Hb 14.5 g/dL ————————
	———————— S. Dellarosa, RMA

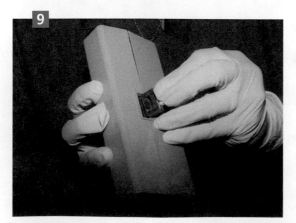

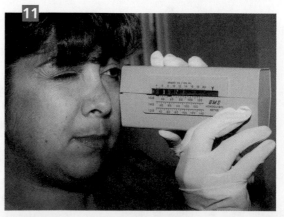

*Photographs from Kinn ME, Woods M: *The Medical Assistant: Administrative and Clinical*, 8th ed. Philadelphia: W.B. Saunders, 1999.

test are waived tests that can be done in any office with a certificate of waiver.

Microhematocrit Determination

When blood is centrifuged at high speeds, it separates, with erythrocytes (red blood cells) settling to the bottom of the tube and leukocytes (white blood cells) and platelets in a thin middle layer and plasma at the top. The microhematocrit method is the procedure used in most POLs. Only a few drops of blood are necessary to perform a **microhematocrit.**

Two capillary tubes containing anticoagulated blood are collected. The samples are spun in a special microhematocrit centrifuge, shown in Figure 25–20, for 5 minutes at 10,000 to 12,000 revolutions per minute (RPM). Using a microhematocrit reader, the packed RBC volumes are measured.

Hematocrit is a measurement of the packed RBC volume, expressed as a percentage of the total blood volume. The sample readings must be calculated within +/− 2 percent. An average of the two samples is reported.

For adult males, normal hematocrit is between 39 and 49 percent. For adult females, normal hematocrit is between 38 and 45 percent. The doctor should be immediately notified of the hematocrit results. Low hematocrit indicates anemia (decreased red blood cells); high hematocrit indicates polycythemia (increased red blood cells).

Procedure 25–9 discusses in detail performing a microhematocrit.

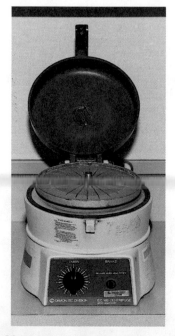

> **Figure 25–20** Microhematocrit centrifuge. (From Stepp CA, Woods MA: *Laboratory Procedures for Medical Office Personnel.* Philadelphia: W.B. Saunders, 1998.)

Erythrocyte Sedimentation Rate

In a well-mixed anticoagulated blood sample left to stand without centrifuging, RBCs will settle to the bottom at a predictable rate. Normal red blood cells are biconcave-shaped and settle at a steady rate. Conditions in which the RBCs are abnormal in shape, such as sickle-cell anemia, or conditions that affect the amount of fibrinogen in the plasma, such as hypofibrinogenemia, can change the sedimentation rate.

Determining the erythrocyte sedimentation rate (ESR)—often referred to as the "sed rate"—is an inexpensive way to check for a number of disease states. Checking the ESR is a good screening tool for inflammatory processes. An increased ESR can be a sign of something as simple and transient as a viral infection. Or it can be a sign of an autoimmune disease such as systemic lupus erythmatosus, rheumatoid arthritis, or Crohn's disease or even the cancer multiple myeloma.

The ESR can also be a good tool to monitor steroid therapy in patients being treated for one of the chronic autoimmune conditions listed above or being treated with chemotherapy. There are automated tools for performing ESR testing; however, the test is usually performed manually using either the Westergren method or Wintrobe method.

In the Westergren method, a venous blood sample is mixed with 3.8 percent sodium citrate solution and left to stand upright for 1 hour. The Sediplast ESR system, shown in Figure 25–21, is a closed system in which laboratory personnel do not have to handle the blood specimen. The ESR is measured in millimeters of sediment that forms in 1 hour (mm/hr).

Normal ranges for ESR using the Westergren method are:

Males: 0–9 mm/hr
Females: 0–20 mm/hr
Children: 0–13 mm/hr.

Potential sources for error using the Westergren method are improperly mixing the solution (less of a problem using the Sediplast prepared system), disturbing the tube during the test, or not placing the stand (and hence the tube) level.

In the Wintrobe method, an EDTA venous blood sample is thoroughly mixed, then transferred to a Wintrobe tube (Figure 25–22). The tube is filled with 1 mL of blood, to the 0 mark on the left, set straight in a rack and left to stand for 1 hour. Again, the reading is mm/hr.

Normal ranges for sedimentation rate using the Wintrobe method are:

Males under 50: 0–15 mm/hr
Males over 50: 0–20 mm/hr
Females under 50: 0–20 mm/hr
Females over 50: 0–30 mm/hr.

The potential sources for error in the Wintrobe method include a dirty Wintrobe tube, disturbances

PROCEDURE 25–9

Performing a Microhematocrit

Performance Objective: The student will be able to perform a microhematocrit test.

- ☑ Wash hands
- ☑ Gloves
- ☐ Eye and Face Protection
- ☑ Lab Coat or Apron
- ☐ Plastic Biohazard Bag
- ☑ Rigid Biohazard Container

Supplies and Equipment: Disposable gloves, alcohol pads, sterile gauze, blood sample containing EDTA (lavender cap) and plain (blue tip) capillary tubes or disposable lancet, heparinized (red tip) capillary tubes and sealing clay, microhematocrit centrifuge and reader, rigid biohazard waste container.

Procedure Steps

1. Wash hands.
2. Assemble supplies and equipment.
3. Identify patient.
4. Explain procedure to patient.
5. Put on disposable gloves.
6. Obtain a venous or capillary specimen of anticoagulated blood in a capillary tube, either by performing a finger stick or heel stick, as appropriate for the age of the patient, and collecting the specimen in a heparinized capillary tube or by using blood from an evacuated tube containing EDTA and collecting the specimen in a plain capillary tube.

Rationale: The blood must contain an anticoagulant to prevent clotting during the test.

7. Hold the tube at an angle to the tube of blood or the second drop of blood that has formed at the site of a capillary puncture and allow the tube to fill by capillary action until three quarters full. If using a finger or heel stick, apply gentle pressure but do not squeeze.

Rationale: The diameter of the tubes is small enough to pull blood into the tubes. Squeezing the finger or heel may cause the blood to be diluted with tissue fluid.

8. Fill two tubes, avoiding bubbles.

Rationale: For accuracy, the hematocrit is calculated as the average of two capillary tubes. Bubbles may cause inaccurate results.

9. Seal one end of each capillary tube with clay sealant.

Rationale: The end of the tube that faces outward in the centrifuge must be sealed to prevent blood from being lost from the tube.

10. Place capillary tubes in microhematocrit centrifuge, clay-sealed end outward. The tubes must be placed opposite each other to balance the centrifuge. Screw centrifuge lid on tight.

Rationale: Placing the sealed end outward and screwing the lid on tightly prevents loss of blood from the capillary tubes.

11. Set timer just past 5-minute mark and centrifuge.

12. After centrifuge has completely stopped, remove lid.

13. Remove the two tubes carefully. Align the top of clay sealant, where red cells begin, on

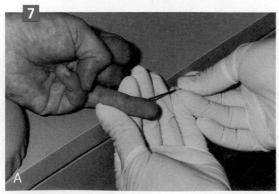

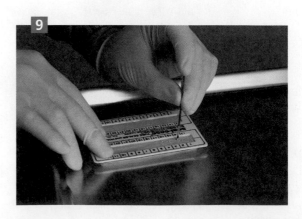

*Photograph from Kinn ME, Woods M: *The Medical Assistant: Administrative and Clinical*, 8th ed. Philadelphia: W. B. Saunders, 1999.

the "0" mark of a microhematocrit reader. Move the outer disk until the reading line is aligned with the meniscus of the plasma. Then rotate the reader until the reading line lies exactly underneath the junction of the

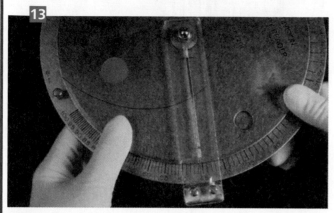

*Photograph from Zakus SM: *Clinical Procedures for Medical Assistants*, 3rd ed. St Louis: Mosby, 1988.

packed red cells and the buffy coat. Read the results on the scale at the outer edge of the reader.

Rationale: The reading for the two tubes must be within ±2% for the test to be valid.

14. Average the readings of the two tubes.
15. Discard tubes and used supplies in biohazard waste container. Remove gloves and discard in biohazard waste container.
16. Wash hands.
17. Document results in the patient's medical record.

Sample Charting	
Date	
6/11/XX	2:15 PM Hct: 40
	S. Williams, CMA

ANEMIA

In anemia, there is a decrease in the amount of hemoglobin or in the number of circulating red blood cells (RBCs). Therefore, anemia can be a manifestation of many physiologic processes. It is helpful to classify anemias by their cause: reduced RBC formation, increased RBC destruction, or blood loss.

Anemias due to decreased RBC formation include those that are due to a nutritional deficiency or a bone marrow failure. Nutritional deficiencies include iron deficiency, vitamin B_{12} or folic acid deficiency, and malabsorption syndromes. Pernicious anemia is the result of a vitamin B_{12} deficiency and is commonly seen in the elderly. Bone marrow problems include endocrine disorders, leukemia, myeloma, and aplastic anemia.

Anemias caused by increased RBC destruction are called hemolytic anemias if due to incompatible blood transfusion or to hemolytic disease of the newborn. Certain drug therapies, autoimmune diseases, infections, and exposure to chemicals can also cause anemia by destroying RBCs.

Abnormally shaped RBCs lead to decreased oxygen-carrying capacity, as well as an increase in RBC destruction. Hereditary hemoglobinopathies include sickle-cell disease (an abnormal hemoglobin S), crystal disease (an abnormal hemoglobin C), and thalassemia.

Acute blood loss after surgery, trauma, obstetrical complications, or gastrointestinal bleeding may cause anemia. Chronic blood loss due to gynecologic or gastrointestinal disorder can also be a cause of anemia.

during testing, the rack and tube not being level, and a blood specimen that was not well mixed.

COAGULATION STUDIES

Coagulation studies measure the ability of blood to clot. All patients on anticoagulant medication therapy need to have the blood monitored regularly for its clotting ability. The goal of anticoagulation therapy is to prolong the amount of time it will take for blood to clot without making that time so long that the person has excessive bleeding. The goal is to make the length of time it takes to clot three times longer than normal.

A prolonged coagulation time makes a person less likely to develop blood clots, especially after heart bypass surgery, heart valve replacement surgery, or any other procedure that disrupts the normal smooth lining of the arterial wall or lining of the heart. Anticoagulation therapy is also used for a person who has a history of blood clots, such as thrombophlebitis, and to prevent heart attack or stroke in individuals with significant risk factors.

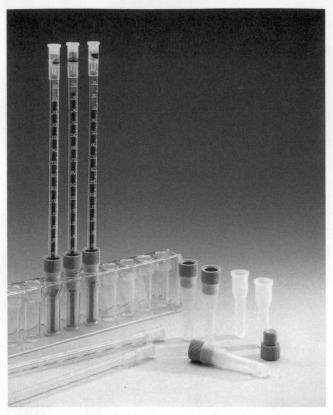

> **Figure 25–21** Sediplast ESR system. (Courtesy of Poly-Medco.)

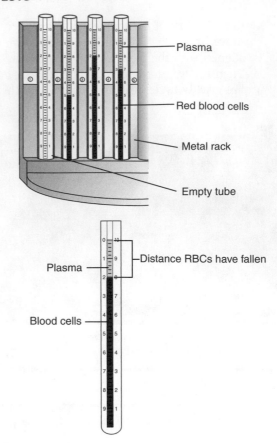

> **Figure 25–22** Wintrobe sedimentation rate system. (From Stepp CA, Woods MA: *Laboratory Procedures for Medical Office Personnel.* Philadelphia: W.B. Saunders, 1998.)

Uses and Types

Coagulation studies measure the ability of plasma to form a clot. There are 12 coagulation factors in human plasma that are involved in clot formation. Formation of a clot has been further subdivided into two pathways. The clotting factors involved in the first pathway, called the extrinsic system, are all dependent on vitamin K for their production. The factors in the second pathway, called the intrinsic system, are not dependent on vitamin K.

The two coagulation studies performed most frequently are the prothrombin time **(PT)**, which measures extrinsic pathway factors, and the partial thromboplastin time **(PTT)**, which measures intrinsic pathways.

Blood for coagulation studies is collected in a tube containing sodium citrate (blue-capped) and sent to a reference laboratory. If the test cannot be performed immediately, it is important to centrifuge the blue-capped tube and separate the plasma from the RBCs. The reference lab may also require that the plasma be placed on ice or refrigerated.

A plain tube of blood must be collected before the blue-capped tube so that any tissue thromboplastin has a chance to be collected separately from the sample to

be tested. If you are only doing a coagulation test, the plain tube can be discarded.

Prothrombin Time

The PT is usually used to monitor patients receiving Coumadin (warfarin) therapy. Because prothrombin is produced in the liver, liver disease can also cause an increase in the PT, which puts patients at risk for bleeding episodes.

The normal PT for patients not taking Coumadin is between 11 and 14 seconds. The range for patients taking Coumadin should be established for the individual lab being used to process the tests.

Some POLs use a machine that can determine PT from a blood sample obtained by a finger stick. Obtain a drop of blood on a reagent strip, insert the strip into the machine, and read the result.

As with any finger stick, the first drop of blood should be wiped away. Make sure the drop used is large enough to completely saturate the square on the strip that has the reagent.

The doctor should be notified immediately of the result, so he or she can decide if the patient's Coumadin dose should be altered.

Partial Thromboplastin Time

The PTT is the screening test for hemophiliacs (people whose blood does not clot or clots slowly, who are prone to excessive bleeding), who are deficient in factor VIII (hemophilia A), or factor IX (Christmas disease). The PTT is also the most common coagulation test for assessment of heparin therapy. Normal ranges should be established for each laboratory, but they are usually between 30 and 45 seconds.

The PTT is a two-stage test, requiring two reagents, contact factor, and phospholipid. The procedure for using each brand of analyzer is different; manufacturer's directions must be consulted before performing the test.

Again, the doctor should be notified immediately of the test results so he or she can decide whether or not to alter the dose of heparin.

Other coagulation studies, such as bleeding time, thrombin time, and fibrinogen assay, measure other parts of the coagulation process.

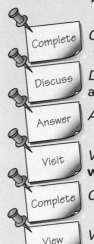

STUDENT STUDY PLAN

To reinforce your understanding of the material in this chapter . . .

Complete the **Review & Recall** questions.

Discuss the situation in **If You Were the Medical Assistant** with your classmates and answer the questions.

Answer the **Critical Thinking Questions** and discuss them with your classmates.

Visit the suggested **Web sites** and search for additional Web sites using **Keywords for Internet Searches.**

Complete the exercises in chapter 25 of the **Student Mastery Manual.**

View the Phlebotomy **Videotape.**

REVIEW & RECALL

1. Describe the composition of blood, including the liquid portion and the cells it contains.

2. Describe the function of erythrocytes, leukocytes, and platelets.

3. What is the purpose of venipuncture?

4. When would you recommend venipuncture using the evacuated-tube method? The syringe method? The butterfly needle method?

5. Why do some evacuated tubes contain additives?

6. Identify the correct order of draw for the evacuated-tube method. What additives are in each tube?

7. What are measures a phlebotomist can take to minimize problems when drawing blood?

8. What are the two sites that can be used for capillary puncture, and when would each be used?

9. Identify at least three blood tests that can be done using blood from a capillary puncture.

10. Identify nine tests that are done in a complete blood count.

11. If a complete blood count includes a differential count, what is being counted?

12. Describe briefly how blood cells are counted manually using a microscope.

13. Discuss the information obtained from measuring the erythrocyte sedimentation rate.

14. How is a blood specimen obtained for coagulation studies?

15. Which patients receive regular measurement of the prothrombin time? The partial thromboplastin time?

IF YOU WERE THE MEDICAL ASSISTANT

Many patients take the anticoagulant medication Coumadin (warfarin) on a regular basis to prevent formation of blood clots after cardiac bypass surgery, after an episode of thrombophlebitis, or for several other reasons. Many receive a monthly prothrombin time, and their Coumadin dosage may be changed based on the results.

Patients often call this medication "my blood thinner." Does Coumadin really make the patient's blood thinner? You may need to look up this medication in a drug reference to answer the following questions:

1. What are signs and symptoms that a patient is taking too much Coumadin? What should a patient be taught to watch for?

2. What is the normal value of the prothrombin time? What values are desired for a patient taking Coumadin?

3. What are the advantages and disadvantages of teaching patients to monitor their prothrombin times at home using a hand-held machine that reads a reagent strip with blood from a finger stick?

 CRITICAL THINKING QUESTIONS

1. Many phlebotomists find it easier to use a butterfly needle to draw blood, and many patients find it more comfortable. Why aren't they used all the time instead of double-pointed needles?

2. Do research to find specific products for safer venipuncture and discuss with your classmates how these products work, how they prevent injury, and the advantages and disadvantages of using them.

3. Usually, waived tests under CLIA must provide "nonsubjective" results, such as those given by a machine. Discuss various blood tests, such as the microhematocrit, hemoglobin, manual blood counts, and the erythrocyte sedimentation rate, and decide if the results are "subjective" or "nonsubjective." Give reasons for your answers.

4. The complete blood count is very often ordered as part of a complete physical examination. Discuss how this test could lead to early diagnosis of different diseases. What should a medical assistant tell a patient who asks why the test is being done?

 EXPLORE THE WEB

INTERNET WEB SITES

capillary puncture tutorial
www.upstate.edu/phlebotomy/pages/cap.htm

venipuncture tutorials

telpath2.med.utah.edu/WebPath/TUTORIAL/PHLEB/PHLEB.html

www.upstate.edu/phlebotomy/

KEYWORDS FOR INTERNET SEARCHES

blood cells
    erythrocyte sedimentation rate
    hematology
    phlebotomy
    prothrombin time
    venipuncture

ANSWERS TO ON THE JOB

1. By asking the patient to spell her name, Craig verified that he is preparing to draw blood from the correct patient.

2. Craig should demonstrate sympathy for Ms. Sanders' concerns. At the same time, he can reassure her that he is competent by making decisions without showing uncertainty. He might reply: "I am going to have you lie down to draw your blood. I see many patients who don't like to have their blood drawn, but most of them say it wasn't so bad when we get finished."

3. Craig will use the evacuated-tube method.

4. Two tubes are needed to collect blood for a chemistry screen and a complete blood count. Usually, Craig would draw a lavender-capped tube for the complete blood count and a red-gray SST (serum separator tube) for the chemistry screen. The lavender-capped tube should be drawn first.

It is also possible for Craig to use a red-capped tube for the chemistry screen. In that case, he would draw the red-capped tube first, and the lavender-capped tube second.

5. Because the blood will be sent to an outside lab, Craig knows that it will not be tested immediately. The blood for the chemistry screen must stand in an upright position until a clot forms (30 to 45 minutes) and then must be centrifuged for 10 to 15 minutes. If the blood was drawn in an SST, after it is centrifuged, the gel in the tube will form a layer between the serum and the clot, preventing the cells from using substances in the serum. If the blood has been drawn in a red-capped tube, the serum must be removed and placed in a separate transfer tube to prevent the cells in the clot from altering the amount of certain chemicals (i.e., glucose) dissolved in the serum.

Chapter 26

Microbiology, Immunology, Chemistry

Instructional Objectives

After completing this chapter, you will be able to do the following:

1. Define and spell the vocabulary words for the chapter.
2. Describe the role of the medical assistant in microbiology testing.
3. Identify equipment used in the microbiology laboratory.
4. Discuss safety measures used when handling microbiology specimens.
5. State the general requirements for obtaining and transporting culture specimens.
6. Describe the process for examining living organisms.
7. Explain why staining procedures are important in identifying microorganisms.
8. List the steps in preparing a slide for staining.
9. Correlate the color obtained for gram-positive and gram-negative organisms to the reagents used to prepare the Gram stain.
10. Describe the different growth media used for culturing.
11. Explain the techniques for inoculating a culture plate and testing for sensitivity.
12. Describe the methods for testing for and identifying parasites.
13. Correlate methods of immunology testing to the antigen–antibody response.
14. List specimens used for immunology testing.
15. Describe methods for pregnancy testing, testing for infectious mononucleosis, and rapid strep testing.
16. Describe how blood testing identifies the four ABO blood groups and the Rh factor.
17. Differentiate between methods of testing specimens for chemical elements.
18. Describe three tests that are useful in the management of diabetes mellitus.
19. Correlate cholesterol and triglyceride testing to the management of risk factors for atherosclerosis and coronary artery disease.
20. Discuss the role of the liver and kidney in the breakdown of protein and removal of urea from the body.
21. Identify other common chemistry tests done in the laboratory.

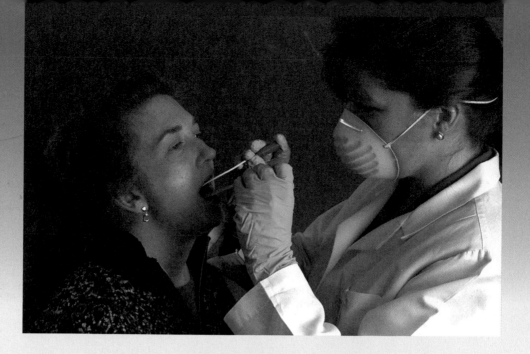

Performance Objectives

After completing this chapter, you will be able to do the following:

1. Obtain a wound specimen for microbiological testing (Procedure 26–1).
2. Obtain a throat specimen and prepare it for processing (Procedure 26–2).
3. Prepare a wet mount and a hanging drop slide (Procedure 26–3).
4. Prepare a dry smear on a microscope slide for staining (Procedure 26–4).
5. Innoculate a culture plate using a throat specimen swab (Procedure 26–5).
6. Prepare a urine specimen for culture using a dip slide kit and read results (Procedure 26–6).
7. Perform a urine pregnancy test and determine the results (Procedure 26–7).
8. Perform a rapid strep test and determine the results (Procedure 26–8).
9. Measure blood glucose using a handheld glucometer (Procedure 26–9).

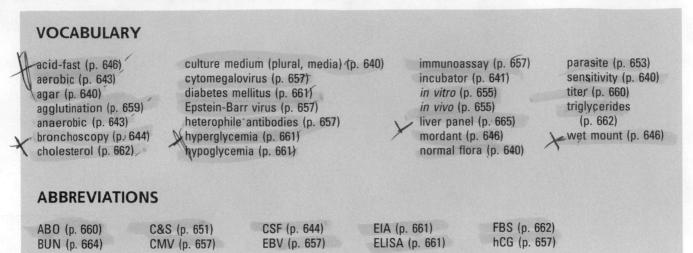

VOCABULARY

acid-fast (p. 646)
aerobic (p. 643)
agar (p. 640)
agglutination (p. 659)
anaerobic (p. 643)
bronchoscopy (p. 644)
cholesterol (p. 662)

culture medium (plural, media) (p. 640)
cytomegalovirus (p. 657)
diabetes mellitus (p. 661)
Epstein-Barr virus (p. 657)
heterophile antibodies (p. 657)
hyperglycemia (p. 661)
hypoglycemia (p. 661)

immunoassay (p. 657)
incubator (p. 641)
in vitro (p. 655)
in vivo (p. 655)
liver panel (p. 665)
mordant (p. 646)
normal flora (p. 640)

parasite (p. 653)
sensitivity (p. 640)
titer (p. 660)
triglycerides
   (p. 662)
wet mount (p. 646)

ABBREVIATIONS

ABO (p. 660)
BUN (p. 664)

C&S (p. 651)
CMV (p. 657)

CSF (p. 644)
EBV (p. 657)

EIA (p. 661)
ELISA (p. 661)

FBS (p. 662)
hCG (p. 657)

INTRODUCTION TO MICROBIOLOGY

Microbiology is the study of organisms too small to be seen without a microscope. Within the field of microbiology are the study of more specific types of microorganisms—bacteria (bacteriology), viruses (virology), fungi (mycology), and parasites (parasitology).

Many microorganisms live in and on the human body and do not cause disease; they are called **normal flora.** A medical assistant needs to know how to collect specimens and test for organisms that are pathogenic—capable of causing infection. These types of microorganisms were discussed in detail in chapter 13.

Medical Assistant Role

The medical assistant performs both clinical and administrative tasks with relation to the collection, testing, and reporting of microbiological specimens.

On the clinical side, the medical assistant is responsible for proper collection of specimens and preparing them so that microorganisms can grow and be identified. Specimens that may contain bacteria are planted on a substance rich in nutrients, called a **culture medium,** and placed in an incubator at body temperature. One common medium is **agar,** a substance obtained from seaweed.

The medical assistant may also be asked to prepare a smear of the sample on a slide or to place antibiotic disks in the culture medium to determine which antibiotic(s) will prevent growth of the offending bacterium. This is called performing a **sensitivity** test.

The medical assistant is also responsible for maintaining safety and standard precautions and for proper cleaning after completing testing.

On the administrative side, the medical assistant is responsible for properly identifying the patient, prop-

erly labeling specimens, and transporting those specimens both within the office lab and/or to outside testing labs.

Three microbiology tests can be performed in a physician's office laboratory (POL) with a certificate of waiver; urine catalase, *Helicobacter pylori*, and rapid strep A. In a POL certified for moderate-complexity testing, many more microbiology tests can be performed.

Equipment

Equipment needed to perform microbiology tests includes equipment for safety, sterilization, inoculation, incubation, visualization, and growing cultures.

Equipment for safety includes germicides for cleaning and containers for biohazardous material and sharps. Personal protective equipment, including gloves, lab coat, goggles, and disposable gown, must be worn when performing microbiology testing. Many

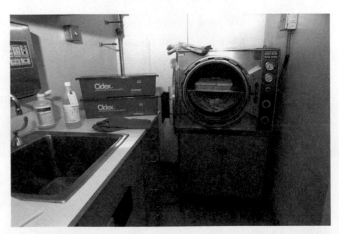

➤ **Figure 26–1** An autoclave is used to sterilize equipment.

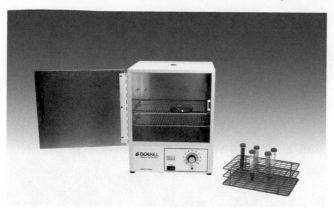

> **Figure 26–2** Table incubator. (Courtesy of Boekel Scientific, Feasterville, PA.)

tests take place on a counter under a laminar flow hood—safety hood—that removes dangerous fumes from the cultures; most POLs do not have laminar flow hoods.

An autoclave, as shown in Figure 26–1 and described in detail in chapter 13, is used to sterilize equipment after use. Many doctors' offices have gone away from using an autoclave and use only single-use, prepackaged sterile materials that are then discarded in the biohazard trash.

An **incubator,** as shown in Figure 26–2, is a cabinet that maintains a constant temperature. Most organisms grow best at a temperature from 35° to 37° C (97° to 101° F). This is body temperature rather than room temperature, and so the cultures need to be grown in an incubator. A few microorganisms need to be tested for by growing cultures at a lower or higher

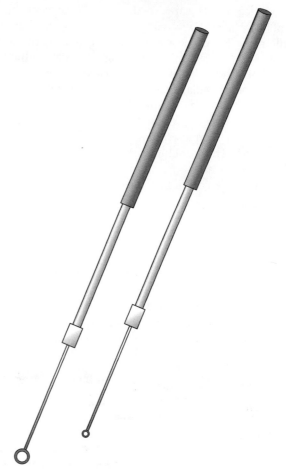

> **Figure 26–4** Inoculating loops.

temperature. Temperature must be tested and recorded daily for quality control.

A brightfield microscope, as described in detail in chapter 23, is used in the microbiology lab. The microscope is used to view organisms too small to be seen with the naked eye.

Bunsen burners and/or electric incinerators are used to sterilize inoculation loops or needles (devices used to plant cultures) immediately before transferring a specimen to an agar plate. Most offices use a loop incinerator like that shown in Figure 26–3, which does not use an open flame, rather than a Bunsen burner.

Inoculation loops, like that shown in Figure 26–4, are either single-use disposable loops made of plastic or metal loops that need to be sterilized immediately before and after each use by passing them through a Bunsen burner flame or an electric incinerator. The loop is used to inoculate, or transfer, cellular material from the sample to a plate or broth medium to grow a culture. Single-use loops reduce the fire hazard and may be preferred in a smaller lab.

Culture media can be categorized as nonselective or selective; within these categories there are many subdivisions.

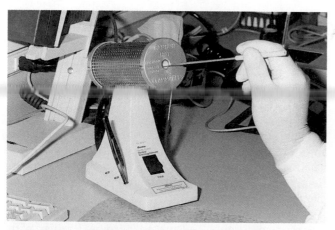

> **Figure 26–3** Loop incinerator. (From Stepp CA, Woods MA: *Laboratory Procedures for Medical Office Personnel.* Philadelphia: W.B. Saunders, 1998.)

Nonselective culture media are 5 percent sheep blood agar. Anything will grow on this type of medium, so it is commonly used. Selective media allow growth of some microorganisms while inhibiting growth of others. These include Hektoen agar for salmonella and shigella, MacConkey agar for some bacilli, and Thayer-Martin medium for gonococci.

Differential media allow a differentiation of bacteria due to colony characteristics (how the colony of bacteria appears). These include EMB agar/MacConkey agar, and Hektoen agar.

Various types of culture media are shown in Figure 26–5.

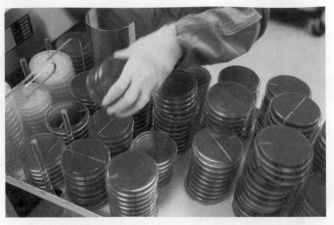

> **Figure 26–5** Various types of culture media.

Safety

Always observe standard precautions while obtaining cultures and performing tests on culture specimens. At all times, wear gloves and a gown or lab coat that cannot be penetrated by fluids at all times. Never mouth pipette (draw material into the pipette by placing the pipette in your mouth and sucking).

Dispose of all glass, needles, and other sharps in the rigid biohazard container. Change the plastic biohazard garbage bags daily even if not full. Clean the blood testing area and centrifuges daily.

Disinfect the work areas that will be used before and immediately after each procedure. Use a 10 percent bleach solution or other acceptable disinfectant to clean work areas. This solution must be prepared fresh daily, using one part bleach and nine parts water. Wash hands before and again after performing each microbiology procedure.

Check culture media and reagent expiration dates, and rotate stock to avoid waste.

Some culture procedures require goggles or laminar flow hoods (these procedures will have specific instructions).

Finally, there should never be any eating, drinking, or smoking in a microbiology lab.

Your employer's exposure control manual documents all safety precautions to be taken for each procedure performed in that specific setting.

Quality Control

Maintaining quality control (QC) is a key to a smooth-running microbiology laboratory. When there are questions about quality control, there are questions about the quality of test results.

When any culture media is received, immediately record the lot number and expiration date in the lab's log. Test each lot number with a known control organism and record the results. Record all QC failures and any corrective action taken. Also record the lot number and expiration date of all reagents when they arrive.

Rotate all stock, with the material that will expire soonest in the front, so it is used and not left on the back of the shelf past its expiration date. Dispose of all outdated materials.

Maintain live known-positive cultures for media control organisms and perform weekly cultures of known control organisms.

Perform daily QC checks of reagents used in test procedures. Record the daily temperature of refrigerators, incubators, and microbiology instruments. Record all routine maintenance and corrective actions performed on all instrumentation.

Maintain accurate and current standard operating procedures for all tests and procedures carried out by laboratory personnel, including specimen collection.

Microbiology testing personnel must have continued training and testing. They must participate in a proficiency testing program in which a third party supplies "unknown" samples to the lab, which performs the specific tests in its facilities on a routine basis. The third party evaluates the results, and the laboratory can compare its responses to other labs participating in the survey.

OBTAINING SPECIMENS

The medical assistant often obtains the specimen and, if it will not be tested in a laboratory at the doctor's office or clinic, also prepares the specimen for transport to the laboratory where the culture procedure will take place. Proper collection is important because an improperly collected specimen can become contaminated and thus yield slow, poor, or inconclusive results, which limits the doctor's ability to provide treatment for the condition.

Before performing any specimen collection, the medical assistant should be sure to become familiar with the protocols for both the office and the lab where the specimen is being sent.

Some specimens are better collected at particular times of the day than others. This is true, for instance, of urine samples to culture for urinary tract infections; the best sample is the first void of the morning, which contains urine that has been incubating in the bladder through the night.

It is also important to make sure sufficient material has been collected in the specimen for the laboratory personnel to run all of the necessary tests.

Cultures are often collected with a sterile swab and put into a container, such as the one shown in Figure 26–6, that has a liquid medium, which maintains the specimen during transport to the lab for testing.

Wound Culture

A wound may contain aerobic or anaerobic bacteria. **Aerobic** bacteria require oxygen to survive, whereas **anaerobic** bacteria thrive under conditions without oxygen. Deep wounds especially are likely to contain anaerobic bacteria. It is important that specimens be collected to perform aerobic and anaerobic cultures. Gram stains should also be performed on all wound specimens.

Use a sterile swab to collect a specimen from a wound that appears to be infected when directed to do so by the doctor. Procedure 26–1 discusses collecting a wound specimen.

Common wound pathogens include *Staphylococcus aureus, Streptococcus pyogenes,* group A beta-hemolytic streptococci, coliform bacilli, *Bacteroides* species, *Proteus* species, and *Pseudomonas* species. Also, anaerobic cocci may be found in wounds; these include *Peptococcus* and *Peptostreptococcus, Clostridium perfringens,* and *Pasteurella multocida,* found most often in animal bites.

Throat Culture

The primary cause of bacterial pharyngitis—sore throat—in North America is group A beta-hemolytic streptococci. Treatment of this infection is important because infection with this microorganism can lead to bacterial endocarditis, rheumatic fever, or acute glomerulonephritis if left untreated.

To obtain a throat culture, use a tongue depressor to hold the tongue down and a sterile swab. Obtain a specimen from the back of the throat without touching the tongue or teeth after the specimen is obtained. The test is performed either by growing a culture in an incubator or by using a rapid strep test kit, which will be discussed in detail later in the chapter. If the rapid strep test is negative, a culture is recommended. To cause the least discomfort to the patient, a medical assistant should take specimens on two swabs simultaneously, rather than having to swab the throat twice.

Procedure 26–2 discusses taking a throat culture in detail.

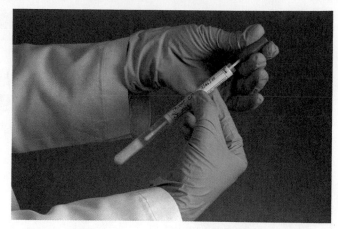

➤ **Figure 26–6** The swab used to take the culture is kept moist by a liquid transfer medium within the container.

Blood Cultures

To obtain a blood sample for culture, the skin must be free of all flora. Blood cultures should be collected from different sites and before antibiotic therapy is initiated.

A blood sample for culture must be collected using sterile technique. After cleaning the area with alcohol, clean again with iodine and allow to air-dry. Collect the specimen in a yellow-capped evacuated tube, then transfer to blood culture bottles, or collect the specimen directly in blood culture bottles that fit the holder, as shown in Figure 26–7. Transport immediately to a laboratory for testing.

Urine Culture

There are three ways to collect urine for a culture:

1. Clean-catch midstream specimen in which the genitals are cleaned, and the urine flows directly into the specimen container; this is described in chapter 24.
2. Catheterized specimen, in which a catheter is inserted into the bladder; this is described in chapter 21.
3. Suprapubic aspiration, an infrequently used method performed by a doctor, in which a long needle and syringe is used to aspirate urine from the bladder.

Other Body Sites

The doctor may collect a vaginal specimen from a female using a cervical swab and a urethral specimen from a male using a small urine cotton swab. Special collection kits are used for gonorrhea and chlamydia testing, which requires carbon dioxide (CO_2) during transport.

PROCEDURE 26–1

Obtaining a Wound Specimen for Microbiological Testing

Performance Objective: The student will be able to obtain a wound specimen for microbiological testing.

☑ Wash hands

☑ Gloves

☑ Eye and Face Protection

☑ Lab Coat or Apron

☑ Plastic Biohazard Bag

☐ Rigid Biohazard Container

Supplies and Equipment: Disposable gloves; sterile culture kits containing tubes, swab, and transport media (both anaerobic and aerobic culture kits may be required); supplies to clean and redress the wound; biohazard waste container.

Procedure Steps

1. Wash hands.
2. Put on personal protective equipment.
3. Identify the patient.
4. Explain the procedure.
5. Remove the old dressing and place in a biohazard waste container.
6. Inspect the wound, observing the wound and any odor, color and amount of drainage, redness, and depth of the wound.
7. Remove the swab from the culture kit and swab the area of the wound where the most exudate is seen. If directed, collect an anaerobic swab first from the deepest part of the wound.
8. Place the swab in the culture tube immediately and crush the transport media ampule by squeezing the sides of the tube firmly.

Rationale: The transport medium keeps the swab liquid, and in an anaerobic culture tube it also releases carbon dioxide.

9. Repeat the procedure using the aerobic collection kit.
10. Label the wound culture tubes with the patient's name, date, time, and doctor's name or apply printed labels prepared for the patient with the encounter form.
11. Change gloves, clean the wound, and apply a fresh dressing as directed by the doctor.
12. Clean the area and discard waste in biohazard waste container. Remove gloves and discard in a biohazard waste container.
13. Wash hands.
14. Document the appearance of the wound, type and amount of drainage, and type and number of specimens sent to the laboratory.
15. Transport the culture tubes to the laboratory immediately.

Charting Example	
Date	
2/16/XX	3:15 PM Raised reddened lesion on Ⓡ
	buttock, 1 inch in diameter c̄ mod
	amt of yellow-green drainage. Aero-
	bic wound culture obtained as
	directed by Dr. Hughes. Sterile
	dressing applied. Patient instructed
	to apply warm, moist compresses
	bid at home and reapply dressing.
	Wound culture transported to
	Memorial Laboratory. ———
	——— S. Dellarosa, RMA

The doctor may also collect specimens from other body parts, such as the eyes, ears, or anus. The procedure for collecting a sputum sample is discussed in detail in chapter 21.

Bronchoscopy is also used for taking lower respiratory tract specimens via bronchial washing, transtracheal aspiration, or lung biopsy.

In addition, a number of body fluids can be collected for microbiology testing.

Cerebrospinal fluid (**CSF**) is collected via a lumbar puncture (discussed in chapter 19). Joint fluid, as well as pleural, pericardial, and peritoneal fluid, can also be collected. Tissue and surgical samples also undergo microbiology testing, as do skin samples.

Labeling and Transporting Specimens

Proper labeling and transport protocols are important for accurate microbiology testing results.

A label must include the patient's correct name and patient identification number, or a bar code; the site of the specimen collection; the type of culture ordered (i.e., throat for beta strep, vaginal for gonorrhea); the date and time of the specimen; the doctor's name; and the initials of the person performing the specimen collection.

All microbiology specimens should be transported as soon as possible to the laboratory. Activate transport media, such as CO_2 ampules or capsules for anaerobic bacteria. Be sure culture tubes have been activated by

---

PROCEDURE 26–2

Obtaining a Throat Specimen for Microbiological Testing

Performance Objective: The student will obtain a throat specimen and prepare it for processing.

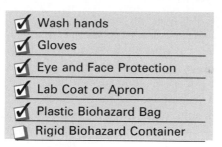

☑ Wash hands
☑ Gloves
☑ Eye and Face Protection
☑ Lab Coat or Apron
☑ Plastic Biohazard Bag
☐ Rigid Biohazard Container

Supplies and Equipment: Disposable gloves, sterile Dacron-tipped throat swabs, or Culturette (swab in container with transport media), tongue depressor, biohazard waste container.

Procedure Steps

1. Wash hands.
2. Put on disposable gloves and other personal protective equipment.

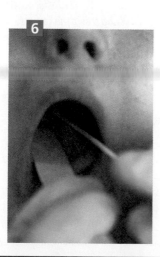

3. Identify the patient.
4. Explain the procedure.
5. Instruct patient to open mouth wide.
   Rationale: You need to be able to visualize the back of the throat.
6. Hold tongue down with a tongue depressor.
   Rationale: The tongue will contract back into the throat if you do not hold it in place.
7. Swiftly and vigorously swab tonsillar areas, especially inflamed or pustular areas, with a Dacron-tipped swab. A figure-of-eight motion allows you to reach all parts of the throat.
   Rationale: Cotton swabs may interfere with bacterial growth; Dacron-tipped swabs should be used to collect throat specimens. Inflamed areas are likely to hold the bacteria that you are looking for.
8A. Place swab in Culturette tube and crush the transport media ampule by squeezing the sides of the tube firmly.
   Rationale: The transport medium keeps the swab liquid and helps preserve the specimen.
   OR
8B. Perform a rapid strep test or plant on agar immediately.
   Rationale: Bacteria need a warm moist environment to survive.
9. Label the culture tubes with the patient's name, date, time, and doctor's name or apply printed labels prepared for the patient with the encounter sheet.
10. Remove gloves and discard in a biohazard waste container.
11. Wash hands.
12. Document that the specimen was obtained and sent to the laboratory.
13. Transport the culture tubes to the laboratory immediately with a completed lab slip.

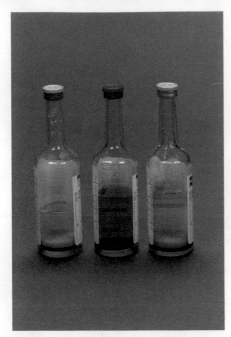

> **Figure 26–7** Blood cultures may be collected in sterile yellow tubes or bottles that fit into the plastic holder.

squeezing the sides of the culture tube to release the holding fluid.

Gynecologic cultures, stool, and blood cultures should be sent to the laboratory immediately. Refrigerate urine if it cannot be transported immediately. Make sure to follow individual laboratories' procedures and policies.

MICROSCOPIC EXAMINATION

Microscopic examination can be done in laboratories certified for physician-performed microscopy and those that are accredited for performing the most complex tests. Chapter 23 discusses using a microscope in detail and lists the various CLIA laboratory levels.

Examining Living Organisms

Usually, the medical assistant in a doctor's office or clinic will prepare slides for viewing, and the doctor or other primary care provider will actually examine the slide. There are two ways to prepare a slide for microscopic examination of living organisms: a wet mount or a hanging drop.

The **wet mount** is used for the examination of a clinical specimen or a colony in the living state. The hanging drop procedure is used for the observation of living specimens on a coverslip over a concave depression, to observe the microorganism's motility (ability to move).

Procedure 26–3 discusses preparing both wet mount and hanging drop slides.

Preparing a Smear

It is usually difficult to see bacteria in the living state. They are small and do not have much color. Because of this, to visualize bacteria under a microscope, a dry smear of the specimen material to be cultured must be prepared, then a stain or dye must be added to color the specimen. Procedure 26–4 describes preparing a dry smear for staining.

The most common staining method is the Gram stain. The Gram stain process differentiates bacteria by their absorption (positive) or nonabsorption (negative) of stain. Gram-positive bacteria have a lower lipid (fat) content than gram-negative bacteria.

The Gram stain differentiates bacteria by their ability to absorb the first stain, or their retention of the second stain, called the counterstain. Gram staining involves several steps.

1. The first reagent, usually crystal violet, is poured on a heat-fixed, dry slide.
2. After a period of time, iodine is added as a **mordant,** a substance that holds the stain.
3. An alcohol-acetone reagent is added as a decolorizer, to remove the purple color.
4. The counterstain, usually safranin, is added.
5. The slide is rinsed with water between each step.

Because of the chemical composition of the cell walls, gram-positive bacteria take up the first reagent and stain purple; gram negative bacteria take on the counterstain and appear pink under the microscope.

Such bacteria as staphylococcus and streptococcus are gram-positive, whereas *Escherichia coli* and many others are gram-negative. Table 26–1 correlates the shape and color of gram-positive and gram-negative bacteria.

Other stain preparations are used often as confirmatory testing, to determine if a specific type of bacteria is present. For example, the bacteria that causes tuberculosis, *Mycobacterium tuberculosis,* and the bacteria that cause leprosy, *Mycobacterium leprae,* are called **acid-fast.** After staining using the Ziehl-Neelsen method, the bacteria retain their red color when treated with a mixture of alcohol and acid. Other bacteria of the same shape are decolorized.

Preparing a Culture

The various kinds of media for growing cultures were discussed earlier in the chapter. Culture media are either in the form of agar, which has the consistency of gelatin and is housed in a petri dish, or broth, which is a liquid and stored in broth tubes or bottles. The medium contains nutrients necessary for growth of bacteria.

A culture is prepared by putting material from the specimen on the proper medium for growing the desired kind of bacteria. This is known as inoculating the medium.

If the material is on a swab, the swab is rolled onto the medium. If the material is liquid or sputum, it is placed onto the medium using an inoculation loop. After the medium has been inoculated, the material should be gently swept across the medium using a flame loop or needle, to dilute the material and make it easier to identify individual colonies.

Procedure 26–5 describes the steps for innoculating a culture plate with a throat swab specimen. After inoculation, the media is incubated for 24 to 48 hours to see what kinds of bacterial colonies grow. Then the appearance and pattern of the colonies is analyzed to identify the bacteria.

First, the specimen is analyzed for gross colony characteristics, such as the size, shape, color, density, elevation, odor, and pigment of the colonies. Also, it is important to determine whether the colonies are pure (a single pathogen) or mixed (many pathogens).

Finally, the specimen is determined to be hemolytic or nonhemolytic—i.e., whether the bacteria break

TAKING ANAL-GENITAL SAMPLES FOR DETERMINATION IN POTENTIAL RAPE CASES

Examination of a sexual assault victim involves both the medical and legal professions. Detailed and carefully documented information is neccessary to aid in police investigation and subsequent prosecution.

The medical record functions as a legal document. It must be complete, detailed, legible, and must not contain any conclusions or judgments about the victim or the circumstances. It is not the doctor's responsibility to determine if a "real" sexual assault occurred but rather to meet the victim's health needs and to observe, describe, collect, and document medical findings.

In many states, the definition of rape is a sexual act engaged in without consent and with the threat or use of force. This means that males as well as females can be victims of rape, because vaginal intercourse is not a condition of rape.

The objective of the anal-genital (and possibly oral) examination of a victim of an alleged rape is to:

1. Diagnose and treat any trauma
2. Collect medical evidence
3. Provide pregnancy prophylaxis if necessary
4. Provide emotional support.

A rape evidence kit should be available in any hospital emergency department and is also available in many public health clinics and community health centers that see urgent walk-in patients. A rape evidence kit comes with explicit instructions, which should be followed exactly in order to collect the evidence necessary to prosecute a sexual assault case.

After the specimens are collected, the evidence box should be sealed and the report on the front filled out. The evidence should then be given to the investigating police officer from the municipality in which the alleged rape took place. The officer will sign for the delivery.

This "hand-off" and "signature" system will be followed at every step of the process from collection to analysis to presentation in court as evidence. This process assures a secure chain of custody, which is imperative to eliminate any chance for a challenge to the evidence by the defense counsel at the time of any future trial.

A doctor will conduct a physical examination of the anal-genital region, as well as the mouth and throat if necessary, both internally and externally, for signs of trauma. Any foreign matter located during the examination will be labeled and "bagged" as evidence.

Laboratory specimens are obtained by the examining doctor in the presence of a witness (possibly a medical assistant). The specimens must be carefully labeled and stored in a locked area until collection for analysis. **They are not to be sent out for routine collection and analysis.**

The following specimens are usually taken:

1. Wet mount for motile sperm, taken from the vagina, cervix, and vulva. The slide should be examined immediately and the results recorded. If this cannot be done, swabs should be placed in separate tubes with a saline solution.
2. A cervical culture for gonorrhea and chlamydia is taken on an appropriate medium, such as Thayer-Martin. Culture should also be taken of the rectum and pharynx if appropriate.
3. A baseline serological test should be taken for syphilis.

PROCEDURE 26-3

Preparing a Wet Mount and Hanging Drop Slide

Performance Objective: The student will be able to prepare a wet mount and a hanging drop slide.

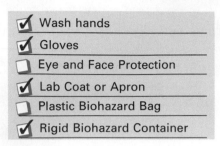

☑ Wash hands

☑ Gloves

☐ Eye and Face Protection

☑ Lab Coat or Apron

☐ Plastic Biohazard Bag

☑ Rigid Biohazard Container

Supplies and Equipment: Disposable gloves, swab and solution containing specimen for examination, glass slide, hanging drop slide, coverslips, bacteriostatic saline and dropper, 10% potassium hydroxide solution, petroleum jelly, microscope, rigid biohazard waste container.

Procedure Steps

1. Wash hands.
2. Assemble supplies and equipment.

Wet mount

3. Roll swab over glass slide.
   Rationale: This places the specimen on the slide.
4A. To prepare a saline mount, add a drop of bacteriostatic saline.

Rationale: This moistens the specimen and suspends microorganisms in liquid.
OR
4B. To prepare a potassium hydroxide (KOH) mount, add a drop of potassium hydroxide.
   Rationale: Potassium hydroxide facilitates examination of a vaginal specimen for yeast.
5. Place a coverslip over the slide. The slide is ready to be examined under the microscope.

Hanging drop slide

6. Place a small amount of petroleum jelly around the edge of a coverslip.
7. Place a drop of solution containing material to be examined on the coverslip.
8. Place the hanging drop slide over the coverslip so that the depression in the slide is centered over the drop of solution and apply pressure.
   Rationale: The petroleum jelly holds the cover slip to the hanging drop slide.
9. Turn the slide over quickly so that the drop of solution hangs from the coverslip into the well of the slide. The slide is ready to be examined under the microscope.
10. After examination, discard the slide in a rigid biohazard waste container. Remove gloves and discard in a biohazard waste container.

PROCEDURE 26-4

Preparing a Dry Smear for Staining

Performance Objective: The student will prepare a dry smear on a microscope slide.

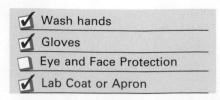

☑ Wash hands

☑ Gloves

☐ Eye and Face Protection

☑ Lab Coat or Apron

☑ Plastic Biohazard Bag

☐ Rigid Biohazard Container

Supplies and Equipment: Clean glass slide with frosted end, container of methanol, cotton swab or dropper, applicator sticks, thumb forceps, biohazard waste container.

Procedure Steps

1. Wash hands.
2. Label slide with pencil on frosted end.
   Rationale: All specimens and tests should be labeled with the patient's name.
3. Put on disposable gloves.
4. Place a thin layer of the specimen onto glass slide using dropper or swab and applicator sticks. The specimen should cover half to two thirds of the slide.
5. Allow specimen to air-dry.
   Rationale: Slow drying of microorganisms on the slide allows them to keep their shape.
6. Hold specimen with thumb forceps by the frosted end.
7. Dip slide into methanol to fix the slide.
   Rationale: Methanol fixation is currently preferred to heat fixation.
8. Allow slide to air-dry again.
9. The slide is now ready to stain.
10. Clean work area and dispose of used equipment in biohazard waste container or bins to be sterilized as appropriate. Remove gloves and discard in biohazard waste container.
11. Wash hands.

Table 26–1	Identification of Bacteria Using Staining Techniques			
Bacteria Shape	**Arrangement**	**Stain Reaction**	**Shape**	**Genus/Species**
Sphere	Pairs and singles	Gram positive		Enterococcus species
		Gram negative		*Neisseria gonorrhoeae*
Sphere	Chains	Gram positive		*Streptococcus pyogenes*
Sphere	Clusters	Gram positive		*Staphylococcus aureus*
Rod (bacillus)	Singles and chains	Gram positive		*Bacillus anthracis* *Clostridium tetani*
		Gram negative		*Escherichia coli*
		Acid-fast		*Haemophilus influenzae* *Pseudomonas aeruginosa* *Mycobacterium tuberculosis* *Mycobacterium leprae*
Spiral	Singles	Gram negative		*Treponema pallidum*

PROCEDURE 26–5

Inoculating a Culture Plate

Performance Objective: The student will inoculate a culture plate using a throat specimen swab.

- ☑ Wash hands
- ☑ Gloves
- ☑ Eye and Face Protection
- ☑ Lab Coat or Apron
- ☑ Plastic Biohazard Bag
- ☐ Rigid Biohazard Container

Supplies and Equipment: Disposable gloves, specimen container containing swabs with bacteria, blood agar plate, loop incinerator, platinum loop (or disposable loop), loop holder, laboratory marker, incubator, biohazard waste container.

Procedure Steps

1. Wash hands.
2. Assemble equipment and supplies.
3. Turn on loop incinerator.
4. Prepare the loop for use by placing it in a loop holder where you will be working.

Rationale: This keeps the tip of the loop from touching anything. It will be sterilized by heating in the loop incinerator.

5. Put on disposable gloves and other personal protective equipment.
6. Remove the cap from the container with the specimen swab and remove one of the swabs. Recap the container and set aside.
7. Place a blood agar plate on the counter, agar side down, and remove the cover.
8. Using the specimen swab, streak approximately one fourth of agar surface.
   Rationale: This transfers some of the specimen to the blood agar plate.
9. Flame inoculating loop in the loop incinerator. If using disposable loops, open a package from the end away from the loops and pull out one loop by the handle.
   Rationale: The inoculating loop must be sterile to avoid introducing bacteria to the agar plate.
10. Go into first streak area at right angles two to three times and spread specimen into second quadrant of plate.
    Rationale: This spreads some of the specimen into the second quadrant of the plate. By

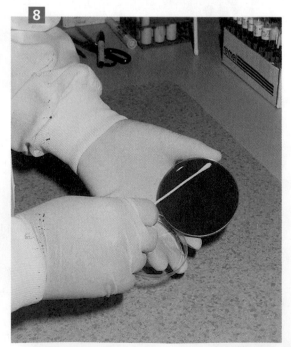

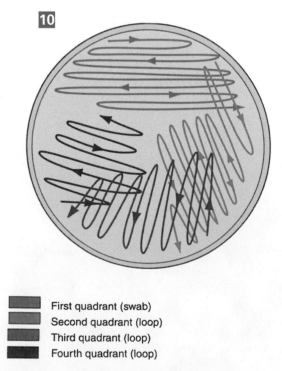

First quadrant (swab)
Second quadrant (loop)
Third quadrant (loop)
Fourth quadrant (loop)

*Figures from Stepp CA, Woods MA: *Laboratory Procedures for Medical Office Personnel.* Philadelphia: W.B. Saunders, 1988.

doing so, this ensures that, if bacteria grow, the colonies will be more isolated.

11. Reflame loop.
12. Go into second streaked area two to three times and at right angles and streak third quadrant of plate.
13. Reflame loop and streak the remainder of plate.
14. Cover the blood agar plate, turn it upside down, and use the laboratory marker to label the plate with the patient's name and date.
15. Reflame the loop and place in the loop holder or discard the disposable loop.
16. Place the blood agar plate in the incubator, agar side up, or place in a plastic biohazard transfer bag with a lab slip and transport to the laboratory immediately.
17. If placed in the incubator, record the date, time, patient's name, and source of the specimen in the laboratory log book.
18. Dispose of waste in the biohazard waste container. Remove gloves and discard in the biohazard waste container.
19. Wash hands.
20. If sent to the laboratory, document the date, time, type and specimen, and laboratory to which it was sent in the patient's medical record.

---

down blood on a blood agar plate. Some bacteria, notably beta-hemolytic streptococci break down the culture medium, creating clear areas in the culture plate, as shown in Figure 26–8, which shows clear areas of hemolysis around colonies of beta-hemolytic streptococci.

Many times, more than one pathogen is growing in a culture. To identify individual organisms, they must be separated from the general culture. This is called creating a pure culture, and is done by picking up the suspicious bacteria colony and streaking it onto a new plate containing an appropriate medium for growth. This plate, which has only one organism present, can be used to set up a number of biochemical tests. This new plate must then be incubated again for an additional 24 hours.

Sometimes the quantity of microorganisms is as important as the type of microorganism present. Streaking for a colony count is usually undertaken with a specimen of body fluid, often urine. A calibrated inoculation loop is needed when performing a streak to determine quantity. The calibrated inoculation loop is used to inoculate a measured amount of fluid onto the culture plate. For a urine specimen, a loop that retains 0.001 mL of fluid is used. Streaking must be done very carefully to get an accurate estimate of the number of bacteria present for a measured sample size.

Cultures should always be incubated according to the growth requirements for the organism being sought. Plates should always be placed agar side up in the incubator to avoid drips from condensation into the media. There are many types of incubators (i.e., aerobic, CO_2, micro-aerophilic), and the proper type should be used to incubate specific cultures.

Additional cultures and/or tests may be necessary to determine the exact type of pathogen present in the culture.

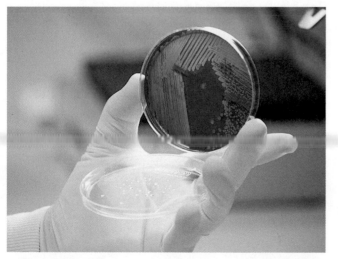

> **Figure 26–8** Clear areas of hemolysis around colonies of beta-hemolytic streptococci. (From Stepp CA, Woods MA: *Laboratory Procedures for Medical Office Personnel*. Philadelphia: W.B. Saunders, 1998.)

Sensitivity Testing

Sensitivity testing is used to determine a microorganism's susceptibility to particular antibiotics. The test is ordered as a culture and sensitivity (**C&S**).

The diffusion method of sensitivity testing shows the ability of any particular antibiotic to inhibit growth of a given organism. The Kirby Bauer method is the most common diffusion method used.

In the Kirby Bauer method, filter disks are impregnated with antibiotics. Organisms are streaked onto plates, and the impregnated disks are placed on top of the plates, using sterile forceps. They are then incubated for 18 to 24 hours and read.

If the antibiotic does not prevent growth of the organism, the organism will have grown close around the disk. If the antibiotic prevents growth, there will be no growth around the disk. Figure 26–9 shows zones of inhibited bacterial growth around sensitivity disks.

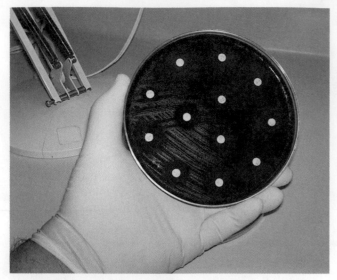

> **Figure 26–9** Zones of inhibition of bacterial growth around sensitivity disks. The greenish lines are bacterial colonies. (From Stepp CA, Woods MA: *Laboratory Procedures for Medical Office Personnel*. Philadelphia: W.B. Saunders, 1998.)

The zones of inhibited growth are measured with a caliper or a template, to the point where there is no growth visible to the eye. The size of the zone is interpreted, and the sensitivity to a particular antibiotic determined, by referring to the National Committee for Clinical Laboratory Standards reference guide.

A few special conditions must be kept in mind when performing this test.

1. Some antibiotics (i.e., sulfonamides) should be interpreted within a margin of heavy growth. Disregard slight growth next to the disk, and measure the zone at the margin of the heavy growth.
2. This method should not be used with fastidious CO_2-requiring organisms (anaerobes).
3. Swarming of *Proteus* into a zone of inhibition should be ignored.

The other major method for sensitivity testing is the dilution method. This is used to measure the minimal

PROCEDURE 26–6

Performing a Urine Culture Using a Dip Slide Kit

Performance Objective: The student will prepare a urine specimen for culture using a dip slide kit and read results.

✓	Wash hands
✓	Gloves
☐	Eye and Face Protection
✓	Lab Coat or Apron
✓	Plastic Biohazard Bag
☐	Rigid Biohazard Container

Supplies and Equipment: Disposable gloves, clean-catch midstream urine specimen either freshly voided or refrigerated, urine dip slide kit (such as Uri✓Check® Plus), incubator, biohazard waste container.

Procedure Steps

1. Wash hands.
2. Assemble equipment and supplies.
3. Put on disposable gloves and personal protective equipment.
4. Open the clean-catch midstream urine specimen without touching the inside of the container. Do not use the slide kit to collect urine.
   Rationale: Touching the inside of the container could introduce bacteria into the specimen.

5. Unscrew the cap of the urine dip slide kit and remove the cap and its attached slide from the vial without touching the slide or the inside of the vial.
   Rationale: Touching the slide or the inside of the vial could introduce bacteria into the specimen.

6. Dip the slide into the freshly voided urine so that the agar surfaces on both sides of the dip slide become totally immersed. If the specimen is of insufficient volume, you can pour urine over the surface of both media using a plastic pipette.
   Rationale: The entire surface of the agar must be exposed to urine to obtain an accurate colony count.

7. Allow excess urine to drain back into the collection container.
   Rationale: Excess urine will cause false high colony counts.

8. Replace agar slide back into the vial. Screw the cap back on but leave the cap about one screw loose.
   Rationale: Urine pathogens require oxygen for growth.

9. Label the collection container with the patient's name, date, and time or use pre-printed labels prepared with the patient's encounter form.

10. Place the dip slide kit in the incubator at 35° to 37° or place in a plastic biohazard transfer bag with a lab slip and transport to the laboratory immediately.

11. If placed in the incubator, record the date, time, patient's name, and source of the specimen in the laboratory log book.

12. Dispose of waste in the biohazard waste container. Remove gloves and discard in the biohazard waste container.

13. Wash hands.

14. If sent to the laboratory, document the date, time, type of specimen, and laboratory to which it was sent.

15. Incubate the slide for 18 to 24 hours. Do not incubate more than 24 hours.
    Rationale: A minimum time period is required to properly enumerate colony counts and characteristics. Incubation longer than 24 hours will cause erroneous results. Most human pathogens grow best at body temperature.

16. Compare growth density to chart supplied by manufacturer.
    - A count of 0–30 colonies is considered nonsignificant.
    - Counts of 31–300 colonies are considered of doubtful significance. Retest patients with specimens in this range, instructing patients to use extra precautions to obtain a clean-catch midstream specimen.
    - Counts of 300 or more colonies per slide indicate a significant level of bacteria in the urine.

17. If results are positive, it is recommended that the doctor review the growth or that the specimen be sent to the laboratory for isolation of the bacteria and drug sensitivity screening.

18. Document the date, time, type of test, and results in the patient's medical record.

amount of antibiotic needed to inhibit or kill a particular organism.

In this method, serial dilutions of antibiotics are inoculated with microorganisms and incubated. The minimal inhibitory concentration is the lowest concentration that inhibits microbial growth. This method is now fully automated.

Urine Culture Using Dip Slide Test Kit

This procedure is used as a screening test for uropathogens. A fresh clean-catch specimen or a catheterized urine specimen is recommended. This test screens for growth of microorganisms; if colonies grow, the culture is sent to a lab for more detailed testing. If there is no growth, the culture is sterile.

Procedure 26–6 describes preparing a urine culture using a dip slide test kit.

TESTING FOR PARASITES

Parasites are organisms that live on or in a host organism. Parasites are of different sizes, from microscopic to the size of insects and visible to the naked eye. They infect blood, feces, tissues, and skin. An examination for parasites includes preparation of slides or wet mounts. See Table 26–2.

Table 26–2	Diseases Caused by Parasites			
Area of Infection	Diseases	Organism	Transmission	Signs and Symptoms
Blood	Malaria	*Plasmodium* species (protozoa)	*Anopheles* mosquito	Chills and fever at regular intervals
Intestine	Amebic dysentery	*Entamoeba histolytica* (protozoa)	Fecal contamination of food and water	Bloody diarrhea, abdominal cramping, fever
Intestine	Giardiasis	*Giardia lamblia* (protozoa)	Contaminated surface water	Diarrhea and cramping; may be asymptomatic
Lungs	Pneumonia	*Pneumocystis carinii* (protozoa)	Common in animals and people with compromised immune systems, such as patients with AIDS	Fever, cough, malaise
Body tissue, including the brain	Toxoplasmosis	*Toxoplasma gondii* (protozoa)	Fecal contamination (cat litter); passed from mother to fetus	Fever, rash; when contracted by the developing fetus causes liver, spleen, and brain abnormalities
Genital area	Trichomoniasis	*Trichomonas vaginalis* (protozoa)	Sexual activity	Vaginal irritation, vaginal discharge
Rectum	Pinworm infestation	*Enterobius vermicularis* (nematode)	Fecal-oral (poor handwashing)	Severe rectal itching, restlessness, insomnia
Intestine	Tapeworm	*Taenia* species, *Diphyllobothrium latum,* and other species of parasitic worms	Undercooked meat or fish	Weight loss, diarrhea, abdominal discomfort
Muscles and tissues	Trichinosis	*Trichinella spiralis* (nematode)	Undercooked pork	Fever, nausea, diarrhea, muscle pain and swelling
Head	Head lice	*Pediculus humanis capitis* (insect)	Direct contact, clothing, bedding	Itching of the head; adult lice and/or eggs (nits) can be seen on hair
Body and/or genital area	Body lice; pubic lice (crabs)	*Pediculus humanis humanus, Pthirus pubis* (insect)	Direct contact, clothing, bedding	Itching of the body and/or pubic area; adult lice and/or eggs (nits) can be seen on body or pubic hair
Under fingernails and/or toenails	Scabies	*Sarcoptes scabiei* (insect)	Direct contact, clothing, bedding	Nocturnal itching, skin burrows seen under fingernails and/or toenails

Collecting Fecal Specimens

A fecal specimen is collected to test for bacteria and/or parasites if a patient's chief complaint is either persistent diarrhea that does not respond to the usual treatment, diarrhea and fever greater than 101° F, or any bloody diarrhea.

A fecal specimen may contain bacteria and/or parasites and should be tested for both.

Fecal collection can be accomplished either by using a rectal swab or by collecting a portion of a bowel movement. The feces should not be exposed to toilet water; therefore, a collection apparatus must be used.

If the patient is hospitalized, this can be done by having the patient use a bedpan. On an outpatient basis, a fecal sample must often be collected at home. The easiest way to do this is to have the patient lay a sheet of clear plastic wrap over the toilet bowl under the seat just before a bowel movement, put a portion of the stool into the sample container, and bring it to the office immediately. The stool should be transported as quickly as possible to the laboratory to avoid pH change.

Any stool specimen that contains visible blood should be tested for hemorrhagic *E. coli* H:027. Unpreserved fecal specimens should be wet mounted in a saline/iodine solution. Other tests may be performed at a laboratory.

Trichomonas

Trichomonas vaginalis are pear-shaped, motile flagellates that cause trichomoniasis, a sexually transmitted disease that affects both males and females. In women, the classic symptom is a yellowish-green vaginal discharge. Men may be asymptomatic for years even if they harbor the parasite. The parasites are identified by microscopic urinalysis, wet mount, or hanging drop. To find *Trichomonas,* the specimen must be examined within 1 hour of being taken, or many of the parasites die out. The specimen should not be allowed to become contaminated with fecal material, which often contains *Trichomonas hominis,* another flagellate.

Pinworm

Pinworms (*Enterobius vermicularis*) are parasites found around the world and are common in children. The worms live in the human intestine, and the female migrates to the anus during the night to lay its eggs. These eggs can cause severe itching during hatching, which can lead to insomnia and irritability. Excessive scratching can also lead to infected wounds.

Sticky cellophane-tape swabs are used to collect samples from around the anus. The tape is placed on a slide and taken to the laboratory for testing. Occassionally, pinworms can be seen on feces or on the skin around the anus.

One negative test should not be taken as conclusive. Tests should be repeated weekly until at least four negative tests have been obtained to say that a patient is free of pinworms.

Checking for Head Lice

Head lice are common among children in all socio-economic categories who attend schools and day-care centers. Head lice cause chronic itching and can lead to infected wounds from excessive scratching if not treated.

Head lice are also highly contagious. Children should be instructed not to share hats or clothing with other children.

Adult lice look like fleas. They also jump, so if one is found on a hair shaft it should be removed with a pair of tweezers and placed under a coverslip on a slide (if removed in a doctor's office) or in a sealable plastic bag (if removed at home). Nits are lice eggs, which attach to the hair shaft.

If one child in a classroom has been diagnosed with lice, all children in the room should be treated prophylactically. This includes examining for living lice and nits, shampooing with a commercial preparation, and delousing the child's environments.

Bedding and hats should be washed in _hot water_. Items that cannot be machine washed, such as pillows and stuffed animals, should be placed in sealed plastic bags for 30 days, as a type of quarantine.

Commercial anti-lice shampoo should be used twice during each treatment, 1 week apart. After the hair is shampooed each time, it should be thoroughly combed with the nit comb that comes as part of the package.

IMMUNOLOGY

Immunology is the study of the immune system and its response to various interruptions by foreign organisms. When harmful microorganisms attack the human body, the immune system responds.

Review of Antigens and Antibodies

Antibodies are produced by B-lymphocytes, transformed into plasma cells, and are found in serum and plasma, the liquid portion of blood after it is either spun in a centrifuge or left to settle. Immunoglobulins are produced in humoral immunity, as discussed in chapter 13.

Each antibody is specific to a target antigen site. An antigen is any particle or substance that can elicit an immune response. Antigens are recognized by the immune system as foreign to the individual, and the immune response is initiated.

Antibodies function both **in vivo** (in the person) and **in vitro** (in the laboratory). This means that the antigen–antibody reaction can be examined in the laboratory—*in vitro*—to simulate what happens in the body.

Methods of Immunology Testing

Immunology testing detects the presence of organisms or antibodies against those organisms or proteins. Immunology testing is also often used to detect viruses, which do not grow in culture.

Specimens Used for Immunology Testing

Some immunology tests require that serum specimens be collected in plain red-capped tubes, not marble-capped tubes. Check with the individual lab being used for the correct protocol for collecting serum for this type of testing. Plasma (blood from a lavender-capped tube) can also be used for some tests.

Other immunology specimens include random-specimen urine (preferably the first morning void), cerebrospinal fluid (CSF), and throat culture for rapid strep testing.

PROCEDURE 26–7

Urine Pregnancy Testing

Performance Objective: The student will perform a urine pregnancy test and determine the results of the test.

- ☑ Wash hands
- ☑ Gloves
- ☐ Eye and Face Protection
- ☑ Lab Coat or Apron
- ☑ Plastic Biohazard Bag
- ☐ Rigid Biohazard Container

Supplies and Equipment: Disposable gloves, urine sample collected in clean container (preferably first morning specimen), minute timer, in-date urine pregnancy test kit containing test cassettes and disposable pipettes, biohazard waste container.

Procedure Steps

The following test procedure is based on the Contrast® hCG-Urine Test. Follow manufacturer instructions for other test kit procedures.

1. Wash hands.
2. Assemble equipment and supplies.
3. Put on disposable gloves and apply personal protective equipment.
4. Remove test kit from pouch.
5. Label each test kit with patient's name and date.

Rationale: All patient lab work should be labeled for accuracy.

6. Aspirate urine with disposable pipette.
7. Drop 3 drops urine in test well from the back of the kit.
Rationale: The correct amount of urine must be used to ensure accurate results.
8. Begin timer.
9. At exactly 3 minutes read results. A positive is indicated by a brown line at the "T" zone. A thicker brown line at the "C" zone must be present on both positive and negative results for the test to be valid.
Rationale: Internal quality control is indicated by the thick brown line at the "C" zone, as outlined in the above procedure, and must be present after 3 minutes. If this line is not present, the test is invalid.
10. External controls should be run when each new test kit is opened. External positive and negative controls may be purchased separately.
11. Dispose of specimen and used supplies in the biohazard waste container. Remove gloves and discard in the biohazard waste container.
12. Wash hands.
13. Record date, time, and brand of test and results in the patient's medical record.

Charting Example	
Date	
11/24/XX	9:15 AM Contrast hCG test: positive.
	C. Johnson, RMA

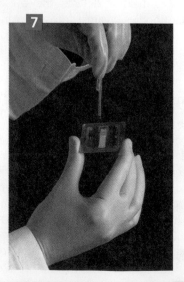

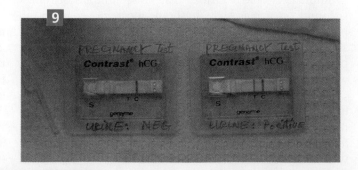

Immunology Tests

Pregnancy Testing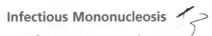

Literally hundreds of urine pregnancy test kits are on the market. Urine pregnancy tests are based on the principle that human chorionic gonadotropin (**hCG**) hormone is produced by the placenta shortly after implantation. An antibody specific against hCG reacts with hCG when it is present in sufficient quantity in the urine. Urine pregnancy tests are sensitive immunoassays or agglutination inhibition tests for the qualitative detection of hCG in urine. Pregnancy testing can also be done on serum using a kit designed for serum.

When performing a pregnancy test, the medical assistant must measure the precise amount of urine using the dropper supplied by the manufacturer. She or he must also time the test precisely according to the directions supplied with the test kit. Procedure 26–7 discusses urine pregnancy testing.

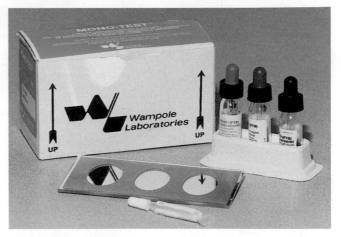

> **Figure 26–10** Mono-Test (Wampole Laboratories) used to test serum or plasma for infectious mononucleosis. (From Stepp CA, Woods MA: *Laboratory Procedures for Medical Office Personnel.* Philadelphia: W.B. Saunders, 1998.)

Infectious Mononucleosis

Infectious mononucleosis is caused by the **Epstein-Barr virus (EBV)** or **cytomegalovirus (CMV)**. The **heterophile antibodies**—specific antibodies seen in infectious mononucleosis—are produced during the infectious episode; these are a group of antibodies that can react with surface antigens on red blood cells. In addition to the presence of heterophile antibodies, infectious mononucleosis also causes an elevation in the number of atypical lymphocytes in the white blood cell count. Several test kits are available to test for infectious mononucleosis. An agglutination or **immunoassay** (a test for the presence of a specific antibody) can also be used.

Figure 26–10 shows a mononucleosis test kit. When using mononucleosis test kits, either serum or plasma from a certified venipuncture specimen may be used. The manufacturer's directions should be followed exactly to determine how much of the specimen to add and how many drops of the developer solution to add.

After reading the correct amount of time, the medical assistant should read the results. As with the pregnancy test, the C (control) line must appear for the test to be valid. A positive result also shows a line at the "T" zone. The results should be recorded in the patient's medical record.

Helicobacter pylori Testing

Several different immunoassays can be used to test serum or plasma for antibodies to *H. pylori,* the bacteria associated with gastric ulcers and other gastrointestinal conditions. The test kits are similar to those used for mononucleosis testing. Serum or plasma is mixed with reagents and observed for agglutination (clumping).

Rapid Strep Tests

Several rapid strep tests are on the market today. Rapid strep tests are based on the principle of the polyclonal anti-strep A antibody–strep A antigen complex. If group A streptococci are present in a specimen, they are placed in solution by adding reagents, and bind to antigroup A streptococcal antibodies present in the test pads. This causes a color change that indicates a positive test.

These rapid tests are beneficial because the doctor can begin treating a positive result immediately. If the test is negative, ideally a second specimen should be sent to a laboratory for a culture. Therefore, when swabbing the throat of an individual in whom strep is suspected, the medical assistant may want to use two swabs—one for the rapid strep test and the other to send for culture in the event of a negative rapid strep test. Procedure 26–8 identifies the steps for rapid strep testing.

Blood Type Antigens

The major blood groups A, B, and O, as well as the Rh factor, are determined by proteins or antigens on the surface of red blood cells. Red cells are therefore classified as blood group A, B, AB, or O. The A and B blood groups have naturally occurring antibodies.

An individual with type A blood has anti-B in his or her serum. Conversely, an individual with type B blood has anti-A circulating in his or her serum. Type O blood individuals have neither A nor B antigens on their red blood cells, so they have anti-A and anti-B in their serum. Finally, individuals with an AB blood type have neither anti-A nor anti-B in their serum, because they have both A and B antigens on their red blood cells.

PROCEDURE 26-8

Performing a Rapid Strep Test

Performance Objective: The student will perform and read a rapid strep test.

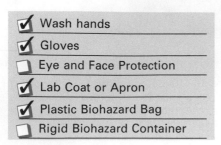

✓	Wash hands
✓	Gloves
☐	Eye and Face Protection
✓	Lab Coat or Apron
✓	Plastic Biohazard Bag
☐	Rigid Biohazard Container

Supplies and Equipment: Disposable gloves, throat specimen (see throat specimen collection procedure), Clearview Strep A test kit containing test unit, extraction tube, and reagents 1, 2 and 3.

Procedure Steps

(This procedure uses the Clearview Strep A test kit; follow manufacturer's directions for other products.)

1. Wash hands.
2. Assemble equipment and supplies.
3. Check the kit expiration date to be sure the kit has not expired.
4. Put on disposable gloves and apply personal protective equipment.
5. Place open plastic tube in tube stand (in test kit box).

6. Place 4 drops of reagent 1 and 4 drops of reagent 2 into the extraction tube.
7. Insert the specimen swab into the tube and mix well. Allow the swab to remain in the tube for at least 2 minutes, but not more than 15 minutes.
   Rationale: This allows bacteria to move from the swab into the solution.
8. Add 4 drops of reagent 3.
9. Use the swab to mix the contents.
10. Express all liquid from swab by rolling swab head against side of plastic tube and pressing slightly while withdrawing swab. Discard the swab.
    Rationale: The reacted liquid from the swab is what will continue to be tested for results.
11. Put the cap on the extraction tube. The test may be performed at any time within the next hour.
12. Remove test cassette from foil pouch.
13. Remove a test unit from the foil package and place on a level surface.
14. Open the extraction tube and drop 3 drops on the paper in the sample window of the test unit (the window at the bottom of the unit labeled STREP A).
15. Begin timing.
16. Read result at exactly 5 minutes. A positive result is the appearance of a pink line in the results window (the larger test window). A

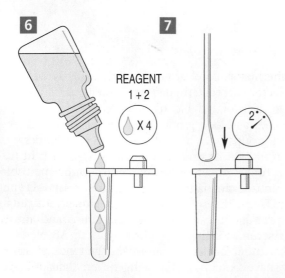

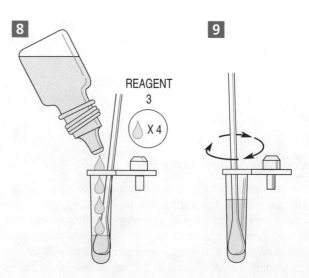

pink line must appear in the control window (the smaller window) for the test to be valid.

17. All negatives should be plated for group A beta hemolytic streptococci using a second specimen swab (see Procedure 26–5).
18. Dispose of used supplies in biohazard waste container. Remove gloves and discard in biohazard waste container.
19. Wash hands.
20. Record date, time, type of test, and results in the patient's medical record.

Quality control

Internal quality control is a red line in the control window, as indicated in the above procedure. Reagent 4 is a positive control included with each test kit. External controls should be run with each new opened test kit; record results.

Charting Example	
Date	
8/14/XX	12:15 PM Clearview Strep A test:
	positive
	S. Williams, CMA

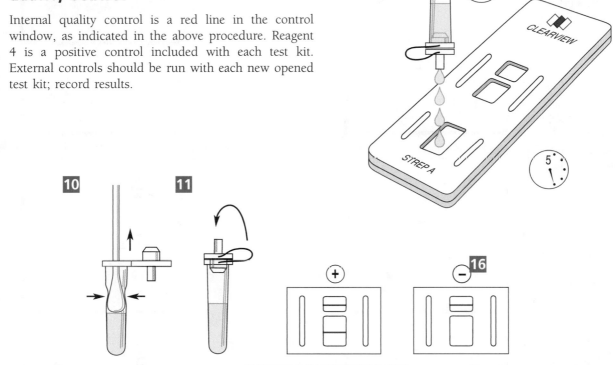

This is why it is necessary to immediately type an individual who needs emergency treatment and provide matched blood from the blood bank for any necessary transfusion. Although medical assistants do not usually perform blood testing, they should understand the principles.

Because type O blood has no antigens present on red cells, blood type O is known as the "universal donor" and can be given to a person with blood types A, B, or AB in an emergency situation. Blood group AB positive is known as the "universal recipient," because a person with AB-positive blood can receive blood from any other donor.

The Rh antigen only elicits an antibody response if a person without the antigen (Rh negative) is exposed to Rh-positive blood. A woman with Rh-negative blood must be given a RhoGam injection at 7 months' gestation, after a miscarriage, after trauma during pregnancy, or when an Rh-positive infant is delivered. If the RhoGam is not given, sensitization may occur with the first Rh-positive fetus, and the second Rh-positive fetus may exhibit hemolytic disease of the newborn. This is discussed in detail in chapter 29, Obstetrics.

Blood types are determined by adding antibodies to serum specimens. If the blood antigen is present, **agglutination** (clumping of blood cells) occurs, as shown in Figure 26–11.

Immunology Tests

Many testing methods are employed in serology testing. The most common tests a medical assistant would use are agglutination, enzyme immunoassay, and chromatographic assays. More complex methods include complement fixation assays and immunofluorescent techniques used in virology testing.

Agglutination tests look for the presence of an antibody (a qualitative test) or the amount of antibody (a

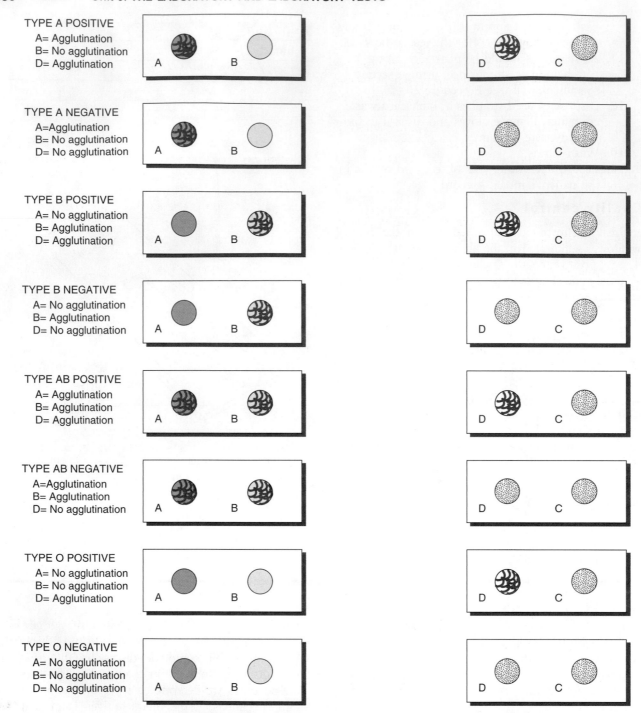

TYPE A POSITIVE
A= Agglutination
B= No agglutination
D= Agglutination

TYPE A NEGATIVE
A=Agglutination
B= No agglutination
D= No agglutination

TYPE B POSITIVE
A= No agglutination
B= Agglutination
D= Agglutination

TYPE B NEGATIVE
A= No agglutination
B= Agglutination
D= No agglutination

TYPE AB POSITIVE
A= Agglutination
B= Agglutination
D= Agglutination

TYPE AB NEGATIVE
A=Agglutination
B= Agglutination
D= No agglutination

TYPE O POSITIVE
A= No agglutination
B= No agglutination
D= Agglutination

TYPE O NEGATIVE
A= No agglutination
B= No agglutination
D= No agglutination

➤ **Figure 26–11** Blood can be tested for blood type by combining a drop of blood with anti-A, anti-B, and anti-D (contains antibodies to the Rh factor) solutions. If antigens are present in the blood, agglutination will result. C is the control (negative).

quantitative test). Quantitative serology tests are also referred to as titer evaluations. A **titer** is a standard of strength per volume of solution. A number of test kits use the agglutination method.

When an antibody–antigen reaction occurs, the complex is not visible to the naked eye. By attaching either latex particles or red blood cells to the reagent,

it is possible to see the antigen–antibody complex in the form of agglutination, or clumping, of the latex or red blood cells.

An agglutination test may be performed on a slide or in a test tube. Agglutination tests are used to detect mononucleosis, rheumatoid factor, the **ABO** blood group, and to identify microorganisms.

Complement fixation tests involve the complement (a series of protein enzymes) in serum that produces lysis of red blood cells when combined with an antibody–antigen complex. Complement fixation tests are done primarily in a reference laboratory. The Venereal Disease Research Laboratory (VDRL) test panel is an example of a complement fixation test. A common test for syphilis, it is performed in a laboratory and is routine during pregnancy and before surgery.

Enzyme immunoassay **(EIA or ELISA)** testing can detect extremely small quantities of antibodies in a person's serum or antigen in a specimen taken for culture.

Enzymes are used to detect particular antibodies or antigens found in certain disease states. A link is formed between the antibody and the antigen, which binds to an enzyme to produce a color reaction.

EIA can be used for qualitative and semi-quantitative evaluation of viral, bacterial, fungal, and parasitic antigens and antibodies. Test kits are common. EIA is used for such tests as serum or urine pregnancy testing for hCG; human immunodeficiency virus; hepatitis A, B, C, D, or E; past or present viral infections such as rubella (German measles) or chicken pox; toxic drugs and chemicals; and thyroid hormones.

Chromatography is a type of test that separates substances in solution by passing them across the surface of an absorbent paper. The process is used in reference labs for specific testing, including drug analysis.

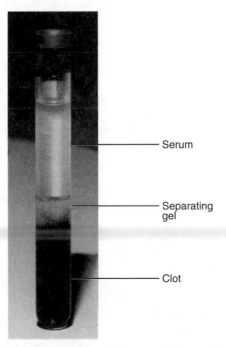

Serum

Separating gel

Clot

> **Figure 26–12** Serum in red/black marbled tube (tiger top) after being centrifuged. (From Stepp CA, Woods MA: *Laboratory Procedures for Medical Office Personnel.* Philadelphia: W.B. Saunders, 1998.)

CHEMISTRY TESTING

Chemistry testing refers to the study of the chemical constituents of the human body.

Types of Specimens

Tubes with different colored tops are used to collect blood that will be used in different tests. The medical assistant must follow the protocol of the particular lab that will perform the tests as to how to prepare samples for testing.

Serum is either collected in a tube with a plain red top, a red/black monojet (for a stat serum, one that must be performed immediately), or a red/gray marbled top (a serum separator tube [SST] or so-called tiger top). In the tiger top tube, allow the blood to sit for 15 to 30 minutes after being drawn so a clot can form, then centrifuge the sample. The gel moves up to separate the serum from the clot, so the serum does not have to be removed immediately. This is shown in Figure 26–12.

Plasma is collected in a tube with a green top for electrolyte testing and in a gray-capped tube for glucose and alcohol testing. Plasma can be used for most chemical tests; because it does not have to stand for clot formation, it is often used for stat tests.

Reminder: All tubes with additives should be gently inverted 8 to 10 times after filling, in order to mix blood with the additives in the tube.

Other specimens also have chemistry testing performed on them, such as urine (usually a sample from a 24-hour collection), cerebrospinal fluid and other body fluids, and whole blood for blood gases and ketones.

Chemistry Analyzers

Often, several tests are done at once, using automated chemistry analyzers. Usually, these complex machines are found in hospitals and reference laboratories. Individual tests can also be done in the analyzers. In the office, where individual tests are usually performed, capillary blood from a finger stick may be used or blood from a venipuncture.

Blood Glucose

Elevated blood glucose, known as **hyperglycemia,** is associated with **diabetes mellitus,** a disorder of carbohydrate metabolism that occurs when the pancreas fails to produce insulin or when the insulin is ineffective in transporting glucose to cells.

Low blood glucose, known as **hypoglycemia,** occurs when a diabetic individual takes too much insulin or when an individual cannot maintain adequate glucose levels.

Although the blood glucose level rises after a person ingests glucose, it should return to normal within 2 hours. Blood glucose testing is used to monitor how quickly a person's blood glucose returns to normal after ingesting a specified amount of glucose over a particular time.

After fasting for 12 hours, normal glucose should be 70 to 110 mg/dl (milligrams per deciliter) of blood. A fasting glucose test or fasting blood sugar **(FBS)** measures a glucose level in the morning after a 12-hour fast.

A glucose tolerance test is more sensitive. In this test, the person is asked to drink a specially prepared, high-glucose drink, and then has blood drawn at regular intervals for 3 to 6 hours, depending on the doctor's orders, to see how quickly the glucose level returns to relative normal. Urine tests are performed simultaneously to monitor the level of glucose and ketones in the urine.

After ingesting the high-glucose drink the patient's blood sugar (glucose level) rises. In a normal individual, the pancreas secretes enough insulin to counteract the high glucose level. Insulin causes cells to absorb the glucose, so the blood sugar level falls to normal limits within 2 hours. A diabetic individual does not produce enough insulin or the insulin may be ineffective, so the blood glucose level remains high.

The renal threshold is usually 175 mg/dl, which means the kidneys will not allow glucose to pass into the urine until the level of glucose in the blood is greater than 175 mg/dl. Glucose over the kidneys' threshold spills into glomerular filtrate and is excreted in the urine. When a person has glucose in their urine, it usually indicates that the blood glucose level is in excess of the renal threshold.

A 2-hour postprandial (after eating) blood glucose level is taken 2 hours after the individual eats a normal meal, and should register less than 140 mg/dl. The medical assistant should be aware of the requirements of the lab that will test the blood; some prescribe a specific meal for this test.

A random blood sugar is a glucose measurement taken at any time during the day. If elevated, the doctor may order an FBS or 2-hour postprandial blood test to investigate further.

Several types of glucose analyzers are available for the office laboratory. They usually use a blood specimen from a finger stick. Diabetics also use a handheld glucometer for their daily glucose measurement. Many brands of glucometer are available. Procedure 26–9 describes glucose testing using a glucometer. This topic will be discussed further in chapter 33, where diabetic teaching is discussed in detail.

Cholesterol

Cholesterol is an unsaturated steroid alcohol that is solid at room temperature. The human body manufactures cholesterol, which is necessary for the production of steroid hormones in both males and females. The body is very efficient at making cholesterol, but it is not as efficient at breaking it down. Therefore, in some people, cholesterol levels rise.

Measuring cholesterol can either be done as part of a chemistry panel or a lipid profile—discussed later in the chapter and conducted at a reference laboratory—or it can be done as a screening test in the office. The specimen of choice for measuring cholesterol is serum, drawn after 8 to 12 hours of fasting.

Total cholesterol level should be below 200 mg/dl of blood.

Office instruments for testing cholesterol operate on a similar principle to those used for testing glucose. The machine should be calibrated and controls should be run daily. The medical assistant should be careful to avoid touching the testing area of the reagent strip. If a finger stick is used to obtain blood, the first drop should be wiped away. The medical assistant should read the instruction manual for the particular instrument he or she plans to use.

Triglycerides

The measurement of triglycerides is also done as part of the lipid profile. **Triglycerides** are a form of lipid that serve as energy. Glycerol and fatty acids from the diet are converted to triglycerides to be used as energy. Triglycerides are transported throughout the body by low-density lipoproteins; when the level of triglycerides in the blood becomes excessive, they settle in the tissues as fat.

Lipid Profile

The lipid profile measures the level of total cholesterol and triglycerides, as well as the level of high-density lipoproteins (HDL) and low-density lipoproteins (LDL).

HDL is responsible for transporting cholesterol to the liver to assist in the manufacture of bile; HDL is sometimes known as "good cholesterol," LDL, which is sometimes known as "bad cholesterol," transports cholesterol to blood vessels and tissues, and is responsible for leaving behind the deposits of cholesterol in arteries.

The levels of HDL, LDL, and cholesterol are partially dependent on age and sex, but should fall within the following "rough normal" ranges:

HDL: 40–70 mg/dl
LDL: 40–130 mg/dl
Chol: 125–200 mg/dl.

PROCEDURE 26-9

Testing for Glucose Using a Glucometer Elite Analyzer

Performance Objective: The student will measure blood glucose using a handheld glucometer.

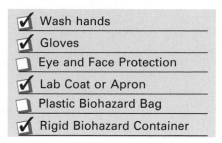

- ☑ Wash hands
- ☑ Gloves
- ☐ Eye and Face Protection
- ☑ Lab Coat or Apron
- ☐ Plastic Biohazard Bag
- ☑ Rigid Biohazard Container

Supplies and Equipment: Disposable gloves, Glucometer Elite blood glucose analyzer with batteries, check strip, code strip for calibration of test strips, test strips, glucose control: normal level, lancet, gauze, bandage, alcohol pads, rigid biohazard waste container.

Procedure Steps

This procedure is based on the Glucometer elite blood glucose analyzer.

1. Wash hands.
2. Gather equipment and supplies.

Check the Meter Performance

3. Check the performance of the meter by inserting the check strip into the meter with the tab toward the top of the meter.
   Rationale: The check strip will only read in one position. If the meter beeps when the strip is in place and again when the result is displayed, the meter is functioning.
4. Compare the result with the check strip range listed on the label inside the check strip box.
   Rationale: This verifies that the meter is functioning correctly. If the result is not within range, refer to the "Problem Solving" chart.

Calibrate the Meter

5. If using a new vial of test strips, use the code strip to calibrate the instrument.
   Rationale: Each vial of reagent strips will contain a code strip that calibrates the instrument to that specific reagent lot number.
6. Insert the code strip into the test slot with the function number face up and the tab at the top.

Rationale: The function number will be printed on the code strip, the code strip packet, and each individual test strip. It is not necessary to calibrate the meter if the new vial of test strips has the same function number as the previous vial of test strips.

7. A beep will sound when the code strip is fully in place. A second beep will sound and the function number will be displayed. If beep does not sound, reposition code strip with a firm motion until it comes to a full stop.
   Rationale: The function number displayed on the meter must match the code strip for accurate results.

Run a control test at the beginning of each day.

8. Remove a test strip from the foil packet by carefully peeling foil to the line to expose the meter end of the test strip.
   Rationale: Touching the test end of the strip will contaminate the test area.
9. Hold the end of the test strip between two layers of foil and insert the test strip fully into the meter. A beep will sound followed by the function number.
   Rationale: The beep tells you that the test strip is properly seated. The function number tells you that the instrument is calibrated to the test strips.
10. Pull the test strip from the meter and quickly reinsert the test strip within 2 seconds. A "C" and the function number will alternately flash on the screen.
    Rationale: This procedure alerts the instrument that a control, not a patient specimen, is going to be tested.
11. Gently squeeze a drop of normal control fluid onto the inside of the foil of the test strip.
    Rationale: The drop of control fluid simulates a patient's blood and should be a rounded drop, not flat.
12. Touch the test end of the test strip to the drop until a beep is heard.
    Rationale: The fluid will fill the test strip end by capillary action.
13. Wait while the timer automatically times the specimen for 59 seconds.

Procedure continued on following page

Rationale: Results are based on a constant test time.

14. When a result appears in the meter screen, compare it to the range listed on the end flap of the test strip container.
    Rationale: If the control strip is within the specified range, the meter is functioning properly. If it is out of range, consult the "Problem Solving" chart in the instruction book. Do not perform testing if the control is out of range.
15. Remove strip and the meter will automatically turn off.
16. Record that the meter was calibrated and the results of the control in the lab log book.

Procedure Steps to Test Glucose

1. Wash hands.
2. Assemble supplies and equipment.
3. Identify the patient and ask when the patient last ate and took insulin (if applicable). The patient should have washed and dried his or her hands thoroughly before the procedure.
4. Explain the procedure.
5. Put on disposable gloves and personal protective equipment.
6. Remove a test strip from the foil packet by carefully peeling the foil to the line to expose the meter end of the test strip.
   Rationale: Touching the test end of the test strip will contaminate the test area.
7. Hold the test end of the strip between two layers of foil and insert the test strip fully into the meter. A beep will sound followed by the function number.
   Rationale: The beep tells you that the test strip is properly seated. The function number tells you that the instrument is calibrated to the test strip.
8. Perform a finger stick with a lancet as described in Procedure 25-4. Wipe away the first drop of blood.

Rationale: The first drop of blood is contaminated with tissue fluid and will dilute the specimen. A false low result could be obtained.

9. Touch the test end of the test strip to the blood and hold until a beep is heard.
   Rationale: Blood is automatically drawn into the test strip by capillary action.
10. After 59 seconds a result will appear on the meter screen. This is the patient's glucose level.
    Rationale: Test results are based on a constant reaction time.
11. The result will be stored when you remove the test strip. If you do not want to save the result, reinsert the strip within 2 seconds and remove.
    Rationale: A single patient may want to store results. Analyzers testing many patients may not want to store this information.
12. Dispose of used supplies and test strip in a biohazard waste container (lancet in a rigid container). Remove disposable gloves and discard in a biohazard waste container.
13. Wash hands.
14. Record patient results in the patient's medical record. You should include the date, time, time of the patient's last meal, and time and amount of the patient's most recent insulin dose or oral hypoglycemic medication.

Charting Example

Date	
8/22/XX	9:15 AM FBS: 92 mg/dL. Pt. has not eaten since snack at 9:00 PM on 8/21/XX. Does not take antidiabetic medication. — C. Johnson, RMA

Blood Urea Nitrogen

Blood urea nitrogen (**BUN**) is a by-product of protein metabolism. The BUN test measures the amount of urea in the blood. Urea is normally broken down in the liver, removed from the blood by the kidneys, and eliminated in urine. Normally, BUN levels are between 8 and 25 mg/dl of blood. BUN is usually measured in a chemical analyzer and is included in general chemistry screens such as the SMA-12 and SMA-20.

The level of urea in the blood indicates the liver's ability to break down protein and the kidney's ability to remove urea from the blood. A high BUN is found in people with kidney disease or conditions in which blood fluid volume is decreased. Low levels of BUN are found in people with liver disease and in cases of malnutrition.

Other Common Chemistry Tests

Many chemistry tests are performed as part of so-called chemistry screening panels.

The **Chem-7** panel measures glucose, creatinine, BUN, and electrolytes including Na$^+$, K$^+$, Cl, and CO_2 (sodium, potassium chloride, and carbon dioxide). Whenever tissue is damaged, enzymes from the cells are released into the bloodstream. The doctor looks for a pattern of elevated enzymes to determine the specific tissue that has been affected.

The **Chem-12** panel measures the above, as well as five other tests. Different laboratories have slightly dif-ferent chemistry combinations for their panels. The **Chem-20** panel adds eight more tests.

A **liver panel** measures liver enzymes such as ala-nine aminotransferase (ALT), gamma-glutamyl transfer-ase (GGT), aspartate aminotransferase (AST), and alka-line phosphatase (ALP), as well as the total and direct bilirubin levels.

A cardiac panel measures lactate dehydrogenase (LDH), alanine aminotransferase (ALT), and creatinine kinase (CK).

Table 26−3 shows normal values for blood chemis-try.

Table 26–3	**Blood Chemistry Normal Values**	
Name of Test	**Abbreviation**	**Reference Range for Adults**
Alanine aminotransferase	ALT	6–37 U/L
Albumin		3.5–5.5 g/dL
Alkaline phosphatase	ALP	0.8–2.0 BLB Unit
Amylase		95–290 U/L
Anion gap (R factor)	AG	10–18 mEq/L
Aspartate transaminase	AST	5–30 U/L
Bilirubin, total		0.2–1.2 mg/dL
Bilirubin, conjugated		0.1–0.3 mg/dL
Blood urea nitrogen	BUN	5–20 mg/dL
Calcium	Ca	8.4–10.2 mg/dL
Carbon dioxide	CO_2	22–29 mEq/L
Chloride	Cl	98–106 mEq/L
Cholesterol, total	CH or Chol	Desirable	< 200 mg/dL
		Borderline	200–239 mg/dL
		High	> 240 mg/dL
Low-density lipoprotein	LDL	Desirable	< 170 mg/dL
		Borderline	170–199 mg/dL
		High	> 200 mg/dL
High-density lipoprotein	HDL	Males	29–60 mg/dL
		Females	38–75 mg/dL
Creatine kinase	CK	Males	15–160 U/L
		Females	15–130 U/L
Creatinine		Males	0.6–1.2 mg/dL
		Females	0.5–1.1 mg/dL
Glucose, fasting	FBS	70–120 mg/dL
Glucose, 2-hour postprandial	PPBS	< 140 mg/dL
Glucose tolerance test	GTT	FBS	70–110 mg/dL
		30 min	110–170 mg/dL
		1 hr	120–170 mg/dL
		2 hr	70–120 mg/dL
		3 hr	← 120 mg/dL
Iron	Fe	40–160 μg/dL
Total iron binding capacity	TIBC	250–400 μg/dL
Lactic dehydrogenase	LD	100–200 U/L
Lipase		0–1.0 U/mL
Magnesium	Mag, Mg	1.3–2.1 mEq/L
Phosphorus	P	2.7–4.5 mg/dL
Potassium	K	3.5–5.1 mEq/L
Protein, total	TP	6.2–8.2 g/dL
Sodium	Na	136–146 mEq/L
Triglycerides	Trig	10–190 mg/dL
Uric acid		Males	3.5–7.2 mg/dL
		Females	2.6–6.0 mg/dL

Measurement of Drugs for Therapeutic Level

The amount of a particular drug in the blood can be measured to check if the level is adequate for therapeutic results. Too low a level may mean the drug is not having the desired effect on the condition being treated. Too high a level can be toxic in some instances. In addition, some medications are prone to abuse, and a number of drugs are commonly found in victims of overdose.

A drug screen for common recreational drugs of abuse includes urine, serum, or gastric content analysis for:

1. barbiturates, either short-, intermediate-, or long-acting;
2. narcotics, such as heroin, morphine, codeine, and synthetics such as meperidine, methadone, propoxyphene, and pentazocine.
3. other drugs, such as cannabinoids (marijuana), LSD, and PCP (angel dust).

Drugs Tested for Therapeutic Levels

acetaminophen	methotrexate
amikacin	phenobarbital
carbamazepine	phenytoin
chloramphenicol	procainamide
desipramine	NAPA
digoxin	quinidine
gentamicin	salicylate
imipramine	theophylline
lidocaine	tobramycin
lithium	valproic acid

Drugs Tested for Overdose

acetaminophen	ethylene glycol
acetone	morphine
barbiturates	phenytoin
codeine	phencyclidine
diazepam	salicylate
ethanol	tricyclic antidepressants

STUDENT STUDY PLAN

To reinforce your understanding of the material in this chapter . . .

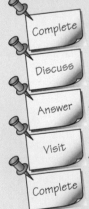

Complete the **Review & Recall** questions.

Discuss the situation in **If You Were the Medical Assistant** with your classmates and answer the questions.

Answer the **Critical Thinking Questions** and discuss them with your classmates.

Visit suggested **Web sites** and search for additional Web sites using **Keywords for Internet Searches.**

Complete the exercises in Chapter 26 of the **Student Mastery Manual.**

REVIEW & RECALL

1. Describe special equipment used to perform microbiological tests.
2. Describe quality control measures used when testing microbiological specimens in the laboratory.
3. Describe how specimens are collected by a medical assistant for wound culture, throat culture, and urine culture.
4. List methods of preparation for examining live and killed organisms under the microscope.
5. How does the Gram stain assist in the identification of microorganisms? the Ziehl-Neelsen stain for acid-fast organisms?

6. Describe how different types of culture media are used to grow microorganisms in the laboratory.
7. Why is a specimen introduced to the culture plate in four quadrants?
8. List common parasites and the diseases they cause.
9. How is the antigen–antibody response used in diagnostic testing? Give several examples.
10. Describe the four ABO blood groups. Describe the Rh factor.
11. What part of the blood contains chemical elements?

12. What is the significance of testing for glucose in the blood?

13. Discuss cholesterol testing in the management of risk factors for atherosclerosis and coronary artery disease.

14. Discuss how the measurement of blood urea nitrogen correlates to normal liver function.

 IF YOU WERE THE MEDICAL ASSISTANT

A patient has called the office with complaints of bloody diarrhea and abdominal cramping for the past 3 days. The patient explains that he has recently returned from a business trip to Mexico. After receiving the patient's message, Dr. Hughes asks you to call the patient and instruct him to collect the next three stools to be tested for ova and parasites.
   Prepare specific instructions for the patient.

 CRITICAL THINKING QUESTIONS

1. Identify as many reasons as you can why it is important for the office laboratory to perform controls daily, to calibrate equipment, and to keep records of the results.

2. Compare and contrast immunologic and chemical testing. Consider what types of specimens are tested, how the tests work, what methods are used for testing, and what units or methods are used to express results.

3. Occasionally, patients come to the medical office with head or body lice. Discuss with your classmates how such a patient should be treated and the measures that must be taken to prevent staff or other patients from contracting lice. Describe your emotional reaction to the idea of a person having lice. How would you want to be treated if you or your child were such a patient?

 EXPLORE THE WEB

INTERNET WEB SITES

Blood type
http://gslc.genetics.utah.edu/basic/blood/types.htm

Gram stain tutorial
www.courses.ahc.umn.edu/pharmacy/5825/GSTutorial.html

Virtual library: microbiology and virology
www.microbiol.org/vl_micro/index.htm

KEYWORDS FOR INTERNET SEARCHES

blood type
cholesterol test
glucose test
Gram stain
Helicobacter pylori
immunology
microbiology
mononucleosis
strep throat
throat culture

6 SPECIAL POPULATIONS

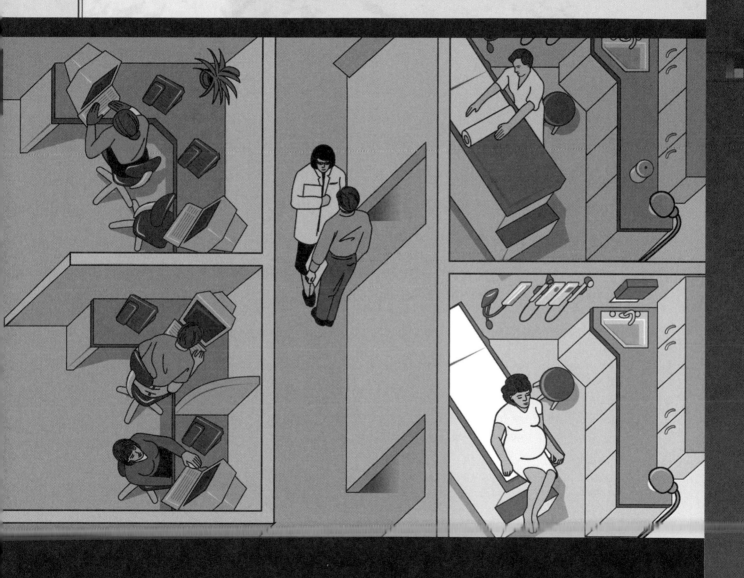

Pediatrics

Instructional Objectives

After completing this chapter, you will be able to do the following:

1. Define and spell the vocabulary words.
2. Describe the normal growth and development of an infant in the first year of life.
3. Explain why regular measurements of length, weight, and head circumference are necessary in childhood and how these measurements are recorded.
4. Describe how the psychosocial development of an infant or child is assessed.
5. Correlate the stage of growth and development of an infant or child to specific actions and/or responses of a medical assistant.
6. Differentiate between well-child visits and sick visits in terms of reason for visit and procedures done during the visit.
7. Describe how to prepare a child for a well-child examination.
8. Compare the procedures for measuring an infant's length and a child's height.
9. Compare the procedures for weighing an infant and a child.
10. Describe how to measure head and chest circumference.
11. Describe the proper method for plotting length or height, weight, and/or head circumference on a growth chart.
12. Identify safe methods to take the temperature of an infant or preschool child.
13. Describe methods to measure an infant's pulse and respiration accurately.
14. Explain how blood and urine specimens may be obtained from infants and young children.
15. Correlate the seven recommended immunizations for children to the diseases they prevent and the usual schedule for administration.
16. Identify special requirements for documentation of immunizations that have been administered.
17. Describe the instructions given to parents about the side effects of pediatric immunizations.
18. Describe three other types of examinations that may be performed during the well-child visit.
19. Describe the medical assistant's responsibilities when assisting with a sick visit for an infant or child.
20. List signs and symptoms of possible child abuse or neglect that should be brought to the doctor's attention.

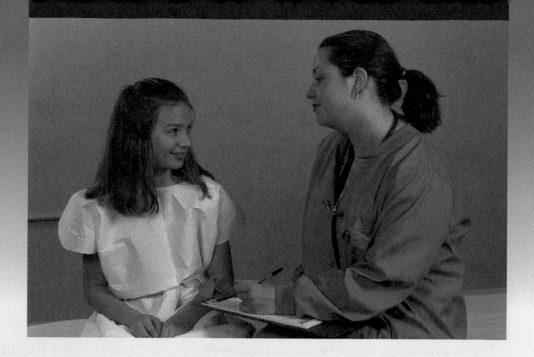

- Prepare patients and assist with routine specialty exams.
- Maintain medication and immunization records.

- Instruct individuals according to their needs.

Performance Objectives

After completing this chapter, you will be able to do the following:

1. Measure an infant's length (Procedure 27–1).
2. Weigh an infant (Procedure 27–2).
3. Measure an infant's head circumference (Procedure 27–3).
4. Measure an infant's chest circumference (Procedure 27–4).
5. Measure an infant's apical pulse (Procedure 27–5).
6. Measure an infant's respirations (Procedure 27–6).
7. Obtain an infant's urine specimen (Procedure 27–7).

VOCABULARY

abuse (p. 694)	growth (p. 673)	neglect (p. 694)	tympanic (p. 683)
aural (p. 683)	hydrocephalus (p. 682)	polio (p. 688)	varicella (p. 689)
circumference (p. 681)	immunization (p. 687)	scoliosis (p. 692)	vaccine (p. 688)
development (p. 673)	mandated (p. 695)	toxoid (p. 688)	

ABBREVIATIONS

DTaP (p. 688)	Hib (p. 688)	MMR (p. 688)	OPV (p. 688)	PCV-7 (p. 689)	Var (p. 689)
HBV (HepB) (p. 688)	IPV (p. 688)				

Pediatrics is the branch of medicine that deals with the normal growth and development of children and adolescents, as well as with childhood illnesses and diseases. Pediatric patients are cared for either by pediatricians or by family practitioners. Those who are cared for by a pediatrician usually stop visiting the pediatrician and switch their medical care to a specialist in adult internal medicine between their 14th and 18th birthdays. Young people with special needs or chronic illnesses may continue to see pediatric specialists until early adulthood (20 to 25 years old).

Pediatric patients are seen regularly from birth through adolescence in what are known as well-child visits. These well-child office visits occur within a few weeks of the baby's birth (the baby will have been examined each day it is in the hospital) and will be frequent for the first 2 years of life—at 2 months, 4 months, 6 months, 12 months, 18 months, and 24 months. From age 2, the American Academy of Pediatrics recommends that each child have an annual well-child physical, although some managed-care plans will only pay for a bi-annual (every 2 years) well-child visit during a child's school-age years.

During the well-child visit, the pediatrician, family doctor, or other provider (nurse practitioner or physician's assistant) will assess the child's growth and development, as well as eating and sleeping habits, social development, and nutritional status. Urine and blood tests will be performed periodically to test for such problems as lead poisoning (many homes and other buildings still have lead paint) and high cholesterol. Regular tests will be taken for tuberculosis.

Immunizations against diphtheria, tetanus, pertussis, polio, measles, mumps, rubella (German measles), *Haemophilus influenzae* (Hib), hepatitis B virus (HBV), chicken pox, pneumococcus and, in some regions of the country, Lyme disease and other viruses, will be given on a prescribed schedule. At each well-child visit, the provider will perform a complete physical exam of all the child's systems.

GROWTH AND DEVELOPMENT

A healthy and normal young child is a virtual growing machine. Between birth and age 6 months, the infant's weight should double; it should triple from birth to 1 year. In the first year of life a normal healthy child should grow 10 to 12 inches in length. From age 1 to 2 years, a normal, healthy toddler should gain 3 to 5 more inches and gain another 5 to 6 pounds. The circumference of the head should continue to grow to accommodate the child's growing brain.

Table 27-1	Milestones of Infant Motor Development
Average Age	**Motor Development**
Birth	Unable to hold head up, prefers position with arms and legs tucked under body.
1 month	Turns head from side to side; grasps adult finger by reflex activity.
2 months	Holds head up when prone; holds object briefly.
4 months	Rolls over; grasps object and brings to mouth; head drops back slightly when pulled to sitting position.
6 months	Sits without support with legs bowed for balance; holds object and transfers from one hand to the other.
8 months	Crawls; pulls self to stand and stands while holding on; grasps objects with thumb and finger.
10 months	Crawls with trunk off the floor; starts to prefer right or left hand; starts to stand alone for short periods.
12 months	Stands alone easily; walks holding on; may take steps independently; uses thumb and forefinger to hold objects, turns pages of book with thick pages.

Table 27–2	Growth and Developmental Stages: Birth through Adolescence		
Age	Growth	Developmental Stage	Psychosocial Development
Infancy (birth to 1 year)	Triples birth weight. Gains control of body. Stands and may walk by first birthday.	Trust versus mistrust	Meeting basic needs helps the infant learn to trust others.
Toddler (1 to 3 years)	Body becomes longer compared to head size, but growth rate slows compared to infancy. Begins to talk and gain coordination.	Autonomy versus shame and doubt	Learning to walk, talk, eat, and dress independently gives the toddler a sense of autonomy. Toilet training gives a sense of being a "big boy" or "big girl."
Preschool (3 to 6 years)	Increase in language and fine motor skills. Becomes longer and leaner.	Initiative versus guilt	The child gains more control of emotions and behavior choices. The child uses imagination freely.
School-age (6 to 12 years)	Grows at a regular rate. Increases coordination through organized sports and other complex activities. Social and intellectual skills develop.	Industry versus inferiority	Achievements give the child a sense of self-worth. Peer group becomes increasingly important in shaping attitudes and values.
Adolescence (12 to 18 years)	Growth spurt and sexual maturation. Changes in hormone levels may cause emotional upset.	Identity versus role confusion	The adolescent develops a sense of personal identity. Has more freedom to make choices and more responsibility for self.

In addition to rapid physical **growth** (increasing in size), infants, toddlers, and preschool children undergo rapid—almost constant—intellectual and emotional **development** (maturation of cognitive and emotional function). Developmental milestones can be noted at every well-child visit. Later in childhood, the child or adolescent will continue to attain physical and intellectual developmental milestones annually, which can be noted at the annual well-child visit. Table 27–1 shows the milestones of infant motor development.

Development Stages

In addition to physical growth, a pattern of cognitive and emotional development begins at infancy and continues throughout the life span. Sigmund Freud, Erik Erikson, and Jean Piaget are among the noted social scientists who have studied patterns of personality and emotional development and have described some of the problems that can arise at different stages. It is important to remember that all aspects of development normally occur together. Problems or limitations in one area affect other areas, and may interfere with the child's ability to meet the normal expectations of his or her age group.

Erikson described in 1950 a reference framework for describing stages of deveveolopment. He theorized that the human progresses through eight stages, each with a key conflict that the individual must master.

If the infant's or child's caregivers and/or environment do not provide enough support for the individual to resolve the psychosocial conflicts in each stage, the individual will have difficulty in similar situations in later years. For example, Erikson identifies the key conflict of infancy as trust. An infant whose basic needs are met in a reasonable time learns to trust the environment as a reasonably safe place to be and feels confident to explore it as motor skills develop. On the other hand, if an infant is neglected and his or her needs are met inconsistently, he or she fails to develop trust and must expend large amounts of psychic energy worrying about being fed and nurtured.

The result may be emotional withdrawal, apathy, and lack of energy to explore the environment and to meet the tasks of the next developmental stage. Table 27–2 summarizes Erikson's developmental stages for children and adolescents.

Tools to Measure Growth and Development

Height (length) and weight are measured carefully at each well-child visit throughout childhood and are charted against statistical norms for girls or boys, depending on the child's gender. Figures 27–1 and 27–2 show growth charts for boys and girls, which were updated by the U.S. Centers for Disease Control and Prevention in 2000 to reflect changing growth patterns.

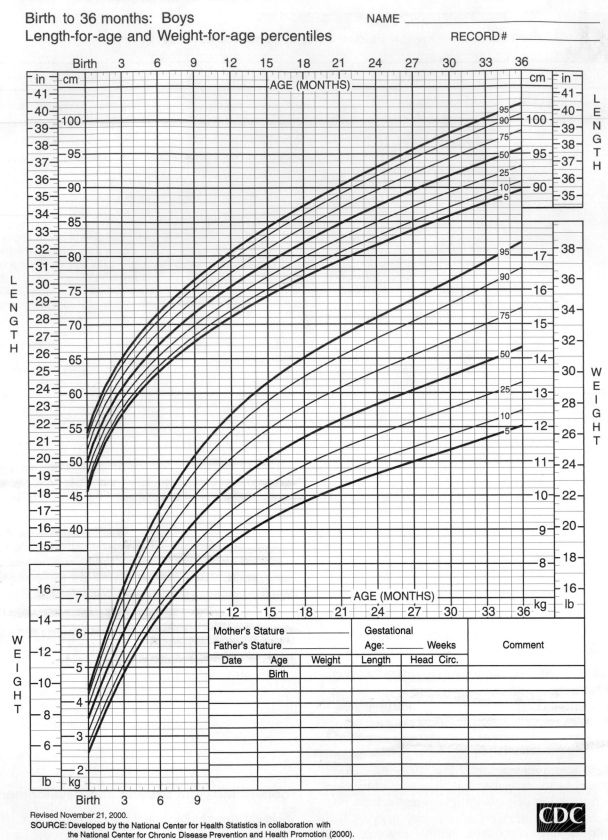

Birth to 36 months: Boys
Length-for-age and Weight-for-age percentiles

NAME _____

RECORD# _____

Revised November 21, 2000.
SOURCE: Developed by the National Center for Health Statistics in collaboration with
the National Center for Chronic Disease Prevention and Health Promotion (2000).
http://www .cdc.gov/growthcharts

➤ **Figure 27–1** Growth chart for boys, birth to 36 months; girls grow at a slightly different rate and have a different chart. (Adapted from the National Center for Health Statistics and the National Center for Chronic Disease Prevention and Health Promotion, 2000.)

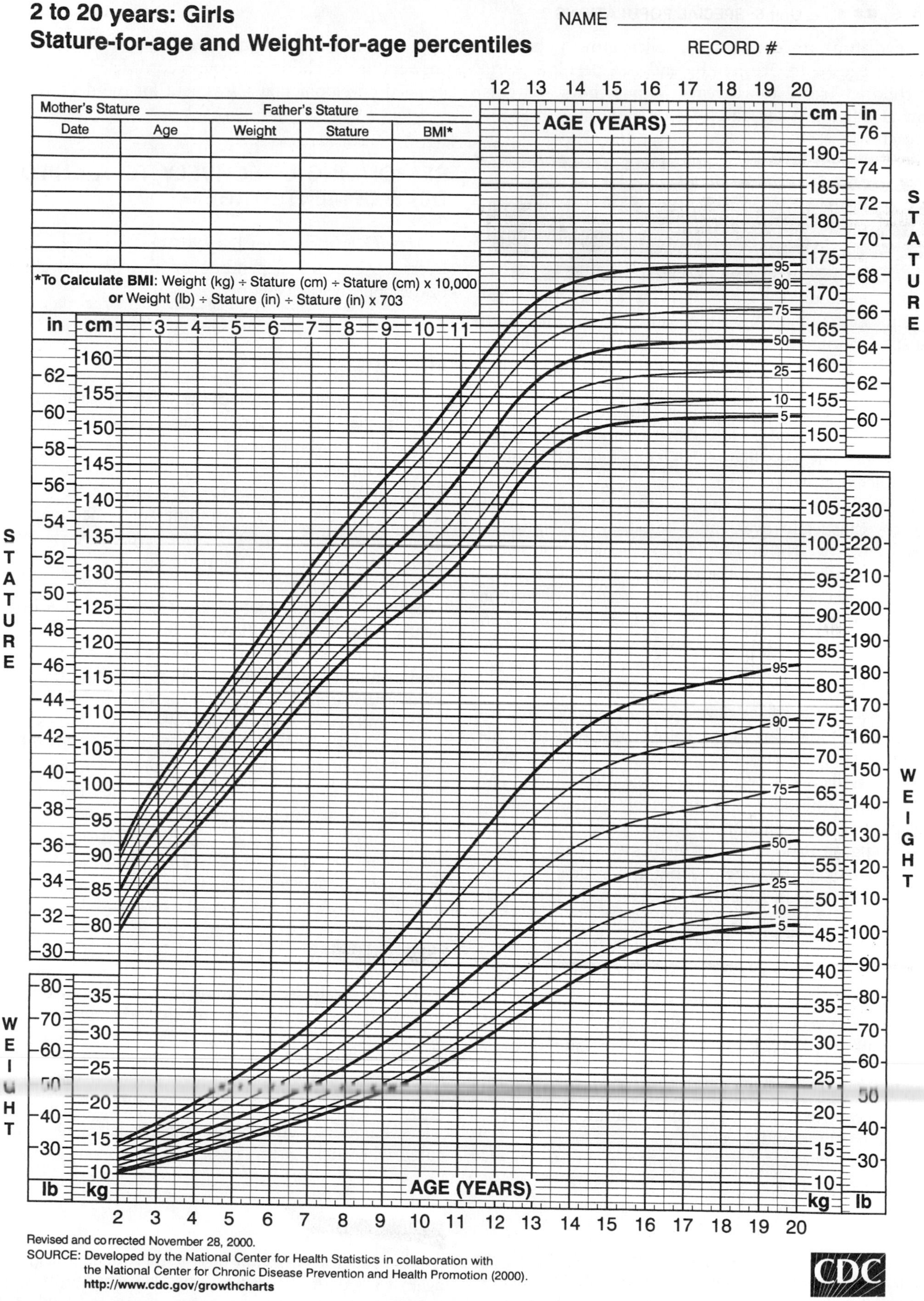

2 to 20 years: Girls
Stature-for-age and Weight-for-age percentiles
NAME
RECORD #
Mother's Stature
Father's Stature
Date
Age
Weight
Stature
BMI*
*To Calculate BMI: Weight (kg) ÷ Stature (cm) ÷ Stature (cm) x 10,000
or Weight (lb) ÷ Stature (in) ÷ Stature (in) x 703
AGE (YEARS)
STATURE
WEIGHT
in
cm
lb
kg
95
90
75
50
25
10
5
2 3 4 5 6 7 8 9 10 11 12 13 14 15 16 17 18 19 20
Revised and corrected November 28, 2000.
SOURCE: Developed by the National Center for Health Statistics in collaboration with
the National Center for Chronic Disease Prevention and Health Promotion (2000).
http://www.cdc.gov/growthcharts
CDC

➢ **Figure 27–2** Growth chart for girls, 2 to 20 years; boys grow at a different rate and have a different chart. (Adapted from the National Center for Health Statistics and the National Center for Chronic Disease Prevention and Health Promotion, 2000.)

The pediatric provider uses a detailed growth chart for children ages 0 to 36 months and less detailed charts for children ages 2 to 16 years. Because boys and girls grow at different rates, there are different growth charts for each.

The solid lines on these charts can be followed to the right margin to identify the percentile of growth into which the child falls. If the child's weight falls on the line of the 25th percentile, it means that out of 100 children, 24 would be expected to weigh less than the child and 75 would be expected to weigh more.

Children tend to grow in such a way that they remain approximately in the same range relative to statistical norms; in other words, a child who is in the 75th percentile at 1 year of age will usually be around the 75th percentile at 5 years of age as well. Because of this, growth charts are useful because they provide a visual record of the child's growth and a comparison with other children. (Figure 10-7 in Chapter 10 shows a completed growth chart.)

If a child's relationship to the statistical norm changes drastically over time—especially a failure to gain enough weight and height to maintain his or her relative position against the statistical norm—the doctor may want to conduct diagnostic tests to determine why this is happening. The medical assistant plays an important role in this process, by making accurate measurements and charting them correctly on the growth chart.

Cognitive and social development also tend to follow patterns that can be predicted and measured. Although each child develops individually, certain behaviors and skills are expected to emerge sequentially. The doctor asks questions and makes observations during the physical examination to identify if the child is developing as expected. The medical assistant may be expected to ask the parent about the child's development, using an assessment tool such as the Denver II Developmental Screening Test, which is shown in Figures 27–3 and 27–4.

This test measures development in four areas:

1. Gross motor skills; the child's ability to control large muscle groups to turn over, crawl, stand, walk, walk backwards, run, jump, and throw a ball.
2. Language; the child's ability to respond to speech, to make and imitate sounds, and later to understand and speak.
3. Fine motor skills; the child's ability to reach, grasp, and later to perform increasingly complex tasks with his or her fingers and hands.
4. Personal and social skills; the child's ability to smile, grab a spoon, drink from a cup, and wash his or her own hands.

Depending on the office setting, the medical assistant may be trained to administer this test or other developmental tests, or ask the parent a series of questions about what the child can do and record the answers in the child's medical record, leaving the more detailed developmental assessment for the doctor.

RESPONDING EFFECTIVELY TO A CHILD'S DEVELOPMENT STAGES

The medical assistant has different priorities and different approaches, depending on the age and abilities of the child being examined.

Infancy

It is important to protect the infant from injury and to keep the infant covered unless performing a procedure. The newborn may be very calm and passive when examined, as seen in Figure 27–5, but an older infant needs to be close to its parent for a sense of security. At this stage, the mother or father may hold the child when he or she is not actually being examined or tested and may help (if agreeable) by holding the child for immunizations.

When an infant reaches about 8 months, he or she clearly knows the difference between parents and strangers and may become anxious and agitated if he or she cannot see mother or father. Although the medical assistant uses a quiet, soothing tone to speak to the infant and avoids sudden movement or noises, it is expected that the infant will cry during parts of the visit. Distraction with lights or brightly colored objects may be an effective way to encourage the infant to stop resisting a procedure or to stop fussing.

The medical assistant should lift and carry the infant safely. For the first 6 months, the infant's neck should be securely supported whenever it is held or lifted.

Cradle Position

The medical assistant holds the infant with one arm under the back and neck, and the other arm supporting the legs and buttocks, as illustrated in Figure 27–6. This position is used when preparing to place the child on a scale.

Because the infant can see the face of the person who is holding him or her, the older infant is reassured when held in this position by someone familiar.

Upright Position

The medical assistant holds the infant's abdomen against his or her body with one hand, supporting the infant's buttocks, and places the other hand behind the infant's head and neck, as illustrated in Figure 27–7. An infant feels very secure in this position.

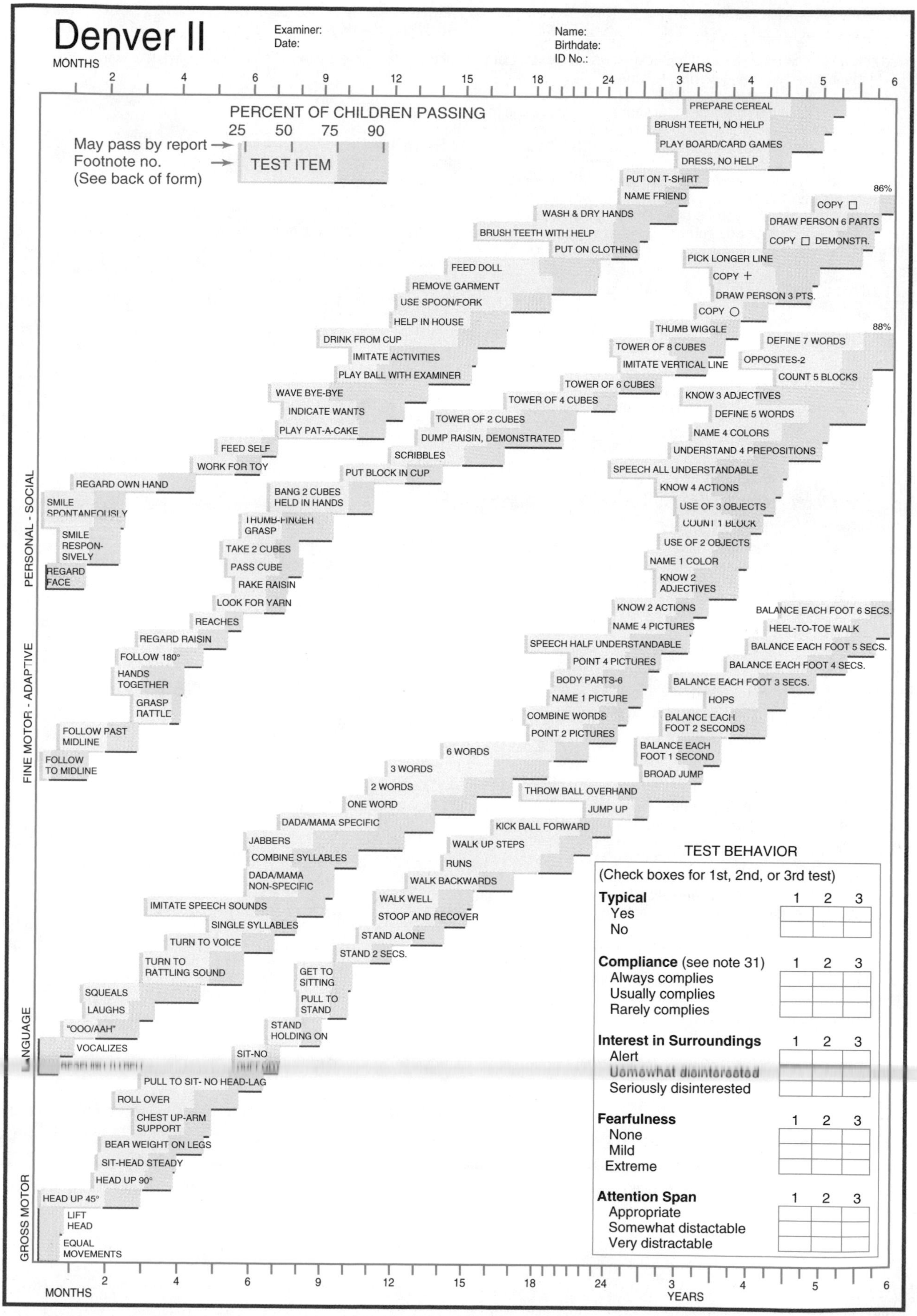

Denver II

Examiner:
Date:

Name:
Birthdate:
ID No.:

MONTHS / YEARS

PERCENT OF CHILDREN PASSING

25 50 75 90

May pass by report →
Footnote no. →
(See back of form)

TEST ITEM

PERSONAL - SOCIAL
- PREPARE CEREAL
- BRUSH TEETH, NO HELP
- PLAY BOARD/CARD GAMES
- DRESS, NO HELP
- PUT ON T-SHIRT
- NAME FRIEND
- WASH & DRY HANDS
- BRUSH TEETH WITH HELP
- PUT ON CLOTHING
- FEED DOLL
- REMOVE GARMENT
- USE SPOON/FORK
- HELP IN HOUSE
- DRINK FROM CUP
- IMITATE ACTIVITIES
- PLAY BALL WITH EXAMINER
- WAVE BYE-BYE
- INDICATE WANTS
- PLAY PAT-A-CAKE
- FEED SELF
- WORK FOR TOY
- REGARD OWN HAND
- SMILE SPONTANEOUSLY
- SMILE RESPONSIVELY
- REGARD FACE

FINE MOTOR - ADAPTIVE
- THUMB WIGGLE
- TOWER OF 8 CUBES
- IMITATE VERTICAL LINE
- TOWER OF 6 CUBES
- TOWER OF 4 CUBES
- TOWER OF 2 CUBES
- DUMP RAISIN, DEMONSTRATED
- SCRIBBLES
- PUT BLOCK IN CUP
- BANG 2 CUBES HELD IN HANDS
- THUMB-FINGER GRASP
- TAKE 2 CUBES
- PASS CUBE
- RAKE RAISIN
- LOOK FOR YARN
- REACHES
- REGARD RAISIN
- FOLLOW 180°
- HANDS TOGETHER
- GRASP RATTLE
- FOLLOW PAST MIDLINE
- FOLLOW TO MIDLINE
- DRAW PERSON 6 PARTS
- COPY ☐ DEMONSTR.
- COPY +
- DRAW PERSON 3 PTS.
- COPY ○
- DEFINE 7 WORDS
- OPPOSITES-2
- COUNT 5 BLOCKS
- KNOW 3 ADJECTIVES
- DEFINE 5 WORDS
- NAME 4 COLORS
- UNDERSTAND 4 PREPOSITIONS
- SPEECH ALL UNDERSTANDABLE
- KNOW 4 ACTIONS
- USE OF 3 OBJECTS
- COUNT 1 BLOCK
- USE OF 2 OBJECTS
- NAME 1 COLOR
- KNOW 2 ADJECTIVES
- COPY ☐

LANGUAGE
- 6 WORDS
- 3 WORDS
- 2 WORDS
- ONE WORD
- DADA/MAMA SPECIFIC
- JABBERS
- COMBINE SYLLABLES
- DADA/MAMA NON-SPECIFIC
- IMITATE SPEECH SOUNDS
- SINGLE SYLLABLES
- TURN TO VOICE
- TURN TO RATTLING SOUND
- SQUEALS
- LAUGHS
- "OOO/AAH"
- VOCALIZES
- KNOW 2 ACTIONS
- NAME 4 PICTURES
- SPEECH HALF UNDERSTANDABLE
- POINT 4 PICTURES
- BODY PARTS-6
- NAME 1 PICTURE
- COMBINE WORDS
- POINT 2 PICTURES

GROSS MOTOR
- WALK UP STEPS
- RUNS
- WALK BACKWARDS
- WALK WELL
- STOOP AND RECOVER
- STAND ALONE
- STAND 2 SECS.
- GET TO SITTING
- PULL TO STAND
- STAND HOLDING ON
- SIT-NO
- PULL TO SIT- NO HEAD-LAG
- ROLL OVER
- CHEST UP-ARM SUPPORT
- BEAR WEIGHT ON LEGS
- SIT-HEAD STEADY
- HEAD UP 90°
- HEAD UP 45°
- LIFT HEAD
- EQUAL MOVEMENTS
- BALANCE EACH FOOT 6 SECS.
- HEEL-TO-TOE WALK
- BALANCE EACH FOOT 5 SECS.
- BALANCE EACH FOOT 4 SECS.
- BALANCE EACH FOOT 3 SECS.
- HOPS
- BALANCE EACH FOOT 2 SECONDS
- BALANCE EACH FOOT 1 SECOND
- BROAD JUMP
- THROW BALL OVERHAND
- JUMP UP
- KICK BALL FORWARD

86%

88%

TEST BEHAVIOR

(Check boxes for 1st, 2nd, or 3rd test)

Typical	1	2	3
Yes			
No			

Compliance (see note 31)	1	2	3
Always complies			
Usually complies			
Rarely complies			

Interest in Surroundings	1	2	3
Alert			
Somewhat disinterested			
Seriously disinterested			

Fearfulness	1	2	3
None			
Mild			
Extreme			

Attention Span	1	2	3
Appropriate			
Somewhat distactable			
Very distractable			

➤ **Figure 27–3** Denver II Developmental Screening Test (DDST). (Copyright 1990 by W.K. Frankenburg and J.B. Dodds)

DIRECTIONS FOR ADMINISTRATION

1. Try to get child to smile by smiling, talking or waving. Do not touch him/her.
2. Child must stare at hand several seconds.
3. Parent may help guide toothbrush and put toothpaste on brush.
4. Child does not have to be able to tie shoes or button/zip in the back.
5. Move yarn slowly in an arc from one side to the other, about 8" above child's face.
6. Pass if child grasps rattle when it is touched to the backs or tips of fingers.
7. Pass if child tries to see where yarn went. Yarn should be dropped quickly from sight from tester's hand without arm movement.
8. Child must transfer cube from hand to hand without help of body, mouth, or table.
9. Pass if child picks up raisin with any part of thumb and finger.
10. Line can vary only 30 degrees or less from tester's line.
11. Make a fist with thumb pointing upward and wiggle only the thumb. Pass if child imitates and does not move any fingers other than the thumb.

12. Pass any enclosed form. Fail continuous round motions.
13. Which line is longer? (Not bigger.) Turn paper upside down and repeat. (pass 3 of 3 or 5 of 6)
14. Pass any lines crossing near midpoint.
15. Have child copy first. If failed, demonstrate.

When giving items 12, 14, and 15, do not name the forms. Do not demonstrate 12 and 14.

16. When scoring, each pair (2 arms, 2 legs, etc.) counts as one part.
17. Place one cube in cup and shake gently near child's ear, but out of sight. Repeat for other ear.
18. Point to picture and have child name it. (No credit is given for sounds only.) If less than 4 pictures are named correctly, have child point to picture as each is named by tester.

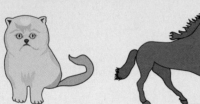 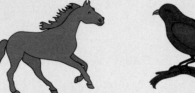 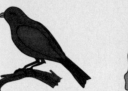   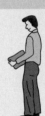

19. Using doll, tell child: Show me the nose, eyes, ears, mouth, hands, feet, tummy, hair. Pass 6 of 8.
20. Using pictures, ask child: Which one flies? . . . says meow? . . . talks? . . . barks? . . . gallops? Pass 2 of 5, 4 of 5.
21. Ask child: What do you do when you are cold? . . . tired? . . . hungry? Pass 2 of 3, 3 of 3.
22. Ask child: What do you do with a cup? What is a chair used for? What is a pencil used for? Action words must be included in answers.
23. Pass if child correctly places and says how many blocks are on paper. (1, 5).
24. Tell child: Put block **on** table; **under** table; **in front of** me, **behind** me. Pass 4 of 4. (Do not help child by pointing, moving head or eyes.)
25. Ask child: What is a ball? . . . lake? . . . desk? . . . house? . . . banana? . . . curtain? . . . fence? . . . ceiling? Pass if defined in terms of use, shape, what it is made of, or general category (such as banana is fruit, not just yellow). Pass 5 of 8, 7 of 8.
26. Ask child: If a horse is big, a mouse is __? If fire is hot, ice is __? If the sun shines during the day, the moon shines during the __? Pass 2 of 3.
27. Child may use wall or rail only, not person. May not crawl.
28. Child must throw ball overhand 3 feet to within arm's reach of tester.
29. Child must perform standing broad jump over width of test sheet (8 1/2 inches).
30. Tell child to walk forward, ⏱⏱⏱⏱⏱ → heel within 1 inch of toe. Tester may demonstrate. Child must walk 4 consecutive steps.
31. In the second year, half of normal children are non-compliant.

OBSERVATIONS:

➤ **Figure 27–4** Instructions for Denver II Developmental Screening Test (DDST). (Copyright 1990 by W.K. Frankenburg and J.B. Dodds)

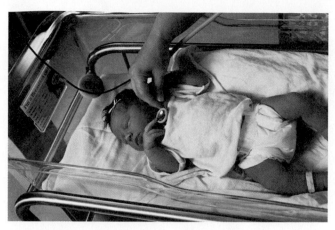

> **Figure 27–5** The newborn may sleep passively through the physical examination.

Early Childhood

A visit to the doctor's office can be very frightening to a preschool-aged child. Crying and negative vocal expressions (shouting "no" for instance) are common in toddlers and preschoolers. The medical assistant needs to help the child feel comfortable by explaining procedures in simple terms the child can understand, by allowing the child to handle equipment such as a stethoscope, and by giving the child reasonable choices, such as asking "Do you want to take off your shirt or your pants first?" Figure 27–8 shows a child handling a blood pressure cuff.

Play is the usual means for learning during early childhood. It may be helpful if the medical assistant makes a game out of a procedure or allows the child to think up a game. Puppets are sometimes used to

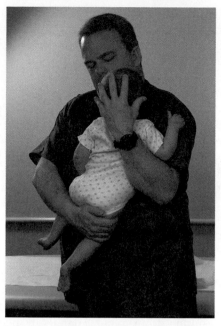

> **Figure 27–7** In the upright position the infant's head should be supported.

instruct toddlers about procedures or upcoming surgeries.

Unpleasant procedures, such as injections, should be performed quickly, even if the child is struggling, protesting, and/or crying. The medical assistant can encourage the child not to cry but should not shame the child for showing emotions or failing to cooperate.

A colorful adhesive bandage helps distract a young child after an injection or injury.

Childhood

Explain procedures to children to gain cooperation. Provide an atmosphere in which the child feels free to

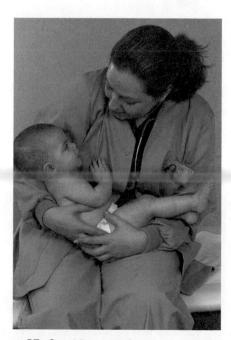

> **Figure 27–6** Holding an infant in the cradle position.

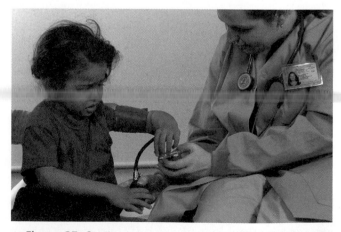

> **Figure 27–8** Allowing a preschool child to handle and use the blood pressure cuff may reduce her anxiety about procedures.

ask questions. Although the mother and/or father usually comes into the examination room with the child, question the child directly and maintain eye contact with him or her.

By age 6 or 7, children do not like to be undressed in front of strangers. Usually they are allowed to wear underpants for the first part of the physical examination. Girls often like to wear a gown over their underpants (and their bras as well as they get older). The medical assistant should leave the room while the child undresses.

Children are still apprehensive about injections and need to express fear and discomfort. Choosing which arm to use for the injection helps the child retain some sense of control.

Adolescence

In adolescence, considerable emotional turmoil is present, resulting from rapid change in body image and hormone levels. As the adolescent copes with body changes and sexual development, he or she may wish to speak to the doctor privately. The medical assistant should identify the adolescent's wishes and encourage the parent to either be present for the examination or wait in the waiting room.

The adolescent may identify more easily with the medical assistant than the doctor. The medical assistant should provide a nonjudgmental atmosphere that allows the teenager to describe behaviors related to possible health hazards such as using drugs or alcohol and risky sexual behavior truthfully. At the doctor's discretion, information about use of tobacco, drugs, alcohol, and possible dangers of unprotected sex may be given without the parent present.

PREPARING FOR THE PHYSICAL EXAMINATION

Children should be prepared for an examination just as an adult should be, except for draping and positioning. The child should be allowed to be in a diaper or underpants for the duration of the examination, until he or she begins to become self-conscious (earlier for girls), when he or she begins using a gown and/or drape.

Young children should be allowed to handle instruments as a way to alleviate fear of the exam, but they should not play with equipment when the medical assistant or doctor is not with them. All tests and procedures should be explained clearly and simply. Children should be given a lot of positive reinforcement when they cooperate with a procedure. Never make light of fear or crying, but explain that this is normal.

On occasion, it is necessary to restrain a child who is agitated, so he or she does not get hurt. This may be as simple as holding the child's arms over the knees or shoulders to prevent motion that could cause an injury. Or it could be as complex as wrapping an infant.

An infant wrap can be made with a sheet folded into a triangle. The long end should be kept even with the shoulders, with more sheet to the left of the child than the right, and the point just below the feet. Bring the longer side over the left arm, then under the body and right arm. Then bring the right side over the right arm and under the body. This restrains the arms but leaves the abdomen available for examination.

Length or Height

Infant length is measured with the child in the supine position, either on a measuring board or on the examination table. A pencil mark is made at the top of the infant's head, then at the bottom of the feet after the legs have been manually extended to their full length. The distance from the marks is then measured. The length is then charted on the growth chart. Procedure 27–1 describes in detail measuring an infant.

As soon as the child can stand unsupported, he or she should be measured standing, using a wall-mounted measuring ruler or a scale with a ruler attached. The measurements should be consistant with regard to whether or not the child wears shoes or not to ensure consistency when plotting height on the growth chart. Measure with the child's back to the bar for accuracy and to avoid accidental eye injury. Figure 27–9 shows a child being measured.

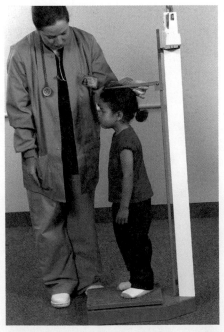

➤ **Figure 27–9** A child may be measured on a wall chart or on a scale with a measuring bar.

PROCEDURE 27–1

Measuring an Infant's Length

Performance Objective: The student will be able to measure an infant's length.

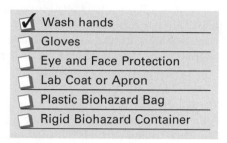

- ☑ Wash hands
- ☐ Gloves
- ☐ Eye and Face Protection
- ☐ Lab Coat or Apron
- ☐ Plastic Biohazard Bag
- ☐ Rigid Biohazard Container

Supplies and Equipment: Examination table covered with paper, marking pen/pencil, measuring tape.

Procedure Steps

1. Wash hands.
2. Assemble supplies and equipment.
3. Identify infant and parent.
4. Explain procedure to parent.
5. Place the infant on his or her back on the table. Some tables have an extender to mark the top of the head, but if one is not present, place a pencil mark on the table paper to mark the top of the infant's head.
6. Holding the infant, stretch the leg and foot down and place a mark at the infant's heel. *Rationale:* This must be done without moving the infant from the original position when the head was marked.
7. Ask the parent to pick up the infant and measure between the two marks. If the office records the measurement in centimeters, have a conversion chart available to tell the parent the length in inches.
8. Wash hands.
9. Document the length in the medical record. Plot the point on the appropriate growth chart.

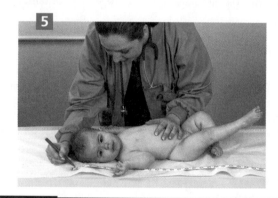

Weight

Infants should be weighed on every visit, whether a well-child visit or a visit due to illness. Illness can often cause an infant to lose weight.

Infants are usually measured either lying or sitting (if they can sit unsupported) in a platform scale. The infants should be weighed without clothes. Balance the scale with a disposable underpad and prepare a new diaper for use immediately after weighing.

Although these scales may use kilograms, weight is usually translated into pounds and ounces for the parents to record in their records. Growth charts contain scales for both kilograms and pounds. Be sure to use the correct scale when plotting the infant's weight on the growth chart.

An uncooperative infant can be weighed being held by a parent or other caregiver. First the adult stands on a scale, holding the infant. Then the adult stands on the scale without the infant. The weight of the adult alone is subtracted from the weight of the adult and the infant to determine the infant's weight.

Procedure 27–2 discusses in detail weighing an infant.

Once a child can stand unattended, he or she should be weighed standing on a scale just as an adult does. Cooperation is important to get an accurate reading. The child should be asked to stand very still for a few seconds, then praised for his or her cooperation. Figure 27–10 shows a child being weighed.

Head Circumference

Head **circumference** measurement (distance around the head) is important because it shows the growth of the skull and by inference the intracranial volume (space inside the skull for the brain). When a child is born, the bones of the skull have not yet fused, so the

PROCEDURE 27-2

Measuring an Infant's Weight

Performance Objective: The student will be able to weigh an infant.

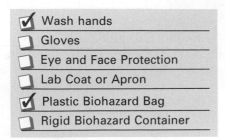

- ☑ Wash hands
- ☐ Gloves
- ☐ Eye and Face Protection
- ☐ Lab Coat or Apron
- ☑ Plastic Biohazard Bag
- ☐ Rigid Biohazard Container

Supplies and Equipment: Scale with platform for infant to lie in supine position, protective underpad, clean disposable diaper, biohazard waste container.

Procedure Steps

1. Wash hands.
2. Place protective underpad on scale and balance the scale at zero.
   Rationale: This allows you to weigh only the infant but have a protective pad on the scale.
3. Identify infant and parent.
4. Explain procedure to parent.
5. Ask the mother to remove all clothes and diaper from the infant.
6. Place the infant on the scale platform in a supine position. Hold a hand on the infant's chest.

Rationale: It is important to hold the infant at all times except for a brief moment when the exact weight is obtained.

7. Slowly move the weights until the scale bar balances. First move the pound weight, then the ounce weight. Remove your hand from the infant just long enough to read the exact weight.
8. Lift the infant up and return to the parent. Provide a clean diaper to place on the infant.
9. If the office charts weights in kilograms, use a conversion chart to tell the mother the weight in pounds and ounces.
10. Discard underpad. If soiled, discard in biohazard waste container.
11. Wash hands.
12. Document weight in the medical record. Plot the point on the appropriate growth chart.

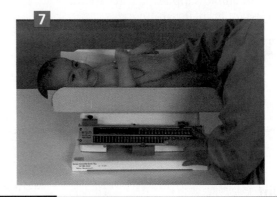

head can expand. Lags or surges in size of the head are indications of serious problems with the brain or the skull.

If the infant's head is too large for its age, it may indicate a condition called **hydrocephalus,** increased cerebrospinal fluid in the brain. This condition must be identified early, before excess pressure destroys brain cells. If the head size is too small, it is equally important for the doctor to follow up and determine if a pathological condition is preventing normal growth.

Head circumference should be measured at each well-child visit from birth until about age 3, and should be plotted on a graph to assure proper growth and to compare with the growth in height and weight over the same period.

Figure 27–11 shows head circumference charts for boys. In the medical office, a slightly different chart is used for girls, whose average head size is the same as a boy at birth but about 1/2″ smaller at age 3. Procedure 27–3 describes in detail measuring head circumference.

Chest Circumference

Measuring chest circumference is done as part of the well-child visit, to assure the proper development of the chest organs and the calcification of the rib cartilage. Generally, head and chest circumference are equal at about age 1 to 2. Before that, chest circumference exceeds head circumference by about 2″ to 3″. Proce-

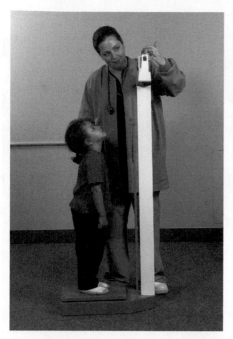

➤ **Figure 27–10** Weighing a child.

dure 27–4 discusses in detail measuring chest circumference.

Temperature

Temperature may be measured in either Fahrenheit or Celsius. Thermometers may be glass, digital, electronic, or tympanic. Electronic and digital thermometers take less than a minute; sensor-based thermometers take only a few seconds.

Oral temperature should only be taken after a child reaches age 5. Like the adult, the child should be instructed to hold the thermometer under the tongue and cautioned not to bite the thermometer.

Taking an **aural** temperature (in the ear)—shown in Figure 27–12—is done using a thermometer with an infrared sensor that measures the temperature of the **tympanic** membrane (eardrum). This method is fast, noninvasive, and accurate when done correctly.

A tympanic or axillary temperature (under the armpit) may be taken for toddlers and preschoolers. The tympanic method is faster. The axillary method is safe and noninvasive, but requires cooperation from the child and takes about 5 minutes. This is shown in Figure 27–13.

A rectal temperature may be taken in infants and toddlers when other methods are not advised. Because it is more accurate, a rectal temperature may be ordered by the doctor to verify a high temperature obtained with a tympanic thermometer. Extreme care must be used when taking a rectal temperature. Never force the thermometer and never let go of the thermometer. A rectal temperature is invasive and requires cooperation and a quiet infant to avoid injury. The infant may lie prone or 'supine, but must be held throughout the procedure. The red probe of an electronic thermometer is used for taking rectal temperature. The procedure for taking a rectal temperature was discussed in Chapter 15 (see Procedure 15-7 specifically).

Other Vital Signs

At each exam, the child's pulse and respirations should be measured. Blood pressure is often measured in school-age children and in infants and toddlers in special circumstances.

The normal pulse for a child varies with age and decreases as the child gets older. A pulse between 100 and 180 beats per minute is to be expected, and a pulse over 200 is not unusual in an infant. By age 2, the child's pulse should be in the range of 70 to 110.

As with an adult, a child's pulse responds to excitement, fever, exercise, temperature, and anxiety and decreases while resting. A child's pulse may also vary with inspiration and expiration. This is called respiratory sinus arrhythmia and is considered normal in children.

The apical pulse is preferred over other sites in children under age 5. As with the adult, the apex of the heart is located to the left of the sternum at the fifth intercostal space. Procedure 27–5 discusses in detail taking an apical pulse in an infant.

When taking a child's respirations, it is not necessary to conceal the fact, as with adults. Count the rise and fall of the chest as you would with adult respirations. Infants breathe with their abdominal muscles more than with their chest; therefore, use abdominal muscles to count. Normal respirations for an infant are 30 to 35 per minute, and for a school-age child 16 to 20. Procedure 27–6 discusses measuring infant respirations.

Blood pressure is not taken all the time at pediatric exams, but may be done in specific circumstances. It is difficult to take a young child's blood pressure, because it is difficult to keep the child still and quiet.

When taking a child's blood pressure, be sure to choose a pediatric cuff and make sure the cuff fits the child.

Children have lower blood pressure than adults, due to the lack of resistance on the walls of the blood vessels. Infant blood pressure may be 90/50 mm Hg. By age 10, 110/60 mm Hg is normal. The school-age child should have his or her blood pressure taken routinely.

Obtaining Specimens—Urine and Blood

Most young children cannot void on command. Therefore, if a urine specimen is needed from a young child, a pediatric urine collection device may be

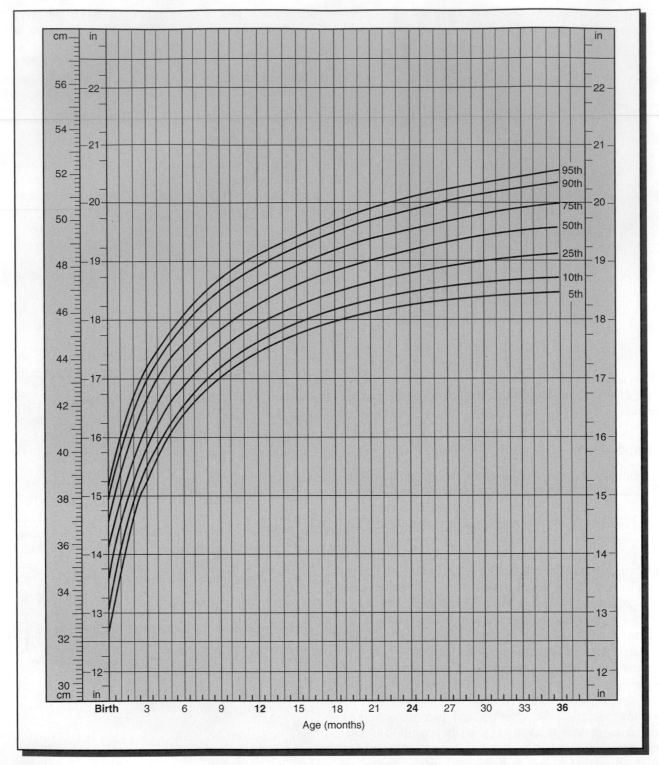

➢ **Figure 27–11** Head circumference chart for boys from birth to 36 months; the girls' chart is similar. (Adapted from the National Center for Health Statistics and the National Center for Chronic Disease Prevention and Health Promotion, 2000.)

needed. Procedure 27–7 discusses obtaining a urine specimen from an infant.

By age 3 or 4, a child should be able to produce a urine specimen, if not at the beginning of the exam then by the end after drinking some water. Once the specimen is obtained, the urinalysis is performed, as discussed in chapter 24.

Blood specimens may be needed to test for blood urea nitrogen (BUN) in newborns who continue to exhibit jaundice after discharge from the hospital. In-

PROCEDURE 27–3

Measuring Head Circumference of an Infant

Performance Objective: The student will be able to measure an infant's head circumference.

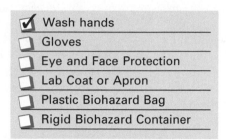

- ☑ Wash hands
- ☐ Gloves
- ☐ Eye and Face Protection
- ☐ Lab Coat or Apron
- ☐ Plastic Biohazard Bag
- ☐ Rigid Biohazard Container

Supplies and Equipment: Measuring tape.

Procedure Steps

1. Wash hands.
2. Identify infant and parent.
3. Explain procedure and the cooperation that may be needed.
   Rationale: Allowing the parent to hold the child while the measurement is taken may help this procedure.

4. Place the measuring tape snugly around the infant's head at the widest part of the head. This is usually called the occipital to supraorbital area.
   Rationale: You want to measure the widest part of the head.
5. Read the measurement to the nearest inch or centimeter.
6. Wash hands.
7. Document the head circumference in the medical record. Plot the point on the head circumference growth chart.

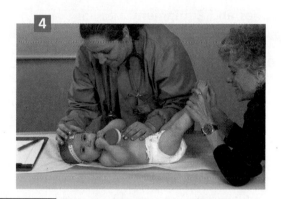

---

fants are also tested for PKU (phenylketonuria) at birth or at the first office visit, as described in chapter 25 (Procedure 25-6). Lead levels are tested routinely in toddlers and preschool children who are at risk for lead poisoning.

A capillary specimen may be obtained from the heel (from birth until the infant is walking) or from a finger, as described in chapter 25. Because the veins are small, venous specimens are more difficult to obtain, and a butterfly needle may be used. Medical assistants who have developed skill in using a butterfly needle may be successful in obtaining venous specimens from children, but they should practice with supervision to develop skill before performing the procedure unsupervised.

WELL-CHILD VISITS

A well-child visit should be carried out every year (many managed-care health insurance plans only pay for a well-child visit every 2 years for school-age chil-dren) to assess the child's development along a number of parameters.

Height and weight are measured. The child's overall appearance and posture are assessed, as well as vital signs and mobility. In addition, it is a chance for the primary care provider to watch the child's interaction with other family members—the parent who brings the child for the visit as well as any siblings who might attend—and to assess the child's intellectual and emotional growth.

Education about health and illness is a regular part of a well-child visit, and once children are old enough to understand, they should be included in these discussions. Topics might include simple concepts such as handwashing and nose blowing for young children to issues of smoking, alcohol use, abuse of prescription and street drugs, and issues of sexuality and sexually transmitted diseases for adolescents. In addition, parents should be instructed to be alert for symptoms of head lice, which are easily contracted in day-care and school. These symptoms include itchy head, presence of egg cases, called nits, or adult lice in the hair.

PROCEDURE 27–4

Measuring Chest Circumference of an Infant

Performance Objective: The student will be able to measure an infant's chest circumference.

- ☑ Wash hands
- ☐ Gloves
- ☐ Eye and Face Protection
- ☐ Lab Coat or Apron
- ☐ Plastic Biohazard Bag
- ☐ Rigid Biohazard Container

Supplies and Equipment: Measuring tape.

Procedure Steps

1. Wash hands.
2. Identify infant and parent.
3. Explain procedure and the cooperation that may be needed.
   Rationale: Have the parent use toys or talk to the infant to distract him or her while performing this procedure.

4 Place the measuring tape snugly around the infant's chest just above the nipple line and under the axillary area.

5. Read the measurement to the nearest inch or centimeter.
6. Wash hands.
7. Document the chest circumference in the medical record. (If the office keeps a chest circumference growth chart, you should plot the point on it.)

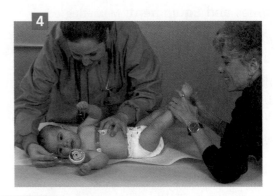

A parent should accompany a child in the exam room until adolescence, at which time the primary care provider and child may conduct part or all of the exam without the parent present. Girls are offered a gown for privacy as soon as they become self-conscious. By

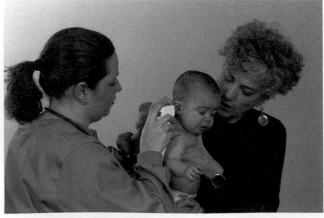

➢ **Figure 27–12** Measuring the temperature of an infant using a tympanic thermometer.

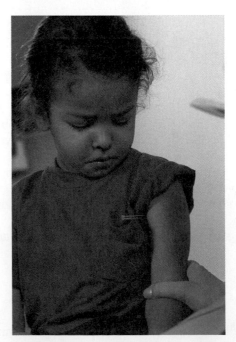

➢ **Figure 27–13** Measuring the axillary temperature of a child.

age 8 or 9, many girls will want to see a woman primary care provider instead of a man.

Immunizations and Immunization Schedule

Immunization is a routine part of well-child visits. The American Academy of Pediatrics has guidelines for a program of preventive immunizations against childhood diseases. Because the child's immune system is poorly developed during the first year, immunizations to prevent disease must be given frequently until the child is 12 to 15 months old.

Parents need to be educated about the possible side effects of each immunization. Many offices provide parents with information booklets about each immunization; these books can be obtained from the U.S. Centers for Disease Control and Prevention (CDC).

An immunization record should also be kept, both by the provider and the parent. The parent record should be filled out by the primary care provider when the vaccine is administered, and the provider should stress to the parent the importance of keeping the vaccination record in a secure place. It is as important as a child's birth certificate.

The medical office record should include the date and lot number of the medication used, the injection site, date of administration, and any immediate side effects reported. Many offices include a space for the parent's signature as part of the immunization record. In addition, the vaccine manufacturer and lot number are recorded to track the origin of a specific dose of vaccine if a problem occurs.

Under the Childhood Vaccination Injury Act of 1986, these records must be kept permanently in the medical office records. In addition, all "adverse events" must be reported to the U.S. Department of Health and Human Services' Adverse Event Reporting System.

PROCEDURE 27–5

Measuring the Apical Pulse of an Infant

Performance Objective: The student will be able to measure an infant's apical pulse.

☑	Wash hands
☐	Gloves
☐	Eye and Face Protection
☐	Lab Coat or Apron
☐	Plastic Biohazard Bag
☐	Rigid Biohazard Container

Supplies and Equipment: Stethoscope, watch with a second hand.

Procedure Steps

1. Wash hands.
2. Identify infant and parent.
3. Explain procedure and the cooperation that may be needed.
   Rationale: Distraction may be necessary to get the infant to lie still during the measurement. Have the parent assist with a quiet toy or talking to the infant during the procedure.
4. Remove the infant's shirt.

5. Sit the infant on the exam table or place in a supine position.
6. Locate the fifth intercostal space. Place the stethoscope at the midclavicular line to the left of the sternum.
   Rationale: You want to place the stethoscope over the apex of the infant's heart to hear the heartbeat clearly.
7. Count beats for 1 minute. Note heart rate at 30 seconds in case the infant becomes too restless to continue for the full minute. If the infant becomes uncooperative, you may double the 30-second heart rate.
8. Wash hands.
9. Document the apical pulse in the infant's medical record. Note any irregular pulse.

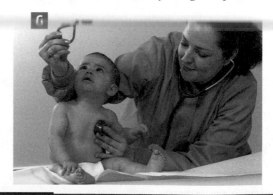

PROCEDURE 27–6

Measuring the Respirations of an Infant

Performance Objective: The student will be able to measure an infant's respirations.

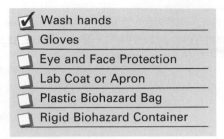

- ☑ Wash hands
- ☐ Gloves
- ☐ Eye and Face Protection
- ☐ Lab Coat or Apron
- ☐ Plastic Biohazard Bag
- ☐ Rigid Biohazard Container

Supplies and Equipment: Watch with a second hand.

Procedure Steps

1. Wash hands.
2. Identify infant and parent.
3. Explain procedure and the cooperation that may be needed.
   Rationale: Have the parent assist to keep the infant from crying with a quiet toy or talking to the infant during the procedure.
4. Remove the infant's shirt.
5. Place infant in supine position.
6. Place hand over infant's chest and count each rise and fall of the chest wall for 1 minute using a watch with a second hand.
   Rationale: Each rise and fall of the chest equals one respiration. If the infant cries, calm him or her and count again.
7. Wash hands.
8. Document the respirations in the infant's medical record. Note any irregularities in sound or rhythm.

This is especially important, not only to comply with the law, but to have records should there be a legal proceeding. Since the 1990s, a movement has come about ascribing a number of problems in childhood and adolescence—from attention deficit disorder to autism—to early childhood immunizations, and a number of lawsuits have been filed against doctors and pharmaceutical companies.

It should be stressed to parents that their children's immunization records should be kept throughout the child's lifetime. Children need a record of their preschool immunizations to attend public school, unless they can show a waiver of immunization requirements for religious or health reasons. In many states, colleges also require a record of immunization, including a booster immunization against measles, because college dormitories provide an environment in which communicable diseases are easily spread.

Currently seven different immunizations are recommended for children. Most are required by state health departments for a child to attend school. In addition, some states recommend or require additional immunizations. Before giving the second or subsequent injections in a series, always ask about reactions to the previous injections.

The substance used to immunize an individual is called a **vaccine.** A vaccine is a suspension of microorganisms or parts of microorganisms that stimulate the production of antibodies against the microorganism.

1. **HBV** (HepB, or hepatitis B vaccine), given intramuscularly three times during the first 18 months, with a booster at age 11 to 12 if any earlier immunizations were late or missed, or if an antibody titer shows incomplete immunity.
2. **DTaP** (diphtheria and tetanus toxoids, and acellular pertussis vaccine), which replaced the DTP (diphtheria and tetanus toxoids, and pertussis vaccine), given intramuscularly four times during the first 18 months, and again at age 4 to 6.
   A **toxoid** is a toxin (harmful substance excreted by bacteria) that has been inactivated but still results in the production of antibodies.
3. **Hib** (*Hemophilus influenzae* type b conjugate vaccine), given intramuscularly four times during the first 15 months. This vaccine prevents pneumonia, meningitis, and septicemia from infection by *H. influenzae* bacteria.
4. **Polio:** two injections of **IPV** (inactivated poliovirus vaccine), given at ages 2 and 4 months, followed by two doses of either OPV (oral polio vaccine) or IPV at age 12 to 18 months and again at age 4 to 6.
5. **MMR** (measles, mumps, and rubella vaccine),

PROCEDURE 27–7

Obtaining a Urine Specimen from an Infant

Performance Objective: The student will be able to collect a urine specimen from an infant.

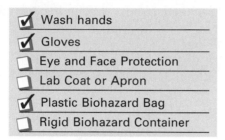

- ☑ Wash hands
- ☑ Gloves
- ☐ Eye and Face Protection
- ☐ Lab Coat or Apron
- ☑ Plastic Biohazard Bag
- ☐ Rigid Biohazard Container

Supplies and Equipment: Disposable gloves, urine collection bag, cleansing cloths, biohazard waste container.

Procedure Steps

1. Wash hands.
2. Identify infant and parent.
3. Explain procedure and the cooperation that may be needed.
4. Remove the infant's diaper.
5. Place infant in supine position.
6. Put on disposable gloves.
7. Clean the perineal area of the infant and dry the area.

Rationale: Cleaning will reduce the number of microorganisms in the area that can cause inaccurate urinalysis results.

8. Remove the paper tabs from the adhesive on the infant urine collection bag.
9. Apply to a male infant over the penis and scrotum. Apply to a female infant over the genitalia with the opening over the urinary meatus.
10. Replace diaper.
    Rationale: The diaper helps hold the bag in place.
11. Remove gloves and discard in biohazard waste container. Wash hands.
12. Check the bag frequently (every 10 to 15 minutes).
13. When the bag is full, put on a new pair of gloves and remove the bag carefully. Gently pull the adhesive away from the infant's skin, holding the bag in an upright position.
14. Place the urine in a container, label, and test or prepare to send it to the laboratory, as discussed in Procedure 24-4.
15. Document the date, time, specimen obtained, results of testing (if done in the office), or that the urine specimen was sent to the laboratory.

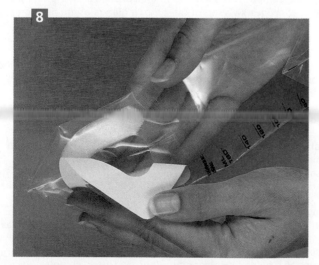

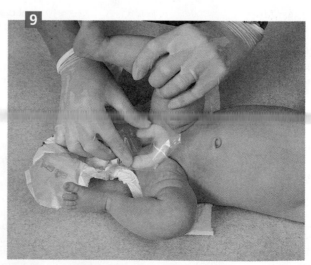

*Photographs from Bonewit-West K: *Clinical Procedures for Medical Assistants,* 5th ed. Philadelphia: W.B. Saunders, 2000.

given subcutanously at age 12 to 15 months and again at age 4 to 6, although the second dose is sometimes given at age 11 to 12. This vaccine should be prepared with a special diluent provided by the manufacturer. Question parents about sensitivity to eggs, because the vaccine is produced using chicken embryos.

6. **Var** (**varicella** vaccine), given at age 12 to 18 months, or to any unimmunized child without a reliable history of chicken pox. This is the most recent vaccine to be required by many states for children entering school and/or day-care.

7. **PCV-7** (pneumococcal conjugate vaccine): Given four times during the first 15 months, this vaccine prevents pneumonia, meningitis, and other diseases caused by pneumococcal bacteria.

Table 27–3 shows immunizations and the diseases they protect against. Table 27–4 gives the ages at which the various vaccines are administered.

Administering Injections to Children

Injection Sites

Because infants receive so many injections during the first year of life, it is very important for the medical assistant to be aware of correct injection technique. The muscles of the lower back and hip, a good choice for injections in adults, are small at birth and do not develop until the child begins to walk. Because of this, the vastus lateralis muscle of the leg is the site of choice for immunization during the first year. (See Chapter 22 for a description of the proper way to locate this site.)

Usually, a 25G 5/8″ needle is used to deliver the medication into the middle of the muscle. If the infant is small, the injection may be given at a 45-degree angle to avoid hitting the bone.

During the period from 12 to 18 months, the child receives several additional immunizations. It is still cor-

Table 27–3	Childhood Immunizations and the Diseases They Protect Against	
Disease	**Immunization**	**Description**
Diptheria	DTaP, Td	A severe bacterial disease that often resulted in death before widespread immunization programs. Toxins produced by the bacteria cause a membrane to be produced in the throat, resulting in respiratory distress.
Hepatitis B	Hep B	A viral disease transmitted by contact with body fluids that causes inflammation of the liver and possible liver damage. Infected individuals may be asymptomatic carriers of the disease.
Measles (rubeola)	MMR	A viral disease that causes fever, photophobia, and a characteristic maculo-papular rash. Although many cases recover without problem, the disease can cause severe complications leading to encephalitis and/or pneumonia.
Mumps	MMR	A viral disease that causes swelling of the parotid glands of the neck on one or both sides. Although children usually recover without problems, the disease can be very severe in adults and cause sterility in sexually mature males.
Pertussis	DTaP	Also called whooping cough because the disease produces severe coughing with a characteristic crowing or whooping sound. This disease is more common and more severe in children.
Pneumonia, or meningitis	Hib	The *Hemophilus influenzae* type b bacteria can cause severe cases of pneumonia and/or meningitis in children that can result in death or brain damage.
Pneumococcal disease	PCV-7	Pneumococcal bacteria can cause severe cases of bacterial meningitis and other infections in children that can result in death or brain damage.
Rubella (German measles)	MMR	A viral disease with a characteristic rash that may resemble rubeola or scarlet fever. The disease itself is usually mild, but it causes spontaneous abortion or birth defects when contracted by pregnant women.
Tetanus (lockjaw)	DTaP, Td	An infection by anaerobic bacilli present in soil, often contracted by a puncture wound. The disease causes painful spasms of the voluntary muscles and usually results in death from asphyxia or exhaustion.
Varicella zoster (chicken pox)	Var	A viral disease that is usually mild but can cause scarring of the skin and can later erupt as a painful skin condition (herpes zoster, shingles) in older adults.

Table 27–4	Recommended Schedule for Immunizations				
Vaccine	1st	2nd	3rd	4th	5th
Hep B	0–1 mo	1–2 mos	6–18 mos	*11–12 yrs	
DTaP	2 mos	4 mos	6 mos	15–18 mos	4–6 yrs
Hib	2 mos	4 mos	6 mos	12–15 mos	
Polio: IPV	2 mos	4 mos			
OPV			6–18 mos	4–6 yrs	
PCV-7	2 mos	4 mos	6 mos	12–15 mos	
MMR	12–18 mos	4–6 yrs	*11–12 yrs		
Var	12–18 mos	*11–12 yrs			

*If earlier vaccines have been missed or were given late or if the child does not have antibody titer showing immunity.

This is the schedule recommended by the Advisory Committee on Immunization Practices (ACIP), the American Academy of Pediatrics (AAP), and the American Academy of Family Physicians (AAFP).

rect to use the leg for these injections, although once the child is walking he or she may experience stiffness or soreness in the muscle from the injection. After age 15 months, if the child is well developed, the doctor may prefer for the medical assistant to use the deltoid injection site on the arm for intramuscular injections to reduce discomfort. The MMR and varicella immunizations are given subcutaneously, usually in the arm.

In older children, all muscles are well developed and injection sites are the same as for adults. Immunizations are usually given in the arm because the volume usually does not exceed 0.5 ml, which can easily be absorbed by the deltoid muscle.

Managing Infants and Toddlers During Injections

Infants and toddlers must be restrained during injections to prevent movement that could cause injury. Even infants learn that doctor visits may involve painful procedures, and the medical assistant should keep the needle and syringe out of the child's direct view. An infant may be held by his or her mother or father in the supine position on the parent's lap, holding both arms and the leg that will be used for the injection, as illustrated in Figure 27–14.

If the parent does not want to assist, the medical assistant should get help from a member of the office staff.

Toddlers between age 15 months and 3 years can be very strong and usually do not have the emotional development to cooperate; it is important to get help holding such a child firmly.

Avoid spending a lot of time trying to talk the toddler into the procedure; instead, simply perform the procedure, explaining that it will prevent the child from becoming sick and will only sting for a short time. An adhesive bandage with cartoon figures often helps distract the child after the procedure and may allay fears triggered by the injection.

Managing Older Children During Injections

By age 4 or 6, when a child often receives additional immunizations, the child should be able to cooperate with the injection without the need for restraint. Allow the child to express that he or she does not want to have the procedure or does not like injections, reminding the child that it only stings or pinches for a short time. Never tell a child that an injection will not hurt,

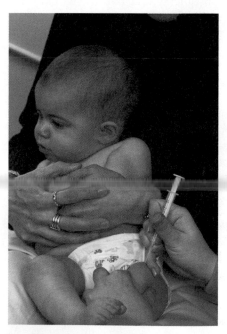

➤ **Figure 27–14** The mother holds the infant securely while the medical assistant administers an injection.

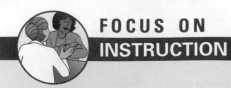

TEACHING PARENTS ABOUT SIDE EFFECTS OF IMMUNIZATIONS

Parents should be educated in the realities of childhood illnesses and vaccinations. The Centers for Disease Control and Prevention publishes a pamphlet called *Parents' Guide to Childhood Immunizations.* The pamphlet is a useful tool to educate parents.

Most offices have parents sign a consent form stating that they have been instructed about immunizations and agree to their child's receiving immunization by injection.

It should be stressed to parents that, although occasional adverse events that can cause permanent disability are associated with vaccinations, far more adverse events, including permanent disability and death, can occur from the diseases themselves. Childhood immunization is, along with sanitary water supplies and sewer systems, the greatest reason for the reduction in infant mortality and the increase in presumed lifespan for people living in industrialized countries.

After any injection, the infant or child may be irritable, have a low-grade fever, and experience stiffness or soreness at the injection site. Parents should follow the doctor's recommendations about using analgesics such as ibuprofen or acetaminophen.

More serious side effects can occur. A progressive neurologic condition can result from the DPT, as well as a fever of 104° F, persistent and uncontrollable crying, and convulsions. For this reason, a new formulation of the vaccine was developed, called DTaP, which includes acellular/pertussis vaccine. It has reduced the incidence of severe side effects in recent years.

Any vaccine, but especially the MMR, may lead to anaphylaxis, a severe respiratory and circulatory reaction.

Oral polio vaccine is made with live polio virus and has occasionally caused polio in unvaccinated adults who care for the child. If the child's parents or grandparents are immigrants, ask if they have been vaccinated against polio. If they have not, notify the doctor, who may wish to use IPV for all polio immunizations.

---

because it does, and telling a child that it will not impairs the child's trust. Once the area is cleaned, give the injection quickly and talk to the child as a distraction. Even older children want to have an adhesive bandage applied after an injection.

Occasionally, an older child or mentally retarded adult cannot cooperate with an injection or with phlebotomy and has become too strong to be safely restrained. There are anesthetic creams, such as Emla cream, that penetrate the skin to decrease pain during such procedures. This type of local anesthetic must be applied several minutes before the injection so it has time to penetrate into deeper tissue layers.

Visual Acuity and Eye Function

Visual acuity testing is usually not performed on infants unless there is suspicion of a problem. If an infant is being tested, the environment should be free of stimulation that can attract the infant's eye.

For young children a children's Snellen Eye Chart with pictures or the letter E can be used rather than the standard chart. Ask the child to identify the pictures or point with his or her hand in the direction in which the E is facing. Make the eye test a game so the

child will cooperate and to try to increase the child's attention span for the exam. When a child can read, the adult eye chart is used.

Figure 27–15 shows the medical assistant explaining how to perform the visual acuity test.

Audiometry

A hearing test is also not usually given to young children but may be performed if impaired hearing is suspected. Infants respond to sound, so sound may be used to produce an expected movement. It is appropriate for a young child to turn toward a sound. A hearing test must be performed in a quiet environment. If there is any question of hearing impairment in a young child, the doctor will refer the child to a specialist.

Scoliosis Examination

Scoliosis (lateral curvature of the spine) can appear in a child of any age, but is more commonly seen at the time a child is having a growth spurt. The scoliosis exam is usually first performed when children are between 8 and 10 (some elementary school nurses perform annual scoliosis exams on all children).

ON THE JOB

Craig Johnson is the medical assistant working with Dr. Hughes at Blackburn Primary Care Associates. Linda Harris has brought her 15-month-old son, Michael, for his well-child visit.

QUESTIONS

1. What measurements will Craig be expected to take before Dr. Hughes examines Michael?
2. Michael weighs 22 pounds, 10 ounces at this visit. His mother asks, "How is his weight compared to other boys his age?" Based on the growth chart shown in Figure 27–1, decide how Craig should answer.
3. When Craig is measuring Michael's head, Mrs. Harris says, "I know someone has explained this before, but I forget why you have to measure his head." What should Craig explain?
4. Using the Denver II Developmental Screening Test shown in Figure 27–3, identify three specific tasks that Michael should be able to perform if his development is on schedule.
5. Craig notes on Michael's immunization record that the baby is up to date on his immunizations. What immunizations should Craig expect Michael to receive today or at the 18-month visit?
6. Before Craig gives Michael any immunizations, what should he ask Mrs. Harris?
7. How does Craig expect Michael to act during the immunizations? What should Craig do to make the immunizations go as easily as possible?

When doing a scoliosis exam, look for a lateral curvature of the thoracic and lumbar spines. Have the child bend over, facing toward you, and examine the bare back to see if one shoulder blade appears higher than the other. Report any findings to the doctor. If treatment is necessary, the medical assistant may need to encourage the child to perform the treatment prescribed.

Figure 27–16 shows a child in the correct position to be examined for scoliosis.

SICK VISITS

Sick visits are made on an as-needed basis. The goal is to treat the injury or illness as promptly as possible and to schedule proper follow-up after treatment has begun. The medical assistant needs knowledge of common childhood diseases and disorders, as well as com-

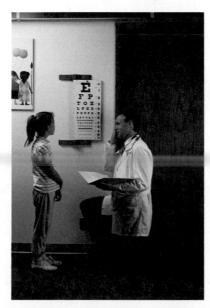

➤ **Figure 27–15** The medical assistant demonstrates how to cover one eye before testing a child's vision.

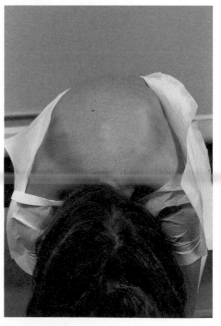

➤ **Figure 27–16** When a child bends over, one shoulder blade may be higher than the other if scoliosis is present.

mon sense about dealing with parents. This is especially important when dealing with first-time parents.

Assessing Chief Complaints

Fever, sore throat, runny nose, and earache can be symptoms of many illnesses. Children with these complaints should be seen by a doctor or a primary care clinician. Pediatric and family practice groups keep many slots open in the daily schedule for "run-in" or "sick kid" appointments, and an appointment should be made for the same day, especially for younger children.

Extremely high fever (over 104° F) should be reported immediately. High fever may trigger convulsions. Children who suffer from such "febrile seizures" usually outgrow them as they get older, but some continue to have them into the school-age years and even adolescence. Also, the tendency to run a fever higher than would be expected with the normal course of illness tends to run in families.

Never recommend aspirin for an ill child because aspirin taken during a viral infection can lead to Reye's syndrome.

■ REYE'S SYNDROME

Reye's syndrome, first described by the Australian pathologist Douglas Reye in 1963, is a rare condition developed by children and adolescents after a viral illness, especially chicken pox or influenza. Reye's syndrome is not contagious but is very dangerous to the child who contracts it. Its cause is unknown.

The symptoms, which usually appear about a week after the onset of the viral illness, include vomiting and mental disorientation. In severe cases, seizures occur that can lead to permanent neurologic damage. Reye's syndrome is fatal in about one case in four.

In the 1970s, it was noted that the incidence of progression of Reye's syndrome to a dangerous level was statistically associated with administration of aspirin or other salicylates to children suffering from viral illnesses, especially chicken pox and influenza. Since the mid-1980s manufacturers of aspirin have included a warning label to this effect on their products sold in the United States, and the incidence of Reye's syndrome in this country has declined since then.

Children are more susceptible to illness than adults because they do not have fully developed immune systems. For some children, sick visits occur very frequently in their early years and decrease as the immune system becomes more developed.

Assisting with the Examination

As with the well-child exam, the medical assistant must have the cooperation of the child during the sick visit. In addition, when dealing with a sick child, the medical assistant needs to follow strict aseptic technique so as not to pass the illness from one child to another.

Basically, the same issues arise as when assisting with a well-child visit. The child may need to be quieted and comforted during the exam so the doctor can hear and look. Distracting the child may be helpful in this regard. As with the well-child exam, any tests or procedures should be explained to the child in a way he or she can understand.

Some pediatric practices have gone to a two-waiting-room system, one waiting room for children making sick visits and the other for children waiting for well-child appointments.

CHILD ABUSE AND NEGLECT

The medical office is one of the places where cases of child abuse and/or neglect are discovered and is also one of the places where it is investigated if suspected.

Different states mandate reporting of particular circumstances to the state's child protection agency.

Abuse vs. Neglect

Abuse always involves physical, emotional, or sexual injury to a child and involves commission of a particular act (hitting, sexually touching) against a child. **Neglect,** on the other hand, involves failure to provide a child with the basic necessities of life and is usually a case of omission by the parent or caregiver rather than commission of a particular act.

Child abuse is the second leading cause of death among children under age 6 months, behind sudden infant death syndrome.

According to U.S. Department of Health and Human Services statistics, in 1998 1,397,000 children received preventive services and an estimated 903,000 children were victims of abuse or neglect. Approximately 50 percent of reports of potential abuse were received from professionals.

Abuse often occurs when the adult is having difficulty adjusting to new circumstances or is coping with such issues as marital problems, economic difficulties, single parenthood, or substance abuse.

Signs and Symptoms of Abuse

The medical assistant should be aware of the signs and symptoms of possible abuse. Some of these signs are behavioral in nature. Also, the medical assistant must listen closely to the versions of events told by the child and caregiver. Signs and symptoms include:

Reports of physical or sexual abuse by the child

Reports of physical or sexual abuse by interested adults (such as teachers)

Frequent visits to the emergency room for injuries, accompanied by stories from those who bring the child in that conflict with the child's description of the injury

Stories of incidents that are inconsistent with the injury

Stories of injuries by siblings, other children, or someone other than the caregiver

"Suspicious" injuries, such as burns in unlikely places, dislocated joints, blunt trauma injuries to the abdomen, and fractures

A child who refuses to make physical contact, or even make eye contact, with a medical professional

Behavioral changes such as a formerly friendly and normally precocious child becoming withdrawn, "too willing to please" a caregiver, or "too compliant with rules"

A child who is suddenly aggressive, demanding, or who has fits of rage

Sudden developmental delays, or regression to previous developmental stages, such as reverting to baby talk or soiling after being toilet trained.

In addition, a pattern of abuse can often be determined through diagnostic tests for a current injury. A child x-rayed for a current possible fracture may have signs of old fractures that were untreated and have healed. Most university-affiliated tertiary care hospitals have a specialist in forensic pediatrics, who specializes in the study and treatment of abuse and neglect. Suspected cases of abuse seen in the office might be referred to such a specialist.

Warning signs of neglect include malnutrition, poor growth patterns, poor hygiene, gross dental disorders, and unattended medical needs. Inadequate clothing is a key indicator—a child wearing clothes that are too small, the wrong season, and/or unwashed.

Other signs of neglect include:

Unusual delay in obtaining medical attention for illness or injury

Excessive punishment while the child is in the medical office

Hesitation by the parent or caregiver to provide information

Little or no observable attachment between the parent/caregiver and child

Comments by the parent or caregiver that the child is unwanted.

Risk factors for children to be abused or neglected include an unhealthy or unsafe home, including the presence of guns, drugs, and frequent visits by nonparent adults; parents or caregivers with criminal records, especially for drug dealing, firearms, or prostitution; inappropriate supervision, including being left with older siblings; and a history of the parent(s) or caregiver(s) having been abused as children.

Mandated Reporting

Reporting of documented abuse or neglect is **mandated** (legally required) by the Federal Child Abuse Prevention and Treatment Act. All cases of threats to children or their physical and mental welfare must be reported to the appropriate child welfare agency in the state.

Some states also require that health care workers report suspected abuse. These reports are kept in confidence, and the reporting party is not disclosed to the parent or caregiver.

A medical assistant should report all suspicions about abuse or neglect to the doctor who is, will be, or has just seen the child. In addition, the telephone number for the state's child abuse hotline should be accessible, as should the number for the local office of the state's child welfare office.

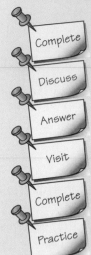

STUDENT STUDY PLAN

To reinforce your understanding of the material in this chapter . . .

Complete

Complete the **Review & Recall** questions.

Discuss

Discuss the situation in **If You Were the Medical Assistant** with your class-mates, and answer the questions.

Answer

Answer the **Critical Thinking Questions** and discuss them with your classmates.

Visit

Visit the suggested **Web sites** and search for additional Web sites using **Key-words for Internet Searches**.

Complete

Complete the exercises in chapter 27 of the **Student Mastery Manual**.

Practice

Practice all activities related to a child's visit in Case 3 on the CD-ROM.

✔ REVIEW & RECALL

1. Identify the appropriate ages at which an infant holds up his or her head, rolls over, sits without support, crawls, pulls to a stand, stands unassisted, and begins to walk.

2. Why is an infant's length, weight, and head circumference measured at each visit during the first year of life?

3. What areas of psychosocial development does the Denver Developmental Screening Test measure?

4. What can a medical assistant do to respond to the psychosocial needs of an infant, a preschool child, a school-age child, and an adolescent?

5. Compare the procedures for weighing and measuring an infant and a child.

6. Why do most doctors keep growth charts on children?

7. Describe how to plot measurements on a growth chart.

8. What methods are recommended to take the temperature of an infant, a toddler, a preschool child, and an older child?

9. What diseases do the following immunizations prevent: HBV (HepB), DTaP, MMR, Hib, PCV-7, Var?

10. How should the medical assistant document any immunization that is given?

11. What are the recommended sites for intramuscular injections in infants? For subcutaneous injections in infants and toddlers?

12. What is the medical assistant's responsibility when assisting with a sick visit?

13. List possible signs of physical abuse, sexual abuse, and neglect of a child.

✔ IF YOU WERE THE MEDICAL ASSISTANT

When you bring Leonie Jacobs, a 10-month-old girl, into the examining room at Blackburn Primary Care Associates, her mother tells you she thinks the child has something wrong with her right ear because she has been fussy and pulling at the ear.

List five questions you would ask Mrs. Jacobs to obtain more information about Leonie's current problem.

What vital signs or measurements would you complete before the doctor sees the baby? Give reasons for your choices.

CRITICAL THINKING QUESTIONS

1. Many parents and doctors are concerned because current recommendations for immunizations require so many injections. Write a paragraph identifying the advantages and disadvantages of giving immunizations from the point of view of the infant, the parent, and society as a whole.

2. Discuss with your classmates how you would feel if you suspected that a family member was abusing a child that came to the office where you worked as a medical assistant. What signs and symptoms might lead you to suspect abuse? How would you feel about the family member that you suspected of the abuse? How do you think you should behave toward the family member? Toward the child?

3. Discuss with your classmates how a pediatric medical practice is different from a medical practice that sees mainly adult patients. Discuss how you would feel working with children. What would you like about it? What might make you uncomfortable? What specialized knowledge would you need?

EXPLORE THE WEB

INTERNET WEB SITES

American Academy of Pediatrics
www.aap.org

National Institute of Child Health and Human Development
www.nichd.nih.gov

National Immunization Program
www.cdc.gov/nip

National Clearinghouse on Child Abuse and Neglect
www.calib.com/nccanch

Virtual Children's Hospital
www.vh.org/VCH/

KEYWORDS FOR INTERNET SEARCHES

child abuse
  immunizations
  pediatrics
  temperature

ANSWERS TO ON THE JOB

1. Craig will expect to measure Michael's pulse and respirations, length, weight, head and chest circumference, and possibly his blood pressure, depending on the doctor's preference.

2. The growth chart shown in Figure 27–1 shows that Michael's weight is at the 25th percentile. Craig can tell Mrs. Harris that Michael is at the 25th percentile for weight; this means that out of every 100 boys his age, about 24 weigh less than he does and about 75 weigh more than he does. Craig can also explain that weight is also related to length (that is, shorter babies tend to weigh less and longer babies tend to weigh more).

3. Until the bones in Michael's skull close completely, his head could expand if there were excess fluid in the brain. The head circumference is measured to make sure that the head is growing normally and there is no extra pressure or other problems.

4. At 15 months, Michael should be expected to be able to feed a doll, remove some of his clothes, use a spoon or a fork, help in the house, make a tower of two cubes, dump raisins from a cup if he is shown how to do it, use three to six words, and walk backwards.

5. Michael needs to receive the DTaP, MMR, and Var immunizations, either today or at his 18-month visit.

6. Craig should ask Mrs. Harris if Michael had any problems after the previous DTaP immunizations. He should also ask if Michael has any allergies and specifically ask about sensitivity to eggs.

7. Craig expects Michael to struggle and cry when receiving an injection. Craig should ask Mrs. Harris or another staff member to help by holding Michael firmly so that he cannot be injured by moving during the injection. Craig should give the injection quickly, without really attempting to convince Michael to cooperate. Immediately after the injection, Craig should apply a bright adhesive bandage to the injection site, remind Michael that it will only sting for a short time, and attempt to distract Michael if possible.

Chapter 28

Geriatrics

Instructional Objectives

After completing this chapter, you will be able to do the following:

1. Define and spell the vocabulary words.
2. Describe the normal changes that are part of the aging process.
3. Differentiate normal physiologic and mental changes from abnormal changes that may indicate disease or a pathologic condition.
4. Describe measures to assist patients with dementia.
5. Describe measures to maintain safety of the patient with decreased mobility.
6. Discuss how to provide effective care and instructions to a patient with decreased eyesight or impaired hearing.
7. List measures to prevent additional health problems in a patient with neuropathy.
8. Assist elderly patients to plan for appropriate safety and support services.
9. Report common signs of elder abuse or neglect to the doctor.

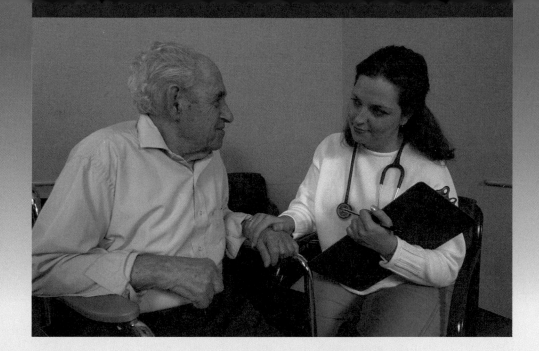

■ Prepare patient for and assist with routine and speciality examinations.

■ Instruct individuals according to their needs.

VOCABULARY

atrophy (p. 701)

cataracts (p. 707)

dementia (p. 704)

exacerbation (p. 704)

gait (p. 701)

geriatric (p. 700)

glaucoma (p. 707)

hypothermia (p. 701)

idiopathic (p. 708)

life expectancy (p. 700)

motility (p. 701)

neuropathy (p. 708)

opacity (p. 703)

orthostatic hypotension (p. 701)

osteoporosis (p. 701)

senile (p. 700)

ABBREVIATIONS

ADLs (p. 709)

Geriatric is a medical term that has a specific meaning—old. Although most people refer to the old as "elderly," geriatric is the proper medical term that defines the older or aged population, as pediatric defines the young population.

The U.S. government defines the geriatric population as those Americans over age 65 years. This population is divided into three categories: the young old, age 65 to 74; the old, age 75 to 89; and the very old, those age 90 and over. Despite these definitions, however, an individual's chronological age is not always a good indicator of physical, social, and emotional well-being.

The geriatric population is the fastest growing group in the United States. According to the U.S. Centers for Disease Control and Prevention statistics, 13 percent of the U.S. population was over age 65 in 2000, and about 2 percent of the population was over age 85. Those who study population trends believe that by the year 2030, 22 percent of the American population will be over 65. The geriatric population is most heavily concentrated in nine states: California, Florida, Illinois, Michigan, New Jersey, New York, Ohio, Pennsylvania, and Texas.

In America, as in most countries, the **life expectancy** of women is higher than men. Life expectancy refers to the expected length of life for a person at a given time. Currently, for an infant born today, life expectancy for a male is 83 and for a female is 90. This life expectancy has increased greatly since 1900, due to advances in medical care, environmental health and safety, and the early detection and prevention of diseases.

Up to 50 percent of adult patients in a primary care medical practice—either adult medicine or family practice—will be over 65. They are often dealing with chronic and degenerative diseases and are feeling the gradual decline of the body's systems. Many older Americans are healthy and vibrant, but sometimes the public's perception is that older people are sick, useless, and even **senile**—having low mental functioning—and generally a burden on the society and the economy.

This attitude often causes fear in many older adult patients. Older people do not always have the same reactions to situations. They are individuals, with individual needs, and different interests. However, they often face common situations and have common concerns. Among the developmental issues facing older adults are:

Adjusting to changes in physical strength and general health

Adjusting to death of life partners, siblings, and long-time friends

Adjusting to retirement and reduced income

Adjusting to the role of elder member of the family.

They must work to develop new routines of daily living and to find activities that are enjoyable and provide them with a feeling of usefulness and self-esteem.

CHANGES IN THE AGING PERSON

The aging person undergoes many changes—some physical, others mental, and still others emotional. Many of these changes are normal, others are abnormal.

Normal Changes

All people do not age at the same rate. Degenerative changes are expected in all people if they live long enough, but some people experience these processes at age 65 and others do not experience them until age 85.

The way in which an individual ages, and his or her particular pattern of degenerative changes, depends on a number of factors, including genetics, nutritional status, personal health habits, the amount of physical activity he or she has undertaken and continues to perform, and even attitude. The box that follows shows some of the physical changes that occur in the geriatric patient.

Physical Changes of the Aging Process

The following changes describe the average individual, but any specific person may vary from these averages.

Brain. Noticeable decrease in memory and reaction time beginning at around age 70.

Eyes. Difficulty focusing begins between age 40 and 50.

After age 50, increased sensitivity to glare, difficulty seeing in dim light, difficulty detecting moving targets.

Difficulty detecting fine detail after age 70.

Ears. Decreased ability to hear high-frequency tones may begin between age 20 and 30.

Decreased ability to hear low-frequency tones begins around age 60.

More hearing loss in men than women from age 30 to 80.

Lungs. Maximum breathing capacity decreased 40% by age 80.

Heart. Maximal heart rate decreased 25% by age 75.

Pancreas. Progressive decrease in glucose metabolism.

Blood vessels. Increase in systolic blood pressure of 20% to 25% by age 75.

Muscles. Muscle mass and oxygen consumption by muscles decreased 5% to 10% every decade.

Strength of hand grip decreased 45% by age 75.

Bones. Loss of bone is greater than replacement of bone beginning at age 35. Greater loss of bone in women, especially after menopause.

Modified from *With the Passage of Time: The Baltimore Longitudinal Study of Aging,* NIH publication No. 93-3685. Bethesda, MD: National Institutes of Health, 1993.

Changes in Vital Signs

Weight and height loss are common in older adults. Loss of sensitivity in taste and smell may cause a decreased interest in eating. If teeth are missing or dentures are uncomfortable, food choices may be limited. Factors like these contribute to weight loss. On the other hand, inactivity decreases caloric requirements, and some older adults, especially those who do not have to shop and work for themselves, such as those who live in assisted-living facilities or nursing homes, may gain weight.

Height decreases both as spinal curvature increases and as intervertebral spaces—the area of soft tissue between the vertebrae in the spine—decreases.

Older people are less likely to develop fever than younger people. Because of this, body temperature is not a reliable indicator of health status. The body's ability to regulate heat also changes, putting older people at greater risk for **hypothermia**—dangerously low body temperature—if not properly clothed in very cold weather and to heat stroke and heat exhaustion in very hot weather.

Pulse rhythm may become slightly irregular and may increase with only slight exertion. Many older people also experience an increase in both systolic and diastolic blood pressure readings, making it difficult to know whether increased blood pressure is due to normal changes or disease.

Musculoskeletal Changes

Muscles **atrophy**—become smaller—and lose mass. Muscle atrophy and bone degeneration cause the chest to increase in size to adjust to loss of lung elasticity. Loss of bone mass of over 2.5 percent is called **osteoporosis.** The condition occurs regularly in old age to both men and women, but is more prevalent and more severe in women because of bone loss that occurs due to hormonal changes after menopause.

Stiffness, muscle spasms, and loss of range of motion in joints is normal and results in a change of **gait**—walking motion. Loss of joint elasticity makes performance of daily living tasks more difficult.

Cardiovascular Changes

The heart muscle itself does not change with age. However, the valves become thicker and more rigid. Blood vessels lose some of their elasticity. This can result in slower response to position changes, especially when getting out of bed. An older person may need to learn how to move from lying down to sitting up for a few minutes before trying to stand up, to avoid dizziness due to **orthostatic hypotension** (decreased blood pressure when changing position).

Gastrointestinal Changes

A decrease in **motility**—muscle movement—within the gastrointestinal tract occurs. This leads to heartburn, constipation, and other forms of gastrointestinal distress.

The gag reflex is diminished, which can cause choking on food or medication. A decrease in stomach capacity leads to less hunger, and lack of taste sensation can lead to less desire to eat. This can, in turn, lead to malnutrition.

Teeth that have been well cared for should remain functional well into old age, but many older adults have partial or full dentures. These should fit well to avoid causing ulceration to the mouth.

Skin Changes

Many changes occur to the skin in old age. The epithelium and subcutaneous tissues thin with age. Skin loses its elasticity and wrinkles, becomes drier, and more fragile. Skin breakdown causes delayed wound healing.

Loss of hair growth on head and body occurs. However, many men experience thickening of the hair on their eyebrows, nose, and ears. Women may experience unwanted hair on their chin and face. See Figure 28–1 for an example of skin and hair changes in an elderly man.

Neurologic Changes

A normal decrease in blood flow to the brain occurs but does not cause any symptoms. The brain shrinks in size, but this should not affect intelligence.

Slower reaction time is expected, and many older people have difficulty adjusting to situational changes. Slowing of motor response is normal—which can be a safety issue for older people who continue to drive cars or operate electrical equipment.

Some loss of memory, especially short-term memory, is expected. Reminder lists, memory aids, and memory exercises can help to alleviate the fear of forgetting, even if they do not actually change the organic process of memory loss. Despite the loss of short-term memory, many older people have an acute sense of long-term memory and love to reminisce and tell stories.

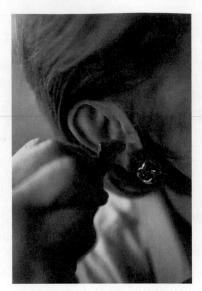

> **Figure 28–2** Inserting a hearing aid.

Sensory Changes

All five senses become less acute in older adults. Because of this, geriatric patients are at greater risk for injury.

Eyesight. Peripheral vision decreases, and sensitivity to light increases.

Hearing. Hearing loss is expected, to one degree or another. Many people are embarrassed to admit a hearing loss. They may not acquire a hearing aid or may not use one they have. Rather than ask people to speak more slowly, to look at them when speaking, or sit on or speak to the side that their "good ear" is on, they may simply withdraw from conversation. See Figure 28–2.

Smell and Taste. These senses are dulled. A decreased sense of smell may cause an older person to eat spoiled food; it is essential to teach them to read "sell by" labels and possibly to label food with the day they opened the container. Decreased sense of taste may cause older people to season food too heavily, making it both unhealthy for themselves and unpalatable for other people.

Sensation/Motor. Senses such as touch/feeling may not be as sensitive, and grip strength may be diminished. This can cause older people to drop objects. Coordination may be decreased and reaction time delayed.

Genitourinary Changes

Kidneys decrease in size, with less ability to filter harmful waste by-products. The bladder also decreases in size, and holds less than 250 mL of urine. Additionally, the bladder walls lose elasticity. Older adults may suffer urinary incontinence to one degree or another.

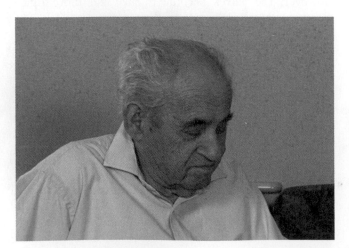

> **Figure 28–1** Skin in the elderly becomes wrinkled and loses moisture.

Eighty percent of men over age 60 have benign prostatic hypertrophy (noncancerous prostate disease). An enlarged prostate gland affects ability to urinate and causes discomfort during urination.

Hormone levels decrease in both men and women, which affects most body systems.

Abnormal Changes

Many of these "normal" changes in the older adult have their parallel abnormal changes. For example, significant increase in blood pressure is not normal. Nor is skin infection. Severe memory loss and difficulty learning is not normal. **Opacity** of the eye lens—cloudy, filmy eyes—or cataracts is not normal. Memory loss that becomes confusion and personality changes are also signs of illness and not normal conditions of aging.

Much loss of tactile sensation is thought to be related to disease processes rather than aging. Diabetes mellitus and thyroid dysfunction are more prevalent in the older person than younger patients.

Older people are prone to fractures due to osteoporosis. Foot problems, due to normal wear and tear as well as chronic diseases such as diabetes, are prevalent. Osteoarthritis may cause joint deformities, posture changes, and fine motor impairment. Geriatric patients are at risk for falls due to loss of vision, strength, and coordination.

Moderate atherosclerotic changes in the blood vessels and heart may lead to heart disease, myocardial infarctions (heart attacks), or strokes. High blood lipids are a result of lifestyle.

Shortness of breath, dyspnea, and fatigue may result from respiratory problems. Pain receptors are diminished in geriatric patients, so pain may not be present during an illness or after an injury. Complications of illness, as well as permanent impairment and disabilities, may result because of this lack of feeling.

The main causes of death in older people are heart disease, cancer, circulatory problems, strokes, and respiratory disorders, including pneumonia and influenza. Because multiple systems are involved with illness, problems in one organ system may ultimately affect the entire body.

Most geriatric patients suffer from one chronic condition, and many have multiple disease processes. Changes in hormone levels and other processes can cause geriatric patients to have adverse drug reactions they would not have had when younger.

Because of skin changes, many older people are susceptible to skin infections, keratosis, pressure sores, dry skin, and skin cancers. Ultraviolet light is more detrimental to older people than younger people because of skin changes.

Medical Assistant Responsibilities Related to the Older Patient

The medical assistant must be sure to have open lines of communication with the older patient. This builds an atmosphere of trust. See Figure 28–3.

Discuss the patient's fears and hopes in real terms. Realize that these patients' medical conditions cause problems with self-image and self-esteem. Such a patient may vent his or her rage at the medical office staff because they see the staff as a safe place for allowing the inner emotion to come to the surface. He or she may also have a decreased ability to control emotions, especially in the early stages of neurologic conditions such as dementia.

Work toward improving the patient's self-image while at the same time assisting the patient to accept his or her physical and mental changes. Allow the person to vent the frustrations that come with the loss of health and independence. Prepare the patient for the fact that previous levels of health may not be an option because of advancing age. Assist the patient and family to make the necessary adjustments to advancing age.

RESPONDING TO SPECIAL PROBLEMS

The geriatric patient's health plan should be based more on maintenance than prevention. To reduce risks, it is important that this plan include exercise, diet modification, and promotion of healthy lifestyle.

In 1995, the most commonly occurring conditions in the geriatric population were arthritis, hypertension, and heart disease. The incidence of stroke, diabetes, arthritis, heart disease, and cancer increased between 1984 and 1995, but the prevalence of hypertension remained fairly constant during that time. Although the incidence of these particular conditions differs by sex, race, and ethnic origin, the general trend is fairly constant across the United States. To maintain health in

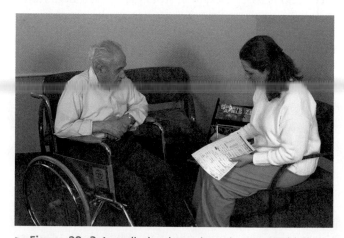

➤ **Figure 28–3** A medical assistant interviewing an elderly patient.

FOCUS ON
INSTRUCTION

INSTRUCTING OLDER ADULTS

1. Always write out the important instructions in steps—short, precise, easy-to-understand terms. Use large print if needed because of visual impairment. A computer-generated checklist is often helpful.

2. Have the patient repeat the instructions you have given, with an understanding of why the procedure is important. Understanding the importance enhances the chances of compliance.

3. If a new procedure has been added to the routine daily tasks, have the patient perform the procedure for you before leaving the office. Be sure to require patient compliance with safety precautions as well as procedural techniques.

4. Provide the patient with aids, such as weekly calendars on which to check off the procedures as they are performed. Suggest medication reminder boxes and so on to help jog memory and facilitate compliance.

5. Help the patient explore ways to incorporate new procedures, medications, and so on, into the daily routine. Routine is important to the elderly, and anything new should be linked to a routine that is already in place to help the elderly person remember to do it.

the older adult, the examination should include an assessment of activities, diet, medications being used, smoking, and alcohol intake.

Any change seen in a geriatric patient may be related to psychosocial factors, as well as to environmental changes, normal age-related changes, acute illness, **exacerbation** (a period when symptoms are increased) of a chronic illness, medication, or a new illness. Assessments can be time consuming because the patient may have multiple health problems, but must be comprehensive to ensure accuracy in diagnosis and to assure that the proper explanation for the patient's current state is offered.

Because of decreased memory and/or the fear of being embarrassed the older adult may answer a question incorrectly or incompletely, rather than admit that he or she cannot remember. In addition, he or she may react with irritation, anger, or other aggressive behaviors.

The medical assistant is the communication link between the patient and the doctor. The medical assistant also often works with family members and others who help care for the geriatric patient. In all of these communications and relationships, the medical assistant must consider the importance of economics and family dynamics when working with an older patient and his or her family. The individual may be living on a fixed income. He or she may lack transportation. Family members may need to take time from work to bring the geriatric patient to appointments. They may be struggling with providing or finding appropriate care and/or an appropriate living situation.

Dementia

Dementia—a condition of memory loss, confusion, and sometimes agitation and aggression—can have many causes. Dementia is normally associated with the loss of memory to recent events.

Sometimes dementia is caused by drug toxicity. This occurs in the older adult because of changes in the liver and kidneys, causing an inability to metabolize medications as efficiently as younger adults. Because of this, a "normal" adult dose of some medications can be toxic to an older patient.

The degree of dementia is proportional to the loss of substance in the frontal lobes of the brain. Dementia in the elderly is often due to Alzheimer's disease, although it may have several other causes. Alzheimer's disease is characterized by the buildup of neuritic plaques and neurofibrillary tangles in the brain as the neurons degenerate. Its cause is unknown.

For many years, Alzheimer's was considered abnormal dementia in the middle-aged or young old; dementia in the old and very old was characterized as simple senile dementia. However, more recently, research using brain scans and other technology has shown that the underlying pathophysiology of most dementia is essentially the same.

ON THE JOB

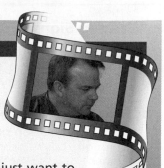

Medication Videotape: "The Follow-Up"

Paul, the medical assistant working with Dr. Lawler, is talking to Mrs. Simon, a patient whose blood pressure was elevated when she saw the doctor last week. It is still elevated at a recheck today. Paul is trying to be sure Mrs. Simon takes her blood pressure medication regularly. Mrs. Simon has brought all her medication with her to the office.

Paul: Yes, two of your pills are important to control your blood pressure, and we just want to make sure that you take them properly. Three times a day for this one (holding up one pill bottle), morning, afternoon, and evening; and this one every other day (holding up the other pill bottle).

Mrs. Simon: Well, I have a pretty good memory. I usually have a piece of paper on the table, and put little numbers down. One, two, three, for blood pressure because I take three. And then I, you know, arrange the others.

Paul: I understand.

Mrs. Simon: I don't have as much trouble with the others because I only take them once a day, but I have a little trouble with the blood pressure pill because three times a day is, well, you know, sometimes I go to bed early.

Paul: Well, it's very important that you do take the pills three times a day, because your blood pressure is still a little high.

Mrs. Simon: You mean, two wouldn't be good enough?

Paul: It's important that you take all the pills as the doctor prescribes. Otherwise they may not work as well as they should, and the numbers show that they are not.

(Paul shows Mrs. Simon a weekly pill organizer, as illustrated below.)

Paul: Perhaps you can use one of these and set the pills in it so you can remind yourself that there are still pills you have to take before you go to bed. Of course, you shouldn't double up, but you should try not to forget to take them either.

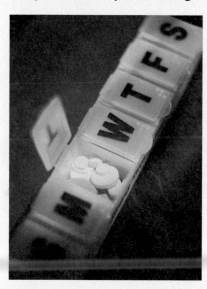

QUESTIONS

1. Why is it important for Paul to find out if Mrs. Simon is taking her blood pressure medication correctly?
2. Does the information in this conversation indicate that Mrs. Simon is or is not taking her afternoon and evening pills?
3. What is the advantage to Mrs. Simon of using a pill organizer in addition to or instead of her current method of marking the pills on paper?
4. Is there any other suggestion Paul could make to help Mrs. Simon?

Warning Signs of Alzheimer's Disease

According to the Alzheimer's Association, the following are warning signs that a person may be developing Alzheimer's disease:

1. Memory loss that affects job skills beyond occasional forgetfulness
2. Difficulty performing familiar tasks. Although busy people may be distracted when cooking or performing other tasks, people with Alzheimer's may not be able to plan a meal or may cook it but forget to eat it.
3. Problems finding words to express ideas or using incorrect words
4. Disorientation to time or place beyond forgetting the date or day of the week for a short time. A person with Alzheimer's may get lost in a familiar location and may not be able to remember the day of the week a short time after being told.
5. Lack of judgment or poor judgment. The person with Alzheimer's may forget to get dressed before going to the store.
6. Problems with abstract thinking. This includes the inability to do things that a person used to be able to do easily, such as multiplication or subtraction.
7. Misplacing things, especially in inappropriate places, such as putting clean dishes in the refrigerator
8. Rapid changes in mood and behavior for no apparent reason
9. Changes in personality that are more dramatic than the usual changes of aging. A person with Alzheimer's may become suspicious, angry, or withdrawn. The person with a formerly easy-going personality may become easily angered.
10. Loss of initiative and lack of interest in former pursuits

Alzheimer's disease is a progressive condition. An individual with Alzheimer's progresses from minor changes in thinking, behavior, and understanding to more severe loss of these abilities. Some individuals stay in one stage longer than others. Eventually, if an individual with Alzheimer's does not die of complications of another disease, such as diabetes, respiratory illness, or heart disease, he or she will lose the ability to consume food.

Tube feeding may be initiated via a nasogastric tube or a gastrotomy tube (a tube placed directly in the stomach). Patients who are unable to chew or swallow without aspirating food particles into their lungs because of other conditions (i.e., stroke or late-stage Parkinson's disease) may also be tube fed.

Medical Assistant Responsibilities Related to the Patient with Dementia

When a medical assistant suspects that an older patient is suffering from dementia, he or she should try to observe the individual's clothing, personal hygiene, and other factors to determine the patient's ability to care for himself or herself. Weight needs to be checked to determine nutritional status. Both short- and long-term memory should be checked. Alertness can be checked by having the patient perform simple calculations or sequencing. Be sure to chart findings appropriately.

The medical assistant should keep in mind the following 13 things when working with a patient suffering from dementia:

1. Use patience and compassion. Help the patient relax.
2. Speak calmly and slowly; act as if you expect the patient to understand.
3. Do not allow your voice to slip into a condescending tone—do not speak to the patient as if he or she is a small child.
4. Repeat necessary medical material as often as needed, and include the family caregiver in the conversation. But never ignore the patient while talking to the caregiver.
5. Keep a list of the caregivers and their roles in the care plan.
6. Introduce yourself as often as necessary.
7. Never threaten the patient. When you sense irritation or frustration, be aware that the patient is beginning to feel frustrated.
8. Use short sentences. Provide ideas one at a time. Sequence the material. Deliver it slowly, and repeat it as often as necessary. Explain what you want done one step at a time.
9. Remind the patient of what you are doing each step of the way when performing a procedure; take the explanation only one step at a time.
10. Accept the fear and anger that comes with memory loss.
11. Do not leave a patient with dementia alone in a waiting room.
12. Use concrete rather than abstract language.
13. Ask questions about medication and general health in such a way that the patient cannot answer simply yes or no, but must actually provide information.

It is important to assist caregivers to understand what is happening to the patient with dementia, so they can be patient and understanding. A frustrated

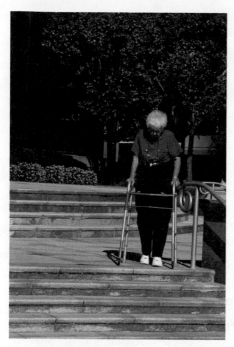

> **Figure 28–4** A walker or other assistive device may be needed for an elderly person to walk safely.

2. Help as needed, but do not give help that is not needed. Make the patient as self-sufficient as possible.
3. Listen to how the patient tells you to handle him or her. The patient knows what will cause further pain and possible injury. Let the patient be in as much control as possible.
4. Schedule appointments at a time the patient has transportation and can be as mobile as possible.
5. Have parking for the patient in an area that is convenient.
6. Encourage the patient to use aids for safety and assistance in living skills.
7. Listen to the patient. His or her intelligence is not affected by limited mobility.
8. Be aware that these patients need continued support from family, medical office staff, and others.
9. Teach safety techniques such as removing scatter rugs in the home and keeping electrical cords out of hallways and other walking areas. Handrails and accessible telephones should be placed throughout the house.
10. Suggest that the patient have a system for calling others, and should have someone to check in on a daily or more frequent basis. Make sure there is safety for those living alone.

The office must be in compliance with all conditions of the Americans with Disabilities Act as it pertains to accessibility for those with impaired mobility.

caregiver only intensifies the fear in the patient with dementia. Have on hand a list of places that provide respite care for families and caregivers of demented patients.

Decreased Mobility

Decreased mobility may come from Parkinson's disease, osteoporosis, arthritis, multiple sclerosis, or other conditions. Heart and respiratory conditions may also severely limit a person's ability to walk or perform other activities. A patient with decreased mobility may use an assistive device such as a cane, crutches, or a walker, or may even use a wheelchair or motorized cart. Figure 28–4 shows a geriatric patient using a walker.

Both gross and fine motor skills tend to decrease with age. Gait speed and step height decrease. Postural changes affect mobility.

Medical Assistant Responsibilities Related to the Patient with Decreased Mobility

The medical assistant should utilize the following 10 guidelines when dealing with geriatric patients with limited mobility.

1. Be careful not to lift or move the individual in a manner that would cause further injury or unnecessary discomfort.

Decreased Eyesight

The senses of sight, hearing, and touch often become impaired in the geriatric patient. This can have an impact on personal safety, as well as on personal relationships. The individual whose senses are impaired often withdraws. Medical assistants can work with these patients to help them cope with their anger and frustration and to create new methods for participating in the world around them.

Those with decreased eyesight often suffer a loss of peripheral vision, visual acuity, and tolerance to glare. Many older adults suffer from **glaucoma**—an increased pressure in the intraocular space—and **cataracts**—growth of tissue over the lens of an eye. Older adults also sometimes lose some of their color vision, with reds and yellows being seen best, and blues and greens fading.

Individuals with vision problems should be scheduled for office visits in morning or early afternoon, because many have night vision problems and should not be driving at dusk. A notation should be made in the chart as to the amount of assistance the patient may need navigating the office space.

Medical Assistant Responsibilities Related to the Patient with Impaired Vision

When dealing with a geriatric patient with impaired vision, the medical assistant should keep in mind the following eight things:

1. Guide patients to where you want them to go. Steer them by letting them hold your arm, shoulder, or elbow so they have some sense of being in control.
2. Give verbal instructions, cues, and warnings. Speak in a normal tone of voice—these patients are not deaf.
3. Speak at a level that ensures their dignity—they are not mentally impaired.
4. Allow the patient to carry all devices he or she uses as aids into the examining room.
5. Always announce yourself when entering a room, so you will not scare the patient.
6. Try to face the patient and speak distinctly.
7. Explain everything you will do and describe where the patient is.
8. Try not to leave the patient alone for any length of time, and check on the patient frequently.

#10 Hearing Impairment

Partial hearing loss is common in older adults. In fact, partial hearing loss is becoming more common in middle age among today's "Baby Boom" generation—those born in the years after World War II. Many researchers believe that this has been caused by the loud popular music many of these people listened to and still listen to, and predict that as this generation ages, partial or total hearing loss will become a more significant problem than ever in the geriatric population.

Hearing loss may be caused by nerve damage, inner ear trauma, or simply by the accumulation of impacted cerumen (buildup of earwax) in the outer ear canal.

Sometimes hearing can be improved by simple ear cleaning. The doctor may direct the medical assistant to perform an ear irrigation (described in Procedure 21–3). If hearing loss is shown to be a permanent problem, the medical assistant should use the following nine techniques when working with a hearing-impaired patient:

1. Always stand in front of the person to talk to him or her. Even if the person does not "read lips," the visual cue of focusing on the speaker's face and the increased concentration that comes from making eye contact with the person who is speaking can help the hearing-impaired individual.
2. Do not shout. This changes the speaker's facial expression and can lead the listener to think the speaker is angry. Older adults with hearing loss

are often embarrassed, fearful, and angry about their condition.
3. Speak slowly and distinctly.
4. If you need to gain the person's attention, gently place your hand on his or her shoulder. Before doing so, walk in front of the person so he or she can see you.
5. Have paper and pencil available so that it can be used to communicate if needed.
6. Treat the patient as an intelligent person.
7. Write important directions so that compliance is assured.
8. Rephrase statements that the patient does not seem to be understanding.
9. Involve family members if possible to be sure that instructions or information is communicated.

Neuropathy

Neuropathy is a lack of sensation due to reduced nerve function. Many older adults suffer from some degree of neuropathy. The condition may accompany diabetes mellitus, circulatory disorders, or be **idiopathic** (of unknown origin). Often a loss of sensation to heat and cold occurs in the extremities—hands and feet. It can also cause uncomfortable sensations such as burning, tingling, or itching.

This can lead to dangerous situations, such as frostbite of the toes from walking in cold, wet shoes or burned hands from touching a hot stove. Minor foot or leg problems may be ignored, leading to infections and/or open lesions that do not heal.

Posture and balance can change if a person is suffering neuropathy of the feet. Neuropathy can be caused by nutritional deficiency (lack of folic acid), medication reaction, or degenerative nerve conditions. It is a common complication of atherosclerosis and diabetes mellitus.

When dealing with a patient with neuropathy, the medical assistant should try to utilize the following nine practices:

1. Provide a safe environment, without dangers of tripping or slipping.
2. Be sure that there is adequate lighting.
3. Teach the patient the dangers related to this impairment of the peripheral nervous system.
4. Check to be sure that the patient is properly clothed for the weather.
5. Give support with walking and assist the patient to and from the exam room.
6. Be patient; these patients need extra time to perform tasks.
7. Be knowledgeable about devices that might help the patient be as independent as possible.
8. Be understanding, and encourage independence.
9. Teach proper care of feet and hands.

Feet should be washed and dried carefully. Use lotion to keep skin from cracking. Nails should be trimmed straight across. If the person has cardiovascular disease or diabetes, he or she is often referred to a podiatrist for regular foot care.

MEASURES TO HELP THE ELDERLY STAY HEALTHY AND PLAN FOR FUTURE HEALTH CARE

The medical assistant must be careful to provide good patient care while also assuring that a geriatric patient's self-image and self-esteem are not damaged. Through cooperation and trust, the medical assistant provides an atmosphere wherein the patient can comply with instructions and maintain dignity and as much independence as possible. If possible, the medical office staff encourages the elderly patient to make decisions and plan a healthy lifestyle before problems occur.

It is imperative to provide full explanations and ask the older patient to repeat instructions to assure understanding. Checking on the patient after the visit may be a way to improve compliance. For the patient with memory problems, the family or caregiver should be aware of any changes in the medical care. Always work to fit new medical care requirements into the normal lifestyle to improve compliance.

Safety Measures

Safety measures are a major concern with older adults. Follow these 10 steps to maximize safety for the older patient:

1. Have the patient and caregiver assess the home for safety.
2. Add safety devices such as grab bars and chairs in the shower when possible.
3. Be sure that water heaters are set at a lower temperature to prevent burns.
4. Eliminate throw rugs, foot stools, and other objects that can cause tripping or slipping.
5. Use arms on chairs and toilets.
6. Be sure that night lights are available.
7. Assist the patient to establish a network of family, friends, and social service agencies that check on him or her on a regular basis.
8. Install smoke and fire alarms in the patient's home and a burglar alarm if appropriate.
9. Assist in finding a link for someone who will assist the patient with the activities of daily living (**ADLs**) and therapy for specific problems when needed.
10. Know the local support groups for assistance, such as Meals on Wheels, the Visiting Nurses

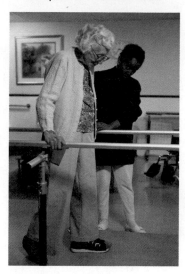

> **Figure 28–5** Exercises to increase strength and mobility may help an aging patient remain independent.

Association, and religious community services (Catholic Family Services, Jewish Family Services, etc.) that can provide respite for caregivers.

Planning for Alternative Living Arrangements

With an increasing older population, there has been an increase in the number and variety of living arrangements—from skilled care nursing facilities (nursing homes) for the frail who need total care—to assisted living and independent living arrangements, retirement villages, and "lifecare" facilities, which provide all levels of care in different wings of the facility.

At some point, the majority of older adults will require some assistance with ADLs, either on a temporary or permanent basis. Most would prefer to receive such care and assistance from family members. Outpatient physical therapy may help increase strength and mobility, as shown in Figure 28–5. But in a mobile society, many must make other arrangements.

Those who plan for and voluntarily move to a new setting tend to experience better emotional and physical health after their move than those who move involuntarily. Relocation is always stressful, as it changes routine, which is especially important to an older adult.

When voluntarily changing living arrangements, the proximity to needed services is a major consideration, as is the size and layout of the living space. The older adult needs to be as close as possible to as many services and amenities as possible, with ample transportation. Although most older adults fight for their independence and are slow to give up trappings of independence such as their car, they may also be relieved to no longer have the burden of providing their own transportation, so long as their new living facility provides a way to get places, from the grocery store to the symphony concert.

The degree to which an older adult is able to maintain his or her previous lifestyle is directly proportional to his or her ability to make the needed adjustments to a new living arrangement. Factors to consider when assisting an older adult in choosing a new living situation include:

1. Cost
2. Who manages the facility, and how it meets residents' needs
3. The staffing level of the facility, staff experience, and staff training, as well as how staff relates to the residents
4. Other services available and proximity of the facility to needed care.

Respecting the Wishes of the Aging Person

The wishes of older patients concerning their current health care, and their plans for when they no longer are able to make decisions about their care both must be respected. An older adult should be encouraged to fill out documents that articulate his or her wishes for future care and name a health care agent to make decisions if he or she becomes unable to do so. A copy of this documentation should be placed in the patient's medical records. Specific types of documents, known collectively as advanced directives, are discussed in chapter 30.

IDENTIFYING AND RESPONDING TO SUSPECTED ELDER ABUSE

The three types of elder abuse are physical, psychological, and material (financial). Elder abuse can occur in members of any race, socioeconomic class, or religious group. In 1994, there were 241,000 reports of elder abuse, 61 percent of which were substantiated.

Some of the symptoms of chronic illnesses may mimic the signs of neglect. Elder abuse is probably as prevalent as child abuse, although this has not been proven. Symptoms of elder abuse may include multiple chronic illnesses, bladder or bowel incontinence, inability to make reasonable requests or decisions, dementia, inability to adjust to the regular routine of the caregiver such as sleep disturbances or eating demands, or total dependence on the caregiver for ADLs.

Neglect may be passive, with the caregiver not giving physical or psychological care, out of ignorance or inability to give the needed care. Neglect may be active, in which the older person is deprived of daily needs such as opportunity to use the toilet, nutrition,

or sleep. Active neglect may also take the form of overmedication to keep the older person passive, non-complaining, and compliant.

Psychological neglect can include physically threatening a person or withholding needed elements or self-dignity and self-esteem.

Material abuse can occur in many ways. A caregiver may be stealing, embezzling, or squandering the older person's money. Or a child or grandchild may take advantage of an older relative by obtaining free housing without providing adequate assistance or care in return.

Physical abuse tends to be more overt than psychological or material abuse, but also may be cleverly hidden from medical providers by the caregiver.

Contributing factors to elder abuse are a history of alcoholism, drug use, or violence in the family (either the older person, a child, or grandchild), and especially in the caregiver; a history of mental illness in the older person or the caregiver; or stressful events in the life of the older person or the abuser. The medical assistant should note the interaction between the caregiver and the patient while getting the patient ready for the examination.

Signs and Symptoms of Elder Abuse

Foul odor on patient (incontinence, lack of bathing)
Poor skin color or tone
Inappropriate clothing for the season and/or soiled clothing
Suspicious wounds in several stages of healing
Extreme concern about finances
Poor hygiene and physical debris on the patient (dried feces, urine, dirt, food)
Poor self-esteem and loss of dignity in previously dignified person
Bruises, burns, etc. on ankles and/or wrists (possible signs of restraints being used)
Poor nutritional state on multiple visits, with no attempt at correction
Large, untreated pressure sores
Untreated medical conditions or injuries
Noncompliance with medical care
Dehydration that is not related to disease processes
Excessive agitation and unwarranted worry while in the office
Apathy.

Reporting

The medical assistant is responsible for bringing suspected abuse to the doctor's attention. If confirmed, it must be reported to the proper authorities—this varies by state. The medical assistant is responsible if abuse is not reported.

It may be necessary to separate the caregiver and the patient during an examination to ensure the proper exam and to gain a full description of suspect signs.

These must be documented. Photographs may be necessary, with permission, for future documentation.

Early intervention usually helps both the patient and the caregiver. Always show a caring attitude and compassion with any patient who has been the victim of elder abuse. Realize that the individual feels dependent on the caregiver and will fear reprisal or abandonment by the caregiver if the abuse is discovered.

STUDENT STUDY PLAN

To reinforce your understanding of the material in this chapter . . .

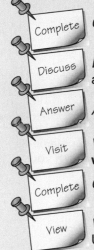

Complete *Complete* the **Review & Recall** questions.

Discuss *Discuss* the situation in **If You Were the Medical Assistant** with your classmates and answer the questions.

Answer *Answer* the **Critical Thinking Questions** and discuss them with your classmates.

Visit *Visit* the suggested **Web sites** and search for additional Web sites using **Keywords for Internet Searches.**

Complete *Complete* the exercises in chapter 28 of the **Student Mastery Manual.**

View *View* the Medication **Videotape,** "Evaluating Medication," and "The Follow-Up."

 ## ✔ REVIEW & RECALL

1. List developmental tasks of the older adult.
2. Describe normal changes in the musculoskeletal system, the skin, and the neurologic system that occur because of aging.
3. How do the senses change in older adults?
4. List common diseases of the elderly.
5. Describe how elderly patients commonly respond when asked for information that they cannot remember.
6. Describe common symptoms of Alzheimer's disease.
7. Discuss measures to prevent injury in a patient with limited mobility.
8. What special measures should a medical assistant take to assist a patient with decreased vision? With impaired hearing?
9. List the ways neuropathy can lead to additional health problems for an elderly person. How can these problems be prevented or minimized?
10. Identify specific symptoms that might lead a medical assistant to suspect elder abuse or neglect.

IF YOU WERE THE MEDICAL ASSISTANT

Mrs. Johnson, a 68-year-old white female, has become increasingly responsible for coordinating care for her husband, Alfred, 76, who has chronic Parkinson's disease. Although Mr. Johnson can still stand and walk about 12 steps with help, he needs a wheelchair when he comes to the doctor's office. In addition, he needs to have his food cut into small pieces, and he needs help with personal care. Mrs. Johnson does not drive. Her daughter is usually available for transportation. Mrs. Johnson asks if you have any suggestions for how she can obtain help.

Investigate community resources and suggest specific resources to help Mrs. Johnson obtain a wheelchair, obtain help with personal care for Mr. Johnson, obtain a raised toilet seat, and arrange for transportation to the medical office if her daughter is not available. Also, find out if there is adult day care available in your geographic area.

CRITICAL THINKING QUESTIONS

1. Discuss how a person can plan for his or her older years before the physical and mental capacity to do effective planning is lost. Why do you think many people neglect to do this? How can the medical office help in this process?

2. Do research to find out if the elderly have special nutritional needs and problems. Are supplements recommended? Discuss your findings with your classmates.

EXPLORE THE WEB

INTERNET WEB SITES

Alzheimer's Association
www.alz.org

Alzheimer's Disease Education and Referral Center
www.alzheimers.org

American Geriatrics Society
www.americangeriatrics.org

Health topic: elderly injuries
www.cdc.gov/health/elderly.htm

National Institute on Aging
www.nih.gov/nia

KEYWORDS FOR INTERNET SEARCHES

aging and health
    Alzheimer's disease
    elderly health
    geriatrics
    hearing loss

ANSWERS TO ON THE JOB

1. To treat Mrs. Simon's hypertension, Dr. Lawler needs to know if her blood pressure is really higher or if she is not taking all of her medications.

2. From this conversation, it appears that Mrs. Simon does not always take her afternoon and/or evening pills, but it is not possible to tell how often she forgets.

3. If Mrs. Simon filled the weekly pill organizer with all the pills she is supposed to take during the week, it would be easy to see if there were pills she forgot to take. This would help the doctor decide whether to change her medication (possibly to another medication that she only needs to take once a day) or to increase her medication. Marking the pills on paper does not seem to be enough for her to be sure that she is taking them all.

4. Paul might suggest a specific activity to link to taking each pill because this can help Mrs. Simon develop an effective routine. For example, she could take her afternoon pill when she watches her favorite television show, and she could take her evening pill when she brushes her teeth just before going to bed. She could place the pill container in a place that would remind her to check it before going to bed. Paul might also suggest that a family member call her each evening to be sure that she has taken all her pills and/or remind her to take the last one.

Chapter 29

Obstetrics

Instructional Objectives

After completing this chapter, you will be able to do the following:

1. Define and spell the vocabulary words for this chapter.
2. Correlate current trends in prenatal care to issues that affect them.
3. Describe physical and psychological changes during pregnancy.
4. Describe the information obtained to complete the menstrual history, past obstetric history, and history of current pregnancy.
5. Explain the lab tests that are normally done at the first prenatal visit.
6. Describe the medical assistant's role in follow-up prenatal visits.
7. Explain special diagnostic tests of pregnancy to a pregnant patient.
8. Correlate the signs of impending labor and false labor to actions a pregnant patient might be advised to take.
9. Discuss the process of postpartum visits.

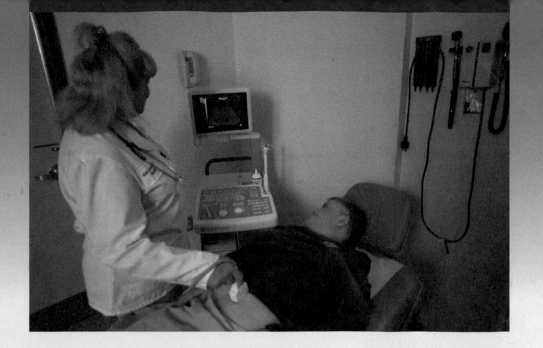

■ Prepare for and assist with routine and specialty examinations.

■ Instruct patients according to their needs.

Performance Objectives

After completing this chapter, you will be able to do the following:

1. Assist a patient during her first prenatal visit (Procedure 29-1).
2. Assist a patient during her follow-up prenatal visits (Procedure 29-2).
3. Assist a patient during her first postpartum visit (Procedure 29-3).

VOCABULARY

abortion (p. 722)	endometrium (p. 716)	Kegel exercise (p. 736)	preeclampsia (p. 727)
albuminuria (p. 725)	episiotomy (p. 736)	labor (p. 733)	premature (p. 721)
amniocentesis (p. 734)	estimated date of	lightening (p. 735)	prenatal (p. 716)
blastocyst (p. 716)	confinement (p. 721)	linea nigra (p. 721)	presumptive signs (p. 718)
chloasma (p. 721)	estimated date of delivery	lochia (p. 736)	probable signs (p. 718)
colostrum (p. 719)	(p. 721)	miscarriage (p. 722)	puerperium (p. 716)
conception (p. 716)	fetus (p. 722)	nonstress test (p. 733)	spontaneous abortion (p. 719)
contraction stress test (p. 733)	fundus (p. 730)	obstetrics (p. 713)	stillbirth (p. 722)
dilation (p. 735)	gestation (p. 721)	ovum (p. 716)	striae gravidarum (p. 719)
eclampsia (p. 727)	glucosuria (p. 725)	para (p. 722)	supine hypotension syndrome
effacement (p. 735)	gravida (p. 722)	pica (p. 720)	(p. 720)
elective abortion (p. 722)	introversion (p. 721)	positive signs (p. 718)	trimester (p. 718)
embryo (p. 721)	in utero (p. 722)	postpartum (p. 736)	viable (p. 716)

ABBREVIATIONS

Ab (p. 722) EDC (p. 721) EDD (p. 721) IUD (p. 739) LMP (p. 721) NST (p. 733)
CST (p. 733)

Obstetrics is the field of medicine that deals with pregnancy, childbirth, and the **puerperium,** the 6-week period immediately after childbirth during which a woman's reproductive organs return to their normal state. Obstetric practice is concerned with the mother-to-be and her fetus, and with the new mother. After birth, the new baby is treated as part of a pediatric practice.

PREGNANCY

Pregnancy is a normal, healthy process and should be seen that way. It is not a disease process. However, a number of circumstances can occur during pregnancy that endanger the mother-to-be as well as her fetus.

Pregnancy begins with **conception.** Conception occurs when a single sperm unites with an **ovum** (egg). There are approximately 50 million to 200 million sperm per milliliter of semen. The average ejaculation contains between 3 and 5 mL of semen. This means there are anywhere from 150 million to 1 billion sperm that have a chance to create conception during a single incident of unprotected intercourse.

Most sperm make their way through the uterus to the fallopian tubes within 1 hour. Sperm remain viable for 48 to 72 hours, but for conception to occur, a **viable** sperm (one that can survive and join with an ovum) must unite with an ovum within 14 to 24 hours after ovulation.

When conception occurs, the fertilized egg multiplies and this ball of cells—known as a **blastocyst**—moves through the fallopian tube and into the uterus, where it implants in the **endometrium**—the uterine wall. This trip takes about five days. Figure 29–1 shows the process of fertilization and implantation.

Aims of Prenatal Care

Prenatal refers to the time before birth. Prenatal care is the care given by obstetric practitioners to a mother-to-be and her fetus. Surveys routinely show that women who receive early and continuous prenatal care have fewer complications during pregnancy and during labor and delivery; they also deliver healthier and higher birthweight babies.

There are seven major aims of prenatal care:

1. Assist every mother-to-be to go through pregnancy, as well as labor and delivery, with a minimum of discomfort and in optimum health.
2. Maintain the fetus in the highest state of health throughout the pregnancy, and labor and delivery.
3. Provide emotional and psychological support for all included in the birth process (this includes fathers-to-be and older siblings).
4. Provide education for the potential parents to develop healthy habits and attitudes toward family relationships; to provide care for their offspring in a responsible, satisfying, and confident

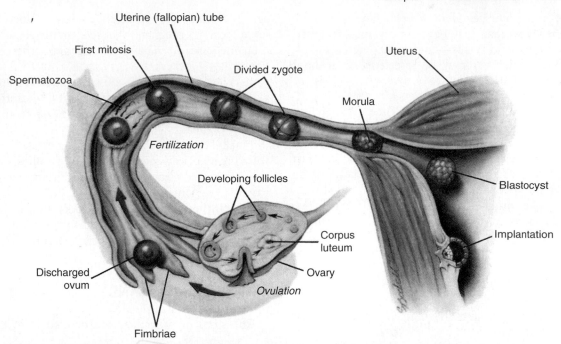

Uterine (fallopian) tube
First mitosis
Spermatozoa
Divided zygote
Uterus
Fertilization
Morula
Developing follicles
Blastocyst
Corpus luteum
Implantation
Discharged ovum
Ovary
Ovulation
Fimbriae

➤ **Figure 29–1** Throughout the menstrual cycle a follicle develops into an ovum, which is released into the fallopian tube at the time of ovulation. If fertilized by a sperm, the single-celled zygote begins to divide, forming a ball of cells called a morula within a few days. Further cell division results in the formation of a hollow ball of cells (called a blastocyst) by the time the developing embryo reaches the uterus and implants in the uterine wall. (From Thibodeau GA, Patton KT: *The Human Body in Health and Disease*. St. Louis: Mosby, 1992.)

manner; and to educate for responsible parenting.

5. Promote family involvement during the pregnancy, labor, delivery, and postpartum periods.
6. Meet the family's cultural, social, and religious needs.
7. Identify families at risk, and provide appropriate intervention or referral.

Current Trends in Prenatal Care

Pregnancy and childbirth are both emotional and dramatic experiences, not just for the mother-to-be, but for the entire family. Prenatal care must include attention to the physical, emotional, and social aspects of the changes in both the mother-to-be and other family members.

Socioeconomic circumstances can greatly affect the care a pregnant woman obtains. If she lives in a household where food and/or necessary medication are not always available, she will have a more difficult pregnancy than a woman whose refrigerator is always well stocked and who can afford necessary medication. If she lacks dependable transportation, she may miss scheduled appointments. If she and/or her partner abuses alcohol, street drugs, or prescription medica-

tion, she may have both physical and emotional difficulties with pregnancy.

Prenatal care must be given with all of these issues in mind.

While the obstetric practice is often being forced to deal with a host of maternal socioeconomic issues, it is also faced with business, insurance, and hospital pressures as well.

Many hospitals and obstetrics practices, in an effort to "market" to particular patients, offer "birthing suites" with all the comforts of home, including a bed for dad and cots for older siblings. Certified nurse-midwives may provide care and delivery in a practice affiliated with a hospital or birth center.

A support person—partner, parent, or friend—is encouraged to participate in the birth, and most hospitals have childbirth classes for the mother-to-be and her support person. Technological advances allow more "high-risk" births to be accomplished today than ever before, with better outcomes for both mother and baby.

At the same time, insurance companies are pushing for early discharge, and few new mothers and baby spend much more than 48 hours in the hospital after birth, except for caesarean section births or babies who must spend time in the newborn intensive care nursery.

There are more choices than ever before about the style of birth a woman may have for an uncomplicated birth, a woman who wants—and sometimes needs—more care after delivery may be forced to do without because of financial contracts between hospitals or birth centers and insurance providers.

Issues That Affect Prenatal Care

Maternal and child health has been of great concern to national and international groups, especially in the past 20 years. The infant mortality rate (usually expressed as the number of deaths per 100,000 live births) has been decreasing steadily in the United States, to an all-time low of 7.1 in 1997. Unfortunately, the infant mortality rate for minority women, women living in poverty, and women with substance abuse problems is still well above the rate for white, middle-class, and wealthy women.

Maternal mortality rates have risen from a low of 6.6 per 100,000 live births in 1987 to 7.5 per 100,000 live births in 1997. Although the maternal mortality rate has not fallen, the number of hospitalizations for severe complications of pregnancy has fallen from 22 per 100,000 live births in 1987 to only 14 per 100,000 live births in 1997.

The single best predictor of infant mortality is poverty. Women who have the least ability to obtain prenatal care have the highest morbidity and mortality rates, both for themselves and for their babies. One of the goals of the federal study *Healthy People 2000* is to increase early prenatal care. In 1997, 82 percent of pregnant women received care in the first trimester of pregnancy.

Teen pregnancy is also an area of concern because of the high potential for low birthweight and at-risk infants. The teen pregnancy rate decreased about 15 percent from 1991 to 1997, and statistics from 1998 and 1999 showed a continued drop. Teens continue to receive less prenatal care in the first trimester than women in their 20s and older (66 percent in 1997). It remains very important to educate teens who become pregnant about the importance of prenatal care.

Teenage mothers are more likely than teenage girls who do not become pregnant to be poor, to leave school before graduating high school, to spend time collecting welfare assistance, to be single mothers, and to have substance abuse problems. Their children are more likely to live their childhood and adolescent years in poverty, and their daughters are more likely to repeat their mother's circumstances in their own teenage and adult lives. Every obstetric practice deals with pregnant teens, and must find ways to help create the most supportive atmosphere possible for both the mother-to-be and the child she will have.

Another issue that obstetric practices are increasingly dealing with is the number of women over age 35 having children. Older women—especially those over age 35 having their first child—are at increased risk for a host of pregnancy-related problems. Their children are also at higher risk for a number of conditions.

In many communities, obstetric practices are dealing with radical changes due to immigration and the cultural differences these immigrants bring to the experience of pregnancy.

Finally, obstetric practices are increasingly dealing with pregnancies among "blended" families, where the new child will have half-siblings from one or both parents, possibly all living together.

All of these realities of 21st-century life have an impact on the way the obstetrics practice performs its role in the health care of American families.

SIGNS OF PREGNANCY

The signs of pregnancy are divided into three categories:

1. Presumptive signs
2. Probable signs
3. Positive signs.

Presumptive signs are those that suggest pregnancy and are usually felt or seen by the pregnant woman. **Probable signs** are usually found by an examiner; when two or more probable signs are present, pregnancy is strongly suggested. **Positive signs** are those that clearly establish the presence of a fetus.

PHYSICAL EFFECTS OF PREGNANCY

A number of physiologic changes occur in the expectant mother during pregnancy, including weight gain, changes to the reproductive organs, and changes in other body systems.

Weight Gain

Weight gain during pregnancy is necessary for the health of both the fetus and the expectant mother. A healthy woman of average weight should gain 25 to 35 pounds during pregnancy, about 2 to 4 pounds in the first **trimester** (3-month period) and more rapid gain in the second and third trimesters. Some of this later weight gain is due to the rapid increase in the fetus's size; the rest is due to fluid retention, increased blood volume, and additional fat deposits.

Changes in Reproductive System

During pregnancy, a woman's reproductive system undergoes significant changes.

Signs of Pregnancy

PRESUMPTIVE SIGNS

1. Amenorrhea (cessation of menses); usually the first sign for a woman who has previously had regular menstrual periods
2. Nausea with or without vomiting; nausea occurs in about one half of pregnancies, vomiting in about one third; often pronounced after waking—hence the term "morning sickness."
3. Breast changes, such as tingling nipples, enlargement, increased sensitivity, and/or tenderness of nipples and/or breasts
4. Urinary frequency; caused by pressure on the bladder from the enlarging uterus, as well as increased plasma filtration in the kidneys
5. Quickening—the mother's first recognition of fetal movement is sometimes mistaken for intestinal gas; usually occurs between 18 and 20 weeks' gestation.

PROBABLE SIGNS

1. Uterine enlargement; can be caused by a tumor and is therefore not a positive sign
2. Hegar's sign, a softening of the lower end of the cervix, which usually occurs around 6 weeks after conception
3. Goodell's sign, a softening of the cervix that occurs 8 weeks after conception
4. Chadwick's sign, bluish or purplish color of the vagina and vulva due to increased vascularity and increases in estrogen
5. Ballottement, a rebounding of the fetus against an examiner's fingers
6. Braxton Hicks contractions, painless uterine contractions in the early stages of pregnancy
7. Positive pregnancy test; most pregnancy tests are accurate 90 to 95 percent of the time
8. Radioimmunoassay test on the woman's serum—again accurate less than 100 percent of the time
9. Chloasma gravidarum, the "mask of pregnancy," a brownish pigmentation to the face that fades after delivery
10. Linea nigra, a dark line on the abdomen from the navel to the pubic hair

POSITIVE SIGNS

1. Fetal heartbeat
2. Funic and uterine souffle; funic souffle is the soft swishing sound of blood as it passes through the umbilical cord; uterine souffle is the swishing sound made by blood passing through the large uterine blood vessels.
3. Presence of fetal movement, felt by the examiner
4. Ultrasonography showing a fetus; very accurate after 13 weeks

---

The uterus becomes 20 times its nonpregnant size. It rises out of the pelvic cavity to become an abdominal organ. Its length increases from approximately 3″ to approximately 14″. Its weight increases from approximately 2 ounces to about 2 pounds.

The cervix shortens and thins. Thick mucus forms a plug in the cervical canal to prevent bacteria from entering the uterus.

In the fallopian tubes and ovaries, the corpus luteum enlarges and produces higher levels of estrogen and progesterone for the first 10 to 12 weeks of the pregnancy.

Estrogen permits the perineum to stretch for childbirth; the vagina becomes more acidic to prevent bacterial growth. There is increased blood flow to the area, along with mucosal thickening and increased vaginal secretions.

The breasts enlarge and become ready for lactation. They are more sensitive to touch, and the erectile tissue of the nipples enlarges. The areolas get darker and **striae gravidarum** (stretch marks) develop in the outer aspects of the breast tissue. **Colostrum** (thick, yellowish fluid that nourishes the baby after birth) is secreted in the later months of pregnancy and immediately after delivery.

Figure 29–2 shows the growth of the uterus during pregnancy.

Changes in Other Body Systems

Other body systems undergo numerous changes as well during pregnancy, including the endocrine system, circulatory system, voice, respiratory system, gastrointestinal system, urinary system, musculoskeletal system, and integumentary system.

In the endocrine system, production and secretion of estrogen and progesterone increase for uterine cell growth and preparation for lactation. This increased hormone production also helps prevent **spontaneous abortions** (miscarriage). Also, secretion of the hormone human chorionic gonadotropin begins, which stimulates the corpus luteum to secrete estrogen and progesterone until the placenta begins to. Human placental lactogen makes more protein and glucose available to the expectant mother and the fetus, and is important in the production of breast milk. Aldosterone from the

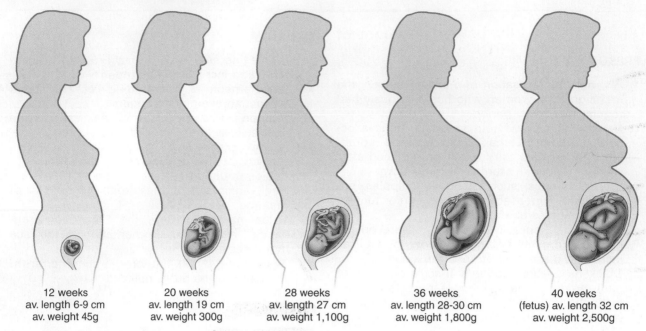

12 weeks	20 weeks	28 weeks	36 weeks	40 weeks
av. length 6-9 cm	av. length 19 cm	av. length 27 cm	av. length 28-30 cm	(fetus) av. length 32 cm
av. weight 45g	av. weight 300g	av. weight 1,100g	av. weight 1,800g	av. weight 2,500g

➤ **Figure 29–2** The fetus increases in length and weight, causing the uterus to enlarge throughout pregnancy.

adrenal glands increases the reabsorption of water and sodium in the kidney tubules.

In the circulatory system, blood volume increases by about 50 percent; because of this, cardiac output also increases. During the first half of pregnancy, blood pressure decreases, but returns to prepregnancy levels during the second half of pregnancy. Heart sounds are strong and regular.

There is a possibility of **supine hypotension syndrome** (low blood pressure when the expectant mother lies on her back). Caused by pressure on the inferior vena cava while in the supine position, this usually occurs during the second half of pregnancy. It can cause dizziness, fast pulse, nausea, and vomiting, as well as a decrease in blood pressure. It can usually be relieved by having the woman lie on her left side with her head slightly elevated.

Pressure on the large veins of the abdomen may interfere with venous return from the legs. This may cause the woman to experience orthostatic hypotension and edema (swelling) in the feet and legs. Also, varicose veins and hemorrhoids may occur as a result of the pressure on the veins of the abdomen and lower extremities.

The voice becomes lower due to an increase in estrogen and the vascularization of the nasopharynx. This may also cause nosebleeds.

In the respiratory system, the need for oxygen increases by about 20 percent. This is caused by progesterone. Also, pulmonary small muscles relax; nasal congestion is common. The woman may experience shortness of breath while lying in the supine position. Shortness of breath in general is common in late preg-

nancy because of the pressure on the thoracic cavity. Vital capacity remains strong.

In the gastrointestinal system, increased estrogen causes gums to be more sensitive and more likely to bleed. There is excessive salivation. A depletion of vitamins may cause lips to crack and peel. Morning sickness in the first trimester is a gastrointestinal reaction to hormonal changes.

A woman may also experience heartburn, due to the pressure on the esophagus and stomach as the uterus moves up into the abdominal cavity. She may also experience constipation, due to the pressure on the intestines. Indigestion is worse in the third trimester, when food is not digested as completely. Flatulence occurs, due to pressure on the colon, especially when the woman lies in the supine position. Some women crave nonfood items such as starch, clay, and even dirt, especially when it is culturally accepted (in some Black and Caribbean cultures). This condition (called **pica**) may interfere with metabolism and nutrient absorption.

In the urinary system, the ability to store urine decreases as the uterus presses on the bladder. This occurs briefly in the first trimester and becomes a persistent problem in the third trimester. Progesterone causes the ureters to dilate, producing a risk of urinary stasis. Kidneys become more efficient at removing waste products because the mother's blood carries fetal waste in addition to her own.

In the musculoskeletal system, changes in a woman's center of gravity require her to adjust posture. The spine curves inward, and maintaining balance is difficult. Relaxin, a hormone secreted by the corpus luteum, causes relaxation of the joints and allows for the widening of joints during labor and delivery.

In the integumentary system, stretch marks are apparent, and the **linea nigra** (dark line on the abdomen) and **chloasma** (brownish pigmentation of the face) may be present.

PSYCHOLOGICAL CHANGES DURING PREGNANCY

As well as encountering physical changes, a pregnant woman also has to deal with many psychological changes, from self-image to anxiety about her own health and the health of the fetus, to changes in sexuality.

Factors That Affect Psychological Changes

General physical health, emotional maturity and stability, educational background, and work status all affect a woman's psychological well-being during pregnancy. Family status and financial considerations play a major role in adaptations to another family member.

The change in body appearance may also affect a woman's feelings about herself. In addition, physical senses become more acute; pregnant women are generally more sensitive to touch. Anxiety is very real throughout a pregnancy.

During the first trimester, an expectant mother often feels ambivalence, fear, fantasies about motherhood, and may dream of her unborn child. She usually has decreased sexual drive, due to fatigue and the discomforts of the early weeks of pregnancy. Strong family support by her partner, parents and/or siblings, and any other children she has plays an important role in her adjustment to pregnancy.

During the second trimester, many women experience rapid mood swings. There is generally more acceptance of the pregnancy as physical discomfort tends to decrease. Adjustment to change in body shape is important. The woman is often introspective, and sometimes evidences **introversion** (a withdrawal into her own thoughts).

During the third trimester, feelings of awkwardness and clumsiness often occur. A women may have fears and apprehension about labor and delivery. She may be concerned about the fetus' physical and mental condition. There is often an increase in "nesting" behaviors with bursts of energy that play themselves out in cleaning the house, preparing the new baby's room, and bursts of creativity.

Developmental Tasks of Pregnancy

During pregnancy, a woman—especially a first-time expectant mother—engages in a number of "developmental tasks" about her new role as mother. These include:

Mimicry. A pregnant woman associates with other pregnant women—especially those who are already mothers—to learn as much as she can about pregnancy and newborns.

Role playing. A pregnant woman finds ways to practice parenting skills; she may read baby books to the dog or cat. This is a good time for educational classes as the woman is interested in learning about herself and her baby at the same time.

Fantasy. Many pregnant women fantasize about the fetus' gender and what it will be like raising a little boy or girl.

Taking-in. A pregnant woman watches the behavior of mothers of young children around her and modifies these behaviors, making them her own.

THE FIRST PRENATAL VISIT

During the first prenatal visit, the obstetrician or nurse-midwife confirms the pregnancy, completes a history and physical examination, and establishes the **estimated date of confinement (EDC)** or **estimated date of delivery (EDD)**. During this exam, the gestational age of the fetus is assessed, as are any risk factors. Laboratory tests are often taken at this time. Time is given to patient education.

The period of **gestation** (the length of time from conception to birth) is calculated from the first day of the last menstrual period (LMP). A normal pregnancy ranges from 259 days (37 weeks) to 287 days (41 weeks). Infants born prior to 37 weeks' gestation are called **premature** (not fully developed). Usually, an infant born before the 20th week of gestation is not viable.

During weeks four through eight, the product of conception is called an **embryo**. From the ninth week

---

Estimated Date of Confinement (EDC)/Estimated Date of Delivery (EDD)

The estimated date of confinement/estimated date of delivery is determined using Nägele's rule, which estimates the date of delivery by taking the first day of the last menstrual period **(LMP)**, subtracting 3 months, then adding 1 year and 7 days. For example:

LMP	October 1, 2001	10/1/01
−3 mo.	July 1, 2001	7/1/01
+ 1 yr, 7 days	July 8, 2002	7/8/02

until birth, the infant *in utero* (in the uterus) is called a **fetus**.

Health History

A detailed health history is very important in the ongoing assessment of a pregnancy. The first order of business is establishing the date of LMP. After that, a thorough and detailed history should be obtained. In addition to general health, gynocologic and obstetric histories of the expectant mother and family and psychosocial histories of both parents are needed. These assist in identifying risk factors for the pregnancy.

This history should be taken in a relaxed environment with no interruptions and with a feeling that the environment is nonthreatening, so the woman will answer questions thoroughly. A feeling of trust must be established. As part of the history, the history of previous pregnancies, deliveries, and abortions and the status of any other children must be obtained.

The following terms are used:

Para. Number of pregnancies that went to the age of viability (Not the number of live births, because multiple births count as only one pregnancy) and **stillbirths** (birth of a dead fetus of the age of viability) is included in this number.

Descriptive Terms Based on Pregnancy History

The following nouns describe women based on their pregnancy status.

Never pregnant
　Nulligravida. Never pregnant and not currently pregnant
Currently pregnant (nouns with the suffix **-gravida**)
　Primigravida. In first pregnancy
　Multigravida. In second or subsequent pregnancy
Not currently pregnant (nouns with the suffix **-para**)
　Nullipara. Never carried a fetus to the age of viability
　Primipara. Has delivered one potentially viable fetus (whether it has survived or not) or one set or twins, triplets, etc.
　Multipara. Has delivered twice or more; each delivery was a potentially viable fetus or multiple birth

These terms are usually used in dictation as in the following example: This 27-year-old white multigravida (Para I, Gravida II, Ab 0) whose EDC is 4/19/XX has been experiencing severe nausea and vomiting since last week . . .

Gravida. Total times pregnant

Abortions (Ab). Number of pregnancies in which the fetus did not reach the age of viability (usually considered to be 20 weeks of gestation). This includes any spontaneous abortions, also called **miscarriages** (natural explusions of the fetus for unknown reasons) and **elective abortions** (intentional termination of a pregnancy).

See the accompanying box for a list of descriptive terms based on pregnancy history.

After the history of previous pregnancies, the history of the current pregnancy is taken, including the LMP, and any medications taken.

Figure 29–3 is a pregnancy health history form and Figure 29–4 is a pregnancy flow sheet.

Physical Examination

A physical examination, complete with a Pap smear and pelvimetry, height, weight, vital signs, and assessment of body systems, must be taken.

For both the physical and the history, it is important to remember that this may be the most complete exam a woman has had in a number of years.

Laboratory Tests

Lab tests are performed to identify any health problems, so they can be treated early in the pregnancy. They include, but are not limited to:

1. Pap test to test for cancer of the cervix
2. Pregnancy test (urine or blood) to verify the pregnancy
3. Blood tests, including:

　Complete blood count (CBC), because the mother must supply iron, B vitamins, and other substances needed to produce blood cells for both herself and the fetus. Many women lack adequate iron stores to maintain desired levels of hemoglobin, the blood protein that carries oxygen to the tissues. Hemoglobin levels are one of the tests included in the CBC.

　Blood type and Rh factor, because incompatibility between maternal and fetal blood can cause problems. This is discussed in detail in the box entitled *Prevention of Hemolytic Disease of the Newborn.*

　Blood test for syphilis, because early treatment of this sexually transmitted disease, which may have no symptoms, will prevent infection of the fetus, which can cause various birth defects and mental retardation.

　Rubella titer (level of antibodies to rubella), to verify the mother's immune status, because rubella also causes birth defects. Once preg-

GYNECOLOGICAL / OBSTETRICAL HISTORY

LAST NAME _____ FIRST _____ MIDDLE _____

PAT. HOSP. # _____

PRENATAL CLINIC / PHYSICIAN _____

PAT. CLINIC # _____

PATIENT - PLEASE COMPLETE SHADED AREAS

Birthplace	Age	Date of Birth	Race	Marital Status	Religion (Optional)

Your Occupation		Education Completed			

Baby's Father's Name	Father's Telephone	Father's Age	Father's Race	Father's Occupation	Father's Education Completed

Person To Contact In Emergency	Telepone	Alternate Telephone	Address

GENERAL HISTORY - SELF & FAMILY

Please check if you *or if* any of your relatives (such as children, brothers, sisters, grandparents, aunts, uncles) have had any of the conditions listed.
CIRCLE ANY CONDITIONS YOU ARE UNSURE OF.

FAMILY	SELF	PHYSICIAN NOTES	CONDITION
No Yes	No Yes		
☐ ☐	☐ ☐		Cancer
☐ ☐	☐ ☐		High Blood Pressure
☐ ☐	☐ ☐		Heart / Valve Disease
☐ ☐	☐ ☐		Rheumatic Fever
☐ ☐	☐ ☐		Lung Disease
☐ ☐	☐ ☐		Stomach / Bowel Problems
☐ ☐	☐ ☐		Kidney Disease
☐ ☐	☐ ☐		Urinary Problems, Infections or Malformations
☐ ☐	☐ ☐		Diabetes Mellitus
☐ ☐	☐ ☐		Anemia / Blood Disorders
☐ ☐	☐ ☐		Other Endocrine / Hormone Disorders
☐ ☐	☐ ☐		Nervous Mental Disorders
☐ ☐	☐ ☐		Convulsive Disorders - Epilepsy
☐ ☐	☐ ☐		Abnormal Babies
☐ ☐	☐ ☐		Genetic Disease
☐ ☐	☐ ☐		Twins

FAMILY	SELF	PHYSICIAN NOTES	CONDITION
No Yes	No Yes		
☐ ☐	☐ ☐		Infertility
☐ ☐	☐ ☐		Blood Clots / Varicose Veins
☐ ☐	☐ ☐		Blood Transfusions
			Sexually Transmitted Diseases:
	☐ ☐		Genital Herpes
	☐ ☐		Condylomata (Warts)
	☐ ☐		Chlamydia
			Infectious Diseases:
	☐ ☐		Hepatitis
	☐ ☐		Tuberculosis
	☐ ☐		PKU
	☐ ☐		DES Exposure
	☐ ☐		Other:

Does the baby's father, or his family, have any history of abnormal babies or genetic disease? ☐ NO ☐ YES

HABITS / ENVIRONMENTAL FACTORS

TOBACCO & CAFFEINE

No	Yes	
☐	☐	Coffee / Tea _____ cups a day
☐	☐	Cola or other caffeinated drinks, _____ a day
☐	☐	Cigarettes - Now ____ a day _____ years
☐	☐	Cigarettes - Ever ____ a day _____ years

When Stopped: _____

ALCOHOL

No Yes
Alcohol ☐ ☐
_____ Drinks per day
_____ Drinks per week

MISC.

		No	Yes
1.	Are you ever around cats?	☐	☐
2.	Do you use a hot tub?	☐	☐
3.	Do you have a regular exercise routine?	☐	☐
4.	Do you, or have you, used drugs (marijuana, cocaine, uppers, downers)?	☐	☐

ALLERGIES / SENSITIVITIES (Detail)

ANTIBIOTICS _____

PAIN MEDICINE _____

ANESTHESIA _____

OTHER _____

_____

Please list all times you have been hospitalized, operated on, or seriously injured.

Year	Operation, Illness, Injury	Hospital and City
_____	_____	_____
_____	_____	_____
_____	_____	_____

LAST CONTRACEPTIVE	MENSTRUAL HISTORY	LMP	Mo.	Day	Year
TYPE _____	CYCLE _____ DAYS ONSET _____ AGE				
DATE STOPPED _____	LENGTH _____ DAYS	EDC	Mo.	Day	Year

Pregnancy History	Grav	Term	Preterm	S.	Abortion E.	Living	C. Sections

No. of Preg.	Mo./ Year	Baby's ...	Wt.	Weeks Gestation	Hrs. Labor	Delivery Type	DETAIL COMPLICATIONS - MATERNAL / NEWBORN ANESTHESIA IF C-SECTION, LIST INCISION TYPE
1							
2							
3							
4							
5							
6							

ORDER # 19-770 • BIBBERO SYSTEMS, INC. • PETALUMA, CA. © 1986
TO REORDER CALL TOLL FREE: (800) BIBBERO (800-242-2376) OR FAX (800) 242-9330 Mfg In U.S.A.

M.D. SIGNATURE _____ DATE _____

➤ **Figure 29–3** Pregnancy health history form. (Courtesy of Bibbero Systems, Inc., Petaluma, CA; (800)272-2376; Fax (800)242-9330; www.bibbero.com.)

PREGNANCY FLOW SHEET

LMP. _____
    MO.   DAY   YEAR

☐ NORMAL   ☐ ABNORMAL

EDC. _____

PRE. PREG. WT. _____

QUICKENING DATE _____

LAST NAME   FIRST   MIDDLE

PAT. HOSP. # _____

PRENATAL CLINIC / PHYSICIAN _____

PAT. CLINIC # _____

DATE	WEIGHT THIS VISIT	BLOOD PRESSURE	URINE PRO-TEIN	URINE SUG-AR	EST. WEEKS GEST. AGE (DATES/ SIZE)	FUNDAL HEIGHT (CMS)	FETAL HEART TONES FHT	PRESEN TATION	FETAL MOVE-MENTS	EDEMA		COMMENTS / COMPLAINTS / TREATMENT	NEXT VISIT	CHECK IF ADDIT. NOTES	INITIALS OF DR.

TELEPHONE CALLS

DATE / PERSON	QUEST.	ADVICE	DATE / PERSON	QUEST.	ADVICE

INITIAL LABORATORY RESULTS   DATE: _____

BLOOD TYPE / RH: PATIENT: _____ / _____   FATHER: _____ / _____

HEMOGLOBIN: HEMATOCRIT: WBC:

URINE: GLUCOSE: PROTEIN: MICRO: CULTURE:

ANTIBODY SCREEN: SICKLE CELL:

SEROLOGY: RUBELLA TITER:

PAP TEST: CERVICAL CULTURE:

TAY SACHS: GC:

CHLAMYDIA: ALPHA FETO PROTEIN:

ULTRASOUND: DATE: RESULTS:

ULTRASOUND: DATE: RESULTS:

GENETIC STUDY

_____ AMNIOCENTESIS   DATE: _____ RESULTS: _____

_____ CHORIONIC VILLI BIOPSY DATE: _____ RESULTS: _____

POST TERM (42 Wks.) MANAGEMENT

_____ NST (date) _____

_____ CST (date) _____

RhoGAM (28 - 32 Weeks)

☐ Indicated   ☐ Given   DATE: _____

GLUCOSE SCREEN (27 - 32 WEEKS)

DATE: _____   RESULT: _____

HERPES CULTURE DATE / RESULT	HEPATITIS DATE / TEST / RESULT
/	/ /
/	/ /
/	/ /
/	/ /

M.D. SIGNATURE   DATE

➤ **Figure 29–4** Pregnancy flow sheets. (Courtesy of Bibbero Systems, Inc., Petaluma, CA; (800)272-2376; Fax (800)242-9330; www.bibbero.com.)

nant, a woman cannot be immunized; but if she discovers that her antibody titer is low, she is aware that she should avoid exposure to rubella and can be immunized after delivery.

Screening for human immunodeficiency virus (HIV), hepatitis B, and possibly hepatitis C antibodies, is recommended. The woman must usually sign a consent form for HIV testing.

Blood chemistry screening, including blood glucose and electrolytes, so that gestational diabetes (diabetes that occurs during pregnancy) can be treated promptly if detected.

4. Urinalysis, looking for problems in general, but especially for **glucosuria** (glucose in the urine) a symptom of gestational diabetes; or **albuminuria** (protein in the urine), which may indicate problems with the kidneys.

5. Vaginal cultures to test for STDs because, like syphilis, early treatment decreases the likelihood of infecting the fetus.

Assisting with the First Prenatal Visit

During this visit, the medical assistant performs a number of tasks. He or she assists in positioning and draping the woman for comfort and privacy, assists with the gynecological exam, and obtains or assists with obtaining vital signs.

The medical assistant should also use the first visit to establish a rapport with the expectant mother. Answer questions and keep up a conversation to relieve the tension. Be sure that the woman has been given explicit instructions and understands exactly what will take place and when.

Be sure that the woman has emptied her bladder, and obtain a urine specimen if that is office policy. Ensure patient safety by helping the woman on and off the examining table, because the changes in her center of gravity make a pregnant patient more awkward than she is used to being.

Explain that the physical exam will include a Pap smear, pelvic exam, breast exam, rectovaginal exam, vital signs, abdominal exam, and pelvic measurements.

Finally, the medical assistant is responsible for scheduling follow-up visits, and for ensuring that needed appointments are made in other areas, as ordered by the doctor. During the discussion, the medical assistant should assure the woman that calling the office with questions is expected and should make sure that instructions are understood and can be followed. If necessary, the medical assistant should write step-by-step instructions and explanations to ensure compliance.

Procedure 29–1 discusses in detail assisting with the first prenatal visit.

Teaching Needs of the Pregnant Patient

Obstetric patients have many teaching needs. The primary care provider (doctor, physician's assistant, nurse practitioner, or nurse-midwife) instructs the patient in detail about possible problems during the pregnancy, such as vaginal bleeding ("spotting"), persistent vomiting, difficulty with urination, abdominal or uterine cramping, dizziness, or blurred vision, and tell the patient what to report to the office. It is helpful if written instructions or a booklet are prepared for the patient—there may need to be separate instructions for each doctor in the practice.

The doctor will also instruct the patient about possible dangers to the fetus from cigarette smoking, drinking alcohol, use of street drugs, or using any medication—even over-the-counter medications—without the doctor's approval. The doctor will also discuss the dangers of pica.

The patient will be cautioned not to have any contact with used cat litter, because of the possible danger of contracting toxoplasmosis (a disease caused by parasites that normally is barely noticed but can cause severe problems for the fetus).

In addition, the primary care provider will instruct the patient about diet, vitamin and mineral supplements, exercise, and recommendations about sexual activity during pregnancy.

These instructions often seem overwhelming to the patient at first. But the medical assistant can go over information again at subsequent visits, following the guidelines of the primary care provider. For example, patients often need support and motivation to follow principles of good nutrition so weight gain remains within the desired range.

FOLLOW-UP PRENATAL VISITS

Return visits provide a time to assess both the expectant mother and the fetus. A pregnant woman is usually seen every 4 weeks through the seventh month, then every 2 to 3 weeks through the next 2 months, and every week after the 36th week of pregnancy. This provides between 10 and 14 visits for a full-term pregnancy.

At each visit, fetal growth and development is assessed, as well as the expectant mother's health.

For the woman, weight, vital signs, history of signs and symptoms of abnormal conditions since the last visit, as well as discussion of the normal discomforts of pregnancy, are all part of the visit. There should also be a discussion of nutritional status, personal adjustments, and psychosocial adjustments.

The medical assistant takes several measures at the beginning of each follow-up visit: weight, vital signs, blood pressure, and dipstick urinalysis (especially for

PREVENTION OF HEMOLYTIC DISEASE OF THE NEWBORN

Hemolytic disease of the newborn, also called Rh disease, can occur when a mother who is Rh negative gives birth to a baby who is Rh positive. Hemolytic disease once affected 20,000 newborns each year in the United States alone. However, since 1968 effective treatment has reduced the incidence substantially; in 2000, the incidence is approximately 4,000 newborns each year, a drop of 80 percent.

Most people produce the Rh factor, a protein found on the surface of red blood cells. About 15 percent of the white population and 7 percent of

FIRST PREGNANCY

At birth some Rh+
fetal blood enters mother

Rh– mother   Rh+ fetus

Blood cell   Blood cell

Mother given **RhoGam**
within 72 hours of birth

Mother immune system
produces Rh+ antibodies

Rh+ antibody   Rh+ blood
(mother)   cell (fetus)

No treatment
second pregnancy

Rh+ antibodies cross the
placenta and destroy fetal RBC's

Rh– mother   Rh+ fetus

Rh+ antibodies   Blood cell
present in mother   (seen as antigen)

Rh+ blood
cell destroyed

Artificial antibodies
destroy cells with Rh+ antigen

Rh+ antibody   Rh+ blood
(artificial)   cell (destroyed)

After Rhogam treatment
second pregnancy

There are no Rh+ antibodies present
in mother for a normal pregnancy

the black population in the United States do not have the antigen, and are called Rh negative.

A problem can occur when an Rh-negative mother and an Rh-positive father conceive a child who is Rh positive. In this instance, there is a possibility that during pregnancy, and especially in the period immediately before birth, Rh-positive blood from the fetus will get into the mother's bloodstream. If this happens and if the mother's body becomes sensitized to the foreign substance, the mother produces antibodies, which can attack and destroy fetal blood cells. This causes hemolytic disease of the fetus the next time the woman becomes pregnant if the fetus is Rh positive.

In 1968, a company introduced RhoGAM, or Rh immunoglobulin, which prevents maternal sensitization to fetal Rh-positive blood in 95 percent of Rh-negative women. If an Rh-negative woman is shown to be carrying an Rh-positive baby, an injection of RhoGAM is given to the woman in the 28th week of pregnancy, and then again about 72 hours before delivery. The artificial antibodies destroy any fetal blood cells in the mother's circulation before her immune system recognizes the "foreign" protein.

Before the development of RhoGAM, the incidence of hemolytic disease increased with each pregnancy, as the mother became increasingly sensitized to the Rh antigen and produced increasing numbers of antibodies to fetal blood cells.

RhoGAM is also given to Rh-negative women following a miscarriage, an ectopic pregnancy, an induced abortion, or any blood transfusion with Rh-positive blood. It is also recommended that it be given after amniocentesis or other invasive tests.

glucose and protein). The results are usually recorded on a flow sheet so that patterns of measurements are easily visible. Hemoglobin and/or hematocrit are tested regularly (such as every 2 weeks or every month) to be sure the woman is not becoming anemic.

The medical assistant should instruct the patient to bring the first morning urine specimen (which is usually a fasting specimen and is highly concentrated) with her at each visit.

Urine that contains glucose may be a sign of gestational diabetes. If glucose is found in the urine lab tests for diabetes will be run, such as blood work and/or a glucose tolerance test.

Urine that contains protein may indicate the onset of **preeclampsia,** a complication of pregnancy characterized by hypertension, albuminuria, and edema of the lower extremities. If untreated, preeclampsia can progress to true **eclampsia,** a serious condition that causes convulsive seizures, coma, and death if untreated.

A fingerstick may be done to obtain blood to measure hemoglobin or hematocrit in the office or blood may be obtained by venipuncture for testing at an outside laboratory. If anemia is present, the woman feels extremely tired; in addition, severe depletion of the mother's iron stores can affect red blood cell production in the fetus.

Further instruction about responding promptly to symptoms of pregnancy complications should occur at each visit. The woman needs to be reminded to call the office if she experiences any of the following:

vaginal bleeding, no matter how little
swelling of hands and/or face
dimness or blurred vision
severe or continuous headache
flashes of light or spots in eyes
persistent nausea and vomiting
dizziness
chills and fever over 100°F
sudden escape of fluid from vagina
irritating or foul discharge
pain in back or abdomen.

Table 29–1 lists complications of pregnancy.

The physical examination includes measurement of the fetal heart rate and measurement of the size of the growing uterus. In addition, a vaginal exam is performed if the woman has experienced symptoms of discharge or spotting and at every visit during the last month before delivery. The woman should be given a paper or cloth drape and instructed to undress below the waist.

Usually, the head of the exam table is elevated about 15 to 25 degrees, but it may be raised higher if the woman becomes clammy or short of breath in the supine position. This may be a result of supine hypotension.

Fetal Heart Rate

The fetal heart rate is normally between 120 and 160 beats per minute, with a regular rhythm. A heart rate that is too slow or too fast is indicative of fetal distress.

Fetal heartbeats can be heard with a Doppler fetal pulse detector between 10 and 12 weeks after conception, and may be auscultated with a handset or heard through amplification. A small amount of gel is placed on the skin or the transducer to improve the conduction of sound waves. The medical assistant moves the hand set over the abdomen until the sound of the fetal pulse is heard clearly.

If the heart rate seems too slow, the pregnant woman's pulse should be counted at the same time,

PROCEDURE 29–1

Assisting with the First Prenatal Visit

Performance Objective: The student will be able to assist a patient during her first prenatal visit.

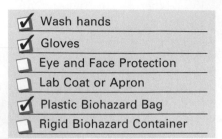

☑ Wash hands
☑ Gloves
☐ Eye and Face Protection
☐ Lab Coat or Apron
☑ Plastic Biohazard Bag
☐ Rigid Biohazard Container

Supplies and Equipment: Disposable gloves, patient gown, drape, water-based lubricant, sphygmomanometer, stethoscope, watch with second hand, measuring tape, Doppler or fetoscope, supplies and equipment for Pap smear (see Procedure 16-2), supplies and equipment for pregnancy test (Procedure 26-7), supplies and equipment for venipuncture (see Procedure 25-1), supplies and equipment for dipstick urinalysis (see Procedure 24-4), biohazard waste container.

Procedure Steps

1. Identify patient.
2. If the patient has not brought a first voided urine specimen, ask patient to empty bladder and collect random urine specimen.
   Rationale: A first voided urine specimen is preferred for pregnancy testing and dipstick urinalysis, but if unavailable, a random specimen will be used for testing.
3. Wash hands.
4. Put on nonsterile gloves.
5. Perform a urine pregnancy test and dipstick urinalysis.
   Rationale: Even if the patient has performed a home pregnancy test, the office usually confirms the test. Urine is checked at each prenatal visit for glucose and protein to monitor for signs of toxemia or gestational diabetes.
6. Remove gloves and dispose of waste in biohazard container.
7. Wash hands.
8. Ask patient to remove shoes and obtain weight.
9. Measure pulse, respirations, and blood pressure.

Rationale: Pulse, respirations, and blood pressure are measured and recorded at each prenatal visit. Temperature is usually not measured unless the patient has complaints that may indicate a fever.

10. Depending on office policy, prenatal blood work may be drawn at this time or the patient may be instructed to visit an outpatient lab after visit.
11. Chart all results in patient record. Record weight, vital signs, and results of dipstick urinalysis on flow sheets.
12. Assist patient to exam room. Be sure equipment and supplies are set up for the physical exam, Pap smear, and bimanual pelvic examination.
13. Ask patient to undress fully, put on a gown, and sit on the exam table. Give patient a gown and a drape.
    Rationale: The doctor will perform a physical exam at the first prenatal visit. The patient should remove all her clothing to allow for a thorough breast, abdomen, and pelvic exam.
14. Assist the patient and doctor as needed with the physical examination and breast examination. Assist the patient to assume the supine position by pulling the table extension out for legs to rest upon.
15. Assist the patient and doctor as needed for the Pap smear and bimanual exam and any cultures that are needed. Assist patient to assume the lithotomy position by pulling out the stirrups, placing the patient's feet in the stirrups, and asking the patient to slide to the end of the examination table.
    Rationale: A Pap smear is taken at the first prenatal visit to be sure the patient does not have cervical cancer. If signs of vaginitis are present, the doctor will test for microorganisms as indicated so that vaginal infections can be treated promptly. A pelvic examination determines presumptive signs of pregnancy.
16. Assist patient to return to supine position. Store stirrups and pull table extension back out.
17. The doctor will measure the height of the fundus of the uterus with a tape measure; if patient is past the first trimester, the doctor will attempt to listen to fetal heart tones with a Doppler or fetoscope.

Rationale: The height of the uterine fundus is measured at every visit to establish fetal growth. Fetal heart tones can be heard early in the second trimester.

18. Instruct patient to dress. Provide tissues to remove water-based lubricant.

19. Wash hands.
20. Chart all procedures and patient concerns in patient record.
21. Schedule follow-up prenatal visit as ordered by doctor.

Table 29–1	Complications of Pregnancy		
Complication	**Description**	**Signs and symptoms**	**Treatment**
Ectopic pregnancy	Implantation of the fertilized ovum outside the uterus (usually in one of the fallopian tubes)	Abdominal pain and cramping, which may become severe; vaginal bleeding; rupture of the fallopian tube may result in fatal hemorrhage	Surgical removal of the ectopic pregnancy; if in the fallopian tube, the tube must usually also be removed. The surgery may be done by laparoscopy.
Hyperemesis gravidarum	Excessive vomiting that can lead to electrolyte imbalances and dehydration	Vomiting beyond what is usually expected, weight loss, poor skin turgor, dizziness, and postural hypotension	Fluid and electrolyte replacement by intravenous infusion
Spontaneous abortion (also called miscarriage)	Natural termination of pregnancy before the age of viability	Abdominal pain and cramping; "spotting" progressing to vaginal bleeding	No treatment may be needed if all products of conception have been expelled; usually a D & C (dilation and currettage) is performed to scrape the uterine wall and remove unexpelled material.
Placenta previa	Low implantation of the placenta on the uterine wall, which makes it difficult to deliver the fetus before the placenta separates from the uterine wall	Painless vaginal bleeding; may be light, progressing to heavy bleeding or hemorrhage	Treated by bed rest if the patient is preterm. Cesarean section may be necessary if bleeding becomes severe.
Abruptio placentae	Premature separation of the placenta from the uterine wall	Profuse vaginal bleeding, which may progress to shock in the mother and fetal distress or fetal death.	Emergency cesarean section is usually necessary to prevent severe hemorrhage in the mother and death of the fetus due to lack of oxygen.
Preeclampsia (pregnancy-induced hypertension)	Condition found in pregnancy in which blood pressure is elevated and protein is lost in urine; low levels of serum proteins result in edema of the lower extremities; risk and severity increase as pregnancy progresses	Edema, headaches, blurred vision, and vomiting; high blood pressure; protein (albumin) is found in the urine	Bed rest, medication to lower blood pressure, restricted sodium and increased protein in diet; requires close monitoring because of potential of developing true eclampsia
Eclampsia	Progression of preeclampsia, with increasing elevations of blood pressure	Symptoms of preeclampsia progress and the patient develops seizures; may progress to coma with uncontrolled hypertension and possibly death	Treatment includes controlling the seizures, lowering blood pressure, and delivering the fetus as rapidly as possible.

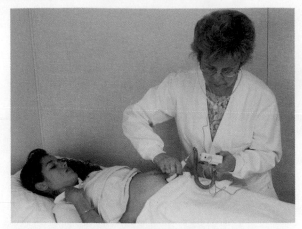

➤ **Figure 29–5** Using a Doppler fetal pulse detector with a headset to measure the fetal heart rate. (From Kinn ME, Woods M: *The Medical Assistant: Administrative and Clinical*, 8th ed. Philadelphia: W.B. Saunders, 1999.)

making sure that the woman's pulse is not what is being picked up by the fetoscope. Figure 29–5 shows measuring fetal heart tones.

Height of the Fundus

The **fundus** is the base of the uterus; it is located opposite the cervix. The height of the fundus is measured and is expected to correspond to the estimated gestational age of the fetus.

It is usually possible to palpate the fundus as an abdominal organ between the 8th and 13th week of pregnancy. By 20 weeks, the fundus should be just below the woman's umbilicus, and between 36 and 37 weeks it should be at the tip of the sternum. Figure 29–6 shows changes in fundal height during pregnancy.

The fundus is measured with the zero end of the tape measure placed at the symphysis pubis, and then pulled over the abdomen to the top of the fundus or to the top of fingers that have been held at right angles to the fundus.

Fundal height using McDonald's rule is used to give an idea of the length of the pregnancy and is considered accurate to within 4 weeks. McDonald's rule states that the height of the fundus of the uterus in centimeters, multiplied by eight, then divided by seven equals the duration of the pregnancy in weeks; or the height of the fundus in centimeters, multiplied by two, then divided by seven equals the duration of the pregnancy in lunar months (28-day periods).

For example, for a fundus with height 25 cm:

$25 \times 8 = 200, \div 7 = 28.6$ weeks

$25 \times 2 = 50, \div 7 = 7.1$ lunar months

During the second trimester, fundal height and weeks of gestation are relatively equal. Because of the

increase in fetal weight during the third trimester, estimation of gestational age using fundal height is difficult.

Fundal height that is not what is expected for the EDD may be used to evaluate variations from normal and allow for assessment of fetal growth, or may be an indication of risks to the pregnancy such as multiple fetuses, polyhydramnios (excess of amniotic fluid), intrauterine death, or poor fetal development. Ultrasound is usually used in such circumstances to make a further assessment.

Procedure 29–2 describes in detail assisting with follow-up prenatal visits. See also *On the Job*.

Special Diagnostic Tests

Special diagnostic tests in pregnancy may be grouped by trimester:

First trimester tests: ultrasonography, chorionic villus sampling

Second trimester tests: amniocentesis, maternal alpha-fetoprotein analysis, ultrasonography

Third trimester tests: fetal heart rate monitoring, ultrasonography, amniocentesis

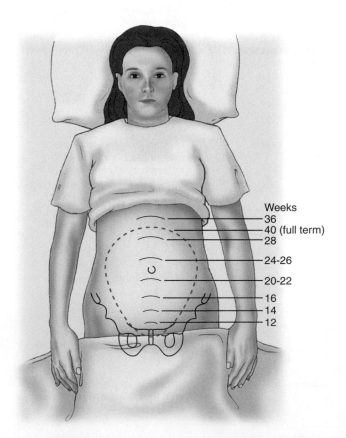

Weeks
36
40 (full term)
28
24-26
20-22
16
14
12

➤ **Figure 29–6** Changes in the height of the fundus during pregnancy.

PROCEDURE 29-2

Assisting with Follow-Up Prenatal Visits

Performance Objective: The student will be able to assist a patient during her follow-up prenatal visits.

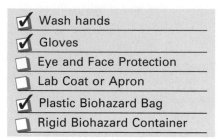

- ☑ Wash hands
- ☑ Gloves
- ☐ Eye and Face Protection
- ☐ Lab Coat or Apron
- ☑ Plastic Biohazard Bag
- ☐ Rigid Biohazard Container

Supplies and Equipment: Disposable gloves, patient gown, drape, water-based lubricant, sphygmomanometer, stethoscope, watch with second hand, measuring tape, Doppler or fetoscope, gel, supplies and equipment for hemoglobin testing (see Procedure 25-8) or microhematocrit (see Procedure 25-9), supplies and equipment for dipstick urinalysis (see Procedure 24-4), biohazard waste container.

Procedure Steps

1. Identify patient.
2. Ask patient to empty bladder and collect random urine specimen.
3. Wash hands.
4. Put on disposable gloves.
5. Test urine for protein, ketones, and glucose using dipstick.
   Rationale: Urine is checked at each prenatal visit to monitor signs of toxemia or gestational diabetes.
6. Remove gloves and dispose of waste in biohazard container.
7. Wash hands.
8. Ask patient to remove shoes and obtain weight.
9. Measure pulse, respirations, and blood pressure.
   Rationale: Pulse, respirations, and blood pressure are measured and recorded at each prenatal visit. Temperature is usually not measured unless the patient has complaints that may indicate a fever.
10. Document weight and vital signs in the patient record. If office policy, question patient

about symptoms such as nausea, vomiting, bleeding, and so on, and document on pregnancy flow sheet.

11. If done in the office, measure hemoglobin or hematocrit levels at regular intervals. The patient may be referred to an outpatient lab to obtain these tests.
12. Chart all results in patient record.
13. Assist patient to exam room.
14. Instruct the patient to undress from the waist down and give the patient a gown and drape.
15. Provide Doppler or fetoscope, gel, and tape measure to doctor to routinely check fetal heart tones and fundal growth measurements.
   Rationale: The doctor will perform this type of assessment at each prenatal visit. Time should be allowed for counseling and listening to concerns from the mother/father.
16. Assist the doctor and patient as needed in positioning in either supine or lithotomy position and recording information such as fetal heart rate and height of the fundus as directed by the doctor.
17. Wash hands.
18. Schedule follow-up prenatal visit as ordered by doctor.

15

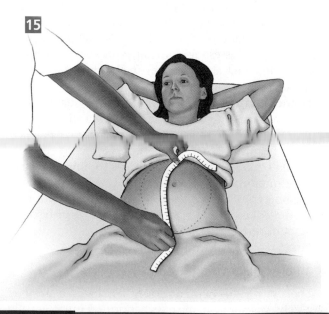

ON THE JOB

Tania Holland, a 26-year-old patient of Dr. Hughes, comes for a visit to Blackburn Primary Care Associates after results of a home pregnancy test indicate she is pregnant. When you interview Tania, you find out that her last menstrual period was on April 3rd of that year (4/3/XX), which was 3 months ago.

Tania tells you that her breasts are tender, she has nausea and vomiting in the morning, and that she has gained 3 pounds over her normal weight. She and her husband have a 3-year-old daughter, born without problems after a vaginal delivery. In addition, she had a miscarriage about 1 year ago.

QUESTIONS

1. What are Mrs. Holland's presumptive signs of pregnancy? Based on the information above, are there any probable or positive signs of pregnancy?
2. Assuming that Dr. Hughes verifies that Mrs. Holland is pregnant, calculate her EDC using Nägele's rule.
3. Describe Mrs. Holland in terms of gravida, para, and abortion. Use Roman numerals. What single obstetric term describes her?
4. Mrs. Holland will be scheduled for monthly visits. List the measurements that will be taken during each visit. What lab tests will be done routinely?
5. When Mrs. Holland returns for her 6-month visit, she asks you, "Why do I have to bring a urine specimen each time I come?" How should you answer Mrs. Holland?

Ultrasonography

Ultrasonography, discussed in detail in chapter 20, uses the echo of sound waves hitting an object and bouncing off to determine the placement and size of the fetus. Sound waves pass through the mother's soft tissue and hit the tissue of higher density (the fetus), which reflects the sound back to the transducer.

In the first trimester, ultrasonography is used to confirm pregnancy and to look for the gestational sac, fetal cardiac and body movements, and uterine abnormalities. In the second and third trimesters, ultrasonography is used to look for intrauterine growth retardation, small gestational age, and large gestational age. It is also used to assess abnormalities of the placenta or uterus, congenital abnormalities in the fetus, as well as multiple fetus pregnancy.

In the third trimester, ultrasonography is used to assess fetal position and size and to locate the placental implantation site. It is also used to rule out cephalopelvic disproportion.

Finally, ultrasonography is used to ensure safety during amniocentesis and chorionic villus sampling. Ultrasonography is noninvasive, safe, painless, and provides immediate results. Figure 29–7 shows ultrasound being performed.

Chorionic Villus Sampling

Chorionic villus sampling may be done as early as 10 weeks gestation. It may be performed intravaginally or transabdominally. A small number of chorionic villi (pieces of the fetal membrane) are aspirated for study of the cells to identify any chemical or genetic abnormalities. The advantage of using this technique is that it can be done early in the pregnancy.

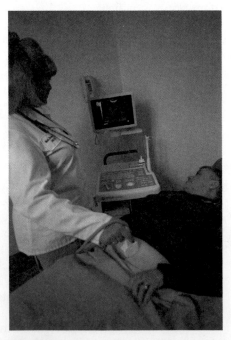

➤ **Figure 29–7** Ultrasound may be performed at any time during pregnancy.

Amniocentesis

Amniocentesis is usually done between the 14th and 16th weeks of gestation. The test looks for congenital abnormalities in the fetus such as Down syndrome and inborn errors of metabolism. It can also determine the fetus' gender.

In the third trimester, amniocentesis is used to assess lung development and fetal distress. See *Amniocentesis* for more detail.

Maternal Alpha-Fetoprotein Analysis

Alpha-fetoprotein is a glycoprotein produced by the fetus that crosses from the amniotic fluid to the mother's bloodstream. If there is a fetal abnormality, the result may be higher or lower than normal, depending on the problem.

Blood is drawn from the mother between the 15th and 18th weeks of gestation. Although this test is nonspecific, it can indicate the need for further testing to rule out Down syndrome, neural tube defects (spina bifida), anencephaly (lack of brain development), and other problems. Ultrasound and/or amniocentesis may be used as follow-up tests.

Electronic Fetal Heart Rate Monitoring

As the pregnancy progresses, a woman usually begins to experience painless uterine contractions every 20 to 30 minutes (called Braxton Hicks contractions). If there is any indication of decreased fetal growth or movement, if the fetus is overdue, or if the mother has certain medical conditions, the doctor may monitor the fetus' heart rate electronically to determine if the heart rate responds normally (becomes more rapid) during its own movement and during Braxton Hicks contractions. An electronic microphone is placed on the woman's abdomen to amplify the fetal heart rate.

In the **nonstress test (NST),** the heart rate is monitored for several minutes to correlate the heart rate to fetal movement and to Braxton Hicks contractions. This test is often done in the doctor's office.

When there is concern about the fetus' ability to tolerate the stress of labor, mild contractions can be stimulated during fetal heart rate monitoring **(contraction stress test, or CST).** Because of the potential for fetal distress, this test is usually performed in a facility with access to more sophisticated medical equipment, such as a hospital or health center.

If the results of these tests indicate fetal distress (such as a heart rate that becomes slower during movement or contractions) labor may be induced or a cesarean section may be scheduled.

LABOR AND DELIVERY

Labor is the process a woman's body goes through immediately preceding birth of a baby. It includes the uterine contractions that allow the baby to be propelled through the birth canal, as well as other changes.

Delivery is the actual period of time when the baby is being born.

Four P's of Labor and Delivery

The 4 P's of labor and delivery are a memory device to remember what is happening to a woman as her body works to give birth. The 4 P's are:

1. Passageway
2. Passenger
3. Powers
4. Psyche.

Passageway

The false pelvis is the area above the imaginary line that runs along the brim of the pelvic basin. This serves as a guide for the fetus toward the true pelvis and supports the growing uterus.

The true pelvis is composed of the inlet, the pelvic cavity or midpelvis, and the outlet.

The pelvis must be of the correct shape and size to allow passage of the fetus to the outside world. If the passageway is not the proper shape and size, the child will need to be surgically birthed in a procedure known as cesarean section (C-section).

Passenger

The passenger in the process of birth is the fetus, which is propelled through the pelvis and the vagina as if on a carnival ride.

Fetal skulls are pliable enough to allow for overlapping and molding during delivery. Five terms are used to describe how the passenger is set for his or her journey: lie, presentation, attitude, position, and station or engagement.

Lie. Lie refers to the position of the fetus in relation to the mother's spine. Lie is described as either longitudinal, with the length of the fetus parallel to the mother's spine, or transverse, with the length at right angles to the spine.

Presentation. Presentation refers to the way the fetus sits as it enters the pelvis. The portion of the fetus that enters the pelvis first is determined by the lie. Presentation can either be cephalic (head first), breech (buttocks first), or shoulder.

■ AMNIOCENTESIS

Amniocentesis is the removal of a small amount of amniotic fluid to test for fetal chromosomal abnormalities and whether the fetus' lungs are maturing properly.

In amniocentesis, fluid is withdrawn through a long needle inserted through the mother's abdomen into the amniotic sac surrounding the fetus. Ultrasound is used to show location of the placenta, fetus, and to make sure that the needle does not penetrate either of them.

Amniocentesis is used to detect chromosomal disorders known as trisomies—chromosomal defects in which there are three chromosomes instead of the usual pair. Three trisomies—trisomy 21, known as Down syndrome; trisomy 18, known as Edward's syndrome; and trisomy 13 are the most common, with Down syndrome accounting for nearly half of all trisomies identified.

The risk of chromosomal abnormality increases as a woman ages, from one in several thousand for women age 18 to 25 to about one in 180 for women age 35 to one in 20 for women over age 45. The procedure carries a risk of miscarriage, about one in 200. This must be balanced against the woman's risk of carrying a fetus with a genetic defect due to age or family history.

Today, trained and certified genetic counselors work with women over age 35 to determine if their particular risk of fetal trisomy justifies the risk of miscarriage from amniocentesis.

The procedure is also performed on women under age 35 when there is a family history of congenital/chromosomal abnormalities or metabolic diseases and on women whose previous pregnancies have resulted in fetal abnormalities.

Other complications of amniocentesis include infection, hemorrhage, and leakage of fluid.

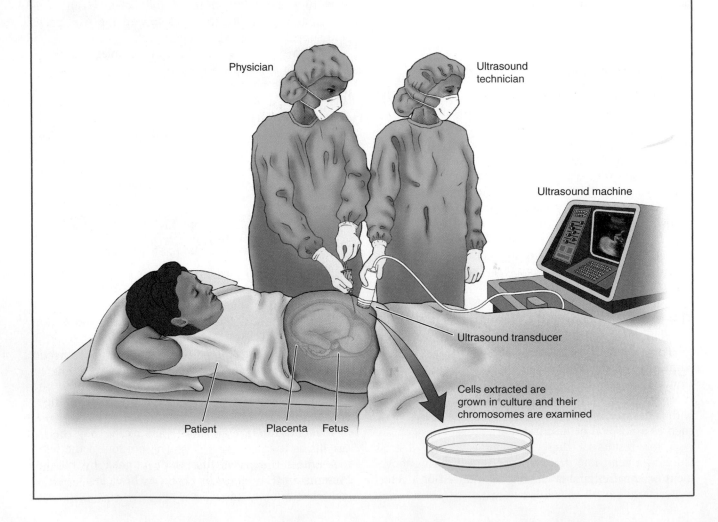

Physician

Ultrasound technician

Ultrasound machine

Ultrasound transducer

Cells extracted are grown in culture and their chromosomes are examined

Patient   Placenta   Fetus

A cephalic presentation occurs when the fetus has been in the longitudinal lie with the head down. A cephalic presentation can either be vertex, with the head flexed to the chin; face, with the head extended and the neck bent backward; or brow, with the head partially extended.

A breech presentation occurs when the fetus has been in the longitudinal lie with the head up. A breech presentation can be either complete breech, with the baby in flexion (knees drawn up to chest); frank breech, with the legs extended; or footling breech (single or double), in which the foot or feet are in the birth canal first.

A shoulder presentation occurs when the fetus has been in the transverse lie.

Attitude. Attitude refers to the relationship of fetal parts to one another. Normal attitude is moderate flexion of the head and the arms and legs flexed.

Position. Position refers to the relationship of the presenting part to the maternal pelvis.

Station (Engagement). Station, or engagement, refers to the relationship of the presenting part to the imaginary line that divides the false and true pelvis. The descent of the fetus into the pelvis may occur during labor or during the last few weeks of pregnancy.

Powers

These are the forces that act to expel the fetus and placenta.

Uterine contractions cause the **effacement** (shortening and thinning of the cervix) and **dilation** (enlargement or opening of the cervical opening) for the delivery of the presenting part. Each contraction begins gradually, builds up to a peak of muscle shortening, and gradually decreases in intensity.

Contractions are described using three measures: frequency, the time between the beginning of one contraction and the beginning of the next; duration, the time from the increment to the decrement; and intensity, the strength of the contraction.

Secondary powers include the mother's voluntary pushing.

Psyche

Psyche is the mother's preparation for labor, which also includes the support system available to help her through labor and delivery.

Signs of Impending Labor

There are seven stages of impending labor:

1. **Lightening,** a descent of the fetal head into the pelvis. This is usually accompanied by pain from the pressure on sciatic nerves, vaginal changes, and increased urinary frequency.
2. Braxton Hicks contractions become more frequent and the mother can feel them more strongly.
3. Vaginal or bloody show, the expulsion of the mucous plug from the opening of the cervix, mixed with blood from the rupturing of cervical capillaries.
4. Rupture of membranes (breaking of the bag of waters). The amniotic sac breaks, with the discharge of clear fluid. The mother will usually call the obstetrical office to report that her water has broken.
5. Cervical changes—effacement, dilation, and softening of the cervix—that may be identified during the pelvic examination. Effacement is the thinning of the cervix, which occurs as the contractions push the fetus against the cervical opening. As the cervix thins, the opening is stretched (dilated).
6. Loss of 1 to 3 pounds due to fluid loss.
7. Burst of energy and nesting instinct.

Stages of Labor

Labor is comprised of four stages: dilation, pushing, birth of the placenta, and readjustment.

The dilation stage begins with the onset of true labor and ends when the cervix is completely dilated and effaced.

The pushing stage begins with complete dilation (at 10 cm) and ends with the baby's birth. Uterine contractions are accompanied by the mother's voluntary pushing.

The placental stage begins with the baby's birth and ends with expulsion of the placenta.

The physiologic readjustment stage begins after expulsion of placenta, when the mother's body begins to adjust to the end of pregnancy. During the first 4 hours, many changes occur, due to physiologic and hormonal effects.

Medical Assistant's Role in Advising Patients During Labor

The medical assistant in an obstetric practice needs to know the signs of onset of labor and the signs of false labor, so he or she can correctly advise the patient. The doctor makes the decisions, but the medical assistant needs to know the questions to ask the woman to get an accurate description of what is occurring.

Also, the woman should have been educated during the course of her prenatal checkups as to the signs of true labor as opposed to the signs of false labor.

Signs of true labor are:

Contractions are regular.

Pain is felt in the back, radiating to the abdomen.

Intervals between contractions shorten.

Duration of each contraction increases.

The intensity of contractions gradually increase; movement by the mother such as walking may help establish effective contractions.

Progressive dilation and effacement occur; this can only be measured through an internal exam by an obstetrician or nurse-midwife.

Signs of false labor are:

Contractions are irregular.

The interval between contractions remains the same.

Each contraction lasts the same amount of time.

Pain is primarily experienced in abdomen.

The intensity of each contraction is the same.

Contractions do not result in cervical effacement or dilation.

After determining that true labor has begun, the mother is instructed to go to the facility she has chosen for her baby's birth.

POSTPARTUM CHECKUP(S)

Postpartum refers to the weeks and months immediately after the birth of a baby. The 6 weeks after birth, during which a mother's reproductive organs return to near prepregnancy state, is known as the puerperium, or involution.

During the postpartum period, the new mother will have one or two follow-up visits with the obstetrical practice. These are usually scheduled during the first and sixth weeks after birth.

Danger Signs in Postpartum

There are 10 danger signs to watch for in the postpartum period:

1. Heavy vaginal bleeding, defined as soaking a pad in 15 to 20 minutes
2. Increased or foul-smelling discharge
3. Recurrence of bright-red bleeding instead of the dark discharge normal in the first few days after delivery
4. Fever
5. Swollen, red, tender, or hot area on a leg, which may be a sign of a blood clot
6. Burning or pain on urination
7. Inability to urinate
8. Persistent pelvic or perineal pain
9. Swollen, tender, hot, or red areas of breasts
10. Persistent feelings of depression, or lack of interest in the baby or self.

Postpartum Visits

When the first postpartum visit occurs depends on the type of delivery (vaginal or cesarean) and the mother's condition. With early discharge from the hospital increasingly common for uncomplicated vaginal deliveries, most postpartum care is now delivered in the medical office.

Those with no complications during pregnancy, labor, and puerperium may be scheduled for one appointment, 4 to 6 weeks after giving birth. Those with less prenatal care or a more difficult delivery will most often have two visits, the first in the first or second week after delivery.

Immediately Postpartum

A new mother should be encouraged during the postpartum period to avoid becoming fatigued, to eat a well-balanced diet, to avoid straining or lifting heavy objects (including older children, which is often a problem), and to perform good perineal care on a regular basis. If the woman has had an **episiotomy** (incision to enlarge the vaginal opening for birth), she needs to clean the area around the stitches and return to the hospital, clinic, or office as directed to have the stitches removed.

The woman also needs to be taught to feed and care for her infant and to identify resources for help if needed.

Kegel exercises (a tightening of the muscles in the pelvic area) should be done to increase muscle tone in the perineum.

Another common topic for the postpartum visit is **lochia**, the discharge that occurs during puerperium. The normal sequence of lochia is:

1. One to three days postpartum, lochia rubra; red, bloody, may have small clots, musty odor, heavy to moderate flow.
2. Four to seven days postpartum, lochia serosa; pink to brown, no odor, no clots, decrease in flow.
3. One to three weeks postpartum, lochia alba; cream to yellow, no odor, little or no flow.

Six-Week Postpartum Visit

The 6-week postpartum visit includes a complete gynecologic and breast exam. The visit should include time for teaching and counseling as needed. New mothers—especially first-time mothers—usually have questions and concerns regarding breastfeeding, contraception methods, resumption of sexual activities, parenting skills, and other issues.

The medical assistant can play a large role in the postpartum exam. In addition to taking height, weight, and vital signs, and helping with draping and position-

PROCEDURE 29–3

Assisting with Postpartum Visits

Performance Objective: The student will be able to assist a patient during her postpartum visit(s).

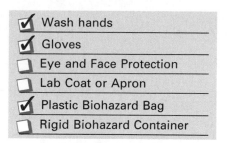

☑ Wash hands
☑ Gloves
☐ Eye and Face Protection
☐ Lab Coat or Apron
☑ Plastic Biohazard Bag
☐ Rigid Biohazard Container

Supplies and Equipment: Sphygmomanometer and stethoscope, supplies and equipment for hemoglobin testing (see Procedure 25-8) or microhematocrit (see Procedure 25-9), supplies and equipment for Pap smear (see Procedure 16-2) if indicated by office policy, biohazard waste container.

Procedure Steps

1. Identify and greet patient.
2. Wash hands.
3. Ask patient to remove shoes and obtain weight.
4. Measure pulse, respirations, and blood pressure.
5. Document weight and vital signs in the patient record. If office policy includes assessment, ask the patient about lochia, cramping or other discomfort, and general concerns, and document.
6. If done in the office, measure hemoglobin or hematocrit level. The patient may be referred to an outpatient lab to obtain these tests. *Rationale:* The hemoglobin or hematocrit is obtained to determine if the mother is replacing blood cells after the delivery.
7. Chart all results in the patient's medical record.
8. Assist patient to exam room.
9. Instruct the patient to undress from the waist down and give the patient a gown and drape.
10. Assist the patient and doctor as needed during the examination, which will include a breast examination and may include a Pap smear if lochia has ceased. *Rationale:* Postpartum drainage or bleeding could interfere with Pap smear results.
11. Instruct the patient to dress. Provide patient with tissues to remove lubricant as needed.
12. Wash hands.
13. Schedule follow-up visit as ordered by doctor.

---

ing, the medical assistant can be a supportive presence and provide counseling and guidance.

A Pap smear may not be included in this exam, if abnormal cells still remain from the healing process after delivery. Procedure 29–3 deals with assisting at the postpartum visit.

Hemoglobin and hematocrit are tested in the postpartum period because anemia is common after delivery. If the mother was shown not to have antibody protection for rubella, the postpartum period is a good time to give her the rubella vaccine.

Assessment of the mother's mental health is essential at the postpartum visit.

By the 6-week checkup, the mother should be physiologically back to her prepregnant state.

Family Planning

During the 6-week postpartum visit, the primary care provider discusses family planning with the woman. Although many women believe they cannot become pregnant while breastfeeding, to avoid pregnancy all women should use an effective birth control method when they resume sexual activity. If the woman has been using a diaphragm, the size must be rechecked after each delivery. Table 29–2 describes methods of contraception, and Figure 29–8 shows a month's supply of birth control pills.

Surgical Procedures: Insertion of Norplant or IUD. If a woman wishes to use Norplant (small rods implanted under the skin on the upper arm that re-

Table 29–2	Methods of Family Planning	

Method—Surgical	Description	Discussion
Vasectomy/tubal ligation	Surgical treatment to cut the path for sperm in the male (vasectomy) or ovum in the female (tubal ligation)	The patient should have considered the decision to have surgical treatment and have consent of his or her partner. This method is used when no more children are desired although there has been some success in reversing both procedures.
Intrauterine device (IUD)	Device placed in the uterus to prevent conception. A string passes into the vagina so that the woman can verify that the device remains in place.	Very effective at preventing pregnancy; sometimes causes uterine bleeding or infection. Can be expelled spontaneously.

Method—Hormonal	Description	Discussion
Norplant (levonorgestrel)	Six small rods implanted in upper arm prevent pregnancy for 5 years	Very effective at preventing pregnancy; rods can be removed at any time if a woman desires to become pregnant.
Depo-Provera injections (medroxyprogesterone acetate)	Injection given every 3 months at doctor's office	Very effective at preventing pregnancy if woman keeps to time schedule. Hormone medication has various side effects, including weight gain, fluid retention, and formation of blood clots.
Oral contraceptive pills	Combination of estrogens and progestins taken orally	Taken daily or for 21 days of each 28-day cycle. Very effective at preventing pregnancy if taken as directed.

Method—Barrier	Description	Discussion
Condom	Sheath fitted over the penis to collect ejaculate and prevent it from reaching the cervix. Female condom is placed into the vagina before intercourse.	Fairly effective at preventing pregnancy, especially if applied before any physical contact and removed immediately after intercourse. Also protects against sexually transmitted diseases (STDs).
Cervical cap	Small latex cup that fits over the cervix; used with a spermicide to prevent sperm from entering the cervix	Fairly effective at preventing pregnancy if used with spermicide. Must be inserted before physical contact and left in place for several hours after sexual intercourse.
Diaphragm	Cup that fits over the cervix that is wider and shallower than a cervical cap; used with spermicide to prevent sperm from entering the cervix	Fairly effective at preventing pregnancy if used with spermicide. Must be inserted before physical contact and left in place for several hours after sexual intercourse. Must be removed after 6 to 8 hours to prevent vaginal infection.
Sponge	Sponge impregnated with spermicide inserted into vagina before intercourse	Less effective than cervical cap or diaphragm at preventing pregnancy. May provide some protection against STDs.

Method—Other	Description	Discussion
Spermicide	Cream or gel inserted into the vagina, which kills or inactivates sperm	Less effective used alone than when in combination with a barrier device. May provide some protection against STDs.
Rhythm or natural methods	Avoiding sexual intercourse during times near ovulation as determined by awareness of menstrual cycle, body temperature, or examination of cervical mucus	High failure rate overall, but may be fairly effective if close track kept of body changes and menstrual cycle. No mechanical or chemical intervention with the natural cycle.

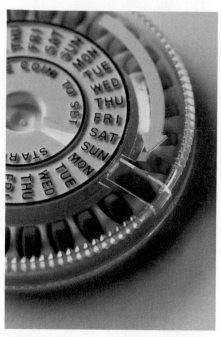

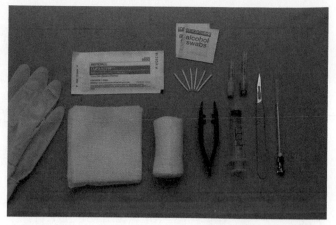

> **Figure 29-9** Supplies needed for Norplant insertion. The Norplant rods are inserted under the skin using a trochar in a fan-shaped pattern.

> **Figure 29-8** If birth control pills are a woman's choice for contraception, she should begin taking them before resuming sexual activity.

lease progesterone for 5 years), the procedure is done either at the 6-week visit or very soon afterward. Figure 29-9 shows the supplies needed for Norplant insertion.*

The woman is placed in a comfortable position, with the upper arm exposed. After preparing and draping the site, the doctor inserts the six small rods using a trochar (a pointed, hollow instrument) to form a tract and an obturator (rod that fits through the trochar) to push the rods into position in a fan-shaped formation under the skin.

The medical assistant sets up a sterile field containing povidone-iodine solution, a syringe and needles for the local anesthetic, a scalpel, hemostats or thumb forceps, and the sterile equipment from the Norplant kit (Norplant rods, trochar, and obturator). In addition,

---

*Norplant was withdrawn by the manufacturer in 2000 and remained unavailable in April 2001.

skin closure strips such as Steri-Strips, gauze squares, and gauze bandages are placed on the sterile field to dress the surgical area.

The medical assistant should follow the principles of sterile procedures discussed in chapter 17. After the procedure, the woman is advised to return for an annual follow-up or if problems occur, such as bleeding from the site, discomfort, or irregular periods.

An intrauterine device (**IUD**) may also be inserted in an office procedure. The woman is placed in the lithotomy position. After cleaning the cervix and using a povidone-iodine solution as a disinfectant, the doctor dilates the cervix and inserts the IUD.

The medical assistant sets up a sterile field containing povidone-iodine solution, a vaginal speculum, a uterine tenaculum (type of forceps with long blades and sharp jaws to grasp the cervix), a uterine sound, sterile scissors, and the IUD kit, which contains the IUD and inserter.

After the procedure, the woman is instructed to check for the IUD string in her vagina every month to be sure it remains in place. She should be evaluated at least annually or if problems occur, such as explusion of the IUD, bleeding, fever, abdominal pain, or pain during intercourse.

STUDENT STUDY PLAN

To reinforce your understanding of the material in this chapter . . .

Complete the **Review & Recall** questions.

Discuss the situation in **If You Were the Medical Assistant** with your classmates and answer the questions.

Answer the **Critical Thinking Questions** and discuss them with your classmates.

Visit the suggested **Web sites** and search for additional Web sites using the **Keywords for Internet Searches**.

Complete the exercises in chapter 29 of the **Student Mastery Manual**.

✔ REVIEW & RECALL

1. How have hospitals and birthing facilities changed in the past 20 years in response to consumer wishes and insurance reimbursement?

2. Identify changes in the reproductive system and other body systems that occur during pregnancy.

3. What specific information is collected during the first prenatal visit regarding the menstrual history, past obstetric history, and history of the current pregnancy?

4. Why are the following laboratory tests done early in pregnancy: CBC, fasting blood glucose, Rh antibody titer, rubella titer, Pap test, blood type, urinalysis, and blood test for syphilis? Identify at least two additional tests that might be done depending on the mother's risk factors.

5. Describe the medical assistant's role during prenatal visits.

6. Identify specific symptoms or conditions that a pregnant patient should report to the medical office.

7. Describe additional lab tests that might be done in special circumstances for the pregnant patient.

8. Compare and contrast the signs and symptoms of true labor and false labor.

9. What diagnostic tests are done during the postpartum visit?

✔ IF YOU WERE THE MEDICAL ASSISTANT

You take a telephone call from a woman who tells you she is in her 24th week of pregnancy and thinks she might be in labor. Identify six specific questions you should ask to obtain information for the doctor. Make a table listing questions and identifying answers to those questions that would indicate true labor and those that would indicate false labor. Describe exactly what you should do if you determine that the caller is probably experiencing true labor.

✔ CRITICAL THINKING QUESTIONS

1. Managed care has been criticized for consistently reducing the length of time a woman may stay in the hospital after a vaginal birth or cesarean section. Find out what insurance plans (including health maintenance organizations) generally available in your area cover. Compare at least three plans. Discuss the implications for women and newborns. Are problems arising because hospital stays are too short? Give reasons for your answer.

2. Discuss the implications of the alpha-fetoprotein blood test and amniocentesis. Why do doctors recommend these tests to their patients, especially women over age 40? What might be discovered by these tests and what are the possible implications for a pregnant woman?

3. Medical assistants are often employed in obstetrical offices. Discuss with your classmates how working in this type of practice would be different from working in a family practice or internal medicine practice. Describe your own feelings about working for a practice that specializes in this area.

 EXPLORE THE WEB

INTERNET WEB SITES

American College of Nurse Midwives
www.acnm.org

birth centers
www.birthcenters.org

Centers for Disease Control-maternal health
www.cdc.gov/nccdphp/drh/

commercial sites for patients
www.epregnancy.com
www.babyonline.com
www.babycenter.com
www.babyzone.com

obstetric ultrasound
www.ob-ultrasound.net

obstetrics and gynecology
www.obgyn.net

KEYWORDS FOR INTERNET SEARCHES

childbirth
childbirth and anesthesia
circumcision
ectopic pregnancy
home birth
midwifery
obstetrics
pregnancy and childbirth
pregnancy complications

 ANSWERS TO ON THE JOB

1. Mrs. Holland's presumptive signs of pregnancy are missed menstrual periods, nausea and vomiting, and breast tenderness. The positive pregnancy test is a probable sign of pregnancy.

2. To calculate Mrs. Holland's EDC, take the date of her last menstrual period (4/3/XX), subtract 3 months (1/3/XX), then add 1 year and 7 days, which results in an EDC of January 10 of the following year.

3. Mrs. Holland is gravida III, para I, and abortion I. Because she is currently pregnant, the obstetric term that describes Mrs. Holland must end in the suffix -gravida. She can be described as multigravida.

4. During routine prenatal visits, the medical assistant measures weight, vital signs, blood pressure, height of the fundus, and fetal heart rate. A dipstick urinalysis is done at each visit. The hemoglobin and/or hematocrit is tested regularly.

5. Two common problems of pregnancy are gestational diabetes (diabetes due to the pregnancy) and preeclampsia (high blood pressure with protein in the urine). If either problem occurs, the primary care provider wants to know about it as soon as possible. If the medical assistant finds glucose (sugar) in the urine, the woman may have diabetes. If the woman's blood pressure is a little high and there is protein in the urine, the doctor has to do more tests to see if the woman is developing a problem. Testing urine at each visit is a simple way to know that everything is going well.

Chapter 30

Patients with Chronic and Terminal Diseases

Instructional Objectives

After completing this chapter, you will be able to do the following:

1. Define and spell the vocabulary words for this chapter.
2. Describe important methods of coordinating care and optimizing rehabilitation for a patient with chronic disease.
3. Correlate descriptions of the common stages of grief, including denial, anger, bargaining, depression, and acceptance, to behaviors seen in those stages.
4. List signs and symptoms of acute grief.
5. Generate ethical questions that arise from the complex relationship of health care to the dying and terminally ill patient.
6. Discuss the principles that govern the use of experimental procedures and medications on the terminally ill patient.
7. Identify the effects of limited medical resources on treatment of the seriously ill and/or elderly patient.
8. Describe how living wills, do-not-resuscitate orders (DNRs), and durable powers of attorney can be used to increase control by a terminally ill patient over his or her medical care.
9. Compare and contrast benign and malignant neoplasms.
10. Describe common classification systems for cancer.
11. Identify groups of risk factors for cancer.
12. Describe tests used in the diagnosis of cancer.
13. Discuss three types of treatment for cancer and how they work together.
14. Describe the signs and symptoms found in the four stages of HIV infection.
15. Discuss the legal implications of HIV testing.
16. List common types of treatments for AIDS and discuss their effectiveness.
17. Identify measures to protect health care workers from HIV infection and to prevent transmission of HIV virus.

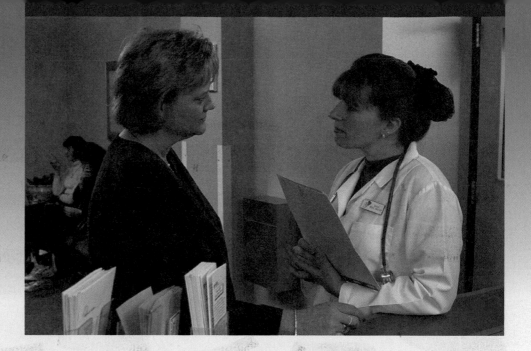

- Manage patients with special and specific needs; patients with chronic disease; and dying patients.

- Instruct individuals according to their needs.
- Perform within clinical and legal boundaries.

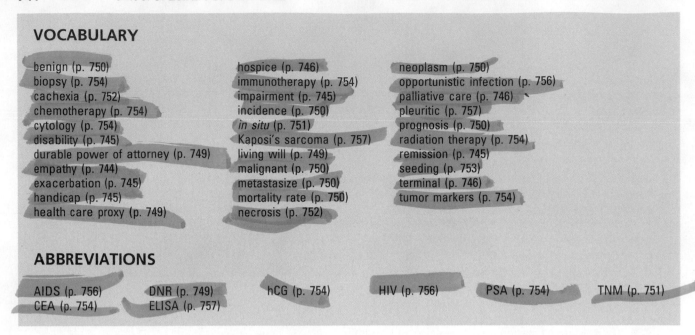

VOCABULARY

benign (p. 750)
biopsy (p. 754)
cachexia (p. 752)
chemotherapy (p. 754)
cytology (p. 754)
disability (p. 745)
durable power of attorney (p. 749)
empathy (p. 744)
exacerbation (p. 745)
handicap (p. 745)
health care proxy (p. 749)

hospice (p. 746)
immunotherapy (p. 754)
impairment (p. 745)
incidence (p. 750)
in situ (p. 751)
Kaposi's sarcoma (p. 757)
living will (p. 749)
malignant (p. 750)
metastasize (p. 750)
mortality rate (p. 750)
necrosis (p. 752)

neoplasm (p. 750)
opportunistic infection (p. 756)
palliative care (p. 746)
pleuritic (p. 757)
prognosis (p. 750)
radiation therapy (p. 754)
remission (p. 745)
seeding (p. 753)
terminal (p. 746)
tumor markers (p. 754)

ABBREVIATIONS

AIDS (p. 756)
CEA (p. 754)

DNR (p. 749)
ELISA (p. 757)

hCG (p. 754)

HIV (p. 756)

PSA (p. 754)

TNM (p. 751)

Chronic diseases have become an expectation as life expectancy has increased during the 20th century. *Healthy People 2000,* an initiative coordinated by the U.S. Department of Health and Human Services, emphasizes vitality and independence for the older adult. Basic health promotion activities can reduce the number of complaints associated with aging, chronic disease, and terminal illness. Exercise, stress management, nutrition, and dealing with substance abuse should be emphasized.

INTRODUCTION TO CHRONIC DISEASE AND TERMINAL ILLNESS

Eighty percent of the elderly have one chronic illness; 50 percent have two or more. The most common chronic diseases of the elderly are arthritis, hypertension, heart disease, hearing impairment, and dementia, a broad impairment of intellectual capacity that is usually progressive.

Older people visit doctors more often than younger people, take more prescription and over-the-counter medications, and experience more functional problems. Chronic conditions require treatment of symptoms and treatment to maximize health status while preventing further disability. Acute conditions must be treated and cured to prevent them from becoming chronic conditions that necessitate lifelong treatment.

Primary care professionals are responsible for coordinating the care of individuals with chronic diseases. The primary care medical office may need to ensure coordination of care among numerous health care providers, including specialists, pharmacists, home health providers, long-term institutional providers, and others.

A medical assistant in a primary care adult medicine or family practice will come in contact with a number of people with chronic and progessive diseases, many of whom have limited life expectancy. When death is a slow process, the medical assistant will be one of the sources of communication and information, as well as a person who provides explanations of the medical treatments being offered both to the patient and his or her caregiver.

The establishment of a professional rapport between the patient and the medical assistant makes this process meaningful. The medical assistant should allow the patient to express his or her fears, as well as hopes for a cure. The medical assistant should never offer false hopes but should be a support that provides a safe handhold in the reality of the situation.

By offering **empathy**—objective insight into the feelings, emotions, and motivation of others—the medical assistant becomes someone who can be trusted with personal feelings and concerns. If a medical assistant maintains this objectivity, the patient may be better able to tolerate the anxiety of facing the unknown without feeling overwhelmed.

Death is a natural process and needs to be confronted as such. At the same time the medical assistant is supporting the dying patient, he or she must remain conscious of personal feelings about death and dying.

COORDINATING CARE

Individuals with disease affecting many organ systems may need a wide range of services, from in-hospital care for acute conditions to home care for chronic conditions. In most instances, the medical assistant in the doctor's office helps to coordinate the medical care because he or she may know the person best.

Chronic illness usually involves permanent disability to one extent or another. A chronic illness is often characterized by periods of **remission,** when symptoms are few if any, and periods of **exacerbation,** when symptoms are many and often debilitating.

Reaction to illness varies among individuals and is affected by their perceptions of the problem, others' perception of the problem, their success or failure in self-care, and their ability to obtain appropriate professional care. Primary care is provided in the doctor's office, with follow-up and continuing care provided by families, home health care teams, or professionals in skilled nursing facilities. Multiple doctors may be required to provide the necessary care.

The medical assistant must be aware of all of the doctors providing care for the individual and all the medications and treatments the individual is using. Through coordination, the patient receives the best possible care.

Coordination Through Documentation

The medical assistant should be sure that all correspondence is readily available in the medical record, that follow-up correspondence has arrived and is ready for the doctor's use, and that the actions of one doctor will mesh with the actions of others.

Coordination Through Appropriate Referrals

Listening closely to the patient allows the medical assistant to help the patient respond to all hints of deterioration, as well as actual problems, as soon as they become apparent. The patient may need to be seen by several health care professionals while receiving additional care at home. The medical assistant can be helpful by being aware of community resources and communicating the needs of the patient and his or her family to the doctor. This requires knowledge of insurance benefits and of the types of insurance the office accepts, as well as other sources of funding assistance the patient may be able to obtain.

Communication on this level must be two-way; if a patient is being seen by visiting nurses, hospice, or other health professionals, the medical assistant may be the person who facilitates communication between the doctor and these other parties.

Coordination Through Cooperation of Health Care Professionals

The medical assistant in the primary care office may ask the patient or caregiver to bring in all medications on a regular basis to maintain updated information. The medical assistant may also ask the patient or care-

giver regularly to go through the list of treatments being received and health care services being used. It can be a big responsiblity to coordinate the efforts of several health care professionals, including specialists, pharmacists, mental health professionals, and staff at acute care and skilled nursing facilities.

Coordination for Maximum Rehabilitation

The goal of care for any patient is restoration to the highest level of functioning possible. This is a process of bringing physical and psychological health, as well as social skills and tasks of daily living, to their highest possible level. The condition of an individual who is less than fully functional is described using one of three terms—impairment, disability, or handicap:

- **Impairment** includes disturbance of functioning that may be physical or psychological, a mild loss of function.
- **Disability** includes measurable loss of function. For example, absent vision in one eye or inability to bend the knees. It may be possible for the affected individual to compensate for the lack of function in most situations.
- **Handicap** indicates the extent to which a person cannot perform normal activities. The extent of handicap may be different in two individuals with similar diability because one may have received training to learn to compensate or may be more highly motivated to overcome his or her disability.

The goal of any program of rehabilitation is to bring the patient to the highest possible level of functioning and maintain that level of functioning with coordinated services.

Problems of Maintaining a Positive Attitude

A patient's personal values, beliefs, and attitudes can become stumbling blocks in the care of a person with chronic disease, especially as these diseases progress and take their toll on the patient.

Medical assistants must remember that their attitude toward patients with progressively declining health is apparent to the patient and his or her family. It is imperative to remember that the chronically ill person is a person first and a patient second. Such a person has a strong desire to be independent even if totally dependent on others for care. This can lead to frustration and anger, which is often expressed against the very people who are doing the most to care for the individual—professional and nonprofessional family caregivers.

People in this situation must learn to control anger, if possible using that anger as a motivation to make decisions and follow through in areas where they can be effective.

As disease processes progress, patient care becomes more difficult for both professional and family caregivers. Illness behavior varies among patients; medical assistant contact must be consistent and caring.

Home Health Care and Hospice

With the increase in hospital costs during the 1980s and 1990s, patients are only able to remain in the hospital for a limited time. A patient whose condition has stabilized or whose active treatment has ended but still requires pain relief, nursing care, and/or comfort measures, must either receive them at home, a nursing home, a rehabilitation center, or a hospice center.

A **hospice** is an organization that provides comfort and palliative care. **Palliative care** is care that relieves symptoms without curing the patient, who is in the **terminal** phase of an illness. The terminal phase is defined as when the patient is not expected to live more than 6 months.

Most hospices provide nursing care, nursing assistants, and volunteers to visit terminal patients in their homes, working with the family to increase the patient's comfort once active treatment is no longer effective or desired. There are also hospice centers, which provide centralized care. In some areas, a patient can receive similar services from home health care agencies and visiting nurse associations.

The medical assistant may serve as a liaison to obtain appropriate referrals from the doctor and assist the patient and/or family to locate providers of needed services.

ISSUES OF DEATH AND DYING

Death is inevitable. For the patient who has progressed to the terminal phase of illness, death can come at any time. Such a death—sudden but not unexpected—can take a toll on both family and professional caregivers. Although much of the grieving process occurs during the illness, there is still a need for appropriate grieving after death.

Everyone in the medical office has "favorite patients," and their deaths hurt. Medical assistants and other professional caregivers must continue providing care for others and work through their grief, but that grief should also be acknowledged, either informally or formally.

Factors That Influence Attitudes of Patients and Health Care Professionals

The manner in which the patient and the medical assistant face imminent death is based on five key factors.

1. Religious belief of both parties. Religion and faith practices play an important role in how death and dying are confronted. The medical assistant should accept the patient's religious beliefs and not try to convert the individual to other religious beliefs. This requires that the medical assistant have a basic understanding of the beliefs of each religion that is prominent in the community from which the patient population is drawn.
2. Personal experiences influence the way both parties respond to the situation. Those patients who have experienced painful and prolonged deaths of loved ones may have special fears that need to be confronted. Likewise, the medical assistant who has experienced the death of a loved one may have more understanding than one who has never confronted death on such a personal level.
3. Cultural responses to death and expectations of death are learned at an early age. Cultural expectations become part of the acceptance or denial of the situation.
4. The patient's age has bearing on how he or she views death. The medical assistant should listen closely to hear what the person has to say. Older people usually are not as afraid of death as a younger person is.
5. Fulfillment of life's ambitions may make death more acceptable. Those who have not accomplished their goals in life are frustrated with the sense they never will.

Stages of Grieving

The grief process has a fairly predictable sequence that includes shock and disbelief; anger, guilt, and hostility; interruptions of normal activities due to the lack of concentration and depression; intense preoccupation with the thought of death or loss of a loved one; and finally acceptance of the impending death, with a resumption of relatively normal activities.

People go through this sequence over varying lengths of time and may move from one stage to another out of the order presented here. Both family and friends of the dying person must grieve for his or her impending death. Although the process is individual, it is important to know that the dying person can come to a type of acceptance and that after death has occurred there is a time when grieving relatives and friends will again be able to engage in loving and fulfilling relationships.

The spiritual author Elisabeth Kübler-Ross argued that each person grieves when death is inevitable in their own way. Each person may experience one or all of the identified stages of grief; an individual may "progress" from one stage to another or "go back" from one stage to another that has previously been experienced.

Finally, she argued, not everyone reaches the stage of acceptance; there are those who never completely accept death or overcome the loss of a loved one. Kübler-Ross also described the kind of grieving that an individual experiences when that person learns of his or her own terminal illness. She defined five discrete stages of this self-grieving process:

 1. Denial. This is the initial response to knowledge that one has a terminal illness; a state of shock and disbelief. Most people simply deny the idea. Denial can be useful; it can provide a period of time to find a way to deal with death.

    When dealing with a patient in denial, a medical assistant should listen to the patient actively without confronting unrealistic statements. Acceptance of the patient's need to deny reality provides support for a patient to accept the diagnosis at his or her own pace.

    Some patients want to get deeply involved in understanding both the disease and the prescribed treatments. It is important to establish trust with the patient by being honest and complete in answering any questions.

2. Anger. Frustration and anger usually follow denial. The patient is in the "why me" mode. The illness seems unfair, and the patient may respond by being belligerent, uncooperative, and critical of those around him or her. Health care providers may become a target of this anger and criticism; it is important for the medical assistant to realize that any such display of anger is not directed at him or her personally but toward the situation and circumstances over which the patient has no control.

3. Bargaining. In this stage, which usually follows anger closely, the patient may try to give something up to gain more time. Most bargaining is done between the patient and his or her personal concept of God. If verbalized, the medical assistant should be accepting of the patient's wish to make a bargain that will prolong his or her life.

4. Depression. The patient recognizes the facts that cannot be denied and becomes depressed. Most people become silent in this stage and prefer to be alone. The patient who is withdrawn is more difficult to deal with than the person who is openly angry. In this situation, a medical assistant needs to be available and present with the patient for companionship and to provide a nonjudgmental listening ear. The medical assistant should always strive to maintain communication with a terminally ill individual in the depression stage.

5. Acceptance. Some people find a degree of peace within themselves when they accept their imminent death. They willingly stop resisting death and rest quietly. This is seldom seen by professionals who work in medical offices, because those who reach this stage may be in a hospital, hospice, or at home. The dying person may want loved ones present at death and may not interact with others at all. Most people fear dying alone and want the comfort of having someone, preferably a loved one, present in the final moments.

A dying person has a number of fears, such as fear of the unknown, fear of pain, and fear of helplessness. It is a challenge for all health care professionals to accept the difficult feelings of fear.

Manifestations of Grief

Signs of acute grief include sleeplessness, loss of appetite, forgetfulness, and absentmindedness. A person experiencing acute grief may repeat the same behavior over and over again. Uncontrollable crying, withdrawal, and unresponsiveness are also signs of acute grief. The grieving person may find someone on whom to place blame and may attempt to run away from the situation. The person may wonder what he or she could have done to prevent the death or be angry at the deceased for dying.

When a person experiences resolution, he or she admits that the death has occurred; that acceptance allows the person to speak of the dead as "gone" or "dead." He or she knows that the death is a reality and stops looking for the deceased's return.

ETHICAL ISSUES OF DEATH AND DYING

Medical assistants can have some influence on the decisions patients make about what treatments to use; this depends on the amount of trust built up in the relationship between the medical assistant and the patient and patient's family. The longer a medical assistant has worked in an office, the more likely he or she is to have developed such relationships to build on.

Advances in medical technology have made it possible to extend the lives of many patients with complex chronic illnesses. But is it always right to do so?

Some treatments used on patients with multiple system disease will add quality to life while not necessarily prolonging life; others will prolong life without necessarily adding quality to that life. The decisions about which of these types of treatments to use are difficult to make. For the medical assistant to be helpful in assisting patients and families make these decisions, he or she must clarify personal feelings about these issues.

Some of the end-of-life questions a medical assistant can help a patient and family work through are:

1. Who should make the decisions about life support?

2. When is it appropriate to allow death to occur?
3. How does the medical team assess the patient's mental ability to make decisions concerning use of life support measures?
4. What values should enter into the decision-making process?
5. Does the patient and/or his or her family have the right to allow a patient to die?
6. What is the normal responsibility of a doctor and a medical office staff regarding dying?
7. Is it always best to act on the side of life?
8. What is the difference between quantity and quality of life?

Experimental Procedures and Treatments

Guidelines for experimental procedures or treatments on living people are based on formalities called the Nuremberg Code, developed after World War II, following the Nuremberg Tribunals of 1946–1949. During these tribunals, medical experimentation undertaken by Nazi doctors during the Holocaust was revealed, and scientists realized a need to agree on procedures to safeguard patients' rights during research. The Nuremberg Code was published as part of the description of *Trials of War Criminals Before the Nuremberg Military Tribunals.*

The Nuremberg Code identifies the need for trained scientists to perform research that can benefit society (as opposed to any imaginable type of research), using measures to ensure that the benefits outweigh the risks. It states that experimental subjects should be fully informed of the research purpose, consent freely to the research, and retain the right to refuse further treatment under the research protocol at any time.

The World Medical Association produced a more detailed set of recommendations, *The Declaration of Helsinki,* in 1964, which was revised in 1975. It made a distinction between pure research and research combined with professional care. This document provides more specific guidelines about research protocols, obtaining consent, publishing results, and preventing harm to experimental subjects.

As scientific research extends into new areas, such as the human genome project, use of fetal tissue, and bioengineering, scientists continue to examine ethical issues in an international forum, and individual institutions establish guidelines and supervisory committees to ensure that patient rights are protected.

Many rules govern human experimentatation in the United States. Universities, medical schools, and hospitals have human investigations committees that approve all research on people. If the research is federally sponsored, the U.S. Department of Health and Human Services also has to approve the research. If the research is being conducted on new pharmaceutical substances in clinical trials, the Food and Drug Adminis-

tration must approve it before the drug company can begin experiments at hospitals, medical schools, or private doctors' offices.

New drugs or other treatments in the very early stages of human studies are sometimes given to patients who are dying. These studies are often designed to determine both therapeutic dose—if very high doses are helpful—and toxicity at varying doses. Usually, the side effects are not known. Deciding whether or not to participate, in such a study or to allow a loved one to participate, is one of the most difficult decisions a dying person and his or her family can make.

Allocation of Resources

Deciding how to distribute available funds to pay for government health care programs is an issue that has become more controversial and open in the United States in the past few years, although decisions about how to allocate scarce resources have been made by doctors and medical administrators throughout the history of professional medical care.

The cost of care for patients in the final months of life is very high. Because a large percentage of care for the dying is paid for by the government under the Medicare and Medicaid programs, end-of-life care has attracted a lot of attention. Information published by the Committee on Care at the End of Life (*Approaching Death: Improving Care at the End of Life,* Washington, DC: National Academy Press, 1997), shows that in 1987, although less than 1 percent of the population died, the health care costs for their last 6 months of life accounted for at least 5 to 7 percent of all personal health care expenditures that year. In addition, their families often experienced serious financial consequences, due to out-of-pocket medical costs and lost time at work, because of the demands of caring for a seriously ill family member.

Oregon was the first state to come to grips with this issue in legislation, making explicit that the state would not use Medicaid dollars to fund certain end-of-life treatments that do more to prolong life than to increase quality of life. With the money saved, the state vastly expanded the routine health services it provides children who are eligible for Medicaid benefits.

A medical assistant must confront these philosophical issues personally before he or she confronts them in practice in the office. Every medical assistant will have to confront resource allocation issues, from organ transplantation to patients' ability to pay for services not covered by insurance, to the cost of transportation to the office or the hospital, to quick hospital discharges.

Too often, the decision on whether to utilize a resource is based on a patient's ability to pay—either out of pocket or through insurance coverage—for the treatment rather than on the patient's ability to truly benefit from the treatment.

LEGAL ISSUES RELATED TO DEATH AND DYING

A dying patient and his or her family can formalize their decisions about what kinds of treatments they would like the patient to have in a number of ways. These include do-not-resuscitate (DNR) orders, living wills, health care proxies, and durable power of attorney documents, which all fall under the heading of "advance directives." A health care proxy or living will may specify care to be given or avoided and name a person to make medical decisions for the individual should he or she become incompetent. This is usually a spouse, child, member of the clergy, or close friend. Medical advance directives should always name a single individual to make decisions, not a committee; this is often a difficult choice, especially for an elderly person who wishes to name all of his or her children.

In addition, the patient may want to provide for donation of any organs that are useful; if the patient does not make this decision ahead of time, the family can do it as part of their decision-making powers under an advance directive document.

Advance Directives

Signed originals rather than photocopies of the advance directives should be held by the named surrogate, and the patient should keep copies with his or her important papers. It should also be noted in the primary care doctor's records, or a copy may be filed, so he or she can contact the surrogate if necessary, especially if the surrogate lives out of town.

Do not resuscitate orders should be in the medical record, and the staff should be informed of the patient's wishes. Facing a DNR is often difficult for medical professionals, who have been taught to heal and cure, while postponing death as long as possible. If the patient is at home, the family must have a copy of the DNR order to show emergency personnel or they will be legally obligated to rescuscitate the patient.

Removal of life support means that no form of support, including mechanical breathing, feeding, or medications to prolong life, should be given. Pain medication and sedation are continued if necessary after removal of life support.

Living Will/Health Care Proxy

A living will is a document executed by an individual that gives medical professionals instructions about how that person wishes to be treated in the event he or she becomes incompetent.

Because a person usually names an agent to carry out his or her wishes if he or she is unable to do so, a living will is also called a health care proxy. It may

Uniform Donor Card

I _____ hereby make this anatomical gift, if medically acceptable, to take effect upon my death. I give:

____ Any needed organs/tissues for any purpose

____ Only the following listed organs/tissues

_____
(Specify the organ(s) or tissue(s)

____ My body for anatomical study if needed

Limitations or special wishes: _____
_____

- -

This is a legal document under the Uniform Anatomical Gift or similar laws, signed by the donor and two witnesses in the presence of each other.

_____
Signature of Donor

_____
Date Signed   Donor's Date of Birth

_____
City   City

_____
Signature of Witness

_____
Signature of Witness

➤ **Figure 30–1** Organ donor card.

detail when treatment should be stopped, and ask that no "heroic" measures be taken.

A living will may also give instructions regarding organ donation, autopsy, or donation of the remains to a medical school for anatomy dissection. Many states allow an individual's wishes to donate organs to be noted on his or her drivers licenses; in this way in the event of a fatal auto accident the police—who usually use the license to make identification—can notify ambulance personnel that the deceased is an organ donor. Figure 30–1 is an organ donor card.

Durable Power of Attorney

A durable power of attorney gives the designated person the ability to make all legal decisions for an individual, including medical decisions. It takes effect when a person becomes unable to make his or her

Table 30-1	**Advance Directives**

Do Not Resuscitate (DNR) Order

   Executed by either patient or health care agent. Allows medical staff to not resuscitate in the event of cardiac or respiratory arrest.

Living Will

   Executed by an individual before or during illness. Gives specific instructions to medical staff about which life-prolonging actions should or should not be taken. Also provides instruction to health care agent as to which treatments he or she should authorize. Provisions for organ donation, autopsy, or donation of remains to a medical school is also usually included in a living will. The living will may be used to name a health care agent (health care proxy).

Durable Power of Attorney

   Executed by an individual before or during illness. Names an individual to execute all legal documents, including a DNR order. The person who is granted power of attorney is often named in the living will and/or health care proxy.

Health Care Proxy

   Executed by an individual before or during illness. Names a health care agent who has the ability to make decisions about care, including signing a DNR. Not as broad as a power of attorney. Becomes effective only when the individual becomes incapable of making his or her own decisions.

Organ Donor Card

   A card that states that an individual wishes to donate organs.

   Many states have done away with a separate organ donor card, preferring to place the organ-donor designation on an individual's driver's license.

own decisions. It may place limits on the designated person's rights and responsibilities and may give specific instructions to the designated person concerning medical issues.

In some states, medical decisions have been carved out so that it is not necessary to execute a durable power of attorney but only to name a health care proxy, a person empowered to make medical decisions on another person's behalf. The person is usually called a health care agent, and any person age 18 or older can execute a health care proxy.

Table 30-1 describes the different kinds of advance directives.

THE PATIENT WITH METASTATIC CANCER

Cancer is the second leading cause of death in the United States, after heart disease. The **prognosis**—outlook for future health—in cancer depends on the type of cancer, how far the cancer has spread (metastasized), and the effectiveness of existing therapies and any experimental treatments for that type of cancer.

More and more treatment of patients with cancer is being undertaken in the oncologist's office on an out-

patient basis. In addition, many people with cancer have other illnesses that are treated in the primary care office or the offices of other specialists.

Overview of Cancer

The **incidence**—frequency of occurrence—of cancer is approximately twice the **mortality rate**—the rate of deaths in a certain number of incidences. Table 30-2 outlines common cancers in men and women. It does not include cases of primary skin cancers (squamous cell and basal cell), which are localized and usually have a good prognosis because of early discovery, but it does include malignant melanoma.

The body is constantly regenerating cells; some cells reproduce abnormally and become **neoplasms**—tumors. These neoplasms may be either **benign**, with relatively harmless cells, or **malignant**, which means the tumors invade nearby tissue, and often spread to other tissue. Figure 30-2 illustrates benign and malignant tumors.

Although benign tumors do not spread to other parts of the body, they may still cause problems, such as pressure on or obstruction of body organs. Benign tumors grow slowly, and as they expand and enlarge the new cells closely resemble the parent cells. They do not recur after removal and do not cause destruction of tissue, except by compression. These tumors can almost always be removed surgically if they become problematic.

Malignant tumors cause some of the same problems but are more threatening because they invade nearby tissue and can even **metastasize**—spread to distant parts of the body via the circulatory or lymph systems. Malignant tumors usually grow rapidly, although they may be slow to invade surrounding tissue. As the tu-

Table 30-2	**Types of Cancer Expected to Cause the Most Deaths in the Year 2000**	
Type of cancer	Estimated new cases	Estimated deaths
MEN		
All sites	619,700	284,100
Lung and bronchus	89,500	89,300
Prostate	180,400	31,900
Colon	43,400	23,100
Lymphoma	35,900	14,400
Pancreas	13,700	13,700
WOMEN		
All sites	600,400	268,100
Lung	74,600	67,600
Breast	182,800	40,800
Colon	50,400	24,600
Pancreas	14,600	14,500
Ovary	23,100	14,000

Statistics from the National Cancer Society

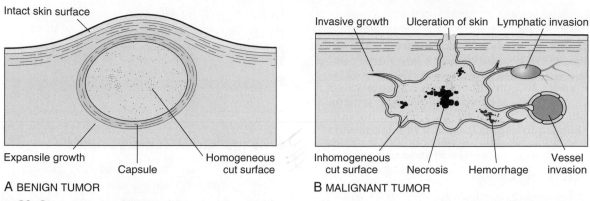

> **Figure 30–2** Appearance of benign (A) and malignant (B) tumors. (From Damjanov I: *Pathology for the Health-Related Professions.* Philadelphia: W.B. Saunders, 1996.)

mor grows, the cells become less differentiated. This means that instead of developing all of the individual characteristics of cells of a particular tissue type, they remain immature and divide rapidly.

Regional invasion may occur as the cells invade the tissues of the area at the original site while metastasizing to other parts of the body. After removal, a malignant tumor may grow back, metastasize, or cause necrosis, ulceration, tissue perforation, and sloughing. Malignant tumors may be fatal.

Classification of Tumors

Tumors are classified by their anatomic site, stage, cell appearance, and amount of differentiation. The suffix *-oma* is used to refer to both benign and malignant tumors.

Tumors are named by the type of tissue from which they develop.

Benign growths are fibromas (from fibrous tissue), lipomas (from fat tissue), and leiomyomas (from smooth muscle tissue).

Malignant growths are carcinomas (from tissues of the skin, glands, and linings of the digestive, urinary, and respiratory tracts); sarcomas (from bone, muscle, and other connective tissue); melanomas (from pigment cells of the skin); leukemias and lymphomas (both of which arise from blood-forming tissues, including lymphoid, plasma cells, and bone marrow). Prefixes may be added to designate the exact type of malignant tissue; for example, osteosarcoma is bone cancer.

Cancers developing from epithelial cells (carcinomas) outnumber nonepithelial cancers by six to one.

Classifying Tumors by Appearance of Tumor Cells (Grade)

One way to classify malignant tumors is by grade. The grade of cancer describes the cancer cells themselves.

A grade I tumor is well differentiated, meaning it is easy to tell what kind of tissue the cancer originated from.

Grade II and III tumors show varying amounts of differentiation; it is less easy to tell the tissue of origin.

Grade IV tumors are poorly differentiated and it is difficult to determine the tissue of origin. The cells are dividing so rapidly that, in effect, Grade IV cancer cells all look alike. In this situation, prognosis is poor.

Classifying Tumors by Extent of Spread (Stage)

The other way to classify cancer is by how extensively the tumor has spread.

In a stage I cancer, the malignant cells are confined to the tissue of origin, and there is no invasion of other tissues.

In a stage II cancer, there is limited spread of the cancer in the local area, usually to the nearby lymph nodes.

In a stage III cancer, the tumor is larger or has spread from the site of origin into nearby tissues, or both. Regional lymph nodes are likely to be involved.

In a stage IV cancer, there is metastasis to distant parts of the body.

Another method of classifying spread of cancer is the TNM system.

T designates the a primary tumor. The stages are T0, Tis, T1, T2, T3, and T4. T0 is used to indicate that after treatment there is no sign of tumor. Tis means cancer ***in situ*** (Latin for *in the place*), meaning that the tumor exists in the epithelial layer and not in the basement membrane of the affected tissue. T1 to T4 reflects the size and extent of the tumor.

N designates the degree of invasion of regional lymph nodes. N0 means no nodes are involved. If regional nodes are involved, they are staged as N1 to N3, showing increasingly distant involvement.

M designates the degree of metastasis to a distant location. M0 means there is no metastasis. M1 represents distant metastasis.

Using this system, the notation Tis, N0, M0 means there is cancer *in situ,* with no evidence of cancer in the regional nodes, and no distant metastasis.

Risk Factors for Cancer

A risk factor is something environmental, genetic, or behavioral that increases an individual's chances of developing cancer. There are genetic, environmental, and behavioral components to the development of cancer.

For instance, cigarette smoking increases the possibility of developing cancers of the lungs, mouth, throat, larynx, bladder, and other organs. As another example, a number of chemicals used in manufacturing have been shown to cause leukemia when they leech into the public water supply—wells or aquifers. Scientific research suggests that up to one third of the over 500,000 cancer death expected in the United States each year could be prevented by changes in diet and other lifestyle factors, not including cigarette smoking.

In addition, age, gender, and site of development play a large part in cancer prognosis. Cancer is more common in older people, with the peak incidence in the 70s. Cancers of the breast and female reproductive tract tend to occur in midlife; lung cancers tend to occur in the 60s and can be prevented by smoking cessation. Prostate cancer incidence rises rapidly in men in their 70s and 80s, and many are not treated if they occur at that age.

The four major risk factors for cancer are:

1. Changes in genetic information in cells caused by carcinogens such as chemicals, radiation, or virus
2. Environmental substances such as asbestos, cigarette smoke, and nitrates
3. Heredity
4. Presence or absence of certain hormones.

Although no single gene has been identified that explains the frequency with which certain cancers appear in families, there are cancers that have a predictable pattern in families.

Public education—and education provided by medical assistants and others in medical offices—includes emphasis on early detection of cancer and early treatment, warning signs of cancer, how to perform self-examinations, and the importance of periodic examinations for common cancers.

Routine—monthly—self-examination and regular examinations by a health care professional can detect cancers of the breast, colon, rectum, cervix, prostate, testes, oral cavity, and skin at an early stage, when treatment is most effective and prognosis is best. The American Cancer Society argues that if all Americans performed self-examination and had routine screenings, the 5-year survival rate for these cancers would improve from the current 80 percent to 95 percent.

Table 30-3 shows recommendations for early detection of cancer.

How Malignant Tumors Spread

Most malignant tumors manifest themselves as an enlarging space-occupying mass. They compress blood vessels, which leads to necrosis and an area of inflammation around the tumor site. Some develop rapidly; others remain *in situ* for a long period. As the mass enlarges, the inner cells frequently are deprived of blood and nutrients, and die. This causes **necrosis** (tissue death) and inflammation.

It also deprives normal cells of nutrients, meaning that they cannot regenerate. Normal tissue is changed to abnormal tissue. Enzymes are secreted by the tumor cells; these break down the proteins and add to the destruction. The breakdown around the tumor allows the abnormal cells to move more easily into the surrounding tissue.

Malignant cells do not adhere to each other but break loose from the mass and infiltrate into the surrounding tissue. This erosion of the area is brought about by pressure and by the secretion of enzymes.

Tumors have both local and systemic effects.

Local Effects

Local effects include obstruction, pain, and necrosis.

Obstruction occurs as the tumor progresses and compresses a duct or passageway or as it surrounds passageways. Blood and lymph supply may be obstructed, leading to necrosis, ulceration, and edema.

Pain is usually not an early symptom, but occurs as the tumor advances. Pain is a warning sign; the severity of the pain depends on the type of tumor and its location. Primary pain may be caused by direct pressure of the mass on the sensory nerves or when the space is restricted. Secondary pain comes from infection, ischemia, and bleeding.

Necrosis may be caused by ulceration and infection, especially when normal flora are opportunistic.

Systemic Effects

Systemic effects of cancer include weight loss and **cachexia** (general wasting), anemia, systemic infections, and bleeding.

Weight loss is caused by anorexia, fatigue, stress, and the increased demands placed on the body by reproducing tumor cells and the nutrients necessary to feed them. Altered carbohydrate and

Table 30–3	**Recommendations for the Early Detection of Cancer (Summarized from the American Cancer Society)**		
Type of cancer	Type of examination or test	Age group	Frequency
Various	Physical examination	20–40	Annual
Breast	Clinical breast exam	20–39; women	Every 3 years
		40 and older; women	Every year
	Self breast exam	20 and older; women	Monthly
Colon/rectum	Fecal occult blood	50 and older	Annual
	Flexible sigmoidoscopy	50 and older	Every 5 years
	OR colonoscopy		Every 10 years
	OR double-contrast barium enema		Every 5 to 10 years
Prostate	Digital rectal exam	50 and older; men	Annual
	Prostate-specific-antigen (PSA) blood test	50 and older; men	Annual
Uterus	Pap test	18 and older; women	Annual until three consecutive normal exams, then every 2 to 3 years
	Pelvic examination	18 and older; women	Annual

protein metabolism leads to fatigue and weakness as well as tissue breakdown.

Anemia, or a decrease in hemoglobin, occurs as a result of the anorexia, decreased food intake, and chronic bleeding and is especially severe in cancers that affect bone marrow cells, such as leukemia and lymphoma.

Systemic infections may occur due to inactivity and are more severe if the immune system is affected by the cancer.

Bleeding occurs because of the erosion of blood vessels, or tissue ulceration.

The spread of a tumor depends on the characteristics of the specific type of cancer. Many spread rapidly before diagnosis; others grow more slowly and are less aggressive.

Tumor cells can erode into a blood or lymph vessel to travel throughout the body to a hospitable site and begin again to divide, producing a new tumor. The first metastasis usually occurs in the regional lymph nodes, which localize the tumor for a time. These can be removed at the time of any surgical treatment.

Many cancers move through the normal venous and lymphatic flow; therefore, the lungs and liver are common sites for secondary tumors. Some tumors spread by seeding, which is the spread of cancer cells in the body fluids and along the membranes. The tumor cells can break away and travel throughout the body easily in body fluids. Other cells might even be transported during surgery or diagnostic procedures. The spread of malignant tumors is shown in Figure 30–3.

Diagnostic Tests for Cancer

Diagnostic tests to detect cancer include screening tests done when a person has no symptoms and more

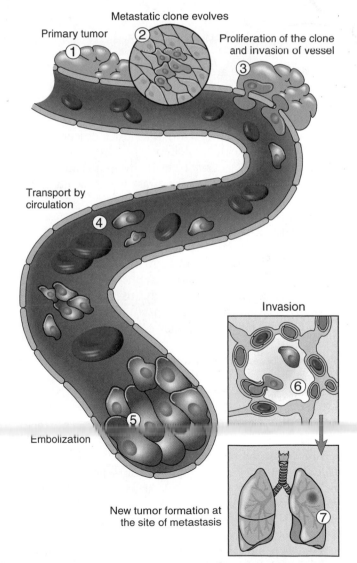

➤ **Figure 30–3** How malignant tumors spread. (From Damjanov I: *Pathology for the Health-Related Professions*. Philadelphia: W.B. Saunders, 1996.)

specific tests done as follow up to abnormal screening tests or suspicious findings on physical examination.

Tissue Examinations

Cells may be examined under the microscope to look for cancerous changes (**cytology**). A Pap smear, which tests cervical tissue, is an example of such a test. Samples can also be obtained from body fluids and from the respiratory and digestive tracts.

For malignancies of blood and blood-forming tissue, the blood cells may be examined microscopically. Other tissue samples may be obtained by **biopsy**, the removal of cells from living tissue for microscopic examination.

Tissue removed may be a whole growth, a sample of a growth, or the removal of cells. Good technique in the removal, handling, and preservation of the sample are imperative for accurate evaluation.

Samples can also be removed during surgery.

Imaging Studies

Imaging studies are used for detecting cancer of the bones and hollow organs.

Routine x-ray studies of areas such as the lungs may provide evidence of lung masses. Low-dosage radiographs are used to do scans for breast cancer (mammography); suspicious calcifications can often be detected before they can be felt by self-examination. Other imaging studies use contrast media taken either orally, rectally, or intravenously to outline organs and look for shadows of abnormal structures. Ultrasound can also detect masses in the breast and abdomen.

Computed tomography (CT) scans may be used for tumors of the head or trunk. A CT scan can be performed with or without contrast media. It provides a three-dimensional view of body tissue, which gives more information than plain-film x-ray studies.

Positron emission tomography scans use nuclear materials that are scanned to reveal patterns of tissue metabolism. This is useful in detecting tumors of the brain and breast and in measuring the effects of cancer treatment.

Magnetic resonance imaging (MRI) scans expose the patient to radiofrequency waves in the presence of a magnetic field. The process causes energy changes that can be measured and converted into computer images. This does not involve x-rays and does not expose the individual to any radiation. MRI is used to diagnose abnormalities of the central nervous system, spinal column, neck, bones, and joints.

Radionuclide scans allow radioactive substances to be taken up by specific body tissues to trace metabolic pathways and functions. The individual is given the radionuclide, then scanned to study the uptake of the substance in target tissue. These studies are used to detect cancer of the thyroid, liver, lung, or breast, or bone metastasis.

Endoscopic Procedures

Endoscopic procedures involve the insertion of a fiberoptic tube with a camera into a hollow organ or body cavity, which allows the doctor to look for tissue abnormalities. Suspicious growths can be removed using forceps threaded down the fiberoptic tube and can then be subjected to tissue studies. The esophagus, stomach, colon, and bronchi can be examined and biopsied endoscopically.

Laboratory Tests

Elevated levels of certain antigens, called **tumor markers,** are associated with certain types of cancer. They can also be used to monitor the effects of treatments for cancer. Hemoglobin and red blood cell counts that are low can be a sign of cancer. Cell characteristics sometimes point to malignancies of blood or blood-making tissues.

Examples of tumor markers include prostate-specific antigen (**PSA**), which when elevated may signal prostate cancer; carcinoembryonic antigen (**CEA**), which may signal colon cancer; or human chorionic gonadotropin (**hCG**), which is normally elevated in a woman during pregnancy but may signal testicular cancer in a man. These markers are used to screen those at risk, to confirm diagnoses made in other ways, and to follow the course of treatment.

Treatments for Cancer

Cancer treatments traditionally have included surgery, **chemotherapy** (treatment using anticancer drugs), and **radiation therapy** (treatment using various types of radiation). **Immunotherapy** (treatment using measures to stimulate the immune system) has been added to the arsenal of cancer-fighting treatments.

Treatments may be used alone or in combination, depending on the site and type of cancer. Treatments may be curative or palliative. Treatments may last from months to years, but monitoring lasts a lifetime.

Surgery

Surgery may be performed for diagnosis, relief of symptoms, maintenance of body function, or to effect a cure. Sometimes later reconstructive surgery is needed as well. In people at particularly high risk, organs are sometimes removed to prevent them from becoming cancerous. Surgery many be extensive or simple; extensive surgery is called a "radical" procedure. Approximately 40 percent of all cancers are treated surgically.

Surgery is likely to be curative if the cancer has not invaded the surrounding tissue and is confined to one place. Surrounding tissue, including nearby lymph nodes, is usually removed to eliminate cancerous cells that have escaped from the tumor mass. Boundaries are checked to confirm removal of the tumor and to confirm the diagnosis.

Chemotherapy

The use of medications to kill tumor cells or prevent cell division is known as chemotherapy. Chemotherapy may be used alone or in conjunction with surgery and radiation therapy. Chemotherapy usually starts 6 weeks after surgery to allow for surgical wound healing.

A combination of two to four drugs from different classifications usually makes up the chemotherapy "cocktail." The drugs act by destroying rapidly dividing cells. In some cases, drug therapy is curative; in other cases it causes the symptoms to decrease. Chemotherapy often enhances quality of life and extends life expectancy, even if it does not cure the cancer.

Types of antineoplastic drugs include antitumor antibiotics, antimetabolites, plant alkaloids, hormonal agents, alkylating agents, and others. They interfere with protein synthesis and DNA replication at different points of the reproductive cycle of tumor cells. As each drug acts at a different point in the cell cycle, the maximum number of tumor cells may be destroyed. These drugs are most effective against the most rapidly reproducing cells and on small tumor masses.

Another reason for giving a combination of drugs is that some drugs have unpleasant side effects; sometimes, the side effects of different drugs used in the combination counteract each other, and the total side effect is less unpleasant than had one drug been used.

Chemotherapy drugs are usually given in cycles, often monthly. Antineoplastics depress bone marrow, which makes the individual susceptible to infections and anemia. The patient's white blood cell count is checked before giving chemotherapy; if it falls too low, the treatment is delayed.

Radiation Therapy

Radiation therapy may be used alone or in conjunction with other therapy to treat radiosensitive tumors. Radiation causes mutation or alteration in the targeted cells' DNA, preventing mitosis or causing cell death. Radiation therapy is most effective on cells undergoing DNA synthesis or mitosis by destroying the rapidly growing cells.

Radiation therapy is sometimes given before surgery to shrink the tumor mass for easier removal. It may also be given after the surgical wound has healed to try to destroy any small seeds of cancer cells that may have begun to grow outside the main tumor.

The therapy itself consists of either electromagnetic waves such, as x-rays or gamma rays (using radium or cobalt) or high-energy penetrating particles, such as electrons or protons.

Radiation may be given externally or internally.

External radiation sources deliver radiation for a short period of time to a specific site and require the patient to have daily treatments for a 6-week period on an outpatient basis.

Internal insertion of radioisotopes is performed by sealing the radioisotope in a seed or a needle and inserting the device at the desired site. Another method is to instill the isotope in a solution in the body cavity to control excessive exudate, blood from the tumor, or infection. Some therapeutic radiation substances that are specific to one organ, such as iodine to the thyroid, are given orally. An individual undergoing internal radiation therapy must be monitored carefully to ensure that the radioactive substances are not causing unwanted exposure to the patient or others.

Hormonal Therapy and Immunotherapy

Hormones may be given in conjunction with the basic treatment for some types of cancer. Glucocorticoids may be given to reduce mitosis and to increase RBC counts while providing a feeling of well-being by decreasing inflammation and swelling around the tumor. Sex hormones may be given when tumor growth is dependent on hormone levels, such as in giving estrogen to slow-growing prostate tumors.

Biologic response modifiers are substances that augment the natural immune response in the body to improve surveillance and remove abnormal cells. Two substances that are being used with some success are interferon (a naturally occurring protein that kills cancer cells) and interleukin 2 (growth factor that increase the effectiveness of the body's immune response).

Other Therapies

Bone marrow transplantation is sometimes used for patients with various types of leukemia, lymphoma, multiple myeloma, and some solid tumors. It carries a high risk of death due to complications and is usually not performed until all alternative therapies have failed to produce a remission.

After the patient's own bone marrow has been destroyed by a combination of chemotherapy and radiation, the patient receives a graft of bone marrow intravenously. This graft may come from a donor or may be the patient's own bone marrow, harvested during an earlier period of remission and stored in case needed. At the time of the transplant and for several weeks after, the patient is unable to produce blood cells and must be supported by transfusions. The patient is also highly susceptible to infection and is usually maintained in a highly controlled environment to prevent exposure to microorganisms.

Therapies that attempt to support the patient's immune system by reducing stress and providing psychological support may also be used as an adjunct to traditional medical therapies. Some such therapies teach patients to use mental imagery to visualize the cells of their immune system attacking and eradicating the invading cancer cells. Although many patients and their families have obtained comfort and a greater sense of control and effectiveness from psychological therapies, there has been little or no accepted scientific evidence that they or other alternative methods (such as vitamin therapy, diet therapy, or energy therapy) are effective on their own as cancer treatments.

THE PATIENT WITH AIDS

When acquired immunodeficiency syndrome **(AIDS)** first appeared on the medical scene in the United States in the 1980s, it was considered a short-term, fatal disease. Today, AIDS and the infection that causes it, the human immunodeficiency virus **(HIV)**, are considered chronic conditions.

Treatments have become more effective, and HIV-positive individuals can live years without ever developing full-blown AIDS. More and more, the patient with HIV disease or AIDS is being treated in an outpatient setting.

But AIDS and HIV disease still carry much social stigma. The 21st century medical office and the personnel who work there must develop a new way of viewing and treating AIDS patients.

Overview of AIDS

No disease carries with it so much legal, social, medical, economic, and psychological baggage as does AIDS and HIV disease.

HIV is a retrovirus that infects cells and copies its RNA into the host cell's DNA. This newly made HIV cell continues to infect other cells in the host and spreads the disease throughout the body.

HIV gradually destroys the T_4 lymphocytes, which are essential for resisting pathogens that invade the body. This makes the HIV-positive individual susceptible to a host of **opportunistic infections,** infections that occur because of the patient's decreased immunity.

HIV is transmitted through the passage of body fluids or blood from an infected individual to another person. There are a few common methods of transmittal.

The first is sexual contact (vaginal, anal, or oral) in which the receiving party has an open wound into which the semen from an infected man—or, less frequently, the vaginal secretions from an infected woman—can go. Anal intercourse is the most danger-

ous in this regard, because tearing of anal tissue is a common occurrence. AIDS first appeared as a public health concern in the United States among the homosexual male community, a large number of whom were engaging in anal sex without using condoms.

The second is through needle sharing on the part of intravenous drug abusers, one or more of whom is HIV positive.

The third is by transfusion of virus-contaminated blood or blood products. This route of transmission has been all but ended in the United States since the early 1990s when the blood supply began to be regularly screened.

The fourth is from mother to child either in utero or through breast milk. Routine AIDS testing for pregnant women and new treatment modalities have greatly reduced this route since the late 1990s.

Today, those most at risk for becoming infected are intravenous drug abusers who share needles and their sex partners, as well as those who have multiple sex partners (heterosexual, male homosexual, or bisexual) and do not use condoms.

Signs and Symptoms of HIV Infection

Years can pass between the time of exposure to HIV and the onset of any clinical symptoms. Early symp-

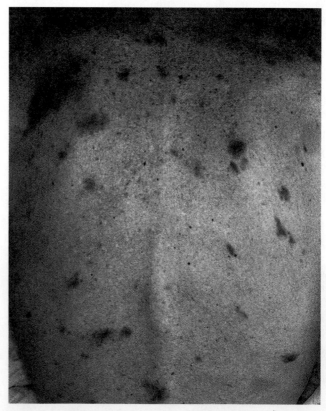

> **Figure 30–4** Kaposi's sarcoma. (From Callen JP, Greer KE, Hood AF, et al: *Color Atlas of Dermatology*. Philadelphia: W.B. Saunders, 1993, p. 220.)

toms are fever, night sweats, weight loss, and anorexia. There may also be burning, numbness, or itchy feet, as well as respiratory problems such as cough or **pleuritic** chest pain (intense pain under the margin of the ribs). Other symptoms may be opportunistic infections.

For women, the first symptom may be vaginal candiasis (fungal infection) that is resistant to topical antifungals but responds to Diflucan or Nizoral.

Skin lesions such as herpes zoster, warts, and **Kaposi's sarcoma** (a rare type of skin cancer) also appear, as shown in Figure 30–4.

HIV can be detected relatively simply. Skin scrapings, cultures, shave or puncture biopsies, and the enzyme-linked immunosorbent assay **(ELISA)** test are used. ELISA detects the presence or absence of an immune response to HIV infection. If the ELISA is positive, the Western blot test is performed for confirmation.

Those who share needles while injecting recreational drugs or who engage in unprotected sex are urged to have blood drawn for testing at least every 6 months.

western blot test

Complications of HIV Infection

Complications include not only opportunistic infections, but secondary cancer, dementia, and wasting.

Stages of HIV Infection

There are four stages to HIV infection:

1. Acute infection
2. Asymptomatic HIV
3. Symptomatic HIV
4. Advanced HIV.

Acute Infection

Acute infection begins about 1 to 3 weeks after infection. The virus undergoes massive replication. Signs and symptoms are fever, sore throat, malaise, headache, and symptoms typical of the flu.

Because these symptoms are common in many conditions and blood tests may not yet be positive for HIV, diagnosis is rare at this stage.

Asymptomatic HIV

After the acute infection subsides, the infected individual is asymptomatic for a period of time lasting from months to years. He or she may possibly experience lymphadenopathy and intermittent headache. The T-cell count drops during this time.

If HIV disease has been diagnosed and appropriate therapy has been started, this phase may last for as much as 10 to 12 years.

Symptomatic HIV

Symptomatic HIV can be broken up into two phases, early and late.

In the early phase, an individual becomes symptomatic, with a variety of symptoms and diseases affecting any and all of the body's organs. There may be fever and oral *Candida albicans,* as well as recurrent herpes simplex. The individual usually experiences night sweats, and chronic diarrhea leading to dehydration and cachexia.

In the late phase, the T-cell count drops below 200 cells per microliter. Common disorders and diseases found at this stage are gastric ulcer, esophagitis, colitis, hepatitis, pancreatitis, fungal infections, neurologic problems, nausea, vomiting, and dermatitis. There is severe weight loss, weakness, persistent diarrhea, and opportunistic infections such as *Pneumocystis carinii* and Kaposi's sarcoma. Figure 30–5 identifies many of the conditions that accompany AIDS.

Advanced HIV

In advanced HIV disease, the T-cell count falls below 50. More virulent and persistent infections occur, which are more resistant to treatment. Symptoms include seizures, confusion, urinary and fecal incontinence, blindness, and coma.

Once an individual is diagnosed with full-blown AIDS, his or her life expectancy is 3 to 5 years. AIDS is 100 percent fatal, with no cure. Vigorous treatment of opportunistic infections can prolong life, but at a certain point quality-of-life issues must be faced by the individual and his or her partner, family, and friends.

Legal Implications of HIV Testing

Testing for HIV is appropriate and should be encouraged to provide early care for those who test positive. An individual must give informed consent specifically for HIV testing. Although patient confidentiality must be respected, the patient must also be made aware of the limits to confidentiality. Exceptions to confidentiality may occur when others are being put at risk.

In most states, pretest counseling is required, so the person being tested is given all information about HIV, is advised about the reason for testing, understands that a positive test means that HIV is present but does not mean he or she has AIDS and that a negative test does not necessarily mean that he or she does not carry HIV.

Retesting is advised if an individual tests negative after a known exposure that occurred less than 12 weeks before the test. AIDS testing identifies antibodies to the virus; it does not identify the virus itself. The development of antibodies may take longer in some individuals than in others. It generally takes 3 to 6 months for antibodies to appear in the blood.

FOCUS ON
INSTRUCTION

TEACHING NEEDS RELATED TO HIV AND AIDS

Prevention of HIV Infection

Target Audience	Adolescents
	Patients with high-risk behaviors (including patients with multiple sex partners or partners, with unknown sexual history and patients who use IV drugs)
Teaching Topics	How HIV is transmitted
	High-risk behaviors
	Effective use of condoms

Signs and Symptoms of HIV Infection

Target Audience	Individuals who may have been exposed to HIV
Teaching Topics	Unexplained symptoms, especially if they last more than 2 to 3 weeks, such as:

    Persistent fatigue
    Fever and sweating at night
    Persistent swollen glands
    Dry cough, shortness of breath
    Difficulty breathing
    Diarrhea or bloody stools
    White patches in the mouth
    Weight loss of 10 to 15 pounds over 2 months
Encourage early testing

Managing Advanced HIV Disease

Target Audience	Patients with AIDS and their families
Teaching Topics	Avoiding infection

    Sterile dressing changes
    Avoiding direct contact with eggs, raw meat, and raw seafood
    Thorough cleaning of utensils and kitchen surfaces
Preventing transmission to others
    Good handwashing by patient and family
    Measures to avoid transmission
    Importance of avoiding reinfection with different strain of HIV
Managing pain
Maintaining adequate nutrition
    Small, frequent meals
    Avoiding liquids with meals
    Eating before taking medications that cause nausea
    Avoiding strong smells; sweet, fried, or fatty foods if they cause nausea and
      vomiting
    Eating slowly, resting in sitting position after meals
    Using soft toothbrush or gauze to clean mouth
    Avoiding spicy or irritating foods
Maintaining support systems, identifying community resources
Preparing for death by making will, planning funeral arrangements, preparing
    advance directives

#23

Treatments for AIDS and HIV Infection

Although there is no cure for AIDS and no vaccine against HIV, a number of drugs have been developed that slow the progress of HIV infection. These include antiviral agents such as zidovudine (Retrovir, formerly known as AZT), didanosine (Videx, ddL), and zalcitabine (Avid, ddC); protease inhibitors; and more recently interleukin 2 and peptide T.

Anti-HIV drugs are often used in combinations, or "cocktails." Some treatment is also done with antiviral

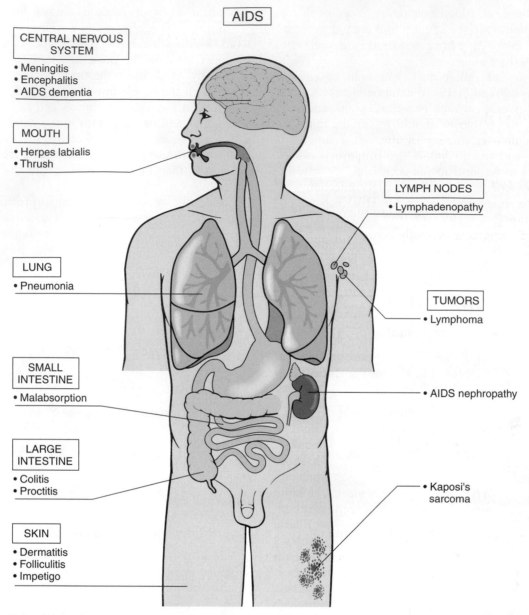

AIDS

CENTRAL NERVOUS SYSTEM
• Meningitis
• Encephalitis
• AIDS dementia

MOUTH
• Herpes labialis
• Thrush

LUNG
• Pneumonia

SMALL INTESTINE
• Malabsorption

LARGE INTESTINE
• Colitis
• Proctitis

SKIN
• Dermatitis
• Folliculitis
• Impetigo

LYMPH NODES
• Lymphadenopathy

TUMORS
• Lymphoma

• AIDS nephropathy

• Kaposi's sarcoma

➢ **Figure 30–5** Conditions that accompany AIDS. (Damjanov, I: *Pathology for the Health-Related Professions*. Philadelphia: W.B. Saunders, 1996.)

drugs used in series, often when the patient is asymptomatic.

The patient must be instructed to take the medications exactly as prescribed. Each patient requires individual monitoring to establish the most effective treatment regimen.

Despite treatment, most individuals will continue to experience opportunistic infections and other complications. HIV and AIDS patients must be watched closely to ensure that these opportunistic infections are not allowed to become overpowering before treatment.

It is considered unethical by the American Medical Association for a doctor to refuse to treat an HIV-positive individual or a person who refuses an HIV test.

Protection of Health Care Workers

Guidelines have been developed by the federal Centers for Disease Control and Prevention for protecting health care workers against exposure to HIV from body fluids. Because it is not always possible to identify an individual with HIV, these standard precautions should be used with all patients.

Gloves should be used when handling any body fluid. Masks, gowns, and goggles should be used when

there is a chance of blood splattering. Needles should be handled with extreme caution and should never be recapped or bent. Puncture-proof biohazard containers should be used for all sharps.

If an accidental spill occurs, it should be cleaned with a dilute solution (1:10) of chlorine bleach.

If a health care worker experiences an accidental needle stick, the employee should report the injury to his or her employer directly or through a supervisor immediately and should follow the employer's written requirements to respond to the accident. This may include prophylactic treatment against HIV infection with one or more drugs and testing for HIV, hepatitis B, and/or hepatitis C at regular intervals.

Hepatitis B virus is more easily contracted than HIV from a single exposure, but immunization with hepatitis B vaccine can eliminate this risk.

Medical assistants should always follow standard precautions, especially when working with sharps, to avoid needle-stick injury. Keep the rigid biohazard container close to the point of use. Never recap used needles by hand; use resheathing devices or the scoop technique if the needle must be recapped.

A resheathing device contains and holds the sheath (instead of holding the sheath in the hand). To use the scoop technique, the medical assistant places the sheath on a table *without* holding it and inserts the needle into the sheath, then raises the needle with the sheath protecting it.

Employers are also encouraged to provide safety devices such as syringes that retract or cover the needle after use or needles that blunt before removal from the patient. Medical assistants should take the time to learn to use these devices comfortably.

STUDENT STUDY PLAN

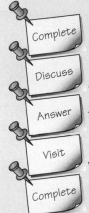

To reinforce your understanding of the material in this chapter . . .

Complete *Complete* the **Review & Recall** questions.

Discuss *Discuss* the situation in **If You Were the Medical Assistant** with your classmates and answer the questions.

Answer *Answer* the **Critical Thinking Questions** and discuss them with your classmates.

Visit *Visit* suggested **Web sites** and search for additional Web sites using the **Keywords for Internet Searches.**

Complete *Complete* the exercises in chapter 30 of the **Student Mastery Manual.**

REVIEW & RECALL

1. What are some ways a medical assistant can help coordinate care for a patient with a chronic and/or terminal illness?

2. Describe the stages of the grieving process, according to Elisabeth Kübler-Ross.

3. What are some of the physical and psychological manifestations of acute grief?

4. Describe how guidelines for use of experimental procedures developed.

5. How can scarcity of medical resources affect treatment of the terminally ill?

6. Identify four types of advance directives that can be used by patients with chronic illness or a disease that may result in death.

7. How are benign neoplasms different from malignant neoplasms in respect to shape, cell type, tendency to invade the surrounding tissue, and tendency to spread (metastasize)?

8. Describe two methods of classifying tumors.

9. Describe risk factors for cancer.

10. List some common tests used to diagnose cancer.

11. Describe the three general types of cancer treatment. How can they work together?

12. List the four stages of HIV infection.

13. What signs and symptoms are seen when a person is HIV positive? When a person is developing full-blown AIDS?

14. What process is required before a person can be tested for AIDS?

15. What types of treatment are used for AIDS? How effective is treatment?

16. Give specific examples of things the medical assistant should do to prevent infection with HIV and to prevent the transmission of the HIV virus to others.

IF YOU WERE THE MEDICAL ASSISTANT

As described in the chapter, the stages most people go through in response to grief or loss are denial, anger, bargaining, depression, and acceptance. Imagine that you are working in a doctor's office and patients or family members make the following statements.

For each statement, identify the stage of grief and formulate a response that demonstrates acceptance and empathy. If a family member is speaking, determine if the family member and the patient are at the same stage of grief.

1. Mr. Wilding, a 57-year-old man with complications from cancer of the pancreas, tells you: "I am following a special diet that my neighbor told me about. I want to hang on until June because my daughter is getting married."

2. A patient says: "Dr. Hughes suggested that I see an oncologist to discuss chemotherapy. I don't see why I need to do that. It was just a little mole that was removed from my arm. I'm tempted to see another doctor."

3. An elderly woman with metastatic cancer says: "I've had a good life. Whatever happens, I've made my peace with God. I even look forward to being with my husband. I only hope my pain doesn't get too bad."

4. A woman whose husband has inoperable lung cancer says: "I don't know what to do for him. He just sits in a chair all day. He won't do anything to pass the time. He doesn't even watch his favorite TV shows. I end up almost yelling at him, and then I wish I hadn't said anything. I cook things he used to like and he won't eat them. Why won't he just try to make the most of the time he has left? Sometimes I just want to shake him."

 CRITICAL THINKING QUESTIONS

1. Patients with chronic diseases like cancer may need narcotics to control their pain. But sometimes patients are reluctant to take narcotics, or family members are reluctant to give them increasing doses out of fear that they will become addicted to them. Research theories of pain relief, and discuss how pain can be effectively managed. Is there a difference in managing pain for patients with terminal illness from pain management for patients who have pain from an acute condition? What can you say to a patient or family member who hesitates to use narcotic analgesics?

2. How do office staff respond when a patient dies? Discuss issues related to feelings and responses of health care professionals who have cared for such a patient.

3. Discuss with your classmates different ways that families treat young children when a parent or grandparent has a poor prognosis. What are some reactions to questions children ask? How much do you think a child should be told when a parent or grandparent is dying? What can happen if the child is not included in discussions about the illness?

4. Discuss your feelings about taking care of patients with AIDS. How do health care professionals manage the fear of infection? Would you feel comfortable drawing blood from or giving an injection to a patient who you know has AIDS? How can you establish a rapport if it is necessary to wear a gown, mask, gloves, and eye protection because of a patient's respiratory and/or skin complications?

 EXPLORE THE WEB

INTERNET WEB SITES

National Institutes of Health
www.nih.gov

National Cancer Institute
www.nci.nih.gov

DeathNet
www.rights.org/deathnet

American Cancer Society
www.cancer.org

Centers for Disease Control and Prevention (CDC)
www.cdc.gov

KEYWORDS FOR INTERNET SEARCHES

advance directive
   AIDS
   cancer
   hospice
   living will

Emergency Care

Instructional Objectives

After completing this chapter, you will be able to do the following:

1. Define and spell the vocabulary words.
2. Describe the purpose of the Emergency Medical Services system and how to activate it.
3. Correlate equipment, supplies, and medications commonly found in a first aid kit and in an emergency box or crash cart to common uses in an emergency.
4. Describe how to survey the scene in an emergency.
5. Compare the components of the primary survey to the secondary survey when dealing with an unconscious individual.
6. Describe how a rescuer assists a person with an obstructed airway.
7. Describe how to perform rescue breathing and cardiopulmonary resuscitation (CPR).
8. Identify safety measures and procedures to ensure proper use of oxygen in the medical office.
9. List various types of allergic reactions, from least to most severe.
10. Describe the proper treatment of a patient experiencing an anaphylactic reaction (anaphylactic shock).
11. Correlate emergency care of burns to the burns' causes and/or classifications.
12. Describe appropriate measures for controlling capillary, venous, and arterial bleeding.
13. Describe the causes and treatments of the six types of shock.
14. Compare and contrast the signs and symptoms, severity, and emergency treatment of angina pectoris and myocardial infarction.
15. Describe the cause, signs and symptoms, and emergency care of diabetic emergencies.
16. Describe how to splint an extremity to prevent movement during transport to an emergency room.
17. Identify the emergency care for a person experiencing a seizure.
18. Describe the causes, signs and symptoms, and emergency care of a person experiencing a cerebrovascular accident (CVA).
19. List four types of head injury.
20. Describe the emergency treatment for ingested, inhaled, and absorbed poisons.

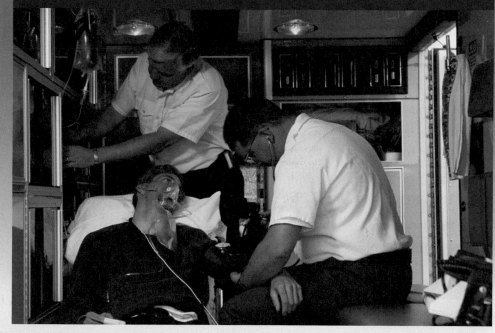

21. Describe poisonous spiders and snakes in the United States, and identify the appropriate care of victims of their bites.
22. Identify the proper emergency care of animal bites and open wounds.
23. Differentiate between the care of a victim exposed to excessive heat and the care of a victim exposed to excessive cold.
24. Describe how foreign bodies are removed from the eye, ear, and skin.

CMA/RMA CERTIFICATION
Content and Competencies

- Obtain CPR certification and first aid training
- Perform within ethical and legal boundaries

- Apply pharmacology principles to prepare and administer oral and parenteral medications

Performance Objectives

After completing this chapter, you will be able to do the following:

1. Check the contents of the emergency box or crash cart (Procedure 31–1).
2. Assist a patient who is choking (Procedure 31–2).
3. Administer oxygen by nasal cannula (Procedure 31–3).
4. Care for a patient with one or more burns (Procedure 31–4).
5. Control a patient's bleeding (Procedure 31–5).
6. Apply a splint (Procedure 31–6).
7. Clean a minor wound (Procedure 31–7).

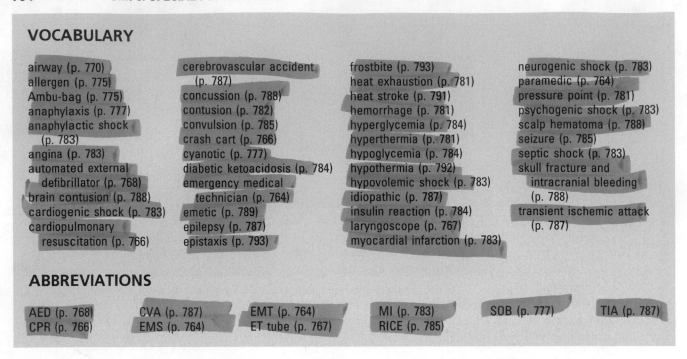

VOCABULARY

airway (p. 770)
allergen (p. 775)
Ambu-bag (p. 775)
anaphylaxis (p. 777)
anaphylactic shock
  (p. 783)
angina (p. 783)
automated external
  defibrillator (p. 768)
brain contusion (p. 788)
cardiogenic shock (p. 783)
cardiopulmonary
  resuscitation (p. 766)

cerebrovascular accident
  (p. 787)
concussion (p. 788)
contusion (p. 782)
convulsion (p. 785)
crash cart (p. 766)
cyanotic (p. 777)
diabetic ketoacidosis (p. 784)
emergency medical
  technician (p. 764)
emetic (p. 789)
epilepsy (p. 787)
epistaxis (p. 793)

frostbite (p. 793)
heat exhaustion (p. 781)
heat stroke (p. 791)
hemorrhage (p. 781)
hyperglycemia (p. 784)
hyperthermia (p. 781)
hypoglycemia (p. 784)
hypothermia (p. 792)
hypovolemic shock (p. 783)
idiopathic (p. 787)
insulin reaction (p. 784)
laryngoscope (p. 767)
myocardial infarction (p. 783)

neurogenic shock (p. 783)
paramedic (p. 764)
pressure point (p. 781)
psychogenic shock (p. 783)
scalp hematoma (p. 788)
seizure (p. 785)
septic shock (p. 783)
skull fracture and
  intracranial bleeding
  (p. 788)
transient ischemic attack
  (p. 787)

ABBREVIATIONS

AED (p. 768)   CVA (p. 787)   EMT (p. 764)   MI (p. 783)   SOB (p. 777)   TIA (p. 787)
CPR (p. 766)   EMS (p. 764)   ET tube (p. 767)   RICE (p. 785)

Some 70 million Americans are treated in hospital emergency rooms each year. One in three Americans suffers a nonfatal injury each year, and more than 150,000 people die from trauma each year. Trauma is the fourth leading cause of death in the United States and the leading cause of death in children under 14. More than 400,000 Americans are permanently disabled each year from injury and trauma. Home accidents cause many injuries that require hospitalization or care in a doctor's office. More than 500,000 children each year are hospitalized because of an accident.

Clearly, accidents and other emergencies happen with such frequency that medical assistants will deal with them on a regular basis. Medical assistants are also instrumental in teaching a medical practice's patients about how to avoid accidents and how to deal with them when they occur.

Medical assistants should teach their practice's patients the rudiments of first aid, and show them how to sustain life in a life-threatening situation. They should also teach their patients about home safety, and about how the patient should respond to an emergency.

Emergencies also occur in the medical office. When such an emergency occurs, a doctor provides care and directs care given by other office personnel, including medical assistants. If an emergency occurs when no doctor is present, the medical assistant must be able to recognize an emergency and know how to call an ambulance or contact a doctor; he or she must also provide emergency care, such as the control of bleeding or beginning cardiopulmonary resuscitation, and try to prevent further injury until Emergency Medical Services personnel arrive to transport the person to an emergency room.

In the medical office, the medical assistant must also be able to deal with incoming phone calls regarding emergencies. He or she must be able to assess the call and advise patients if no doctor or other licensed caregiver is in the office when the call comes in. This is covered in detail in chapter 9.

The medical assistant should also know about the applicable Good Samaritan laws for the state in which he or she is working. These laws release healing professionals who assist in an emergency from liability, provided they act with reasonable prudence.

EMERGENCY MEDICAL SERVICES SYSTEM

Most cities and towns today have 911 capabilities together with a well-trained staff of **emergency medical technicians (EMTs)** who have the ability to provide life support and transport to the nearest hospital. **EMTs** are professionally trained providers of pre-hospital emergency care; they provide this care both at the scene of the accident or illness and during transport to the hospital. Many members of local police and firefighting forces are trained as EMTs.

EMTs are part of the Emergency Medical Services **(EMS)** system, a community resource of equipment and personnel trained to care for emergencies. Often, the first hour following an emergency is the most important.

In addition to EMTs, the EMS includes **paramedics,** who are trained in advanced life-support techniques such as advanced airway maintenance, placing an intravenous line and maintaining IV fluids, cardiac monitoring and interpretation, and cardiac defibrillation. Like

FOCUS ON
LAW: GOOD SAMARITAN LAWS

Most states have one or more laws called Good Samaritan laws, which protect health care personnel who provide emergency care at the scene of an accident from civil liability. These laws usually protect doctors and nurses; sometimes they also protect those certified to perform CPR, such as ski patrol members and school volunteers, depending on the state and the particular circumstances of the emergency.

The purpose of Good Samaritan laws is to encourage health professionals to stop and give care at the scene of an accident without fear of being sued for any adverse outcome the injury victim might suffer. In France, all people are obliged to help any accident victim they come upon; but in the United States, doctors, nurses, and private citizens are not required to give assistance.

A person who gives care at the scene of an accident in good faith is protected from legal liability unless his or her actions reflect gross negligence or willful misconduct. Lack of equipment and facilities, combined with unsterile conditions, may make it impossible to provide the same level of care as that available in an emergency room or a medical office. In addition, the injured person's condition may require intervention that goes beyond the usual daily responsibilities of the person who is trying to assist.

The medical assistant is not covered in most states by a specific Good Samaritan law, but some states do have a statute (law) relating to people who perform CPR at the scene of an emergency. Medical assistants who retain current CPR certification should not hesitate to perform CPR if necessary.

It is recommended that all health professionals carry a respirator (in a purse or in their cars) to protect themselves if they need to give life support to an accident victim.

EMTs, paramedics may be members of the local fire department; or they may be part of a private ambulance service that works under contract to the municipality.

Activating the 911 system is an important step for a medical assistant to take in an emergency. Usually, the call is taken by a dispatcher who relays the call to the EMS. Dispatchers are trained to handle emergencies. The dispatcher asks a series of questions concerning the emergency and listens to the caller's answers; then he or she determines what help is needed and sends the appropriate personnel and equipment. The same dispatcher routes calls to police, fire, and emergency medical personnel. The dispatcher may also relay information from the emergency medical personnel to the caller about how to maintain the situation until professional assistance arrives.

If an emergency occurs in the medical office and a medical assistant calls 911, he or she needs to provide the dispatcher with as much detail as possible to ensure prompt and appropriate care. The box "If You Call an Ambulance. . . " lists information to give to an emergency dispatcher. Also, while waiting for the emergency personnel to arrive, the medical assistant must maintain proper infection control, using personal protective equipment (PPE) as necessary.

During an emergency, the office staff should stay calm, act in a confident and organized manner, and reassure the patient. But staff members must never say that "everything will be all right."

PREPARATIONS FOR AN EMERGENCY IN THE MEDICAL OFFICE

Policies and Procedures

The office procedure manual should supply guidelines for dealing with an emergency. Responsibilities for dealing with an emergency should be assigned to each office staff member.

If You Call An Ambulance . . . Be Prepared with the Following Information . . .

1. Exact location of the victim(s)
   street name and house number
   floor and room number (if applicable)
2. Number of victims involved
3. Condition of the victim(s)
   - complaints
   - symptoms
   - progression of symptoms
4. Name of caller, relationship to the victim(s)
5. Care that has already been given

Staff Training

The emergency plan described in the office procedure manual should be practiced to ensure smooth handling of emergency situations. In addition, all members of the office staff should be current in **cardiopulmonary resuscitation (CPR)**, which is a technique used to manually pump the heart of an individual whose heart has stopped.

Incident Reports

As with any medical incident, documentation of the emergency in the office is very important. An incident report should be filed as soon as possible, with a complete description of the emergency situation and how it was handled. Such a report is a part of the patient record and, as such, is a legal document. It must be complete and accurate.

A printed form should be available for use in such an instance. This form should be approved by the practice's liability insurance carrier.

It is impossible to keep patients from becoming suddenly ill in the office—and possibly needing to be treated as an emergency. But it is possible to prevent many office accidents that cause injuries. The office should have no scatter rugs that a patient could trip over. Whenever a floor is mopped to clean up a spill, the area should be marked with "wet floor" signs. All medications should be stored away from patients in a locked cabinet. All spills should be wiped up immediately, and all dropped objects should be picked up immediately.

EMERGENCY EQUIPMENT

Every office should have a first aid kit for treatment of minor injuries, as well as an emergency box or crash cart for treating any person who goes into cardiac or respiratory arrest.

First Aid Kit

A first aid kit holds supplies for dealing with minor injuries. Such supplies include adhesive bandages (e.g. Band-Aids), tape and gauze, prepackaged antibacterial solutions to clean a cut, a chemical ice pack, and possibly a pressure bandage. No medicines are kept in a first aid kit. First aid kits should be available in all work areas of public buildings, including medical offices.

Emergency Box/Crash Cart

Unlike a first aid kit, an emergency box or **crash cart** is found in medical settings only. The crash cart gets its name from the slang term describing a person

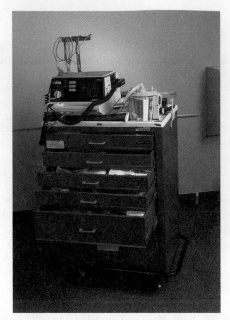

➤ Figure 31–1 Many medical offices and clinics have a crash cart for use in emergencies.

who has gone into cardiac or respiratory arrest as "crashing." An emergency box in a medical office may be a large tool or tackle box, or it may be a small tool cart like the one found in an auto repair shop. Figure 31–1 shows a crash cart.

The box or cart should contain the basic supplies, drugs, and emergency equipment necessary to sustain life. Most carts contain first aid supplies for minor injuries as well as more sophisticated life-saving equipment.

Every medical assistant should be familiar with the materials in the emergency box in the office where he or she works. He or she should also know where the box is. Office policy should mandate that no supplies be removed from the cart for other purposes, as "borrowing" from the emergency supplies puts the office at risk of not having the necessary supplies in the event of an emergency.

In addition, the supplies in the box must be checked regularly for completeness and expiration dates.

Medications Commonly Used for Emergencies

Medications found on the crash cart vary from one medical specialty to another, and each crash cart should have all medications necessary for the types of emergencies a particular office is most likely to encounter. But regardless of specialty, all crash carts should have all the medications necessary for emergencies that might occur in any medical office. See the boxes "Medications That Should Be in Every Emergency Box/Crash Cart" and "Emergency Supplies."

Medications That Should Be in Every Emergency Box/Crash Cart

1. Epinephrine (Adrenalin): A vasoconstrictor used to improve circulation; also for use in coronary conditions or as a bronchodilator to relieve respiratory distress. Crash carts often contain preloaded syringes for intracardiac administration.
2. Atropine: May be used to decrease body secretions while increasing respiratory and heart rates. Also a smooth muscle relaxer, it relieves hypermotility of the intestinal tract and gastrointestinal cramps.
3. Digoxin (Lanoxin): A cardiotonic with a fairly rapid action, used for congestive heart failure
4. Xylocaine (Lidocaine 0.5 percent or 1.0 percent): Used as a local anesthetic. Lidocaine in various strengths is also given intravenously or intramuscularly to prevent cardiac arrhythmia. Crash carts often contain preloaded syringes for use in a cardiac emergency.
5. Syrup of ipecac: An emetic
6. Apomorphine hydrochloride: A rapid-acting emetic
7. Isoproterenol (Isuprel, Medihaler-Iso, and other brands): An antispasmodic for bronchospasm; also a cardiac stimulant. Should be kept in both injectable and inhalable forms.
8. Diphenhydramine hydrochloride (Benadryl): An antihistamine to relieve the effects of histamines, or for mild to severe allergic reactions
9. Metaraminol (Aramine): For shock
10. Amobarbital sodium (Amytal): A sedative for anxiety; also given to relieve convulsions
11. Diazepam (Valium): A sedative and anticonvulsant
12. Activated charcoal: Binds with some poisons to prevent absorption
13. Furosemide (Lasix): Diuretic for congestive heart failure
14. Methylprednisolone or prednisone: Corticosteroids used for allergic reactions and for respiratory symptoms
15. Nitroglycerin tabs: Vasodilator
16. Dilantin: Anticonvulsant
17. Glucagon, orange juice, glucose paste, sugar packets, Dextrose 50 percent: Used for hypoglycemic reactions
18. Insulin: To reduce elevated blood sugar
19. IV dextrose in saline or water, as well as lactated Ringer's solution: For intravenous hydration
20. Sodium bicarbonate: Injectable, used to restore acid/base balance in cardiac arrest
21. Sterile saline and sterile water: For injection
22. Aromatic spirits of ammonia: To revive after fainting

Emergency Supplies

First Aid Supplies

1. Adhesive tape
2. Hot and cold packs
3. Slings, triangle bandage, tourniquets
4. Sterile and unsterile dressings in various sizes
5. Alcohol wipes
6. Bandages, gauze, bandage scissors
7. Tongue blades
8. Personal protective equipment such as gloves and goggles
9. Splints
10. Elastic bandages and gauze bandages
11. Stethoscope
12. Penlight

Additional Supplies Usually Found on a Crash Cart

1. Airways (plastic devices to maintain an open airway) in various sizes
2. Manual resuscitator (Ambu-bag)
3. Endotracheal tubes (**ET tubes**) in various sizes
4. **Laryngoscope** (instrument to view the larynx during intubation)
5. Oxygen and supplies for administering it (This equipment is all part of the setup for maintaining an airway so a patient can breathe. Figure 31–2 shows this equipment for emergency airway management.)
6. Syringes and needles in various sizes
7. Medications in cartridges, with holders for the cartridges
8. Sphygmomanometer
9. IV equipment, including bags, tubing, tourniquets, boards, pole, butterfly needles, and/or intracaths to start an IV
10. A defibrillator and/or cardiac monitor is usually kept on top of the crash cart.
11. Suction catheters and suction equipment

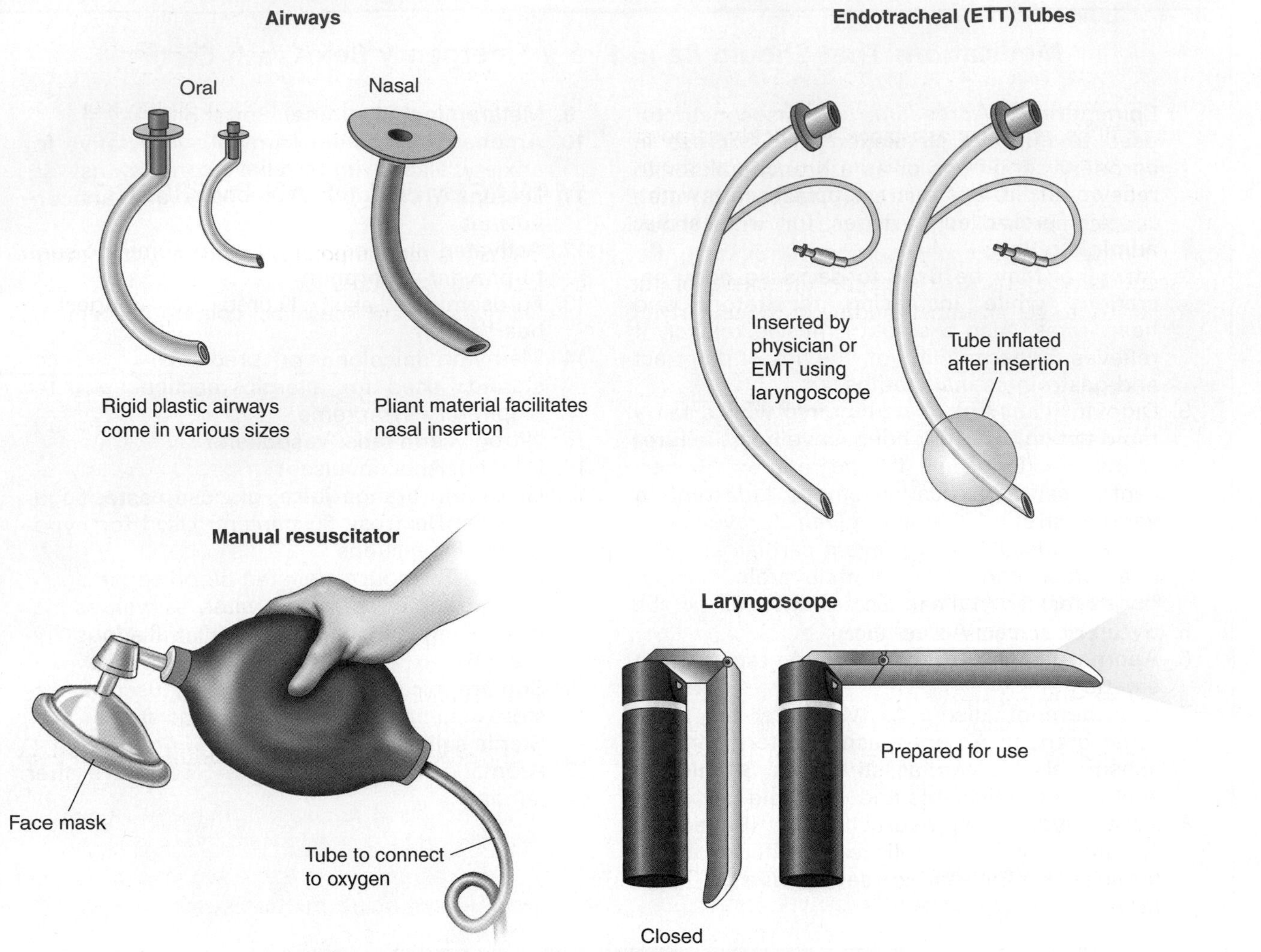

Airways

Oral   Nasal

Endotracheal (ETT) Tubes

Inserted by
physician or
EMT using
laryngoscope

Tube inflated
after insertion

Rigid plastic airways
come in various sizes

Pliant material facilitates
nasal insertion

Manual resuscitator

Face mask

Tube to connect
to oxygen

Laryngoscope

Prepared for use

Closed

> **Figure 31–2** Equipment for emergency airway management.

Checking the Contents of the Emergency Box/Crash Cart

Each crash cart should have a list of the medications and supplies that are supposed to be on it. One person should be assigned to make sure the cart is always ready and available for use in an emergency.

The medications and supplies on the cart should be checked regularly against the list. All used or expired medications and supplies should be replaced. Be sure the sterile items have not been opened and contaminated. Check equipment to make sure it is in working order. See Procedure 31–1.

Use of Automated External Defibrillator

Most individuals who go into sudden cardiac arrest are in ventricular fibrillation (VF or Vfib), discussed in detail in chapter 18. If defibrillation is provided in the

first 5 minutes after onset of sudden cardiac arrest, chances are about 50:50 that the individual's life can be saved. After 10 minutes, virtually no chance of resuscitating the individual remains.

Automated external defibrillators (AEDs) are small, battery-powered defibrillators that can be used by individuals trained in CPR for emergencies. The American Heart Association, in an effort to promote the most rapid defibrillation possible of individuals who suffer sudden cardiac arrest, is promoting a program of what it calls Public Access Defibrillation (PAD).

Under PAD programs, AEDs are being placed with "nontraditional" users, such as police and firefighters, who often respond to medical emergencies and are often trained as "first responders" but not as EMTs. AEDs are also being placed in worksites, public gathering spaces, and even in the homes of individuals at high risk of sudden cardiac arrest.

FIRST RESPONSE TO AN EMERGENCY

In the event of an emergency, the first medical personnel to arrive should survey the scene, put on appropriate PPEs, and give assistance as quickly as possible. The person responding to an emergency should quickly determine if it is safe to approach the victim. For example, fire and exposed electrical wires should be responded to before placing yourself in danger. If the scene is safe, try to determine the cause of the injury, or try to get an understanding of the underlying medical condition of the ill person. You may be able to get important information from the patient, from a person who has accompanied the patient to the doctor's office, or from another person on the scene.

MANAGEMENT OF AN EMERGENCY

First aid is the temporary, immediate care given to a person who is injured or becomes suddenly ill. The person giving care must be able to recognize life-

---

PROCEDURE 31-1

Checking Contents of Emergency Box/Crash Cart

Performance Objective: The student will be able to check the contents of an emergency box or crash cart for completeness.
Supplies and Equipment: Crash cart or emergency box, inventory control sheet, disposable sealing or locking mechanism.

Procedure Steps

1 Using an inventory control sheet, open the crash cart and check each drawer (or all the contents of an emergency box) to make sure that each item is present. This is usually done monthly or as soon as possible after a crash cart has been used for an emergency.

2. After identifying each item, check the expiration date. Replace expired items.

3. Record findings and check off the inventory control sheet.

4. Contents should include, but not be limited to, the following first aid/emergency supplies:
   a. airways—various sizes
   b. manual resuscitator, such as an Ambu-bag
   c. pocket mask, oxygen mask
   d. IV supplies—tubing, needles, fluids
   e. suction tubing
   f. alcohol wipes
   g. sterile gauze—2 × 2, 4 × 4
   h. bandaging materials, including dressings
   i. tape—various types
   j. penlight or flashlight with spare batteries
   k. hot and cold packs
   l. blood pressure cuff and stethoscope
   m. gloves—nonsterile and sterile
   n. diabetic gel or candy
   o. tourniquet or constricting band
   p. obstetric delivery instruments—bulb syringe, umbilical cord clamp, scissors
   q. sterile water
   r. activated charcoal
   s. diphenhydramine (Benadryl)
   t. epinephrine
   u. nitroglycerin tablets
   v. ammonia ampules
   w. syrup of ipecac
   x. Xylocaine, lidocaine
   y. needles and syringes—various sizes

5. Secure the crash cart using an easily opened disposable locking mechanism to prevent casual use of supplies. If supplies are used from an emergency box, replace immediately.
   Rationale: If supplies are used and not replaced, they will not be available in an emergency.

6. Keep cart in easy-to-access area.
   Rationale: Some crash carts end up in a tight area or one that is hard to access; then when an emergency arises, the cart is not readily available.

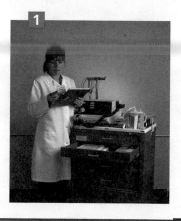

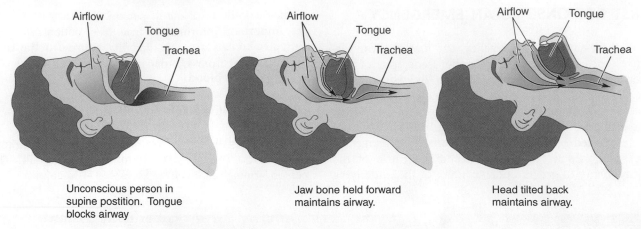

Unconscious person in supine postition. Tongue blocks airway

Jaw bone held forward maintains airway.

Head tilted back maintains airway.

➤ **Figure 31–3** Opening a blocked airway in an unconscious patient.

threatening situations and take effective actions to keep the person alive and in the best possible condition.

An individual providing first aid should know what *not* to do as well as what to do. He or she should know how to care for a life-threatening situation; how to minimize further injury and complications; how to make the injured person as comfortable as possible, and how to help him or her conserve energy, how to minimize infection; and how to assist in transporting an injured person to a medical facility for further care if necessary.

Patient Assessment

The medical assistant should assess the emergency to see if there is a life-threatening condition. This primary assessment should take about 5 seconds. Whenever possible, the rescuer should put on gloves before attempting to assess an unconscious patient.

Primary Survey: Airway, Breathing, Circulation

The first thing to check for is responsiveness. Ask "Are you okay?" Be careful not to jar or move the person. The responsive person is one who has a heartbeat, is conscious, and is breathing. If a person can speak, he or she is breathing and has circulation.

If the person is unresponsive, further evaluation of pulse and breathing is necessary.

Airway

The three issues to concentrate on are the ABC of the primary response—airway, breathing, circulation.

When unconscious, a person's tongue may relax and obstruct the **airway**—the route of passage of air into the lungs. If not corrected, this obstruction can lead to

cardiac arrest and death. Getting the tongue out of the airway is called establishing an airway, as shown in Figure 31–3.

To establish an airway, place one hand on the patient's forehead and the other under the patient's chin. Gently lift the jaw while pushing the head back, as shown in Figure 31–4. If there is any chance that a neck injury has occurred, open the airway by grasping both sides of the jaw and pushing the jaw forward.

Breathing

The rescuer should carefully examine for ABC by looking, feeling, and listening, as shown in Figure 31–5.

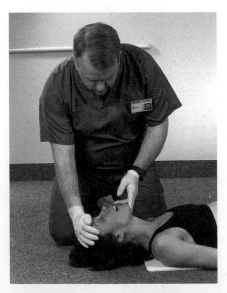

➤ **Figure 31–4** Establishing an airway by the head-tilt, chin-lift method.

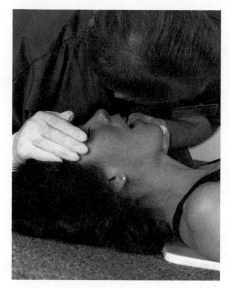

➢ **Figure 31–5** Look, listen, and feel for breathing.

Look at the rise and fall of the chest as the person breathes.

Feel for a pulse and the movement of air as the person breathes.

Listen for air moving through the nose and mouth.

If the individual is not breathing, the airway should be cleared and rescue breathing begun. If the heart is not beating, blood is not circulating to the body's tissues. In that case, irreversible brain damage may occur after 4 to 6 minutes; death may occur in 10 minutes.

Circulation

To assess circulation in an adult feel the carotid artery; in an infant or young child, check the brachial artery (see Figure 31–6).

If there is no circulation, start CPR immediately.

Remember, the first step in supplying oxygen is to establish an open airway. The second step is to begin supplying oxygen to the lungs for circulation of oxygenated blood.

After breathing and circulation have been established, the person should be assessed for trauma and severe bleeding. Severe bleeding is bleeding that is uncontrollable, that spurts rather than oozes (which signifies that an artery has been damaged). Bleeding must be controlled to prevent shock and death.

Secondary Survey: Other Body Systems

After making sure the individual is breathing and not bleeding excessively, the secondary assessment of other body systems can take place. A full assessment should be performed by moving down the body from superior to inferior, and from medial to lateral.

The individual should be assessed for possible damage to the spine. He or she should not be moved until potential damage has been assessed. The individual's level of consciousness also needs to be established. An individual's level of consciousness can be described in one of four universally recognized ways:

1. Awake and alert
2. Responds to voice
3. Responds only to pain
4. Unresponsive or unconscious.

If the individual is fully conscious, is he or she oriented and aware of the surroundings? The three questions typically asked to establish orientation are:

"What is your name?"
"What day is today?"
"Who is the president of the United States?"

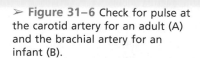

➢ **Figure 31–6** Check for pulse at the carotid artery for an adult (A) and the brachial artery for an infant (B).

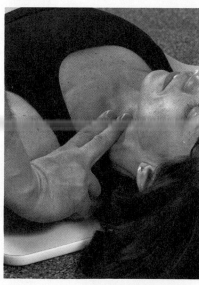

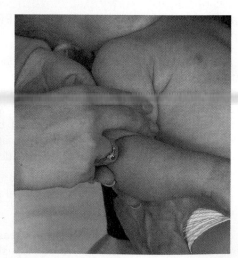

A

B

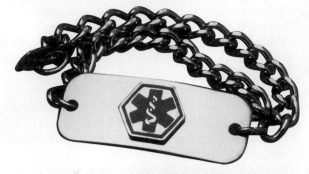

> **Figure 31–7** It is recommended that patients with diseases or severe allergies wear a bracelet identifying their medical condition.

It is important to establish if the individual has voluntary movement of arms and legs, and if he or she has any sensation of pain or pressure. It is also important to see if there is paralysis or weakness on one side, or if the individual's speech is slurred. These are signs of a cerebrovascular hemmorhage (stroke).

Potential fractures are assessed by seeing if any limb is out of its proper anatomic position. Extremities should be palpated for bruises, depressions, and other irregularities.

Vital signs should be taken as soon as possible, with variations from normal noted to all concerned. Skin temperature should be assessed for signs of vasoconstriction or vasodilation.

Look for medical alert necklaces or bracelets that identify a particular medical condition or medications to which the individual is allergic. Figure 31–7 shows a Medic-Alert bracelet, one of many different brands of medical alert jewelry.

In addition to questioning the injured or ill individual, it is important to get as much information as possible from others at the scene who may have information about the injured or ill person.

Cardiopulmonary Resuscitation (CPR), Rescue Breathing, and Blocked Airway

The information that follows summarizes emergency care. But health professionals should become certified in CPR and first aid, maintaining their certification by taking courses from the American Red Cross or the American Heart Association. (Because all health professionals should maintain current certification, CPR is only described, and procedures are not included in this book.)

Choking

Choking is a serious problem. It is easily recognizable: The stricken individual cannot speak or breathe. Choking is one of the most common medical emergen-

cies. With adults, choking most often occurs when food becomes lodged in the trachea; in children non-food objects such as toy parts, buttons, coins, and candy can also be the cause of choking. Also, pieces of food such as a hot dog or slices of raw carrot are more likely to cause choking in children than in adults.

If a person is coughing forcefully in an effort to dislodge the object in the trachea, the medical assistant should not do anything. Being able to cough means that the airway is only partially obstructed. In that case, the medical assistant should observe the individual: He or she may be able to dislodge the object; or the object may become more tightly lodged, so that the individual becomes unable to speak or breathe.

The universal sign for choking is a hand held up to the throat. If the person choking signals that he or she cannot breathe, the Heimlich maneuver should be attempted.

To perform the Heimlich maneuver, stand behind the choking person. Make a fist with one hand and place that side of your body against the person's abdomen, below the ribs. Reach around the person and grab the fist with the other hand; the two hands should now be in front of the person. Using both hands, compress the abdomen rapidly. Rapid, jerky motions, aimed at the person's spine about 6 inches above the hands, are most effective; this uses pressure from the person's own lungs to push the blockage out of the trachea. Procedure 31–2 describes how to assist the choking patient.

Rescue breathing provides an individual with oxygen and allows the removal of carbon dioxide from the lungs. Rescue breathing is used to keep an individual alive until more advanced techniques can be instituted.

Rescue breathing is used for respiratory arrest when there is no or minimal movement in the chest. If available, a respirator should be used to protect the rescuer from touching the individual's mucous membranes.

Figure 31–8 shows a respirator used in rescue breathing.

If rescue breathing is attempted and air cannot be blown into the individual's lungs, the airway is said to be blocked or obstructed. Before rescue breathing can be resumed, the obstruction must be cleared. Training to breathe for a patient and to clear a blocked airway of an unconscious patient is included in CPR courses for certification.

CPR is a method of providing manual pumping of a heart to bring about blood circulation. CPR combines chest compressions with rescue breathing to provide oxygen to body tissues, in order to sustain the function of cells within the body. Figure 31–9 shows the proper position for chest compressions for an adult and an infant.

Brain cells will die within 4 to 6 minutes without oxygen. Although CPR delivers only about one-third of the necessary oxygen to the brain and cannot sustain

PROCEDURE 31-2

Assisting the Choking Victim

Performance Objective: The student will be able to assist a choking patient.
Supplies and Equipment: None.

Procedure Steps

1. Identify that patient is choking by watching for universal sign—clutching the neck and not getting air exchange.

2. Place the thumb side of your fist against the patient's middle abdomen, just above umbilicus.

3. Grasp your fist with opposite hand and provide quick, upward thrusts on patient's abdomen.

4. Continue thrusts until the object is dislodged or until the patient loses consciousness.
   Rationale: Should the patient lose consciousness, assist him or her to the floor or ground and continue choking assistance by giving five abdominal thrusts and performing a tongue-jaw lift. Sweep mouth for object and attempt to give two breaths. Continue with abdominal thrusts and breaths until help arrives or object is dislodged.

5. Assist patient to a sitting position once object is dislodged and patient is breathing freely, or position the patient on his or her side if unconscious.

6. Wash your hands.

7. If this incident happened in the medical office, record a description of the event in the patient's medical record. If the choking victim was not a patient, complete an incident report.
   Rationale: Any unusual incident that threatens the health or safety of an individual in a medical office should be documented in case questions arise at a later date.

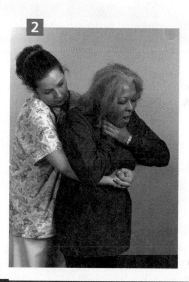

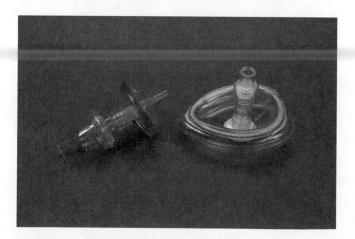

life indefinitely, it can keep brain cells from dying in the first few critical minutes after cardiac arrest.

Also, medical professionals need to remember that CPR's success is dependent on the underlying amount of damage or disease to the heart muscle, and that CPR is often unsuccessful. CPR failure should not be seen as personal failure on the part of the individual performing the CPR.

➤ **Figure 31-8** Equipment to protect rescuer from contact with mucous membranes of a victim during artificial respiration.

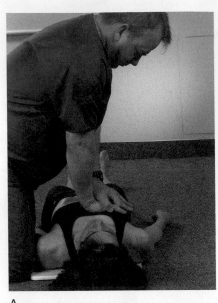

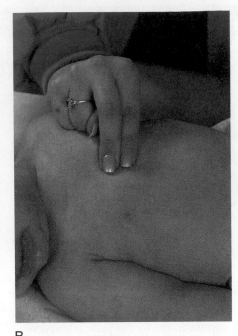

A   B

➤ **Figure 31–9** Proper position for chest compressions during CPR for an adult (A) and an infant (B).

Administering Oxygen

Oxygen is a colorless, odorless gas that comprises about 21 percent of the air at the earth's surface at sea level. At higher altitudes, there is less oxygen in the air.

Oxygen for medical use comes in green steel cylinders, as shown in Figure 31–10. No other medical product comes in green cylinders; thus oxygen is immediately recognizable to medical personnel. An oxygen tank should always be secured in the upright position, with the fittings on the top. Fittings, hoses, regulators, and cylinders should be checked regularly to ensure that oxygen is available in an emergency.

No smoking should be allowed in any area where oxygen is in use. Although oxygen itself does not burn, it supports combustion; in the presence of oxygen, a spark can cause any flammable material to burst into flame. When the oxygen is not in use, the cylinder's valves should be closed whether the tank is full, partially full, or empty.

A variety of systems are available to deliver oxygen from the tank to an individual in need of oxygen. The office staff should be trained in how to use each system, and they should know where the office's oxygen supply is kept. The two most common oxygen-delivery systems, as shown in Figure 31–11, are nasal cannula and face mask, with or without a breathing bag.

Procedure 31–3 describes administering oxygen with either a nasal cannula or a face mask. The doctor orders both the method of administration and the flow rate (expressed in liters per minute, L/min). The medical assistant must be sure to regulate the oxygen correctly.

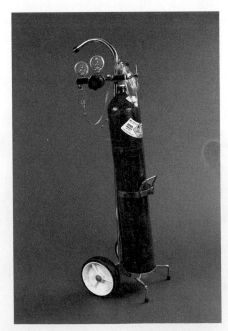

➤ **Figure 31–10** Oxygen tank.

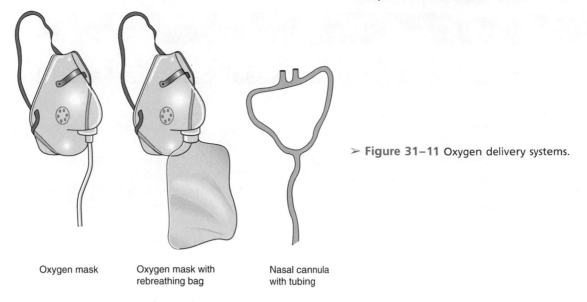

Oxygen mask   Oxygen mask with   Nasal cannula
              rebreathing bag   with tubing

> **Figure 31–11** Oxygen delivery systems.

Nasal Cannula

A nasal cannula is used for low-flow oxygen delivery, where room air mixes with oxygen from the tank. The cannula is two soft plastic tips inserted a short way into the nostrils and attached to the cylinder by thin tubing. One disadvantage of using a nasal cannula is that the nasal membranes become dry, which can cause nosebleeds.

Face Mask

A face mask is used for delivery of 50–55 percent oxygen. There are various types of masks. Some have an attached bag so that exhaled carbon dioxide mixes with the oxygen being administered. A mask allows a medium to high concentration of oxygen. The greatest disadvantage is that some people feel suffocated when they use an oxygen mask.

Manual Resuscitator

The manual resuscitator (**Ambu-bag**) consists of a bag with a mask that fits tightly over the individual's face. It can be used with room air, or it can be connected to oxygen by tubing. It is used to force air into the individual's lungs. A valve between the mask and the bag prevents exhaled air from entering the bag.

The manual resuscitator eliminates direct contact with the person's face while ventilating the individual, but it is only effective if the seal between the mask and the person's face is airtight. It must be used only by someone who is trained to maintain an airtight seal.

Allergic and Anaphylactic Reactions

An allergic reaction occurs when a normally inoffensive foreign substance stimulates an atypical immune response—that is, an allergy. An antigen that causes the hypersensitive response is called an **allergen.** An allergic response begins with sensitization to the foreign substance. An allergen is produced by this primary encounter with only a small amount of the offending substance; the body begins to react to the allergen on subsequent encounters, as more and more antibodies are formed. This triggers the release of histamine whenever the body comes into contact with the allergen.

Some allergic reactions come from contact with skin-contact poison plants, such as poison ivy, poison sumac, or poison oak. Most people are sensitive to such plants, and contact creates a mild to severe dermatitis. Such allergic reactions appear as red raised rashes with blisters, pain, and itching.

Other allergic reactions come from insect bites or stings. For most people, bites and stings cause local reactions, with swelling, redness, and pain. But those who are allergic to stings can become severely ill, with generalized edema, headache, shortness of breath, and a mottled blue appearance.

Individuals who are allergic to insect stings should carry an allergic response kit with them. Such a kit should contain epinephrine, as shown in Figure 31–12. Usually, the device in such a kit is designed for easy self-injection.

Drug allergies may also cause reactions, including respiratory problems with swelling of the vocal cords.

Allergy treatment is dependent on the specific allergen. In general, antihistamines are used to reduce his-

PROCEDURE 31–3

Administering Oxygen by Nasal Cannula/Face Mask

Performance Objective: The student will be able to administer oxygen by nasal cannula or face mask.

Supplies and Equipment: Oxygen in portable tank or wall unit, oxygen mask with elastic strap or nasal cannula with elastic head strap, tubing, flowmeter; optional—humidifier bottle.

Procedure Steps

1. Identify the patient.
2. Evaluate doctor's order and explain procedure to patient.
   Rationale: Doctor will determine which method of delivery (cannula or mask) would best supply the oxygen required for the patient.
3. Assemble equipment.
4. Wash hands.
5. Assess patient before beginning oxygen therapy by measuring pulse, respiratory rate, quality of respirations, and color. Pulse oximetry may be performed if there is an oximeter in the office. Record observations.
   Rationale: The most accurate means of determining respiratory status is to measure the oxygen concentration of the blood. Normal oxygen saturation measured by pulse oximetry is 95–100 percent.

6. Place mask comfortably on patient's face, covering mouth and nose. If using a nasal cannula, place prongs into the patient's nose, loop the tubing behind the patient's ears, and regulate the adjustable portion to hold securely below the patient's chin. If the device is irritating the ears, pad the device with a commercial foam padding. Do not use tissue paper or gauze; such materials are abrasive and will aggravate the irritation.
   Rationale: To promote comfort for the patient.
7. Connect the tubing to the oxygen tank, turn on the oxygen, and adjust the flowmeter to the level ordered by the doctor.
   Nasal cannula—flow rate 1–6 L/min. For a flow rate greater than 2 L/min, a humidifier bottle should be added.
   Mask—flow rate 6–10 L/min. A humidifier bottle should be added. The flow rate for an oxygen mask should be at least 6 L/min to provide adequate oxygenation.
   Rationale: When ordering oxygen for a patient, the doctor should specify the optimum flow rate to meet the needs of the patient.
8. Reassess the patient after 5 minutes. Notify the doctor if the patient still appears to have respiratory difficulty. The doctor may order adjustments to the oxygen flow rate.
9. Document procedure in patient record.

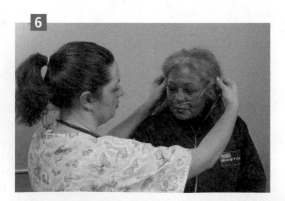

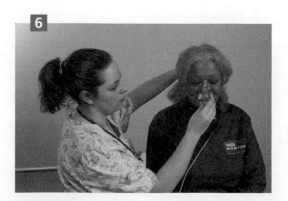

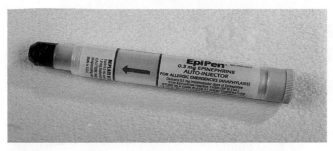

➤ **Figure 31–12** Epinephrine for use in an anaphylactic reaction. (From Bonewit-West K: *Clinical Procedures for Medical Assistants;* 5th ed. Philadelphia: W. B. Saunders, 2000)

tamine release for mild to moderate reactions and epinephrine is used for severe reactions. Glucocorticosteroids may also be used for their anti-inflammatory properties.

Asthma is a reaction to an allergen that causes constriction of the lungs' brochi. Symptoms include wheezing, coughing, choking, and shortness of breath (**SOB**). A severe attack may require the use of epinephrine as a brochodilator.

Some individuals with asthma have chronic constriction of the bronchioles that allows them to move only a small amount of air to their lungs, even under the best of circumstances. If such an individual comes into contact with an allergen, he or she may become **cyanotic** (exhibiting a bluish skin color) and have labored breathing—clear signs of respiratory distress.

If an individual is having a severe asthma attack, it is of the utmost importance to keep the airway open, administering oxygen and any medication the doctor orders. The person should be kept as calm as possible because stress exacerbates such an attack. Vital signs must be monitored carefully.

Anaphylaxis is an acute, life-threatening allergic reaction that can occur within minutes of exposure to an allergen. The situation can deteriorate into shock, coma, and death.

The chain of events set in motion in an anaphylactic reaction are intended for self-preservation. However, the individual actually experiences physiologic changes that can be fatal. Massive amounts of histamine released in anaphylaxis cause bronchospasm, vasodilation, and the release of certain fluids into circulating body fluids, causing blood pressure to fall dramatically. Signs and symptoms of anaphylaxis include anxiety, wheezing, and shortness of breath; cyanosis, hives, and edema—especially of the face; and hypotension.

Symptoms of a less severe allergic reaction to medications include anxiety; flushed, dry skin; hives and itching; swollen lips and tongue, with cyanosis of the lips; nasal congestion, with sneezing or rhinorrhea; and nausea and stomach cramping.

If the decreased blood pressure results in hypoxia (lack of oxygen flow) to the brain and vital organs, the person may experience shock, cardiac irregularities, respiratory and/or cardiac failure, renal failure, and death.

Anaphylaxis is an emergency, and must be treated promptly. The office should have a protocol for anaphylaxis treatment, with different responsibilities assigned to various personnel. Breathing must be assessed constantly by a staff member dedicated to that task; this individual should assess breathing and report symptoms of poor oxygenation and increased respiratory effort. Vital signs should be assessed constantly by a second staff member. These individuals must communicate vital information to the doctor in charge of the emergency response.

Epinephrine should be used according to the doctor's orders. It is given subcutaneously, and the site of the epinephrine injection should be massaged vigorously to enhance absorption. If the patient's breathing and blood pressure do not stabilize, an ambulance should be called.

The potential for life-threatening anaphylactic shock is present whenever medication is administered. Office personnel should regularly practice the protocol for treating anaphylaxis.

Medication reactions can be prevented by listening closely to patients' descriptions of previous medication reactions and by observing the site of all injections for redness and swelling following administration. Any signs of medication reaction should be noted in the patient's chart in such a way that any personnel dealing with the patient in the future will be alert to possibilities for medication reactions.

Burns

Burns are painful and traumatic, emotionally as well as physically. Treatment of burns can be painful, and rehabilitation of severe burns is a long, slow, and painful process. Many burns cause permanent physical disfigurement, which can cause long-term or permanent emotional difficulties.

Types of Burns

There are three types of burns:

1. Thermal
2. Chemical
3. Electrical.

Thermal Burns. Excessive heat causes thermal burns, which are the most common burns. Individuals can suffer thermal burns in building fires, cooking accidents, or fiery automobile accidents. Many thermal burns occur in the home. For first aid, use cool water or ice packs immediately to cool and soothe the burning sensation.

ON THE JOB

Videotape: Legal, Ethical, and Professional Concepts: Scene 2.1A, "Antibiotic Reaction"

Keith McAllister, an 18-year-old male, was seen by Dr. Hughes at Blackburn Primary Care Associates, with symptoms of an infection. Dr. Hughes ordered Rocephin (ceftriaxone), a cephalosporin antibiotic, to be given intramuscularly.

Before the injection was given, Keith was asked if he was allergic to Rocephin or any other antibiotic. Keith replied that he was not allergic to anything.

About 3 minutes after receiving the injection, Keith complained that his mouth and lips were swelling, and he began to have difficulty breathing, with wheezing and a respiratory rate of 34 labored breaths per minute. His pulse was 120, and his blood pressure was 84/54.

Dr. Hughes immediately ordered an injection of epinephrine subcutaneously, and oxygen by face mask at 8 L/min. After receiving the epinephrine, Keith began to breathe more easily, and his blood pressure rose to 96/66.

While Keith was being cared for by the doctor and other staff members, Kevin, the medical assistant, took Keith's mother into an exam room and informed her about the problems her son had had. Mrs. McAllister informed Kevin that Keith had a known allergy to Ceclor, a related drug, and asked how the office could have given her son a drug that he was allergic to.

In this situation, the allergic reaction to Ceclor was later found to have been recorded in the record by a doctor who had seen Keith once when Dr. Hughes was not available. Unfortunately, no sticker had been placed on the chart to alert personnel in the future. Keith, who was very young at the time of the previous reaction, did not remember the incident. Since he was 18, no one questioned his mother about possible allergies.

1. Which of Keith's signs and symptoms were typical of a severe reaction to medication? What other signs and symptoms might Keith have experienced?
2. Did office staff take all possible precautions to find out if Keith was allergic to Rocephin?
3. What is the reason for giving epinephrine to a patient experiencing an allergic reaction to a medication? (You may need to look up this medication in a drug reference.)
4. Why should someone stay with a patient who has received epinephrine to monitor vital signs?
5. What steps should be taken to prevent Keith from having another (and perhaps more severe) reaction to cephalosporins?

Chemical Burns. Chemical burns occur as a result of contact with, ingestion of, or inhalation of acids or alkalies. Chemical burns are most likely to occur on a worksite, often in an industrial facility. For first aid, the area should be immediately flooded for at least 15 minutes, and for 20 minutes or more if the burn is to the area around the eye. Any dry chemicals should be brushed off the skin before using water.

Electrical Burns. Electrical burns occur when the body comes into contact with electric current from faulty wiring, high-voltage power lines, or lightning. An electrical burn is usually life-threatening; in addition to the burning, the electrical impulses can interfere with the body's own electrical mechanisms—most notably those that control the beating of the heart.

Before first aid can be administered, the victim should immediately be removed from the source of electricity. This can pose a risk to the rescuer, especially if the victim is in a wet area, because water conducts electricity very well. Tissue damage caused by electrical burns may take a few days to manifest itself completely, so first aid will often focus more on treating the victim for shock.

Classification of Burns

Although burns are classified in several ways, the most important classification systems focus on the amount of body surface involved and the penetration of skin layers.

A description of the amount of body surface burned can be made utilizing the Rule of Nines, as shown in Figure 31–13.

The level of penetration into the skin's layers is expressed as the "degree" of the burn.

First-degree burns, or superficial burns, primarily damage the epidermis. The skin reddens, and there is moderately severe pain. Treatment includes cool-water dressing or immersion in cool water, followed by a gentle patting to dry the area.

Adult

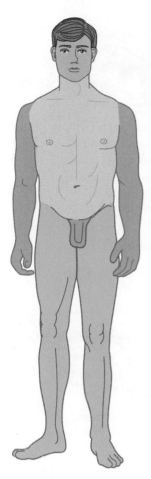

Head 9%

Chest 18%

Back 18%

Right arm 9%

Left arm 9%

Right leg 18%

Left leg 18%

Genital area 1%

100%

Child

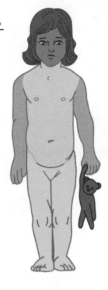

Head 18%

Chest 18%

Back 18%

Right arm 9%

Left arm 9%

Right leg 13.5%

Left leg 13.5%

Genital area 1%

100%

➤ **Figure 31–13** Rule of nines for assessing the extent of burns. Note that the head contains proportionately more skin surface in a child than in an adult.

Second-degree burns, or partial-thickness burns, involve the epidermis and part of the dermis. Leakage of plasma and electrolytes from capillaries damaged by the burn causes blisters and results in moderate edema and pain. Such a burn should be immersed in cool water, patted dry, and covered with sterile dressing. Do not burst the blisters. Antiseptic ointment should be applied only at the doctor's request. If the patient is wearing jewelry on the affected area, it should be removed promptly because the area will swell, making later removal difficult.

Third-degree burns, or full-thickness burns, involve the epidermis, dermis, and subcutaneous tissue, including fat and muscle and even bone and nerve. No blisters appear, but white, leathery tissue and thrombosed vessels are apparent. Usually, there is no pain immediately after the burn because nerve endings have been damaged and destroyed. The burned area can appear charred black, brown, or cherry red, with the underlying tissue appearing pearly white. Tissue involvement in different types of burns is shown in Figure 31–14.

All third-degree burns should receive immediate professional medical care. If more than 10 percent of the body surface area is involved, surgical intervention is usually required, as well as IV fluids, pain medication, and protection from tetanus.

The only first aid for third-degree burns is to cover the burn with sterile dressings and treat the patient for shock. No attempt should be made to remove clothing or other adhering materials, as this will only deepen the burn.

Procedure 31–4 describes the care of burns. See also the "Estimating Burn Severity" box.

Cardiovascular Emergencies

The four cardiovascular emergencies that may need attention in the medical office are:

1. Bleeding
2. Shock
3. Angina
4. Myocardial infarction (heart attack).

Controlling Bleeding

Excessive bleeding is traumatic both to the victim and to others around the incident. The medical caregiver must remain calm in order to control the bleeding quickly and effectively.

Bleeding occurs when a vein or artery is punctured or torn. Direct pressure applied to the site of the

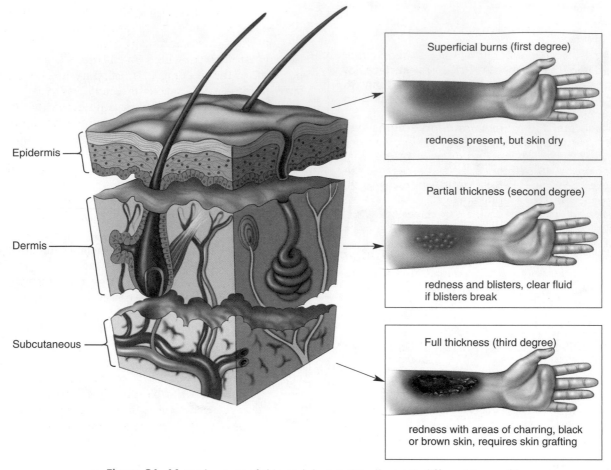

Superficial burns (first degree)

redness present, but skin dry

Partial thickness (second degree)

redness and blisters, clear fluid
if blisters break

Full thickness (third degree)

redness with areas of charring, black
or brown skin, requires skin grafting

Epidermis

Dermis

Subcutaneous

➤ **Figure 31–14** Involvement of skin and deeper tissue layers in different types of burns.

PROCEDURE 31–4

Caring for Burns

Performance Objective: The student will be able to perform burn care to a patient.
Supplies and Equipment: Cotton cloth, water (sterile if available).

Procedure Steps

1. Remove source of burn and stop the burning process.
2. Assess severity of burn and the patient's breathing status.
3. Call 911 or emergency number for moderate or major burns (i.e., third-degree burns that cover more than 2 percent of body surface or extensive second-degree burns).
4. Flush chemical burns and thermal burns that have not penetrated the dermis with copious amounts of cool water. Use sterile water if available.
5. If burns have penetrated the dermis, cover burn with cotton, nonadhering cloth.
6. Continue to monitor breathing status of a person with moderate to severe burns.
7. As burn heals, do not apply ointments, lotions, or antiseptics. Do not break or drain blisters, and do not use materials to cover that may leave fragments in burned area.

Estimating Burn Severity

Minor burns are third-degree burns that cover less than 2 percent of body surface, or second-degree burns that cover less than 15 percent of an adult's body surface or less than 10 percent of a child's body surface.

Moderate burns are third-degree burns that cover between 2 percent and 10 percent of body surface, or second-degree burns that cover from 15 percent to 25 percent of an adult's body surface or from 10 percent to 20 percent of a child's body surface.

Major burns are third-degree burns that cover more than 10 percent of body surface area, or second-degree burns that cover more than 25 percent of an adult's body surface or more than 20 percent of a child's body surface.

Burns to the hands, feet, or genitalia are always considered major burns. Burns to individuals who are poor risks or have associated fractures are always considered major burns. Electrical burns are always considered major burns.

bleeding compresses the blood vessel and the blood, allowing a clot to form and seal off the bleeding area.

When bleeding is severe, it is called a **hemorrhage.** Hemorrhage can cause hypovolemic shock—low blood volume that leads to low blood pressure. This can be life-threatening. The amount of blood loss necessary to become life-threatening varies with each individual, depending on age, size, and general health. Hemorrhage is usually the result of an injury, but may also be caused by an illness.

External Bleeding. External bleeding can be seen coming out of an open wound in the skin or from an orifice such as the nose, mouth, or anus.

Symptoms of excessive external bleeding are obvious bleeding, restlessness, cold clammy skin, thirst, rapid and thready pulse, rapid and shallow respirations, a drop in blood pressure, and a decrease in the level of consciousness.

Capillary bleeding, which is the most common type of external bleeding, involves a slow oozing of red blood. Scratches, minor cuts, and scrapes result in capillary bleeding.

Venous bleeding occurs when a vein is punctured. It is characterized by a slow but steady leak of dark red blood.

Arterial bleeding is the most serious type of bleeding. Fortunately, it is also the least common type. It occurs when an artery is punctured. Arteries lie deep in the body and are usually protected by bone. Arterial bleeding is characterized by spurts of bright red blood; the spurting occurs because the blood is pumping through the artery each time the heart beats.

The best way to control external bleeding is to apply pressure to the site. This can stop or at least slow the flow of blood. Pressure usually controls capillary bleeding and most venous bleeding. If direct pressure does not control the bleeding it is necessary to find a **pressure point**—a site where an artery lies close to the skin. When a pressure point is compressed, the flow of blood to a wider area can be slowed, giving the bleeding site a chance to form a clot. Pressure points are shown in Figure 31–15.

A pressure bandage may be used to control bleeding. But once the bandage has been applied, it should not be removed. Elevating the bleeding body part above the level of the heart can also help slow the blood flow. If these measures do not control bleeding, grasp the pressure point that is proximal to the injury and apply firm pressure with the hands.

In the past, using a tourniquet over a pressure point was recommended. Today, however, tourniquets are not recommended, because they interfere with blood supply to an entire extremity. This can lead to tissue death. Tourniquets should never be used in the medical office or in any populated area where a medical facility is a short ride away. A tourniquet should be applied only when the bleeding is occurring in a remote area (e.g. a campsite) and the choice is between bleeding to death or suffering localized tissue death.

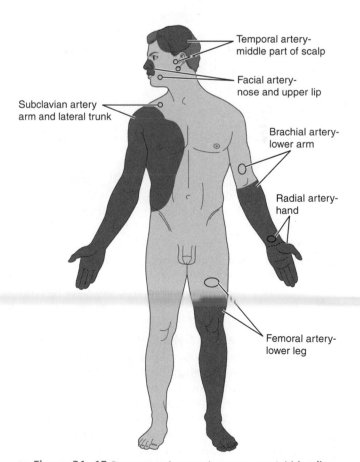

> **Figure 31–15** Pressure points to decrease arterial bleeding.

PROCEDURE 31-5

Controlling Bleeding

Performance Objective: The student will be able to control bleeding from an open wound.

Supplies and Equipment: Gloves, sterile dressing, gown and eye protection, mask, biohazard waste container.

Procedure Steps

1. Identify the patient.
2. If bleeding appears severe, call 911 or emergency number.
3. Wash hands (if possible); if available, put on PPE (personal protective equipment), including gloves, eye shield, mask, gown.
4. Assemble equipment and explain procedure to patient when applicable.
5. Apply dressing over open wound and press firmly. Use a sterile dressing if available. In an emergency when bleeding is profuse, use a clean piece of woven (not knit or fuzzy) cloth, white if possible.
   Rationale: The need to control bleeding may take priority over the need to preserve sterility.

6. If the wound is on the arm or hand, elevate above heart level.
   Rationale: Gravity helps to decrease bleeding.
7. Continue pressure for several minutes to assure that clotting has occurred and bleeding has stopped.
8. If bleeding persists and seeps through dressing, continue holding pressure. If blood is flowing with pulsations and is bright red, suspect arterial bleeding. Apply firm pressure with the hands to the nearest pressure point, as shown in Figure 31-15, and maintain pressure to slow bleeding until emergency help arrives.
9. Wash hands. If the bleeding occurred in the medical office, document the circumstances in the patient's medical record, or fill out an incident report if the person bleeding was not a patient.
   Rationale: Any unusual incident that threatens the health or safety of an individual in a medical office should be documented in case questions arise at a later date.

Procedure 31-5 describes how to control external bleeding.

Internal Bleeding. Internal hemorrhage is often a medical emergency and requires rapid transport to a hospital. The individual suffering from internal hemorrhage shoud be kept calm, quiet, and warm to minimize shock.

Internal bleeding flows into body cavities, an organ, or between tissues. A **contusion**—or bruise—is technically internal bleeding, where the bleeding is occurring into the space between skin layers. Bruises on arms or legs are not usually emergencies. However, a bruise on the trunk, neck, or groin, may be a symptom of more severe internal bleeding, which can be flowing into the peritoneum or into the internal organs of the abdomen, such as intestine, liver, spleen, or kidneys. In addition to bruising at the site, an individual suffering internal bleeding usually has a rapid weak pulse, cold and clammy skin, nausea and vomiting, excessive thirst, a drop in blood pressure, and decreased conciouness.

Shock

Shock is a life-threatening state brought about by failure of the cardiovascular system to bring oxygen and nutrients to the vital organs. This brings the body's metabolic processes to a stop.

Early symptoms of shock are restlessness, irritability, fear, rapid pulse, cool clammy skin, lethargy, pallor, and increased respirations. Unless the shock was caused by a head injury, these symptoms should be treated by raising the individual's legs 8 to 10 inches above the head, so more blood flows to the head and less to the extremities. In the case of head injury or suspected head injury, the individual should be kept flat, or with the head slightly raised, to prevent increasing pressure to the brain. In the office setting, a doctor may order oxygen to be administered to an individual in shock.

Monitoring the ABCs of emergency care is critical. Shock is progressive. Once it reaches a certain point, it is irreversible. The organs most affected by shock are the heart, brain, and lungs. Irreparable damage may be done in as little as 4 to 6 minutes.

Without immediate treatment, shock can progress to a significant loss of blood pressure, cyanosis, unconsciousness, and death. The goals of treatment include raising the individual's blood pressure, increasing circulating blood volume and oxygen concentration, and treating the underlying cause of the shock. When shock is suspected, the person should be transported to a hospital emergency room for monitoring and treatment.

Hypovolemic shock is caused by loss of blood or other body fluids. It usually occurs with external or internal hemorrhaging; plasma loss from severe burns; or dehydration from vomiting, diarrhea, or profuse sweating. First aid for hypovolemic shock is to control the loss of body fluids and replace lost body fluids using intravenous fluid replacement and transfusions. Often, surgery is necessary to remove or repair bleeding organ(s).

Cardiogenic shock occurs when the heart fails to pump an adequate blood suppy to the vital organs. It is caused by injury or damage to the heart. Cardiogenic shock is usually seen with myocardial infarction, but may also occur in individuals with congestive heart failure, arrhythmias, valve disease, or a pulmonary embolus. Cardiogenic shock is difficult to reverse, and is fatal in 80 to 90 percent of instances.

Neurogenic shock occurs with damage to the nervous system, which causes an inability to control the diameter of blood vessels. When the nervous system loses the ability to tell the vessels to dilate or contract, the blood pools in the peripheral areas of the body, away from vital organs. Blood pressure cannot be controlled when this occurs. Neurogenic shock occurs with spinal and brain injuries.

Anaphylactic shock is an acute, life-threatening allergic reaction, as discussed earlier.

Septic shock results from widespread infection that affects blood circulating in the body. Urinary tract infections (particularly in older adults), postpartum infections, and a variety of infections in individuals with depressed immune systems can lead to septic shock.

Psychogenic shock is caused by unpleasant physical or emotional stimuli such as pain, fright, or the sight of blood. In such cases a sudden dilation of the blood vessels causes blood to pool in the abdomen and extremities. This keeps blood from the brain and temporarily deprives the brain of oxygen. A loss of consciousness (fainting) occurs. An individual experiences sudden light-headedness, weakness, nausea, and blurred vision. The individual also begins to sweat, becomes pallid, feels warm, and yawns.

If a person looks about to faint, place him or her in a position where the feet are higher than the head to facilitate blood flow to the brain. A supine position is preferred; but if the patient is sitting in a chair, place his or her head between the knees.

Angina

Angina is a clinical syndrome that accompanies arteriosclerotic cardiovascular disease.

Chest pain is caused by narrowing of the arteries, resulting in arteriospasm. Angina attacks may be caused by any condition that increases myocardial oxygen demand, such as exercise, eating, extremes in temperature, high humidity, and stress.

Signs and symptoms of angina include severe substernal pain or a feeling of tightness, squeezing, burning, or pressure. There may be nausea, vomiting, and/or shortness of breath. The pain is in the left side of the chest and may radiate to the left jaw and into the left arm.

Angina attacks usually last about 15 minutes and no longer than 30 minutes. Increase in muscular activity tends to increase the intensity of pain, and rest may relieve pain. Angina attacks are reversible and do not damage the heart muscle. But they do indicate cardiac problems, so they should be evaluated immediately.

It is almost impossible for an untrained person to tell the difference between an angina attack and a myocardial infarction. Risk factors for angina include smoking, obesity, hypertension, stress, and family history.

Treatment of angina includes keeping the individual quiet, in a semi-reclining position. Nitroglycerin, a vasodilator, is used sublingually for rapid relief; it can be administered three times at five-minute intervals. Constricting clothing should be loosened, vital signs should be monitored closely, and oxygen should be administered as needed.

If an individual who is known to experience angina attacks continues to have pain after two or three nitroglycerin pills, activate the emergency medical system.

Myocardial Infarction

Myocardial infarction (MI) is the technical term for a heart attack. It occurs when blood flow to the heart is severely reduced or completely cut off. This usually occurs because of blockage of a major vein leading to the heart. Lack of oxygen flowing to the heart causes destruction of heart muscle tissue.

The cardinal sign of a heart attack is midline chest pain that is described as crushing, burning, heavy, aching, or similar to indigestion. Pain may radiate down the left arm or into the jaw, throat, or both shoulders. There may be shortness of breath, nausea and vomiting, and profuse sweating. An individual suffering a heart attack is pallid, has an irregular pulse, and may experience a "feeling of doom." Heart attack pain will not be relieved at all by nitroglycerin.

Some patients, especially women, have less severe symptoms and may not realize they are having a heart attack. Stimulation of the vagus nerve may cause gastrointestinal symptoms, leading the patient to believe he or she has heartburn. If the patient contacts the office, advise him or her that it is always best to have the condition checked, because it may signal cardiac problems.

In the event a patient has a heart attack in the office, activate the emergency medical system immediately; give the patient any heart medication he or she has on hand, and be prepared to administer CPR. Administer oxygen if directed by the doctor. Monitor vital signs, place the patient on a cardiac monitor if available (or obtain an EKG), and prepare the crash cart.

Diabetic Emergency

Diabetes mellitus is a disease in which the body is unable to utilize glucose either because the body does not make insulin or because the body cannot use the insulin it does make. Because diabetes affects the blood sugar level, a person with diabetes might encounter two types of emergency: hypoglycemia (low blood sugar) and hyperglycemia (high blood sugar).

The teaching needs of a patient with diabetes are discussed in chapter 33; a patient who understands his or her diabetes is often vigilant to signs of a possible emergency situation.

Hyperglycemia (Diabetic Coma)

If an insulin-dependent diabetic does not receive enough insulin, the blood glucose level rises. This is called **hyperglycemia.** If the blood glucose level becomes high enough, the person will fall into a coma and eventually die.

When glucose cannot be used, fats break down and acid waste products—known as ketones—build up in the blood. Therefore, this condition is also called **diabetic ketoacidosis.**

Signs are polyuria (excessive urination), polyphagia (excessive eating), polydipsia (excessive thirst), vomiting, abdominal pain, warm dry skin, rapid and deepsighing respirations, sweet or fruity odor to the breath and body, and eventually a rapid weak pulse, disorientation, confusion, and possibly death.

Hyperglycemia has a gradual onset over 12 to 18 hours. It may be caused by an illness or infection, overeating, not administering medications, or insufficient amounts of insulin.

Hypoglycemia (Insulin Reaction)

Hypoglycemia (low blood sugar) occurs in diabetes when there is too much insulin and not enough glucose in the body. Because it occurs in individuals who are taking insulin injections, it is usually called an **insulin reaction.**

Symptoms include rapid respirations, pallor, cold clammy skin, sweating, dizziness, and headache. There may also be a rapid pulse, high blood pressure, and extreme hunger. Aggressive behavior may occur, with lack of coordination, followed by fainting, seizure, or coma as the blood sugar continues to fall. This condition is also sometimes called insulin shock. These symptoms usually occur quickly, in 5 to 20 minutes after the beginning of symptoms.

Treatment for hypoglycemia requires rapid intake of sugar or glucose. For a conscious individual, fruit juice, candy, sugar, or soft drinks may be given to get sugar into the bloodstream immediately. In addition, foods like peanut butter may be given. Such fat-laden foods assure that the glucose level will be maintained for a longer time as the fat is broken down into sugars. An unconscious individual needs to be treated with intravenous fluids that contain glucose or an injection of glucose.

When blood sugar falls in a diabetic individual, it is usually caused by an excess of insulin—the result of eating too little or exercising too much.

Hypoglycemia and hyperglycemia have some of the same signs and symptoms, so it is often difficult to distinguish between the two conditions. Observation of respirations and the odor of acetone (fruity odor) are the best distinguishing characteristics.

Hypoglycemia occurs more rapidly than hyperglycemia, and it can cause permanent brain damage. So the first response to a comatose diabetic should be to give sugar and observe the response. There is little risk from giving a little extra sugar. The body can handle high sugar levels for a lot longer than it can handle low sugar levels. If the individual is actually having a hypoglycemic episode, he or she should regain consciousness quickly.

Many diabetic people can tell the subtle differences between hypoglycemia and hyperglycemia by the way they feel, even if medical personnel cannot distinguish the external signs and symptoms. If the individual is conscious, listen to what he or she is saying. The person may also be able to help the medical personnel determine the situation by describing what he or she has done earlier in terms of eating and activity, and any acute illness that may be influencing the ability to utilize glucose. Table 31–1 provides a comparison of hypoglycemia and hyperglycemia.

Musculoskeletal Injury

Musculoskeletal injuries were discussed in detail in chapter 21.

First aid for musculoskeletal injuries includes the following steps:

1. Immobilize.
2. Apply cold to reduce swelling.
3. If there is no obvious fracture or dislocation, use an elastic wrap to provide compression.
4. Elevate.

Table 31–1	Comparison of Diabetic Coma and Insulin Reaction	
	Diabetic Coma	Insulin Reaction
Cause of the condition	Lack of insulin	Too much insulin
Onset	Gradual	Rapid
Skin	Warm, dry	Cool, clammy
Breath	Fruity or acetone odor	Unremarkable
Respirations	Deep	Shallow
Pulse	Rapid, thready	Rapid, bounding
Thirst	Intense	Not marked
Hunger	May or may not be present	Intense
Vomiting	Common	Rare
Abdominal pain	Common	Rare
Blood glucose level	Hyperglycemia: >200 mg/dL	Hypoglycemia: <60 mg/dL
Urine glucose	Present	Absent

The acronym **RICE** (rest, ice, compression, elevation) is used to help remember the four steps.

Musculoskeletal injuries should be immobilized to prevent motion that can cause pain and further damage. A splint made of wood, plastic, rolled newspaper, cardboard, or other available material can be used in an emergency.

The body part should be splinted in the position in which it was found. The splint should be held in place by gauze if possible, but neckties or other wide wrapping material may be used if necessary. The splint should be applied snugly, but not tightly. Once the injury is immobilized, the individual should be taken to a hospital emergency room.

Air splints are found in some prepackaged first aid kits, or they can be included in a kit made up in the medical office. An air splint is clear plastic that is blown up until the skin whitens. It usually has a zipper for easy removal at the hospital emergency room.

Procedure 31–6 describes in detail applying a splint.

Neurologic Emergency

The three most common neurologic emergencies are:

1. Seizure
2. Stroke
3. Head injury.

Seizure

A **seizure** is a sudden violent series of involuntary muscle contractions caused by abnormal electrical discharges from neurons in the brain. It may be called a **convulsion.** The abnormal impulses lead to involun-

---

PROCEDURE 31–6

Applying a Splint

Performance Objective: The student will be able to apply a splint to an extremity.

Supplies and Equipment: Straps for securing— could be material such as cotton or a leather belt; a flat surface, such as a board or branch, to immobilize; padding, such as rolled towels; pillow or newspaper to assist when needed.

Procedure Steps

1. Assess the patient who has experienced a musculoskeletal injury. Indications that a fracture

has occurred include an extremity at an abnormal angle, visible bone fragments, shortening or abnormal rotation of the extremity, and severe pain and swelling.
2. If possible, call 911 or emergency number.
3. Assemble equipment and explain what you will attempt to do to patient when applicable.
4. Depending on the area of injury, attempt to immobilize the area to decrease pain and prevent further injury during transport:

Procedure continued on following page

PROCEDURE 31–6 *(continued)*

a. Place padded boards along a leg or arm and hold in place by tying with cloth strips.

b. Immobilize a foot or hand by tying a rolled-up towel or small rug around the extremity. Leave shoe or clothing in place.

c. Wrap several layers of newspaper or magazines around an upper or lower extremity and tie in place with cloth strips.

d. After splinting, an injured arm can be supported with a triangle bandage. An extra tie around the chest prevents movement. Legs may be tied together with cloth strips to prevent movement.

5. Assure that extremity is not movable and transport patient to nearest medical facility or wait for emergency help to arrive.

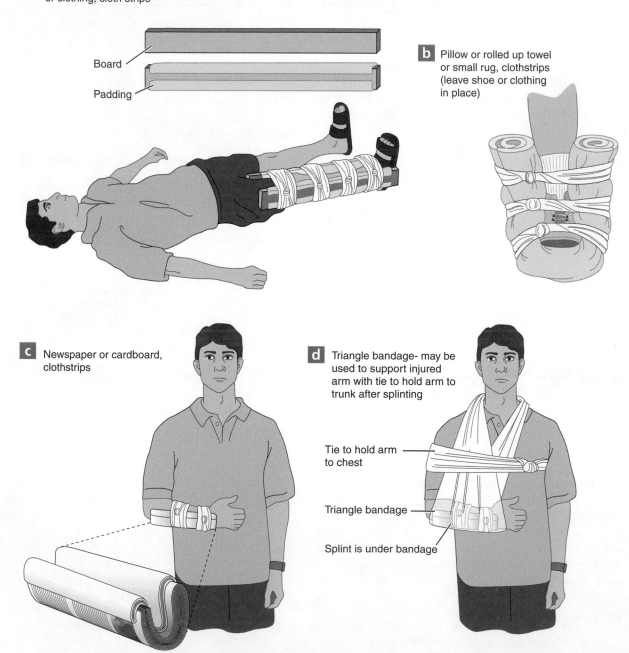

a. Boards padded with fabric or clothing, cloth strips

Board

Padding

b. Pillow or rolled up towel or small rug, clothstrips (leave shoe or clothing in place)

c. Newspaper or cardboard, clothstrips

d. Triangle bandage- may be used to support injured arm with tie to hold arm to trunk after splinting

Tie to hold arm to chest

Triangle bandage

Splint is under bandage

tary movement of various body parts and/or abnormal sensations or loss of consciousness.

A seizure can be a manifestation of many disease states that overstimulate the brain cells. The cause can be a high fever caused by a virus or bacterial infection (febrile seizure), meningitis (a swelling of the lining surrounding the brain or spinal cord), diabetes, or certain prescription or street drugs. **Epilepsy** is a chronic condition characterized by frequent seizures. Epilepsy may occur after injury to the brain; more often, however, it is **idiopathic** (meaning it appears for no reason).

Seizures can begin in a certain part of the brain and affect only a portion of the body (partial seizure), or they can affect the entire body (generalized seizure). During a seizure, in addition to the involuntary muscle contractions that cause "jerking" or "twitching," the individul may have a glassy stare, become confused, be unable to speak, and even lose consciousness. Generalized seizures result when abnormal electrical activity spreads throughout the brain.

The best known form of seizure is the generalized major motor seizure (also called a tonic-clonic, or grand mal, seizure). During the tonic phase, the individual loses consciousness and has generalized rigid muscular contraction, with absent respiration that causes cyanosis and loss of bladder and bowel control. This phase usually lasts less than 30 seconds. It is followed by the clonic phase, during which the body jerks violently and the jaw muscles tighten and release. This phase usually lasts less than a minute. Following these two brief stages is a postictal phase—a 10- to 30-minute period during which the individual has a depressed state of consciousness, headache, and disorientation.

Individuals with epilepsy who suffer tonic-clonic seizures regularly report an "aura" (an early warning that the seizure is going to happen), which allows them to find a safe spot before the actual seizure occurs.

Emergency care of seizures includes assuring the individual's safety by removing furniture or other hazards in the immediate area. In Figure 31–16, for example, a medical assistant is moving a chair out of the way of a person having a seizure. Help the individual to lie down gently. If necessary, lay a towel or jacket down to protect the individual's head if it is banging on the floor during the clonic phase.

Do not restrain the person. After the seizure has started, do not attempt to put an object between the clenched teeth; this may interfere with breathing, damage teeth, and initiate a gag reflex that would cause vomiting. After muscle contractions have stopped, assist the person to lie on his or her side to maintain an open airway, to allow drainage of excess saliva, and to prevent aspiration should vomiting occur. Loosen any clothing that might interfere with breathing; unbutton the upper buttons on a shirt, for example, and loosen belts.

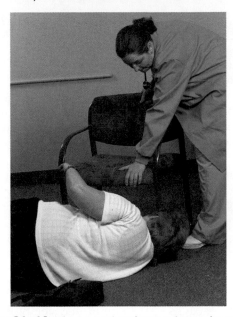

> **Figure 31–16** When a patient has a seizure, the medical assistant moves items away but does not restrain the individual in any way.

After the seizure is over, allow the person to rest or sleep, and obtain help if the person does not regain consciousness in 10 to 15 minutes. Monitor the individual's vital signs following the seizure. If the person is known to have a seizure disorder, it may not be necessary to call an ambulance. Assess the patient's condition and support system before deciding how the patient's needs are best met. If the individual has never had a seizure before, he or she should undergo a full neurologic evaluation to determine the reason for the seizure. If a seizure occurs in the medical office, the medical assistant should document any care given.

A medical assistant should be careful to preserve the individual's dignity at all times.

Stroke

Stroke, or **cerebrovascular accident (CVA)**, occurs when an artery in the brain is blocked or ruptures and blood flow to the brain is interrupted. One third of all people who suffer a CVA will die or have permanent disability.

Individuals who are prone to strokes include those with hypertension; a history of **transient ischemic attacks (TIAs)**, which are small interruptions of blood flow to the brain; diabetes; high cholesterol; arteriosclerosis; or autoimmune diseases such as gout. The three most common causes of strokes are:

1. Thromboses accompanying conditions such as atherosclerosis, where plaque builds up and

blood flow to an area of the brain is either slowed or stopped. Interruption of blood flow results in necrosis (death) of the brain tissue that has been deprived of oxygen. TIAs usually precede this type of stroke.

2. Emboli (blood clots) that travel through the bloodstream to the brain. This type of stroke has rapid onset; it occurs in people who have heart disease or blood clots in the leg or other parts of the body.

3. Hemorrhaging into the brain from the rupture of a blood vessel, or aneurysm. This type of stroke has a rapid onset, and is accompanied by severe headache and vomiting. Eighty percent of those who have a major hemorrhage into the brain will die from it.

Signs and symptoms of TIAs include blindness in one eye, dizziness, personality changes, fainting, temporary paralysis of the face or one side of the body, difficulty with speech, or the inability to recognize familiar objects. These transient changes can last from one hour to one day.

An individual may have a mild stroke, with little or no permanent damage, or a more extensive stroke, with immediate paralysis and lasting disability.

Signs and symptoms of stroke include sagging muscles on one side of the face and inability to move the arm, leg, or both extremities on that side; unequal pupils; headache; respiratory distress; confusion and slurred speech; nausea and vomiting; loss of bladder and bowel control; visual and sensory changes; difficulty in communicating (difficulty finding the words with which to express a thought); and an altered level of consciousness.

Even if an individual having a stroke is unable to speak, he or she can almost always hear. Loosen clothing and position the individual to prevent choking. Assess respiration and remove dentures if necessary. Take vital signs, using both carotid and radial pulses. If the individual is unconscious, put him or her on the side, preferably with the paralyzed side down. Keep the individual quiet by speaking in a relaxed and reassuring tone. Do not give the individual anything to eat or drink. Call an ambulance and have the individual transported to the hospital emergency room.

Head Injury

The four most common head injuries are concussion, brain contusion, skull fracture and intracranial bleeding, and scalp hematoma.

Concussion is a jarring injury to the head in which the brain is shaken. Whenever a person loses consciousness following a blow to the head, even for a minute, the injury is called a concussion. The individual may also have a temporary loss of vision and memory. He or she is pallid and listless, and may be unable

to answer questions or follow commands appropriately. The individual may vomit. These symptoms can resolve rapidly or last up to a full day; however, recent research has shown that the effects of concussion can last many weeks.

Individuals who suffer repeated concussions, such as athletes who play in contact sports such as football, hockey, or boxing, often take longer to recover from successive concussions. Concussions often go unrecognized in children, but can later prove dangerous if the child is not given several days to rest and heal after any head injury with loss of consciousness.

If a person has suffered an apparent concussion, keep the individual quiet. Give him or her time to get reoriented. Observe pupils for equality and responsiveness. If the individual does not regain orientation within a couple of hours or vomits repeatedly, call an ambulance to transport him or her to the hospital emergency room.

Brain contusion is bleeding into the brain caused by injury to one or more blood vessels at the time of the head injury. This can be very dangerous. The individual usually experiences a loss of consciousness and paralysis (one-sided or total) and exhibits unequal pupils, forceful repeated vomiting, and a marked alteration in vital signs.

A person who has suffered a brain contusion needs immediate neurologic care in a hospital and should be transported to the emergency room by ambulance.

Skull fracture and intracranial bleeding is caused by some sort of blunt trauma to the skull. A skull fracture is a depression or a crack in the skull. Intracranial bleeding frequently occurs with a skull fracture, but not always. Bleeding from a skull fracture is not usually as severe as that from a brain contusion, but the symptoms are similar. There may be leakage of cerebrospinal fluid from the ears or nose, seizures, and/or respiratory distress.

A person who has suffered a skull fracture needs immediate neurologic care in a hospital and should be transported to the emergency room by ambulance.

A **scalp hematoma** is a swelling under the skin on the skull. This can be caused by a laceration or trauma to the head. Scalp lacerations usually bleed profusely because blood vessels in the head are close to the skin.

Apply ice immediately to prevent further swelling. Apply direct pressure to the laceration site. A pressure bandage may be used to reduce swelling or slow bleeding.

Poisoning

Poisons can be ingested, absorbed, inhaled, or injected. They can also enter the body through bites and stings (discussed under allergies). Poisons can cause acute illness, permanent injury, or even death.

Most poisonings occur at home. Poisoning often occurs in children under age five because of the combination of their natural curiosity, their lack of repulsion to strong odors, and their tendency to put things in their mouths. Poisoning is also more dangerous to the young than to the old.

If someone calls the office with a possible poisoning, you should ask what the substance was, how much was taken, and when it was taken. The telephone number of the local or regional poison control center should be kept near every telephone in the office, so anyone who receives the call can either call the poison control center or direct the caller to the center.

There are more than 500 poison control centers in the United States; these centers, which are staffed 24 hours a day, have information about nearly every poison.

Ingested Poisoning

If a poison is swallowed, it usually stays in the stomach for just a short time. Drugs, cleaning products, contaminated food, petroleum products, and poisonous plants are the most common types of ingested poisons. Alcohol and other drugs, either separately or together, may also result in poisoning.

Signs and symptoms of poisoning include open bottles of medicine or chemicals; stains on clothing; burns around the hands and/or mouth; nausea, vomiting, abdominal pain, and excessive salivation; difficulty breathing; profuse sweating; dilated or constricted pupils; dizziness, drowsiness, unconsciousness, and possible convulsions; and changes in skin color.

If you take a telephone call regarding a possible poisoining, ask the following seven questions:

1. Where is the person calling from (address and phone)?
2. What is the name, age, and size (weight) of the person who ingested the poison?
3. What is the name of the poison ingested?
4. How long ago was the poison ingested?
5. How much was ingested?
6. Has any vomiting occurred?
7. Has any first aid been given?

Keep the caller on the line, and tell him or her not to leave the victim alone. Call the poison control center. Forward all information and directions from the center to the individual attending the victim. Then call and arrange transportation to the hospital emergency room.

Treatment for poisonings must be quick. Speed can prevent absorption of the poison into the bloodstream.

For some poisonings, vomiting should be induced. For instance, if the individual has ingested an excess of an edible substance such as contaminated food, plant material, alcohol, or medication in liquid or pill form, it is safe for the person to vomit. The poison control center will be able to advise on other substances for which vomiting is indicated.

However, vomiting should not be induced if the poison is caustic (likely to injure the mucous membranes of the esophagus or mouth) or if the poison contains petroleum products, which can easily be aspirated. The poison should be diluted with milk or water, but the individual needs to be transported to a hospital emergency room as soon as possible. Vomiting should not be induced in an unconscious person or a person having a seizure.

When instructed to induce vomiting by the poison control center, use syrup of ipecac as an **emetic** (a substance used to cause vomiting). Mix one tablespoon and one cup of water. If vomiting has not occurred within 20 minutes, repeat. It may also be necessary to force the person to gag by touching the back of the tongue lightly. Encourage the victim to drink fluids until emesis is reasonably clear. It is recommended that syrup of ipecac be kept in the home where young children are living, because immediate vomiting is often the preferred treatment.

After the individual has vomited, collect some of the vomitus to be analyzed at the hospital. Also take a container or a sample of the suspected poison to the hospital. Activated charcoal may be administered in the hospital emergency room. It binds to the poison and prevents the poison from being absorbed in the gastrointestinal tract.

Parents of young children should always be instructed to store medication and cleaning supplies in cupboards with child-proof latches or in high cupboards out of the reach of children. Gasoline or other petroleum products, paint, insecticides, and cleaning solutions should be stored on high shelves or in locked cupboards in garages or sheds, where children cannot gain access to them.

Inhaled Poisoning

Some poisons can be inhaled in the form of gas, spray, or vapor. The most common is carbon monoxide, which can come from car exhaust, a malfunctioning heater, or a fire. Others are carbon dioxide issuing from sewers or wells, and fumes from household products. If ammonia and chlorine bleach are mixed when cleaning, the combination forms ammonium chloride, which is corrosive to lung tissue.

Signs and symptoms of an inhaled poison are severe headache; nausea and vomiting; respiratory distress, including shortness of breath, coughing, wheezing, rales, and cyanosis; chest pain and tightness; burning eyes, nose, and throat; confusion or dizziness; and even unconsciousness.

Carbon monoxide poisoning can cause headaches, skin flushing, and flulike symptoms without a fever. This gas is especially dangerous because carbon monoxide replaces oxygen in the blood. Carbon monoxide is odorless, so the victim often falls asleep and lapses into unconsciousness without being aware that he or she is being poisoned.

When trying to help an individual who has been poisoned by inhalation, be sure the area is safe; make sure there are no fumes that can cause poisoning to any potential rescuer. Move the individual into fresh air as quickly as possible. Loosen tight-fitting clothing. Keep the individual quiet and monitor vital signs. Seek medical assistance immediately.

Absorbed Poisoning

Many poisons—from fertilizers or pesticides—can enter the body through the skin. This usually occurs through a burn, a lesion, or an inflammatory process. An individual can also come into contact with a poisonous plant.

Signs and symptoms of absorbed poisoning include irritated, burning, and itching skin; irritated, burning, and itching eyes; headache; abnormal pulse, respiration, or both; and/or generalized swelling.

To treat absorbed poisoning, remove all clothes that have come into contact with the poison. Wash the affected skin area thoroughly with soap and water, and rinse thoroughly. Check creases in the skin (inside elbows, behind knees, under arms, and so forth) to make sure that the toxin has been removed. Use calamine lotion, colloidal baths and soaks, and corticosteroid ointments to relieve the itching. Seek medical attention, since systemic toxic effects may occur.

Injected Poisoning

Poison can be injected through bites, stings, or needle puncture. Signs and symptoms of injected poison include an altered state of awareness; evidence of a sting, bite, or puncture mark on the skin; mottled skin; localized pain or itching; burning, swelling, or blistering at the injection site; difficulty breathing; abnormal pulse rate; nausea and vomiting; and anaphylaxis.

Spider Bites. Two particular spiders have life-threatening bites: black widow spiders and brown recluse spiders. Both prefer dark, out-of-the-way places. Bites usually occur on the hands or arms, when a person reaches into the spider's hiding place. Often, the individual does not know that he or she has been bitten until the area becomes red and swollen, and the person begins to feel ill.

The black widow spider, which is approximately 1″ long, is black with a red hourglass pattern on its abdomen. Its venom is toxic to the central nervous system.

Signs and symptoms of a black widow bite include swelling and dull pain at the injection site, nausea and vomiting, a rigid abdomen, fever, rash, difficulty breathing, difficulty swallowing, headache, and high blood pressure. The symptoms usually last about a day, but the headache and malaise can last for months.

Treatment includes applying ice to the area and monitoring vital signs. Take the spider to the medical facility for confirmation of its species if at all possible.

Brown recluse spiders are usually brown, but their color may range from yellow to dark chocolate brown. They also have a brown violin-shaped marking on the upper back. The bite does not heal, and requires surgical grafting to repair.

Signs and symptoms of a brown recluse bite are redness, tenderness, and swelling at the injection site. Most people do not realize they have been bitten at first because the bite is initially painless. But within a few hours, the bite has a bluish area with a white periphery, which gradually becomes surrounded by a red halo. Within 24 hours, the person may have a fever, joint pain, nausea and vomiting, and chills. Within 7 days, the bite becomes larger and ulcerates.

If the bite is noticed soon after it occurs, put ice on the area. If possible take the spider to the medical facility for testing.

Snake Bites. Poisonous snakes that live in the United States include the rattlesnake, copperhead, cottonmouth, and coral snake. There are poisonous snakes in every state except Hawaii, Alaska, and Maine. Fifty-five percent of poisonous snake bites in the United States are from rattlesnakes, 34 percent from copperheads, 10 percent from cottonmouths, and 1 percent from coral snakes. Any unidentified snake should be considered poisonous. Snake bites are usually treated in an emergency room.

Animal Bites. Animal bites can range from minor to serious and life-threatening. In most areas of the country, an animal bite must be reported to the local board of health. A bite from an animal that may have rabies poses a serious threat, because rabies is always fatal. Rabies vaccination is available. This vaccination produces antibodies to fight the rabies virus. A person will be given a series of immunizations if there is any question of a bite by a rabid animal. If the animal can be identified, it will be tested and quarantined for observation (if a pet). A rabid animal will be euthanized.

Minor animal bites should be washed with soap and water. An antibacterial ointment should be applied, and a sterile dressing. If the individual has not had a tetanus shot in more than 10 years, he or she should receive one after any animal bite.

For serious animal bites, stop the bleeding by applying direct pressure. Because it might cause more bleeding, cleaning the wound should wait until the individual arrives at a hospital emergency room for treatment.

Wounds

Because wounds and wound healing are described in detail in chapter 17, this section only discusses general guidance for immediate wound treatment. Wounds can be classified as either open or closed.

Open Wounds

An open wound is a break in the skin or mucous membrane that exposes the underlying tissue. Because the skin is broken, the main goals of treatment are to control bleeding and reduce the possibility of infection. If an individual has not had a tetanus shot in more than 10 years, he or she should have one after any serious open wound, especially a puncture wound. Tetanus bacilli are widespread, so the risk of infection is high. Also, they prefer to grow at the inside portion of a wound after the skin has closed it, so puncture wounds are particularly susceptible to tetanus.

The following five first aid steps should be taken for open wounds:

1. Control the bleeding, but allow any puncture wound to bleed freely for a time to cleanse the inner portion of the wound and rid it of bacteria.
2. Clean the wound with soap and water. Go to an emergency room for treatment of a severe wound or to remove any embedded debris.
3. Allow the wound to dry.
4. Cover the wound with a dry sterile dressing. Small wounds do not require a dressing, unless they are in areas where clotting is difficult.
5. Seek medical attention if there is discharge, swelling, or profuse bleeding; if the incision is more than one 1″ long, or if foreign material is embedded in the wound.

When there is embedded material, apply pressure with a sterile gauze dressing, but do not remove the embedded object because that will cause further bleeding. Transport the individual to the hospital emergency room for further treatment.

In the case of a traumatic amputation, use sterile dressing to control bleeding. Take the individual to a hospital emergency room immediately. Bring the amputated part to the hospital for possible reattachment. Keep the amputated part cool, but do not freeze it or immerse it in water.

Closed Wounds

Closed wounds involve injury to the underlying tissues without a break in the skin. They are usually caused by a sudden blow or force from a blunt object.

A contusion occurs when the tissue under the skin is injured, with blood vessels leaking blood into the tissues. This results in a bluish discoloration of the skin and swelling. Cold compresses reduce the swelling and discoloration, and relieve pain. After several days, the contusion changes from bluish to green and then to yellow as oxidation of the blood pigments takes place.

A hematoma is a collection of blood beneath the skin, with ecchymosis—a lump with bluish discoloration. The best treatment is rest, ice, compression, and elevation (RICE).

Procedure 31–7 discusses cleaning minor wounds.

Other Emergencies: Exposure, Foreign Bodies, and Nosebleeds

Exposure

Exposure to excessive environmental heat or cold can result in local tissue damage or systemic disorders. The elderly, infants and young children, those who work outdoors, people with poor circulation, and individuals under the influence of alcohol or drugs are susceptible to environmental injuries.

Hyperthermia is a heat-related injury that is likely to occur on very hot days with high humidity and little breeze. Hyperthermia can manifest itself either as heat stroke or as heat exhaustion. It is important to differentiate between heat stroke and heat exhaustion because the treatment differs.

Heat stroke is a life-threatening emergency that occurs after prolonged exposure to high temperature and humidity. It includes excessive loss of fluids (dehydration) and insufficient volume of blood in the circulatory system (hypovolemic shock), leading to an inability to regulate body temperature. If body temperature becomes too high, tissues and organs become damaged. If left untreated, a person can die from heat stroke.

Signs and symptoms of heat stroke are hot, dry skin; high body temperature; altered state of mind; rapid pulse and breathing; dizziness and weakness; and pupils that are equal but dilated.

Treatment for heat stroke is to move the person to a cool spot and remove outer clothing unless it is made of light cotton. Cool the person by any means possible, such as spraying with a hose or applying a cold washcloth to the forehead. Place ice packs in groin and armpits—areas where the body gets rid of heat through perspiration. Keep the person's head and shoulders slightly elevated. Transport to a hospital emergency room as quickly as possible.

Heat exhaustion is a less severe condition. An individual suffering from heat exhaustion has a pale, cool, moist face. The skin is cool and clammy. The individual is sweating profusely. Other signs and symptoms include a headache, confusion, and a sense of "giddiness"; weak and rapid pulse; quiet and shallow respirations; muscle cramping; and thirst, nausea, and vomiting. The pupils are equal but dilated.

For treatment, put the individual in the recumbent position, with head lowered to maintain warmth and fight shock. Give salt tablets and large amounts of

PROCEDURE 31–7

Cleaning Minor Wounds

Performance Objective: The student will be able to clean minor wounds using aseptic technique.

Supplies and Equipment: Sterile dressing(s), sterile gauze, sterile gloves, sterile water, or other sterile solution as ordered by doctor, sterile basin, sterile drapes, biohazard waste container.

Procedure Steps

1. Identify the patient and visually assess wound site.
   Rationale: Visual inspection of the wound size, depth, and type of wound determines supplies needed.
2. Assemble supplies needed for wound cleaning depending on size and depth of the wound and solution that will be used to clean the wound.
   Rationale: The wound should be cleaned with sterile water or other solution ordered by the physician.
3. Wash hands.
4. Prepare to clean wound by:
   a. Pouring sterile solution into sterile basin.
   b. Soaking gauze in solution. (You may use commercially prepared swabs.)
   c. Opening packaged dressings, or other bandaging materials.
   d. Draping wound area if needed.
   e. Positioning biohazard container close by for waste disposal.
5. Put on sterile gloves.
   Rationale: To prevent introducing microorganisms into a break in the patient's skin.
6. Clean wound site using one swipe per gauze pad or swab using a downward motion. If the wound is rounded, start cleaning from the inside of the wound and work outward in a circular fashion. Do not go over the same area twice with the same gauze/swab, or recontamination will occur. Clean area thoroughly, then go back over it again with another clean gauze/swab if necessary. Clean with gentle strokes so abrasion does not occur.
   Rationale: Working from a cleaner area to a less clean area prevents introducing microorganisms into cleaner areas.
7. Cover with sterile dressing as directed by the doctor. Use nonirritating adhesive tape to anchor dressing.
8. Document the appearance of the wound and the treatment provided in the patient's medical record.

---

liquid if the individual is conscious. Loosen tight clothing.

Another condition arising from exposure to heat is heat cramps. With heat cramps, the person may perspire profusely, and will lose body salt. He or she will complain of severe muscle cramping in the abdomen and legs, and may feel faint, dizzy, and exhausted.

Treatment includes salt tablets and a lot of fluid. Electrolyte drinks like Gatorade™ or Powerade™ can be helpful. Have the person lie down in a cool place.

Sunburn is another condition that should not be treated in a trivial manner. It can result in redness, tenderness, pain, swelling, blisters, and peeling skin. A severe sunburn, or continuous sunburn, can lead to skin damage and predispose the person to develop skin cancer later in life.

Sunburned skin should be soaked in water to reduce the heat. Legs and arms should be elevated to relieve swelling. Oils or lotions should not be used if the skin is warm, since they hold heat in; wait until the skin has dried and begun to flake before using lotions. A person who has been sunburned should drink plenty of fluids.

Hypothermia

Hypothermia is a life-threatening emergency when the body temperature falls dangerously low. This may occur rapidly if a person falls through ice into cold water, or may occur more slowly from prolonged exposure to cold temperature. In hypothermia, the body loses its ability to regulate its temperature and to generate body heat.

Signs and symptoms of hypothermia include shivering, numbness, drowsiness, apathy, a glassy stare, and a decreased level of consciousness.

Treatment focuses on warming the patient and preventing further heat loss. Remove the person from the cold, especially any cold or wet clothing, and wrap in a blanket. Warming should be done gradually. The individual should be taken to a hospital emergency room.

Frostbite is localized tissue freezing. The severity depends on the environmental temperatures, the duration of the exposure, and the wind-chill factor. Frostbite is usually not life-threatening, but it may cause tissue damage that requires amputation.

Signs and symptoms of frostbite include numbness followed by loss of feeling in the affected area; skin redness; burning and itching; cold, waxy skin; and white, yellow, or blue discoloration of the skin.

To treat frostbite, slowly rewarm the area by placing it in water between 103 and 105° F. **Never rub a frostbitten area.** Give the person hot beverages to act as a stimulus to dilate blood vessels and increase circulation. Place the frozen area in contact with another body part for gradual rewarming.

Foreign Bodies

A foreign body is a substance that becomes lodged in any part of the body where it does not belong.

Foreign bodies in the eyes can usually be seen fairly easily. Always wash your hands before touching the eyes. The foreign body may be removed with a bit of cotton or a fold of moistened facial tissue.

It may be necessary to evert the upper lid to remove the foreign matter. If the foreign matter is on the cornea, it is necessary to flush the eye with irrigating solution. If it is embedded in the cornea, it will be necessary for a doctor to remove it. The individual should be told not to rub the eye. An eye patch is placed loosely over the eye until the patient can receive instillation.

A doctor should promptly assess any patient with an object lodged in the ear or nose. Food, such as a pea or a bean, may swell if it becomes wet, and become more difficult to remove.

Splinters can generally be removed at home or with splinter forceps in the office. Wash the area with soap and water and gently pat dry. Lift the exposed end of the splinter with a needle that has been held over a flame or cleaned with alcohol. Grasp the splinter with tweezers and remove. Splinters that are deeply embedded or lodged under the fingernail should be removed by a doctor.

Nosebleeds

A nosebleed (**epistaxis**) may be caused by blunt trauma, or may be the result of an upper respiratory infection, hypertension, strenuous activity, or high altitude.

Have the person sit with the head tilted slightly forward to prevent blood from running down the back of the throat, which may cause nausea. Apply direct pressure by pinching the nostrils together—it usually takes about 15 minutes to get a clot to form. An ice pack can also be applied to the bridge of the nose or the back of the neck to help stop the bleeding. Advise the person not to blow the nose for several hours, because this will dislodge the clot.

If bleeding cannot be controlled, have the individual transported to an emergency room for further treatment.

STUDENT STUDY PLAN

To reinforce your understanding of the material in this chapter . . .

Complete the **Review and Recall** questions.

Discuss the situation in **If You Were the Medical Assistant** with your classmates, and answer the questions.

Answer the **Critical Thinking Questions** and discuss them with your classmates.

Visit the **Web sites** suggested and search for additional Web sites using **Keywords for Internet Searches.**

Complete the exercises in chapter 31 of the **Student Mastery Manual.**

View Legal, Ethical, and Professional Concepts; **Videotape:** "Antibiotic Reaction"

REVIEW & RECALL

1. What are the differences between equipment contained in a first aid kit and that found in the emergency box or crash cart in a medical office?

2. Differentiate between the problems encountered by a rescuer if the airway is blocked in a person who is conscious and in a person who is unconscious.

3. How soon should artificial respiration and/or cardiopulmonary resuscitation be started in order to prevent death of brain cells?

4. Describe two methods to administer oxygen to a patient. How does the medical assistant decide which method to use?

5. Describe the tissue layers involved in superficial burns, partial-thickness burns, and full-thickness burns.

6. Describe capillary, venous, and arterial bleeding, and give appropriate measures to control each.

7. What is the underlying problem in the medical condition called shock? Describe the underlying physiologic problem in six different types of shock.

8. What is the emergency care for a person complaining of chest pain?

9. Differentiate between the cause, signs and symptoms, and treatment of diabetic coma (diabetic ketoacidosis) and insulin reaction.

10. Identify information that should be available when calling the poison control center.

11. Describe the possible consequences to a victim of a bite by a poisonous spider or snake, or the victim of a wild animal bite.

12. Describe the emergency care of a victim of heat exhaustion, heat stroke, and hypothermia.

13. How should a splinter be removed from the skin?

IF YOU WERE THE MEDICAL ASSISTANT

On the way home from work, a medical assistant stops to assist a person who is lying on the ground after falling off a bicycle. The victim is a young woman who is lying on her side, unconscious. She appears to have a head injury, and is bleeding from the head, as well as from a wound on her left leg. A friend of the medical assistant goes immediately to call for help.

1. After assessing that it is safe to approach the person, what is the first action the medical assistant should take?

2. The victim is bleeding profusely from the wound on her left leg, above the knee. If she had injured an artery, what might the bleeding look like? If she had injured a large vein, what might the blood look like?

3. If direct pressure does not control the leg bleeding, to which artery should the medical assistant apply pressure?

4. If the victim is going into shock, what might the medical assistant observe? What should the medical assistant do?

5. Is there any other care the medical assistant should begin while waiting for an ambulance to arrive?

CRITICAL THINKING QUESTIONS

1. Why is it recommended that you give glucose to a diabetic who is confused, falling asleep, and not able to give an adequate history if you do not have the equipment available to perform a blood test?

2. Discuss why a parent is advised to call the poison control center immediately if he or she suspects that a child has ingested a poisonous substance. Why should the parent not immediately induce vomiting?

3. The American Heart Association has begun a plan to place automated external defibrillators (AEDs) in places where they are readily available in case of a cardiac emergency. If you have not already been trained in the use of an AED with your CPR training,

do research to find out how they work. What are the advantages and disadvantages of placing several AEDs in each community?

4. When should you call an ambulance if a person has had a seizure? Suppose a patient calls your office asking what to do if she sees a person she does not know having a seizure. Prepare a list of questions to ask the caller.

5. In France, there is a law that requires passers-by to stop and assist at the scene of an accident. Discuss the implications of this law with your classmates. Should such a law be adopted in the United States? Support your position with several reasons.

EXPLORE THE WEB

INTERNET WEB SITES

American Heart Association
www.americanheart.org

AHA Emergency Cardiovascular Care Program
www.cpr-ecc.org

American Red Cross—CPR Information
www.redcross.org/services/hss

Find Your Poison Control Center
www.aapcc.org/findyour.htm

First Aid and Poison Control Section
www.medicinet.com

First Aid and Self-Care Guide (Mayo Clinic)
www.mayohealth.org

KEYWORDS FOR INTERNET SEARCHES

automated external defibrillator (AED)
    CPR
    first aid
    emergency care
    good samaritan laws
    poison control

ANSWERS TO ON THE JOB

1. Typical symptoms of a medication reaction include swelling of the mouth and lips; difficulty breathing, wheezing, and increased respirations; increased pulse; and decreased blood pressure. Other signs and symptoms include anxiety, cyanosis, hives, edema of the face, flushed dry skin, nausea, and stomach cramping.

2. By asking the patient about allergies both to the specific medication and to antibiotics in general, office staff assumed that they had taken adequate precautions to identify allergies. Since Keith is 18, he is responsible for decisions about his own health care. In this case, however, asking his mother (with Keith's permission) and/or a more careful review of the medical record would have given more information to prevent the reaction.

3. Epinephrine is used as a bronchodilator and vasoconstrictor during anaphylactic reactions. It facilitates breathing and helps raise blood pressure to improve circulation.

4. After receiving epinephrine, the patient's pulse rate or blood pressure may rise to a higher level than is desired. If the epinephrine wears off, or if the dose was not high enough, the patient's symptoms may recur.

5. An allergy sticker should immediately be placed on Keith's chart. Any referrals or correspondence about Keith should note that he has a history of severe reaction to cephalosporins. Keith should be instructed to inform any health care providers about his allergy, noting that there are many different cephalosporin antibiotics and he is probably allergic to all of them. Keith should also be encouraged to wear a medical identification bracelet, since he might not be able to give information if he were injured in an accident.

Patient Teaching and Follow-up

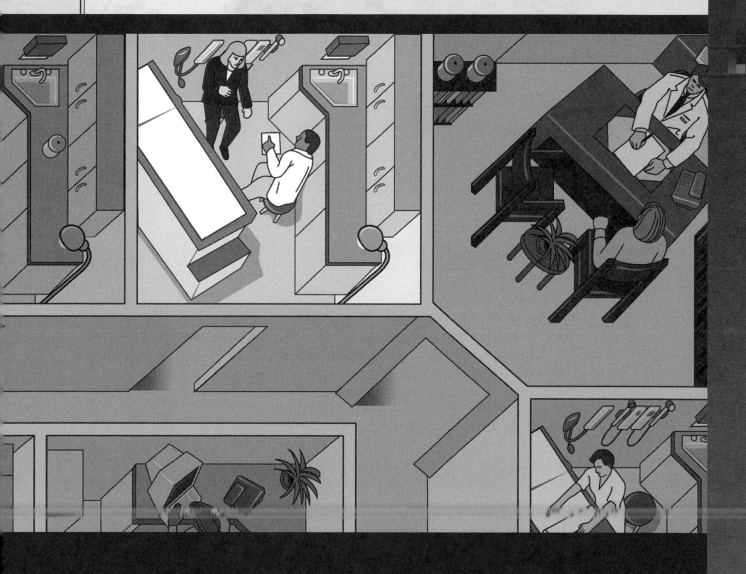

Chapter 32

Teaching Patients in the Medical Office

Instructional Objectives

After completing this chapter, you will be able to do the following:

1. Define and spell the vocabulary words.
2. Describe principles that are important for effective teaching and learning.
3. Differentiate between the three domains for learning and the implications for teaching and learning.
4. List the six steps of the teaching process.
5. Identify factors that require adaptation of teaching and may pose barriers to learning.
6. Discuss various teaching strategies and their appropriate use.
7. Prepare a written teaching plan, including learning objectives, topics, teaching methods, and evaluation methods.
8. Describe two methods of documenting planned teaching.
9. Describe the important information to teach a patient with a cast.
10. Differentiate between indications for and use of a cane, crutches, and a walker.
11. Describe the following gaits used with crutches: four-point, two-point, three-point, swing-to, and swing-through.
12. Identify the general areas of teaching needed to prepare patients for diagnostic tests and surgery.
13. Explain the kinds of teaching that the medical assistant may initiate about medications and medication regimens.

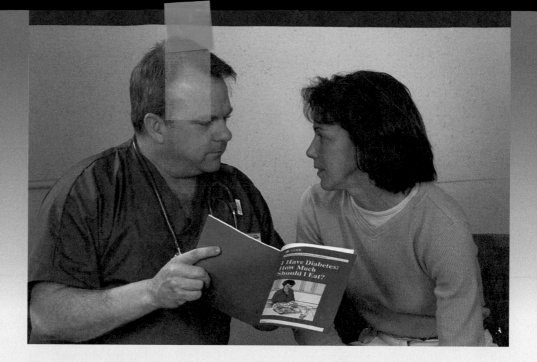

CMA/RMA CERTIFICATION
Content and Competencies

- Recognize and respond to verbal communications
- Recognize and respond to nonverbal communications
- Document appropriately

- Explain general office procedures
- Instruct individuals according to their needs
- Provide instructions for health maintenance and disease prevention
- Identify community resources

Performance Objectives

After completing this chapter, you will be able to do the following:

1. Teach a patient to use a cane (Procedure 32–1).
2. Teach a patient to use crutches (Procedure 32–2).
3. Teach a patient to use a walker (Procedure 32–3).

VOCABULARY

affective (p. 801)
axillary crutches (p. 811)
cognitive (p. 801)
forearm crutches (p. 812)

four-point gait (p. 812)
learning objective (p. 803)
platform crutches (p. 812)
psychomotor (p. 801)

swing-through gait (p. 813)
swing-to gait (p. 813)
three-point gait (p. 812)
two-point gait (p. 812)

weight-bearing status (p. 812)

ABBREVIATIONS

ADL (p. 805)

NSAIDs (p. 818)

OTC (p. 818)

INTRODUCTION TO TEACHING AND LEARNING

Changes in the nature of medical care are increasing the importance of patient education. More than ever before, patient education is now being conducted in office-based medical practices. Today, we see

1. Shorter hospital stays: This means more visits to the doctor's office by individuals who, a generation ago, would have remained in the hospital.
2. Increasingly portable medical devices: This means the ability to treat more chronic conditions in an out-patient or even a home environment rather than a hospital.
3. An aging population: This means a larger percentage of the patient population who live with chronic illnesses.

At the same time, payment methods such as capitation and productivity-based bonuses, as well as high overhead costs, are forcing doctors, nurse practitioners, and physician assistants to see more patients per day in the office, reducing the time they have to provide all of the teaching necessary.

These trends have combined to push an increasing amount of the patient education load onto medical assistants. Although this can seem a daunting task to some, patient education is one of the more fulfilling aspects of medical assisting today. Working continuously with a patient and his or her home-based caregivers (usually a life partner, parent, or child) to educate them about day-to-day care of a medical condition can lead to a satisfying ongoing relationship.

The medical assistant has two roles in patient education. One is to engage in an ongoing process to give all patients information about health, and to encourage them to make lifestyle choices that will improve their general health. The medical assistant also provides information or answers questions about procedures, diagnostic tests, and follow-up care for acute illness or injury. The second patient-education role is to provide intensive one-on-one education for self-care and self-management of chronic illnesses such as asthma, diabetes, or hypertension.

Principles of Teaching and Learning

People learn in a holistic manner. This means that they respond to all of the various aspects and stimuli of a situation, not merely to what is said or written. The consequence of this is that the teacher's tone of voice, body language, and general demeanor are as important as the information the teacher is trying to impart to the learner.

When learning, a person internalizes new information, ideas, emotions, and behaviors. Providing information is not enough; a patient educator must stimulate the learner, and get the learner to work with the new information, take ownership of that information, and work through feelings triggered by the material being learned.

An individual interacts with information in many ways: by seeing words written on a page; by hearing words coming from an educator; by watching a demonstration of a particular technique or process, either in person or on video; by performing the particular technique or process with assistance, either in person or in a simulation using educational technology; and performing the particular technique or process alone, then receiving feedback to improve performance.

Learning occurs when a person finds personal meaning that motivates him or her to learn. Many factors can inhibit this process, including lack of interest and failure to see the personal relevance (including denial of the underlying medical issue that necessitates the learning). Distractions—preoccupation with the physical, psychological, or social concerns that are more important at the time—or distaste for the teacher, learning environment, or particular activities being learned can also interfere with learning.

Retention of information improves when it is provided at the appropriate level for the learner to grasp and when it is presented in a clear, well-organized fashion that builds new learning on old learning, so that the learner sees how new learning fits with what has already been accumulated. Retention is also improved when the same information is presented through more than one modality (seeing, hearing, doing) and when it is repeated on more than one occasion. It is also reinforced when the learner is able to use the information to achieve personal goals.

Allowing the learner to become the teacher is also an effective way to get the learner to internalize and feel ownership of information. Having to articulate newly learned information is one of the most effective ways of learning. Children know this intuitively—they love nothing more than to teach their parents something they have recently learned in school, be it a new arithmetic technique or a new word. Doctors in training after medical school learn new information and skills through the "see one, do one, teach one" method. Even the first-year doctor in training is put in the position of supervising medical students so that he or she can teach what may have been learned only a few weeks earlier.

Domains for Learning

Individuals learn holistically; but for the purpose of educational theory, learning is divided into three areas, or domains. When planning a teaching exercise, the patient educator needs to make sure that he or she is presenting material so that all three domains will be stimulated. The three domains are:

1. Cognitive (thinking, reasoning, and remembering)
2. Affective (feeling)
3. Psychomotor (doing).

Cognitive

The **cognitive** domain covers what a person knows as information, expressed primarily in words. This includes knowledge or information, comprehension or understanding, and the use of knowledge as a basis for action.

Cognitive processes are intellectual processes. The processes used in the cognitive domain are *memory,* the ability to remember and recall information in the proper context; and *thinking,* the ability to use knowledge to analyze, plan, synthesize, and evaluate.

Memory is divided into short-term and long-term. An individual remembers items in short-term memory long enough to process it. After a short time, the information is either stored in long-term memory or forgotten. Repetition, restatement, and recasting of the information to take advantage of other senses helps refresh short-term memory and allows the information to become stored in long-term memory.

Affective

The **affective** domain refers to feelings, emotions, values, and attitudes. Although emotions occur naturally, each person learns how to respond to them differently, depending on life circumstances. Emotions and values are very important because they affect motivation, confidence, and how important things seem.

A medical assistant in a patient education environment must determine how much an individual's feelings or emotions are influencing his or her behavior, as well as his or her ability to retain, internalize, and take ownership of the learning.

A patient's emotions and attitudes can either facilitate or hinder effective learning of information important to maintaining health or caring for chronic illness.

Psychomotor

The **psychomotor** domain concerns motor skills and the ability to perform tasks and processes. In this domain, an individual learns through doing—watching and imitating, observing and practicing. Finally, the individual is able to perform the task or process independently. A teacher demonstrates, and a learner does a return demonstration.

Barriers to Learning

There can be barriers to learning in all three domains.

In the cognitive domain, impaired memory or poor cognition due to dementia, mental illness, or mental retardation can hinder learning. Language barriers also fall in the cognitive domain.

In the affective area, anxiety, failure to see a need for learning, and denial can be barriers. Different personal values can reduce motivation to learn. Other affective barriers include previous experiences, personal habits, cultural customs, poor coping skills, pain, and fatigue.

In the psychomotor domain, barriers include physical limitations such as tremor, paralysis, muscle weakness, and decreased vision or hearing. Some individuals have better coordination and fine motor control than others, allowing them to learn motor skills more easily.

Barriers to learning can also be created by external factors, such as distractions, noise, excessive heat or cold, and other environmental conditions.

THE TEACHING PROCESS

There are six steps in the process of creating and providing appropriate patient education, as illustrated in Figure 32–1.

1. Identify a need for teaching.
2. Assess the learner.

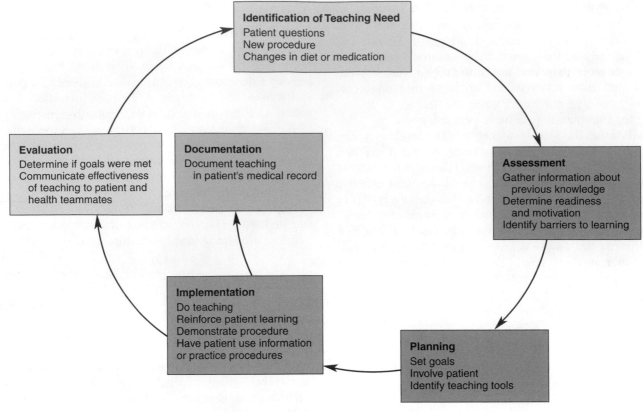

> Figure 32–1 The patient teaching process.

3. Plan activities to meet learning needs.
4. Implement teaching.
5. Evaluate effectiveness of teaching and learning.
6. Document learning outcomes.

Steps in the Teaching Process

Identify the Teaching Need

Identification of a teaching need comes from something the patient does or says. For example, a patient who has just had a Mantoux test asks "What happens next?"

If it seems that the patient does not fully understand what is occurring but is too shy or embarrassed to ask, the medical assistant may prompt the patient to admit he or she needs more information. For example, a patient may answer in the affirmative when asked if she knows how to provide a clean-catch urine specimen, but look puzzled when given the package of wipes and the specimen cups.

Finally, when a patient is newly diagnosed with a chronic illness, it is assumed that the individual needs education about the condition, daily care of the condition, and the medical regimen for treating the condition. For example, a newly diagnosed diabetic needs to learn about diet; taking medication; managing an exer-

cise regime; and caring for his or her skin, especially on the feet.

Assess What the Patient Knows and Feels

Before planning and implementing an appropriate education program for a particular patient, the medical assistant must assess not only what the patient knows about the subject, but also how motivated the patient is to learn, what particular learning skills the patient has, and what barriers might inhibit learning. From this, the medical assistant can utilize teaching tools that work well with the patient's strong skills (e.g. learning by doing, learning from pictures) while downplaying the patient's weaker learning skills (e.g. low reading comprehension).

In addition to speaking with the patient, the medical assistant can gather information about the patient's learning skills and potential from the doctor, from the patient's medical record, from family, and from other members of the health care team.

Plan the Learning Experience

The key to good learning is good planning on the part of the patient educator. The best patient educators are always planning, although their planning may be imperceptible to others and may be second-nature to themselves.

A plan can be as simple as deciding to give a particular patient a two-sentence response to a question. Or it can be as complex as the outlining of a multi-session education plan for a patient to learn to manage all aspects of care for his diabetes.

Planning involves identifying goals (desired outcomes), the actions that will be taken to meet those goals (teaching strategies), and the particular tools that will be used in conjunction with the teaching strategies. These might include brochures, information sheets, flip charts, videotapes, and (increasingly) CD-ROM-based simulation exercises.

The teaching plan should be broken down into discrete learning objectives that can be measured and evaluated.

One objective for a patient whose doctor has prescribed a low-cholesterol diet would be that the patient can identify 10 specific foods that are included in the diet and 10 specific foods that should be avoided. An additional objective would be that the patient can verbalize why adherence to this diet is important to manage cholesterol.

Implement the Learning

The actual teaching may be a verbal explanation or discussion; reviewing with the patient a sheet of written instructions, a pamphlet, or a brochure; demonstrating a procedure or process, then having the patient do a return demonstration; arranging to have a patient watch a videotape or use a simulation tool; or any combination of these techniques.

Teaching sessions are most effective when they are short and focus on a discrete set of tasks or activities. Material from the previous session can be repeated briefly at the beginning of the next session, then the session should move on to a new set of materials. If the patient needs to learn to perform a procedure, several sessions should be scheduled so the patient can practice, with coaching and encouragement from the medical assistant.

Whenever possible, standardized material should be used to promote consistency and accuracy of information. However, teaching of the information should be personalized for the particular patient. Personalization can be as simple as using the word "you" where the words "the patient" appear on a sheet of written material. Or it might mean explaining a particular piece of information using the patient's particular family characteristics as an example.

Whenever possible, use simple, straightforward language, brief descriptions, and short presentations. Use familiar words rather than technical terms, even to patients with above-average reading level and vocabulary. Ask the learner to rephrase what has been learned to see if he or she has grasped the concepts. Presenta-

tions should be friendly and sensitive, but given with confidence so the learner appreciates your expertise.

Evaluate Patient Retention

Goals and objectives need to be measurable so they can be evaluated.

Consider, for instance, the example of the patient on a low-fat, low-cholesterol diet. Here, the goal is for the patient to be able to follow the prescribed diet. If the teaching was appropriate, and the learner retained the information, he or she should be able to identify foods that are allowed and foods that should be avoided. If the patient's blood cholesterol falls from an elevated level to a normal level, there is evidence that the patient has benefited from the diet teaching.

In the more complex case of self-management of diabetes, the learning is divided into objectives, and each objective should be evaluated and measured individually in order to determine that the patient has mastered the goal of self-management.

Document the Learning

After instructing a patient, the medical assistant should document any teaching done, and identify statements and activities indicating that the patient has mastered the subject.

The bottom line is: "If it wasn't documented, it wasn't done."

Using Learning Objectives

The goal of patient education is to improve health, usually by changing behavior. Within the framework of this overall goal, it is helpful to describe specific, measurable behavior changes that demonstrate the learner's progress toward meeting the goal. Statements that describe these behavior changes are called **learning objectives,** sometimes referred to as instructional objectives, performance objectives, or behavioral objectives.

In this book, for example, a list of instructional objectives is introduced at the beginning of every chapter. These objectives describe what the student should be able to do after learning the material in the chapter. In addition, each procedure throughout the book includes a performance objective, which describes the task to be performed. In the *Student Mastery Manual,* additional information is given about performance objectives, namely the conditions under which a task will be performed and the criteria used to determine satisfactory performance.

Use of learning objectives helps the learner to know exactly what is expected, and helps the educator evaluate how effective his or her teaching has been. When preparing to teach, it is helpful to develop a set of learning objectives first. This will be demonstrated in practice later in the chapter.

Adapting Teaching to the Individual Learner

A number of factors go into adapting standard material to be used with a particular learner. These include the learner's age and developmental stage, level of education, culture, and any physical or mental impairment.

Developmental Stage

People learn in different ways as they pass through different stages of growth and development. For instance, young children learn by experiencing and by incorporating learning into play. The learner's develop-mental stage has a profound effect on the teaching methods that should be used for the most effective learning. Table 32–1 provides a summary of how people learn at different developmental stages.

Level of Education

An individual's level of education affects the type of written information that should be used. Highly educated individuals may prefer detailed written material; but those with lower educational attainment may need brief written materials cast in simple language, with many illustrations to reinforce the written message.

Table 32–1	Teaching and Learning at Different Stages of Development
Ways of Learning	**Effective Teaching Methods**

Infant

Uses senses to explore environment

Learns to trust when held securely, when changes are introduced slowly, and when shown love and acceptance

Help the infant learn to trust his or her environment by holding securely, speaking softly, and allowing time for visual and tactile exploration.

Toddler

Learns to use language to communicate but still tends to express feelings through behavior

Uses play to explore environment and imitation to learn new behavior

Use simple words and brief explanations.
Use play to teach a procedure.
Allow for imitation and play.
Praise reinforces desired behavior.

Preschooler

Still learning to use language correctly

Still tends to express feelings through actions rather than words

Asks questions to learn about environment

Use role playing, imitation, and play to teach.
Use short sentences but reinforce with demonstration.
Encourage questions.

School-Age Child

Learning to think about information abstractly

Can memorize facts, safety rules, and procedures

Judgment improves

Learns from observation, discussion, reading, and experimentation

Discussion can be reinforced by pamphlets, videos, and other visual aids, but level of language must not be too complex.
Allow time for questions.
Evaluate learning by having child summarize information or demonstrate skills.

Adolescent

Can analyze, compare, make decisions, and solve abstract problems

Emotionally challenged to adapt to body image changes and manage intense feelings

Wants to be responsible for self, but judgment may need development

Demonstrate problem-solving skills.
Provide privacy and autonomy.
Help to learn about feelings; demonstrate acceptance of intense feelings.
Encourage responsible decision making about health issues.

Young and Middle-Aged Adult

Has reached full cognitive development, but may be overwhelmed by family, occupational, and social responsibilities

Allow participation in setting goals and determining appropriate learning activities.

Older Adult

May have decreased vision, hearing, mobility, and strength.

Ability to think, remember, and control emotions may be decreased

Usually needs longer time to respond and more repetition to remember

Treat with dignity; but use simpler language and louder and slower speech if necessary, and allow time to respond.
Teach in short sessions and observe for signs of fatigue such as irritability or failure to pay attention.

Cultural Factors

Cultural factors include both the issue of English as a second (or foreign) language and the ways in which different cultures look at the experience of obtaining medical care as well as the lifestyle effects of various cultures.

Written patient education materials should be available in any language spoken by a significant proportion of the office's patient population. Of course, it is difficult for any medical practice to have materials in every conceivable language a patient may speak. But if more than 10 to 15 percent of the patient population speaks a particular language other than English, at the very least basic patient education materials on nutrition, smoking, and hypertension should be available. In addition, the office should have either bilingual educators or access to translation services for patient education.

As important as language is the issue of cultural impact on lifestyle. This is especially important with regard to nutrition and hypertension. Food is a distinguishing factor in many cultures, and dietary changes that mean moving away from cultural "comfort foods" can have a profound effect on the dynamics of an entire household. The family cook may agree to reduce salt, cook with vegetable oil instead of butter or fat, and substitute chicken and fish for red meat. But all of the food consumers, not just the patient, may resent the changes, both for the loss of cultural distinction in the new diet and for the changes in family power structure the changes may signal.

Physical or Mental Impairment

Physical impairment affects the way in which patient education is conducted; and in many instances, it also necessitates education in ways to adapt to impairment.

Adaptive devices are available to assist the physically impaired perform many activities of daily living (**ADLs**). Occupational therapists and occupational assistants teach patients with severe physical impairments. However, medical assistants can help patients with minor physical impairments adapt their activities or learn to use adaptive devices.

Consider, for example, the patient with severely arthritic hands. A medical assistant can help such a patient learn how to use Velcro-fastened shoes or elastic shoe laces. (Elastic laces are tied once, after which the patient can simply slip the shoes on.) Or think about a diabetic patient with failing vision. The medical assistant can help such a patient learn how to use a device that attaches to a syringe and magnifies the markings.

A medical assistant may work with a patient with failing memory, teaching him or her how to keep track of pills using a weekly pill container, as shown in Figure 32–2. The individual, or a caregiver, can set up the week's regimen of pills in the container. If the pills are still in the slot for Tuesday, and it is Tuesday

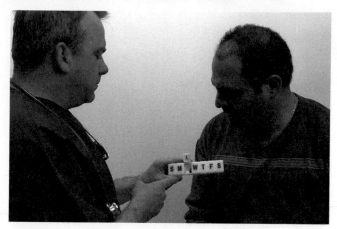

> **Figure 32–2** Medical assistant demonstrating the use of a weekly pill container.

night, then the patient knows he or she needs to take that day's medication.

Teaching Strategies

A good teacher is a good learner. As a medical assisting student, you can watch your teachers closely to pick up particular teaching strategies they are using and try to think about how those strategies can be utilized for educating patients in the medical office. Seven specific teaching strategies may be useful:

1. One-on-one instruction
2. Group instruction, or lecture
3. Discussion
4. Demonstration
5. Role playing
6. Watching a videotape or film
7. Using programmed study materials.

One-on-One Instruction

One-on-one instruction should be brief and focused. It might be a one-time interaction about diagnostic tests, or it might be a series of structured sessions explaining a new dietary regime.

Multi-session one-on-one instruction should be supplemented with written materials, such as posters, pamphlets, instruction sheets, and fact sheets. These materials form the basis for the session's teaching, and they give the patient something to take away for reinforcement. Figure 32–3 shows a medical assistant using brochures as teaching aids.

Group Instruction

Group instruction is an efficient use of an instructor's time when a number of learners need the same information. Group instruction also gives learners an

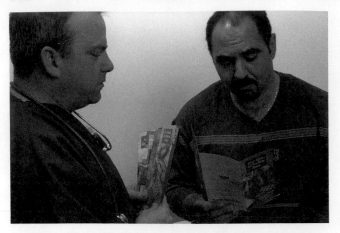

➤ **Figure 32–3** Medical assistant using brochures to teach a patient.

opportunity to meet others having the same interests or facing the same issues.

Although group instruction may reduce the amount of individualization—unless one-on-one sessions are also scheduled with the group participants—it offers learners a chance to learn from one another as well as from the instructor.

Discussion

Discussion encourages active participation by the learner. It also facilitates emotional adaptation to the particular issues being addressed in the learning, as the learner works out issues for him- or herself.

Demonstration

Demonstration is important for the psychomotor domain of learning. Usually, the teacher demonstrates a particular skill or task, then the learner practices and demonstrates for the teacher while the teacher coaches and corrects.

Demonstration is a technique widely used in the education of medical assistants to learn particular skills, from taking a blood pressure to entering patient information into a computer. During your own education, pay attention to how teachers use demonstration. Notice especially how they make demonstration a one-on-one activity and how they utilize discussion in conjunction with demonstration, so students can ask questions and understand the reasons for each step involved in the task or activity.

Role Playing

Role playing allows individuals to prepare for a particular situation by acting out the roles of different participants in the interaction, and by acting out various solutions to the situation as various responses are made. Many people are uncomfortable using role play-

ing, but it should be utilized whenever possible to help an individual try out more than one way to respond to a given situation.

Role playing is used in medical assisting education when one student plays the medical assistant and another plays the patient.

Watching a Videotape or Film

Watching a videotape or film can provide information. But more importantly, it helps put information into the context of real-life events. Watching a video or film allows the student to see what something looks like, or how a particular task is undertaken in the real world.

Follow-up is imperative when using visual presentations. The best videos are the ones that prompt the viewer to want to ask questions or discuss elements of the video. The videos that accompany this text were developed specifically to be paused at particular points for follow-up class discussion.

Using Programmed Study Materials

Programmed study materials come either as paper-and-pen kits or as software, delivered either as a CD-ROM or, increasingly, downloaded directly from educational Web sites. Programmed study materials are designed for the individual learner to move at his or her own pace. The best materials are designed to engage the learner in forwarding his or her own learning. The potential weakness of programmed study materials is that they do not give learners answers to individual questions.

Computer study materials are becoming ever more sophisticated. Many include text, video clips, animation, and activities that reinforce learning.

Obtaining Written Materials to Give to Patients

Written materials for patient education are available from a host of sources. National organizations that advocate for treatment of particular diseases—such as the American Heart Association, Juvenile Diabetes Society, or Crohns and Colitis Foundation of America—usually distribute their educational materials free or at minimal cost to doctors' offices. In addition, many commercial companies produce patient education materials and sell them to health-care facilities. These companies sometimes provide comprehensive materials that include instructor materials, fact sheets and brochures, videos, and self-instruction software.

Many offices have a display in the waiting room that contains general patient education materials. More specific materials are usually kept in a set of patient-education-material files. If you see a good piece of

ON THE JOB

Kathy Anderson, a medical assistant at Blackburn Primary Care Associates, has been asked to teach Warren Blake, a 23-year-old newly diagnosed insulin-dependent diabetic, to measure his blood sugar using a glucometer.

QUESTIONS
1. State an overall goal for this teaching in patient terms.
2. List each skill Mr. Blake must learn in order to measure his blood sugar (psychomotor domain).
3. Identify the information Kathy has to teach Mr. Blake so he understands why he must test his blood and how he should interpret the results (cognitive domain).
4. What does Mr. Blake need to understand in order to motivate him to follow up and test his blood glucose level at home?
5. How will Mr. Blake's emotions affect his ability to learn and assume responsibility for managing his illness (affective domain)?

---

patient education material in another office or in a library, take one for your office if you can, or at least note the sponsoring organization and try to obtain some copies.

Preparing a Written Teaching Plan

Because the time for teaching a patient is often very limited, it is important that a medical assistant have a written teaching plan. Such a plan gives you a reference for complex teaching needs rather than having to remember all of the teaching plan steps. In addition, you may be involved in planning for teaching that is to be carried out by other members of the health care team.

The better the planning—and the clearer the written teaching plan—the more effective the teaching can be, because all individuals involved with teaching will be working from the same planning document and presenting the patient with the same material.

A written teaching plan need not be a complex document. If the time for teaching is limited, and all the material is to be presented at one patient visit, the plan may simply be a set of points that need to be made. If the teaching will take more time, and will be undertaken over many visits, the plan should be developed so that new material presented to the patient at each visit expands upon material presented at earlier visits.

Although parts of a teaching plan are generic— meaning they are used for every patient—the plan should be individualized based on the patient's level of education, previous knowledge about the subject, and specific teaching needs.

Parts of a Written Teaching Plan

A written teaching plan has five parts:

1. The general goal. The goal may be anything from total self-care to assisting a caregiver, to recognizing signs and symptoms that would necessitate a telephone consultation with the doctor's office.
2. Topics to be covered. This lists all the topic areas that will be covered and the order in which they will be covered.
3. Learning objectives. This describes what the patient should know and/or be able to do after the teaching is completed.
4. Teaching methods and resources. Resources can include discussions, written patient education, demonstrations by the medical assistant and practice by the patient, as well as other techniques.
5. Evaluation methods. This answers the question of how the patient and medical assistant know if the teaching has been effective.

A teaching plan is summarized in the box, "Teaching Plan for a Patient with Right Leg Cast."

Documenting Planned Teaching

The teaching plan may contain a section for documentation, or the documentation may be entered as a note in the patient's medical record. For the example of the patient with the lower-leg cast, (Box 32–1), teaching should be documented at the time the cast is applied, at the time the patient is scheduled for cast removal, and again when the cast is removed.

Teaching Plan for a Patient with Right Leg Cast

Patient information: Henry Folger, 22-year-old male with closed fracture of distal right fibula. Fiberglass cast applied to right lower extremity. To be discharged on crutches, non-weight-bearing for 48 hours, partial weight-bearing for 2 weeks.

Teaching goal: Patient will manage fracture by caring for cast correctly and using ambulatory aids properly, so that bone healing occurs without complications.

Material to be taught: Process of bone healing, cast care, proper use of crutches, follow-up care, cast removal, skin care following cast removal, strengthening exercises.

Learning Objectives	Teaching Method/ Audiovisual Aids	When Teaching Planned	Evaluation Methods/ Indications That Teaching Effective
Patient demonstrates understanding of fracture and process of bone healing	Instruction Patient's x-ray(s) Picture of bone healing	Before discharge with cast	Patient explains how healing occurs
Patient demonstrates understanding of cast and fracture care instructions during first 24 hours: a. Elevation b. Use of ice packs c. Non-weight-bearing d. S & S to report	Instruction using Cast Care Instruction sheet	Before discharge with cast	Patient able to verbalize that instructions have been understood Patient does not return with excessive swelling under cast Patient does not require stronger pain medication than take-home prescription
Patient demonstrates knowledge of cast care: a. Keep dry; use plastic bag to shower b. Keep elevated if possible c. Do not varnish or paint d. Do not poke sharp objects under cast	Instruction using Cast Care Instruction sheet	Before discharge with cast	Patient verbalizes understanding of instructions Patient does not return with broken, wet, painted cast or drainage from under cast Patient's skin is not excoriated when cast removed
Patient demonstrates understanding of progressive weight-bearing status	Instruction Demonstration/return demonstration of non-weight-bearing, partial weight-bearing, and full weight-bearing	Before discharge with cast After follow-up x-ray and doctor's permission to advance	Patient demonstrates non-weight-bearing and partial weight-bearing Follow up x-ray shows healing as expected Patient demonstates full weight-bearing
Patient demonstrates correct use of crutches	Instruction Demonstration/return demonstration	Before discharge with cast After progression to full weight-bearing	Patient demonstrates ability to use crutches correctly No complications due to incorrect use of crutches
Patient describes timing and process for removing cast	Instruction	At follow-up visit when cast removal is planned	Patient returns for cast removal as scheduled without undue apprehension
Patient demonstrates understanding of proper skin care after cast removal	Instruction	When cast removed	Patient's skin regains normal elasticity and color after cast removed
Patient demonstrates understanding of exercises to regain mobility and strength after cast removal	Instruction Instruction sheet with recommended exercises Demonstration/return demonstration	When cast removed	Patient regains normal mobility and strength in right lower extremity

Another method of documentation is a checklist that identifies areas of teaching and allows for documentation that teaching has been performed. Such checklists are often used in hospitals, especially when a patient requires extensive teaching. After the teaching has been completed, the checklist is incorporated into the patient's medical record. Figure 32–4 shows such a checklist, which might accompany the teaching plan outlined in the box on the previous page.

Evaluating Teaching Effectiveness

A checklist is a useful tool if it includes a section for evaluating teaching effectiveness.

One common method of evaluating teaching effectiveness is to have the patient or other learner verbalize understanding. Ideally, this should be more than a simple statement of understanding or not understanding. If the learner can repeat the directions or explana-

---

CAST CARE AND CRUTCH WALKING

Patient Name __Henry Folger__

Family Member __Ø__

Date Teaching Initiated __8/16/XX__

PI = Patient instructed
D = Demonstration by staff
PI = Family member instructed
V = Patient verbalizes understanding
RD = Patient returns demonstration

Topic	PI	D	FI	V	RD	Comments
Understanding of Condition Fracture	JH 8/16			SR8/16		
Bone Healing	JH 8/16			SR8/16		
Cast Care - first 24 hours elevation	SR8/16			SR8/16		
Use of ice packs	SR8/16	SR8/16		SR8/16	SR8/16	
Circulation checks	SR8/16	SR8/16		SR8/16	SR8/16	
S&S to report	SR8/16					
Cast Care - general Keep dry	SR8/16			SR8/16		Seems to have good understanding
Plastic bag to shower	SR8/16			SR8/16		
Elevate if possible	SR8/16			SR8/16		
Don't varnish or paint	SR8/16			SR8/16		
Don't poke anything under	SR8/16			SR8/16		
Weight bearing status None (24 hours)	SR8/16	SR8/16		SR8/16	SR8/16	
Partial (until MD orders)	SR8/16	SR8/16		SR8/16		
Full (when MD orders)						
Crutch walking 3-point gait	SR8/16	SR8/16		SR8/16	SR8/16	has used crutches before
Stairs	SR8/16	SR8/16		SR8/16	SR8/16	
Use of 1 crutch						
Cast removal Process						
Timing						
Follow up after cast removed Skin Care						
Exercises						

➤ **Figure 32–4** Checklist to document teaching for cast care and crutch walking.

tion, the teacher can be more certain that the learner truly understands the concepts.

If a skill has been taught, the learner should perform the skill for the teacher. This is called a return demonstration. When a learner is able to demonstrate how to do something, the teacher can be sure that learning has occurred.

Documentation of teaching should include the results of the evaluation, both for the sake of good patient care and as part of an effective risk-management program. The health care team is responsible for providing effective instruction to promote healing and prevent injury following diagnostic procedures and treatments, or when patients are discharged with casts or ambulatory aids.

Documentation that indicates understanding of instructions and ability to perform skills before discharge helps the medical office avoid liability if the patient for some reason fails to follow instructions, resulting in injury or complication.

DISCHARGE INSTRUCTIONS FOR CAST CARE

Memorial Hospital

Patient Name

Casts are applied to keep your extremities protected, stable, and immobile so that your injury can heal properly. There are two types:

- Plaster (durable, strong, and hardens in 48 hours)
- Fiberglass (strong, lightweight, hardens in 2 hours, cannot be walked on for 24 hours)

Dos and Don'ts

1. DO elevate the injured extremity. Keep your cast raised on pillows, above the level of your heart.
2. DO apply an ice bag to reduce the swelling and pain.
3. DO NOT stand on your cast or rest it against a hard surface until it is completely dry.
4. DO NOT get cast WET under any circumstances.
5. DO NOT scratch under the cast. Scratching can irritate skin and may cause bleeding and infection.
6. DO NOT decorate and seal your cast. Coverng the cast with paint or varnish prevents air from circulating. When air circulation is impaired, the skin under the cast can break down.

Excercises and Activities

1. Wiggle your fingers or toes back and forth to maintain circulation. This will promote healing and reduce swelling and stiffness.
2. Use a sling or crutches as instructed by your doctor.
3. Check with your doctor before resuming normal and strenuous activities or returning to work or school.

Special Instructions

If you encounter any problems in following these instructions, or if any of the following conditions occur, please report to your physician.

1. Extreme pain or tightness requiring more medication than was prescribed at the time of discharge.
2. Numbness, swelling, or tingling of the toes or fingers.
3. Fingers or toes that are cold to the touch or dark in color.
4. A skin rash or open sore that is oozing from the edges of the cast and creating a strong odor.
5. A fever.
6. Sharp edges on the ends of the cast.
7. A wet, broken, or cracked cast.

➤ Figure 32–5 Cast care instruction sheet.

TEACHING A PATIENT TO CARE FOR A CAST

Cast-care instructions are important for several reasons. If the cast is too tight, it may impair circulation. If this occurs, fingers (in the case of an arm cast) or toes (leg cast) may be uncomfortable at first. But once circulation has been interrupted, the nerve endings no longer transmit impulses and stop hurting, although tissue damage due to lack of oxygen and nutrients continues.

The patient, or a family member, needs to check circulation, especially in the first 24 hours after the cast has been put on, by checking for movement of fingers or toes, and for color (pink is good, but blue or a dark color should be reported to the doctor immediately).

A family member should be enlisted to remind the patient to keep the extremity elevated, to keep ice packs around the cast, and to encourage the patient to wiggle the fingers or toes.

For a cast on an ankle or leg, the patient must be told when he or she can put weight on the cast, and how much weight can be put on the extremity. The patient should also understand how to care for the cast, and when to return for follow-up care. After the cast has been removed, the patient may need physical therapy or an exercise plan to help strengthen muscles and improve joint mobility.

Figure 32–5 is a cast-care instruction sheet.

TEACHING A PATIENT TO USE ASSISTIVE DEVICES FOR AMBULATION

A number of musculoskeletal diseases and conditions, as well as traumatic injuries, can force a patient to use an assistive device for walking.

Whenever an assistive device is to be used, the patient and a family member should be taught how to use the device safely and effectively.

Cane

A cane is the least cumbersome of the assistive devices for ambulation. It also offers the least support. Canes are useful to assist an individual to maintain balance, or when one leg is weak.

There are two types of canes—a standard cane and a quad cane.

A standard cane may be made of wood or aluminum. A wooden cane must be properly matched to the individual's height in order to provide proper support. Aluminum canes are usually adjustable. The bottom of the cane is covered with a rubber tip, so the cane does not slip on smooth surfaces.

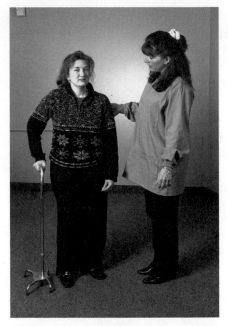

> **Figure 32–6** Patient being taught to use a quad cane.

A quad cane has four feet at the base. This makes the cane more stable, and offers the individual more support. It also makes the cane heavier. Quad canes are aluminum and adjustable. They have a rubber tip at the bottom of each foot. Figure 32–6 shows a patient using a quad cane.

Whether a single-footed cane or a quad cane is used, the cane should be sized by making sure the top of the cane is even with the patient's hip. Metal canes can usually be adjusted at the bottom.

An individual should hold the cane in the hand opposite from the affected leg. The elbow should be bent 20 to 30 degrees for best support. With each step, the affected leg should advance 12 to 18 inches. Then the unaffected leg should be brought forward slightly ahead of the cane.

Procedure 32–1 describes in detail teaching a patient to use a cane.

Crutches

Crutches are devices that have handgrips. They are made of aluminum or wood, and are usually used in pairs. There are three types of crutches: axillary, forearm, and platform.

Axillary crutches can be made of aluminum or wood. They are adjustable. The top of each crutch rests under the axilla, and they are held with handgrips. This is the most common type of crutch used by people who have suffered an injury to the leg, and who will use crutches for a period of weeks or perhaps months.

PROCEDURE 32-1

Teaching a Patient to Use a Cane

Performance Objective: The student will be able to teach a patient to use a cane.
Supplies and Equipment: Cane.

Procedure Steps

1. Identify the patient and explain the procedure
   Rationale: Understanding the need for teaching increases motivation.
2. Instruct the patient to hold the cane on the strong side of the body, opposite the weak extremity.
   Rationale: It will improve the patient's base of support to have the cane on the side opposite the weakest leg.
3. Be sure the top of the cane reaches to the patient's hip (so that the elbow is slightly flexed). If the height is incorrect, adjust the cane.
4. Instruct the patient to move the cane forward about 6 inches.
   Rationale: Moving the cane before the affected leg provides more support. The patient can also move the cane with the affected leg, which allows for a more normal gait.
5. Instruct the patient to move the affected leg forward to be parallel to the cane.
6. Instruct the patient to move the unaffected leg forward about 6 inches ahead of the cane.

7. Ask the patient to demonstrate walking with the cane, following Steps 4 to 6, and make corrections after observing the patient if needed.
   Rationale: By observing how the patient uses the cane, the medical assistant can assess the patient's understanding of the instructions.
8. Document in the patient's medical record that the patient was instructed in the proper use of a cane.

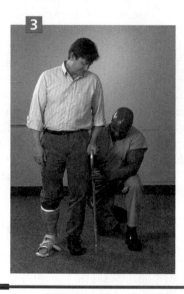

Forearm crutches—also called Canadian or Lofstrand crutches—are always made of aluminum. They are adjustable. They are held in the hands, and have a metal cuff that fits around the forearm. Forearm crutches are usually used by people who always need crutches for balance and support. Figure 32–7 shows a patient using forearm crutches.

Platform crutches have a shelf-like device, with straps to support the forearms, and handgrips. Platform crutches are used by people with poor arm strength.

Figure 32–8 illustrates the different types of crutches.

Crutches can be used in several different ways. A medical assistant needs to know what is appropriate to teach each patient. This is usually based on the doctor's orders, as well as the patient's **weight-bearing status,** meaning whether the patient must keep the affected leg completely off the floor (non-weight-bear-

ing), or whether he or she may put some weight on the affected leg (partial weight-bearing).

Crutches can be used in a four-point, three-point, or two-point gait:

Four-point gait: Each crutch and each leg is moved separately. This method is used for partial weight-bearing on both legs, when both legs need some support.
Three-point gait: Both crutches are moved along with the affected leg. The affected leg can be either non-weight-bearing or partial weight-bearing.
Two-point gait: Each leg is moved along with the opposite crutch. This method is also used when both legs need some support. The two-point gait provides less support than the four-point gait, but is a much faster method of ambulation.

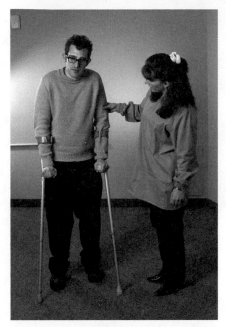

➤ **Figure 32–7** Medical assistant teaching a patient to use forearm crutches.

Two other methods for using crutches are the swing-to and swing-through gaits. In the **swing-to gait,** both crutches are moved forward, then both legs are swung up to a position even with the crutches. In the **swing-through gait,** both crutches are moved forward, then both legs are swung through, to a position ahead of the crutches.

In either the swing-to or the swing-through gait, both legs must be weight-bearing. Figure 32–9 shows the various gaits for crutch use.

When using stairs, an individual can either hold the handrail and place both crutches under one arm, or can use both crutches. When going up stairs, the individual should use the crutches and/or rail for support, move the unaffected leg up, then bring up the crutch and the affected leg. Going downstairs, the crutches and affected leg move down first, followed by the unaffected leg.

Procedure 32–2 describes in detail teaching a patient how to use crutches.

Walker

Walkers are made of aluminum. They provide excellent support. They have either two wheels or two rubber-tipped feet in front, about 2 feet apart, and two rubber-tipped feet in the rear, a little wider apart. At the top, there is either a grab bar or two handgrips to hold onto.

Most walkers are adjustable. The individual's elbows should be bent 20 to 30 degrees for maximum support. Either picking up the rear legs and rolling forward or picking up the entire walker and placing it forward, the patient should move the walker about 18 inches to 2 feet ahead, then, holding the grips, step forward toward the walker.

Procedure 32–3 describes in detail teaching a patient to use a walker.

Text continued on page 818

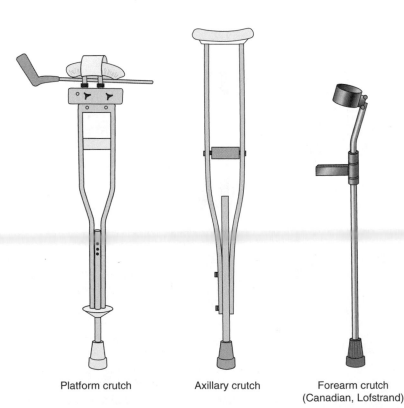

Platform crutch   Axillary crutch   Forearm crutch
(Canadian, Lofstrand)

➤ **Figure 32–8** Types of crutches.

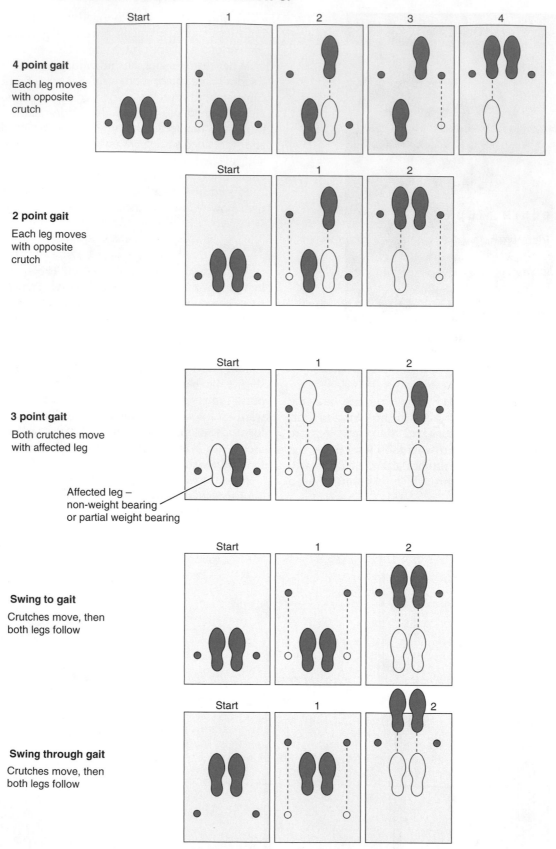

➢ **Figure 32–9** Gaits for use with crutches.

PROCEDURE 32-2

Teaching a Patient to Use Crutches

Performance Objective: The student will be able to teach a patient to use crutches.
Supplies and Equipment: Crutches.

Procedure Steps

1. Identify the patient and explain the procedure
   Rationale: Understanding the need for teaching increases motivation.
2. Adjust the crutches to fit the patient. When the patient is standing in normal footwear with the crutches about 2 inches in front of the feet and about 4 inches to the side of the feet, the shoulder rests should come to a point approximately 11/2 to 2 inches below the axilla. The elbow should be slightly bent when the patient grasps the handgrips. Both the length of the crutches and the height of the handgrips can be adjusted by removing the wingnuts and bolts, inserting the bolts into lower (or higher) holes and replacing the wingnuts.
   Rationale: The top of each crutch should be supported by the side of the chest. If the crutch is too long, it can put pressure on the brachial plexus (a concentration of nerves under the axilla), possibly causing paralysis. The handgrip should be at the proper height for the patient to use the crutches without fatigue.
3. Check the height of the crutches after they have been adjusted. You should be able to insert two fingers above the top of the crutch below the patient's axilla.
4. Instruct the patient to stand with the crutches about 4 inches to the side of the legs and 4 to 6 inches ahead of the foot. Verify that the patient is placing the correct amount of weight on the affected leg according to the doctor's orders: none if non-weight-bearing; less than 50 percent if partial weight-bearing, and as desired if full weight-bearing.
   Rationale: Placing the crutches out to the side and somewhat ahead of the center of the foot provides a wide base of support.
5. Instruct the patient to move the crutches and legs to achieve the proper crutch gait, as illustrated in Figure 33–9. The four-point gait or the two-point gait is used for partial weight bearing on two weak extremities. The three-point gait is used for non-weight-bearing or partial weight-bearing on one extremity. The swing-to and swing-through gaits are used for patients wearing braces on the lower extremities and/or patients with severe prob-

Procedure continued on following page

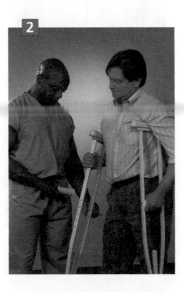

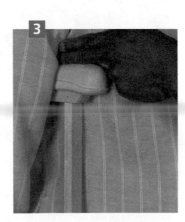

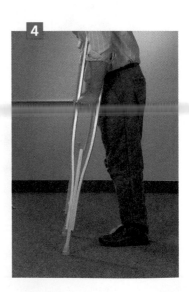

PROCEDURE 32–2 *(continued)*

lems of both lower extremities (such as paralysis.)

6. Demonstrate the gait for the patient; then guide the patient to use the gait, coaching the patient through each step.
   Rationale: Demonstration helps the patient form a mental picture of the activity. Performing the activity with coaching allows the patient to learn the correct steps.

7 As an example, if teaching the three-point gait for a patient who is non-weight-bearing on the right extremity, instruct the patient to move the crutches about 6 to 8 inches ahead of the body and to move the right knee forward while holding the right foot elevated.

8 Then instruct the patient to support his/her weight with his/her hands on the handgrips of the crutches and bring his/her good leg even with the crutches.

9. Allow the patient to practice using crutches until the patient is able to ambulate correctly. Correct the patient if necessary.
   Rationale: Supervised practice allows a person to master a motor skill.

10 When the patient can ambulate comfortably, teach the procedure for going up and down stairs. To ascend, the patient should support his or her body weight on the crutches on

the lower stair, place the good leg on the upper stair, and raise the body on the good leg.

11. To go down stairs, the process is reversed. The crutches and bad leg go down first and support the body weight while the good leg is lowered.

12. Document the patient's weight-bearing status, the crutch gait taught, and that the patient was able to demonstrate the gait correctly.

Charting Example	
Date	
11/28/XX	2:00 PM Pt. with Ⓡ leg cast,
	non-weight-bearing, instructed in
	crutch walking using 3-point gait
	on level surfaces and stairs. The pa-
	tient verbalized understanding that
	he should keep all weight off of the
	right leg, and he was able to demon-
	strate correct use of the crutches.
	—————— Kevin Jones, RMA

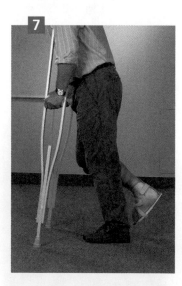

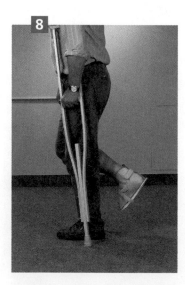

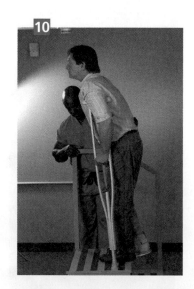

PROCEDURE 32–3

Teaching a Patient to Use a Walker

Performance Objective: The student will be able to teach a patient to use a walker.
Supplies and Equipment: Walker.

Procedure Steps

1. Identify the patient and explain the procedure
   Rationale: Understanding the need for teaching increases motivation.
2. Adjust the height of the walker so that the patient can hold it comfortably when standing with the walker slightly ahead of his or her body. The elbows should be slightly bent.
   Rationale: When the handgrips of the walker are at a comfortable height for the patient, the walker can be used to greatest advantage.
3. Instruct the patient to pick up the walker using the handgrips and move it forward about 6 inches.
4. After setting the walker down securely, the patient should walk forward into the cage of the walker. He or she holds onto the handgrips for support.
5. While standing, the patient should pick up the walker and move it ahead again. Caution the patient to be sure that he or she has good

balance before picking up the walker to move it.
   Rationale: It takes a certain amount of strength to advance the walker, and the patient must be careful not to lose his or her balance when the walker is off the ground.
6. If the patient does not have the strength to lift the walker, obtain the type of walker that has wheels at the two front supports. To advance this type of walker, the patient must only lift the two back legs and push the walker forward.
7. Observe the patient practicing with the walker.
   Rationale: By observing how the patient uses the walker, the medical assistant can assess the patient's understanding of the instructions.
8. If the walker folds for storage, demonstrate how to fold it and ask the patient to return the demonstration.
   Rationale: A return demonstration helps the medical assistant to determine that the patient knows how to fold the walker for storage.
9. Document in the patient's medical record that the patient was instructed in the proper use of a walker.

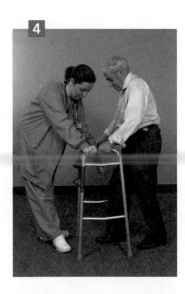

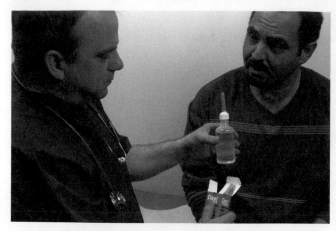

➤ **Figure 32–10** Medical assistant showing a patient how to use a Fleet enema.

PREPARING FOR DIAGNOSTIC PROCEDURES

Generally, before a diagnostic procedure, the patient must be instructed as to what the procedure is, where it will be performed, how long it will take, how to prepare for the test, and what will happen after the test. Often, the medical office schedules the test and keeps preparation instruction sheets on hand to give to patients. The medical assistant needs to become familiar with preparation for frequently ordered tests, but should check with the testing facility if he or she is unsure about that facility's particular preparation protocols.

Preparation for x-rays often requires dietary or bowel preparation, especially when they involve the gastrointestinal or urinary tract. The patient needs to understand what diet to follow and how to prepare the bowel, including what supplies are needed and where to purchase them. Various laxatives used in bowel prep are available without a prescription at the drugstore. Single-use hypotonic enemas, under the brand name Fleet enema, are also available at the drugstore without a prescription. Figure 32–10 shows the medical assistant explaining the use of a Fleet enema to a patient.

Sometimes a prescription tablet or suppository is used. Figure 32–11 shows a bowel preparation sheet for a barium enema, which can be used as a model for teaching.

See Instructing Patients for Procedures That Require Dietary Restrictions and/or Bowel Preparation.

Preparation for blood tests may require that a patient fast. For example, a lipid profile usually requires an 18-hour fast, and an overnight fast is standard for a fasting blood sugar. Other blood tests are repeated at regular intervals; for example, a prothrombin time is repeated monthly for patients taking the anticoagulant Coumadin. Patients on anticoagulants need to know where, when, and how to follow up to find out if the test showed that their medication level is appropriate, or if the dosage needs to be changed. A patient having a strep test should not be taking any antibiotics, or the test results will not be accurate. Patients should be taught about how your office follows up on their tests, and when they should call for results.

Instructions for imaging tests vary. For a pelvic ultrasound, the bladder needs to be full. For an MRI (magnetic resonance imaging) or mammogram, the patient needs to be reminded not to wear any metal products. For an MRI, a woman cannot even wear makeup that may contain metal flakes. For mammograms, the woman should not use any antiperspirant on the underarm or under her breasts.

Some tests require that the patient stop any medications or avoid certain foods in the days before the test, and patients need specific instructions when these tests are scheduled.

TEACHING RELATED TO MEDICATION

The medical assistant plays an important role in management of patient medications. Although the doctor or other primary care provider instructs the patient about medications, the medical assistant may need to reinforce these instructions, and may need to act as a liaison by informing the doctor if the patient has any questions regarding the medication regimen and by relaying prescriptions to a pharmacy. The medical assistant also reinforces information about proper use of medication, such as continuing to take the entire prescription even after feeling better, as is the case with antibiotics; taking with food, as is the case with some antibiotics and most nonsteroidal anti-inflammatory drugs (**NSAIDs**); or eating foods high in potassium, as is necessary when taking diuretics.

Also, the medical assistant may work with a patient to establish a method for making sure medication is taken as prescribed; the medical assistant may even be involved in helping the patient find assistance to pay for expensive medication.

When giving a patient a medication sample or a prescription the doctor has written, the medical assistant needs to remind the patient about any possible side effects that should be reported to the office. He or she should know if there are over-the-counter (**OTC**) medications that can cause medication interactions and warn the patient not to use them while taking the prescription. In addition, the medical assistant should also know about OTC medications the doctor recommends in particular situations.

INFORMATION FOR PATIENTS SCHEDULED FOR TESTS AT MEMORIAL HOSPITAL:

PATIENT'S NAME: _____

PROCEDURE: BARIUM ENEMA

DATE: _____

PREPARATION: CHECK IN AT OUTPATIENT REGISTRATION 15 MINUTES
                      BEFORE TEST.

BARIUM ENEMA WITH AIR

1. 12:00 NOON – LUNCH – Eat only the following:

   1 cup of boullion soup with crackers.
   1 chicken or turkey white meat sandwhich (no
   butter, mayonaise, lettuce or other additive).
   1/2 glass clear apple juice or clear grape juice.
   1 serving plain Jello (no cream, fruit, or other
   additive).
   1 glass of skimmed or nonfat dry milk.

2. 1:00 PM   Drink at least one full glass or more of water,
                    clear juice or soda.

3. 3:00 PM   Drink at least one full glass or more of water,
                    clear juice or soda.

4. 4:00 PM   Drink one 11 ounce bottle of Magnesium Citrate (cold).
                    Can be purchased from your local Pharmacy.

5. 5:00 PM – DINNER – Eat only the following:

   1 cup of boullion soup
   1 glass of clear apple juice or clear grape juice.
   1 serving of plain Jello (no cream, fruit or other
   additive).

6. 7:00 PM   Drink at least one full glass or more of water, clear juice
                    or soda. Take 3 biscodyl tablets (can be purchased from
                    your local pharmacy) with at least one full glass or more
                    of water.

7. Before Bed   Drink at least one full glass or more of water, clear juice
                    or soda.

8.   Nothing to eat or drink after midnight.

Take 1 ounce of Milk of Magnesia after all barium studies (UGI, BE, Small
Bowel) unless otherwise indicated by M.D.

➤ **Figure 32–11** Sample preparation sheet for barium enema.

Before making any recommendations regarding medication, the medical assistant should review the procedure manual and any other written guidelines the office has. Some medical offices and other facilities have instruction sheets for their medical assistants to use with specific medications. These sheets, prepared by a licensed health care professional, include specific points for instruction, including the patient's understanding of the medication's proper use, the medication's actions, coping with side effects, adverse reactions to report to the office, and how to assure understanding of follow-up lab work that may be necessary.

Pharmacies also have instruction sheets they often give to patients when a prescription is filled. The medical assistant should encourage patients to read these instruction sheets.

FOCUS ON
INSTRUCTION

INSTRUCTING PATIENTS FOR PROCEDURES THAT REQUIRE DIETARY RESTRICTIONS AND/OR BOWEL PREPARATION

Many diagnostic tests and surgical procedures require the patient to follow special instructions the day before. If the procedure is scheduled by the medical office, the office must also give any necessary instructions to the patient. The patient should understand what the test or surgery is for, how long it is expected to take, where to check in, and what kind of preparation is required. Diet sheets, bowel preparation sheets, and general information sheets can be obtained from the facility that will give the test and be reproduced to give to patients. The patient also needs to be told where to purchase laxatives, enemas, or other supplies. Any female patient scheduled for X-ray must be questioned about the possibility of pregnancy, and instructed to delay X-ray examination if she might be pregnant.

Common Terms

NPO (nothing by mouth)	Nothing to eat or drink
Clear liquids only	Only liquids such as water, clear broth, soda, apple juice, and sports drinks such as Gatorade; no milk or juices with visible residue such as orange juice
Fat-free meal	A meal made with food that contains very little or no fat and no added butter, margarine, or cooking oil, such as baked or boiled potato without butter or margarine, broiled white meat of chicken with skin removed before cooking, vegetables without butter or margarine, fruits, juice, or soda
Laxative	A medication that loosens the bowels and causes the bowels to evacuate. As a preparation for a gastrointestinal X-ray, the goal is to empty the bowels completely. *Examples* *Magnesium citrate*—the patient drinks an entire 8-ounce bottle, which can be purchased at the drugstore. It tastes better chilled or with ice. *Castor oil*—two tablespoons (30 cc); small containers can be purchased at the drugstore. Mix in orange juice for better taste. *Dulcolax tablets*—take one or two as directed. *Milk of magnesia*—sometimes the patient is instructed to take one or two tablespoons in the evening after the test was performed to help remove barium from the GI tract.
Suppository	A medication administered by rectum; glycerine suppositories and Dulcolax suppositories cause the rectum to contract and evacuate its contents.
Enema	A solution introduced into the rectum. As a preparation for a gastrointestinal procedure, usually the patient purchases one or more Fleet enemas which can be self-administered. The enema, which should be retained for 10 to 15 minutes, draws fluid into the rectum and stimulates evacuation.

Summary of the Process for Instructing Patients

1. Schedule the test or surgery for the patient (or assist the patient to schedule).

2. Give patient the instruction sheet used by the facility where the test has been scheduled

3. Discuss how to obtain laxatives, enemas, suppositories, and other supplies needed as part of the bowel preparation. The patient should verbalize understanding of how to obtain needed medications or supplies and how to use them properly.

4. Go over dietary restrictions. The patient should verbalize understanding of dietary restrictions.

5. Answer any questions the patient has about preparation for the diagnostic test or surgery.

STUDENT STUDY PLAN

To reinforce your understanding of the material in this chapter . . .

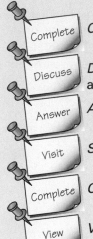

Complete the **Review & Recall** questions.

Discuss the situation in **If You Were the Medical Assistant** with your classmates and answer the questions.

Answer the **Critical Thinking Questions** and discuss them with your classmates.

Search for **Web sites** using **Keywords for Internet Searches**.

Complete the exercises in chapter 32 of the **Student Mastery Manual**.

View Patient Education with Special Populations **Videotape,** Part 2: "Cast Preparation and Cast Care".

REVIEW & RECALL

1. Identify six principles that promote effective learning.

2. Describe the three domains for learning: cognitive, affective, and psychomotor.

3. Identify specific ways the three domains for learning affect the teaching and learning process.

4. Give an example of each of the six steps in the learning process.

5. Describe how to adapt teaching for patients of different developmental stages.

6. Give examples of factors that may make teaching and learning difficult in the medical setting.

7. Describe seven teaching strategies and give one example when each might be used.

8. Identify the parts of a written teaching plan.

9. Describe two ways planned teaching can be documented.

10. List the key points to teach a patient who is going home with a cast.

11. Describe the correct use of a cane and a walker.

12. Compare the following crutch gaits: two-point, three-point, four-point, swing-to, and swing-through. What kind of support and weight-bearing status does each involve?

13. Explain the medical assistant's role in teaching patients about diagnostic tests and following medication regimes the doctor prescribes.

IF YOU WERE THE MEDICAL ASSISTANT

You have been asked to prepare a teaching plan for Julie Herman, a 22-year-old woman whose right knee has been immobilized in a removable lower-leg brace following an injury. There was no fracture, but tendons and muscles supporting the knee have been torn and/or strained.

The doctor has asked you to provide Julie with crutches to support ambulation. She can bear weight on the right leg as tolerated. The doctor wants Julie to wear the leg brace at all times when out of bed (except for a daily shower) for the next four weeks, when she should return to the office.

Prepare a detailed teaching plan. Include instructions about wearing the brace and about using both the four-point and two-point crutch gait. Also include teaching activities and ways you will evaluate the effectiveness of the teaching.

Finally, identify what you will chart in the medical record after teaching Julie.

CRITICAL THINKING QUESTIONS

1. Describe your own learning style. Do you learn best in the cognitive, affective, or psychomotor domain? Discuss your learning strengths and weaknesses with your classmates.

2. Discuss the following statement. "Learning occurs when a person finds personal meaning that motivates him or her to learn." Agree or disagree with the statement, and give examples and reasons to support your position.

3. Discuss the advantages and disadvantages of creating written teaching plans for patients with teaching needs.

4. Why is it important to be sure that any patient using an ambulatory aid such as a cane, crutches, or walker has been given complete instructions?

5. What could happen if a patient using crutches did not understand their correct use, or his or her weight-bearing status?

EXPLORE THE WEB

KEYWORDS FOR INTERNET SEARCHES

teaching
> learning
> ambulatory aids
> crutches

ANSWERS TO ON THE JOB

1. The overall goal describes what you want the patient to be able to do after the teaching is complete. The goal might be formulated as follows: The patient will be able to test his/her blood sugar using a glucometer, and modify daily insulin doses and/or food intake, based on accurate results.

2. The patient must learn the following skills: How to perform a fingerstick; how to transfer a drop of blood to the reagent strip; how to insert the reagent strip into the glucometer; how to time the reading; how to read the result; how to keep records of results; how to verify the calibration of the glucometer; and how to care for the glucometer and strips.

3. Warren Blake needs to learn how diabetes affects blood glucose levels and how insulin helps lower blood glucose. He also needs to know the normal values of blood glucose and the amount of insulin his doctor wants him to take if his blood glucose is low, normal, and high.

4. To motivate Warren to monitor his blood sugar at home, he needs to understand why good control of blood sugar is crucial to prevent diabetic ketoacidosis, hypoglycemia, and the complications of diabetes. In addition, he has to accept that he must be responsible for managing his diabetes for the rest of his life.

5. If Warren cannot accept his diagnosis (if he is in denial), he may not pay close attention to the teaching, and he may forget to carry out the steps he has been taught. If he is very anxious, he will be unable to focus on details of the teaching, and will not be able to retain information. If he becomes depressed, he may show lack of interest in teaching, and also lack the energy to push himself to test his blood sugar and/or give himself insulin regularly. If Warren is highly competitive, he may try to learn everything as well, and as fast, as possible to bolster his self-image as a person who is extremely capable.

Maintaining Health: Nutrition, Exercise, and Self-Examination

Instructional Objectives

After completing this chapter, you will be able to do the following:

1. Define and spell the vocabulary words for this chapter.
2. Identify components of a healthy diet and sources of nutrition.
3. Discuss types and contents of restricted and modified diets.
4. Identify recommendations for exercise in the healthy individual.
5. Explain how to perform range-of-motion exercises.
6. Describe how to teach breast self-examination and testicular self-examination.
7. List teaching needs of patients with diabetes mellitus.
8. Compare and contrast learning needs of patients with insulin-dependent diabetes mellitus (IDDM) and non-insulin-dependent diabetes mellitus (NIDDM).

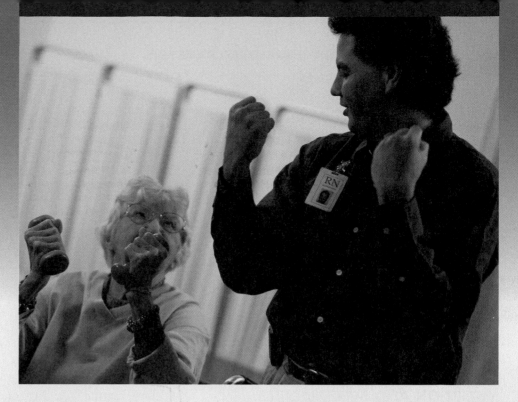

- Recognize and respond to verbal communications
- Recognize and respond to nonverbal communications

- Document appropriately
- Instruct individuals according to their needs
- Provide instructions for health maintenance and disease prevention

Performance Objectives

After completing this chapter, you will be able to do the following:

1. Teach patients and/or family members to perform range-of-motion exercises (Procedure 33–1).
2. Teach female patients to perform breast self-examination (Procedure 33–2).
3. Teach male patients to perform testicular self-examination (Procedure 33–3).

VOCABULARY

abduction (p. 834)
active exercise (p. 833)
active-assistive exercise (p. 835)
adduction (p. 834)
adipose (p. 829)
aerobic (p. 833)
beta cells (p. 842)
calorie (p. 831)

diabetes mellitus (p. 837)
eversion (p. 834)
extension (p. 834)
glucometer (p. 840)
flexion (p. 834)
hypoglycemia (p. 840)
hyperextension (p. 834)

insulin reaction (p. 842)
inversion (p. 834)
isometric (p. 833)
isotonic (p. 833)
ketoacidosis (p. 840)
oral hypoglycemic (p. 842)
passive exercise (p. 833)

polydipsia (p. 840)
polyphagia (p. 840)
polyuria (p. 840)
pronation (p. 834)
range of motion (p. 833)
rotation (p. 834)
supination (p. 834)

ABBREVIATIONS

HDL (p. 828)   IDDM (p. 840)   LDL (p. 828)   NIDDM (p. 840)   ROM (p. 833)

NUTRITION AND SPECIAL DIETS

The medical assistant needs basic knowledge in order to instruct patients on the many facets of a healthy lifestyle. Patients need teaching in five common areas: nutrition and special diets, exercise, self-examination, preparation for diagnostic procedures, and taking medication.

In May 2000, the U.S. Department of Agriculture released the fifth edition of its booklet *Nutrition and Health: Dietary Guidelines for Americans*, which makes the following recommendations:

1. Aim for fitness. This means maintaining a healthy weight and being physically active each day.
2. Build a healthy base. This means using the food pyramid as the guide for food choices; eating a variety of grains daily, especially whole grains; and eating a variety of fruits and vegetables daily.
3. Choose sensibly. This means choosing a diet low in saturated fat and cholesterol, and moderate in total fat; choosing beverages and foods to moderate sugar intake; and choosing and preparing foods with less salt.
4. Use alcohol in moderation, if at all.

Food Guide Pyramid

The food pyramid is designed in the following manner. The number of servings recommended is based on a mature man weighing approximately 175 pounds. Smaller adults and children should adjust these suggestions accordingly. The food pyramid is illustrated in Figure 33–1.

Grains are on the bottom of the pyramid, forming the base. Grains, which should make up the base of a healthy diet, include bread, rice, cereal, and pastas. An individual should have 6 to 11 servings of grain daily.

One serving is a slice of bread, one cup of ready-to-serve cereal, or one-half cup of cooked cereal, rice, or pasta.

The next tier of the pyramid is fruits and vegetables. An individual should have three to five servings of vegetables and two to four servings of fruit each day. A vegetable serving is one cup of raw leafy vegetables; one-half cup of other vegetables, either cooked or raw; or three-quarters of a cup of vegetable juice. One fruit serving is a medium apple, pear, orange, or banana; one-half cup of chopped, cooked, or canned fruit; or three-quarters of a cup of fruit juice.

At the third tier of the pyramid, an individual should have two to three servings of dairy products and two to three servings of meat, poultry, or other protein. A dairy serving is one cup of milk or yogurt; 11/2 ounces of natural cheese, such as cheddar or swiss, or 2 ounces of processed cheese. A protein serving is 2 to 3 ounces of cooked lean meat, poultry, or fish. One-half cup of cooked dry beans or tofu, a 21/2-ounce soyburger, one egg, or two tablespoons of peanut butter are equivalent protein servings.

At the top of the pyramid are fats, sweets, and oils, which should be consumed sparingly.

Major Nutrients Needed by the Body

The body needs nutrients from six different classes to function:

1. Carbohydrates
2. Fats/lipids
3. Proteins
4. Vitamins
5. Minerals
6. Water.

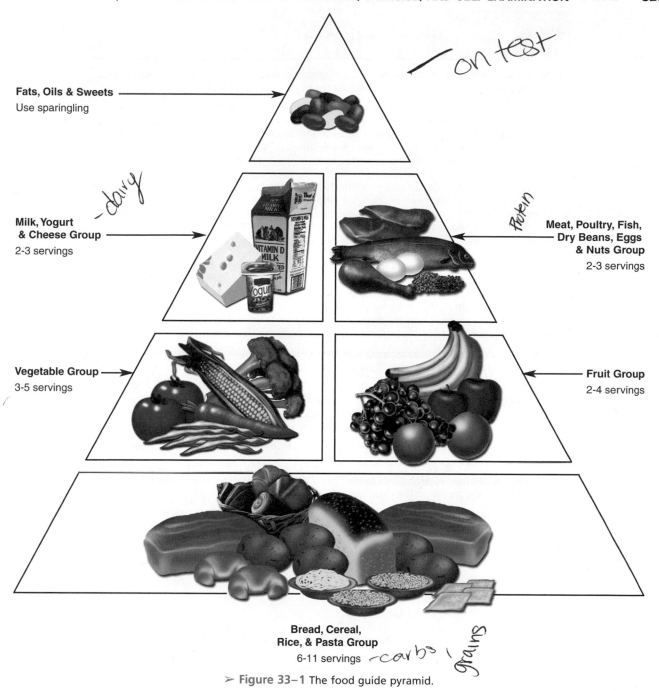

Fats, Oils & Sweets
Use sparingling

on test

dairy

**Milk, Yogurt
& Cheese Group**
2-3 servings

Protein

**Meat, Poultry, Fish,
Dry Beans, Eggs
& Nuts Group**
2-3 servings

Vegetable Group
3-5 servings

Fruit Group
2-4 servings

**Bread, Cereal,
Rice, & Pasta Group**
6-11 servings *carbs* *grains*

➤ **Figure 33–1** The food guide pyramid.

Carbohydrates

Carbohydrates provide 4 calories per gram (a calorie is a unit of measure for heat energy).

Carbohydrates are found in two forms—sugars and starches—which are the easiest foods for the body to break down into usable energy. Simple sugars, such as glucose or fructose, can be used without further digestion. Disaccharides (two simple sugars joined together) are easily broken down. Lactose (found in cow's milk) and sucrose (table sugar) are disaccharides. Starches are complex carbohydrates composed of many sugar molecules joined together.

Carbohydrates can be thought of as the basic fuel for the body, like gasoline for a car. Carbohydrates are also needed to metabolize fats. When consumed in the proper quantities, carbohydrates power the body while proteins are used for building and rejuvenating tissues. Without enough carbohydrates, proteins must be used to supply energy.

Healthy sources of carbohydrates are milk, fruits, vegetables, and grains. Fruits and vegetables provide many simple carbohydrates, while whole grain breads and cereals provide many of the complex carbohydrates. Foods high in sugar, such as candy, syrups, and

Table 33–1	Fats, Cholesterol and Lipoproteins

Names for different types of fats refer to the chemical structure of the fatty acids, which are combined with glycerol to form the most common types of dietary fat.

Saturated fats contain fatty acids with single bonds between the carbon atoms. These fats come from animal products and are usually solid at room temperature.

Unsaturated fats contain fatty acids with at least one double bond in the carbon chain. These fats come from plant products and are usually liquid at room temperature.

    Monounsaturated fats contain one double bond in the fatty acid chain. Examples are olive oil, peanut oil, and canola oil.

    Polyunsaturated fats contain two or more double bonds in the fatty acid chain. Examples are sunflower oil, soybean oil, corn oil, and safflower oil.

Hydrogenated fats have hydrogen atoms pumped into unsaturated oils; this saturation makes the resulting compound more solid at room temperature. Hydrogenated fats, such as margarine behave like saturated fats in cooking and in the body, but do not contain cholesterol.

Trans fatty acids are hydrogenated fats in which the hydrogen atoms have moved to the opposite side of the carbon chain. From 17 to 25 percent of the fatty acids in margarine are trans fatty acids. Trans fatty acids tend to raise blood cholesterol.

Omega-3 family of fatty acids is a group of polyunsaturated fatty acids found in fish such as halibut, herring, salmon, and mackerel. These fatty acids are being studied for their possible role in reducing blood cholesterol and diminishing the risk of heart disease.

Cholesterol is a natural body substance. It causes problems when it forms deposits on the arterial walls; these deposits, called plaques, can narrow or block arteries, especially those that supply the heart muscle.

Cholesterol belongs to a class of compounds known as sterols, which are present in all animal fats. Cholesterol is synthesized by the body, but it is also eaten in food from animal sources. Foods obtained from plants never contains cholesterol.

Lipoproteins carry fats in the bloodstream, both those from dietary sources and those manufactured by the liver.

HDL—high-density lipoproteins (also called "good" cholesterol)—collect cholesterol throughout the body and transport it to the liver for excretion in bile

LDL—low-density lipoproteins (also called "bad" cholesterol)—carry cholesterol to body cells. This activity is needed for formation of hormones and cell membranes, but a high level of LDL predisposes to excessive deposits of cholesterol within the walls of arterial cells, where it tends to form atherosclerotic plaques.

---

desserts, supply carbohydrates, but often without other essential nutrients. If eaten beyond an individual's caloric needs, the extra calories are stored as fat.

An inadequate intake of carbohydrates forces the body to use fat and protein for energy. This can impair proper metabolism and reduce body fat and/or protein to an unhealthy level.

Fats/Lipids

All fats, whether saturated or not, provide 9 calories per gram. Table 33–1 describes the chemical structure and characteristics of different types of fats, cholesterol, and lipoproteins.

Fats are essential in a healthy diet, and should not be totally eliminated. If all fats are removed from the diet, linoleic acid deficiency results, because the body does not manufacture linoleic acid.

Fats are classified based on their degree of saturation. Most saturated fats are solid at room temperature, while unsaturated fats (both monounsaturated and polyunsaturated) are liquid at room temperature. A large intake of saturated fats has been linked to heart disease and stroke.

Cholesterol is a lipid that is manufactured by the body; it is also consumed in foods. The body uses cholesterol to make bile and certain hormones.

Some fats exist inside the body as compound lipids. Lipoproteins, for example, are made up of a lipid and a protein. Because lipoproteins have been linked to heart disease, a lipid panel is one of the common blood tests performed during adult physicals.

Low-density lipoproteins (**LDLs**) are the main transporter of cholesterol; thus, they are considered "bad" because they raise the level of cholesterol in blood serum. High-density lipoproteins (**HDLs**) serve to lower cholesterol levels in blood serum by carrying cholesterol to the liver. Hence, HDLs are considered "good."

Fats provide a concentrated form of energy, either for use or for storage. Adequate intake of fat allows proteins to be used for building and rejuvenating tissue, rather than for energy. A healthy amount of fatty (**adipose**) tissue provides protection for internal organs against blunt trauma injury and insulates the body against rapid temperature changes.

Most saturated fat is consumed via beef, hard yellow cheese, butter, and oils that contain saturated fats such as palm and coconut oil. Monounsaturated fats are found in oils such as peanut or olive oil. Polyunsaturated fats are found in oils made from safflower, corn, or sunflower. Cholesterol is found only in animal products, especially in organ meats and egg yolks.

Diets too low in fat can lead to sensitivity to cold, an increase in infections, and amenorrhea in women. Long-term fat deficiency can lead to metabolic problems and fat-soluble vitamin deficiency.

Diets too high in fat have been linked to breast and colon cancer as well as heart disease and stroke. It is recommended that dietary fat provide less than 30% of daily calories and that saturated fats and hydrogenated fats be avoided because they tend to raise serum cholesterol levels.

Proteins

Proteins provide 4 calories per gram. After water, protein is the substance that makes up the bulk of the human body. Proteins are formed from amino acids, which are classified as either essential or nonessential. Essential amino acids must be brought into the body through food intake because the body does not manufacture them on its own.

Foods that have enough essential amino acids to support body growth are said to have proteins that are high-quality, high-biologic-value, or complete. Eggs, dairy products, meat, fish, and poultry all have complete proteins. Foods that do not have all the essential amino acids are called incomplete protein foods. Legumes, grains, and nuts are incomplete protein foods. It is recommended that foods containing incomplete proteins be combined in a meal, as in a recipe for rice and beans.

Protein is a component of all cells in the body; as such, the basic job of proteins is to build and repair body tissue. When the diet is deficient in protein, it is difficult for the body to maintain itself.

Vitamins

Although it has been known for centuries that certain diseases were related to dietary nutrients, the first chemical isolation of organic nutrients (vitamins) occurred in the early part of the 20th century.

The first substance isolated, thiamine, was called a "vitamine" because it was necessary for life (from the Latin *vita*, meaning "life giving") and had the chemical structure of an amine, a nitrogen-containing compound. Some of the additional essential organic compounds that were discovered were not amines, so the name of this entire group of nutrients was changed to vitamin.

Each vitamin is necessary in very small amounts, but a deficiency can prevent normal body function. Table 33–2 identifies the dietary sources and major functions of vitamins.

Fat-soluble vitamins, such as vitamins A, D, E, and K, are stored in fatty tissues and the liver. Vitamin A contributes to vision and healthy nerve sheaths. Vitamin K is important in blood clotting. Either a deficiency or an excess can cause physical abnormalities.

Water-soluble vitamins (B vitamins and vitamin C) are not stored in the body, so they must be ingested daily. B vitamins are important for blood and nerve cell formation. Vitamin C is required for healthy skin and is an important factor in the formation of connective tissue, such as muscles and cartilage, as well as for the maintenance of healthy blood vessels.

Minerals

Minerals are inorganic elements needed by the body in large or small amounts for proper function. Minerals needed in large amounts, sometimes called macronutrients, include calcium, magnesium, phosphorus, potassium, sodium, and sulfur. These macronutrients are important for the development of teeth and bones, for body structure, and as electrolytes for body functions such as nerve transmission.

Table 33–3 shows the minerals needed by the body.

The recommended intake of calcium depends on age and gender. Women need more calcium than men do, especially adolescent girls and post-menopausal women.

Calcium is naturally found in dairy products such as milk, yogurt, and natural cheese; in dark green leafy vegetables such as spinach and kale; and in canned fish with soft bones such as sardines and salmon. Many products today also have calcium added artificially, including fruit juices, breakfast cereals, and tofu made with calcium sulfate.

Another important mineral is iron. Although the body does not need a large amount of iron, iron deficiency is one cause of anemia. Iron-rich foods include shellfish, lean meats, dark-meat turkey, sardines, and spinach. Some foods have iron added in their preparation, including enriched and whole grain breads, and ready-to-eat cereals with added iron.

Table 33–2	Fat-Soluble and Water-Soluble Vitamins	
Vitamin	**Dietary Sources**	**Major Functions**
Fat-Soluble Vitamins		
Vitamin A (carotene)	Yellow and green leafy vegetables; milk, cheese, butter	Component of visual pigment; maintenance of epithelial tissue
Vitamin D	Cod liver oil, eggs, fortified dairy products	Increases absorption of calcium; promotes growth of bones
Vitamin E	Seeds, green leafy vegetables, margarine	Acts as an antioxidant to prevent cell membrane damage
Vitamin K	Green leafy vegetables; pork	One of the factors that help blood clot
Water-Soluble Vitamins		
Vitamin B_1 (thiamine)	Pork, organ meats; whole grains, legumes; yeast, wheat germ	Helps the body release energy from metabolism of amino acids and fats
Vitamin B_2 (riboflavin)	Whole grains, green leafy vegetables; milk, eggs; organ meats	Helps the body release energy from metabolism of carbohydrates, amino acids, and fats
Niacin	Liver, lean meats; grains, legumes	Combines to act as a coenzyme in metabolic reactions
Vitamin B_6 (pyridoxine)	Meats; vegetables; whole grain cereals	Helps build body tissue; helps in protein metabolism
Pantothenic acid	Lean meats; vegetables, fruits; whole grains, legumes	Helps the body release energy from metabolism of carbohydrates and fats
Folacin (folate, folic acid)	Legumes, grains; green vegetables	Helps in the production of genetic material and red blood cells
Vitamin B_{12} (cobalamin)	Muscle meats; eggs, dairy products	Helps in the production of genetic material, functioning of the nervous system, and metabolism of amino acids and fats
Biotin	Legumes, vegetables; meats	Helps in fat synthesis, amino acid metabolism, and formation of glycogen
Vitamin C (ascorbic acid)	Citrus fruits, tomatoes, green peppers	Essential for the structure of bones, cartilage, muscle, and blood vessels. Helps maintain capillaries and gums

Water

Water makes up 50 to 60 percent of adult body weight. As such, it is the most important nutrient. Water acts as a solvent for nearly all the chemical reactions that take place in the body. It maintains the balance of all body fluids. Water between cells reduces friction. Finally, water helps regulate body temperature by evaporating through the skin as perspiration.

All liquid foods contain water, as do solid foods. Meats are half water, and fruits and vegetables are more than half water. The body's metabolic processes also produce water.

Water deficiency is called dehydration. Dehydration occurs when the individual is not taking in enough water; it can also occur because of vomiting, diarrhea, hemorrhage, or profuse sweating.

Restricted and/or Modified Diets

Every medical office should have on hand instruction sheets for commonly prescribed diets. These should be available in English and whatever other languages are spoken by a large percentage of patients in the practice. There are five common diets for which instruction sheets should be available:

1. Liquid diet

2. Low-calorie, low carbohydrate, weight-loss diet

3. Sodium-restricted diet

4. Low-fat, low-cholesterol diet

5. Fiber (restricted-fiber and high-fiber) diets.

Table 33–3	**Minerals Needed by the Body**	
Minerals	Dietary Sources	Functions
Major Minerals		
Calcium	Milk, cheese, dark green vegetables	Bone and tooth formation, blood clotting, nerve transmission
Phosphorus	Milk, cheese, meat, poultry, grains, fish	Bone and tooth formation, acid-base balance
Potassium	Leafy vegetables, cantaloupe, lima beans, potatoes, bananas, milk, meats, coffee, tea	Acid-base balance, fluid balance, nerve transmission
Sodium	Table salt	Acid-base balance, body water balance, nerve function
Sulfur	Present in dietary protein	Acid-base balance, liver function
Chloride	Table salt	Important part of extracellular fluids
Magnesium	Whole grains, green leafy vegetables	Acts in protein synthesis
Minor Minerals		
Iron	Eggs, lean meats, legumes, whole grains, green leafy vegetables	Hemoglobin formation
Iodine	Marine fish and shellfish, iodized salt, vegetables	Formation of thyroid hormone
Trace Minerals		
Zinc, copper, selenium, fluorine, chromium		

Liquid Diet

A liquid diet is necessary before certain diagnostic tests of the gastrointestinal tract, and for a period of time after diarrhea or other medical problems.

Clear liquids include water, apple juice, and clear broth. Sports drinks (not red-colored) are also considered clear liquids, and are often prescribed after diarrhea to increase intake of electrolytes.

Full liquids include cranberry juice and juices with pulp (orange or grapefruit).

After a diarrheal illness, an individual will make a transition from clear liquids to full liquids to soft foods to solid food.

Special liquid diets are also sometimes used for weight loss, using commercial preparations to provide maximum nutrition while restricting calories. Long-term liquid diets should be monitored by a doctor.

Low-Calorie, Low-Carbohydrate, Weight-Loss Diet

A **calorie** (in scientific terms, a large calorie or kilocalorie) is the amount of heat needed to raise the temperature of 1 kilogram of water (a little more than 1 quart) by 1 degree Celsius.

When calorie consumption exceeds metabolic needs, excess nutrients are converted to fat, which is stored in the body. When calorie intake decreases below the body's needs, fat is burned for energy, resulting in weight loss. A traditional method of promoting weight loss has been by counting calories of foods consumed and maintaining intake at a level low enough to result in continued weight loss.

Recently, diet management has been moving away from counting calories. Rather, food intake is managed by increasing the amount of whole grains, fruits, and vegetables consumed and decreasing sugars and fats.

Sodium-Restricted Diet

A sodium-restricted diet can vary from a no-salt-added diet to a complete restriction on using sodium for food preparation. A specific sodium-restricted diet would be ordered by the doctor.

Moderate sodium restriction is recommended as part of an overall plan to control high blood pressure. Sodium is an element in table salt, but it is also found in many other foods. Thus a patient must not only refrain from adding salt to food, but must also avoid foods containing salt, especially fast foods and prepared foods.

Reducing sodium involves careful shopping, careful cooking and eating at home, and extreme care when eating away from home.

At the store, fresh, plain frozen, or salt-free canned vegetables are best, as are fresh or frozen fish, shellfish, poultry, and meats, rather than canned or processed varieties.

At home, in addition to reducing the amount of salt used in cooking and not using extra salt at the table, use of condiments such as soy sauce, ketchup, mustard, pickles, and olives should be reduced, and spices should be used instead of salt.

In restaurants, entrees should be ordered grilled or roasted, along with baked potatoes, and salad with oil and vinegar.

An abundance of fruits and vegetables, which are low in salt, should be consumed, and water should be consumed freely.

Low-Fat, Low-Cholesterol Diet

The current recommendation is to reduce fat to less than 30 percent of total daily calories, with no more than 10 percent of daily calories from saturated fats.

A doctor may also prescribe a low-cholesterol diet, lower than the standard recommendation of less than 300 milligrams per day. Foods that are high in cholesterol are organ meats such as liver, shellfish, egg yolks, and dairy foods. However, simply restricting dietary cholesterol is often not enough to lower blood cholesterol to recommended levels; thus, a doctor may prescribe medication to be taken as well.

Fiber (Restricted/High) Diets

Fiber is the indigestible material found in plants. Often composed of cellulose, fiber adds bulk to the diet and promotes healthy bowel function. An increase in fiber is often recommended to relieve constipation and as a preventative against colon cancer. High-fiber foods include whole grains, fruits, and most vegetables.

However, certain intestinal diseases, including diverticulitis, ulcerative colitis, and Crohn's disease, may necessitate a reduced-fiber diet.

EXERCISE

Benefits of Exercise

Exercise increases muscle tone, strengthens the heart and lungs, and burns calories. Exercise has been shown to lower the risk of heart disease, high blood pressure, and diabetes, as well as to reduce bone loss due to osteoporosis.

The brain chemicals released during exercise even reduce the desire to eat. All weight-loss studies show that dieting in conjunction with increased exercise is a better way to lose weight than adjusting diet alone or using diet medications. Studies done in the elderly have found that a moderate amount of exercise three or four times a week helps reduce blood pressure, improves sleep, and generally adds quality to life.

ON THE JOB

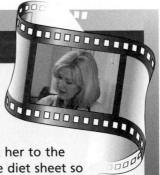

Videotape: Patient Education with Special Populations Scene 5.1 B; "Communicate & Motivate, Part II"

Sandra, a medical assistant at Blackburn Primary Care Associates, has been asked by Dr. Lopez to go over a low-salt, low-cholesterol diet sheet with Aida Hernandez, a 54-year-old Hispanic woman who has recently been diagnosed with hypertension and elevated serum cholesterol.

Mrs. Hernandez does not speak English. Her daughter, Maria, who has brought her to the office, needs to translate. Sandra tells Maria and Mrs. Hernandez to look over the diet sheet so she can answer questions for them. When Mrs. Hernandez was first diagnosed, the office did not have a Spanish instruction sheet, but since the last visit, Sandra has had the standard instruction sheet translated.

QUESTIONS
1. Why is it important for Sandra to have some knowledge of Mrs. Hernandez's dietary patterns in order to help her adhere to these new dietary restrictions?
2. What specific recommendations should Sandra give to avoid saturated fat and foods high in cholesterol?
3. Why is it important to provide Mrs. Hernandez with a diet sheet in Spanish? Since her daugher can translate for her, isn't that good enough?
4. How will Sandra know if Mrs. Hernandez understands and is following the diet Dr. Lopez has prescribed?

The important things to tell patients about exercise are:

1. Find exercises you enjoy. Lap swimming or running on a treadmill may be boring, but riding a bicycle for 20 minutes or walking briskly around a nature trail may not be, and may be equally beneficial.
2. Make exercise a part of daily life. Walk up two or three flights or stairs instead of taking the elevator. Walk or ride a bicycle to work if the distance is not great and the climate allows. Use a walk-behind lawnmower instead of a riding mower.
3. Exercise regularly and moderately, rather than irregularly and extensively.
4. Always warm up by stretching and starting slow; cool down slowly rather than simply stopping.

Types of Exercise

Aerobic and Isometric

Exercising can generally be classified as aerobic, isotonic, or isometric. **Aerobic** exercise includes walking, jogging, rowing, bicycle riding, and swimming. **Isotonic** exercise involves applying tension against muscle groups during motion. Isotonic exercise includes weight training, which utilizes free weights or machine-weight exercises, as well as joint mobility, or flexibility, exercises such as gentle stretching. **Isometric** exercise is contraction of muscles without movement.

Range of Motion Exercise

Range of motion (ROM) exercises are passive exercises designed to keep joints, muscles, and supporting structures supple and able to move. Each joint should move through its normal range of motion daily. If the patient has normal muscle function, he or she can perform **active exercises**—exercises performed without assistance.

For individuals with weakness due to paralysis, nerve damage, or joint injury, these movements are performed via **passive exercise**—exercise accomplished without muscular effort, using either a machine or human assistance. Figure 33–2 shows and the "Normal Range of Motion" box defines normal range of motion for various body joints.

When an individual has decreased mobility, the doctor may recommend performing ROM exercises, either independently or with the help of a family member or friend. Procedure 33–1 describes how to teach a patient or family member to do this.

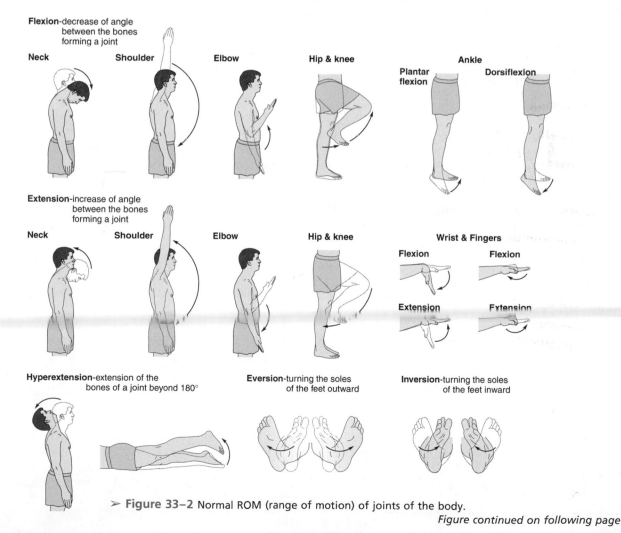

> **Figure 33–2** Normal ROM (range of motion) of joints of the body.

Figure continued on following page

Abduction-movement away from the median plane
of the body (Latin *ab* = away from)
Adduction-movement toward the median plane
of the body (Latin *ad* = to, toward)

Neck

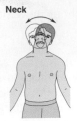

Shoulder

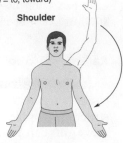

Hip

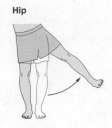

Fingers

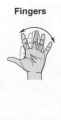

Pronation -turning palm of hand up
Supination-turning palm of hand down

Rotation-turning the bones of a joint
inward or outward

Supination

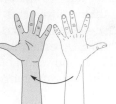

Pronation

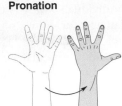

Neck

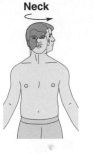

Hip: external rotation   **Hip: internal rotation**

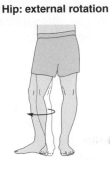
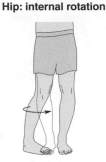

➤ **Figure 33–2** (*Continued*)

Normal Range of Motion

Abduction: Lateral movement away from the body's midline

Adduction: Lateral movement toward the body's midline

Eversion: Turning soles of feet outward

Extension: Increase in the angle between the bones of a joint

Flexion: Decrease in the angle between the bones of a joint

Hyperextension: Extension of the bones of a joint beyond 180°

Inversion: Turning the soles of the feet inward

Pronation: Turning the wrist so the hand faces down

Rotation: Turning a bone on its axis

Supination: Turning the wrist so the hand faces up

SELF-EXAMINATION

Many cancers can be detected early through self-examination. Patients should be taught to perform these examinations on a regular basis.

Skin Examination

Skin should be examined for any mole that changes color, shape, or size, and for any sore that does not heal in a reasonable time. Individuals should be taught to examine their skin, especially where it is exposed to sun, and to have another person examine the places they can not see, such as the back, neck, and top of the head (especially bald men).

Squamous cell and basal cell carcinomas are the most common types of skin cancers. They are also the most easily treated. Because they are usually confined to the tumorous growth itself, they can simply be excised by a dermatologist or plastic surgeon. A painless sore that does not heal may be a squamous or basal cell cancer.

Melanomas can be more dangerous because they will metastasize (spread) if not treated. Malignant melanomas are the leading cause of death due to skin disease. Melanomas usually appear as moles, and can be white, blue, purple, or red. About one-third of melanomas grow on a pre-existing nevus (mole or birthmark).

Over time the melanoma may change color and shape, and the edges often become irregular. Melanomas can grow quickly, both in radius and in depth into the dermis; this is what makes them so dangerous. Figure 33–3 shows a malignant melanoma.

Breast Examination

Women should be taught to do a monthly breast exam, because most lumps are found by women themselves and not by their doctors. The self-exam should take place one week after the woman's menstrual period. Breasts may be tender immediately before and during her period.

A good time to teach breast self-exam is during the annual physical exam. A number of good brochures are available, but teaching has more impact if it includes an actual self-exam conducted under teaching and coaching. It is helpful to use a model that contains the type of lump a woman should be looking for.

The exam includes two parts. First, lying on her back with a pillow under the same side as the breast being examined, the woman should examine and palpate the breast. Second, the procedure is repeated while standing. Tumors are usually hard and painless, but any lump should be reported. In addition, swelling and tenderness should be reported if it persists. The doctor will examine any self-reported problem.

Most irregularities of the breast discovered on self-examination are benign. However, the incidence of breast cancer is on the rise. A condition called fibrocystic breast disease, in which painful lumps develop in the breast, is common. Although these lumps are usually benign, women with this condition have a 2–5 times greater chance of developing breast cancer and should be particularly careful to perform monthly self-examination.

Procedure 33–2 describes how to teach female patients breast self-examination.

Testicular Examination

Testicular self-exam is especially important for boys and men between 15 and 34, when the incidence of testicular cancer is highest. Early diagnosis is essential for effective treatment.

Testicular self-exam should be performed monthly. During a shower or after a bath is a convenient time, because warm water relaxes the scrotum. Each testicle should be rotated between the thumb and forefinger, looking for hard, painless lumps. The cordlike structure behind the testes and the vas deferens—the narrow tube that runs up the scrotum—should also be felt for lumps.

As is the case with breast self-examination, most lumps or swelling found on self-exam are not cancerous, but should be followed up by a doctor.

It may be difficult for a medical assistant, especially a female medical assistant, to get a male patient to do a return demonstration self-exam under coaching. In fact, many men are uncomfortable performing testicular self-exam or thinking about testicular cancer.

Procedure 33–3 describes how to teach male patients testicular self examination.

PROCEDURE 33–1

Teaching Range-of-Motion Exercises

Performance Objective: The student will be able to teach a patient and/or family member to perform range of motion (ROM) exercises.
Supplies and Equipment: Treatment table, pillows.

Procedure Steps

1. Wash hands.
2. Identify the patient and the family member or other person to be included in the teaching; explain that ROM exercises help keep joints moving freely and are especially important when a person has paralysis or partial paralysis.
   Rationale: Understanding the need for teaching increases motivation.
3. Explain that ROM exercises are usually done in sequence from the head down. If a person performs the motions in his or her daily activities, the exercises do not always need to be done as special exercises, although going through all exercises may provide a suitable exercise program for an elderly person. For muscle groups that are weak or paralyzed, the joint should be moved through its full range of motion to the extent that can be done without pain or excessive force. The patient may perform the exercises without assistance (active exercise) or with assistance: The patient may use an unparalyzed extremity or an assistant to help move a weak extremity (**active-assistive exercise**), or an assistant may move a paralyzed extremity (passive exercise). Each exercise is performed

Procedure continued on following page

PROCEDURE 33–1 *(continued)*

at least three times. Refer to Figure 33–2 for illustrations of the motions of various joints.
Rationale: The patient and family member need to understand that every joint should be moved, even if the patient is unable to move it voluntarily.

4. Begin with the patient in a sitting position if possible.
Rationale: Although most ROM exercises can be done when the patient is lying down, the sitting position is more closely related to normal movement and is easier for the patient to learn.

5. Ask the patient to move the head and neck through normal motion without straining or stretching excessively. Normal motions of the head include turning the neck from side to side; tilting each ear toward the shoulder; and rolling the head gently around from a forward position (neck bent), to the side, back, and to the other side. If the patient cannot do these exercises actively, do not include them in the exercise program.
Rationale: Head motions are generally done only by the patient because the cervical spine can be injured by overstretching if head motions are done passively.

6. Ask the patient to move each shoulder through normal range of motion. If one arm is weak, the patient can use the other to assist or the family member can move the weak extremity for the patient. Instruct the patient to reach toward the ceiling from the front and side and to make arm circles using the shoulders. The patient should also reach behind his or her body with the arms.
Rationale: The shoulder is a ball-and-socket joint capable of flexion, extension, hyperextension, abduction, adduction, and rotation.

7. Ask the patient to move the elbow, forearm, wrist, and the fingers of each hand through normal range of motion. The patient should bend and straighten the arms at the elbows with palms facing up, then down. The patient should bend and straighten the wrists, then the fingers. The patient should make circles with the wrists in both directions; then, holding the fingers straight, spread and close the fingers. The patient should make circles with the thumb and touch the thumb to each finger.
Rationale: The elbow is a hinge joint capable of flexion and extension. The wrist joint contains many bones, allowing several types of motion including flexion, extension, rotation,

pronation, and supination of the hand. The fingers allow flexion, extension, abduction, and adduction. The thumb is a saddle joint allowing for circular motion and opposition to the fingers.

8. While in a sitting position, have the patient arch the back (leaning the head back) and round the back (bringing the head toward the chest). This moves the vertebrae of the back.

9. Have the patient move the joints of the knees and feet through their full range of motion. From the sitting position, straighten the leg, raising the feet. Make circles with the ankles. Turn the soles of the feet toward each other. Turn the soles of the feet away from each other. Bend, straighten, and spread the toes. The knees and feet can also be exercised with the patient lying down.
Rationale: The knees and toes are hinge joints capable of flexion and extension. The toes can also perform abduction and adduction. The ankles are capable of flexion, extension, and rotation. The feet can be inverted or everted.

10. Have the patient lie down on the treatment table to exercise the hip joints. Lying on the back, lift each leg as high as possible with the knee straight and/or bent. With the leg straight, move each leg to the side, back to the middle, and across the opposite leg. Turn each leg from the hip so that the feet point away from each other, then toward each other. The hips can also be rotated by bending the knees and allowing them to fall away from each other. Lying on the stomach (if the patient can tolerate this position), raise the leg in a straight position. If one of the patient's legs is weak, he or she can use the other to assist by placing the foot of the opposite leg under the ankle or knee. If the patient is not strong enough to do this, the family member should support each leg at both the knee and the ankle to perform the exercises.
Rationale: The hip joint is a ball-and-socket joint capable of flexion, extension, hyperextension, abduction, adduction, and rotation. The weight of the leg requires support of the knee and ankle, either by the patient's own muscles or those of an assistant during exercise.

11. For each exercise, ask the patient to demonstrate the exercise. If the patient needs assistance, ask the family member to demonstrate how to help the patient. Make suggestions and corrections if necessary.

Rationale: Having the learner do a return demonstration provides feedback about the effectiveness of teaching.

12. If you notice that the patient has problems with the exercises—such as decreased mobility of a joint, pain in a joint, excessive weakness or difficulty learning to do the exercises—consider asking the doctor to refer the patient to a physical therapist for individualized therapy.

    Rationale: A physical therapist is able to assess muscle and joint function and provide therapeutic exercises to increase strength and mobility.

13. Wash hands.

14. Document all teaching done and its effectiveness.

Charting Example	
Date	
8/12/XX	2:45 PM Patient instructed in performance of range of motion exercises, especially for the right lower extremity, which has some weakness. Instructed to use both hands to assist in extension of the knee and ankle, flexion of the toes, inversion and eversion of the foot. The patient was able to demonstrate all exercises, including those done as passive-assistive exercises. The patient verbalized understanding of the need to keep all joints mobile, even those of the of the weak right lower extremity.
	Paul Dean, RMA

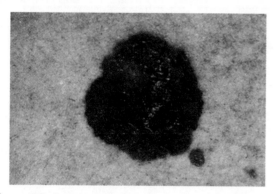

➤ **Figure 33–3** Malignant melanoma: This growth demonstrates the irregular border, irregular coloration, irregular elevation, and dark color of melanoma. (From Thibodeau GA, Patton Kevin T: *The Human Body in Health and Disease.* St. Louis: Mosby, 1992.)

HELPING THE PATIENT WITH DIABETES MELLITUS TO MAINTAIN HEALTH

Diabetes Mellitus

Diabetes mellitus is a chronic illness. A lack of insulin in the body, or the body's inability to use insulin effectively, leads to altered carbohydrate, fat, and protein metabolism. The major symptom of diabetes mellitus is persistent hyperglycemia (abnormally high blood sugar) because of the body's inability to break down sugars.

Estimates are that more than seven million Americans are diagnosed diabetics, and that an equal number of diabetics have never been properly diagnosed. Diabetes is a major cost to the American health care system—representing over 10 percent of the total cost of health care in the United States—and an enormous

PROCEDURE 33–2

Teaching Breast Self-examination

Performance Objective: The student will be able to teach a woman to perform breast self-examination.
Supplies and Equipment: Treatment table, pillows, model of the breast containing abnormal lump.

Procedure Steps

1. Wash hands.
2. Identify the patient and explain that monthly breast self-examination is important for early detection of breast cancer.

Rationale: Understanding the need for teaching increases motivation.

3. Instruct the patient to perform the examination each month, about one week after the beginning of the menstrual period, so that breasts are not swollen or tender. If the patient no longer menstruates, instruct the patient to perform the examination on the same day each month.

Rationale: It is recommended to perform

Procedure continued on following page

PROCEDURE 33–2 *(continued)*

breast self-examination monthly from the on-set of menstruation until a woman dies.

4 Instruct the patient to begin the examination lying down with a pillow under the right shoulder and the right arm lifted above the head. Encourage the patient to demonstrate this position.
Rationale: The position allows the patient to palpate the entire breast easily. Demonstrating the position helps the patient remember the correct position.

5 Instruct the patient to use the pads of the index finger, middle finger, and ring finger of the left hand to feel all parts of the breast in a pattern, such as a circular pattern, up-and-down pattern, or wedge pattern. Encourage the patient to choose one pattern and make a habit of always palpating the entire breast in the same way. The patient will probably be less shy if allowed to practice palpation on a model of a breast.
Rationale: The entire breast should be palpated systematically to identify lumps if present.
Building a habit facilitates effective examination. Using a model to practice will be less embarrassing for the patient. In addition, most models have lumps for the patient to find, making it clearer what an abnormal finding feels like.

6. Instruct the patient to repeat on the left side using the right hand.

7 Instruct the patient to repeat the examination standing up, placing the hand on the side being examined on the shoulder and examining with the other hand. This part of the examination may be done in the shower.
Rationale: The upright position makes it easier to palpate the part of the breast near the underarm. Palpation may be easier when the breast is wet and soapy.

8. Wash hands.

9. Document all teaching done and its effectiveness.

Charting Example	
Date	
6/22/XX	10:15 AM Patient instructed how to perform breast self-examination using a model. The patient was able to demonstrate the supine and standing positions for self-examination and to demonstrate effective palpation on the breast model. The patient identified the reason for monthly examination and that the exam should be done regularly after the menstrual period. ————
	———— Kathy Anderson, RMA

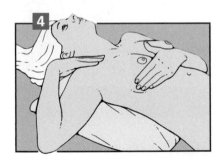

Circular

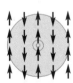

Up & down

Wedge

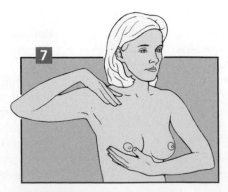

Teaching Testicular Self-examination

Performance Objective: The student will be able to teach a man to perform testicular self-examination.
Supplies and Equipment: Model of the testes containing abnormal lump.

Procedure Steps

1. Wash hands.
2. Identify the patient and explain that monthly testicular self-examination is important for early detection of testicular cancer. Remind the patient that testicular cancer is commonly found between the ages of 15 and 34 and can be very serious.
   Rationale: Understanding the need for teaching increases motivation.
3. Instruct the patient to perform the examination each month on the same day.
   Rationale: It is recommended to perform testicular self-examination monthly beginning at age 15.
4. Instruct the patient that symptoms of testicular cancer may include a feeling of heaviness in the scrotum, a dull ache in the scrotum, accumulation of fluid without injury, or a change in the consistency of any part of the scrotum.
   Rationale: Cancer of the testes may be present without a palpable lump.
5. Instruct the patient to use the pads of the thumb and fingers to roll each teste gently, feeling for evidence of a small lump or thickening. The best time to do the examination may be during a shower or after a bath.
   Rationale: Warmth relaxes the structures of the scrotum.
6. Instruct the patient to locate the epididymis and spermatic cord just above the teste and continue palpating up along the spermatic cord for each teste.
   Rationale: A tumor may grow above the teste along the spermatic cord.
7. Ask the patient to demonstrate the technique on a model or on himself. The patient may be less shy using a model.
   Rationale: Most men find this technique embarrassing to discuss and even more embarrassing to demonstrate. Using a model also allows the man to identify the feeling of an abnormal area that should be reported.
8. Wash hands.
9. Document all teaching done and its effectiveness.

Charting Example	
Date	
10/05/XX	11:15 AM Patient instructed how to perform testicular self-examination using a model. The patient was able to demonstrate effective palpation on the testicular model. The patient identified the reason for monthly examination and that the exam should be done on the same day each month. ———————— K. Jones, CMA

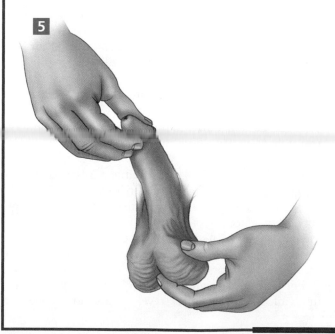

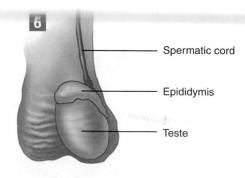

Spermatic cord

Epididymis

Teste

economic cost due to lost work time and permanent disability. Diabetes is one of the most common causes of new cases of blindness, and foot and partial-leg amputations.

Diabetes is characterized as either Type I, also known as insulin-dependent diabetes mellitus **(IDDM)**, or Type II, also known as non-insulin-dependent diabetes mellitus **(NIDDM)**. While individuals who suffer from Type I diabetes are treated with insulin injections or constant-infusion insulin via an insulin pump, those who suffer from Type II diabetes can often be treated through modifications in diet and exercise, with oral diabetic medication if necessary.

Initial instruction to a patient newly diagnosed with diabetes is usually carried out by a teaching specialist. However, the medical assistant is often responsible for reinforcing teaching throughout the patient care, as well as for repeating teaching of specific points if and when it becomes necessary.

Signs and symptoms of diabetes differ by type, as does the usual age of onset.

Type I diabetes is usually diagnosed in individuals under 40 years of age, and often in children and teens. (Type I diabetes used to be called juvenile onset diabetes, and the organization that raises private funds for diabetes research is still called the Juvenile Diabetes Foundation.) Individuals usually show a number of symptoms, including **polyuria** (frequent urination), **polydipsia** (extreme thirst), and **polyphagia** (extreme hunger). The individual may have had a precipitous weight loss, despite the increased appetite and food intake. He or she is often fatigued, and may be experiencing an extreme itching sensation. Women may have vaginal itching.

Type II diabetes is usually diagnosed in individuals who are over 40 and obese. The individual may show none of the classic symptoms of diabetes; if these symptoms do occur, they are usually less pronounced and less severe than in an individual with Type I diabetes. The diabetes is usually discovered on a routine blood test, or when the person has an open sore that fails to heal, most often on the foot or ankle.

Individuals with either Type I or Type II diabetes may also suffer from blurred vision; pain, tingling, or numbness in one or more extremities; and/or slow-healing skin infections.

The goal in treating diabetes mellitus is to keep blood sugar within normal limits, or not more than 6–8 percent above 120 mL/dL, which is the highest level considered normal. Such maintenance greatly reduces complications. In order to maintain blood sugar within this range, patients must be taught to monitor their blood sugar by using a fingerstick to obtain a drop of blood to test in a **glucometer** (a blood glucose monitoring device). Patients who need insulin must be taught how to administer an insulin injection, or how to monitor and maintain their constant-infusion pump equipment.

Managing Diet and Exercise

Diet

The so-called diabetic diet is the primary tool for management of diabetes mellitus. Most doctors refer their diabetic patients to a dietitian or nutritionist for regular semiannual (every 6 months) visits.

Management of diet in diabetes has five goals:

1. To help the patient attain, then maintain, his or her appropriate body weight. Although "weight loss" is not necessarily communicated to the patient as the primary goal, adherence to an appropriate diet, when combined with exercise, usually does reduce weight.
2. To provide adequate nutrition. The diet must provide enough nutrition for growth and development in children and adolescents, and for fetal growth and development in pregnant women.
3. To achieve and maintain blood glucose levels within normal ranges, or as close as possible.
4. To prevent acute episodes of diabetic complications—most importantly, **ketoacidosis** (acidity of the blood due to the buildup of ketones, the breakdown products produced when fat is burned for energy) and **hypoglycemia** (acutely low blood sugar).
5. Preventing, or at least delaying, long-term degenerative complications—most importantly, diabetic retinopathy (a degeneration of the retina of the eye) and diabetic neuropathy (a degeneration of the nerves in the extremities, leading to a lack of sensation).

The American Diabetes Association (ADA) recommends that individuals with diabetes consume 55 to 60 percent of their calories from carbohydrates, preferably complex carbohydrates; 15 to 20 percent from protein; and less than 30 percent from fat. Cholesterol should be limited to under 300 mg per day, and sodium to less than 3 g per day.

It is important to coordinate meals and snacks with medication, especially if insulin is being used. Once insulin has been injected, it continues to transport glucose from the blood to the cells. If enough glucose is not available, the blood sugar may fall dangerously low, a condition called hypoglycemia. It is also important to try to eat meals at the same time each day whenever possible.

A dietitian can help in planning meals and snacks, using appropriate "exchanges" to provide variation in the diet. Exchanges are alternative foods that supply equivalent amounts of carbohydrate, protein, or fat as the major item listed on the diet. For instance, two starch exchanges can be provided by two slices of bread, one hamburger roll, or one pita bread pocket.

For individuals who cannot often eat at the same time, or who frequently travel across time zones on business, a dietitian or nutritionist can help create a strategy for maintaining blood sugar at a constant level.

Exercise

Exercise helps to lower blood sugar and blood cholesterol. Daily exercise is a part of any weight-reduction or weight-maintenance plan. For the diabetic patient, it helps if exercise can be undertaken at the same time every day in order to coordinate the exercise with diet and medication.

Anti-diabetic Medication

Insulin

Individuals with Type I diabetes must take insulin, usually two or three times a day by injection, or by a continuous-infusion pump.

For an individual newly diagnosed with diabetes, the amount of insulin to be taken with each injection is a matter of trial and error. The doctor prescribes a particular amount of insulin to be taken in each injection, based on the blood glucose level. However, it takes weeks, and sometimes months, to find the optimal level of insulin per injection, based on the patient's diet, level of exercise, and general metabolism.

Once the basic level has been determined, the patient then needs to be taught to adjust the dose based on blood sugars in the frequent blood samples he or she takes to monitor the blood sugar level. A full discussion on the procedure for measuring blood glucose using a glucometer appears in chapter 26.

Figure 33–4 shows the equipment and record sheet for a patient who must test blood sugar. Figure 33–5 shows a patient performing a fingerstick.

There are many types of insulin, and insulin is sold by many pharmaceutical companies. Each type has some distinctive characteristics. Most commercially sold insulin is genetically engineered human insulin, al-

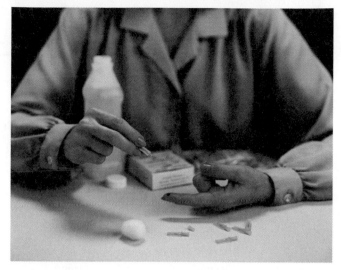

> **Figure 33–5** A patient performing a fingerstick to test blood for glucose.

though insulin from pigs (porcine insulin) is still available. Some types act rapidly, but only for a short time; others contain substances that delay the action so the insulin is longer acting.

Insulin is measured in U.S. Pharmacopeia units (U), which refers not to volume but to a measure of insulin activity. Insulin comes in doses of either U-100 or U-500. Most individuals respond to U-100 insulin (100 units per milliliter); U-500 insulin (500 units per milliliter) is used only in cases of severe insulin resistance. U-100 insulin syringes are marked in units, and have orange needle covers.

Table 33–4 lists the types of insulin.

Many patients take two types of insulin: regular insulin, which begins to act within one-half to one hour after administration, and a longer-acting preparation to cover insulin needs throughout the day. The solution for regular insulin is clear, and the solution for the longer-acting types is cloudy.

Figure 33–6 shows the medical assistant teaching the patient how to draw up the two types of insulin in the same syringe. Notice that the dose of regular insulin is drawn up first, followed by the longer-acting type. This way, the patient avoids the problems that can occur if the regular insulin is contaminated by the longer-acting insulin. If a small drop of regular insulin is accidentally introduced into the longer-acting insulin bottle, the patient is less likely to experience problems.

An individual with insulin-dependent diabetes mellitus, who must take numerous injections of insulin every day, must rotate the sites of the injections, so as not to overburden any one area. The injections should be given using the subcutaneous route, usually in the abdomen, thighs, buttocks, or the backs of the arms. Figure 33–7 shows a patient injecting himself with insulin.

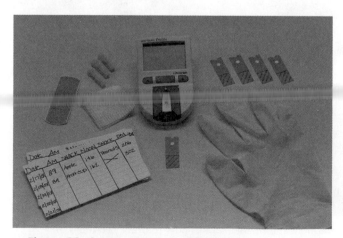

> **Figure 33–4** Equipment for a diabetic to perform a fingerstick and record results.

Table 33-4	Types of Insulin		
Category	**Onset**	**Peak Action**	**Duration**
Rapid-acting			
Lispro insulin (Humalog®)	10–15 minutes	30–60 minutes	4 hours
Regular insulin	1/2–1 hour	2–3 hours	5–7 hours
Concentrated regular insulin (500 U/mL)	1/2–1 hour	2–5 hours	5–7 hours
Semilente insulin	1–2 hours	2–5 hours	12–16 hours
Intermediate-acting			
Lente insulin	1–2 1/2 hours	7–15 hours	12–24 hours
NPH (isophane insulin suspension)	1–2 hours	4–12 hours	18–24 hours
Long-acting			
Ultralente insulin	4–8 hours	10–30 hours	7–36 hours
Lantus insulin	4–6 hours	No peak	24 hours
Mixtures			
NPH/Lispro 75/25	10–15 min	Varies	14–24 hours
NPH/regular insulin 50/50 or 70/30	1/2–1 hour	Varies	14–24 hours

It is important for patients to be able to recognize and respond appropriately to the signs of hypoglycemia, also called **insulin reaction** when the blood glucose level falls too low because there is more insulin in the bloodstream than the patient needs. Figure 33–8 shows a medical assistant teaching a patient to respond to hypoglycemia. The signs and symptoms of hypoglycemia were discussed in chapter 31. An insulin-dependent individual should wear a medical identification bracelet, as shown in chapter 31.

Oral Hypoglycemics for Type II Diabetes

Individuals with non-insulin-dependent diabetes mellitus are often treated with diet, exercise, and oral medical called **oral hypoglycemics**. They act by stimulating the insulin-producing cells, called **beta cells**. Beta cells reside on the pancreatic islets, or islets of Langerhans, which are tiny clumps of cells (islands) that appear randomly in the ocean of pancreatic cells. Oral hypoglycemics are usually taken once a day.

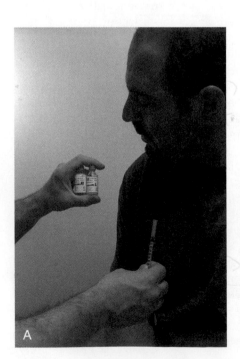

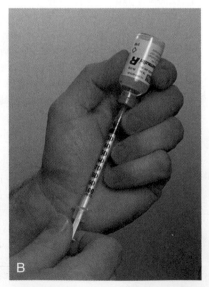

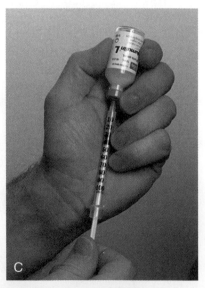

➤ **Figure 33–6** A medical assistant demonstrates how to draw two types of insulin in one syringe. (A) Holding both bottles of insulin and the insulin syringe; (B) drawing up the regular insulin; (C) adding the Lente insulin.

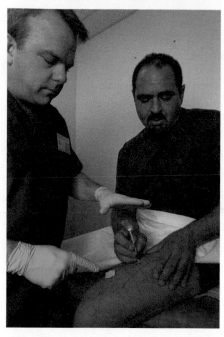

➤ **Figure 33–7** Diabetic patient demonstrating self-injection.

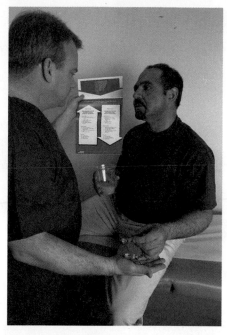

➤ **Figure 33–8** Medical assistant showing a patient how to identify and respond to an insulin reaction (hypoglycemia).

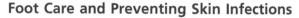

Foot Care and Preventing Skin Infections

Because of diabetic neuropathy, many individuals with diabetes have a lack of skin sensation. This can be very dangerous, as they do not feel the pain caused by skin irritations or abrasions, which can become infected over time. If infections are not treated until they are serious, gangrene can infect the wound, requiring amputation of the toes or lower leg. The height of the amputation depends on the circulation to the skin and deeper leg tissues.

Diabetic patients should receive regular care from a podiatrist. In addition, for the best continuous quality of life, they should be taught proper foot self-care, and this teaching should be reinforced by the medical assistant at every visit.

Diabetic foot self-care has three aspects: assessment, hygiene, and skin softening.

Each day, the diabetic patient should do a thorough examination of his or her feet and ankles. This means a visual examination of the entire foot, top and bottom, each toe, and between toes. Any scrapes, cuts, or nicks should be noted, washed, and treated appropriately. If an area is infected, the doctor should be consulted.

To keep the feet from becoming dry, cracked, and infected, the feet should be soaked daily in a warm soak. They should be dried thoroughly by patting dry, not rubbing. Nails should be clipped straight across (often, podiatrists perform nail clipping for diabetic patients).

Finally, softening lotion should be applied daily.

The diabetic patient should also examine his or her shoes daily to make sure the inner portion has not been damaged in any way that could cause irritation or abrasion to the foot. Special diabetic shoes provide extra protection, and have been shown to help maintain good foot health over time.

Commercial kits are available for diabetic teaching; they contain booklets, diet guides, and a checklist like the one shown in Figure 33–9 to validate that all areas of teaching have been covered.

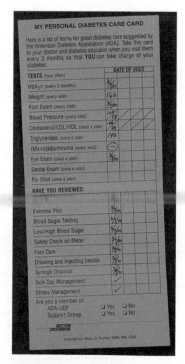

➤ **Figure 33–9** Card to document diabetic teaching.

STUDENT STUDY PLAN

To reinforce your understanding of the material in this chapter . . .

Complete the **Review & Recall** questions.

Discuss the situation in **If You Were the Medical Assistant** with your classmates, and answer the questions.

Answer the **Critical Thinking Questions** and discuss them with your classmates.

Visit the **Web sites** suggested and search for additional Web sites using **Keywords for Internet Searches.**

Complete the exercises in chapter 33 of the **Student Mastery Manual.**

View Patient Education with Special Populations **Videotape**: Part I—Diet Teaching.

REVIEW & RECALL

1. List the four main guidelines for maintaining health, as recommended by the U.S. Department of Agriculture.

2. Identify the food groups on the food guide pyramid, and the recommended daily number of servings for each group.

3. Describe the six major types of nutrients (including water) in a healthy diet.

4. Identify five types of restricted diets and describe the dietary restrictions in each.

5. Define the term "range of motion" and describe the normal range of motion of each joint in the body.

6. Identify the reasons and procedure for breast self-examination, and testicular self-examination.

7. Describe modifications to diet and exercise that are needed to maintain health in a person with diabetes mellitus.

8. Identify the teaching needs of a diabetic who must give him- or herself daily insulin injections.

9. Discuss why good foot care and infection prevention are especially important to maintain health in a diabetic patient.

IF YOU WERE THE MEDICAL ASSISTANT

Develop a detailed teaching plan for teaching Warren Blake, the newly diagnosed insulin-dependent diabetic patient described in On the Job in chapter 32. Add the new information to your plan to teach Warren how to administer insulin, and how to follow a regular exercise program. Include methods to evaluate the effectiveness of your teaching with respect to exercise and self-administration of insulin.

CRITICAL THINKING QUESTIONS

1. Information about the components of a healthy diet is widely available, but most people will admit that they eat many foods they do not believe are healthful. Identify as many reasons as you can why people fail to follow dietary recommendations they believe would be good for them. Discuss why people's dietary patterns are difficult to change.

2. Identify ways to introduce the topic of breast self-examination and testicular self-examination to minimize embarrassment for yourself and the patient. How can patients be motivated to perform these examinations regularly?

3. Discuss how you would teach a patient with partial paralysis of the right lower leg to do range-of-motion leg exercises on himself. What if it was the arm that was paralyzed? How could a family member help the patient in both cases?

4. Compare and contrast the teaching needs of patients with IDDM and NIDDM. What is the same? What is different?

EXPLORE THE WEB

INTERNET WEB SITES

American Cancer Society
www.cancer.org

American Dietetic Association
www.eatright.org

American Heart Association
www.americanheart.org

Cholesterol Interactive Site
www.nhlbi.nih.gov/chd

National Institute of Diabetes and Digestive and Kidney Diseases
www.niddk.nih.gov

U.S. Department of Health and Human Services
www.os.dhhs.gov

KEYWORDS FOR INTERNET SEARCHES

diabetes mellitus
    exercise
    nutrition

ANSWERS TO ON THE JOB

1. It is important to have knowledge of dietary patterns to help patients understand how to substitute for foods they are accustomed to eating. In many Hispanic cultures, the diet tends to be high in fat and sodium. Rice (a staple food) is usually cooked with lots of salt and oil. Meat and other foods are usually fried, and seasoned with salt. Beans (another staple) are also cooked with salt and oil.

    Sandra needs to understand this in order to instruct Mrs. Hernandez to gradually cut down on the amount of salt used in cooking; to avoid frying meat and other foods, such as plantains (a type of cooking banana) or yucca (a vegetable); and to choose a polyunsaturated vegetable oil such as canola oil.

    She should explain to Mrs. Hernandez that if salt is reduced gradually, all family members will become accustomed to food with less salt; this will be a healthy benefit for everyone.

2. Sandra should tell Mrs. Hernandez to choose vegetable oils rather than solid fats; to trim fat from all meat and remove skin from poultry; to avoid high-fat processed meats; to avoid organ meats such as liver; to limit the intake of egg yolks and, if possible, substitute egg whites or commercial egg substitutes made from egg whites; to avoid shellfish; to avoid cheese or use low-fat cheese; and to check labels of prepared foods to be sure they do not contain high amounts of saturated fat or cholesterol.

3. Since Mrs. Hernandez does not speak English, she needs to be given these dietary instructions in Spanish. Translation should not be provided by her daughter, since this can cause a struggle within the family about who is in control of food preparation and food intake.

4. Mrs. Hernandez should be able to tell Sandra specific ways she is supposed to change her diet. If she and Sandra have established a good relationship, on follow-up visits Mrs. Hernandez will tell Sandra if she is following the diet some of the time, most of the time, or all of the time. If the patient's blood pressure and serum cholesterol are lower on follow-up visits, Sandra will also know that the treatment regime Dr. Lopez has prescribed is being followed and is effective.

Chapter 34

Oral Follow-up

Learning Objectives

After completing this chapter, you will be able to do the following:

1. Define and spell the vocabulary words for this chapter.
2. Correctly make a follow-up appointment.
3. Add patients to a recall list.
4. Schedule patients for diagnostic tests.
5. Give instructions to a patient for a diagnostic test.
6. Schedule a patient for hospital or surgery-center surgery.
7. Complete a referral form for managed care.
8. Obtain a managed care preauthorization
9. Complete an appointment card.
10. Describe how to obtain results for diagnostic tests.

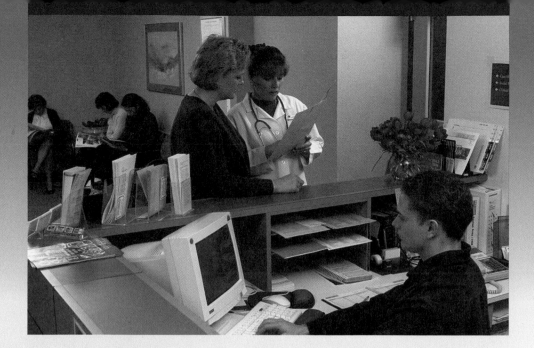

- Schedule and manage appointments
- Schedule inpatient and outpatient admissions and procedures
- Obtain managed care referrals and preauthorizations

Performance Objectives

After completing this chapter, you will be able to do the following:

1. Schedule a diagnostic test (Procedure 34–1).
2. Schedule surgery for a patient (Procedure 34–2).
3. Complete a referral form (Procedure 34–3).

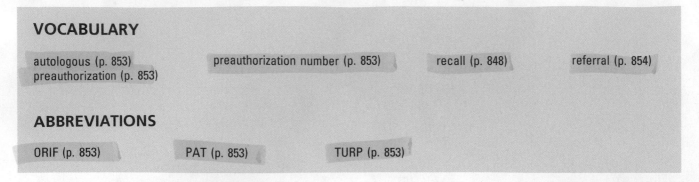

VOCABULARY

autologous (p. 853)   preauthorization number (p. 853)   recall (p. 848)   referral (p. 854)
preauthorization (p. 853)

ABBREVIATIONS

ORIF (p. 853)   PAT (p. 853)   TURP (p. 853)

Medical assistants who work in primary care offices spend a large amount of time making follow-up appointments for patients and assisting patients to schedule follow-up with other health care providers.

SCHEDULING A FOLLOW-UP APPOINTMENT

A follow-up appointment can be scheduled when the patient leaves the office, or the patient can be told when to call the doctor's office to schedule the appointment.

When scheduling the follow-up as the patient leaves, the medical assistant must remember to provide the patient with all the information he or she needs for the appointment, in addition to putting the necessary information into the appointment schedule.

Information Necessary for Scheduling a Follow-up

A number of pieces of information are necessary to schedule a follow-up appointment. These are the patient's full name, telephone number, and the reason for the follow-up visit, as well as how much time the follow-up visit will take. The doctor usually indicates when the patient should return on the charge slip (encounter form).

· Some follow-up appointments must be made on a particular day. For instance, a dressing may need to be changed two days after it is first put on, or a person who has just been put on a new medication must have the medication level in the bloodstream checked after a specific number of days. ·

◂ In other cases, a follow-up appointment can occur within a period of one or two days. In the case of a person with a chronic illness, for instance, the doctor may want to see that person every four weeks—the day of the week that person comes in during the fourth week since the last visit does not really matter. For physical examinations or check-ups, the patient's insurance may not pay for the visit unless a specified time period has elapsed (e.g. 12 months) since the last physical. ·

· Other follow-up visits must be scheduled at a particular time of day. For instance, if the doctor wants a fasting blood test at the next appointment, the appointment must be early in the morning before the patient eats breakfast. Figure 34-1 shows a medical assistant making a follow-up appointment with a patient. ·

◂ In addition to entering the appointment into the office schedule and making an appointment card for the patient, the medical assistant may need to give the patient some instructions to follow to prepare for the appointment, such as when to eat or for how long not to eat before the appointment, whether to bring a first-void of the day urine specimen from home, and so on. ·

◂ Finally, the medical assistant may need to provide the patient with instructions about treatment to be followed between appointments, what to expect of the injury or illness, and what symptoms might occur that would cause the patient to call the doctor's office. For instance, the medical assistant might tell a patient with a burn on the arm that a small area of the dressing will become stained, which is to be expected; but if fluid oozes out from under the dressing, the doctor needs to be informed. Most offices have sheets with written instructions for common problems to help remind patients once they have left the office. ·

Documenting a Follow-up

·If the patient is in the office when the follow-up appointment is made, the appointment should be noted both on the office schedule and on an appointment card that is given to the patient. Figure 34-2 shows a completed appointment card. ·

·If the follow-up appointment is scheduled for many months later, make sure to place the patient's name and the appointment time in the **recall** file (a file of reminders to recall patients), a type of tickler file. The recall file—which can be paper notes in a file folder, a system of tabs on a calendar, or a notation system in a computerized calendar program—reminds the staff to

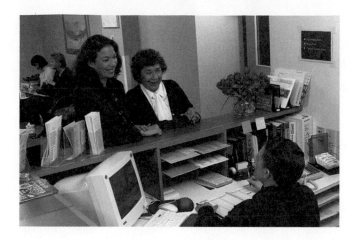

> **Figure 34–1** The medical assistant often makes follow-up appointments before the patient leaves the office.

call or send a postcard to remind the patient of the appointment.

If the appointment is made over the phone, the medical assistant may prepare a letter, appointment card, or postcard to mail to the patient as confirmation of the appointment. Many offices use telephone reminders a day or two before the appointment. Working from the list of appointments, the medical assistant calls each patient and reminds him or her of the date and time of the appointment, or leaves a voicemail message with the information. Figure 34–3 shows a medical assistant calling patients using a computerized appointment schedule.

SCHEDULING A DIAGNOSTIC TEST

It is often easier for a doctor's office to schedule a diagnostic or laboratory test for a patient than to have the patient schedule the test. Again, this can be done while the patient is in the office or when the patient is at home. The details of the appointment and any special instructions for the patient can be sent to the patient in the letter that confirms the appointment, and followed up with a telephone call.

Information Necessary for Scheduling a Diagnostic Test

To schedule a test, the medical assistant needs to know the patient's name, telephone number, the type of test being performed, the reason for the test, the time frame within which the test must be performed, and insurance information including any need for a written referral. Procedure 34–1 describes in detail how to schedule a diagnostic test for a patient.

Giving a Patient Instructions for Preparing for a Diagnosic Test

Patients often need particular instructions about what to do to prepare for a diagnostic test or procedure. After an appointment has been made, the medical assistant should call to inform the patient when and where the test will be performed. The medical assistant may also need to provide directions to the testing facility, as well as instructions for preparing for the test. If there are written instructions available, these should be given or sent to the patient. Document in the patient chart the fact that this material was provided.

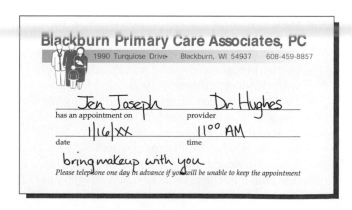

> **Figure 34–2** A completed appointment reminder card reminds the patient of the date and time of the appointment and any special instructions.

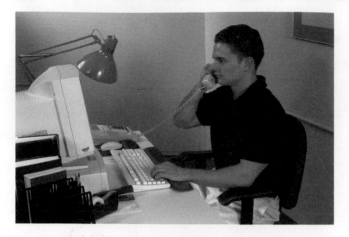

➤ **Figure 34–3** The medical assistant may call patients daily to remind them of appointments.

Documenting an Appointment for a Diagnostic Test

Many offices keep a log to track diagnostic tests, the results, and when the patient was notified of the results. An example is shown in Figure 34–4. Such a log helps office staff verify that each step of the process has taken place.

All verbal and written follow-up instructions to the patient about the test should be documented in the patient chart. You should document when patients are notified of the test results as well. Precise documentation in patient charts is necessary to avoid later claims of malpractice or abandonment.

Calling a Patient with the Test Results

The patient should be informed of all diagnostic test results as soon as possible after they are received in the doctor's office. Many offices send letters for routine tests. The medical assistant may be asked to prepare them for the doctor to sign.

The medical assistant may also be asked to place calls to patients for the doctor to discuss test results with a patient, or to schedule a follow-up appointment

---

PROCEDURE 34–1

Scheduling Diagnostic Tests

Performance Objective: The student will be able to schedule a diagnostic test for a patient.
Supplies and Equipment: The patient's medical record and insurance information, name of the test or procedure to be scheduled, telephone, name and telephone number of the department of the facility that will perform the test.

Procedure Steps

1. Assemble information necessary to schedule the test, including the patient's name, address, telephone number, and insurance information.

2. From the patient's medical record or a diagnostic test requisition filled out by the physician, determine the test or procedure to be performed.
   Rationale: To diagnose a patient correctly, the proper procedure must be scheduled. Clarify with the doctor if necessary.

3. Determine the time frame for performing the test and, if possible, discuss with the patient preferred days and times.

4. Determine what facility the test will be performed at and locate the telephone number.
   Rationale: For insurance reimbursement, a fa

cility that participates in the patient's insurance plan must be used.

5. Obtain preauthorization from the patient's insurance if necessary by calling the toll-free number provided by the insurance company. *Rationale:* Some diagnostic tests require preauthorization. If unsure, you must check with the insurance company to avoid unexpected expense for the patient. If preauthorization is needed, the facility will need the preauthorization number.

6. Call the facility to schedule the test. Determine a date and time for the procedure to be performed and provide information about the patient as requested by the facility.

7. Confirm the date and time with the patient.

8. Provide verbal and written instructions to the patient, including preparation for the test, special instructions, and dietary restrictions. *Rationale:* If preparation is required, the patient must know what to do. Written instructions reinforce verbal explanations.

9. Document the scheduled procedure and instructions given to the patient in the patient's medical record.

10. Record the scheduled test on the diagnostic test tracking log.

11. If requested by the hospital, send the test requisition to the appropriate department.

Charting Example	
Date	
9/22/XX	3:45 PM Barium swallow scheduled at Memorial Hospital for 9/28/XX at 9:15 AM. Pt. instructed to remain NPO after midnight and given directions to Memorial Hospital X-ray department. Pt. verbalizes understanding that she cannot eat or drink anything (including water) after midnight. ———————
	——————— Diane Cabot, RMA

DIAGNOSTIC TRACKING LOG

BLACKBURN PRIMARY CARE ASSOCIATES, PC
1990 Turquiose Drive
Blackburn, WI 54937
608-459-8857

Date of test	Patient	Test to be performed	Place of test	Date and when results received.	Called patient with results

➤ **Figure 34–4** Log for tracking diagnostic tests.

PROCEDURE 34-2

Scheduling a Surgical Procedure

Performance Objective: The student will be able to schedule a surgical procedure for a patient.

Supplies and Equipment: The patient's medical record and insurance information, name of the surgical procedure to be scheduled, telephone, name and telephone number of the department of the facility that will perform the surgery.

Procedure Steps

1. Assemble information necessary to schedule the surgical procedure, including the patient's name, address, telephone number, and insurance information.
2. From the patient's medical record, determine the surgical procedure to be performed and the patient's diagnosis.
   Rationale: To diagnose a patient correctly, the proper procedure must be scheduled. Clarify with the doctor if necessary.
3. Determine the time frame for performing the surgery and, if possible, discuss with the patient preferred days and times.
4. Determine the facility where the surgery will be performed and locate the telephone number.
   Rationale: For insurance reimbursement, a facility that participates in the patient's insurance plan must be used.
5. Obtain preauthorization from the patient's insurance, if necessary by calling the toll-free number provided by the insurance company.
   Rationale: Surgical procedures usually require preauthorization. If unsure, you must check with the insurance company to avoid unexpected expense for the patient. If preauthorization is needed, the facility will need the preauthorization number.
6. Call the facility to schedule the surgery. Determine a date and time for the procedure to be performed and provide information about the patient as requested by the facility. Determine the type of preadmission testing required.

Rationale: The type of preadmission testing depends on the facility where surgery will be performed, the age and general health of the patient, and the type of surgery.

7. Confirm the date and time with the patient.
8. Perform preadmission testing (PAT) or arrange with the hospital or laboratory accepted by the patient's insurance.
   Rationale: Preadmission testing must be done at a location that participates in the patient's health insurance program for reimbursement.
9. Provide verbal and written instructions to the patient, including preparation for the surgery, dietary restrictions, and any special instructions. If general anesthesia is to be used, the patient will be NPO after midnight.
   Rationale: If preparation is required, the patient must know what to do. Written instructions reinforce verbal explanations.
10. Document the scheduled surgery and instructions given to the patient in the patient's medical record.

Charting Example	
Date	
5/7/XX	11:15 AM Pt. scheduled for laparoscopic cholecystectomy at Memorial Hospital on 5/15/XX at 7:00 AM. CBC, SMA-24, and VDRL drawn and sent to Memorial Laboratory. EKG done. Pt. to have chest X-ray at Memorial Hospital today. Pt instructed to bathe with Phisoderm soap the night before the procedure and to remain NPO after midnight. Pt. verbalizes understanding that she cannot eat or drink anything (including water) after midnight. —————————— John Stiles, CMA

when test results have come in. Results should never be given to the patient until the doctor sees them.

SCHEDULING SURGERY

In addition to scheduling diagnostic tests and procedures, the medical assistant may also be responsible for scheduling surgery. Just as with a diagnostic test, it is important to have the proper information when scheduling the surgery, to instruct the patient about any special pre-surgery activities, and to document all of the interactions both between the medical assistant and other health care providers and between the medical assistant and the patient.

Information Necessary for Scheduling Surgery

More information is necessary to schedule a patient for surgery properly than for a diagnostic test. In addition to the patient's name, date of birth, and telephone number, the medical assistant must also know the type of surgery to be performed (e.g. **ORIF**, open reduction, internal fixation of (r)ight wrist; or **TURP**, trans-ure-thral resection of the prostate), the time frame within which the surgery is to be performed, who the surgeon and any assistant surgeons will be, who the anesthesiologist will be, and what hospital or day-surgery center at which the surgery will be performed.

Before scheduling the surgery, the medical assistant should call the patient's insurance company and obtain **preauthorization** (prior approval by the insurance company). The **preauthorization number** obtained from the insurance company must be given when scheduling surgery, since it facilitates payment by the insurance company for the procedure. The patient's insurance may restrict where surgery or diagnostic tests can be performed to specific institutions.

Finally, the medical assistant also needs to know who is to perform the pre-admission testing, known as **PAT.** PAT includes blood tests, an EKG, and a chest X-ray. Some hospitals do all of their own pre-admission testing; in other communities, the surgeon who will perform the surgery does it; and in still others, the patient's primary care doctor is responsible.

A patient may also need to be scheduled to donate one or more units of his or her own blood to provide an **autologous** (to one's self) blood transfusion during the surgery.

Procedure 34–2 describes scheduling surgery in more detail.

Giving a Patient Instructions Before Surgery

It is often necessary to give the patient specific instructions prior to surgery. If general anesthesia is being used, the patient should not eat for a period of time before the surgery. The patient may need to wash with antibiotic soap or need to take a particular medication before the surgery, such as an antibiotic or a sedative.

Patients are often instructed not to bring valuables with them to the hospital. If they are having day surgery, they need to arrange to have someone pick them up after surgery, since they usually are not allowed to drive. If the patient is NPO (not to eat or drink) after midnight before the surgery, it is important to check with the doctor about whether the patient should take his or her daily medications before the surgery. Sometimes the surgeon allows the patient to take morning medication with a sip of water.

Figure 34–5 shows a medical assistant discussing surgery with a patient.

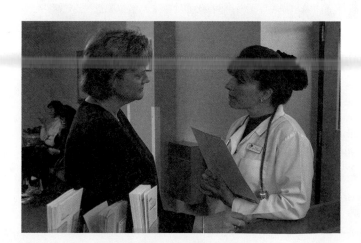

➢ **Figure 34–5** The medical assistant discusses preparation for surgery with the patient.

Documenting an Appointment for Surgery

As in the case of scheduling a test, the medical assistant should make sure to document in the patient's file all of his or her interactions with surgical team members and facilities, as well as interactions with the patient about the surgery.

SCHEDULING AN INPATIENT HOSPITAL ADMISSION

If the doctor wants to admit a patient to the hospital, the medical assistant must call the hospital's admitting department to arrange the admission. Before sending the patient to the hospital, it is also necessary to call the patient's insurance company to obtain a preauthorization.

The medical assistant gives the admitting department the patient's name, address, date of birth, admitting diagnosis, and the patient's insurance information and preauthorization number. The hospital usually asks when the doctor is coming to see the patient (who must be seen by his or her own doctor within the first 24 hours after admission.)

If the patient goes to the emergency room and is determined to require admission, the hospital obtains the information from the patient and calls the doctor to obtain admitting orders.

REFERRALS AND PREAUTHORIZATIONS

Especially for patients who have managed-care insurance, every referral must be documented closely and often justified to the insurance company's utilization review personnel. Medical assistants play an important role in facilitating the referral process.

A **referral** is made by the patient's primary care doctor. It is an authorization for a specific number of visits to or treatments by a specialist or other health care practitioner. Usually, the primary care provider can initiate a referral to a doctor who participates in the patient's managed care plan without preauthorization, consistent with his or her role as "gatekeeper," or person responsible for deciding what care is medically necessary for the patient. An exception is patients covered by Medicaid, where all care except visits to the primary care provider must be preauthorized.

Preauthorization may be required for therapy (such as physical therapy, occupational therapy, or speech therapy), certain diagnostic tests or procedures, consultations by a doctor who does not participate in the insurance plan, and procedures that cost more than a specific amount of money. If preauthorization is required, the medical assistant usually calls the insurance company and sends a follow-up written referral request.

Referrals are generally made for one of three reasons: to a specialist for a consultation on a particular disease, condition, or injury; to a provider of ongoing therapy, such as physical therapy, occupational therapy, or psychological therapy; or to a provider of community-based services, such as home health care, visiting nurses, or respite care for a care giver. The doctor determines the type and amount of service needed, but the medical assistant usually completes the referral form(s). A sample referral form was shown in Figure 12–6.

Referrals for Consultations

For a consultation referral, the medical assistant needs to know the following information: the patient's full name; the insurance information necessary, to-

ON THE JOB

In the office of Blackburn Primary Care Associates, you are filling in for Sandra, a medical assistant. You need to schedule a patient of Dr. Joanne Hughes for surgery, to take place in two weeks.

QUESTIONS
1. What information do you need from the patient in order to schedule the surgery?
2. What information do you need from Dr. Hughes about the surgery?
3. Once the arrangements are made, and you have given the patient information about the arrangements as well as special instructions, how will you verify that the patient understands the instructions?
4. What needs to be documented in the medical record?
5. Why is documentation so important?

PROCEDURE 34-3

Completing a Referral Form for Managed Care

Performance Objective: The student will be able to complete a referral form for managed care.

Supplies and Equipment: The patient's medical record and insurance information, information about the service to be provided, paper referral form or computer terminal, telephone, telephone number of the patient's insurance company.

Procedure Steps

1. Assemble the information necessary to complete the referral form, including the patient's name, address, telephone number, and insurance information.
2. From the patient's medical record or the doctor, determine the service for which the patient will be referred, including the specialist or service provider, the reason for the referral, and the number of visits.
   Rationale: This information is required to complete the referral form.
3. Obtain preauthorization from the patient's insurance, if necessary by calling the toll-free number provided by the insurance company. Describe the service requested, the reason for the referral, and the number of visits requested.
   Rationale: The patient's medical condition must justify the service requested. Preauthori-

zation, if granted, will be for a specific number of visits.
4. Complete a referral form, including the requested information about the patient, referring physician, specialist or facility to which the patient is being referred, reason for the referral, preauthorization number (if verbal preauthorization was obtained), and amount of service authorized.
5. If preauthorization is required, submit the form to the patient's insurance company for approval. In some cases, the patient will not be able to obtain service until written preauthorization is received from the insurance company.
6. Retain a copy of the referral for the patient's medical record and give the remaining copies to the patient to submit when service is received. You may also choose to send the referral forms directly to the specialist or facility to whom the patient has been referred.
7. Instruct the patient how to make the appointment (or assist the patient to make the first appointment).
8. File the copy of the referral form in the patient's medical record.

---

gether with any particular referral authorization forms to use; the doctor who is making the referral; the doctor or other provider to whom the patient is being referred, the reason for the consultation; and the number of visits that will be made to the specialist. Procedure 34–3 describes completing a referral form in more detail.

Referrals for Therapy

The same information is necessary when making a referral for therapy. It is especially important to know the number of visits, and if preauthorization is required by the patient's insurance company.

Referrals to Community Resources

For a referral to a community resource, the medical assistant must know the patient's name, address, and telephone number, as well as the particular resource needed, the diagnosis, and the reason for the service.

Some community agencies do an intake evaluation of the patient, but others depend on the primary care or other doctor and staff to tell them what resources the patient needs. These resources can go from the simple, such as meals on wheels—a daily hot meal delivered to the patient's home—to complex hospice care, which involves a range of services provided to an individual who is going to die in a reasonably short period of time.

STUDENT STUDY PLAN

To reinforce your understanding of the material in this chapter . . .

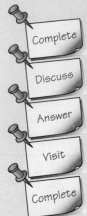

Complete the **Review & Recall** questions.

Discuss the situation in **If You Were the Medical Assistant** with your classmates, and answer the questions.

Answer the **Critical Thinking Questions** and discuss them with your classmates.

Visit the **Web sites** suggested and search for additional Web sites using the **Keywords for Internet Searches**.

Complete the exercises in chapter 34 of the **Student Mastery Manual**.

✔ REVIEW & RECALL

1. What information do you need to schedule follow-up appointments?

2. How do you schedule a diagnostic test for a patient?

3. What is the purpose of a diagnostic tracking log?

4. What information do you need to schedule surgery for a patient?

5. What instructions must be given to a patient when surgery is scheduled?

6. Define and state the purpose of a referral.

7. Differentiate between a referral and a preauthorization.

✔ IF YOU WERE THE MEDICAL ASSISTANT

You are reviewing the diagnostic tracking log and notice that you have not received the results of tests on three patients. What steps should you follow to determine why they have not been received? What legal issues are at stake?

✔ CRITICAL THINKING QUESTIONS

1. Contact several large practices in your area to research the insurance companies that require referral forms. Report on each company and the procedures they follow.

2. Contact the hospitals in your area and make a chart of their requirements for admission to a hospital.

3. Discuss the implications for the medical assistant when different insurance companies require lab tests, diagnostic procedures, and surgery to be performed by specific labs or hospitals.

4. What is the impact on patient care if the doctor's ability to make a referral is limited by the patient's insurance company? Give examples to support your answer.

EXPLORE THE WEB

INTERNET WEB SITES

Managed care links
www.managedhealth.com

Information about diagnostic tests for patients
www.healthwatch.medscape.com/
  select library, then medical tests

KEYWORDS FOR INTERNET SEARCHES

[Your local hospital] (Local hospital Web sites often contain information about preparation for surgery or admission.)
  managed care referrals
  preoperative teaching

 ANSWERS TO ON THE JOB

1. To schedule surgery, you need to know the patient's name, date of birth, and insurance information.

2. The information you need from the doctor is the name of the procedure, the diagnosis, the urgency for the surgery, the surgeon, and any assistants.

3. You can verify patient understanding by asking the patient to repeat the instructions to you.

4. Document the date, time, place, type of surgery scheduled, and the specific instructions given to the patient. Include that the patient was able to express understanding of the instructions and had no further questions.

5. Documentation is used as evidence that care was given—in this case, that the patient was given pre-operative instructions.

Written Follow-up

Instructional Objectives

After completing this chapter, you will be able to do the following:

1. Define and spell the vocabulary words for this chapter.
2. Obtain previous medical records for a patient.
3. Complete consent for release of information.
4. Describe how to prepare envelopes and business letters.
5. List steps to sort incoming mail.
6. Describe the process of transcribing medical reports and correspondence.
7. Identify how to use a fax machine or e-mail to send information.
8. Describe how to open, sort, and organize incoming mail.

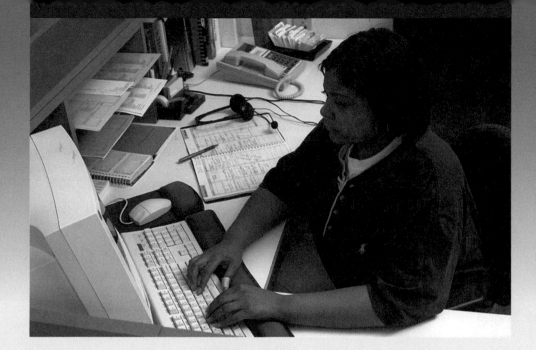

CMA/RMA CERTIFICATION
Content and Competencies

- Obtain a "release of information" for medical records
- Compose a letter

- Address a business envelope
- Complete a fax cover sheet
- Process incoming mail for office personnel

Performance Objectives

After completing this chapter, you will be able to do the following:

1. Compose and key a business letter (Procedure 35–1).
2. Address an envelope for mailing (Procedure 35–2).
3. Transcribe a dictated letter or report (Procedure 35–3).
4. Prepare outgoing mail (Procedure 35–4).
5. Send a fax (Procedure 35–5).
6. Prepare copies of multiple-page documents (Procedure 35–6).

VOCABULARY

block style (p. 863)	left-justified (p. 863)	proofread (p. 867)	simplified letter style (p. 863)
collate (p. 873)	modified block style (p. 863)	right-justified (p. 863)	template (p. 867)
e-mail (p. 871)	postage meter (p. 870)	semi-block style (p. 863)	transcription (p. 867)
fax (p. 870)			

Written follow-up can be provided to a patient, to the party that is paying for the treatment, or to another doctor who has referred the patient to your practice.

Until 20 years ago, all written follow-up was provided by letter, and mailed through the U.S. Postal Service. Today, much written follow-up is provided by fax and even by e-mail. Regardless of how the written material is transmitted, however, it is still important that the follow-up correspondence or reports be presented in the proper format.

Finally, when written follow-up is provided to a party other than the patient, it is necessary to acquire the patient's permission to release his or her medical information regarding the visit, procedure, or treatment provided in your office.

FOLLOW-UP THAT REQUIRES A PATIENT'S WRITTEN RELEASE OF INFORMATION

The patient must give permission for the office to release information or seek information from another party in two instances. One is obtaining hospital records or records from the primary care doctor the patient previously saw. The other instance occurs when the current medical provider must send information to a third party, such as an insurance company (in order to be paid) or an attorney (in the case of a lawsuit, worker's compensation claim, or other matter).

This permission is usually provided on a standard form used by the office, as illustrated in Figure 35–1.

Medical Records

If the patient is new to the office, he or she should be asked to give permission for the office to seek his or her medical records from the primary care doctor who previously took care of the patient.

In addition, from time to time it becomes necessary for the doctor to retrieve information from a hospital where the patient has been treated. In this case, again, you can ask the patient to sign a form giving permission for the hospital to release medical records to your office.

Insurance/Legal

If a patient is new, or if the patient has changed insurance, it is necessary for the patient to sign a new form allowing the office to forward records of all visits, treatments, tests, and procedures to the patient's insurance company in order to substantiate bills to the insurance company.

Also, if the patient has been treated for an injury caused by an incident that is the subject of a lawsuit, or one that is subject to worker's compensation, the patient must sign a form allowing information regarding the treatment to be sent to the attorney and liability insurance company involved in the suit, or the insurance company that holds the worker's compensation policy.

Reports to Other Doctors or Health Care Facilities

When a doctor sees a patient for a consultation, he or she sends a written consultation report to the primary care provider. If a patient moves, copies of his or her medical record are often sent to the new primary care provider, after permission has been obtained from the patient. Medical records may also be sent to nursing homes or other health care facilities to provide continuity of care.

WRITTEN CORRESPONDENCE AND REPORTS

Letters leaving the medical office that pertain to a patient visit—whether sent to a referring physician, an attorney, or an insurance company—require proper formatting. The letter may be dictated by the doctor and transcribed by the medical assistant; or in some cases, the medical assistant can compose the letter based on the doctor's guidelines.

Letters should be single-spaced, typewritten or word-processed, and use one of four styles: block, modified block, modified block with indented paragraphs, or simplified. (These styles are described immediately after the description of parts of the letter.)

AUTHORIZATION FOR RELEASE OF MEDICAL INFORMATION
please complete in ink

Date _____

PATIENT IDENTIFICATION   Name _____

    Address _____

    _____

MEDICAL FACILITY   Telephone _____

    Doctor _____

    Address _____

    _____

    _____

I hearby authorize and request you to release the complete medical records in your possession, concerning my illness and/or treatment during the period from _____ to _____

I understand that if my medical record contains information in reference to drug and/or alcohol abuse, psychiatric, venereal disease, social service and/or sensitive information, hepatitis testing/treatment, I agree to its release.

_____   _____
Signature of patient/legal guardian   Date

Note:
In ADDITION to the signature above, if you want your HIV/AIDS testing/treatment records released you MUST sign and date below:

I agree to the release of HIV/AIDS testing/treatment information found in my medical record:

_____   _____
Signature of patient/legal guardian   Date

➤ Figure 35–1 Permission form signed by patients authorizing the medical office to release information.

The Business Letter

A business letter has nine parts, which fall within four sections:

Section	Part
Heading	Sender's name and address
Opening	Date line
	Inside address (of receiver)
	Salutation
Body	Body text
Closing	Complimentary close
	Signature
	Signature line
	Reference notation
	Enclosure notation
	Distribution notation

The heading is the name of the individual sending the letter (even if a staff person is actually physically typing or keying the letter) and the return address. If

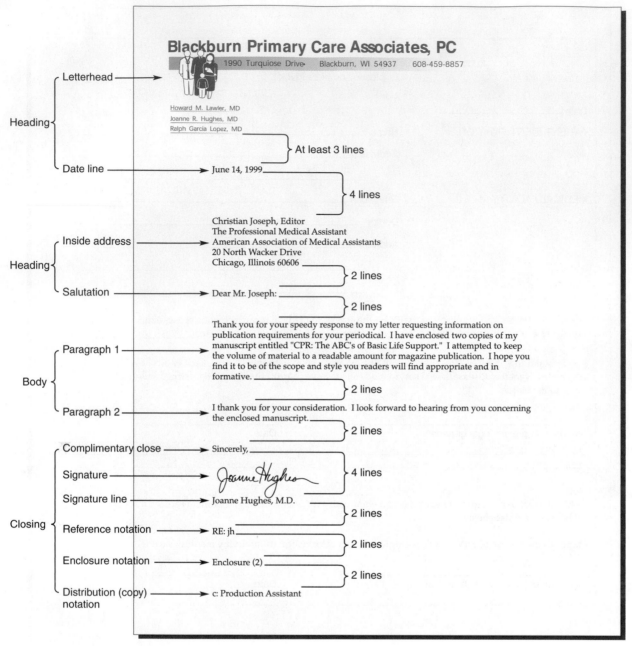

Blackburn Primary Care Associates, PC

1990 Turquiose Drive   Blackburn, WI 54937   608-459-8857

Howard M. Lawler, MD
Joanne R. Hughes, MD
Ralph Garcia Lopez, MD

Letterhead

Heading

At least 3 lines

Date line — June 14, 1999

4 lines

Inside address
Christian Joseph, Editor
The Professional Medical Assistant
American Association of Medical Assistants
20 North Wacker Drive
Chicago, Illinois 60606

2 lines

Heading

Salutation — Dear Mr. Joseph:

2 lines

Paragraph 1
Thank you for your speedy response to my letter requesting information on publication requirements for your periodical. I have enclosed two copies of my manuscript entitled "CPR: The ABC's of Basic Life Support." I attempted to keep the volume of material to a readable amount for magazine publication. I hope you find it to be of the scope and style you readers will find appropriate and in formative.

2 lines

Body

Paragraph 2
I thank you for your consideration. I look forward to hearing from you concerning the enclosed manuscript.

2 lines

Complimentary close — Sincerely,

4 lines

Signature — Joanne Hughes

Signature line — Joanne Hughes, M.D.

2 lines

Reference notation — RE: jh

2 lines

Enclosure notation — Enclosure (2)

2 lines

Distribution (copy) notation — c: Production Assistant

Closing

➤ **Figure 35–2** The parts of a letter in block format.

office letterhead is used, no heading needs to be composed.

The date line is the date the letter is composed. The month is written out in full on the date line.

The inside address is the address of the party to whom the letter is being sent.

The salutation is the greeting.

Together, the date line, inside address, and salutation are known as the letter's opening.

The body of the letter contains the substance, which should be presented clearly and concisely. Doctors, attorneys, and insurance claims adjusters (worker's compensation or liability claims) all receive much mail, and the information they need about an interaction between the staff in your office and the patient is very specific. It will be placed in the patient's medical records.

The complimentary close is the line with which the letter's personal communication to the party receiving the letter is ended. It is a sign of respect, and can be adjusted depending on how well the letter's author and the party being addressed know each other. "Sincerely" is the standard close; "Cordially" is considered a little less formal by many people. "With my best regards" should be used only when the individuals know each other well. A more formal closing is "Yours truly" or "Very truly yours."

The signature is the actual written signature of the individual sending the letter.

The signature line is the name of the individual sending the letter, typed out, sometimes with credentials (e.g. M.D.) or a job title in the office (e.g. Office Manager).

The reference notation notes the initials of the person who composed the letter (in uppercase) followed by the initials of the person who typed or keyed the letter (in lowercase). If the letter contains enclosures, such as a log of visits or billing records, this is noted in the enclosure notation, two lines below the reference notation. Distribution notation (copy notation) identifies the recipient(s). The letter "c" followed by a colon signifies that one copy was distributed; "cc" followed by a colon is used for more than one copy.

Business letters can be written using one of the following four styles.

In **block style** (full block), all lines are **left-justified** (starting all lines flush to the left margin on the page). A double space is left between the end of one paragraph and the beginning of the next. A business letter using block style is shown in Figure 35–2.

Modified block style starts all lines in the body of the letter flush left, and double-spaces between paragraphs. However, the date line, complimentary close, and signature lines begin in the center of the letter, or are sometimes **right-justified** (flush right margin).

Modified block style with indented paragraph (**semi-block style**) is the same as modified block style, except that the first sentence of each new paragraph is indented five spaces.

Simplified letter style resembles a memorandum. Instead of a salutation, a subject line typed all in capital letters is placed three lines below the inside address, and the complimentary close and signature lines are replaced by an all-capital-letter signature five lines below the letter's body.

See Procedure 35–1 for a full description of the proper method for composing and keying a business letter.

The Envelope

The business envelope, shown in Figure 35–3, has three parts.

The business envelope is most often a size 10 enve-

PROCEDURE 35–1

Composing a Business Letter

Performance Objective: The student will be able to compose and key a business letter.

Supplies and Equipment: Letterhead stationery; blank stationery; typewriter, word processor, or computer and printer.

Procedure Steps

1. Assemble materials, determine the address of the recipient, and decide on a format for the letter.

2. Formulate the content for the business letter. Write a rough draft of the content to be sure all necessary information is included.

3. Insert the date on the third line below the letterhead. For block format, the date is at the left margin. For modified block format, the date begins at the center of the line.

4. Place the inside address four to ten lines below the date at the left margin. If using a computer, this space can be adjusted after the letter has been keyed so that the body of the letter is centered on the page.

5. Place the salutation two lines below the inside address. The salutation should include a title and the person's last name (e.g. Dear Dr. Gordon, Dear Mrs. Wilson, Dear Rev. Meyers) unless the recipient of the letter is a person you routinely call by his or her first name.
   Rationale: A business letter is usually more formal than personal correspondence.

6. If desired, place a subject line two lines below the salutation. A subject line begins with the Latin word re (meaning about) followed by a colon. It is usually capitalized (e.g. Re: AAMA meeting on Thursday, June 12, 200X.)
   Rationale: Although optional, a subject line helps the recipient identify the subject of the letter before reading it.

7. Begin the body of the letter two lines below the salutation (or subject line, if used.) The body of the letter is single-spaced with two spaces between paragraphs. In block and modified block letter styles, the paragraphs

Procedure continued on following page

PROCEDURE 35-1 *(continued)*

begin at the left margin. If modified block style with indented paragraphs is used, indent the first line of each paragraph five spaces.

8. The final paragraph of the letter should summarize the contents and/or most important ideas.

9. Place the complimentary close two spaces below the final paragraph of the body of the letter. For the block letter style, the complimentary close begins at the left margin. For the modified block letter style, it begins at the center of the line. "Yours truly" and "Very Truly Yours" are normal; "Sincerely yours" is less formal and most commonly used.

10. Drop down four lines and type your name, beginning at the same place as the complimentary close. (If you are composing a letter for someone else, type that person's name.) *Rationale:* Typing the name under the handwritten signature facilitates a response, since the signature may be difficult to read.

11. If necessary, add a reference line, enclosure notation, and/or distribution notation, placing each two lines below the others at the left margin. If you compose and key your own letter, a reference line is unnecessary. If you compose and key a letter for someone else, place your initials in lowercase letters. If you key a letter that was dictated by the person signing the letter, place his or her initials (uppercase) followed by your initials (lowercase) separated by a colon. The enclosure notation may be written out or abbreviated "Enc." The number of enclosures may be placed in parentheses if there is more

than one. The distribution notation identifies individuals who receive a copy of the letter. The letter "c" followed by a colon is usually used if one copy is distributed and, "cc" followed by a colon is used if more than one copy is distributed (e.g. c: Dr. Sam Gardner.) *Rationale:* The person who receives the letter is entitled to know who keyed the letter and who received copies. If the number of enclosures is indicated, it is easier to tell if all intended material is enclosed with the letter.

12. If the letter is longer than one page, the second page should be printed or typed on stationery of the same quality and weight as the letterhead stationery, beginning one inch from the top. Space the letter so that at least two lines of the body of the letter continue to the second page.

13. Spell-check the letter and proofread it carefully. If using a computer, print the letter. *Rationale:* A business letter should not contain errors. If errors are present, the credibility and professionalism of the sender may be doubted.

14. Sign the letter below the complimentary close, or have the person for whom you prepared the letter sign it.

15. Make a copy of the letter *Rationale:* Copies of all business letters are retained in case there are questions or further correspondence is necessary.

16. Prepare an envelope (Procedure 35–2) and send the letter. If the letter concerns a patient, a copy of the letter is filed in the patient's medical record. Other letters are usually filed in folders by subject (e.g. letters to suppliers).

---

lope, measuring 4⅛ inches from top to bottom and 9½ inches from side to side, or a size 6¾ envelope, measuring 3⅝ inches from top to bottom and 6½ inches from side to side.

In the upper left-hand corner of the envelope is the sender's return address, either printed to match the office letterhead, or typed or keyed beginning 1/2 inches from the envelope's upper left edge. The address of the person to whom the letter is being sent is centered on the envelope. For a size 10 business envelope, the address begins 14 lines from the top, with a left margin of four inches; for a size 6¾ envelope, the address begins 12 lines from the top, with a left margin of two inches. The U.S. Postal Service (USPS) recommends keying the address in capital letters without punctuation, except for a hyphen in the zip + 4 (nine-character) zip code. (See the box on page 865 for a list of two-letter abbreviations for states.)

The postal service web site, which can be used to determine the zip code, is found at the end of this chapter.

In order for postal scanning equipment to work properly, nothing should be placed below the address. If the letter is directed to the attention of a specific individual, the postal service recommends placing the attention line directly above the address (e.g. ATTN: Joan Collins, Midwest Collections . . .) Other special directions, such as "personal" or "confidential," should be placed on the left side of the envelope below the return address, but above the mailing address. Mailing directions, such as "Via Air Mail" or "Priority Mail,"

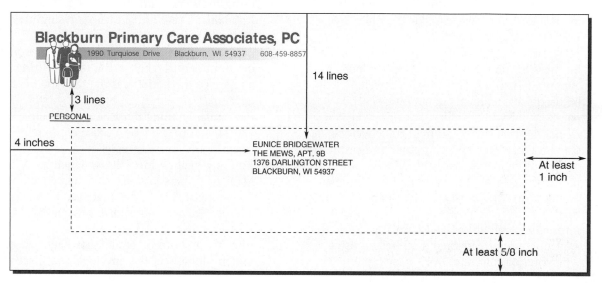

➢ **Figure 35–3** Addressing a business envelope.

Two-Letter Abbreviations for States and Territories

AL	Alabama	IL	Illinois	NC	North Carolina	RI	Rhode Island
AK	Alaska	IN	Indiana	ND	North Dakota	SC	South Carolina
AZ	Arizona	IA	Iowa	NE	Nebraska	SD	South Dakota
AR	Arkansas	KS	Kansas	NH	New Hampshire	TN	Tennessee
CA	California	KY	Kentucky	NJ	New Jersey	TX	Texas
CO	Colorado	LA	Louisiana	NM	New Mexico	UT	Utah
CT	Connecticut	ME	Maine	NV	Nevada	VT	Vermont
DE	Delaware	MD	Maryland	NY	New York	VI	Virgin Islands
DC	District of Columbia	MA	Massachusetts	OH	Ohio	VA	Virginia
FL	Florida	MI	Michigan	OK	Oklahoma	WA	Washington
GA	Georgia	MN	Minnesota	OR	Oregon	WV	West Virginia
GU	Guam	MS	Mississippi	PA	Pennsylvania	WI	Wisconsin
HI	Hawaii	MO	Missouri	PR	Puerto Rico	WY	Wyoming
ID	Idaho	MT	Montana				

PROCEDURE 35–2

Addressing an Envelope

Performance Objective: The student will be able to address an envelope for mailing.

Supplies and Equipment: Envelope, pen, typewriter, or computer and printer.

Procedure Steps

1 Determine the exact address to be used to address the envelope. Addresses may be kept in an index card box, circular card file (e.g. Roladex), or computer file.

2. Select an envelope of the appropriate size. For business letters a No. 10 envelope is most commonly used. A large manila envelope may be used for documents containing several pages.

3. Decide on a means to address the envelope, using a typewriter or a computer and printer, or writing by hand. The address may be placed directly on the envelope or on a label. Avoid addressing business correspondence by hand.
   Rationale: Standard business correspondence appears more professional if addressed using a typewriter or computer.

4. Key the address in capital letters near the center of the envelope with the name of the re-

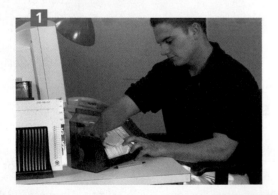

cipient on the first line; the apartment number or suite (if any) on the second line; the street address on the next line; and the city, state, and nine-number zip code on the bottom line. Do not use punctuation, except for a hyphen after the first five numbers of the zip + 4 code. If using an envelope without letterhead, key the return address in the upper left corner using the same guidelines.
   Rationale: These are guidelines recommended by the U.S. Postal Service.

5. Add any special notations, such as "Personal" or "Confidential," below the return address and above the address at the left side of the envelope.
   Rationale: Nothing must be placed below the address in order for post office equipment to read the envelope correctly.

6. Add any mailing instructions (such as "Via Air Mail" or "First Class" for a manila envelope) on the right side of the envelope above the address, leaving room for a postage label above them.

7. After the item to be mailed has been placed in the envelope, seal the envelope and place the correct amount of postage in the upper right corner. Weigh the piece of mail if it contains more than two sheets of paper. Consult a chart for postage if a manila envelope is used because large envelopes require additional postage if sent first class.
   Rationale: The letter will be delayed if inadequate postage is used.

8. Take the item to the post office if it should be sent by certified mail, registered mail, or return receipt requested; complete the required forms. If using priority mail, a pickup can be requested, or the item can be taken to the post office.

should be placed above and to the right of the mailing address, leaving space above them for a label from a postage meter.

See Procedure 35–2 for a description of how to address an envelope for mailing.

The address should include the street address, any post office box number, city, state, and the postal code (zip + 4 code in the United States). The return address contains the same information, and is necessary in case the letter cannot be delivered.

Transcription

The purpose of **transcription** is to produce any verbal notes the doctor makes about the patient interaction in typed or word-processed format. While some doctors still handwrite their notes about the patient encounter, many more use some form of dictation and transcription system.

Modern transcription systems include a small, handheld dictation recorder into which the doctor dictates his or her notes, and a desktop unit with a foot pedal that the transcriber uses to listen to the dictation tape. The recorder and the transcription machine must take the same size tape cassettes (standard or microcassette). The transcriber keys the dictation, using word-processing software. Dictation equipment is shown in Figure 35–4.

Word-processing software allows the transcriber to create a **template** (an incomplete document that serves as a pattern) that presets the format for the transcription.

The reports doctors most often dictate in an office setting are progress notes, history and physical examination, consultation reports, and correspondence.

Progress notes may be set up in SOAP format (see Chapter 10, Figure 10–1B) or using other headings (such as CC: Chief Complaint; PE or Px: Physical Examination; Dx: Diagnosis; Rx or Plan: Treatment). Each note should include the patient's name, clinic number or birthdate, and the date of the office visit. Progress notes are single-spaced, with two spaces between paragraphs or headings. Entries under Diagnosis (Assessment) and Plan are usually numbered. A signature line is usually included for the doctor to sign the note.

Each office has a preferred format for progress notes. The progress note for each visit may be printed on a separate piece of paper, or paper with adhesive backing may be used so each note can be mounted in chronological order in the medical record. When a doctor dictates progress notes, the findings of tests and interviews done by the medical assistant are often incorporated into the dictated notes.

There is no standard format for dictated history and physical examination reports, so the medical assistant should determine the preferred format for the office where he or she is working. Usually, the report is divided into identifying information (patient, clinic number or birthdate, doctor, and date of examination), the sections of the history (described in chapter 14), and sections of the physical examination (described in chapter 16), with each heading keyed in all capital letters followed by a colon. The text of each section may be lined up flush with the left margin, or to a tab placed to make a separate column beside the headings. The physical examination usually includes a section for each body system examined. The final section of the physical examination usually includes the impression (Diagnosis) and Plan. The report of a physical examination was presented in chapter 16, as shown in Figure 16–16.

A consultation report may be dictated as a letter or in a format similar to the history and physical examination report. Medical assistants who work for specialists are more likely to transcribe consultation reports than those who work for primary care practitioners.

While transcribing the report, the medical assistant should look up any unfamiliar words in order to spell them correctly. It is helpful to use medical spell-check software, which is available from several companies. An ordinary spell-check program can also be personalized over time by adding medical words and abbreviations that the program does not recognize; however, additions should always be checked for correctness. After the report has been keyed, the transcriber should print a copy, **proofread** it (read it carefully and make corrections), then correct it and print out a final copy. If there is an unintelligible word, a space can be left and marked in pencil for the doctor to fill in before signing the report. Figure 35–5 is a list of proofreader's marks.

Today, a few doctors are beginning to use voice-recognition software, which allows them to dictate into a microphone and have the computer immediately produce the written dictation. Either the doctor or the transcriptionist then goes through the text to write out abbreviations, put in proper punctuation and paragraph breaks, and make any other changes needed for proper format of the voice-recognition produced transcript.

Some medical transcriptionists fear that voice-recognition software will end the practice of transcription,

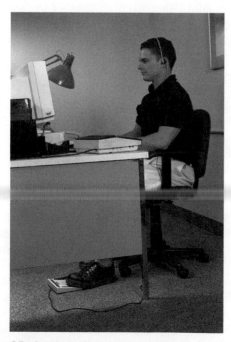

➤ **Figure 35–4** The medical assistant uses a transcribing tape recorder with a foot pedal.

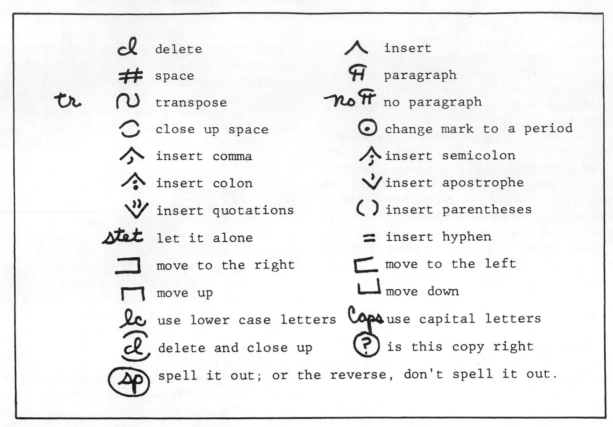

> **Figure 35–5** Standard proofreader's marks. (From Diehl MO, Fordney MT: *Medical Typing and Transcription: Techniques and Procedures*, 3rd ed. Philadelphia: W.B. Saunders, 1991.)

but others feel that voice-recognition will force transcriptionists to upgrade their skills, focusing more on editing than simply keying and proofreading. See Procedure 35–3 for a description of transcribing dictated letters and reports.

WAYS TO SEND WRITTEN FOLLOW-UP

There are three ways to forward written follow-up to the party who needs to receive it: mail, fax, and electronic mail (e-mail).

The U.S. Postal Service

The United States Postal Service provides a variety of ways for mail to be transported from sender to receiver. The cost of these various services depends on the urgency with which mail must be received, and any special handling services provided.

Classification of Mail

Express Mail. Express mail is delivered within 24 hours, and by noon to most major cities. It includes letters and packages up to 70 pounds. Envelopes and packing materials are available from the post office.

Priority Mail. Priority mail is used for mail weighing more than 11 ounces that is to be treated as first-class mail. Envelopes and packing materials are available from the post office.

First-Class Mail. First-class mail is used for letters or other light-weight items to be delivered within 2 to 4 days. The postage for items up to 11 ounces is based on weight, in 1-ounce increments.

Bound Printed Matter. This type of mail is used for advertising material and magazines up to 15 pounds.

Media Mail (Book Rate). This type of mail includes books, printed material, sound recordings, and other types of media material.

Parcel Post. Parcel-post mail is used for items that weigh more than 16 ounces that are not urgent. Items may weigh up to 70 pounds, or total 100 inches in combined length and circumference. Packages should be securely wrapped in sturdy boxes to avoid damage.

Combined Mail. If a letter is sent with a catalogue or package, it should be placed in an envelope that is attached to the package. The letter is charged for first-class postage, and the package is charged for the appropriate class.

Special Services

Additional services are available with most classifications of mail, to insure or track items sent:

Return Receipt. A postcard addressed to the sender is attached to the mail. When the item is received, the postcard is signed by the recipient and sent back to the sender by the postal service. The sender then has a copy of the signature of the person who signed for the piece of mail.

Registered Mail. Registered mail is available for first-class and priority mail, to insure the contents. The cost depends on the value of the item being sent. The sender receives a receipt that is kept until the recipient receives the item. The recipient must sign a form acknowledging receipt. For an additional fee, the sender can receive a return receipt.

Certified Mail. Certified mail requires the recipient to sign upon delivery. This service can also be combined with a return receipt for an additional fee.

Insured Mail. Insurance can be purchased on the contents of packages. The cost depends on the value of the contents. If the mail is lost or damaged, the post office will pay the declared value.

Most medical office correspondence is sent by first-class mail, using a stamp placed on the envelope by hand, by postage meter, or by computer printer through e-stamping.

When proof is needed that a particular letter arrived and was accepted, it can be sent by certified mail or registered mail, with a return receipt requested.

Other Package Delivery Services

There are several other companies that deliver letters or packages. Some, like FedEx, Airborne Express, or United Parcel Service (UPS), have next-day and two-day delivery service for letters or small packages. Larger packages that are not time-sensitive can be shipped via UPS or FedEx ground service. These companies will pick items up from your office, and offer item tracking either through an 800 telephone number or over the company's Web site. This ability may justify the higher cost for these services than typical postal rates.

Using a Postage Meter

Offices that send out a steady volume of mail regularly often use a mechanical postage meter or a computerized e-postage system.

PROCEDURE 35-3

Transcribing a Dictated Letter or Report

Performance Objective: The student will be able to transcribe a dictated letter or report.

Supplies and Equipment: Letterhead stationery, blank stationery or paper, transcription machine, headphones, tape containing dictation, typewriter, word processor or computer and printer.

Procedure Steps

1. Assemble materials, and decide on a format for the letter or report.
2. Set up the transcription machine and plug in headphones.
3. While listening to the dictation, key the letter following the guidelines given in Procedure 35–2 or key the report.
4. For a letter, be sure to include a reference line using the initials of the person who dictated the letter (uppercase) followed by your initials (lowercase) separated by a colon.
   Rationale: The person who receives a letter is entitled to know who keyed the letter and who received copies.
5. Spell-check the letter and proofread it carefully. Check the letter or report for consistency of style, grammar, and overall appearance.
   Rationale: Business letters and medical reports must be as accurate as possible.
6. Prepare an envelope (Procedure 35–2) for a letter and place the letter or report for the person who dictated it to sign.
7. After a letter has been signed, make a copy of the letter.
   Rationale: Copies of all business letters are retained in case there are questions or further correspondence is necessary.
8. Place the original letter in the envelope and send it. If the letter or report pertains to a patient, file the copy in the patient's medical record. Other correspondence is usually filed in folders by subject.

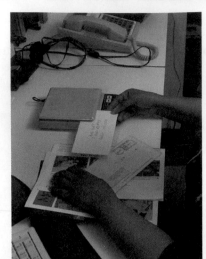

➤ **Figure 35-6** A postage meter can facilitate preparation of outgoing letters.

A mechanical **postage meter** is a machine that weighs and automatically stamps outgoing mail with the proper postage. A postage meter can be rented from the postal service or one of its approved vendors or purchased from an approved vendor. The amount of postage that can be stamped with the meter is predetermined and prepaid, either on a regular basis (e.g.

monthly) or when the amount remaining is getting low.

When using a postage meter, the date is changed each day to the correct day. The postage can be stamped directly on the envelope by passing the envelope through the meter (which may also automatically seal the letter), or by printing a premoistened label to be placed on the envelope. If the postage meter does not include a scale, the office should have an accurate scale and chart to calculate the amount of postage to place on each item. Figure 35-6 shows the medical assistant using a postage meter.

To refill the meter, it is taken to a postal service branch, where a postal service worker opens it, accepts payment, and sets the machine's internal metering system to the amount of postage that has been paid for.

E-postage systems use either an electronic meter attached to a computer or software installed on the computer to do the weighing and stamping. The stamping can be done right from the computer printer. Software allows payment to be made directly through the computer using a credit card, and the new authorized stamping amount is downloaded into the computer.

Procedure 35-4 details the preparation of outgoing mail.

Fax

When a **fax** (facsimile) is being sent, a cover sheet is attached. The cover sheet has information about the

---

PROCEDURE 35-4

Preparing Outgoing Mail

Performance Objective: The student will be able to prepare outgoing mail.
Supplies and Equipment: Letters, other items to be mailed, stamps or postage machine.

Procedure Steps

1. Assemble all letters and other items to be mailed.
2. Be sure each letter has been inserted in a properly addressed envelope and sealed.
3. Sort envelopes according to size.
4. Separate any items with special mailing instructions that must be taken to the post office. If necessary, add instructions to the envelopes. If the office does not have a postal

scale, include any letters that may need extra postage.
5. Place appropriate postage on envelopes to be mailed from the office using stamps or a postage meter.
6. Place items with postage in a mailbox.
7. Take special items to the post office. This includes items that are to be sent return receipt, certified mail, registered mail, or insured mail as well as items weighing more than 1 pound. Items to be sent priority mail (up to 1 pound) can be mailed from the office if appropriate postage is placed on them.
   Rationale: Mail weighing more than 1 pound will not be accepted from a mailbox even if proper postage is attached.

Blackburn Primary Care Associates, PC

1990 Turquiose Drive • Blackburn, WI 54937 • 608-459-8857

Howard M. Lawler, MD
Joanne R. Hughes, MD
Ralph Garcia Lopez, MD

DATE: _____ TIME: _____ NUMBER OF PAGES: _____

TO: _____
(name of authorized receiver)

_____
(name of authorized receiver's facility)

TELEPHONE: _____ FAX: _____
(of receiver)   (of receiver)

FROM: __BLACKBURN PRIMARY CARE ASSOCIATES - DR._____
(name of sender)

TELEPHONE: __608-459-8857__ FAX: __608-459-8342__
(of sender)   (of sender)

Comments:

******CONFIDENTIALITY NOTICE******

The documents accompanying this telecopy transmission contain confidential information, belonging to the sender that is legally privileged. This information is intended only for the use of the individual or entity named above. The authorized recipient of this information is prohibited from disclosing this information to any other party and is required to destroy the information after its stated need has been fulfilled, unless otherwise required by state law.

If you are not the intended recipient, you are hereby notified that any disclosure, copying, distribution, or action taken in reliance on the contents of these documents is strictly prohibited. If you have received this telecopy in error, please notify the sender immediately to arrange for return of these documents.

> **Figure 35–7** A fax cover sheet is often created on office letterhead.

sender, such as the office address, the name of the individual sending the fax, the total number of pages in the fax, a return fax number, and a return voice phone number in case the fax does not come through clearly. A fax cover sheet is shown in Figure 35–7.

It is important to realize that fax is not a secure means of communication. Information that can be compromising to a patient should not be faxed.

Information in a fax travels over the telephone line; the machine translates the written symbols on the page into analog or digital signals to transmit over the phone lines, then the machine at the other end retranslates the analog or digital signals into the written symbols to appear again on the paper. Just as a telephone can be tapped to listen to a conversation, a fax line can be tapped to extract the signals. In addition, in spite of the confidentiality notice, the fax may be viewed by unauthorized individuals at the receiving location. Procedure 35–5 describes sending a fax.

E-Mail and Other Forms of Electronic Data Transmission

E-mail (electronic mail) is rapidly becoming the preferred means of communication throughout the business world. A computer with modem is used to send e-mail; the modem translates the digital signals from the computer into analog or digital signals for the telephone, and the modem at the other end of the communication retranslates the signals.

PROCEDURE 35-5

Sending a Fax

Performance Objective: The student will be able to send a fax.

Supplies and Equipment: Fax machine, cover sheet, document to be faxed.

Procedure Steps

1. Prepare the cover sheet including the name, address, and fax number of the recipient; fax number of the sender; and number of pages (including the cover sheet.) If there is a message to the sender, include it on the bottom of the cover sheet.
2. Organize all pages to be faxed with the cover sheet first.
   Rationale: Pages should be in order and all facing the same direction.
3. Place pages in the fax machine, face up or face down as is correct for the machine being used.
4. Enter the fax number. Include any extra digits as required such as a "9" to obtain an outside line, a "1" for long-distance, and/or an area code if required.
   Rationale: Some areas of the country have introduced so-called "overlay" area codes requiring all telephone numbers to be dialed with an area code.
5. Verify the fax number as it appears in the window or on the computer screen to be sure the number is correct.
   Rationale: To maintain confidentiality, always be sure the fax number has been entered correctly.
6. Press the correct button to send the fax.
7. Check back to be sure the fax has been sent. Some machines print a confirmation for every fax, and some only print a written report if the fax does not go through.
   Rationale: If the fax does not go through, you must determine the reason and resend it.
8. File the original document appropriately.

As with the fax, there are security issues since the information is sent over the telephone lines. However, e-mail and other computer communications using telephone lines can be encrypted to increase security.

Currently, electronic methods are commonly used to submit insurance claims. This topic is discussed in detail in chapter 38, which covers insurance claim submissions.

PROCESSING INCOMING MAIL

Another task of the medical assistant is to process incoming mail. Processing mail involves both routing mail to the appropriate individual to handle the correspondence, as well as knowing which mail the medical assistant can open and deal with and how to set up the incoming mail for the doctors and various other specialists to deal with.

ON THE JOB

Stacey, a medical assistant for Blackburn Primary Care Associates, is planning to send an order to a medical supply company using the fax machine.

QUESTIONS
1. What other ways could she have sent the information?
2. What are the advantages and disadvantages of using the fax machine?
3. Is it important to maintain confidentiality in this case? If it is, how can Stacey maintain confidentiality?
4. What information should be on the fax cover sheet?

Sorting Mail to the Appropriate Person

Incoming mail should be sorted in the following way.

If the mail is addressed to a particular doctor, it goes into that doctor's box or pile. Mail from another doctor's office that is not addressed to a particular doctor should go into the box or pile of the managing partner, medical director, or office manager.

Mail from insurance companies should go to the insurance specialist, or medical assistant who handles insurance matters. Mail from pharmaceutical companies, medical supply companies, medical equipment companies, and other vendors should go to the office manager, or the medical assistant who manages the office. The same is true of mail from the office's other vendors, such as office equipment vendors, liability insurance carrier, attorney, or accountant.

Once the mail is sorted, it must be opened. The medical assistant must know which mail he or she is to open, and which is to go unopened to the individual who must deal with it. Some doctors like to open their own mail, but others like to have the mail opened, organized, and ready for them to read and respond to. Clearly, any mail marked "personal" or "confidential" should not be opened.

Usually, the person who sorts the mail is empowered to open all of the office's business mail, which then goes to the business manager and/or insurance specialist.

Procedure for Organizing Opened Mail

If the doctor or doctors prefer mail to be opened, use a letter opener to open each piece carefully at the top edge. Stamp each letter with the receipt date and alphabetize by the patient's last name. The pages of each report should be stapled together if they are not already that way. If the letter concerns patient information, find the patient's medical record and clip the letter to it.

Many offices put a cover sheet on the top of each report, on which the doctor can check off the action he or she wishes to occur with regard to the report— such as file, respond, call the patient, and the like. Reports will be filed in the patient's medical file only after the doctor has had a chance to look at them, and any action indicated has been taken.

Non-patient-related items are stacked together to be dealt with by the appropriate member of the staff. Medical journals addressed to a particular doctor can be put in his or her mail pile; those addressed to the practice can be put into the medical library or staff lounge. If the office is large, each staff member may have a cubicle in a central location, as shown in Figure 35–8.

When a doctor is on vacation, someone on the office staff is delegated to review his or her mail and

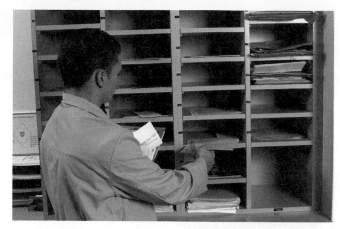

➤ **Figure 35–8** In a large office, each staff member may have a mailbox at a central location.

refer any urgent mail either to the doctor by telephone or e-mail at the vacation location, or to a covering doctor. Arrange nonurgent mail by date received for the doctor to review when he or she returns to the office.

Professional magazines for medical assistants, nurses, and others can be routed to the appropriate person. General-interest magazines can be placed in the waiting room for patient use.

COPYING MULTIPLE-PAGE DOCUMENTS

The medical assistant may need to copy documents using a copy machine. It may be necessary to copy documents of several pages (such as a patient's medical record) or to make several copies of a document (such as a report to be discussed at a staff meeting).

In order to copy efficiently, the medical assistant should become familiar with special features of the available copy machine. Before copying, staples should be removed from the document to be copied, the pages should be arranged in order, and the copy machine should be checked to be sure it has enough paper.

When several copies of a multiple-page document are needed, the machine should be preset to **collate** (arrange each copy in sequence) if the machine has this feature. Some machines will also staple documents.

For a machine that copies only single pages, the desired number of copies of each page must be copied, arranged in order, and stapled manually. The medical assistant should avoid distractions when copying, and should be careful to copy each page correctly and place pages in the correct order.

Procedure 35–6 describes this process in detail.

PROCEDURE 35–6

Preparing Copies of Multiple-Page Documents

Performance Objective: The student will be able to prepare copies of documents with multiple pages.
Supplies and Equipment: Photocopy machine, paper, document to be copied, stapler, staples, staple remover.

Procedure Steps

1. Assemble all pages of the document or report. If it is stapled, remove all staples.
   Rationale: Staples may damage the glass or the feeder of the copier.
2. Be sure that the copy machine is on and warmed up.
3. If the report to be copied includes all or part of a patient's medical record, verify that there is a signed release of information.
4. Place the originals in the machine according to the directions for the individual machine.
   Rationale: Depending on the size and com-plexity of the machine and the type of docu-ment to be copied, it may be necessary to copy one page at a time or the machine may accept the entire document. The original may have to be placed face down on the glass (single sheet copying) or the document may be loaded face down or face up into a feeder.
5. Set the size, number of copies, and if the machine allows, press buttons so that copies will be collated and/or stapled.
6. Press the "start" button.
7. After the copies have been made, if necessary, arrange the pages in the correct order and staple.
8. If the patient will be charged for copying large sections of the medical record (which is com-mon when the patient requests personal cop-ies or an attorney requests copies), verify the number of pages and submit to the person responsible for billing.

STUDENT STUDY PLAN

To reinforce your understanding of the material in this chapter . . .

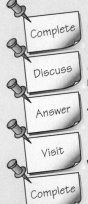

Complete the **Review & Recall** questions.

Discuss the situation in **If You Were the Medical Assistant** with your class-mates, and answer the questions.

Answer the **Critical Thinking Questions** and discuss them with your classmates.

Visit the **Web sites** suggested, and search for additional sites using the **Key-words for Internet Searches.**

Complete the exercises in chapter 35 of the **Student Mastery Manual.**

 REVIEW & RECALL

1. What instances require a patient's written permis-sion to release information?
2. What are the nine parts of a business letter?
3. Describe the different styles of business letters.
4. Describe the different methods doctors use for tran-scription.
5. What types of services does the U.S. Postal Service provide?

6. What is the difference between a mechanical postage meter and an electronic postage meter?

7. What are the different ways of sending and receiving information?

8. Describe the type of mail that is sorted to each of the personnel in the office.

IF YOU WERE THE MEDICAL ASSISTANT

Today's mail has arrived. Your job is to sort it for the office staff. The mail includes insurance information, a letter from an attorney, a consultation report on a patient, a flyer from a medical supply company, and a request from a patient to release information to a new doctor.

1. What mail goes to the doctor?

2. What mail goes to the insurance specialist?

3. What mail goes to the medical assistant?

4. How do you process the release?

CRITICAL THINKING QUESTIONS

1. Describe the pros and cons of the different ways to send information—traditional mail, fax, and e-mail.

2. Discuss the confidentiality issues pertaining to the different ways of sending and receiving information.

3. Look in the local classified section of the newspaper and discuss the job opportunities for medical assistants who can perform transcription.

4. Go to the local post office and gather materials necessary to send mail via certified mail, registered mail, and express mail, and to request a return receipt.

5. Research the cost of each method of sending mail.

EXPLORE THE WEB

INTERNET WEB SITES

American Association for Medical Transcription
www.aamt.org

MT daily (Medical Transcription Networking Center)
www.mtdaily.com

Postal address standards
http://pe.usps.gov

Zip codes
www.usps.com/ncsc/lookups/lookup_zip+4.html

KEYWORDS FOR INTERNET SEARCHES

medical transcription
medical office forms
US Postal Service

ANSWERS TO ON THE JOB

1. Stacey could send the order by standard mail, or she could telephone the order.

2. Faxing the order is a rapid way to place the order, and avoids the possibility of misreading numbers. It saves time for Stacey, especially if several items are being ordered. The disadvantage is that the supplier will not be able to tell Stacey if certain items are not in stock.

3. Confidentiality is not an important issue when placing an order. Some level of confidentiality could be maintained by checking the fax number for accuracy, and by using a cover letter directing the information to the particular party.

4. The fax cover sheet should include the name and fax number of the party to whom the information is going, the name and telephone number of the person sending the fax (in case the fax does not come through clearly), the number of pages, a brief message, and a statement of confidentiality.

UNIT 8

Financial Management and Health Insurance

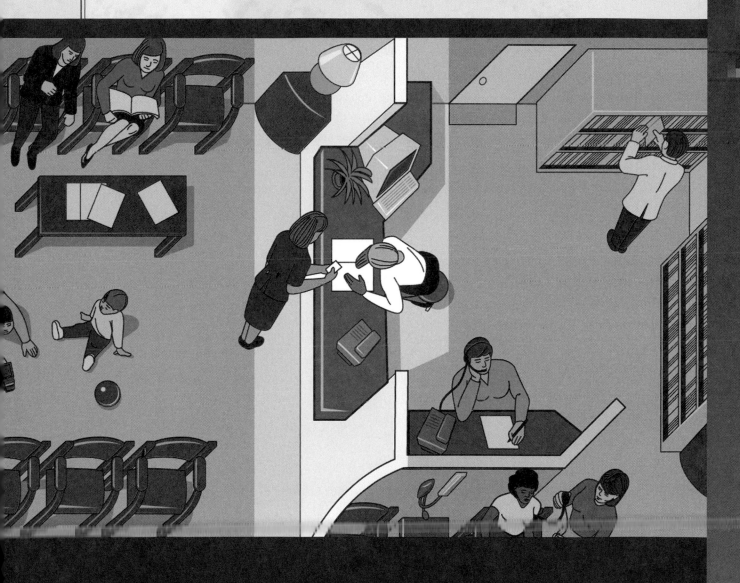

Chapter 36

Managing Practice Finances

Instructional Objectives

After completing this chapter, you will be able to do the following:

1. Define and spell the vocabulary words.
2. Describe three ways to maintain patient accounts.
3. Differentiate between a simple charge slip and an encounter form (superbill).
4. Describe how a charge slip and an encounter form are completed.
5. Identify the information contained on a fee schedule and describe how it is used.
6. Describe the information contained in a patient account ledger.
7. List the information recorded on a day sheet.
8. Identify various types of bank accounts.
9. Discuss the information printed on a check.
10. Describe various methods to write checks.
11. Describe how a bank deposit is prepared and made.
12. Identify reasons why it is important to reconcile every bank statement.
13. Describe the components of accounts payable.
14. Describe how entries are made in the cash disbursement journal.

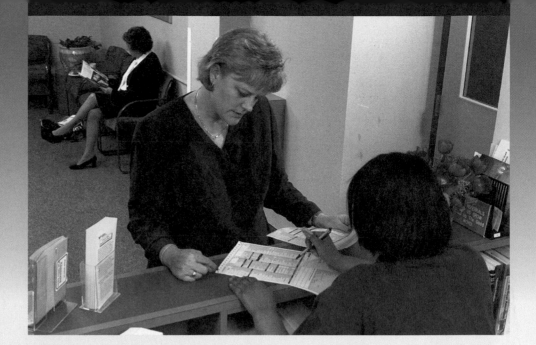

CMA/RMA CERTIFICATION
Curriculum and Competencies

- Prepare a bank deposit
- Reconcile a bank statement
- Post entries on a day sheet
- Perform accounts receivable procedures
- Perform accounts payable procedures

- Prepare a check
- Establish and maintain a petty cash fund
- Post adjustments
- Use a physician's fee schedule

Performance Objectives

After completing this chapter, you will be able to do the following:

1. Prepare charge slips (Procedure 36–1).
2. Prepare an encounter form (Procedure 36–2).
3. Post charges to a patient ledger using a charge slip (Procedure 36–3).
4. Post payments and/or adjustments to a patient ledger (Procedure 36–4).
5. Record information related to a patient visit on a day sheet (Procedure 36–5).
6. Balance a day sheet (Procedure 36–6).
7. Prepare a bank deposit (Procedure 36–7).
8. Reconcile a bank statement (Procedure 36–8).
9. Prepare a check (Procedure 36–9).

VOCABULARY

ABA number (p. 893)   credit (p. 890)   fee schedule (p. 884)   petty cash (p. 896)
accounts receivable (p. 880)   day sheet (p. 880)   ledger (p. 884)   reconciling (p. 895)
accounts payable (p. 896)   debit (p. 890)   payee (p. 893)   restrictive endorsement (p. 895)
adjustments (p. 885)   disbursements (p. 896)   pegboard system (p. 881)   superbill (p. 882)
charge slip (p. 881)   encounter form (p. 882)

ABBREVIATIONS

MICR (p. 893)   NSF (p. 899)

A medical office is a business. That is a fact of life, one that some doctors wish were not true but one that all doctors come to accept and appreciate over time. The business of a medical office is providing medical services to people in need—one of the most important services in the entire economy.

Because the medical office is a business, daily management of the practice's finances is key to the doctors' ability to provide the best services possible for patients. If the practice's bills are not paid and fees are not collected, the practice will cease to be a viable business and the patients will suffer.

Managing the daily finances is a task that usually falls to a medical assistant in smaller practices. In larger practices, a business manager or office manager often assumes this duty.

Many people feel overwhelmed by the challenges of bookkeeping and accounting. Although a number of tasks are involved in bookkeeping and accounting, a set of rather simple principles can facilitate understanding. Once the concepts are clear, the tasks become manageable.

This chapter focuses on the parts of the daily financial activities involved in charging patients for the services provided on that day, maintaining patient accounts and other accounts receivable (money owed to the practice), paying bills incurred by the practice, and managing the accounts payable (money the practice owes).

PATIENT ACCOUNTS OR ACCOUNTS RECEIVABLE

Patient accounts make up the bulk of the medical practice's income. Some income might come from rental of space—for instance, to a particular laboratory for a blood-draw station or to a social worker, psychologist, or other specialist who consults to the practice. Other income may come from royalties—on a particular medical instrument that one or more of the doctors developed, for instance, or for a book written by the professionals in the practice. But the bulk of the practice's income will be earned on a daily basis from the charges for services to patients.

Some medical services are paid for at the time they are performed. Others are paid over a period of time by the patient or by an insurance company. Because each patient has a separate account, the total amount of money owed for services performed is called the **accounts receivable.**

Methods of Maintaining a Patient Account

Patient accounts may be recorded in one of three ways: manually, on a computer, or by a combination of the two.

A manual system utilizes:

1. A daily journal, sometimes called a **day sheet,** to record one day's services rendered, charges, and payments made on that day
2. An accounts receivable ledger card for each patient, to record the charges and payments made to pay for current or prior charges for services performed
3. A record of monthly financial activity of individual doctors in the practice, which is kept using the day sheet.

In a computerized billing system, when the procedures performed for individual patients are entered, charges are automatically posted to the patient's account and the daily record of charges. In a similar way, payments made by the patient (or an insurance company) are posted to both the patient account and the daily record of charges. The computer program can access data to generate a variety of reports, including monthly statements, activity of individual doctors, number of specific procedures billed, and so on.

4/5/xx	Intermediate Exam, EKG	110	100		110		100	Darla Sissle
DATE Family member	**DESCRIPTION**	**TOTAL FEE**	**PAYMENT** CREDITS	**ADJ.**	**BALANCE**		**PREVIOUS BALANCE**	**PATIENT'S NAME**

This is your RECEIPT for this amount ⸻
This is a STATEMENT of your account to date ⸻

BLACKBURN PRIMARY CARE ASSOCIATES, PC
1990 Turquiose Drive
Blackburn, WI 54937
608-459-8857

B–Biopsy	INJ–Injection
C–Consultation	LAB–Laboratory
CPX–Complete Physical	N.C.–No Charge
EKG–Electrocardiogram	O.V.–Office Visit
E.R.–Emergency Room	L–Limited
H.A.–Hospital Admit	C–Comprehensive
H.V.–Hospital visit	ROA–Rec'd on Acct.
IOV–Initial Ofc. Visit	S–Surgery
	X–X-Ray

Please present this slip to receptionist befor leaving office

OFFICE VISIT	55
CONSULTATION	
EKG	
INJECTION	55
LABORATORY	
X-RAY	
SURGERY	
TOTAL	110

Thank You

YOUR NEXT APPOINTMENT WILL BE

Darla Sissle	6	2	3:00
PATIENT NAME	DATE	DAY	TIME

1000   1000   ___ DAYS ___ WKS ___ MO.

> **Figure 36–1** Simple charge slip for pegboard system.

Components of a Patient Account

There are four components to maintaining a patient account:

1. The charge slip
2. The fee schedule
3. The patient account ledger
4. The day sheet.

Charge Slip

A **charge slip** is a means of keeping track of charges for services and payments made at the time of the patient visit. A charge slip can be individually prepared by hand, generated from a pegboard system, or computer generated.

The charge slip is usually prepared before the patient visit and completed after the patient is seen. In its simplest form, the charge slip contains the patient's name, the date of the service rendered, any procedures performed (including the visit itself), and a diagnosis.

Many offices that use manual accounting systems utilize a "one-write" or "write-it-once" system, where all necessary forms are held in place on a metal or plastic board that has a row of pegs across the left side to hold the forms in place (leading to another common name, a **pegboard system**).

The forms have strips of dark waxy pigment on the back (like carbon paper) so information is transferred to the form below when entries are made. The information is entered once and generates a charge slip and receipt, entry on the ledger card, and a journal entry. Figure 36–1 shows a simple pegboard charge slip.

A pegboard system eliminates the need to write separate postings to patient accounts. In addition, the pegboard can be used to record daily income, make bank deposits, and write checks. Figure 36–2 shows a medical assistant using a pegboard system.

Procedure 36–1 details the steps necessary to prepare a charge slip using a pegboard system.

When insurance companies began requiring numerical codes for procedures and diagnoses, these codes were standardized and made uniform. Consequently, a

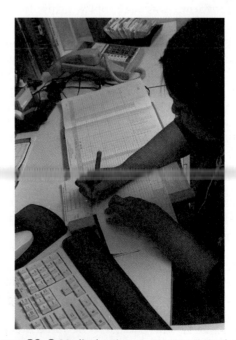

> **Figure 36–2** Medical assistant using pegboard system.

PROCEDURE 36–1

Preparing Charge Slips for the Day's Patients

Performance Objective: The student will be able to prepare charge slips for patients using the daily schedule.

Supplies and Equipment: Blank charge slips, patient ledger cards, daily patient schedule, and medical record for each patient scheduled.

Procedure Steps

1. Using the daily appointment schedule, place the patients' medical records in order of appointment times.

   Rationale: Most offices schedule patients with designated times for effective utilization of time. Organizing the files or charts in that order promotes better time management.

2A. For an office using the pegboard system of accounting, using the daily appointment schedule, pull the ledger card for each patient from the ledger file and place in the order of the appointments.

   Rationale: The ledger card is the source of information on a patient's previous balance in the pegboard system.

2B. If the office uses a computerized accounting system, for each patient on the schedule, print a charge slip that contains the patient's information.

   Rationale: In a computerized billing system, the computer program generates charge slips, but it may be necessary to enter the patient's balance manually.

3. For each patient on the appointment schedule, write the patient's name and previous balance on a charge slip. Locate the balance from the patient's ledger card. If computer-generated charge slips are used, only the outstanding balance is entered. It is found in the patient's account in the computer program. Once complete, attach the charge slip to the front of the patient's medical record with a paper clip for the physician to complete with the service and diagnosis after the patient's visit.

---

new type of charge slip, often called a **superbill** or **encounter form,** was developed. This form, which usually has three parts, contains codes that are commonly used by an individual office, as well as blank spaces to add codes for less commonly used procedures and/or diagnoses. Coding (the process of selecting correct codes) is discussed in detail in chapter 37.

The superbill, or encounter form, can have holes on the left side so it can be combined with a pegboard charge slip; but, if the office uses a computerized billing system, it does not have holes. One copy of the superbill is given to the patient as a receipt, one copy is retained by the office, and one copy may be sent to the insurance company to verify services and charges. Figure 36–3 shows an example of a completed encounter form (superbill).

Although some providers still use a simple charge slip (especially providers whose services are often not reimbursed by insurance, such as chiropractors and podiatrists), most medical offices use an encounter form as a charge slip. The computer may generate information about the patient to be printed on the top of the form before the visit.

When the patient is seen, the doctor or other provider who sees the patient checks off the boxes next to the correct code for the type of visit (problem-focused/straightforward, detailed/low-complexity, comprehensive/moderately complex, and so forth) as well as any other procedures performed and the correct diagnosis.

Using the fee schedule, charges are added and any payments made by the patient are entered. For an office that uses a computerized billing system, the encounter form is used to update the patient's account and generate computer claims. For this reason, it is extremely important to be sure that the encounter form is filled out completely at the time of the patient visit.

Figure 36–4 shows the medical assistant clarifying charges with the doctor before submitting the encounter form to the billing department.

Computerized medical office accounting systems can generate a simple charge slip (sometimes called a walk-out receipt).

➤ Figure 36–3 Completed encounter form (superbill) used as a charge slip.

Blackburn Primary Care Associates, PC
1990 Turquoise Drive
Blackburn, WI 54937
(608) 459-8857

Howard M. Lawler, MD   11
Joanne R. Hughes, MD   21
Ralph Garcia Lopez, MD   31
TAX ID NO. 00-00000000

GUARANTOR NAME AND ADDRESS	PATIENT NO.	PATIENT NAME			DOCTOR NO.	DATE
Darla Sissle 468 Maple Street Blackburn, WI 54937		Darla Sissle			21	6/5/XX

	DATE OF BIRTH	TELEPHONE NO.	INSURANCE			
			CODE	DESCRIPTION		CERTIFICATE NO.
	2/17/32	459-2075		CPC		21 - 58624

OFFICE - NEW				OFFICE - ESTABLISHED				OFFICE - CONSULT				PREVENTIVE CARE - ADULT			
X	CPT	SERVICE	FEE	X	CPT	SERVICE	FEE	X	CPT	SERVICE	FEE	X	CPT	SERVICE	FEE
	99201	Prob Foc/Straight			99211	Nurse/Minimal			99241	Prob/Foc/Straight			99385	18-39 Initial	
	99202	Exp Prob/Straight			99212	Prob Foc/Straight			99242	Exp Prob/Straight			99386	40-64 Initial	
	99203	Detailed/Low			99213	Exp Prob/Low	(55)		99243	Detailed/Low			99387	65+ Initial	
	99204	Compre/Moderate			99214	Detailed/Moderate			99244	Compre/Moderate			99395	18-39 Periodic	
	99205	Compre/High			99215	Compre/High			99245	Compre/High			99396	40-64 Periodic	
													99397	65+ Periodic	

GASTROENEROLOGY				CARDIOLOGY & HEARING				INJECTIONS & IMMUNIZATION				REPAIR & DERMATOLOGY			
X	CPT	SERVICE	FEE	X	CPT	SERVICE	FEE	X	CPT	SERVICE	FEE	X	CPT	SERVICE	FEE
	45300	Sigmoidoscopy Rig			93000	EKG (Global)	(55)		86585	TB Skin Test			17110	Warts: #	
	45305	Sigmoid Rig w/bx			93015	Stress Test (Global)			90716	Varicella Vaccine				Tags: #	
	45330	Sigmoidoscopy Flex			93224	Holter (Global)			90724	Flu Vaccine				Lesion Excis	
	45331	Sigmoid Flex w/bx			93225	Holter Hook Up			90732	Pneumovax				Lesion Destruct	
	45378	Colonoscopy Diag			93227	Holter Interpretation			90718	TD Immunization			SIZE CM:	SITE:	
	45380	Colonoscopy w/bx			94010	Pulm Function Test							MALIG:	PREMAL/BEN:	
	46600	Anoscopy			92551	Audiometry Screen			90782	Injection IM*				(Check One Above)	

OTHER			SUPPLIES/DRUGS*		INJECTIONS			REPAIR		
			DRUG NAME:			90788	Injection IM Antibiot*		Simple Closure	
							Injection joint*		Intermed Closure	
			UNIT/MEASURE:			SM MED MAJOR		SIZE CM:	SITE:	
			QUANTITY			(circle one)				
						FOR ALL INJECTIONS, SUPPLY DRUG		10060	I&D Abscess	
						INFORMATION		10080	I&D Cyst	

DIAGNOSTIC CODES: ICD-9-CM

- [ ] 789.0 Abdominal Pain
- [ ] 795.0 Abnormal Pap Smear
- [ ] 706.1 Acne Vulgaris
- [ ] 477.0 Allergic Rhinitis
- [ ] 285.9 Anemia, NOS
- [ ] 281.0 Pernicious
- [ ] 411.1 Angina, Unstable
- [ ] 427.9 Arythmia, NOS
- [ ] 440.9 Arteriosclerosis
- [ ] 714.0 Arthritis, Rheumatoid
- [ ] 414.0 ASHD
- [ ] 493.90 Asthma, Bronchial W/O Status Ast.
- [ ] 493.91 Asthma, Bronchial W/Status Ast.
- [ ] 466.1 Bronchiolitis, Acute
- [ ] 466.0 Bronchitis, Acute
- [x] 727.3 Bursitis
- [x] 786.50 Chest Pain
- [ ] 574.20 Cholelithiasis
- [ ] ~~414.01 Communicable Unmodified~~
- [ ] 564.0 Constipation
- [ ] 496 COPD
- [ ] 692.9 Dermatitis, Allergic
- [ ] 250.01 Diabetes Mellitus, ID
- [ ] 250.00 Diabetes Mellitus, NID
- [ ] 558.9 Diarrhea
- [ ] 562.11 Diverticulitis
- [ ] 562.10 Diverticulosis

- [ ] 782.3 Edema
- [ ] 492.8 Emphysema
- [ ] V16.0 Family History Of Diabetes
- [ ] 780.6 Fever of Undetermined Origin
- [ ] 578.9 G.I. Bleeding, Unspecified
- [ ] 727.41 Ganglion of Joint
- [ ] 535.0 Gastritis, Acute
- [ ] V72.3 Arythmia, NOS
- [ ] 748.0 Headache
- [ ] 550.90 Hernia, inguinal, NOS
- [ ] 054.9 Herpes Simplex
- [ ] 053.9 Herpes Zoster
- [ ] 708.9 Hives/Urticaria
- [ ] 401.1 Hypertension, Benign
- [ ] 401.0 Hypertension, Malignant
- [ ] 402.90 Hypertension, W/O CHF
- [ ] 244.9 Hypothyroidism, Primary
- [ ] 380.4 Impacted Cerumen
- [ ] 487.1 Influenza
- [ ] 564.1 Irritable Bowel Syndrome
- [ ] 464.0 Laryngitis, Acute
- [ ] 454.9 Leg Varicose Veins
- [ ] 424.0 Mitral Valve Prolapse
- [ ] 412 Myocardial Infarction, Old
- [ ] 715.90 Osteoarthritis, Unspec. Site
- [ ] 620.2 Ovarian Cyst

- [ ] 614.9 Pelvic Inflammatory Disease
- [ ] 685.1 Pilonidal Cyst
- [ ] 462 Pharyngitis, Acute
- [ ] 627.1 Postmenopausal Bleeding
- [ ] 625.4 Premenstrual Tension
- [ ] 782.1 Rash
- [ ] 569.3 Rectal Bleeding
- [ ] 398.90 Rheumatic Heart Disease, NOS
- [ ] 431.9 Sinusitis, Acute, NOS
- [ ] 782.1 Skin Eruption, Rash
- [ ] 845.00 Sprain, Ankle
- [ ] 848.9 Sprain, Muscle, Unspec. Site
- [ ] 785.6 Swollen Glands
- [ ] 246.9 Thyroid Disease, Unspecified
- [ ] 463 Tonsillitis, Acute

- [ ] 474.0 Tonsillitis, Chronic
- [ ] 465.9 Upper Respiratory Infection, Acute
- [ ] 599.0 Urinary Tract Infection
- [ ] V03.9 Vaccination/Bacterial Dis.
- [ ] V06.8 Vaccination/Combination
- [ ] V04.8 Vaccination, Influenza
- [ ] 616.10 Vaginitis, Vulvitis, NOS
- [ ] 780.4 Vertigo
- [ ] 787.0 Vomiting, Nausea
- [ ] _____ _____
- [ ] _____ _____
- [ ] _____ _____

RETURN APPOINTMENT	BALANCE DUE			
	DATE OF SERVICE	CPT CODE	DIAGNOSIS CODE(S)	CHARGE
_7_ Days				
_____ Weeks				
_____ Months				
Authorization Number: ▶ _____				

Place of Service:
( ) Office
( ) Emergency Room
( ) In Patient Hospital
( ) Out-Patient Hospital
( ) Nursing Home

TOTAL CHARGE	$ 110
AMOUNT PAID	$ 100
PREVIOUS BAL	$ 100
BALANCE DUE	$ 110

Check #: _____
(Circle Method of Payment)
CASH   CHECK   MC   VISA

Physician's Signature
▶ _____

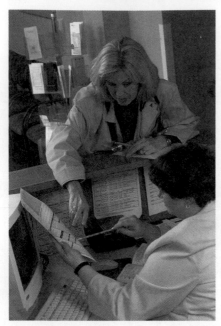

➤ **Figure 36–4** Medical assistant clarifying patient charges with the physician.

Fee Schedule

A **fee schedule** is a list of charges for the various procedures a doctor performs. Years ago, a doctor had one set of fees that he or she charged patients for office visits, procedures and/or treatments. Patients were charged for the service, and paid what they could over whatever period of time it took them. Eventually, the doctor got paid or wrote the bill off as an uncollectable debt.

Today, however, a medical practice may have to accept different levels of payment for each service it performs, depending on which insurance provider is paying for the service.

With most fee-for-service (indemnity) insurance plans, as long as the doctor's charge is "usual, customary, and reasonable," the plan will pay a fixed percentage (often 80 percent) of a doctor's charges.

However, most HMOs have created schedules of what they will pay doctors for various treatments, procedures, and types of office visits.

In addition, if the doctor treats patients covered under the federal Medicare program (for the elderly and disabled) and/or the federal/state Medicaid program (for the poor), the practice will receive a different amount for patients covered by these programs. Finally, the practice may treat patients covered by TRI-CARE (formerly CHAMPUS), the program for dependent family members of military personnel, or CHIP, the federally mandated and state-run children's health improvement programs that pay for treatment of children in families that earn too much to be Medicaid-

eligible but who have no private health insurance. These programs, too, have different payments.

Figure 36–5 shows a medical office fee schedule.

The fee schedule is used to fill out charges on the charge slip and/or encounter form. Procedure 36–2 details how to complete a superbill for a patient using the charge slip and fee schedule.

Patient Account Ledger

In addition to the journal day sheet or accounts receivable record, an account card, usually called a **ledger** card, is kept on each patient, on which charges and payments are entered and from which periodic bills are generated. Each patient account has the five pieces of general information, and four pieces of financial information. The general information is:

1. Patient's name
2. Patient's address
3. Patient's telephone number
4. Name, address, and telephone number of the person responsible for payment.
5. Insurance identification (if any), including the name of the plan, group number, and/or subscriber number.

The financial information is:

1. Previous balance
2. Charges by date
3. Payments by patient or insurance carrier
4. Adjustments to the balance due.

Figure 36–6 shows a patient account ledger.

Payment for services performed can be received in three ways:

1. The patient pays at the time of service, in full or in part (such as a copayment for an HMO); or the patient pays the bill in full, then seeks reimbursement from an insurance provider (if the patient has indemnity insurance).
2. The patient may make a payment through the mail in response to a bill.
3. An insurance company may make a payment—either by mail or, increasingly, by electronic transfer. These payments are entered on the patient's ledger in slightly different ways, as described in Procedures 36–3 and 36–4.

Table 36–1 identifies common terminology used in relation to entering charges and payments.

Day Sheet

The day sheet keeps a running tally of the practice's income for that day. Medical offices utilize the *cash method* of accounting, meaning that they record income when it is received and expenses when bills are paid.

FEE SCHEDULE

BLACKBURN PRIMARY CARE ASSOCIATES, PC
1990 Turquiose Drive
Blackburn, WI 54937
608-459-8857

Federal Tax ID Number: 00-0000000   **BCBS Group Number:** 14982
Medicare Group Number: 14982

OFFICE VISIT, NEW PATIENT

Focused, 99201	$45.00
Expanded, 99202	$55.00
Intermediate, 99204	$60.00
Extended, 99204	$95.00
Comprehensive, 99205	$195.00
Consultation, 99245	$250.00

OFFICE VISIT, ESTABLISHED PATIENT

Minimal, 99211	$40.00
Focused, 99212	$48.00
Intermediate, 99213	$55.00
Extended, 99214	$65.00
Comprehensive, 99215	$195.00

OFFICE PROCEDURES

EKG, 12 lead, 93000	$55.00
Stress EKG, Treadmill, 93015	$295.00
Sigmoidoscopy, Flex; 45330	$145.00
Spirometry, 94010	$50.00
Cerumen Removal, 69210	$40.00
Collection & Handling	
Lab Specimen, 99000	$9.00
Venipuncture, 35415	$9.00
Urinalysis, 81000	$20.00
Urinalysis, 81002 (Dip Only)	$12.00
Influenza Injection, 90724	$20.00
Pneumococcal Injection, 90732	$20.00
Oral Polio, 90712	$15.00
DTaP, 90700	$20.00
Tetanus Toxoid, 90703	$15.00
MMR, 90707	$25.00
HIB, 90737	$20.00
Hepatitis B, newborn to age 11 years, 90744	$60.00
Hepatitis B, 11-19 years, 90745	$60.00
Hepatitis B, 20 years and above 90746	$60.00
Intramuscular Injection, 90788	
Penicillin	$30.00
Cephtriaxone	$25.00
Solu-Medrol	$23.00
Vitamin B-12	$13.00
Subcutaneous Injection, 90782	
Epinephrine	$18.00
Susphrine	$25.00
Insulin, U-100	$15.00

COMMON DIAGNOSTIC CODES

Ischemic Heart Disease	414.9
w/o myocardial infarction	411.89
w/coronary occlusion	411.81
Hypertension, Malignant	401.0
Benign	401.1
Unspecified	401.9
w/congest. heart failure	402.91
Asthma, Bronchial	493.9
w/ COPD	493.2
allergic, w/ S.A.	493.91
allergic, w/o S.A.	493.90
Kyphosis	737.10
w/osteoporosis	733.0
Osteoporosis	733.00
Otitis Media, Acute	382.9
Chronic	382.9

➤ **Figure 36–5** Fee schedule.

Manufacturing and other businesses usually utilize the *accrual method* of accounting, which records income when goods are shipped, even if they are not paid for at that time, and records expenses when materials arrive, even if the company does not pay for them at the time of arrival (see Bookkeeping Systems).

The day sheet, shown in Figure 36–7, records five items for each patient seen that day, as well as a couple of other items for the practice in general. For each individual patient seen, the day sheet records:

1. Charges
2. Payments
3. Previous balance
4. Adjustments
5. New balance.

Adjustments (alterations to the patient account balance) are usually discounted payments made by

Completing an Encounter Form (Superbill) for a Patient

Performance Objective: For each patient who has an appointment correctly complete an encounter form (superbill) with information from the charge slip and the fee schedule.

Supplies and Equipment: Charge slips, encounter forms, fee schedule, pen.

Procedure Steps:

1. Using charge slips that contain the patient's name and previous balance, the date, and indications of service provided, add fees using the fee schedule.
2. Fill in the superbill by writing the fee for each service provided beside the line containing the correct code (if the physician has not already done so). All items in the accounts receivable system need to have identical information, so it is important to check each superbill against the charge slip, patient ledger, and chart for accuracy.
3. Complete the remainder of the superbill by:
   a. inserting payments made and calculating the new balance
   b. inserting correct diagnosis code(s)

Example: See Figures 36–1, 36–2, and 36–5

The charge slips both relate to the services provided to the patient Darla Sissle. She was charged $55.00 for the office examination and $55.00 for the EKG (electrocardiogram). The charges are taken from the fee schedule (Figure 36–5). The patient had a previous balance of $100. The patient paid $100. The diagnosis was chest pain. Note how the information on the completed encounter form (Figure 36–2) relates to the information on the simpler charge slip (Figure 36–1).

PATIENT LEDGER

BLACKBURN PRIMARY CARE ASSOCIATES, PC
1990 Turquiose Drive
Blackburn, WI 54937
608-459-8857

Darla Sissle
468 Maple Street
Blackburn, WI 54937

Previous Balance				$100.00
Date	**Service**	**Charge**	**Payment**	**Balance**
6/5/xx	Intermediate, EKG	$110.00		
	payment by patient check no. xxx		$100.00	$110.00

➤ **Figure 36–6** Patient account ledger.

PROCEDURE 36-3

Posting Charges to the Patient Ledger

Performance Objective: Using the information from the completed charge slip, the student will post charges to a patient ledger.
Supplies and Equipment: Patient charge slip, patient ledger, fee schedule, calculator or adding machine, pen or computer.

Procedure Steps

1. After a patient's service or appointment is complete, remove the charge slip from the chart and check that the name of the patient on the charge slip matches that on the chart or file as well as the ledger card or computer account.
   Rationale: To ensure accuracy in billing and later submission to third-party carriers, charges must be entered to the correct patient account.
2. Refer to the fee schedule for correct charges for the service(s) provided.
   Rationale: There may be different fee schedules for different insurance carriers within an office,

so it is important to check that you are using the correct one.
3. If using a manual system, post the charges on the patient ledger using one line for one day's services. Place the total charge for the service in the column labeled charges. If using a computer program, post each charge separately. For most computer programs entering the procedure code will prompt the computer to automatically generate the correct charge for the patient's insurance.
   Rationale: You may need to add up several charges if the patient had more than one service during one appointment.

Example: See Figure 36–6
The patient had an intermediate office exam for $55.00 and an EKG for $55.00. Both services from the charge slip are placed in the column labeled Services on the ledger and added together. The amount of $110 is placed in the Charge column.

PROCEDURE 36-4

Posting Payments and/or Adjustments

Performance Objective: The student will be able to post payments and/or adjustments to a patient account.
Supplies and Equipment: Patient ledger card or computer, check or cash from the patient or check from the insurance carrier, calculator or adding machine.

Procedure Steps

1. When a payment has been made, select the correct patient ledger card(s) or locate the patient account in the computer.
   Rationale: Checks received in the mail will need to have the correct patient ledger pulled from the ledger file or selected in the computer. For payments at the end of a patient

visit, just check that you have the correct ledger or account in front of you.
2. Compare the amount of the payment against the total amount owed.
   Rationale: The total amount owed will be the balance due and charges for new services.
3. Record the payment in the column labeled Payment. Identify if the payment is cash or a check and if it is from the patient or insurance. If it is a check, record the number of the check.
   Rationale: Recording information about the payment is useful if there are inquiries at a later date.
4. Do the math calculations to complete the ledger:
   a. Determine if there is a previous balance.

Procedure continued on following page

PROCEDURE 36–4 *(continued)*

b. If payment is at time of service, add all charges.

c. Add the previous balance to the total charges for services.

d. Subtract payment.

e. Record any new balance due. (A computer program does the calculations for you.)

5. Enter adjustments in the Adjustment column (or if there is no Adjustment column, enter adjustments that reduce the bill in the Payments column and adjustments that increase the bill in the Charge column) on the ledger card or designated as Adjustments in a computer program. An adjustment would be necessary if the insurance contract requires that the in-surance payment be accepted as payment in full.

6. Calculate the balance. (A computer program does all calculations.)

7. Endorse the check using a stamp containing the practice name, the statement "For deposit only," and the number of the checking account.

Rationale: This type of endorsement only allows the bank to deposit the check and prevents anyone from cashing the check or using it in any other way.

8. Place cash or the processed check in the designated drawer or money box for later deposit.

Example:

On the ledger in Figure 36–6 the patient paid $100.00 using check number XXX. After this payment, the patient's balance is $110.00.

HMOs, Medicare, Medicaid, CHAMPUS, or CHIP according to the contract provisions. Suppose, for instance, the charge for an extended office visit is $125, the patient pays a $10 copayment, and the HMO pays $79.50 for the visit. Then the record of charges and payments will look something like this:

Date	Charge	Payment	Adjust	Source	Balance
1/1/2002	$125				$125
1/1/2002		$10		Co pay	$115
2/15/2002		$79.50		Insurance	$35.50
2/28/02			–$35.50		$000

In addition, the day sheet has columns labeled "distribution" that can be used by the practice to itemize charges under several headings, commonly by the doctor who generated the charge. However, it can also be used to track the type of procedure performed.

Procedure 36–5 details recording a patient visit on the day sheet, and Procedure 36–6 details balancing a day sheet.

BANKING ACTIVITIES

If the medical practice is to pay its bills, including salaries for medical assistants and other employees, it

---

Table 36–1	Common Terminology Used in Relation to Entering Charges and Payments

Account balance	The amount remaining in the account after all entries have been totalled
Accounts receivable control	A summary of all unpaid accounts
Adjustment	Entry to change an account, often to include a discount
Credit	The record of a payment received
Credit balance	An amount when payments exceeds charges
Debit	The record of a charge or debt incurred
Day sheet	The record of daily financial transactions (daily journal in a pegboard accounting system)
Disbursements	Money paid out
Invoice	A written statement describing a purchase or service and the amount due
Journal	The original record of financial transactions that identifies the accounts to which they belong
Ledger	A card or book to which records of financial transactions are transferred
Payables	Amounts owed to others
Posting	Transferring information from one record to another
Proof	Validation of calculations
Receivables	Amounts of money owed by others
ROA (received on account)	Designation used for payments which reduce the amount owed but are not payment in full
Trial balance	A method of checking the accuracy of calculations of accounts

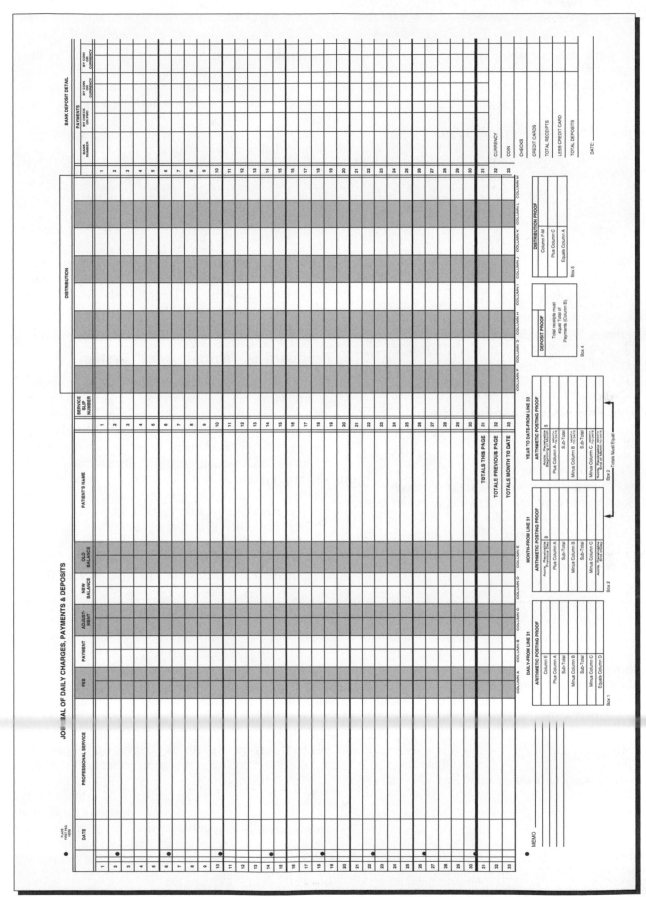

➢ Figure 36–7 Day sheet. (Courtesy of Bibbero Systems, Inc., Petaluma, California, (800) 272-2376. Fax (800) 242-9330; www.bibbero.com.)

▬ BOOKKEEPING SYSTEMS

The three most common systems for keeping records of accounts in the medical office are single-entry, double-entry, and pegboard or "write-it-once" systems.

Single-Entry Bookkeeping System

This is the simplest system; it requires at least three records:

1. A journal that keeps track of all charges, such as a daily journal
2. A journal that keeps track of payments, such as a checkbook
3. A ledger that keeps track of individual patient accounts. These may be recorded on pages of a book, index cards, or ledger cards.

Although the single-entry system is simple, it lacks methods for cross-checking to prevent and/or detect errors. Each entry is made separately, and bills to patients and insurance companies are generated manually.

Double-Entry Bookkeeping System

This is the most complete type of bookkeeping system. However, it usually requires a trained bookkeeper or accountant in order to be used effectively.

Every transaction is posted into two different records, as a credit in one and a debit in the other. Records of money and property owned by the business and of money owed to the business are balanced against records of liabilities—money owed to others by the business.

A charge for service to a patient, for example, is a **credit** (positive number) in the records of assets because it increases the total assets; but it is a **debit** (negative number) in the records of liabilities because it decreases the amount owed by the business.

A common formulation of the accounting principle is as follows:

$$\textbf{Assets} = \textbf{liabilities} + \textbf{owner's equity}$$

where assets are property owned by the business, liabilities are debts, and owner's equity is the amount by which the owner's assets exceed liabilities.

When a double-entry bookkeeping system is used by a medical practice, the medical assistant is usually responsible only for keeping the daily journal and/or entering charges in the computer. The actual books are kept by an accountant.

Pegboard or "Write-It-Once" System

The pegboard system is similar to the single-entry system. However, the day sheet used as a daily journal contains sections at the bottom to facilitate checking the totals in a section called "arithmetic posting proof." In addition, fewer entries are made manually, because the pegboard system uses a duplicating system so that one entry is posted to the daily journal, patient ledger card, and charge slip or daily journal, payable ledger, and check.

Most computer systems are based on the pegboard system because this was the most common bookkeeping system used in medical offices when computerized accounting systems were developed.

must have money in the bank. Part of the responsibility of the individual who handles the office's financial management is maintaining the practice's bank accounts.

Types of Accounts

Businesses such as medical practices will generally have one or more of the following types of bank accounts—checking, savings, or money market savings.

Checking Account

A checking account is an account in which the money held can be drawn by simply writing a check against the funds available. Many banks allow businesses to earn interest on their checking accounts as long as a certain amount of money remains in the account (the minimum balance). The minimum balance can range from as little as $500 to as much as $2,500. Interest is the payment the bank makes to the owner of the money on deposit for the privilege of being able to use the depositor's money to make loans to other bank customers.

If the checking account balance falls below the minimum, the account does not earn interest. In addition, there is usually a monthly service charge and a charge for each check written against the account for the entire monthly reporting period in which the balance was below the minimum.

A practice that does not want to maintain a minimum balance can open a checking account that pays

PROCEDURE 36–5

Recording a Patient's Visit on the Day Sheet

Performance Objective: The student can post charges and payments on a day sheet using information from the superbill, ledger, and charge slip.

Supplies and Equipment: Day sheet or accounts receivable record, encounter form, charge slip (if separate from encounter form), patient ledger, patient medical record, pen.

Procedure Steps

1. Prepare the day sheet by reviewing the appointment schedule. If using a pegboard billing system, set up the pegboard with the day sheet on the bottom and shingled charge slips aligned with the lines of the day sheet.
   Rationale: Some practices record names of scheduled patients and previous balance on the day sheet prior to beginning the day, while other practices place the name as the visit is completed. The advantage of recording the names before the start of the day is that it saves some time and provides some means of quality control or cross-checking patients recorded against patients actually seen. The disadvantage is that if the patients cancel or miss appointments, there are blank lines on the day sheet.

2. As each patient completes his or her appointment, the charge slip, encounter form (if separate), and patient ledger are completed. The identical information is to be placed on the day sheet or accounts receivable record. This happens automatically if using a pegboard system because the information is transferred to the patient ledger and day sheet when the top of the charge slip is completed. If using a computerized billing system, the information

is also entered automatically in the daily journal. The process can be done manually, however.
   Rationale: The day sheet is the journal of original entry, which is a running record of charges and payments made during the day.

3. Complete the columns on the right side of the day sheet or account receivable record manually by entering information tracked by the practice. This may include entering charges and payments for each doctor in the practice or it may include entering information about specific procedures performed.
   Rationale: This enables a practice to accumulate data about the financial activity of each doctor or about specific procedures. If a computer billing program is used, this type of information can be tracked through the report features of the program.

4. Record payments received in the mail on the day sheet and patient ledger when the mail is processed.
   Rationale: Payments made at the completion of the visit are recorded at the same time as the charges. Payments made through the mail are to be recorded on the ledger and day sheet only.

5. Record all payments on the deposit slip when they are received or processed. The deposit slip can be totalled at the end of the day. A record can be made for the practice by filling out a duplicate deposit slip or by photocopying the deposit slip when it is complete.
   Rationale: The practice should keep a copy of each deposit slip in case questions arise at a later date.

PROCEDURE 36–6

Balancing the Day Sheet

Performance Objective: The student will verify the accounts receivable daily by balancing the day sheet entries.

Supplies and Equipment: Day sheet, completed for one day, calculator or adding machine, pencil, pen.

Procedure Steps

1. Determine if all entries have been entered in a given day. Names can be checked against the appointment book as well as copies of the charge slips.

Procedure continued on following page

PROCEDURE 36–6 (continued)

Rationale: Entries cannot be added after a day sheet has been proofed, or results will be inaccurate.

2. Add up each column with a calculator and place the total in pencil in the bottom row labeled "TOTALS THIS PAGE."

   Rationale: Changes can be made more easily if totals are made in pencil and the proofs are calculated to be sure the day sheet balances before entering the totals in pen.

3. Add the totals from the current day to totals from the previous day and totals from previous months. These figures have usually been entered from the previous day's day sheet by the person who prepared the day sheet for the current day; if not, they can be transferred from the day sheet of the previous day.

4. To proof (verify the correctness of) entries, add the total of the column labeled Old Balance or Previous Balance plus the total of the column labeled New or Current Balances. To further proof entries:

   a. The amount in the Payment column should equal that in the Bank Deposit column.

   b. The amount in the Total Fee column should equal that of all charges in the right-hand columns sometimes called the distribution section(s).

   The day sheet usually contains a section at the bottom to assist with completing the proofs.

   Rationale: Accuracy in bookkeeping is necessary for financial audits and accounting.

5. When the day sheet balances, rewrite all totals with a pen. Once the day sheet is complete, it must not be altered. If mistakes have occurred, they must be corrected by making adjustments on a subsequent day.

   Rationale: The day sheet is a legal document and must be completed in ink.

---

no interest and has no monthly maintenance fees. Sometimes a bank will waive the minimum balance in the practice's checking account if the practice agrees to keep a higher minimum balance in either a savings account or a money market savings account.

Savings Account

A practice may want to keep cash that is not needed to pay expenses in a savings account, which usually earns interest at a slightly higher rate than an interest-bearing checking account. A savings account does not have any check-writing privileges, but money can be withdrawn or transferred to the checking account if necessary.

Money Market Savings Account

A money market account offers features of both savings and checking accounts. Money market accounts usually require a fairly high minimum balance (often $2,500). However, they may earn interest at the money market rate—the rate at which major corporations lend to or borrow from one another for 10- to 30-day periods.

Money market accounts let the owner draw a specified number of checks per month without a processing fee. They often require checks to be for at least $500.

A medical practice might want to maintain a money market account in order to hold money for regular but infrequent expenses, such as quarterly, semi-annual, or annual payments for malpractice insurance, licenses for

ON THE JOB

Linda, who works for Blackburn Primary Care Associates, is getting ready to begin the day. After reviewing the schedule for the day's patients, she pulls the ledgers, prepares the day sheet, and attaches a superbill to each patient chart. She notes that there are 10 Medicare patients, three fee-for-service patients, and the rest are assorted HMO patients.

QUESTIONS

If you had a job similar to Linda's . . .

1. How could you determine how much to charge each patient?
2. Where would you record the charges and payments?
3. If the three fee-for-service accounts had a balance forward, or previous balance, how would you handle that?
4. For which patients' accounts would you need to show an adjustment?

doctors and other licensed professionals on the staff, or dues to the state, county, or local medical association or chamber of commerce.

Types of Checks

About Checks

Checks, sometimes called "drafts," are slips of paper by which a checking account owner authorizes the bank to pay to the person presenting the check the amount of money written on the check. Paying by checks allows the medical practice to maintain a permanent record of the payments it makes for goods and services.

In addition to the checks from the practice's checkbook or money market account, the practice may have occasion to ask its bank to prepare a cashier's check or to certify one of its own checks to assure the **payee** (person or company who is being paid) that funds are available. This might be the case if the office were purchasing a large piece of equipment for which the seller is unwilling to accept a simple business check.

At the top right of each check, under the check number, is the **ABA number,** the number assigned by the American Bankers' Association. This number designates the federal reserve bank zone, the state or territory, and the unique identification number for the bank on which the check is drawn. Across the bottom of checks is a set of numbers written in magnetic ink, which contain the account number and the routing number. When checks are processed and "cleared" for payment from the issuing bank to the account of the individual making the deposit, this set of numbers is read by a magnetic ink character recognition **(MICR)** system.

Business Checkbook with Stubs

The business checkbook most commonly used, as shown in Figure 36–8, has three checks to a page, with check stubs on the left on which to record the same information that is recorded on the check when it is written. The checks and matching stubs are preprinted in order. In addition, the stubs have room in which to write in the amount of deposits made; the stubs therefore act as a running checkbook ledger.

Computer-Generated Checks

A number of business accounting software programs will generate checks and immediately post the payment to the accounts payable ledger. To use these systems, the practice will need to buy blank checks for computer printing. The software also generates the ABA and MICR numbers.

Pegboard System for Check Writing

In addition to entering charges, a write-it-once or pegboard system allows for checks to be written. The check overlays the accounts payable ledger on the pegboard; and, using carboned checks, the "pay to the order of" and "amount" lines are copied from the check to the underlying ledger.

On-Line Payment

The Internet has made it possible to make payments on-line by establishing a relationship with a bank that has a computerized banking capability. This is becoming an increasingly popular method with suppliers, who invoice on-line and accept (some even expect) payment to be transferred from the practice's account directly to the supplier's account using a pay-by-computer system.

Because some businesses still do not accept on-line payment, a medical practice will still need to maintain a checking account for the next few years, especially if the practice writes out its own payroll checks. In the near future, some highly automated practices will do all of their bill paying to regular suppliers, medical associations, liability insurance carriers, and other creditors on-line, and have their payroll checks written by an outside service provider.

Preparing a Check

Checks are produced on watermarked paper to make it difficult for people to erase and then overwrite part of the check. The bank has the right not to honor a check with erasures, overwrites, or other alterations. This protects the account holder from having people to whom checks are written cross out the amount and write in a larger amount. However, this also makes it important that checks be written carefully.

Most checks have at least one memo line—a line on which to write the purpose of the check. If the check is for payment of an invoice, the invoice number or the account number for that particular vendor would go on the memo line.

If a mistake is made on a check, write "void" on the check and check stub. Do not throw the incorrect check away; rather, file it with canceled checks so it is available for the practice's auditors. When writing a check, begin the amount in numbers immediately after the printed dollar sign, and write the amount in words at the left side of the check. Legally, the amount in words is accepted as the amount for which the check is written if there is a discrepancy. Figure 36–9 shows a check that has been completed properly.

After all of the checks for a particular period (week or month) have been written, attach them to the supporting invoices and place them in a folder or envelope on the desk of the doctor who is to sign the checks

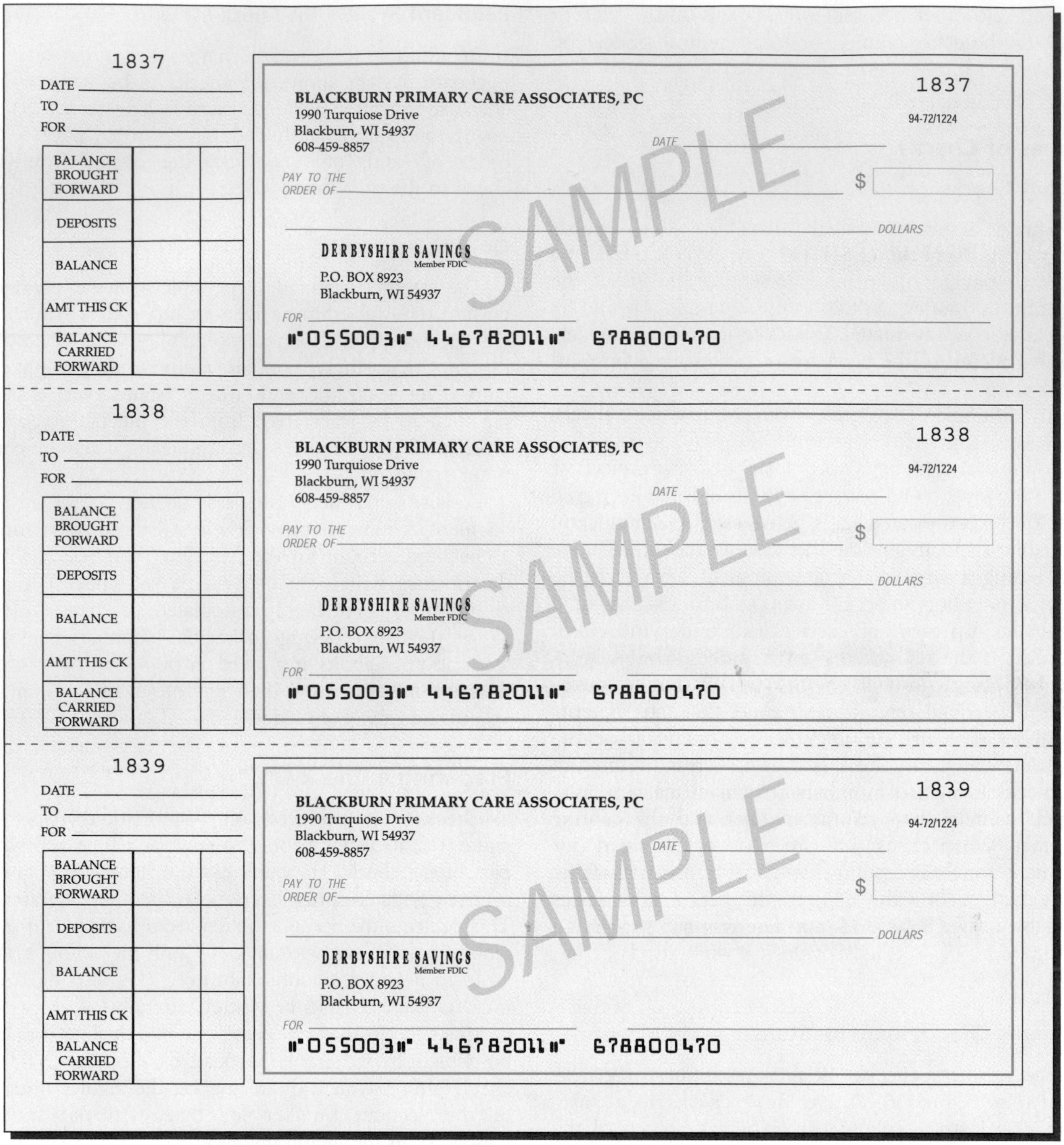

➤ **Figure 36–8** A business checkbook is often arranged with three checks per page and check stubs to record transactions.

that week. In many practices, two doctors have check-signing privileges so that one can sign if the other is on vacation. Also, in some practices, checks exceeding a certain amount—such as $500 or $1,000—must be signed by two people; this is often a provision of that part of the practice's general liability insurance policy that covers employee theft.

Preparing a Bank Deposit

Every time a deposit is made at the bank, it must be recorded on a deposit slip. A deposit slip is an itemized listing of the cash or checks being deposited. Deposit slips, such as those shown in Figure 36–10, are found at the far right side of the day sheet. Deposit

➤ **Figure 36–9** A properly filled in check.

slips are also located in the back of the practice's checkbook; these deposit slips are preprinted with the practice name and the account number into which the deposit is being made. When making a deposit, the amount of the total cash being deposited is written on the cash line, followed by an itemized listing of the checks being deposited. The first part of the ABA number (e.g., 921–72) should be entered on the deposit slip to identify each account.

Each check being deposited must have an endorsement on its back. The endorsement is either handwritten or stamped with an ink stamp. It is recommended to stamp checks with a **restrictive endorsement** (an endorsement that limits the power of the bank) such as "for deposit only" with the account number. Procedure 36–7 discusses how to fill out a deposit slip properly.

Figure 36–11 shows the medical assistant preparing a deposit slip.

Making a Deposit

Deposits can be made either in person or by mail. Deposits in person can be made at a teller station in the bank, through the drive-through window, via the ATM, or via the night-deposit box usually located by the bank's front door. The night deposit box may require a key, which is supplied by the bank to customers who use it. (This prevents tampering or unauthorized use of the deposit slot.)

If depositing by mail or using the night-deposit box, use one of the bank's special mailing deposit slips and envelopes, which the bank will give to a customer on request. Do not send cash in a mail deposit.

Reconciling the Bank Statement

Reconciling a bank statement means making sure that the balance in the checkbook and the balance on

the bank statement equal each other after adjusting for checks that were written but have not yet cleared through the bank and deposits recorded after the statement period ended.

Each month the bank will send the practice a statement of account activity. The account balance at the end of the statement period will almost always be different from the account balance in the office's checking account ledger.

There are five reasons for this discrepancy. First, it usually takes about a week from the time the statement period ends until the office receives the statement, during which time more checks have been written. Second, checks written near the end of the statement period usually will not have cleared the account when the period ends. Third, some vendors and others do not promptly deposit or cash checks; thus, some checks will not clear the account for a month or more. Fourth, bank charges are added to the statement for such things as checks returned for insufficient funds on a payor's account, per-check fees, lockbox fees, and so on. Finally, interest may accrue on the balance during the month.

For this reason, it is important to reconcile the bank statement with the office's checkbook as a double-check of the arithmetic used by those who have written checks. Most banks have a preprinted reconciling page on the back of the statement. This form allows you to take the statement period-end balance, subtract from it the dollar amount of checks that have been written since the end of the period, subtract any bank charges, add the dollar amount of checks that have not cleared, and add any interest earned, to get a true balance. This true balance should match the balance in the office's checking-account ledger. Figure 36–12 shows a bank statement reconciling form, and Procedure 36–8 discusses how to reconcile a bank statement.

BANK DEPOSIT DETAIL

BANK NUMBER	PAYMENTS			CREDIT CARD
	BY CHECK OR PMO	BY COIN OR CURRENCY		
TOTALS				
CURRENCY				
COIN				
CHECKS				
CREDIT CARDS				
TOTAL RECEIPTS				
LESS CREDIT CARD $				
TOTAL DEPOSITS				

DEPOSIT DATE: _____ FIRM: _____

➤ **Figure 36–10** Bank deposit slip of the type found with a pegboard system. (Courtesy of Bibbero Systems, Inc., Petaluma, California, (800) 272-2376. Fax (800) 242-9330; www.bibbero.com.)

OTHER FINANCIAL ACCOUNTS

In addition to taking money in, a practice pays money out. Some of this is done on a regular basis, taking care of weekly or bi-weekly salaries, mortgage or rent, equipment leases, and utilities. Other payments are made in relation to specific invoices for materials or equipment.

Unless a bill is paid immediately when presented, it becomes part of the **accounts payable** (money owed by the business). A complete bookkeeping system notes each month any outstanding accounts payable as well as the **disbursements** (payments) made during the month.

In addition, many offices keep a petty cash drawer, a small amount of cash available for everyday expenses. Again, petty cash must be recorded.

Accounts Payable or Record of Cash Disbursements

The record of cash disbursements is called the cash disbursement journal, as shown in Figure 36–13. In a one-write or pegboard system, the cash disbursement journal is automatically recorded at the time each check is written out. In a computerized bookkeeping system, the cash disbursement journal is also automatically updated, or posted, when a check is drawn. In a single- or double-entry system, the cash disbursement journal must be separately maintained by hand.

Each line of the cash disbursement journal has seven columns to record seven specific pieces of information, followed by a series of columns to track expenses by type:

1. Check number
2. To whom the check is written
3. Date
4. Amount of the check
5. A bank deposit
6. Beginning bank balance
7. Columns for the account against which the payment is charged.

Each time money is deposited for an accounts payable, the amount is recorded in the column labeled bank deposit.

Procedure 36–9 describes how to write checks to pay bills for the medical office and record them on the cash disbursement record.

Petty Cash

Petty cash is the cash kept on hand to pay for small, miscellaneous items, such as tips for a delivery, postage due, reimbursement to a staff member for parking at a meeting, or even a box of Girl Scout cookies for the office break room.

PROCEDURE 36–7

Preparing a Bank Deposit

Performance Objective: The student will prepare a bank deposit.

Supplies and Equipment: Deposit slip, cash and checks received as payments, calculator or adding machine, envelope or bank deposit envelope or bag.

Procedure Steps

1. Obtain a practice deposit slip and place today's date on it.
   Rationale: Every practice has a bank account and a number. This number should be the same as that which was placed on the back of each check received on a patient's account as endorsement when payments were received.

2. Total all the cash and place the total on the line that says *Cash.*

3. Insert the amount of each check on the Bank *Deposit Detail* with a reference number, which is usually the ABA number. This information may have already been recorded on the deposit section of the day sheet.
   Rationale: This allows the bank to verify individual items if questions arise.

4. Total all the checks and place that total where it indicates for checks.

5. Total the cash and total amount of checks for the total amount of the bank deposit. The total amount of this deposit should be equal to the amount in the *Payments* column on the day sheet or accounts receivable record for the given day.

6. Copy the deposit slip if a duplicate deposit record has not been made when creating the day sheet.
   Rationale: The office should keep a copy of the checks and cash included in a deposit in case there are questions at a later date.

7. Place the deposit in a bank envelope or bank deposit bag and take or send it to the bank.

8. A receipt should be given after deposit. Record the amount of the deposit on the accounts payable record or record of disbursements (see Figure 36–13).
   Rationale: This provides information on the amount of money in the checking account against which checks can be written.

9. File the bank deposit receipt and copy of the bank deposit detail in a labeled file folder.
   Rationale: All bank records must be saved for a period of time for tax and accounting purposes.

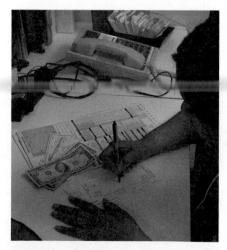

> **Figure 36–11** Medical assistant preparing deposit slip.

A check for a small amount—usually $50 to $100 at a time—is drawn to cash or petty cash in order to maintain the cash box. (It is important to keep accounts receivable separate from accounts payable. Thus, cash should never be taken from any patient payment and put into petty cash—petty cash should always be funded via a check drawn on the practice's account.)

A petty cash journal should be located near the cash box, so that each disbursement can be recorded. Also, a pad of petty cash receipts should be available, so that a receipt can be filled out each time a person receives money from the petty cash account.

THIS WORKSHEET IS PROVIDED TO HELP YOU BALANCE YOUR ACCOUNT

1. Go through your register and mark each check, withdrawal, Express ATM transaction, payment, deposit or other credit listed on this statement. Be sure that your register shows any interest paid into your account, and any service charges, automatic payments, or Express Transfers withdrawn from your account during this statement period.

2. Using the chart below, list any outstanding checks, Express ATM withdrawals, payments or any other withdrawals (including any from previous months) that are listed in your register but are not shown on this statement.

3. Balance your account by filling in the spaces below.

ITEMS OUTSTANDING		
NUMBER	**AMOUNT**	
TOTAL	$	

ENTER

The NEW BALANCE shown on
this statement_____$

ADD

Any deposits listed in your register $
or transfers into your account $
which are not shown on this $
statement.   +$ _____

TOTAL

CALCULATE THE SUBTOTAL_____$

SUBTRACT

The total outstanding checks and
withdrawals from the chart at left_____-$

CALCULATE THE ENDING BALANCE

This amount should be the same
as the current balance shown in
your check register_____$

➢ **Figure 36–12** Bank statement reconciliation form.

PROCEDURE 36–8

Reconciling a Bank Statement

Performance Objective: The student will be able to reconcile a bank statement.
Supplies and Equipment: Monthly bank statement, checkbook and/or record of disbursements, pen, calculator.

Procedure Steps

1. Examine the record of disbursements or checkbook ledger and determine which portion applies to the current bank statement.

2. Open the current bank statement and locate the ending balance and the list of checks and deposits.
   Rationale: Reconciling a bank account necessitates comparing the bank statement to the checkbook record of deposits and checks written for the same time period.
3. Check your checkbook register or record of disbursements against the bank statement and place a checkmark against each check and deposit on your record that has been recorded on the bank statement.
4. Note those checks and deposits in your record that have not cleared the bank (i.e., do not appear on the statement).
   Rationale: There are several days from the bank closing date on the statement until the statement is received in the office or practice. During that period, additional checks could be written and deposits made.
5. Note any additional charges such as service charges, ATM charges, or charges for returned checks. If there are additional charges, include them in the check ledger or record of disbursements.

6. Note any additional deposits such as interest. Include them in the check ledger and calculate the new balance.
   Rationale: To calculate the correct balance, it is necessary to include any charges or deposits that do not already appear in the check ledger.
7. Calculate the balance using the worksheet provided on each bank statement by:
   a. starting with the bank's ending balance,
   b. adding any deposits listed on your check register to that ending balance not listed on bank statement, and
   c. subtracting any outstanding checks from that subtotal.
   See Figure 36–12 for a sample worksheet to reconcile an account. The balance on the bank statement should now equal that of your check ledger or record of disbursements. If the balance does not equal, recheck all calculations in the check ledger. If the check ledger still does not balance with the bank statement and you suspect an error, contact the bank.

PROBLEMS WITH CHECKS

From time to time, the office may encounter a problem either with a check it has written or with one that has been written to the office by a patient.

Insufficient Funds in the Office Account. It is illegal to write a check for more than the amount of money in the account. However, this occasionally happens because of an arithmetic error in calculating the balance while writing checks or because of failure to reconcile a bank statement. If the office's account accidentally becomes overdrawn, the bank may refuse to honor any check written after the account is overdrawn. The check will be returned to the person or company that deposited it marked **NSF** (not sufficient funds) in the payer's account to cover the check.

If the office has a long-standing relationship with the bank, a bank officer may call to notify the practice that it is overdrawn, and the bank may honor the check or checks that are drawn against insufficient funds while the discrepancy is accounted for. In addition, it is possible to create a line of credit with the bank. A line of credit allows the practice to continue writing checks on an account with no funds, or to link a checking account to a savings account. The bank will charge interest on all the money borrowed against a credit line.

Stopping Payment. From time to time, it may become necessary to ask the bank to stop payment on a check. A check might have been lost and a new check issued; or there may be a dispute between the practice and a vendor about a purchase or a previous payment. Banks charge a fee for stopping payment, so this practice should be used sparingly.

Insufficient Funds in a Patient Account. The bank may not honor a check deposited by the practice because the patient's account has insufficient funds. If a check is returned marked NSF, do not hesitate to call the patient and tell him or her of the problem; this may be the first of many checks that are being returned, and it is important for the person to find out why he or she is writing checks against insufficient funds.

DISBURSEMENT RECORD FOR PRACTICE

Check No.	Name	Date	Amount	Deposit	Beg. Bal. 10,000 — Bank Balance	1 Supplies	2 Salary	3 Rent	4 Misc.
1837	Dustin E Dobblins	3/12/xx	1000		9000	1000			

➤ **Figure 36–13** Cash disbursements journal.

PROCEDURE 36–9

Writing Checks to Pay Bills

Performance Objective: The student will be able to write checks to pay bills for a medical office and record them in the checkbook or check register and on the disbursement record.

Supplies and Equipment: Checkbook or checks for pegboard system, monthly bills to be paid, cash disbursement record (record of accounts payable), pen.

Procedure Steps

1. Assemble supplies.
2. Organize bills to be paid by opening envelopes and/or arranging invoices. Use a pen to prepare a check for each bill or invoice.
   Rationale: This prevents alterations after the check has been written.
3. Write the name of the payee on the line of the check that says "Pay to the order of."
4. Write the date on the line that says "Date." If the check does not have a preprinted number, write the number of the check in the top right-hand corner, using the next unused number according to the check register.
   Rationale: Each check is numbered to assist in keeping records and discussing a specific check if questions arise.

5. Write the amount of the check in numbers next to the dollar sign and in words on the line below the name of the payee. Begin writing at the beginning of the line. When writing the numbers, use a decimal after the dollar amount and write the number of cents at a different level (*Example*: $1,568.^{42}). When writing the words, remember that the word "and" is only used before the number of cents. Write the number of cents as a fraction over 100. Draw a line from the end of the fraction to the word dollars (*Example*: One thousand five hundred sixty-eight and 42/100————dollars).
   Rationale: This helps prevent an unauthorized person from altering the check.
6. Write the invoice number, account number, and/or purpose of the check on the line marked "for" or "reference."
   Rationale: If the check is separated from the invoice, this helps the payee identify what the check is for. It may also assist in record keeping after the check is returned by the bank.
7. Record the date, check number, payee, amount of the check, and reason the check was written on the check stub in the checkbook or in the check register.

Rationale: A record is kept of every outstanding check.

8. Record the information about the check on the cash disbursement record as it was recorded on the check. If you are using a pegboard system, this step is unnecessary because a carbon on the back of the check automatically transfers the information to the cash disbursement record.

Rationale: The cash disbursement record is a running record of financial activity for accounts payable.

9. Subtract the amount of each check from the balance in the check register and on the disbursement record as you write it.

Rationale: Keeping a running balance makes it possible to determine easily how much money is present in the checking account.

10. If you make a mistake, draw a single line through the mistake, correct the error, and initial the correction.

11. If the check cannot be used, write the word "Void" across the check and enter the word "Void" in the check register. Place the voided check in the folder where accounts payable records are kept.

Rationale: Keeping voided checks instead of destroying them facilitates accurate record keeping and provides proof that the check was voided.

12. Prepare an envelope to mail the payment or use a window envelope supplied by the vendor. Enclose the payment slip or a copy of the invoice. If using a window envelope, be sure that the payee's address is visible through the window.

Rationale: The payment slip or invoice assists the recipient of the check to identify the account to be credited with the payment.

13. If deposits were made to the checking account, enter the date and amount of the deposit and add the amount to the checking account balance in both the check register and on the cash disbursement record.

14. Check all entries for accuracy. To proof entries, the total amount of each column of expenditures should equal the total amount of the column labeled *Amount.* The ending bank balance can also be proofed by adding the total of deposits to the beginning bank balance and subtracting the total amount of the checks written. This should equal the ending balance.

15. Place all invoices, bills, deposit slips, and voided checks in the accounts payable folder.

STUDENT STUDY PLAN

To reinforce your understanding of the material in this chapter . . .

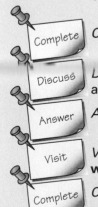

Complete the **Review & Recall** questions.

Discuss the situation in **If You Were the Medical Assistant** with your classmates and answer the questions.

Answer the **Critical Thinking** questions and discuss them with your classmates.

Visit the **Web sites** suggested and search for additional Web sites using **Keywords for Internet Searches.**

Complete the exercises in chapter 36 of the **Student Mastery Manual.**

REVIEW & RECALL

1. Where does practice income come from?
2. How can patient accounts be maintained?
3. What are the five components of a patient account?
4. What is the purpose of a fee schedule?
5. What is a superbill used for?
6. What information does a day sheet have?

7. What are three types of bank accounts, and what are their differences?
8. What is the purpose of reconciling an account? What steps do you perform to accomplish this task?
9. What information can you find on a cash disbursement record?

 ## IF YOU WERE THE MEDICAL ASSISTANT

As a medical assistant, you have been entrusted with the responsibility of making daily bank deposits. What steps would you follow to double-check your deposits and ensure accuracy?

 ## CRITICAL THINKING QUESTIONS

1. Research the pros and cons of maintaining financial accounts within the practice or utilizing an outside accounting firm or medical management company. To do this, contact both large and small practices as well as accounting firms and medical management companies.

2. What would you do if the accounts receivable or day sheets consistently did not balance?

3. Discuss the process of maintaining a cash disbursement record, addressing the problems of a positive cash flow. What problems and solutions can you identify?

 ## EXPLORE THE WEB

INTERNET WEB SITES

Health Care Financing Administration (HCFA)* Physician fee schedule by state
www.hcfa.gov/stats/carrpuf.htm

KEY WORDS FOR INTERNET SEARCHES

    billing
    fee
    fee schedule
    medical billing software

---

*Effective 6/2001, the name of this agency has been changed to the Centers for Medicare and Medicaid Services (CMMS). A new web site address will probably be created.

ANSWERS TO ON THE JOB

1. Refer to the fee schedule.

2. The charges and payments would be recorded on the ledger, superbill, and day sheet or accounts receivable record.

3. The previous balance needs to be placed on the service or charge slip, if used. It will need to be added to the charges for completing the ledger, superbill, and day sheet.

4. Adjustments would be shown on accounts of the HMO patients.

Coding

Instructional Objectives

After completing this chapter, you will be able to do the following:

1. Define and spell the vocabulary words.
2. Describe the history and usage of the three most common coding systems.
3. List the six sections of the CPT manual.
4. Describe the type of codes included in each section of the CPT manual.
5. Describe how to look up CPT codes properly.
6. Describe the three levels of HCPCS codes.
7. Identify when HCPCS codes should be used.
8. Describe the format and use of ICD-9-CM codes.
9. Discuss how to look up ICD-9-CM codes in the list of diseases (Volume 2).
10. Identify the meaning of parentheses, brackets, the term "excludes," and instructions to code first the underlying condition.
11. Describe how fourth and fifth digits are used with ICD-9-CM codes.

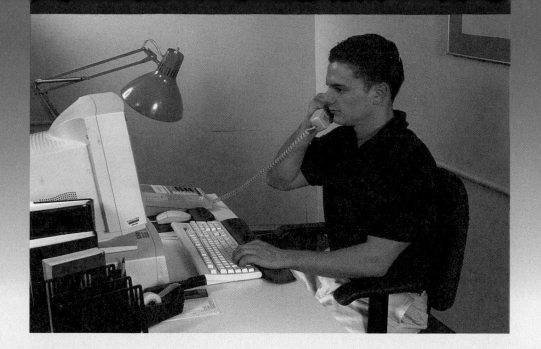

■ Perform procedural coding

■ Perform diagnostic coding

Performance Objectives

After completing this chapter, you will be able to do the following:

1. Look up the proper CPT-4 code for a procedure (Procedure 37–1).
2. Look up the proper HCPCS code for a service or piece of equipment (Procedure 37–2).
3. Look up the proper diagnostic code for a patient (Procedure 37–3).

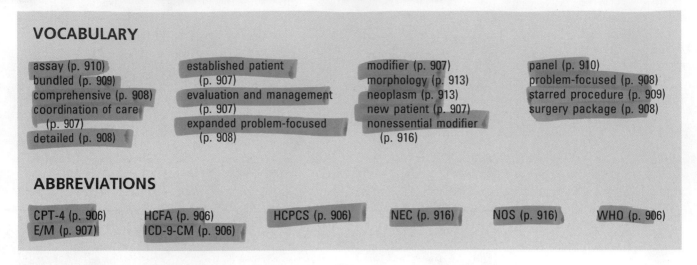

VOCABULARY

assay (p. 910)
bundled (p. 909)
comprehensive (p. 908)
coordination of care
   (p. 907)
detailed (p. 908)

established patient
   (p. 907)
evaluation and management
   (p. 907)
expanded problem-focused
   (p. 908)

modifier (p. 907)
morphology (p. 913)
neoplasm (p. 913)
new patient (p. 907)
nonessential modifier
   (p. 916)

panel (p. 910)
problem-focused (p. 908)
starred procedure (p. 909)
surgery package (p. 908)

ABBREVIATIONS

CPT-4 (p. 906)   HCFA (p. 906)   HCPCS (p. 906)   NEC (p. 916)   NOS (p. 916)   WHO (p. 906)
E/M (p. 907)   ICD-9-CM (p. 906)

For hundreds of years, medical researchers have been interested in collecting statistics related to health and disease, including the number of individuals who contract certain diseases and the number of deaths caused by those diseases. As a starting place, it was necessary for doctors to agree on a system to classify diseases. The first such disease classification system was published in 1869 as the *American Nomenclature of Disease* by the American Medical Association. (The word *nomenclature* means what things are called; in essence, this book was a dictionary of diseases.)

Turning a classification system into a coding system requires systematic replacement of names with numbers or combinations of numbers and letters. This allows information to be standardized, written in abbreviated form, and more easily managed and manipulated by computers.

In 1948 the World Health Organization (**WHO**) published the first edition of the *International Classification of Diseases*, which used numbers to describe diseases. This system was developed so more accurate statistics could be collected about the incidence (occurrence) and treatment of disease. But it proved to be useful for health care review and for insurance claims processing as well.

The WHO has revised the *International Classification of Diseases* several times since then, and is currently using the tenth edition (IDC-10). For insurance coding and review of medical records, a modified version reflecting "clinical manifestations" is used, and this version is still in the ninth edition (the tenth is being prepared). The acronym for this coding system is **ICD-9-CM,** which stands for *International Classification of Diseases* (9th edition) *Clinical Manifestations.*

ICD-9-CM became the system of choice for diagnostic coding after 1989, when the United States Health Care Financing Agency (**HCFA**), an arm of the Department of Health and Human Services, began requiring its use on all Medicare Part B insurance claims forms.

In addition to diagnostic codes, several attempts have been made to classify the care given to patients. The three main reasons for developing what have come to be called procedure codes are:

1. to justify medical services by correlating procedures to diagnosis
2. to collect statistics about the outcome and effectiveness of treatments
3. to help doctors and hospitals set fees based on the amount of time, and the amount of skill, required to provide a specific service.

In 1966 the American Medical Association published the first edition of the *Current Procedural Terminology* (CPT) coding system. The original version focused primarily on surgical procedures, and was one of many attempts to translate medical and surgical procedures into numerical codes.

The fourth edition (**CPT-4**), which is currently in use, was first published in 1977 and is updated annually. It became the standard for insurance billing in the early 1980s, when HCFA decided to use it as the basis for its own procedure coding system, the HCFA Common Procedure Coding System (**HCPCS**), pronounced "hic-pics." The first level of HCPCS codes (95 to 98 percent of codes used for Medicare Part B) includes the current CPT codes. In addition, there are additional HCPCS codes for procedures, injections, and durable medical equipment covered by Medicare Part B that are not included in the CPT system.

Each medical office must purchase updated versions of the ICD-9-CM, CPT, and HCPCS code books or computer files every year. The CPT codes are available only from the American Medical Association, but ICD-9-CM and HCPCS codes can be purchased from several publishers and are available at some locations on the Internet.

CPT CODING

The CPT manual provides both a narrative description and a five-digit code for each procedure or service a doctor or other licensed provider may perform for a patient. When entering codes on insurance claims (as discussed in chapter 38), the five-digit code is sufficient for most procedures, but a **modifier** (a two- or five-digit addition to a CPT code) may be necessary to indicate a more extensive or unusual procedure.

The two-digit modifier is added to the main code after a hyphen. The modifier can also be written as an additional five-digit code for electronic billing. The five-digit modifier is composed of "099", meaning plus the two-digit modifier.

Sections of the CPT Manual

The fourth revision of *Current Procedural Terminology* (CPT-4) is currently used for procedure coding. It is divided into six sections, each of which defines the procedures and services provided for specific types of medical services. The six sections, and the range of codes for each, are as follows:

- Evaluation and Management 99201 to 99499
- Anesthesiology 00100 to 01999
- Surgery 10040 to 69979
- Radiology 70010 to 79999
- Pathology and Radiology 80000 to 89399
- Medicine 90701 to 99199

In each annual update of the CPT-4, new codes may be added for new procedures, old codes may be dropped for procedures no longer in use, and modifications may be made to current procedures. A darkened circle in front of a code indicates that the code is new. A darkened triangle in front of the code indicates that the description for the code has been changed or modified. The medical assistant must familiarize him- or herself with the important revisions each year when the new code book is purchased.

The main body of the CPT manual is organized by section, then subsection, subheading, and finally category, each providing a finer level of detail. There is also an alphabetical index of procedures at the back of the manual. The most common procedures performed in a given office are usually found on the encounter form and in the computer billing program.

Evaluation and Management

The Evaluation and Management section is where the medical assistant responsible for coding finds codes for office visits provided by primary care practitioners and specialists. **Evaluation and management (E/M)** codes cover the service-oriented, rather than the procedure-oriented, parts of medical care.

While procedures are fairly easy to define—for instance, incision and drainage of a cyst—the amount of service provided by a doctor during a routine visit is more difficult to describe. One doctor may consider 20 minutes an appropriate amount of time for a routine visit, while another may consider 30 minutes the minimum amount of time to spend with a patient. One doctor may focus strictly on the problem the patient presents with, while another may want to examine the patient more completely, especially if he or she has not been seen for several months.

The codes in the Evaluation and Management section attempt to link reimbursement to the completeness of the examination and the amount of skill required to manage the patient's problems. Unfortunately, this tends to limit the doctor's discretion to practice in his or her own style. If the patient does not have well-defined, complex medical problems, the visit is reimbursed as uncomplicated, no matter how much time the doctor spends with the patient.

When determining the proper code for evaluation and management services, the medical assistant must consider a number of factors.

1. For coding purposes, the patient is either an **established patient** (one who has been seen in the previous three years) or a **new patient** (one who has not had services performed by the provider in the previous three years). There are separate groups of codes for each type of patient. New patients are expected to take longer to examine and are reimbursed at a higher rate.

2. There are separate groups of codes, depending on where the service is provided and whether the doctor is the patient's primary care provider or a consultant. A medical service could have been provided in the office, in a nursing home, in a hospital to a patient who has been admitted, or in a hospital emergency room.

3. The level of service provided can vary, depending on seven factors:

   - The history, which can be problem-focused, detailed, or comprehensive.
   - The physical examination, which can be problem-focused, detailed, or comprehensive.
   - The complexity of medical decision making (which can be straightforward, or have a low, moderate, or high level of complexity).
   - The amount of time spent with the patient.
   - The nature of the patient's problem.
   - The need for **coordination of care** (discussion and/or planning with other health care providers).
   - The need for counseling with the patient and/or family regarding test results, treatment instructions, and so forth.

History and Examination

There are four levels of history taking and examination: problem-focused, expanded problem-focused, detailed, and comprehensive.

For histories:

A **problem-focused** history addresses the chief complaint, with a brief history of the illness or problem.

An **expanded problem-focused** history addresses the chief complaint, a brief history of the present illness or problem, and a review of systems that have to do with the chief complaint.

A **detailed** history addresses the chief complaint, an extended history of the present illness, and a review of body systems in which additional body systems may be reviewed. Family history is also reviewed as it relates to the present problem.

A **comprehensive** history includes a chief complaint; an extended history of the present illness; a review of all body systems, especially those directly related to the problem; and a complete family history.

For examinations:

A **problem-focused** examination is limited to the affected body system or organ.

An **expanded problem-focused** examination is related to the affected body system, as well as other symptomatic or related organs or systems.

A **detailed** examination includes the affected body systems or organs, and other related systems or organs.

A **comprehensive** examination is a multisystem examination, or a complete examination of one system.

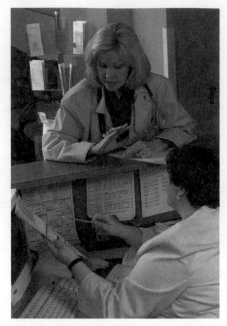

➢ **Figure 37–1** The medical assistant may discuss what code to use for an office visit with the physician.

See the accompanying box for more detail about the criteria for determining the level of care of the history and physical examination.

When coding for evaluation and management services, it is important to have documentation that supports the code chosen. Often, the doctor or other primary care provider checks the appropriate box on the encounter sheet at the time of the patient visit. Other times, the medical assistant may ask the doctor about the level of service immediately after the visit, as shown in Figure 37–1. Or the medical assistant may have to review the medical record when completing the insurance claim, and decide which of the categories is supported by the doctor's progress note.

Anesthesia

Anesthesia is the administration of a drug that causes a total or partial loss of sensation. Anesthesia can be administered to provide analgesia (comfort and absence of pain) for a patient during a surgical procedure, wound closure, removal of a foreign body, childbirth, or for a diagnostic test, including radiology, as well as for therapeutic radiology.

Anesthesia can be general, regional, or local. CPT codes for anesthesia are specified by the anatomic region affected, as well as the type of anesthesia provided. Anesthesia services are often provided by the time, in hours and minutes, that the anesthetist or anesthesiologist was present.

There are two types of modifiers in the anesthesia section—standard modifiers and physical status modifiers. Standard modifiers are those used throughout the CPT code manual; physical status modifiers indicate the patient's condition at the time anesthesia was administered. Patient condition can influence the level of complexity of administering anesthesia in the proper dose over the proper time frame.

In the office setting, most anesthesia will be local, provided by the doctor performing the procedure.

Surgery

The surgery section is the largest section of the CPT manual. This section is organized by body parts or organ systems. Many minor or simple surgical procedures are coded as a **surgery package.** In a surgery package, all of the areas—including the surgery itself, anesthesia, and "normal" uncomplicated follow-up care—are bundled for the purpose of reimbursement.

The term **bundled** means grouped together. This means that one code covers all the services in the bundle. If complications occur, however, either during the surgery or during follow-up, treatment of the complications can be coded separately.

Within the surgery section of the CPT manual, it is assumed that the code is a surgery package unless the code is a **starred procedure,** a surgical procedure that is not bundled and submitted as a surgery package. Some minor surgical procedures that might be performed in the medical office may be starred procedures. In cases where the patient came to the office for a routine visit and a minor procedure with a starred code was performed, the patient can be charged for the visit, for the surgical procedure, for anesthesia, and so on, separately.

For example, if the patient had several lacerations, the manual would show the appropriate code for the repair of one of them as 20001*. If the appointment was scheduled specifically for the surgery, however, the patient cannot also be charged for the office visit.

There are several modifiers that apply to the codes for surgical procedures. The modifiers applying to multiple surgical procedures are shown in the accompanying chart, CPT Modifiers for Surgical Procedures.

Radiology

The radiology section of the CPT manual is divided into four major subsections:

- diagnostic radiology
- diagnostic ultrasound
- radiation oncology
- nuclear medicine.

Most standard radiologic procedures are found in the diagnostic radiology subsection, including plain x-ray films, computed tomography (CT or CAT), magnetic resonance imaging (MRI), magnetic resonance angiography (MRA), and standard angiography. The codes for diagnostic radiology correspond to the anatomic site of the radiographic image, starting with the head and moving down. Some codes indicate a single view, while others indicate multiple views.

The subsection on diagnostic ultrasound is divided into eight subheadings by body area. In addition, there are four different modes for ultrasound. *A-mode* (A for amplitude) is a one-dimensional display for mapping structure; it reflects the time it takes a sound wave to reach a structure that is being mapped, then return. *M-mode* (M for motion) is the one-dimensional display of structural movement. *B-scan* (B for brightness) is a two-dimensional display of organ and tissue structure. And *real-time scan* is a two-dimensional scan of both structure and motion.

The subsection on radiation oncology includes the three categories of services necessary for utilizing radiation as a treatment for shrinking or destroying cancerous tumors. These are clinical treatment planning; medical radiation physics, dosimetry, treatment devices, and special services; and radiation treatment delivery. Radiation oncology services and procedures are billed in an unbundled manner.

There are three different levels of clinical treatment planning: simple, intermediate, and complex. Within any of these treatment planning levels, there are deci-

---

CPT Modifiers for Surgical Procedures

Examples of codes for surgical procedures include:

- -20 Microsurgery
- -22 Unusual procedural services
- -26 Professional component
- -47 Anesthesia provided by surgeon (not including local anesthesia)
- -50 Bilateral procedure—This code is added to the second (bilateral) procedure performed at the same operation
- -51 Multiple procedures performed on the same day or at the same session
- -54 Surgical care only—This code is used when another doctor provides preoperative and postoperative care
- -55 Postoperative management only
- -56 Preoperative management only
- -57 Decision for surgery (added to an E/M code)—This code is used when the doc-

tor makes the decision for surgery during an E/M visit
- -58 Staged or related procedure by the same doctor during the postoperative session
- -59 Procedure that was distinct or independent from other services on the same day
- -62 Two surgeons
- -66 Surgical team
- -76 Repeat procedure by the same doctor
- -77 Repeat procedure by another doctor
- -78 Return to operating room for a related procedure during the postoperative period
- -79 Unrelated surgical procedure by the same doctor during the postoperative surgery
- -80 Assistant surgeon
- -81 Minimum assistant surgeon
- -82 Assistant surgeon (when qualified resident surgeon not available)

sions that need to be made about the treatment modality to be used, dose calculations, and development of individualized treatment devices. Then there is the actual delivery of the radiation treatments. Clinical treatment management is coded separately.

Nuclear medicine, the placement of radionuclides into the body for diagnosis or treatment, is coded by body areas and organ systems.

Pathology and Laboratory

The pathology and laboratory section of the CPT manual is organized by the type of tests performed, such as individual tests, panels, or assays. A **panel** is a group of laboratory tests, usually ordered together for diagnosis or screening, such as a cardiac panel (a group of tests ordered for a patient with cardiac symptoms).

If all tests in the panel are done, only one code is used. If individual tests are done, each test is coded separately. An **assay** is ordered to test for the presence and amount of a specific drug in the patient's blood, such as a digoxin level.

Different codes are used for laboratory tests performed by automated equipment and tests performed manually. When coding for a medical office, the medical assistant must distinguish between those tests actually performed in the office (such as a dipstick urinalysis), for which the office bills the patient, and tests sent to an outside laboratory (such as an automated urinalysis) that performs its own billing.

Pathology testing, such as Pap tests and biopsies, are usually done by a special laboratory. The medical office charges for the visit or surgery where the specimen is collected, but the laboratory bills for the actual specimen testing.

Medicine

The medicine section of the CPT manual gives the proper codes for noninvasive diagnostic and treatment services, many of which are performed in the offices of primary care doctors and specialists. (Invasive services, those that enter a body cavity, generally fall in the surgical section.)

The medicine section is organized according to body system.

A number of highly specialized types of testing and treatment, ranging from electrocardiograms (EKGs) to ophthalmologic tests, are found in the medicine section. In addition, the medicine section contains the codes for immunizations and infusion therapies, including chemotherapy.

Codes for procedures from this section that are performed frequently (such as EKGs in the office of an internist or cardiologist) are usually found on the encounter form or in the medical billing software. In a pediatrician's office, the codes for all standard immunizations are found on the encounter form.

When a medical procedure is performed infrequently, the doctor usually writes it in on the encounter form, and the medical assistant may need to look up the code for billing. In the case of injections, it is important to identify the current code for the specific injection if it is listed in the CPT manual as immunizations are. Many drugs given by injection do not have specific codes, and are identified by the route given (i.e., subcutaneous, intramuscular, intravenous). The medication name should be included with the documentation sent to the insurance company. Note that there are different codes for injections of antibiotics and injections of other medications.

Guidelines to Find the Correct CPT-4 Code

The first step in coding is to look up the procedure that is to be coded in the alphabetical index at the back of the CPT manual.

Never code directly from the index, because it does not contain descriptions of the code, and may result in use of an incorrect code.

It may be necessary to look up the procedure in several ways before determining that you have found the correct code. For procedures, you may need to look under the name of the procedure and/or the anatomic location—for example, if you are trying to locate a procedure for the application of a cast to the lower arm. In some cases, looking up the diagnosis may lead to the code for the procedure used to treat it.

There are several pieces of information that may be significant when choosing the correct code for a procedure:

- location
- size of lesion or repair
- method of performing the procedure, or test, or surgery
- complexity of the procedure or service.

It is important to review information from the patient's medical record carefully before choosing the code that best describes the service.

The CPT manual itself contains information at the beginning of each section entitled *Guidelines* to help locate the current codes. In addition to specifying which code to use for what kind of service, there are general guidelines about what substantiating documentation must be submitted in order for the claim to be approved for payment.

Information about modifiers for each section is contained in the guidelines for each section, as well as in Appendix A. Directions about how to use the modifiers are included for each.

Appendix B is a complete list of changes and deletions from the previous year's manual. When the new manual is published, you may not be able to find a code that you have used in the past. Appendix B gives you a fast way to find out if the code has been deleted, changed, or bundled as part of another procedure.

Clinical examples of different codes are given in Appendix D. Reading these can be very helpful in learning how to decide what code to use, especially for evaluation and management codes.

Procedure 37–1 discusses how to look up the proper CPT-4 code.

HCPCS CODING

HCPCS coding is used by insurance companies that administer Medicare claims for the federal government's Health Care Financing Agency (HCFA),* which runs the program. Medicare is the federal health insurance program for the elderly, disabled, and certain other specific groups. Part A covers hospitalization, and part B covers outpatient services. As an insurance program, Medicare is discussed in detail in chapter 38.

HCPCS is a five-digit alphanumeric coding system. As the AMA does with CPT codes, HCFA updates the HCPCS codes annually.

Description

HCPCS codes, which begin with a letter, are used by Medicare primarily for certain suppliers, materials, injections, and procedures. There are three levels of coding.

Level I coding includes most procedures paid for under Medicare Part B, which covers doctors' services. Level I codes are identical to CPT-4 codes.

Level II codes are consistent across the country and designate specific services and equipment not included in Level I. Level II codes start with a letter from A to V.

Level III codes are used for procedures that are not common to all Medicare administrative carriers across the country. They are designated by regional carriers. They start with a letter from W to Z.

* Effective 6/2001, the name of this agency has been changed to the Centers for Medicare and Medicaid Services (CCMS).

PROCEDURE 37-1

Looking Up a CPT-4 Code

Performance Objective: The student will be able to look up the proper CPT-4 code for a procedure.

Supplies and Equipment: Patient's medical record, charge slip, CPT-4 manual.

Procedure Steps

1. Find the name of the procedure to look up and information about the procedure (if necessary) using the patient's charge slip and/or medical record.
   Rationale: The charge slip usually identifies the procedure(s) performed, but the medical record may be needed to identify the appropriate level of service.
2. For evaluation and management (E/M) services, identify if the patient is a new patient or an established patient.
   Rationale: Different codes are used for new patients and established patients.
3. For E/M services, identify if the patient was seen in the medical office or at another location such as the hospital, emergency room, or nursing home.

Rationale: Different E/M codes are used depending on the location where the patient was seen. The coding and billing for visits provided by a doctor to a hospitalized patient, nursing home resident, or patient in the emergency room are often done by staff at the physician's medical office.

4. Using the index at the back of the manual, locate the section in which the category of codes will be found.

Examples:
A. To locate an initial office visit for a new patient, look in the index under New Patient, Initial Office Visit (99201–99215) or under Evaluation and Management, Office and Other Outpatient (99201–99215, 99211–99215.)
B. To locate a hepatitis B immunization, look under Immunization, Active, Hepatitis B (90748). At the beginning of the section on immunizations, you are informed that when immunization is the only service performed, a minimal service may be listed in addition to the injection. You may not add an additional charge for the injection or supplies.

Procedure continued on the following page

PROCEDURE 37–1 *(continued)*

5. Look in the manual at the code or range of codes to read the description and determine the correct code. Do not code from the index. *Rationale:* You cannot be sure that you have identified the correct code without reading the description of the code. You may also find additional information in the section to help you code properly.

6. If the service is unusual or does not seem to fit the description of the code completely, check the list of modifiers for the section of the manual to see if a modifier is needed.

Example:

A patient has presented with an abscess of the skin in the right axillary area on which another doctor performed an incision and drainage two weeks ago, but which required incision and drainage again today. You look up Incision and Drainage, Abscess, Arm Upper, which refers you to 23930–23931. When you look at those codes, you notice that they are for deep abscesses and you should look at codes 10040–10160 for superficial abscesses. The code 10060* (incision and drainage of abscess: simple or single) appears to be the best

description of the procedure done. The code is starred, which means it is not a surgical package; but because the patient came for an office visit specifically for treatment of the abscess and no other evaluation and management services were provided, you do not charge for a separate office visit. When you check the list of modifiers in the surgery section, you realize that this is a repeat procedure by another doctor, so you add the modifier, -77, to the code or use the separate five-digit modifier code 09977.

7. Enter the correct code(s) on the charge slip, encounter form, and if applicable in the patient's record in the computer so that it can be used for insurance billing. *Rationale:* Reimbursement is made by insurance companies based on the codes submitted. They must be accurate and reflect the service or procedure performed. In the example given above, the insurance company might refuse to pay for the service (as already provided) without the modifier, which indicates that it is in fact a repeat service of a procedure performed by another doctor.

Sections

The level II and level III codes cover categories of services that are paid for by Medicare but usually are not covered by traditional health insurance. Some examples are transportation services, chiropractic services, medical and surgical supplies, durable medical equipment, prosthetic devices, and vision and hearing services. Figure 37–2 shows codes from the HCPCS manual.

Level II codes are needed to specify exactly which medications were administered. The CPR manual has separate codes for immunizations, but other injections are distinguished only by routes of administration, and if they are antibiotics.

Guidelines for determining the proper code for a particular service or procedure are listed at the beginning of each section. Modifiers are found in an appendix. Another appendix shows the changes and additions from the previous edition. Procedure 37–2 discusses how to look up HCPCS codes.

ICD CODING

In addition to coding procedures, it is also necessary to code diagnoses. Diagnostic coding was originally developed to fulfill four purposes: to track disease pro-

cesses, to classify the causes of death, for medical research, and for evaluation of hospital service utilization.

Today, it is necessary to use ICD-9-CM coding for diagnosis to have an insurance claim approved for the proper amount of reimbursement. If the proper ICD coding format is not used, many insurance companies will "code down" a claim, translating a written diagnosis to an ICD code that is close and pays less than a more specific code.

ICD-9-CM coding is also necessary to participate in government-financed programs such as Medicare and Medicaid, as well as in a number of professional review organizations.

Format of ICD-9-CM Manuals

The ICD manual has three volumes.

Volume I contains a tabular list of diseases, arranged numerically by disease classification. Volume II contains an alphabetic listing of diseases. Volumes I and II are used primarily in doctors' offices.

Volume III, which has both a numeric tabular listing and an alphabetic listing of procedures, is primarily used in hospitals.

ICD-9-CM codes consist of three digits (from 001 to

999) that can be preceded by a letter and/or followed by a decimal point plus one or two additional digits. Digits after the decimal point make a given diagnosis more specific. Letters before the number are used for codes that are not a diagnosis, but that give information about why a medical service was provided.

V codes list the factors influencing health status or an encounter with health services when there is no disease or injury, such as to receive an immunization. If a person schedules an office visit because he or she has a family history of diabetes, the ICD-9-CM code for diabetes (V18.0) is used. The person may (or may not) be found to be healthy, but the medical history justifies an examination.

E codes cover external causes of injury or poisoning, such as injury due to collision of a motor vehicle with another motor vehicle. E codes are used in combination with diagnosis codes to give more information about the cause of a medical problem.

For example, an open wound of the cheek without complications is given the code 873.41. In addition, an E code is assigned to identify the cause of the wound

(e.g., E 828.2, an accident to the rider of an animal, such as a horseriding accident). E codes facilitate the collection of statistics about causes and severity of injuries.

M codes describe **morphology** (structure and form) of **neoplasms** (an abnormal growth of tissue), and whether they are benign or malignant (cancerous). These are also used to compile statistics.

Tables are included for hypertension, neoplasms, and adverse effects of drugs; these tables organize information, making it easy to find codes for these problems.

Guidelines to Find the Correct ICD-9-CM Code

Using Volume 2 (Index)

The first step in coding a patient's diagnosis is to find the diagnosis in Volume 2, which is an alphabetic index. Some terms in the index may be marked with a symbol that indicates that the diagnosis requires a fifth digit (placed in the second position, after the decimal point.)

⊙	J1561	Injection, immune globulin, intravenous, 500 mg MCM 2049
	J1562	(Deleted 12/31/00)
▶ ⊙	J1563	Injection, immune globulin, intravenous, 1 g MCM 2049
⊙	J1565	Injection, respiratory syncytial virus immune globulin, intravenous, 50 mg MCM 2049
⊙	J1570	Injection, ganciclovir sodium, 500 mg MCM 2049
⊙	J1580	Injection, Garamycin, gentamicin, up to 80 mg MCM 2049
⊙	J1600	Injection, gold sodium thiomalate, up to 50 mg MCM 2049
⊙	J1610	Injection, glucagon HCl, per 1 mg MCM 2049
⊙	J1620	Injection, gonadorelin HCl, per 100 mcg MCM 2049
⊙	J1626	Injection, granisetron HCl, 100 mcg MCM 2049
⊙	J1630	Injection, haloperidol, up to 5 mg MCM 2049
⊙	J1631	Injection, haloperidol decanoate, per 50 mg MCM 2049
⊙	J1642	Injection, heparin sodium, (Heparin Lock Flush), per 10 units MCM 2049
⊙	J1741	Injection, hydroxyprogesterone caproate, 250 mg/ml MCM 2049
⊙	J1742	Injection, ibutilide fumarate, 1 mg MCM 2049
⊙	J1745	Injection, infliximab, 10 mg MCM 2049
⊙	J1750	Injection, iron dextran, 50 mg MCM 2049.5
	J1760	(Deleted 12/31/99) Cross Reference J1750
	J1770	(Deleted 12/31/99) Cross Reference J1750
	J1780	(Deleted 12/31/99) Cross Reference J1750
⊙	J1785	Injection, imiglucerase, per unit MCM 2049
⊙	J1790	Injection, droperidol, up to 5 mg MCM 2049
⊙	J1800	Injection, propranolol HCl, up to 1 mg MCM 2049
⊙	J1810	Injection, droperidol and fentanyl citrate, up to 2 ml ampule MCM 2049
⊙	J1820	Injection, insulin, up to 100 units MCM 2049, CIM 60-14
⊙	J1825	Injection, interferon beta-1a, 33 mcg (Code may be used for Medicare when drug administered under the direct supervision of a physician, not for use when drug is self-administered.) MCM 2049

➤ **Figure 37–2** A sample of codes from the HCPCS level II codes for medical services, supplies, and equipment. (From Buck C: W.B. Saunders ICD-9-CM and 2000 HCPS. Philadelphia, W.B. Saunders, 2001.)

PROCEDURE 37–2

Looking Up a HCPCS Code

Performance Objective: The student will be able to look up the proper HCPCS code for a service or piece of equipment.

Supplies and Equipment: Patient's medical record, charge slip, HCPCS manual.

Procedure Steps

1. Refer to the charge slip or the patient's medical record to locate the service, supplies, or equipment requiring a HCPCS code.
   Rationale: The charge slip usually identifies the procedure(s) performed, but the medical record may be needed to identify more detail about the service, supplies, and so on.

2. Using the index at the back of the manual, locate the section in which the category of codes will be found.

3. Look in the manual at the code or range of codes to read the description and determine the correct code. Do not code from the index.
   Rationale: You cannot be sure that you have identified the correct code without reading the description of the code. You may also find additional information in the section to help you code properly.

4. If the service is unusual or does not seem to fit the description of the code completely,

check the list of modifiers for the section of the manual to see if a modifier is needed.

5. Enter the correct code(s) on the charge slip, encounter form, and if applicable in the patient's record in the computer so that it can be used for insurance billing.
   Rationale: Reimbursement is made by insurance companies based on the codes submitted. They must be accurate and reflect the service or procedure performed. In the example given above, the insurance company might refuse to pay for the service (as already provided) without the modifier, which indicates that it is in fact a repeat service of a procedure performed by another doctor.

Example:

To locate the code for an injection of diphenhydramine hydrochloride 25 mg, look up the drug in the index. (This medication may be given intramuscularly for an allergic reaction.) The code given is J1200. When you look at the code in the manual, you are told that the code J1200 covers injections up to 50 mg. It would therefore be the correct code for the example above. Other medications may have different codes for different amounts of medication.

Even though the categories of the fifth digit subclassification may be listed in the index, you should never code directly from Volume 2 without looking up the code in Volume 1, because you may overlook important information that can help you choose a more specific code.

You must always keep in mind that insurance companies will be using the diagnosis code to determine if the procedure for which you have billed the patient is medically justified. If the diagnosis codes are incorrect or incomplete, the insurance carrier may refuse to pay for the services provided.

To find the diagnosis in Volume 2, you may look under the main word of the diagnosis or impression identified by the doctor, or you may start from the anatomic location of the medical problem. If there are two problems, you may need to identify two codes.

If the doctor identifies a medical symptom, followed by the term "rule out" or "possible" with a possible diagnosis, use the symptoms to find the code, since that is the most specific problem that is currently established. Figure 37–3 is an example from Volume 2.

Examples

1. If the progress note describes the patient's problem as "recurrent right shoulder pain, rule out bursitis," you look in the index under *Pain, joint, shoulder (region)*, which directs you to code 719.41. If you look first under *shoulder*, you are instructed to "see condition."

2. If the patient's diagnosis is given on the charge slip as diabetic neuropathy, you look in the index under *Diabetes, neuropathy*, where you find two codes: 250.6 (additional digit required) and 357.2. You should look up both codes as part of the process of selecting the correct code.

➤ **Figure 37–3** In the ICD-9-CM index to diseases (Volume 2), diseases and conditions are arranged alphabetically. (From Buck C: W.B. Saunders ICD-9-CM and 2000 HCPCS. Philadelphia, W.B. Saunders, 2001.)

Diabetes, diabetic (*Continued*)

Note   Use the following fifth-digit subclassification with category 250:

0   type II [non-insulin dependent type] [NIDDM type] [adult-onset type] or unspecified type, not stated as uncontrolled

Fifth-digit 0 is for use for type II, adult-onset diabetic patients, even if the patient requires insulin

1   type I [insulin dependent type] [IDDM type] [juvenile type], not stated as uncontrolled

2   type II [non-insulin dependent type] [NIDDM type] [adult-onset type] or unspecified type, uncontrolled

Fifth-digit 2 is for use for type II, adult-onset diabetic patients, even if the patient requires insulin

3   type I [insulin dependent type] [IDDM type] [juvenile type], uncontrolled

with
  coma (with ketoacidosis) 250.3
    hyperosmolar (nonketotic) 250.2
  complication NEC 250.9
    specified NEC 250.8
  gangrene 250.7 [785.4]
  hyperosmolarity 250.2
  ketosis, ketoacidosis 250.1
  osteomyelitis 250.8 [731.8]
  specified manifestations NEC 250.8
acetonemia 250.1
acidosis 250.1
amyotrophy 250.6 [358.1]
angiopathy, peripheral 250.7 [443.81]
asymptomatic 790.2
autonomic neuropathy (peripheral) 250.6 [337.1]
bone change 250.8 [731.8]
bronze, bronzed 275.0
cataract 250.5 [366.41]
chemical 790.2
  complicating pregnancy, childbirth, or puerperium 648.8
coma (with ketoacidosis) 250.3
  hyperglycemic 250.3
  hyperosmolar (nonketotic) 250.2
  hypoglycemic 250.3
  insulin 250.3
complicating pregnancy, childbirth, or puerperium (maternal) 648.0
  affecting fetus or newborn 775.0
complication NEC 250.9
  specified NEC 250.8
dorsal sclerosis 250.6 [340]
dwarfism-obesity syndrome 258.1
gangrene 250.7 [785.4]
gastroparesis 250.6 [536.3]
gestational 648.8
  complicating pregnancy, childbirth, or puerperium 648.8
glaucoma 250.5 [365.44]
glomerulosclerosis (intercapillary) 250.4 [581.81]
glycogenosis, secondary 250.8 [259.8]
hemochromatosis 275.0

Diabetes, diabetic (*Continued*)
hyperosmolar coma 250.2
hyperosmolarity 250.2
hypertension-nephrosis syndrome 250.4 [581.81]
hypoglycemia 250.8
hypoglycemic shock 250.8
insipidus 253.5
  nephrogenic 588.1
  pituitary 253.5
  vasopressin-resistant 588.1
intercapillary glomerulosclerosis 250.4 [581.81]
iritis 250.5 [364.42]
ketosis, ketoacidosis 250.1
Kimmelstiel (-Wilson) disease or syndrome (intercapillary glomerulosclerosis) 250.4 [581.81]
Lancereaux's (diabetes mellitus with marked emaciation) 250.8 [261]
latent (chemical) 790.2
  complicating pregnancy, childbirth, or puerperium 648.8
lipoidosis 250.8 [272.7]
macular edema 250.5 [362.01]
maternal
  with manifest disease in the infant 775.1
  affecting fetus or newborn 775.0
microaneurysms, retinal 250.5 [362.01]
mononeuropathy 250.6 [355.9]
neonatal, transient 775.1
nephropathy 250.4 [583.81]
nephrosis (syndrome) 250.4 [581.81]
neuralgia 250.6 [357.2]
neuritis 250.6 [357.2]
neurogenic arthropathy 250.6 [713.5]
neuropathy 250.6 [357.2]
nonclinical 790.2
osteomyelitis 250.8 [731.8]
peripheral autonomic neuropathy 250.6 [337.1]
phosphate 275.3
polyneuropathy 250.6 [357.2]
renal (true) 271.4
retinal
  edema 250.5 [362.01]
  hemorrhage 250.5 [362.83]
  microaneurysms 250.5 [362.01]
retinitis 250.5 [362.01]
retinopathy 250.5 [362.01]
  background 250.5 [362.01]
  proliferative 250.5 [362.02]
steroid induced
  correct substance properly administered 251.8
  overdose or wrong substance given or taken 962.0
stress 790.2
subclinical 790.2
subliminal 790.2
sugar 250.0
ulcer (skin) 250.8 [707.9]   ◄▥
  lower extremity 250.8 [707.10]   ◄
    ankle 250.8 [707.13]   ◄
    calf 250.8 [707.12]   ◄
    foot 250.8 [707.15]   ◄
    heel 250.8 [707.14]   ◄
    knee 250.8 [707.19]   ◄
    specified site NEC 250.8 [707.19]   ◄
    thigh 250.8 [707.11]   ◄
    toes 250.8 [707.15]   ◄
  specified site NEC 250.8 [707.8]
xanthoma 250.8 [272.2]

Diacyclothrombopathia 287.1
Diagnosis deferred 799.9
Dialysis (intermittent) (treatment)
  anterior retinal (juvenile) (with detachment) 361.04
  extracorporeal V56.0
  peritoneal V56.8
  renal V56.0
    status only V45.1
  specified type NEC V56.8
Diamond-Blackfan anemia or syndrome (congenital hypoplastic anemia) 284.0
Diamond-Gardener syndrome (autoerythrocyte sensitization) 287.2
Diaper rash 691.0
Diaphoresis (excessive) NEC 780.8
Diaphragm - *see* condition
Diaphragmalgia 786.52
Diaphragmitis 519.4
Diaphyseal aclasis 756.4
Diaphysitis 733.99
Diarrhea, diarrheal (acute) (autumn) (bilious) (bloody) (catarrhal) (choleraic) (chronic) (gravis) (green) (infantile) (lienteric) (noninfectious) (presumed noninfectious) (putrefactive) (secondary) (sporadic) (summer) (symptomatic) (thermic) 787.91
achlorhydric 536.0
allergic 558.3   ◄▥
amebic (*see also* Amebiasis) 006.9
  with abscess - *see* Abscess, amebic
  acute 006.0
  chronic 006.1
  nondysenteric 006.2
bacillary - *see* Dysentery, bacillary
bacterial NEC 008.5
balantidial 007.0
bile salt-induced 579.8
cachectic NEC 558.9
chilomastix 007.8
choleriformis 001.1
coccidial 007.2
Cochin-China 579.1
  anguilluliasis 127.2
  psilosis 579.1
Dientamoeba 007.8
dietetic 558.9
due to
  achylia gastrica 536.8
  Aerobacter aerogenes 008.2
  Bacillus coli - *see* Enteritis, E. coli
  bacteria NEC 008.5
  bile salts 579.8
  Capillaria
    hepatica 128.8
    philippinensis 127.5
  Clostridium perfringens (C) (F) 008.46
  Enterobacter aerogenes 008.2
  enterococci 008.49
  Escherichia coli - *see* Enteritis, E. coli
  Giardia lamblia 007.1
  Heterophyes heterophyes 121.6
  irritating foods 558.9
  Metagonimus yokogawai 121.5
  Necator americanus 126.1
  Paracolobactrum arizonae 008.1
  Paracolon bacillus NEC 008.47
    Arizona 008.1
  Proteus (bacillus) (mirabilis) (Morganii) 008.3
  Pseudomonas aeruginosa 008.42
  S. japonicum 120.2

Excludes | *that with mention of hypertension (642.0–642.9)*

● **646.3 Habitual aborter**
[0–1,3]
Excludes | *with current abortion (634.0–634.9)*
without current pregnancy (629.9)

● **646.4 Peripheral neuritis in pregnancy**
[0–4]

● **646.5 Asymptomatic bacteriuria in pregnancy**
[0–4]

● **646.6 Infections of genitourinary tract in pregnancy**
[0–4]   Conditions classifiable to 590, 595, 597, 599.0, 616
complicating pregnancy, childbirth, or the puerperium
Conditions classifiable to 614–615 complicating
pregnancy or labor
Excludes | *major puerperal infection (670)*

● **646.7 Liver disorders in pregnancy**
[0,1,3]   Acute yellow atrophy of liver (obstetric) (true) of
pregnancy
Icterus gravis of pregnancy
Necrosis of liver of pregnancy
Excludes | *hepatorenal syndrome following delivery (674.8)*
viral hepatitis (647.6)

☐● **646.8 Other specified complications of pregnancy**
[0–4]   Fatigue during pregnancy
Herpes gestationis
Insufficient weight gain of pregnancy
Uterine size-date discrepancy   ◄

☐● **646.9 Unspecified complication of pregnancy**
[0,1,3]

● **647 Infectious and parasitic conditions in the mother classifiable elsewhere, but complicating pregnancy, childbirth,
or the puerperium**

Use additional code(s) to further specify complication

Requires fifth digit; valid digits are in [brackets] under
each code. See beginning of section 640–648 for definitions.

Includes: the listed conditions when complicating the
pregnant state, aggravated by the preg-
nancy, or when a main reason for obstetric care

Excludes | *those conditions in the mother known or sus-
pected to have affected the fetus (655.0–655.9)*

● **647.0 Syphilis**
[0–4]   Conditions classifiable to 090–097

● **647.1 Gonorrhea**
[0–4]   Conditions classifiable to 098

● **648 Other current conditions in the mother classifiable elsewhere, but complicating pregnancy, childbirth, or the puerperium**

Use additional code(s) to identify the condition

Requires fifth digit; valid digits are in [brackets] under
each code. See beginning of section 640–648 for definitions.

Includes: the listed conditions when complicating the
pregnant state, aggravated by the preg-
nancy, or when a main reason for obstetric care

Excludes | *those conditions in the mother known or sus-
pected to have affected the fetus (655.0–665.9)*

● **648.0 Diabetes mellitus**
[0–4]   Conditions classifiable to 250
Excludes | *gestational diabetes (648.8)*

● **648.1 Thyroid dysfunction**
[0–4]   Conditions classifiable to 240–246

● **648.2 Anemia**
[0–4]   Conditions classifiable to 280–285

● **648.3 Drug dependence**
[0–4]   Conditions classifiable to 304

● **648.4 Mental disorders**
[0–4]   Conditions classifiable to 290–303, 305–316, 317–
319

● **648.5 Congenital cardiovascular disorders**
[0–4]   Conditions classifiable to 745–747

☐● **648.6 Other cardiovascular diseases**
[0–4]   Conditions classifiable to 390–398, 410–429
Excludes | *cerebrovascular disorders in the puerperium
(674.0)*
venous complications (671.0–671.9)

● **648.7 Bone and joint disorders of back, pelvis, and
[0–4] lower limbs**
Conditions classifiable to 720–724, and those classifiable to 711–719 or 725–738, specified as
affecting the lower limbs

● **648.8 Abnormal glucose tolerance**
[0–4]   Conditions classifiable to 790.2
Gestational diabetes

☐● **648.9 Other current conditions classifiable elsewhere**
[0–4]   Conditions classifiable to 440–459
Nutritional deficiencies [conditions classifiable to
260–269]

ICD-9-CM

600-699

Vol. 1

➤ **Figure 37–4** In the ICD-9-CM tabular list (Volume 1), similar conditions are grouped together. (From Buck C: W.B. Saunders
ICD-9-CM and 2000 HCPCS. Philadelphia, W.B. Saunders, 2001.)

Using Volume 1 (Tabular List)

—Once you have identified one or more specific
codes to look up, find the correct section and determine the best code to match the information on the
patient's charge slip or in the medical record. Be sure
to look at the additional information given relating to
the diagnosis. See Figure 37–4 for an example of a
section from Volume 1. The abbreviation **NOS** means
"not otherwise specified," and is used only when a
more specific code cannot be identified. The abbreviation **NEC** means "not elsewhere classified," and de-

scribes codes that are used when a more specific one
cannot be identified. ◄

The first three digits of the code are called the
category, and are helpful in locating the general area
where the code can be found. The category code, followed by a decimal point and one digit, identifies a
subcategory.◄

Parentheses used around words in a subcategory
identify what are called **nonessential modifiers,** words
that may occur in the diagnosis but are not required.
For example, the code 250.0 is used for diabetes melli-

PROCEDURE 37–3

Looking Up an ICD-9-CM Code

Performance Objective: The student will be able to look up the proper ICD-9-CM code to describe a patient's diagnosis

Supplies and Equipment: Patient's medical record, charge slip, ICD-9-CM manual

Procedure Steps

1. Refer to the patient's charge slip and/or medical record to identify the diagnosis. In the medical record, the physician may use the term "impression."
   Rationale: The charge slip usually identifies the diagnosis, but the medical record may be needed for additional information to select the correct code.

2. Decide on the key word or phrase to look for the code in the list of diseases (Volume 2).

3. Locate the key word and look for the body part or other distinguishing factors. Identify the possible code number(s).

4. Locate the number(s) in the tabular list (Volume 1).
   Rationale: You cannot be sure that you have identified the correct code without looking at the tabular list. You may also find additional information in the tabular list to help you code properly.

5. Review the information given in the tabular list and select the four-digit code that most correctly corresponds to the information on the charge slip and/or in the medical record. Add a fifth digit if required.

6. Enter the correct code(s) on the charge slip, encounter form, and if necessary in the patient's record in the computer, so that it can be used for insurance billing.
   Rationale: Reimbursement is made by insurance companies based on the codes submitted. Diagnosis codes must be accurate and justify the service provided.

Example:

To locate the code for a patient with the diagnosis "chest pain, possibly angina pectoris," first locate *pain,* then *chest* in the list of diseases (Volume 2). You will find entries similar to the following:

Pain(s)
    cervicobrachial 723.3
    chest (central) 786.50
        atypical 786.59
        midsternal 798.51
    ....
    coccyx 724.79

Look up the code 786.50 in the tabular list (Volume 1).

786.5 Chest pain
    786.50   Chest pain, unspecified
    786.51   Precordial pain
    786.52   Painful respiration

When you review other codes in the category, you decide that 786.50 relates best to the information given by the physician.

---

tus without mention of complications, or diabetes (mellitus) NOS. The parentheses mean that the word *mellitus* does not have to appear in the doctor's diagnosis.

Brackets are used to identify synonyms or alternative wording, as in diabetes type II {non-insulin-dependent type} {NIDDN type} {adult-onset type}.

Certain codes require a fifth digit added after the subcategory code. If the diagnosis is diabetes mellitus, for example, a fifth digit is always required. The use of the fifth digit varies for each category where it is required, and it is necessary to review the instructions carefully before choosing the fifth digit.

Use of the fourth and fifth digits is not optional.

If a certain code may not be used for a condition (usually a similar or related condition) the word "excludes" is placed in a box under the code, and the correct code is identified. If the code cannot be used as a primary diagnosis, instructions are given to code the underlying disease first.

If you look up the code 357.2 for polyneuropathy (multiple nerve dysfunction) in diabetes, you are instructed to code the underlying disease, diabetes mellitus, first. If the patient has the secondary condition, it is important to include both diagnoses, because the specific treatment given may be related to the secondary diagnosis (which cannot be used independently).

Procedure 37–3 describes how to look up a correct ICD-9-CM code.

ON THE JOB

You are new to Blackburn Primary Care Associates. You are being oriented to each aspect of the office, and today you are working with Linda, who handles the front-office part of the practice. She has asked you to review three new patient files and determine the procedures and diagnoses performed.

QUESTIONS

1. The first patient is a new patient who came to the office with shortness of breath. After taking a comprehensive history, performing a physical examination, and having the medical assistant perform a spirometry test, the doctor diagnosed the patient with chronic obstructive pulmonary disease. Which section of the CPT manual should you look in to find the doctor's examination? to find the spirometry test? What should you look under to find the diagnosis in the ICD-9-CM manual?

2. The second patient is also a new patient, who saw Dr. Hughes for a routine checkup and to have his blood pressure checked. Dr. Hughes performed a problem-focused history and physical examination, and adjusted the patient's medication. The diagnosis is essential hypertension. What section of the CPT manual should you look in to find the doctor's examination? to find the blood pressure check? What should you look under to find the diagnosis in the ICD-9-CM manual?

STUDENT STUDY PLAN

To reinforce your understanding of the material in this chapter . . .

Complete the **Review & Recall** questions.

Discuss the situation in **If You Were the Medical Assistant** with your classmates and answer the questions.

Answer the **Critical Thinking Questions** and discuss them with your classmates.

Visit the **Web sites** suggested and search for additional Web sites using the **Keywords for Internet Searches**.

Complete the exercises in chapter 37 of the **Student Mastery Manual**.

REVIEW & RECALL

1. What are the differences among the three types of coding systems?
2. What are the six sections or categories of codes within the CPT manual?
3. What is a modifier?
4. What factors must be considered when determining a code in the Evaluation and Management section of the CPT manual?
5. What does the surgery package mean in the surgery section of the CPT manual?

6. When is a HCPCS code to be used?
7. What is the primary purpose for using ICD codes?
8. When looking up a diagnosis in the ICD manual, which volume do you begin with?
9. How do you select a fifth digit if required for an ICD-9-CM code?
10. What relationship are insurance companies looking for between diagnosis codes and procedure codes?

IF YOU WERE THE MEDICAL ASSISTANT

For each of the following descriptions, look up the correct procedure codes in the CPT-4 manual and the correct diagnosis codes in the ICD-9-CM manual.

1. An established patient had a complete physical examination (including a comprehensive history and comprehensive physical examination), an electrocardiogram, blood work (general health panel), and a stool specimen for occult blood. Identify the correct procedure codes (4) and diagnosis code (1). (*Hint:* Remember that V codes are used for physical examinations.)

2. A new patient is seen for acute bronchitis. The doctor performs an expanded problem-focused history and physical examination, and decides to treat the

patient with medication. No laboratory testing is done. Identify the correct procedure code (1) and diagnosis code (1).

3. A 12-month-old infant (established patient) is seen for a well-baby visit. The doctor performs a detailed history and examination, and also removes two skin tags from the baby's neck. The baby is given the following immunizations: MMR and Varicella (chicken pox). Identify the correct procedure codes (4) and diagnosis codes (2).

CRITICAL THINKING QUESTIONS

1. Research the different coding certifications available and describe the qualifications necessary to take the exam.

2. Work with your classmates to look up codes and discuss the proper selection of codes. When learning to code, learning about code selection is more important than getting the correct code.

3. Review changes in procedure coding from the previous year in your current version of the CPT-4. Discuss with your classmates why revisions may have been made.

4. What can happen to a medical assistant who codes for services and procedures that were not performed? who codes incorrectly?

5. Obtain information about ICD-10, and find when the ICD-10-CM is expected to be placed in use.

EXPLORE THE WEB

INTERNET WEB SITES

American Medical Association CPT codes
www.ama-assn.org/ama/pub/category/3113.htm

American Health Information Management Systems
www.ahima.org

Central office on ICD-9-CM of the American Hospital Association
www.icd-9-cm.org

ICD-9-CM codes on line
www.mcis.duke.edu/standards/termcode/icd9

ICD-10
www.hcfa.gov/stats/icd10/icd10.htm

National Center for Health Statistics
www.cdc.gov/nchs/icd9.htm

KEYWORDS FOR INTERNET SEARCHES

coding
   Federal Register
   HCFA
   medical coding

ANSWERS TO ON THE JOB

1. For this patient, the code for the office visit is found in the Evaluation and Management section of the CPT manual. The spirometry is found in the Medical section of the CPT manual. To find the diagnosis, look first under disease, then under pulmonary.

2. The code for the office visit is found in the Evaluation and Management section of the CPT manual. Monitoring blood pressure is included in the office visit. You must look for the diagnosis code under *hypertension, essential,* or *blood pressure, high.*

Health Insurance

Instructional Objectives

After completing this chapter, you will be able to do the following:

1. Define and spell the vocabulary words.
2. Describe eight different types of health insurance.
3. Determine patient eligibility for insurance reimbursement.
4. Identify information contained on an insurance form.
5. Recognize potential errors in a completed insurance form.
6. Describe the process for submission and payment of health insurance claims.

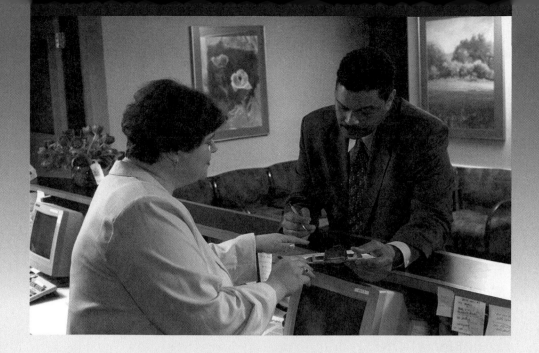

- Apply managed care policies and procedures
- Apply third-party guidelines

- Obtain managed care referrals and pre-certifications
- Complete insurance claim forms

Performance Objectives

After completing this chapter, you will be able to do the following:

1. Complete an HCFA-1500 form for insurance reimbursement (Procedure 38–1).

VOCABULARY

assignment of benefits (p. 924)
authorization (p. 930)
benefit (p. 923)
birthday rule (p. 924)
capitation (p. 927)
carrier (p. 930)
CHAMPVA (p. 923)
coinsurance (p. 924)
coordination of benefits (p. 924)
copayment (p. 924)

crossover claim (p. 929)
deductible (p. 923)
diagnostic related groups (p. 928)
exclusive provider organization (p. 927)
explanation of benefits (p. 936)
fee for service (p. 922)
fiscal intermediary (p. 928)
group practice model HMO (p. 926)
independent practice association (p. 926)

insured (p. 930)
managed care (p. 922)
Medicaid (p. 923)
Medicare (p. 922)
Medigap (p. 924)
network model HMO (p. 926)
point-of-service plan (p. 927)
prefered provider organization (p. 927)
premium (p. 923)
primary care physician (p. 926)
primary insurance (p. 924)

reimbursement (p. 936)
resource-based relative value scale (p. 928)
secondary insurance (p. 924)
signature on file (p. 930)
staff model HMO (p. 926)
subscriber (p. 926)
TRICARE (p. 923)
workers' compensation (p. 929)

ABBREVIATIONS

CHIP (p. 923)	EOB (p. 936)	HMO (p. 922)	PCP (p. 926)	PPO (p. 927)	SOF (p. 930)
DRG (p. 928)	EPO (p. 927)	IPA (p. 926)	POS (p. 927)	RBRVS (p. 928)	UCR (p. 922)

INTRODUCTION TO HEALTH INSURANCE

The growth and change in the structure of health insurance has affected American health care since the end of World War II. At the time when many other industrialized countries, mostly in western Europe but including Canada, were beginning to experiment with government-provided health care, the United States was turning to the private market to provide insurance coverage for Americans.

Today, despite the variety of health insurance plans and opportunities to obtain health insurance, many Americans still do not have health insurance. Market-based, regulatory, and legislative measures all failed to solve this problem throughout the 1990s.

History of Health Insurance

Health insurance had its beginnings in accident insurance, which was first sold in the mid-1800s. In exchange for a monthly payment of a premium by a customer, the insurance company agreed to replace lost income due to accident, and later due to a few specific illnesses such as smallpox, diphtheria, typhoid, and scarlet fever.

In the 1930s, a group of Dallas school teachers made an arrangement with Baylor Hospital to have any necessary hospital care provided in exchange for monthly premiums. This arrangement was the precursor to the Blue Cross and Blue Shield programs, which were incorporated by each state as not-for-profit companies. These programs provide **fee for service** insurance, where the insurance company reimburses all or part of the costs of services provided, as long as that cost is usual, customary, and reasonable (**UCR**) for that particular procedure in that part of the country.

During World War II, Henry Kaiser created clinics in California to provide both in-patient and out-patient care for the workers in his shipyards. These clinics later opened themselves to other employers and individuals, and became the Kaiser Permanente program, for many years the country's largest health maintenance organization (**HMO**). Over time, the HMO model broadened, from one in which doctors were salaried employees and worked in a central facility to one in which HMOs contract with limited numbers of private doctors in each community. The various HMO models, collectively, are known as **managed care,** because the HMO administrators manage the care patients get by predetermining the doctors who can be seen, the procedures that can be performed in different circumstances, and the medications that can be prescribed.

Each patient chooses a primary care provider, who then "manages" the patient's care by approving referrals to specialists and additional services.

By the 1960s, many larger and even medium-sized businesses were providing company-paid health insurance benefits as a fringe benefit instead of increased wages or salary. Health care costs began to increase faster than the general rate of inflation, with doctors beginning to earn large incomes. But certain groups of Americans—most notably the poor, the elderly, and the permanently disabled—were unable to obtain medical insurance.

The federal government created two programs to try to close these large gaps in medical coverage. One was **Medicare,** the health insurance program for the elderly, disabled, and those with end-stage kidney disease. Medicare is paid for with federal taxes paid by employers and workers. The other was **Medicaid,** the health insurance program for the poor and those whose health care needs would force them into poverty if they had to pay those costs out of pocket. Medicaid is administered by each state; the federal government pays for the majority of required care and a smaller percentage of optional care, such as dental care, while the states pay for the rest.

Many senators, congress persons, and doctors were against Medicare and Medicaid at the beginning, calling it "socialized medicine." But there were precedents for the government's involvement in paying for medical care. The Veterans Administration department offered medical care for life for any man or woman who had seen active duty in the military, provided he or she wished to use the VA facilities. In addition, the CHAMPUS program had been developed to provide medical care in the private sector at government expense for dependent spouses and children of active-duty military personnel. Today, the former CHAMPUS program is called **TRICARE** (because there are three different plans); and a companion program, **CHAMPVA,** covers dependent spouses and children of military veterans with service-connected disabilities.

At the beginning of the 21st century, American society is still trying to resolve insurance issues, among them providing prescription drug benefits for the elderly under Medicare and expanding health care insurance to children living in homes with incomes too high to be eligible for Medicaid but too low to afford private insurance. This has been an increasing problem for some time as low-wage workers often do not get health insurance through their employers, or have insurance only for themselves and not their dependents. State programs, called Children's Health Insurance Programs (**CHIPs**), were established in 1998, funded by the federal government, and available to children in families earning up to 200 percent of the income for Medicaid eligibility.

Obtaining Health Insurance

There are basically three ways for individuals and families to obtain health insurance coverage: through a group plan, by purchasing an individual policy, or through one of the government plans described above.

Most group plans are available through an employer. Larger employers generally have several different plans available. Often, they will pay the full cost of the lowest-priced plan for the employee, with the employee paying for coverage for other family members, or to purchase a more expensive plan.

Unionized workers often have very good health insurance, since this has been a focus of much contract negotiation, especially in years when employers were unable to pay larger wage increases.

Many small business owners are able to purchase insurance through group plans sponsored by the local chamber of commerce or a trade organization. Individuals sometimes have access to group plans through professional associations, or even college alumni associations. The self-employed are allowed to deduct a portion of their health insurance costs from their business income, as companies do.

As part of the process of gaining the right to sell health insurance in a particular state, most insurance plans are required to offer individual policies to individuals or families who are not covered under a group plan. There is usually an open-enrollment period at least once per year, when individuals can purchase coverage. There is discussion at the federal level about allowing individuals or families who purchase their own insurance to claim a tax credit, or a larger tax deduction, for the cost.

Taxpayer-funded, or government, health insurance is usually provided as an entitlement when other conditions are met. For instance, when an individual reaches age 65, he or she is entitled to Medicare benefits. However, the individual must still file an application because the benefits do not begin automatically. An individual is eligible for Medicaid if certain income and asset conditions are met.

Paying for Health Insurance

With all insurance, the amount of money paid by the consumer is called the **premium.** This premium can be paid monthly, quarterly, semi-annually, or annually. In exchange for the payment of a premium, the insurance company or HMO agrees to provide payment to doctors, hospitals, laboratories, and other health care providers for specific services. A specific service paid for by the insurance company is called a **benefit.**

When the premium is paid by a person's employer, even if the employee is responsible for part of the cost, that premium is often paid with before-tax dollars. This means that the amount of the premium payment is deducted from the employee's paycheck before taxes are computed; this in effect gives the employee a tax deduction for the portion of his or her insurance cost not paid by the employer.

The amount the employee pays for your health insurance and whether the portion the employee pays is tax-advantaged is an important question to ask when looking for a job; the savings can be substantial.

Depending on the type of policy, the patient may have to make certain payments for medical services. Traditional, fee-for-service insurance usually has a **deductible,** an amount of money that must be paid for services provided to an individual or a family member in a group plan every calendar year before insurance begins to pick up the payments. After the deductible is met, the cost of services is usually split, with the insurance company paying 80 percent of the bill, and the patient paying 20 percent; this is called **coinsurance.** Managed care plans do not have deductibles, but they usually require the patient to make a small **copayment,** a fixed dollar amount, every time he or she obtains medical services or fills a prescription.

Coordination of Benefits

Many households have two working adults, both of whom are covered under separate employer health benefits. **Coordination of benefits** is a term for the rules insurance companies use to coordinate the payments for medical services so that no provider is paid more than 100 percent of the charge for any service provided.

Coordination of benefits can become complex because each state writes its own rules and some policies have no coordination of benefits provisions. In addition, some people—especially those who work for large corporations with many offices or plants across the country—are often covered by insurance written outside of the state in which they live.

If both members of a couple have insurance with coordination of benefits provisions, the following rules apply.

If the employee who holds the policy is the patient, his or her insurance is the **primary insurance** for any services obtained. The spouse or partner's insurance becomes the **secondary insurance,** and can be used to pay for any portion of the charge not covered by the primary insurance.

If a child is the patient, in most states the "birthday rule" applies. Under the **birthday rule,** the primary insurance is the insurance belonging to the working adult whose birthday comes first in the year, and the insurance of the adult whose birthday is later is the secondary insurance.

If a child of divorced parents who both have medical insurance is the patient, the rules can get somewhat complicated. If a court has decreed that one parent is the "responsible party," that parent's policy provides the primary insurance. A responsible party ruling is often made in cases of joint custody, although the responsible party can also be a noncustodial parent. If no court ruling is in place, the custodial parent's policy is primary if the custodial parent has remarried. If there is no court ruling in place and the custodial parent has not remarried, the birthday rule remains in effect. If one plan is written in a state without a coordination of benefits law, the plan from the state with a coordination of benefits law determines the primary and secondary policies.

Coordination of benefits issues can be avoided if individuals in households with two working adults make modifications in their benefits. In order to reduce premium costs, some employers allow employees to take cash instead of health insurance if the family already has insurance. In cases where the company only pays for individual coverage, only one person needs to pay for family coverage. Of course, available plans should be compared for cost and benefits when deciding which policy to extend to family coverage.

If the patient is a Medicare recipient who also is covered by an employer's policy, the employer's policy is the primary insurance, and Medicare is the secondary insurance. If the patient is a Medicare recipient who does not work but has purchased a **Medigap** insurance plan—which covers medical costs that Medicare does not—Medicare is the primary insurance and the Medigap policy is the secondary insurance.

Assignment of Benefits

Assignment of benefits allows the medical provider to bill the insurance company and receive payments directly, rather than having the patient pay for the service, then file for reimbursement with the insurance company. In early health insurance plans, the patient submitted a claim form (often partially completed or signed by the doctor) and was reimbursed by the insurance company after paying the bill. The current trend is for the medical office to submit the bill and accept assignment of benefits in order to be paid directly. The patient must sign a form allowing the insurance company to pay the doctor directly. This is usually part of the new patient information form (see Figure 12-4).

In many instances, however, if the doctor or other medical provider agrees to accept assignment, he or she cannot bill the patient for any portion of the charge not paid by the insurance company except the deductible and copayment or coinsurance.

TYPES OF INSURANCE

There are eight different types of insurance that pay for medical services:

1. Fee for service
2. HMOs
3. Other managed care plans
4. Medicare
5. Medicaid
6. Children's Health Insurance Plans (CHIPs)
7. Workers' Compensation
8. TRICARE/CHAMPVA.

Fee for Service

Fee-for-service insurance provides payment, either to the doctor or to the patient, for each medical service provided. Up until the late 1980s, fee-for-service dominated the health care industry, through private insurance companies and also through the Blue Cross and

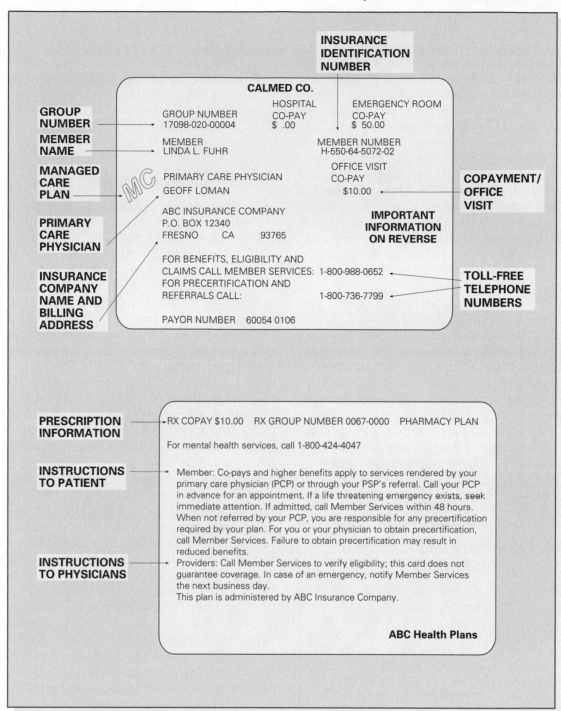

INSURANCE IDENTIFICATION NUMBER

GROUP NUMBER

MEMBER NAME

MANAGED CARE PLAN

PRIMARY CARE PHYSICIAN

INSURANCE COMPANY NAME AND BILLING ADDRESS

COPAYMENT/ OFFICE VISIT

TOLL-FREE TELEPHONE NUMBERS

CALMED CO.

GROUP NUMBER
17098-020-00004

HOSPITAL
CO-PAY
$ .00

EMERGENCY ROOM
CO-PAY
$ 50.00

MEMBER
LINDA L. FUHR

MEMBER NUMBER
H-550-64-5072-02

MC

PRIMARY CARE PHYSICIAN
GEOFF LOMAN

OFFICE VISIT
CO-PAY
$10.00

ABC INSURANCE COMPANY
P.O. BOX 12340
FRESNO   CA   93765

IMPORTANT INFORMATION ON REVERSE

FOR BENEFITS, ELIGIBILITY AND
CLAIMS CALL MEMBER SERVICES: 1-800-988-0652
FOR PRECERTIFICATION AND
REFERRALS CALL: 1-800-736-7799

PAYOR NUMBER   60054 0106

PRESCRIPTION INFORMATION

INSTRUCTIONS TO PATIENT

INSTRUCTIONS TO PHYSICIANS

RX COPAY $10.00   RX GROUP NUMBER 0067-0000   PHARMACY PLAN

For mental health services, call 1-800-424-4047

Member: Co-pays and higher benefits apply to services rendered by your
primary care physician (PCP) or through your PSP's referral. Call your PCP
in advance for an appointment. If a life threatening emergency exists, seek
immediate attention. If admitted, call Member Services within 48 hours.
When not referred by your PCP, you are responsible for any precertification
required by your plan. For you or your physician to obtain precertification,
call Member Services. Failure to obtain precertification may result in
reduced benefits.

Providers: Call Member Services to verify eligibility; this card does not
guarantee coverage. In case of an emergency, notify Member Services
the next business day.
This plan is administered by ABC Insurance Company.

ABC Health Plans

➤ **Figure 38–1** Sample insurance card showing front (top) and back (bottom). (From Fordney MT: Insurance Handbook for the Medical Office, 7th ed. Philadelphia WB Saunders, 2002.)

Blue Shield plans, which were established in each state as not-for-profit, quasi-governmental agencies. Figure 38–1 shows a sample patient insurance card.

Since the late 1980s, the percentage of individuals covered under fee-for-service plans has steadily decreased. Today, fewer than 25 percent of Americans are covered by fee-for-service plans.

There are three ways an insurance company may determine the amount it will pay for specific services under a fee-for-service plan.

1. Some plans pay through a fee schedule. A fee schedule says the insurance company will pay a specified percentage of a particular amount for a particular procedure; anything above that is the patient's responsibility.

2. Other plans pay service benefits, which defines the services they will pay for but not the payments they will make. Under service benefit plans, the insurance company agrees to pay a specified percentage of charges that are usual, customary, and reasonable for the procedure and for the state or region of the country in which it was performed. The patient is responsible for coinsurance or copayment and for any charges above those approved by the insurance company. The insurance policy outlines the amount of the patient's deductible and coinsurance or copayment for medical services.

   Under a fee-for-service plan, a patient can make an appointment with any doctor, in any specialty, he or she wishes, and the insurance will pay the designated amount for the services. Some plans have lists of approved providers for whom they pay 100 percent of charges, and pay only a percentage of charges for other providers (similar to a preferred provider organization [PPO] discussed in more detail later in the chapter). See the box below for further information about usual, customary, and reasonable charges.

Usual, Customary and Reasonable (UCR) Fees

Usual fee	The amount that a doctor usually charges or charges most often; that is, the amount the doctor most frequently charges to the majority of patients
Customary fee	The fee charged by doctors in the same specialty in the same geographic area (usually the 90th percentile amount of the charges of all doctors in the area)
Reasonable fee	The fee that meets the two criteria described above or is justifiable if there are special circumstances

Based on statistics kept by the insurance company, the fee actually charged by the doctor is reviewed. The insurance company's payment is based on its own determination of what is usual, customary, and reasonable.

---

3. A third method of establishing allowable charges is to use the resource-based relative value scale, the fee schedule developed for Medicare in 1992, on which Medicare bases its payments to doctors and other health care providers. This will be discussed in greater detail later in the chapter in the discussion of Medicare.

Health Maintenance Organizations

Health maintenance organizations (HMOs) were introduced around the time of World War II, when the Kaiser plan was formed. Today, HMOs are the dominant form of medical insurance in America, covering more than 75 percent of all Americans who have private health insurance. There are HMOs for Medicare and TRICARE. An individual insured by an HMO is considered a **subscriber** rather than a policy holder.

Under the HMO concept, all medical care is provided for one year for a fixed premium, with no deductibles or coinsurance. Usually, the HMO requires a small copayment for each visit or prescription. HMOs have always practiced preventive medicine, on the theory that much of the cost of medical care can be eliminated through routine care by primary care providers. Also to reduce the cost of specialty care, **primary care physicians** (PCPs) and other primary care providers such as nurse practitioners and physician assistants in HMOs act as "gatekeepers," seeing patients first for nearly all illnesses and referring them to specialists only when necessary.

An HMO can be organized in one of four ways:

Staff Model HMO. The health plan hires the doctors directly and pays them a salary for providing health care to members. This type of plan was more common when HMO first began, and is rare today.

Group Practice Model HMO. The doctors form an independent group and contract with the health plan for medical treatment for plan members. The doctors are employees of the group practice, which is organized as a corporation; they are not employees of the HMO. This gives the doctors more autonomy than the staff model.

Network Model HMO. The health plan contracts with two or more group practices to provide health services. This is a type of expanded group practice model.

Independent Practice Association (IPA). The doctors work independently in the community, but formally organize a physician association. They are paid from funds collected from subscribers of the health plan minus administrative costs, marketing and sales costs, and other overhead costs.

IPAs often have a "hold back"—a portion of the agreed fee that is not paid to the doctors until after the end of the association's fiscal year, when the HMO determines if it has earned a profit or had financial losses. This way, the HMO requires member doctors to share some business risk.

Other HMOs ask primary care providers to share even more of the risk through a system known as **capitation.** Capitation (meaning literally "per head," or per person) can work in one of two ways.

Under some capitation plans, the primary care provider can be paid an annual fee for providing all routine care, with payments for other services being paid for directly by the HMO. In these plans, the primary care provider shares risk because he or she may have to provide more services to a patient than are being paid for. Suppose, for instance, the primary care practice or clinic is paid $900 per adult male to provide all primary-care services, including lab work. This may be fine to cover care for a healthy 40-year-old, but may be less than what it really costs the practice to treat a 55-year-old diabetic. The medical practice is caught in the middle; it has no power to set rates as an insurance company or HMO does, and it has no power to limit patients to healthy, and therefore profitable, individuals.

Under a more all-encompassing form of capitation, the HMO contracts with a primary care provider to manage all of the medical services for a patient, and pays the provider the subscriber's premium minus administration, marketing, and other costs. The primary care provider then subcontracts with any specialists, laboratories, hospitals, and other providers to provide other services to the patient. Under such a plan, if a few of the practice's patients were to need very expensive medical services, the practice could actually lose money.

Needless to say, doctors have rebelled against total capitation, and few HMOs use that methodology today. However, HMOs retain some ability to keep a lid on costs. They do this primarily in three ways: precertification of hospitalizations and emergency room visits, referrals from primary care doctors to specialists, and the ability to audit the medical records of any patient and provider.

Under precertification, the patient's primary care doctor, or another doctor covering the patient's doctor outside of normal office hours, has to approve any hospital admission or visit to the emergency room. This keeps patients from using the emergency room unnecessarily when they could be treated in the doctor's office.

Referrals keep patients from visiting specialists without having first been seen by, or at least speaking with, the primary care doctor.

Medical record audits allow the HMO to check the records of any doctor's patients to make sure the doctor is not performing unnecessary procedures or ordering unnecessary tests.

Each HMO works in its own way, and each one has a procedure book for providers. The medical assistant should familiarize him- or herself with the various requirements of each particular HMO, including such things as whether a referral to a specialist must be in writing or can be given over the telephone. Each precertification and some referrals must be authorized by the HMO, and the authorization number should be noted on all of the certification or referral paperwork.

The medical assistant must also know which laboratory can do lab work and where patients can be referred for diagnostic follow-up. Most HMOs have contracts with a limited number of laboratories and/or medical facilities, and will pay only for services provided by an approved facility.

Other Managed Care Plans

Other types of managed care plans combine features of the HMO with features of traditional plans. These organizations do not have HMO licenses and are subject to the laws that regulate insurance companies rather than those that regulate HMOs.

Exclusive Provider Organization (EPO). In this type of plan, the organization pays providers on a fee-for-service basis and maintains contracts with a network of providers. EPOs resemble HMOs in that members are restricted to the plan's network (except in certain cases, when they are traveling or for serious emergencies). EPOs function in a similar way to network HMOs.

Preferred Provider Organization (PPO). This type of plan maintains a similar philosophy to an HMO, but does not limit its subscribers to a certain network of providers; instead, patients are free to choose any provider or hospital. The amount of coverage is lower, however, when the patient seeks service outside the network of designated preferred providers. These plans often include deductibles, copayments, and coinsurance.

The PPO may pay 80–100 percent (after copayment) for services received from a preferred provider; the insurance payment may drop to 60–80 percent for out-of-network services. The amount of the bill the patient is responsible for often cannot be determined until after the insurance payment has been made.

Point-of-Service (POS) Plan. This type of plan is either a hybrid of an HMO and PPO or of an HMO-like network and a PPO. If members stay within the primary network, their costs are usually limited to a copayment. But if they choose medical services in the secondary network, they are required to assume a greater share of the financial responsibility for payment through higher copayments and deductibles. Members may have more choices than with an HMO, but less expense than with a PPO.

Medicare

Medicare is a federally funded plan administered by the Health Care Finance Administration (HCFA).* It pays for health care services for retired individuals over 65 who are on Social Security, retired railroad employees, and some retired federal employees; individuals who have been permanently disabled for two years; blind individuals; individuals with chronic renal disease who require dialysis or kidney transplant; and kidney donors.

The Medicare plan has two parts. Medicare Part A provides coverage of hospitalization services. Medicare Part B covers physician and other provider services. Each individual's Medicare enrollment card, shown in Figure 38–2, states whether the enrollee is covered by Part A alone or by Part A and Part B.

Individuals 65 and older on Social Security, those younger than 65 but who collect Social Security disability benefits, and those who receive railroad retirement benefits are automatically enrolled in Medicare Part A. There is no premium for participation in Medicare Part A. The first day of each hospital admission is not paid by Medicare; this is the Part A deductible. Medicare Part A is funded through a tax paid by working individuals on all of their earned income.

Anyone eligible for Medicare Part A may also obtain Part B coverage. However, they must apply and pay a premium for Part B. Former federal employees, who receive federal employee pensions rather than Social Security and are not covered by Medicare Part A, can purchase Medicare Part B coverage.

Medicare claims are handled by insurance companies that contract with HCFA. A different **fiscal intermediary** (insurance company that contracts to review and pay claims for HCFA) processes claims in each state for Medicare Part A and Medicare Part B. The amount of payment for any service is standardized nationally.

Payment to hospitals for claims under Part A are based on **diagnostic related groups** (**DRGs**), a system that classifies patients according to the diagnosis, treatment, and length of hospital stay. The patient is assigned a DRG based on the primary diagnosis, and the payment made by Medicare to a hospital is determined by the DRG rather than the length of time the patient remains in the hospital.

Since 1992, payments for services under Part B have been based on a **resource-based relative value scale** (**RBRVS**) developed by researchers at Harvard University. This system establishes relative value units for each procedure, based on the amount of work involved, overhead expenses, and cost of malpractice insurance. The amount Medicare pays for each relative value unit is then adjusted annually; it is also adjusted for different geographic areas (because overhead and malpractice cost may vary). The Medicare local carrier sends each doctor an annual fee schedule for the geographic area, identifying the amount Medicare pays for specific procedures.

If a doctor participates in the Medicare program, the office must bill for the patient, accept assignment of benefits, and accept Medicare's determination of the allowable charge for the service. Under Part B, after paying an annual deductible for $100, the patient is responsible for 20 percent of the allowable charge.

If a doctor does not participate in the Medicare program, usually he or she does not accept assignment of benefits, but collects the bill from the patient up to a limiting charge (percent limit on fees above the fee-schedule amount) set by legislation.

Many patients purchase additional insurance (known as Medigap insurance) that covers the annual deductible and 20 percent coinsurance for Part B, as well as the charge for the first day of a hospital stay (the deductible for Part A). They may also be covered by employment plans after retirement. In this case, Medicare is the primary insurance, and the Medigap or employment retiree plan is secondary. If a person continues to work after 65 and obtains insurance through employment, that insurance is the primary insurance for that individual, and Medicare is the secondary insurance.

---

*Effective 6/01, this agency has been renamed the Centers for Medicare and Medicaid Services (CMMS).

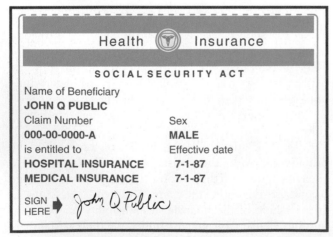

> Figure 38–2 Medicare identification card (From Kinn ME, Woods M: The Medical Assistant: Administrative and Clinical, 8th ed. Philadelphia, W.B. Saunders, 1999.)

Medicaid

Medicaid, formally Title XIX (Title 19) of the 1965 amendments to the Social Security laws, provides for the federal government to give each state a grant to be used toward care of the medically indigent—either the poor or those whose medical costs would force them into poverty. Along with the federal government's basic funding comes an obligation for the states to provide basic health care; states may add coverage for other care to their Medicaid laws, but must pay for most of those costs, with the federal government paying a portion. The name of the Medicaid program, as well as procedures for gaining access to the program, varies from state to state.

Doctors may agree or decline to provide services to Medicaid patients. If they agree to treat Medicaid patients, doctors must agree to accept the state's payment for services, without billing patients for the difference between the state's payment and the actual charge.

Adults and children receiving basic welfare grants from a state are automatically eligible for Medicaid. Also, the children in many working households are eligible for Medicaid benefits if the parents' pay is low enough to put the family below the poverty line and employee-provided medical insurance, if there is any, covers only the employed parent.

In addition to paying for medical services, Medicaid also covers the cost of long-term nursing home care for poor elderly and disabled individuals, which can be $50,000 or more per year. Because of these costs, 80 percent of Medicaid beneficiaries in many states—children and poor adults—account for 20–30 percent of all Medicaid costs, while 20 percent of Medicaid beneficiaries—the elderly poor living in nursing homes—account for 70–80 percent of the cost of the Medicaid program.

Beginning in the mid-1990s, some states tried to move Medicaid patients into a system of managed care, even going so far as to put them under capitation. Often, children were the first beneficiaries moved into managed care. HMOs bid for the right to cover Medicaid managed care beneficiaries. States often chose their Medicaid managed-care providers on the basis of which company asked for the lowest payment.

Reimbursements were set so low that many doctors refused to participate in these companies' plans because they would have had to accept Medicaid patients and reimbursement that was lower than the actual cost of providing the care. States and managed care companies were forced to increase their reimbursements to keep medical practices in poor communities that treat the bulk of Medicaid patients from going bankrupt. By the year 2000, many of these managed care companies had dropped their Medicaid managed care contracts after losing millions of dollars.

If a patient has both Medicare and Medicaid insurance, Medicare is the primary insurance. After processing, it will automatically be sent to Medicaid. For this reason, it may be called a **crossover claim**—a claim that automatically crosses over from Medicare to Medicaid.

Children's Health Insurance Plans (CHIPs)

In 1998, the federal government provided funding for states to establish children's health insurance plans (CHIPs) to further assist children living in "working poor" families. CHIPs provide health insurance to children in families whose household income is up to 200 percent of the income level at which the family would normally be eligible for Medicaid.

Workers' Compensation

Workers' compensation insurance covers lost wages and the cost of medical treatment for workers injured on the job or who fall ill due to workplace hazards or disease. Each state has its own workers' compensation programs, and the cost of workers' compensation insurance is paid by employers. The premium for a given employer depends on how many previous employees have made claims under workers' compensation.

Workers are required to make a prompt claim for workers' compensation coverage after an accident or the onset of an illness. In many states, the employer and the insurance company issuing the policy have the right to choose the doctor who treats the patient.

If a patient visits his or her regular primary care doctor and says the illness or injury is workplace-related, the medical assistant should check promptly with the employer to verify that the employee has made a report and that the care will be covered by the company's workers' compensation plan.

If a patient of the medical practice is seen for a workers' compensation case, separate medical and financial records should be established for that patient. Laws require that requests for medical records for compensation cases must contain only information associated with the work-related injury. If work-related injury records are needed by a workers' appeal board, it is very important that no other medical information about the patient be released.

For a workers' compensation case, the doctor must file a Doctor's First Report of Injury; in most states this must be done within 72 hours of the patient's initial visit for a workplace injury. Four copies are prepared: one for the employer's compensation insurance carrier, one for the employer, one for the state compensation board, and one for the patient's medical record.

In addition to the report, the doctor submits a statement of services to the insurance carrier. The doctor must sign all forms, because for workers' compensation cases a stamped signature is not accepted. As in most government programs, the doctor must accept the payment provided as payment in full. The doctor submits a report and a statement monthly until care is completed.

TRICARE/CHAMPVA

The Civilian Health and Medical Program of the Uniformed Services (CHAMPUS) was established by the federal government in 1966 to provide health benefits for the dependent spouses and children of active military personnel when receiving care from civilian doctors and health facilities. The name has been changed to TRICARE with the addition of managed care services, because there are three plans available to members of the armed services: TRICARE Standard (formerly CHAMPUS), TRICARE Prime, and TRICARE Extra.

TRICARE Standard benefits are available to dependent spouses and children of active-duty military personnel, dependent spouses and children of military personnel who died while on active duty, and military retirees (and their dependents) who are not old enough to be eligible for Medicare.

TRICARE Prime is an HMO-type plan with optional participation. In addition to the services covered by TRICARE Standard, it includes preventive and primary care services. There is an annual enrollment fee for families whose member of the armed forces is not on active duty. Some doctors are contracted to provide service to TRICARE beneficiaries at discounted rates to TRICARE Prime members.

TRICARE Extra allows an individual to seek care from a network provider on a visit-by-visit basis, receiving a discount on medical services provided and a lower copayment than when using TRICARE Standard.

In 1973, the federal government created CHAMPVA to provide both inpatient and outpatient medical benefits for the dependent spouses and children of veterans who have suffered total, permanent, service-connected disabilities, and for surviving spouses and children of veterans who have died as a result of those service-connected disabilities. The nearest Veterans Administration Medical Center determines eligibility and issues an identification card; but the CHAMPVA-covered patients are allowed to choose their own doctors and other medical service providers.

THE INSURANCE FORM

Since the 1950s, the Health Insurance Association of America has sought to have all medical insurance claims filed on a common form. Although no universally accepted form has yet been created, most insurance companies will accept the HCFA-1500 form, either alone or as an attachment to the company's own form.

Whether the HCFA-1500 or an insurance company's own form, all health insurance forms have four sections:

1. The patient section
2. The subscriber section
3. The carrier section
4. The provider section.

The Patient Section

The patient section contains the patient's basic demographic information. This includes the patient's name, address, date of birth, and sex as well as the patient's signature allowing the doctor's office to release medical information to the insurance company for purposes of verifying the services provided (known as **authorization**).

It also identifies whether the doctor accepts assignment of benefits, which is authorized by the patient's signature. The abbreviation **SOF** which stands for **signature on file**, is often used to indicate that the office maintains a copy of the patient's signature. The patient, subscriber, and carrier portion of the HCFA-1500 form are shown in Figure 38–3.

The Subscriber Section

The subscriber section has information pertaining to the individual who is the beneficiary or subscriber of the insurance policy. For a private policy, this is usually the head of the household; for an employer-sponsored policy, this is the employee.

This section includes the following information about the subscriber (sometimes called the **insured**, or the guarantor): the subscriber's name, address, and relationship to the patient. In addition, for employer-sponsored plans, the employer's name is listed. For all plans, the name of the insurance carrier and the identification numbers of both the policy and the patient must be listed. For a family, there is a basic identification number, often the policy holder's Social Security number, followed by a one- or two-digit number. The subscriber usually gets 1 or 01, the spouse 2 or 02, and children get succeeding numbers.

The Carrier Section

The **carrier** section includes the name of the insurance company. It also identifies whether the insurance company is the primary or secondary provider for the particular claim, and whether the claim is for other than general reasons (e.g., auto accident, workers' compensation, or disability).

When the patient is covered by more than one insurance plan, you will need to fill out a claim for each insurance company, and state whether that company is the primary or secondary insurer.

The Provider Section

The provider section is where the information about the medical service provided is noted. In addition to information about the medical problem, the ICD-9-CM code for each diagnosis (up to four) is listed. On the lower lines, information about each procedure is given,

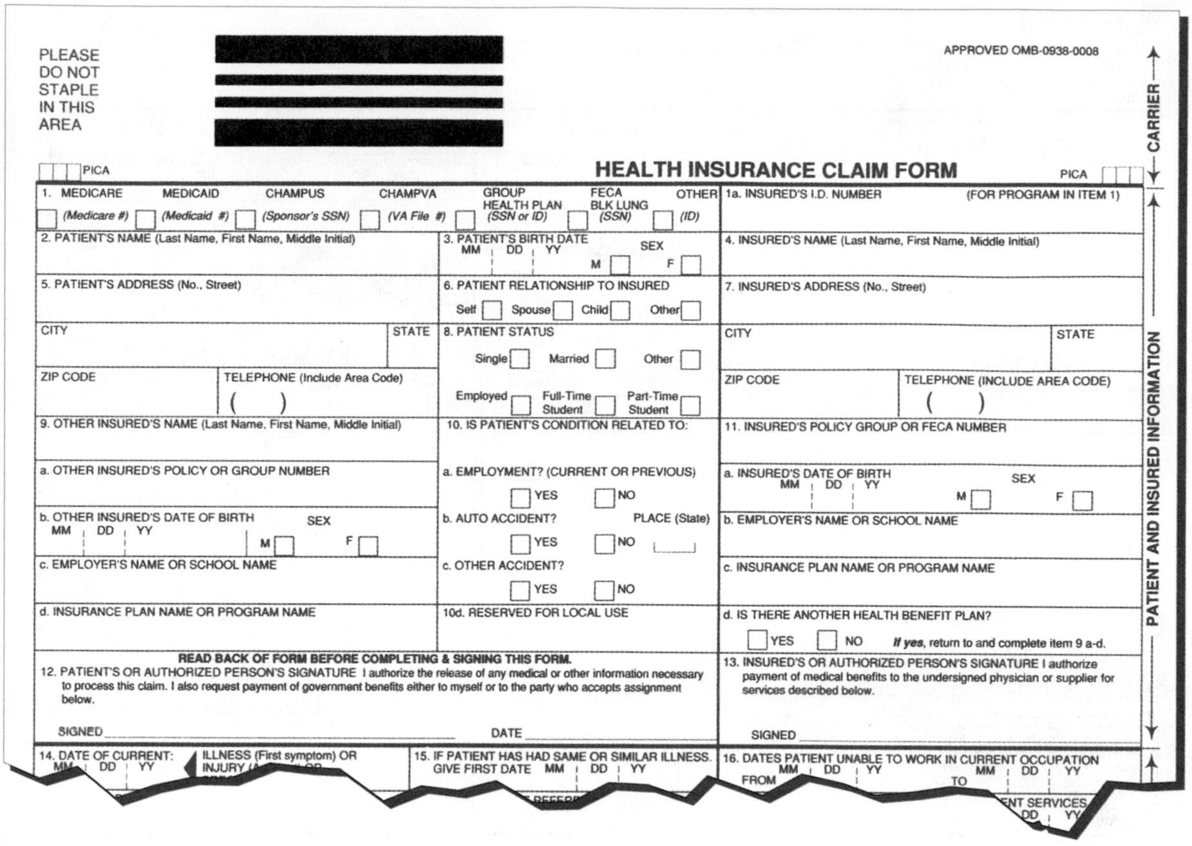
PLEASE DO NOT STAPLE IN THIS AREA

APPROVED OMB-0938-0008

CARRIER

PICA **HEALTH INSURANCE CLAIM FORM** PICA

1. MEDICARE (Medicare #) MEDICAID (Medicaid #) CHAMPUS (Sponsor's SSN) CHAMPVA (VA File #) GROUP HEALTH PLAN (SSN or ID) FECA BLK LUNG (SSN) OTHER (ID)

1a. INSURED'S I.D. NUMBER (FOR PROGRAM IN ITEM 1)

2. PATIENT'S NAME (Last Name, First Name, Middle Initial)

3. PATIENT'S BIRTH DATE MM DD YY SEX M F

4. INSURED'S NAME (Last Name, First Name, Middle Initial)

5. PATIENT'S ADDRESS (No., Street)

6. PATIENT RELATIONSHIP TO INSURED Self Spouse Child Other

7. INSURED'S ADDRESS (No., Street)

CITY STATE

8. PATIENT STATUS Single Married Other

CITY STATE

ZIP CODE TELEPHONE (Include Area Code) ( )

Employed Full-Time Student Part-Time Student

ZIP CODE TELEPHONE (INCLUDE AREA CODE) ( )

9. OTHER INSURED'S NAME (Last Name, First Name, Middle Initial)

10. IS PATIENT'S CONDITION RELATED TO:

11. INSURED'S POLICY GROUP OR FECA NUMBER

a. OTHER INSURED'S POLICY OR GROUP NUMBER

a. EMPLOYMENT? (CURRENT OR PREVIOUS) YES NO

a. INSURED'S DATE OF BIRTH MM DD YY SEX M F

b. OTHER INSURED'S DATE OF BIRTH MM DD YY SEX M F

b. AUTO ACCIDENT? PLACE (State) YES NO

b. EMPLOYER'S NAME OR SCHOOL NAME

c. EMPLOYER'S NAME OR SCHOOL NAME

c. OTHER ACCIDENT? YES NO

c. INSURANCE PLAN NAME OR PROGRAM NAME

d. INSURANCE PLAN NAME OR PROGRAM NAME

10d. RESERVED FOR LOCAL USE

d. IS THERE ANOTHER HEALTH BENEFIT PLAN? YES NO *If yes, return to and complete item 9 a-d.*

READ BACK OF FORM BEFORE COMPLETING & SIGNING THIS FORM.

12. PATIENT'S OR AUTHORIZED PERSON'S SIGNATURE I authorize the release of any medical or other information necessary to process this claim. I also request payment of government benefits either to myself or to the party who accepts assignment below.

SIGNED DATE

13. INSURED'S OR AUTHORIZED PERSON'S SIGNATURE I authorize payment of medical benefits to the undersigned physician or supplier for services described below.

SIGNED

PATIENT AND INSURED INFORMATION

14. DATE OF CURRENT: MM DD YY ILLNESS (First symptom) OR INJURY

15. IF PATIENT HAS HAD SAME OR SIMILAR ILLNESS. GIVE FIRST DATE MM DD YY

16. DATES PATIENT UNABLE TO WORK IN CURRENT OCCUPATION MM DD YY FROM TO MM DD YY

➢ **Figure 38–3** The top half of the HCFA-1500 health insurance claim form contains the patient section, the subscriber information, and insurance carrier information.

including the date of service, place of service, procedure code, charge for the service, and number of units being billed.

Each procedure must be linked to a primary diagnosis code to justify the procedure. The number (one to four) of the line that identifies the primary diagnosis for each procedure is entered in box 21 of the form. See the box below for a list of codes commonly used for place of service when billing from the medical office. Figure 38–4 illustrates the provider section of the HCFA-1500 form.

Common Types of Forms

As mentioned earlier, the most commonly used insurance form is the HCFA-1500. This form began life as the Health Insurance Claim Form, which was approved for use by the American Medical Association (AMA) in 1975. It was gradually accepted by various insurance plans for payment of claims by those plans. Because of its acceptance by HCFA, the form has been dubbed the HCFA-1500. In 1990 this form was revised and printed in red. It became the required form for Medicare claims in 1992.

Another commonly used form is the UB92, also known as the HCFA-1450. This form is used by hospitals and other institutions to submit insurance claims. It is a summary document, supported by a detailed bill.

Some medical insurers do not accept the HCFA-1500, insisting rather that the claim be made on a form used only by the company. Other companies will accept the HCFA-1500, but ask that it be attached to the company's form, with the patient and subscriber portions of the company form being filled out.

Place of Service Codes Commonly Used for Billing in the Medical Office

11	Office
12	Home
21	Inpatient hospitalization
22	Outpatient hospitalization
23	Emergency room—hospital
24	Ambulatory surgical center
25	Birthing center
36	Military hospital or clinic
31	Skilled nursing facility
32	Nursing facility
33	Custodial care facility

➤ Figure 38–4 The bottom half of the HCFA-1500 health insurance claim form contains information about the health care provider and the care provided.

Optical Scanning

The HCFA-1500 form is printed in red to facilitate optical scanning when paper forms are submitted. The bar code in the upper left-hand corner is read by the electronic scanner as the beginning of a new claim. If paper claims are submitted, insurance companies prefer those prepared by word processor or computer to be printed forms purchased from a medical supply company or a company that provides medical billing computer programs.

For the optical character reader to scan the claim, it is recommended to use all capital letters and no punctuation, to be sure that all information is within the required box, and to proofread for typographical errors that might cause the claim to be rejected. A space is used in many locations instead of a hyphen:

between the five-digit zip code and the additional +4 numbers

after the area code and the first three numbers of a telephone number

after the first two numbers of the federal tax identification number

within numbers identifying policy and group number of the insured.

Procedure 38–1 discusses how to fill out an insurance claim form properly.

Submission of Insurance Forms

Forms can be submitted in two ways, either by mail or electronically.

If the office submits claims by mail, the frequency of submission depends on the size of the office, the number of personnel devoted to processing claims, and the number of patients the office sees who are covered by any particular insurance plan. Submission is usually done daily or weekly.

Electronic submission speeds things up enormously. Submission is instantaneous, instead of taking a few days to move through the mail. The office may submit insurance claims directly to the insurance company, or submit them to a clearinghouse that processes the data and submits it to the appropriate carrier. The procedure for submission depends on the computer software

PROCEDURE 38-1

Completing the HCFA-1500 Form for Insurance Reimbursement

Performance Objective: The student will be able to complete an HCFA-1500 form for insurance reimbursement.

Supplies and Equipment: Patient information; patient account or ledger card; copy of the patient's insurance card; insurance claim form; typewriter, word processor, or computer and printer.

Procedure Steps

1. Assemble information needed to prepare an insurance claim, including a claim form, information about the patient, the patient account or ledger card, a copy of the patient's insurance card or insurance information.

2. Enter information as required on the HCFA-1500 form using capital letters and no punctuation.
   Rationale: Most insurance companies use optical scanning to digitize information on paper claims, and the equipment works best following the guidelines outlined above.

3. Enter the name and address of the insurance company to whom the claim will be sent on the top of the form above the words "Health Insurance Claim Form."

4. Complete the patient portion of the insurance form from information on the new patient registration form or from the patient's computer information form.

   Box 2—The patient's last name, first name, middle initial.

   Box 3—The patient's date of birth in the format MM DD YYYY and the patient's sex (M or F).

   Box 5—The patient's address using the two-letter state code and the nine-digit zip code with a space between the fifth and sixth digits; the telephone number with a space between the area code and number and another after the first three digits of the number (instead of a hyphen).

   Box 6—Put an X in the box that defines the patient's relationship to the insured (i.e., person whose name is on the insurance policy). The choices include
   self ☐   spouse ☐   child ☐   other ☐.

   Box 8—Check the boxes that best describe the patient's marital status and employment status. If the patient has insurance through the employer, assume that he or she is employed. If the patient is a college student (over 18), it is important to determine if he or she is a full-time student. The choices include
   single ☐   married ☐   other ☐
   employed ☐   full-time student ☐
   part-time student ☐

   Box 10—Identifies information related to the cause of the patient's condition(s). Check the correct box (Yes or No) to answer the questions. If the patient's condition is caused by an automobile accident, identify the state where the accident occurred using the correct two-letter code.

   Box 12—If the office has on file the patient's signature on a similar permission form, place the initials SOF (signature on file) in this box. Otherwise, the patient must sign the form.

   Box 13—If the doctor accepts assignment of benefits and the office has on file the patient's signature on a similar permission form, place the initials SOF (signature on file) in this box (or have the patient sign the form). If the physician does not accept assignment of benefits, leave the box blank.

5. Complete the subscriber (insured) portion of the claim form from information found on the copy of the patient's insurance card and/or the new patient information sheet.
   Rationale: If incomplete or incorrect information about primary and secondary insurance plans is given, the claim will be denied.

   Box 1—Place an X in the type of insurance being billed. If the patient is covered by insurance obtained from employment, check Group Health Plan.

   Box 1a—Enter the identification number of the insured person, often the Social Security number which may have additional letters or additional digits to identify a spouse or child of the insured.

Procedure continued on following page.

Box 4—Enter the name of the insured person. If the patient is the insured person, enter SAME.

Box 7—Enter the address of the insured person. If you entered SAME in Box 4, leave Box 7 blank. If you entered the name of a person other than the patient in Box 4 who lives at the same address as the patient, enter SAME in Box 7.

Box 9—If the patient is covered by a second insurance policy, enter the name of the insured, policy or group number (9a), insured's date of birth (MM DD YYYY) and sex (9b), employer's name (9c), and insurance plan or program name (9d). If the insured is not covered by secondary insurance, leave this box blank.

Box 11—Enter information about the primary insurance, including the insured's group or FECA number (of patient in federal Black Lung program), insured's date of birth (MM DD YYYY) and sex (11a), employer's name (11b) and insurance plan or program name (11c), and if there is another health benefit plan (11d). Many patients do not have a group insurance number. Box 11c may be left blank if the name of the insurance plan is given at the top of the form.

6. Complete the physician or supplier information on the bottom half of the form.

Boxes 14–16—Not usually required for Medicare, Medicaid, TRICARE, CHAMPVA, and most private insurance. If they must be filled in, use dates obtained from the patient's medical record and/or the doctor.

Box 17—Enter the name of the doctor who referred the patient.

Box 17a—Enter the ID number of the referring doctor. For Medicare, use the NPI or UPIN number.

Box 18—If the patient's claim is for a hospitalization, either a visit or surgery performed when the patient was hospitalized, enter the dates of hospitalization. Otherwise, leave the box blank.

Box 19—Leave blank unless instructed by a specific insurance carrier to use this box for information specific to that carrier.

Box 20—Check No unless billing Medicare for outside lab charges, when you should check Yes and enter the amount of the charges.

Box 21—Enter the ICD-9-CM code for up to four diagnoses.

Box 22—Leave blank unless the claim is a Medicaid resubmission, when the code and original reference number should be entered.

Box 23—Leave blank unless you were given a preauthorization or precertification number by the insurance company.

Box 24A—Enter the date service began under the From section in the format MM DD YYYY. If the service occurred on one day only, leave the To section blank; otherwise, enter the date service ended.

Box 24B—Enter the code for the place of service. The code for the medical office is 11.

Box 24C—For medical service leave this box blank. For other types of service (e.g., anesthesia), enter the correct numeric code.

Box 24D—Enter the procedure code and modifier (if any).

Box 24E—Enter the number (from 1 to 4) that identifies which diagnosis code justifies the procedure.

Box 24F—Enter the charges, leaving a space between the number of dollars and the number of cents instead of using a decimal point.

Box 24G—If charging for more than one of the same procedure (for example, visits to a hospitalized patient on three consecutive days), enter the number of units of the procedure charged. Otherwise, enter 1.

Box 24H—Leave blank unless the patient is enrolled in the Medicaid program for early, periodic, screening, diagnosis, and service (EPSDT).

Box 24I—Leave blank unless service took place in a hospital emergency room, when an X should be placed in the box.

Box 24J—Leave blank unless there is coordination of benefits. If an individual doctor in a group practice has performed the service, place the first two digits of the doctor's NPI number in this box.

Box 24K—This box may be used for the last seven digits of a doctor's NPI number as described above.

7. Enter information in Box 24 on lines 1–6 for each procedure that is being billed to the insurance company. For more than six procedures, complete an additional HCFA-1500 form.

8. Complete the remaining boxes on the HCFA-1500 form.

> Box 25—Enter the tax identification number. Indicate by checking the correct box if this is the Social Security number of an individual doctor (check box SSN) or the employer identification number of a group practice (check box EIN).
>
> Box 26—Enter the patient account number; leave blank if there is no patient account number.
>
> Box 27—Check Yes if the doctor accepts assignment of benefits or No if assignment of benefits is not accepted.
>
> Box 28—Enter the total charges with a space between the number of dollars and the number of cents.
>
> Box 29—Enter the amount paid toward the current charges, including any co-payment. If the amount is zero, leave the box blank.
>
> Box 30—Enter the balance due with a space between the number of dollars and the number of cents.

> Box 31—Either have the doctor sign the form or use a stamp with the doctor's signature. Enter the date.
>
> Box 32—Enter the name and address of the facility where the services were provided. If services were provided at the same address as the billing address, enter SAME.
>
> Box 33—Enter the name, address, and telephone number of the physician group or supplier of services. Do not use punctuation. Leave a space between the city and two-letter state code and within the nine-digit zip code after the fifth digit. Leave spaces between the area code and digits three and four of the telephone number. Enter the NPI number for a group practice after GRP# or the PIN number for an individual physician after PIN#.

9. Copy and proofread the form before mailing. Keep the copy in an insurance claims file.

used by the office or the clearinghouse. There is no chance that insurance company personnel will make errors inputting the information into the company's computer system, since the transmission is computer-to-computer.

Faster delivery, and faster and more accurate processing, means faster reimbursement. If electronic claim submission is coupled with electronic payment from the company to the practice's operating account, the entire turnaround time from submission to money in the bank can be days instead of weeks.

Regardless of how claims are submitted, an insurance claims log, as shown in Figure 38–5, needs to be kept, either manually or by computer.

INSURANCE CLAIM REGISTER

BLACKBURN PRIMARY CARE ASSOCIATES, PC
1990 Turquoise Drive
Blackburn, WI 54937
608-459-8857

Claim number	Service	Insurance and ID and group no.	Date and amount of claim	Date and amount paid	Difference	Follow-up action

➤ **Figure 38–5** Insurance claims log.

REIMBURSEMENT

Reimbursement is the payment received by the medical practice from the insurance company for the services performed.

Types of Reimbursement

There are two basic types of reimbursement: capitation and fee-for-service.

Under capitation, the primary care doctor receives a monthly, quarterly, semi-annual, or annual payment from the managed care company. This payment may just cover primary care services or may be larger if the primary care doctor must also pay for specialists and/or diagnostic services. The reimbursement for each patient is the same, regardless of the amount of care the patient receives.

As discussed earlier, capitation moves some of the risk away from the managed care company and onto the primary care doctor who treats the patient. If the capitation is for primary care services only, the doctor's risk is reduced. In most circumstances, there will be enough healthy patients who cost the doctor less to treat than the amount being paid by the company to make up for the few sick patients who cost more to treat.

If the doctor has to manage and pay for all specialists as well as hospital, laboratory, and other treatments and procedures, he or she carries essentially all the risk. The managed care company essentially acts as a broker, acquiring patients, collecting premiums, and keeping a portion of the premium for marketing and sales costs and profit.

Under fee-for-service reimbursement, the doctor is reimbursed for each treatment or procedure performed. In this case, the only difference between traditional fee-for-service insurance and managed care is that managed care companies usually negotiate to pay lower fees for procedures than traditional indemnity plans pay.

All specialists are paid essentially on a fee-for-service basis; the only issue is whether the fee is being paid for by an insurance company or by a primary care doctor out of the money received under capitation.

Using a Claims Register

Every insurance claim filed should be logged into the insurance claims register. An insurance claims register can be kept either manually or on the computer.

The claims register includes the claim number (the number you have given the claim as part of the office's tracking system); the patient's name and insurance group or policy number; the insurance company's name; the date and amount of the claim; a column for any follow-up actions taken (by mail or telephone); the date and amount of the paid claim; and any difference between the amount submitted and the amount paid.

Explanation of Benefits Forms

After payment has been made by the insurance company to the doctor, or if a claim is being denied, both the doctor and the patient receive an **explanation of benefits** (EOB) form. Although each provider has its own form, the type of information contained on any

BLACKBURN PRIMARY CARE ASSOCIATES, PC
1990 Turquoise Drive
Blackburn, WI 54937
608-459-8857

Patient name and ID no.	Date of service	CPT/ HCPCS codes	Total submitted	Excluded or denied	Copay	Amount paid by carrier	Reasons for denial	Subscriber responsibility

➤ Figure 38–6 Typical information that would be contained on an EOB (explanation of benefits) form.

STANDARD HEALTH CARE EOB
1500 SUMMIT AVENUE
WESTERN XY 45000

Blackburn Primary Care Associates, PC
1990 Turquoise Drive
Blackburn, WI 54937

Practice ID # 01-1234567

Date Prepared: 8/15/XX

Patient's Name	Dates of Service	POS	Proc	Qty	Charge Amount	Eligible Amount	Patient Liability	Amt. Paid Provider
St. Cyr, June	7/22/XX–7/22/XX	11	99212	1	$48.00	$43.00	$10.00	$33.00
St. Cyr, June	7/22/XX–7/22/XX	11	90703	1	$15.00	$10.00	00	$10.00
St. Cyr, Mary Ann	7/14/XX–7/14/XX	11	99212	1	$48.00	$48.00	$10.00	$38.00
St. Cyr, Mary Ann	7/14/XX–7/14/XX	11	94010	1	$50.00	$50.00	00	$50.00

******************************** Check #288 is attached in the amount of $131.00 ********************************

> **Figure 38–7** A sample EOB (explanation of benefits).

EOB is largely the same, as shown in Figure 38–6. If the insurance company is denying the claim, the doctor may also receive a remittance advice form, showing why the claim was disallowed. See Figure 38–7 for a sample explanation of benefits.

Claims are usually denied for one of the following reasons: wrong patient; wrong subscriber; wrong insurance company; wrong patient or doctor identification number; confusing the primary with secondary insurance; incomplete diagnosis; inaccurate procedures and/or diagnosis codes; the procedures and diagnosis do not justify each other; or no preauthorization was received from the managed care company to perform the procedures. See the box on this page for a list of common errors in submitting insurance claims.

Follow-up and Resubmission of Claims

If a claim is denied, it should be resubmitted immediately, following any advice given by the company on the remittance advice form. Any questions about a denial should be discussed with a provider relations representative at the company.

If claims are not being paid or denied in a timely fashion, follow-up is in order. Follow-up can be made via letter or over the telephone. Instead of following up individual claims, use the claims log to find all claims to any company that are becoming delinquent and include them in the follow-up call or letter.

Common Errors on Insurance Claim Forms

- Reversing the name of the patient with the subscriber (guarantor)
- Reversing the primary insurance with the secondary insurance
- Transposing numbers in one of the identification numbers
- Missing signatures or signature stamps
- Diagnosis inconsistent with patient gender
- Incorrect diagnosis code or not coded to the fourth or fifth digit (ICD-9-CM)
- Inaccurate procedure or service codes (CPT-4 or HCPCS)
- Missing modifier
- No preapproval or preauthorization
- Diagnosis does not justify procedures performed
- Total amount of billing does not agree with services provided
- No physician NPI or PIN number
- Required attachments missing (such as a pathology report)
- Incomplete boxes
- Place of service inconsistent with procedure code

ON THE JOB

Claire Johnson just retired. Her primary insurance is through her former employer and her secondary insurance is through her husband's employer. Claire visits Blackburn Primary Care Associates, and a small nodule is discovered on her breast. She has a mammogram, which shows a marble-sized nodule. Dr. Smithson performs a breast biopsy. The specimen is sent to the lab. It is found to be benign.

Her insurance claim for the breast biopsy is denied.

QUESTIONS

1. List all the reasons a claim might be denied for payment by an insurance carrier.
2. What can you do as a medical assistant to prevent these errors?
3. What can you do when a claim is denied?

STUDENT STUDY PLAN

To reinforce your understanding of the material in this chapter . . .

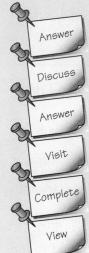

Complete the **Review & Recall** questions.

Discuss the situation in **If You Were the Medical Assistant** with your classmates and answer the questions.

Answer the **Critical Thinking Questions** and discuss them with your classmates.

Visit the **Web sites** suggested and search for additional Web sites using the **Keywords for Internet Searches.**

Complete the exercises in chapter 38 of the **Student Mastery Manual.**

View the **Insurance Videotape,** "The HCFA Files."

REVIEW & RECALL

1. Describe how health insurance evolved over the years.

2. How may a person acquire health insurance?

3. How do you decide which insurance is primary, and which secondary, for each member of a family of four in which both parents work and have insurance through their employer?

4. Describe the eight different types of insurance and what each provides.

5. What are some of the differences between HMOs and other types of managed care plans?

6. Who is eligible for Medicare? Medicaid? CHIP? TRI-CARE?

7. When is a person eligible for workers' compensation?

8. What are the major portions of the insurance claim form?

9. How are insurance forms submitted to an insurance company?

10. What is the purpose of a claims register?

11. What information is contained on an explanation of benefits?

IF YOU WERE THE MEDICAL ASSISTANT

You have processed the mail and the office has received several explanation of benefits (EOB) forms. How will you handle these forms? Where will you record the information? How do you follow up on denials of claims?

 CRITICAL THINKING QUESTIONS

1. Identify the fiscal intermediary for Medicare in your state. Contact the local Medicare office and arrange for a speaker to come to your class to discuss the different types of Medicare programs in your area, so that you can answer patient questions.

2. Arrange to tour a medical billing company that sends claim forms and receives EOBs electronically; discuss how this process is different from that in a doctor's office where such forms are handled manually.

3. Research the primary insurance carriers in your area and explore their similarities and differences.

4. Compare and contrast traditional indemnity insurance plans and managed care plans in relation to cost and services from the point of view of the insurance company, the doctor, and the patient.

 EXPLORE THE WEB

INTERNET WEB SITES

Health Care Financing Administration (HCFA) training site
www.medicaretraining.com

Health Information Management Supersite
www.himinfo.com

American Medical Association (AMA)
www.ama-assn.org

KEYWORDS FOR INTERNET SEARCHES

Blue Cross
HCFA
health insurance
Medicare
reimbursement

 ANSWERS TO ON THE JOB

1. The reasons a claim form can be denied are:
   a. wrong patient
   b. wrong IDs
   c. wrong primary and/or secondary insurance
   d. no preauthorization
   e. all required information not filled in

2. To prevent these errors, check with the patient at the time of the appointment that you have the most up-to-date information in your records. Check the insurance card and confirm all diagnoses and procedures with the medical record.

3. When a claim is denied, locate the reason, correct the error, and follow the carrier's instructions for resubmitting a claim.

Billing and Collections

Instructional Objectives

After completing this chapter, you will be able to do the following:

1. Define and spell the vocabulary words.
2. Describe the process of billing and collections.
3. Develop a collection system.
4. Identify past-due accounts and the actions needed.
5. Describe the information to include in a collection letter.
6. Identify legal requirements that affect collections for the medical office.

940

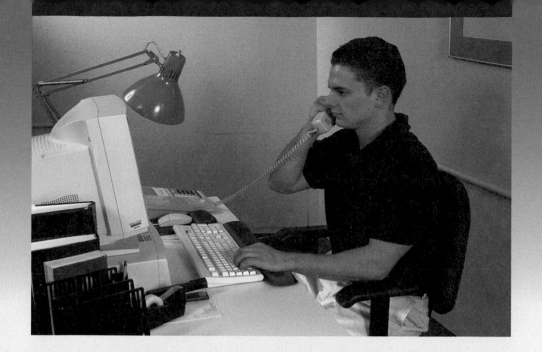

- Perform billing and collection procedures
- Perform within ethical and legal boundaries

- Post collection agency payments

Performance Objectives

After completing this chapter, you will be able to do the following:

1. Create and examine an accounts aging record to determine collection activity (Procedure 39–1).
2. Write a collection letter (Procedure 39–2).

An increasing amount of patient care is being funded through HMO-type insurance, where the patient makes a small copayment at the time of service and the doctor bills the managed care company for the balance. But there is still a need to maintain patient financial accounts and for collecting money owed by patients who have coinsurance, patients who are responsible for amounts not paid by insurance, or patients without insurance.

BILLING

Most doctors' offices request that payment be made at the time a medical service is provided in order to minimize billing. A large number of medical offices also accept payment by credit card, which makes payment at the time of service possible and convenient for many patients. However, a number of patients still need to make arrangements to pay for their medical services over a period of time. In this case, the office must establish an account for the patient and send periodic bills. These bills can be generated by photocopying the patient ledgers and sending those in an envelope, but it is more common for a computer software program to produce the bills.

Even if the patient is not being billed directly, a billing record should be kept for that patient, showing the amount billed to the insurance company.

Types of Billing

Bills can be sent to patients every two weeks, monthly, or at any regular period, such as once every three months (quarterly). The time between bills is called the billing cycle. A bill sent out at the end of a cycle will show the **balance due** (the amount of money owed) at the beginning of the cycle, any payments made during the billing cycle, any new charges for new services that occurred during the billing cycle, and the balance due at the end of the cycle.

Often, the patient accounts are divided into equal parts, usually alphabetically. Each week a different section of the patient accounts is billed. For instance, on the first week of the month, patients with a last name

beginning with the letters A–E may be billed; the second week, F–L; the third week, M–S; and the fourth week, T–Z. The same cycle is followed each month. This process is called **cycle billing**.

Bills can be produced manually, by computer, or by utilizing a billing service.

Manual bills are usually typewritten on a billing form, with a copy sent to the patient and a copy kept in the patient's financial file. Computer-generated bills are usually produced by the office's computerized bookkeeping software. A billing service can either send a paper record of all of the bills sent out at the end of each cycle, or can transfer billing information from its computer to the office's computer, linking the information into the patient's financial record and the office's bookkeeping software.

Beginning the Billing Process

At regular intervals, patient financial accounts should be examined, and the accounts that must be billed should be processed. Billing insurance companies and billing patients are both straightforward transactions. However, you should be aware of some special situations.

A patient may have been treated for a final illness just before dying. In this case, any charges will have to be billed to the patient's estate. (Billing an estate is discussed in more detail at the end of this chapter.)

A patient may be a minor who sought treatment without his or her parent's knowledge. When minors are brought to a doctor by a parent or guardian for treatment, the parent or guardian acknowledges that he or she is the responsible party for financial purposes. However, if a minor is treated without the parent's knowledge, the minor is responsible for fees as well. Because of confidentiality, the doctor may not try to collect payment from the parent or guardian.

A patient may have a **credit** agreement with the practice, which allows the patient to pay bills off over time, along with interest on the balance due. This is important because, in such situations, even though a fee may become very old, it should not be considered delinquent and sent out of the office for collection.

Enter credits in parentheses ( ) and subtract when totaling columns and P

ACCOUNTS RECEIVABLE AGING RECORD

| Name | | As of Date | Prepared by | | | | | | Page of Page | |

NO.	ACCOUNT NAME / Amounts brought forward	Insurance Information — Date Claim Filed	Amount of Claim	Date of Last Payment	Current 1 to 30 days	31 to 60 days	61 to 90 days	91 to 120 days	121 days and over	TOTAL
1	Mary Smith			8/8/XX	120					120 -
2	John Payne			7/6/XX		250 -				250 -
3	Jack Desmonde			5/25/XX			500			500 -
4	Jill Jayne			4/2/XX		80 -				180 -
5										

A

Blackburn Primary Care Associates
Patient Aging

NAME	CURRENT 0 - 30	PAST 31 - 60	PAST 61 - 90	PAST 91 - 120	PAST over 120	Total Balance
Mary Smith Last Payment on 08/08/XX	$120.00					$120.00
John Payne Last Payment on 07/06/XX		$250.00				$250.00
Jack Desmonde Last Payment on 05/25/XX			$500.00			$500.00
Jill Jayne Last Payment on 04/02/XX		$80.00		$100.00		$180.00
Report Aging Totals Percent of Total Aging	$120.00 11.4%	$330.00 31.4%	$330.00 47.6%	$100.00 9.5%		$1,050.00 100.0%

B

➤ **Figure 39–1** Sample accounts aging record: (A) Prepared by hand; (B) prepared by computer.

ACCOUNT AGING

Account aging is the process of determining how long specific accounts/balances have been outstanding. An **account aging record** is kept in which accounts that are overdue are recorded. Accounts are aged in 30-day intervals. Figure 39–1 shows a sample account aging record.

Examining Accounts for Those Overdue

An account is considered overdue (i.e., an account is aged) if it is not paid within 30 days of the date billed unless there is an outstanding credit agreement. Accounts for which all the charges are from the previous billing period are considered 30 days. Overdue accounts are categorized as 60 days, 90 days, and 120 days.

An account with an outstanding balance after 120 days requires collection activity, such as sending the account out to a collection agency or writing a demand letter informing the account holder that a lawsuit will be brought if the account is not brought up to date. Most of the time, the balance of medical office accounts is small enough to permit legal action in small claims court. (Small claims court will be discussed in more detail at the end of the chapter.)

Procedure 39–1 describes how to create and examine an account aging record to determine the appropriate collection activity.

Organizing Collection Activities

Many people who owe money have every intention of paying their bill but are unable to do so in the short term because of some emergency. As accounts age, it is

PROCEDURE 39–1

Creating and Examining an Accounts Aging Record

Performance Objective: The student will be create and examine an accounts aging record.
Supplies and Equipment: Patient account ledgers, accounts aging record analysis form, pen or computer.

Procedure Steps

1. Assemble all ledgers with outstanding balances. A good time to do this is when monthly billing is done.
   Rationale: The accounts with an outstanding balance are the ones that will be "aged," that is, recorded to determine the length of time that the account balance is overdue.

2A. For each account with an outstanding balance, record the amount still owed and the length of time it has been owed since the first bill was sent. A single account may have amounts owed for different lengths of time.
   Rationale: If the patient received additional service before the bill for service received earlier was paid, there can be amounts due for different lengths of time.

2B. If the office uses a computerized accounting system, direct the computer to compile an accounts aging report for patients and for insurance companies.
   Rationale: In a computerized billing system, the computer program can generate the report of all overdue accounts.

3. Separate bills with unpaid insurance claims from bills that insurance has already paid.
   Rationale: Patients usually do not pay on bills with outstanding insurance claims until they find out how much the insurance will pay. These bills, if overdue, need to be followed up with the insurance company.

4. For accounts that are 31–60 days old, attach a note or sticker to the bill to remind the patient that payment is due.

5. For accounts that are 61–90 days old, place a note or sticker to indicate that the bill is now overdue and should be paid.

6. For accounts that are 91–120 days old, place a telephone call to the patient. Follow up with a letter confirming any agreement made.

7. For accounts over 120 days old, review previous collection attempts. Unless there are known circumstances that warrant a delay in collection activity, send a collection letter stating that if payment is not received by a certain date the account will be given to a collection agency or pursued in small claims court (depending on the procedure used by the office to collect delinquent accounts).
   Rationale: After 120 days without activity, especially if the person owing money has been contacted by telephone and letter, it is unlikely that the bill will be paid without more aggressive collection measures.

8. Record all action taken on the back of the ledger.
   Rationale: This provides a written record of actions taken and results of telephone conversations.

9. Review actions with the doctor or billing manager.

10. Write follow-up letters to document in writing any agreements made during telephone conversations.
   Rationale: A written record of verbal communications regarding bills and payments provides evidence in case further legal action is necessary.

---

appropriate to increase the forcefulness of any message to the patient that the account is overdue. Patients should always be invited to call the office and make arrangements to pay over time if they have had a true emergency. Sometimes, it is medical bills themselves that are piling up, especially in the case of a patient

with a chronic illness who does not have any or adequate insurance.

Patients are also encouraged to discuss accounts for which insurance payment is expected but delayed. By working with the insurance company, the patient can more easily determine whose responsibility the bill is.

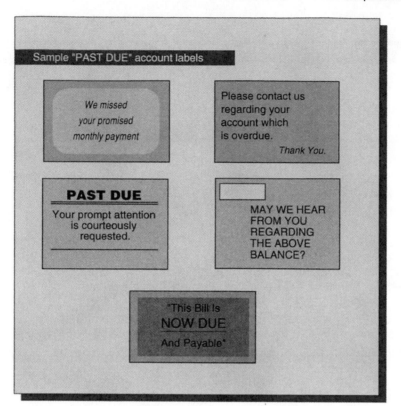

> **Figure 39–2** Stickers for overdue accounts.

Messages encouraging payment of the bill (often called **claim messages**) can be attached to bills or included in the billing envelope. Some computer programs will print message on the bill itself.

Bills that are 60 days overdue should be accompanied by a note or sticker reminding the patient that the bill is overdue. Examples of such stickers are shown in Figure 39–2. Many offices use a series of messages that become more forceful as time passes without payment.

Bills that are 90 days overdue should be followed up with a telephone call. The medical assistant must be careful to follow legal guidelines when discussing accounts with patients, as discussed in Guidelines for Telephone Collections. By contacting patients directly, the medical assistant can determine why there is no activity related to the account.

Bills that are aged 120 days should either be accompanied by or followed up by a collection letter, such as the one seen in Figure 39–3. Procedure 39–2 describes how to write a collection letter.

When writing a collection letter, the medical assistant should gather information related to the account before composing the letter. The recipient should be clearly informed what action is expected, and the deadline for action. The letter should not threaten consequences that will not be carried out (i.e., do not threaten legal action unless you are prepared to take it).

If the collection letter does not receive a response, another letter should be sent stating either that the account is being turned over to a **collection agency** (a company that collects overdue bills for other companies) or that a lawsuit will be filed in small claims court if the account is not paid by a certain date. This letter should also ask the patient to find a new health care provider and ask the patient to request that his or her medical records be forwarded to that provider.

The process for ending a relationship with a patient was discussed in chapter 4. In this case, the letter should be sent certified, with a return receipt requested. The letter should allow the patient at least two weeks to arrange to find another health care provider.

CREDIT AGREEMENTS

Credit agreements are documents that allow patients to set up a schedule to pay off their bills as long as they make the specified monthly payments. If a patient decides independently to pay his or her bill in installments (i.e., without discussing it with the medical office), no credit agreement is necessary. If the office and patient make an agreement regarding installment payments, even if no interest is charged, the agreement must be in writing. An interest charge is often added to the balance due at the end of each billing cycle when a written agreement exists.

FOCUS ON
GUIDELINES FOR TELEPHONE COLLECTIONS

THINGS TO DO

1. A **creditor** (person or company who is owed money) may contact the person who owes money by telephone during reasonable hours. Be sure to gather accurate information before placing the telephone call:
   a. Who owes the money?
   b. How much money is owed?
   c. How long has the money been owed?
   d. Is there any insurance claim pending?
   e. Has the insurance company processed the claim and/or made any payment?

2. A creditor may take measures to locate a person, but may not divulge that he or she is trying to collect a bill to anyone other than the person who owes money. Identify the person with whom you wish to speak when placing the call—the patient or the person responsible for the account.

3. A creditor may not misrepresent him- or herself in order to trick the person who owes money into taking the call. After asking for the person responsible for the account, identify yourself and the office for which you are placing the call.

4. A creditor may not harass or intimidate a person who owes money. Speak calmly and professionally. Discuss the different options for payment, including full payment, partial payment, and monthly installments. If possible, obtain a verbal commitment for a date and amount of at least a first payment and/or a payment plan.

5. Although a verbal agreement is legally binding, a written agreement is easier to enforce if legal action becomes necessary. Follow up any verbal agreement with a letter referring to the conversation and the agreement. If an arrangment was established for monthly payments, include a truth-in-lending statement, even if the patient will not pay interest.

6. Although you may not harass the patient, you may contact him or her if payments are not made as agreed. Often, the knowledge that attention is being paid to the account will encourage the patient to adhere to the repayment schedule.

THINGS NOT TO DO

1. Do not call too early in the day or too late at night.

2. Do not divulge to employers, neighbors, or other third parties that you are trying to collect a bill from the patient.

3. Do not threaten.

4. Do not end the conversation on vague terms.

5. Do not call repeatedly.

A credit agreement with a medical office is a type of revolving credit, like a department store or gasoline company charge card. As long as the monthly minimum is paid, the account is considered in good standing.

Truth-in-Lending Agreements

Because a credit agreement is a type of revolving credit, it falls under federal and state government fair lending practices. Thus, a truth-in-lending statement must be supplied to the patient when the agreement is made.

This **truth-in-lending** statement includes facts about such things as the maximum amount the patient may charge to the account, the interest rate, how the interest is computed (i.e., average daily balance, or balance at the end of the billing period), and how the minimum monthly payment is computed (i.e., percentage of outstanding balance). Figure 39–4 shows a sample credit agreement.

Policy for Patients with Outstanding Balances

Most medical offices insist that a patient close out any current balance due before writing a credit agreement with that patient. If the practice has had trouble collecting bills from a patient in the past, it may write the credit agreement for a lower maximum balance. But the practice cannot charge a different interest rate or compute the minimum payment in a different way for different patients depending on past payment history.

OTHER COLLECTION TECHNIQUES AND SPECIAL CIRCUMSTANCES

Five collection activities can be classified under special circumstances:

1. Tracing skips
2. Sending an account to a collection agency
3. Filing a lawsuit in small claims court
4. Billing an estate
5. Collecting from a patient who has filed for bankruptcy.

Tracing Skips

Occasionally, a bill is returned to your office from the post office with the notation "address unknown." This may be an innocent mistake—the result, perhaps, of an incorrect address by your office or the patient's

---

Blackburn Primary Care Associates, PC
1990 Turquoise Drive
Blackburn, WI 54937

04/02/01

Dear Patient,

Your account in this office is more than 120 days overdue. We have made previous attempts with you to set up a mutually agreeable payment schedule but you have not as yet followed through on your commitment. This will be your final notice. If you do not contact this office within 7 days of receipt of this letter we will have no choice but to turn over this account to the collection agency. Please contact this office if you wish to avoid collection activity.

Yours truly,

Joanne Hughes MD
Joanne Hughes, MD

➤ **Figure 39–3** Sample collection letter.

PROCEDURE 39-2

Writing a Collection Letter

Performance Objective: The student will compose a collection letter.

Supplies and Equipment: Accounts aging record, patient ledgers for patients with accounts that are 90–120 days old, letterhead stationery, envelope, word processor, computer and printer or typewriter.

Procedure Steps

1. After the accounts aging record has been created, determine which accounts need a letter. In general, this will be the accounts that are 90–120 days old.

   Rationale: A letter is usually sent after reminders and a telephone call have been made to the person responsible.

2. Review each account for the amount due, how long it has been due, any previous activity, and special situations. If the account is due from the estate of a deceased patient, insurance, or if there is a known reason why delayed payment is acceptable, do not take action on the account.

   Rationale: There may be circumstances that justify the delay in payment.

3. Otherwise, prepare a letter for each outstanding account. The letter should state clearly the amount of the outstanding balance, the date that the charges were incurred, the service provided, and the amount paid by insurance. It should also describe any previous conversations and/or agreements. The letter should clearly state that the outstanding balance is due and identify the date by which it is expected to be paid (usually in 10 days).

   Rationale: Even though the bill is overdue, the recipient of the letter is given a reasonable amount of time to respond to this letter.

4. The letter should be signed by the doctor, office manager, or person responsible for billing and collection. Place this person's name in the written signature line and prepare a reference line using your own initials.

   Rationale: The letter should be signed by a person who is authorized by the medical practice to collect outstanding accounts.

5. Prepare an envelope.

6. Place a copy of the letter in the patient's medical record. Place a notation that a letter was sent on the patient's ledger card or in the computer account. You may also file a copy of the letter in a collection follow-up file.

   Rationale: Future activity to collect on the account should be based on a review of your current activity.

7. Mail the letter.

---

failure to notify the office after moving. On the other hand, it may be a deliberate attempt to "skip out" on your bill and the bills of other professionals and/or merchants.

A potential **skip** (account for which no billing information is available) should be followed up immediately. First, call the patient's phone number: He or she may have moved within the same town and still have the same telephone number, or may have had the phone company use a "new number" message to forward calls.

If there is no new number listed, call the patient's place of business and ask to speak with the individual. You can also try to get in touch with the person by contacting professional associations, unions, or other organizations with which the person is associated.

Never tell a third party that the person owes you money, only that you wish to speak with the person.

Also, it is illegal for you to call a third party more than once in an attempt to trace a skip unless that person asks you to call back (e.g, the person you reach says he or she will speak to the person you are looking for and asks that you call back the next day).

You can also try sending a letter by registered or certified mail, with a return receipt requested, to the individual at the old address. Even if the person did not ask the post office to forward all mail, he or she may have asked for mail requiring special handling to be forwarded. Make sure to send a registered or certified letter in a plain envelope, with just the return street address and no office name; this minimizes the chances that the individual will refuse to accept the mail.

If all of these efforts fail, you should turn the bill over to your collection agency as soon as possible. Most collection agencies handle far more skips than

━ LAWS AFFECTING CREDIT AND COLLECTION ACTIVITIES

Equal Credit Opportunity Act	Federal law that prevents discrimination when offering credit based on (A) sex, marital status, race, national origin, religion, age (B) the fact that applicant receives public assistance income (C) the fact that applicant has exercised rights under consumer credit laws An applicant must be informed if credit is denied and has 60 days to request, in writing, the reason for denial of credit.
Fair Debt Collection Practices Act	Federal law that requires the fair treatment of debtors and prevents unfair debt collection measures, including harassment, false statements, and threats. The debt collector may not make frightening, verbally abusive, or threatening calls. The debt collector may not call before 8 AM or after 8 PM. The debt collector may not threaten action that cannnot legally be taken or is not intended to be taken.
Federal Truth-in-Lending Act	Governs installment agreements of more than four payments (or fewer if interest is charged). Administered by the Federal Trade Commission (FTC). Requires creditors to provide applicants with a form disclosing in a clear and obvious way all finance charges and terms.
Fair Credit Reporting Act	Requires credit bureaus to supply correct and complete information to businesses to use in evaluating a person's application for credit, insurance, or employment

individual medical offices do, and sometimes utilize other, more aggressive techniques. The sooner the collection agency receives the account, the better chance it has to collect the bill.

Sending Accounts to a Collection Agency

Collection agencies are in business specifically to collect accounts that have "aged out." This means that by the time a collection agency receives a delinquent account, the business such as a medical office has given the person who owes the money fair warning that the bill is overdue, and that a professional collector is going to become involved.

Each state has specific laws under which collection agencies must work. These laws define when collection agency personnel can call, what they can say, and what other tactics they can use to collect the bill.

Collection agencies generally charge between 20 and 40 percent of the amount they collect. They are not

ON THE JOB

At Blackburn Primary Care Associates, Linda, the medical assistant, is assigned to the front office, doing the monthly billing. As she reviews the monthly billing and accounts aging record, she notes that ten patients have accounts overdue by more than 90 days, two have accounts overdue by more than 120 days, and the majority of accounts are aged between 30 and 60 days.

QUESTIONS
1. How should Linda handle the accounts aged between 30 and 60 days?
2. What should Linda do with accounts 90 days overdue?
3. What should Linda do with accounts 120 days overdue?
4. What legal issues does Linda need to remember?

Blackburn Primary Care Associates, PC
1990 Turquoise Drive
Blackburn, WI 54937
608-459-8857

Federal Truth in Lending Statement

Patient _____

Address _____

    1. Fee for service of   _____

    2. Amount down   _____

    3. Amount financed   _____

    4. finance charge   _____

    5. total of payments 3 + 4 _____

    6. number of payments   _____

    7. amount of each payment _____

    Total no. of payments _____ payable over _____ monthly installments

    In the amount of $_____. The first payment is due _____.

Date _____ Signed_____

➤ **Figure 39–4** Sample credit agreement.

allowed to "cut a deal" with a patient and accept less than full payment unless the medical office has agreed to the arrangement for payment.

When a check is received from a collection agency, it should be recorded on the daily ledger. In addition, it should be posted to the account for which it was collected. The patient account (ledger) must be reduced by the amount actually collected by the collection agency (including the agency's collection fee). The difference between the amount collected and the amount paid to the office is entered on the day sheet as a negative adjustment; it will be entered as an expense by the practice accountant.

Small Claims Court

Small claims courts exist in each state. They are special sessions of the local district court that deal only with civil lawsuits involving small amounts of money. Most small claims lawsuits involve disputes over payments. Each state has its own rules for the maximum claim that can be brought in small claims court. This maximum amount runs from about $500 in some states to as much as $10,000 in others.

The question for a medical practice when choosing to use the court system is always whether it will sacrifice more in "good will" than it will gain in money if the collection is successful. Many offices bring suits in court only after a patient has left the practice without paying a bill in full. Furthermore, winning a judgment in small claims court is only the first step. The office must still collect the judgment.

Small claims courts are set up to reduce the legal fees for those seeking to collect relatively small amounts of money. Because there is no lawyer, the plaintiff must represent him- or herself (or business, in the case of an office administrator or medical assistant who handles the office's small claims). A collection agency cannot represent the office.

The clerk of the court has all of the documents necessary to file a small claim, and can usually walk a first-time claimant through the process, explaining how to fill out the forms and which documentation to submit to back up the claim. Only the defendant can appeal a small claims court judgment; for the plaintiff, a negative judgment is final.

Billing an Estate

Patients do sometimes die without having paid their medical bills in full. In this instance, the office will have to collect the balance due from the estate. Estates fall into an area of the law known as probate, and probate law is administered by a special section of the court system in each state.

It is not appropriate to send a bill to a deceased patient's estate immediately after the death while the family is grieving; however, the bill should be sent within 30 days so the account does not become "cold." The bill should be sent to "The Estate of" the patient at the patient's address rather than to a family member or other individual unless that person has made a written promise to cover the deceased's medical costs.

If the deceased patient had a will, it usually has a provision that the costs of the patient's final illness be paid by the estate outside of the probate process. In such a case, the bill will probably be paid promptly. The will should be filed within 30 days, and the clerk of the probate court should then be able to furnish you with the name of the executor or administrator (the person responsible for handling the estate's business dealings). An itemized final bill should then be sent to this individual by certified mail with a return receipt requested.

If the patient did not have a will, the medical practice's bill will be put in with other creditors' bills, and be paid only when payment is approved by the probate court and the administrator appointed by the court.

Bankruptcy

Bankruptcy laws are federal laws, meaning that they apply equally regardless of the state in which the bankrupt person lives. Bankruptcy is a means for an individual or business to "get out from under" a crushing load of debt, either by reorganizing the debt or by liquidating assets and dividing the funds among all of the creditors.

Individuals file for personal bankruptcy either under Chapter VII or Chapter XIII of the bankruptcy code.

A Chapter VII bankruptcy is a liquidation of assets. Under such a bankruptcy, only secured creditors will be paid from the proceeds from the sale of any assets. If the bankrupt patient had a credit agreement, the medical office is a secured creditor. But if the office is merely trying to collect a bill, the office is an unsecured creditor and will not receive payment.

A Chapter XIII bankruptcy is an "Adjustment of Debts" bankruptcy. In such a bankruptcy, the debtor (patient) pays a particular amount determined by the bankruptcy court to the court-appointed trustee, who then distributes the money to creditors. The debtor, if he or she has a regular income, can be required to make payments from that income into the trustee account for three years, and the trustee makes payments to creditors under payment plans he or she works out.

During the period the debtor is under the jurisdiction of the bankruptcy court, no creditor may try to collect a debt outside the bankruptcy process. However, a medical office can demand payment in full for any additional service it provides to a patient from whom it is collecting old debts under a bankruptcy agreement.

■ STUDENT STUDY PLAN

To reinforce your understanding of the material in this chapter . . .

Complete the **Review & Recall** questions.

Discuss the situation in **If You Were the Medical Assistant** with your classmates and answer the questions.

Answer the **Critical Thinking Questions** and discuss them with your classmates.

Visit the **Web Sites** suggested and search for additional Web sites using the **Keywords for Internet Searches**.

Complete the exercises in chapter 39 of the **Student Mastery Manual**.

REVIEW & RECALL

1. What are the different methods a practice can use for billing patients?

2. Describe the collection activities that should be performed at each level of account aging.

3. What is the correct technique when using the telephone to assist in collections?

4. What information must be in a truth-in-lending statement?

5. Describe the steps one can take if a patient has "skipped" on a bill.

6. What steps do you have to take if a claim is to be brought in small claims court?

7. How is a claim collected from a patient's estate?

IF YOU WERE THE MEDICAL ASSISTANT

Mrs. Jay Smith has an overdue balance of $1,200 and her account is 120 days old. There is no activity and no outstanding insurance claim pending. Prepare a collection letter.

CRITICAL THINKING QUESTIONS

1. Contact a lawyer to speak to your class concerning collection practices, and discuss ethical and unethical collection practices.

2. Research local collection agencies and explore their collection techniques, both those that are the same and those that are different. Determine how many provide monthly reports, contracts, and so on.

3. Explain the Fair Collection Act of 1977 and how it applies to the collection practices of a doctor's office.

EXPLORE THE WEB

INTERNET WEB SITES

Medscape Medical Office Management
www.medscape.com/Home/network/MOM/MOM.html

KEYWORDS FOR INTERNET SEARCHES

medical bill collecting
medical billing

ANSWERS TO ON THE JOB

1. For accounts aged between 30 and 60 days, Linda may attach notes or stickers to the statements reminding patients to pay the bill or call the office to discuss the bill.

2. For accounts 90 days overdue, Linda should call the person responsible for the bill. She should identify why the bill is overdue and, if possible, obtain a verbal commitment to pay a specific amount by a specific date. This enables her to follow up easily.

3. Linda should write a collection letter demanding payment to the person responsible for each account that is 120 days overdue.

4. Linda needs to remember not to call patients too early in the morning or too late at night, not to disclose to anyone but the patient that she is calling about a bill, and not to call repeatedly once an agreement has been made. She also needs to remember that if an agreement is made for installment payments, the office must provide a written agreement for the patient to sign that includes the amount and frequency of payments as well as the amount of interest that will be charged.

From Student to Professional Medical Assistant

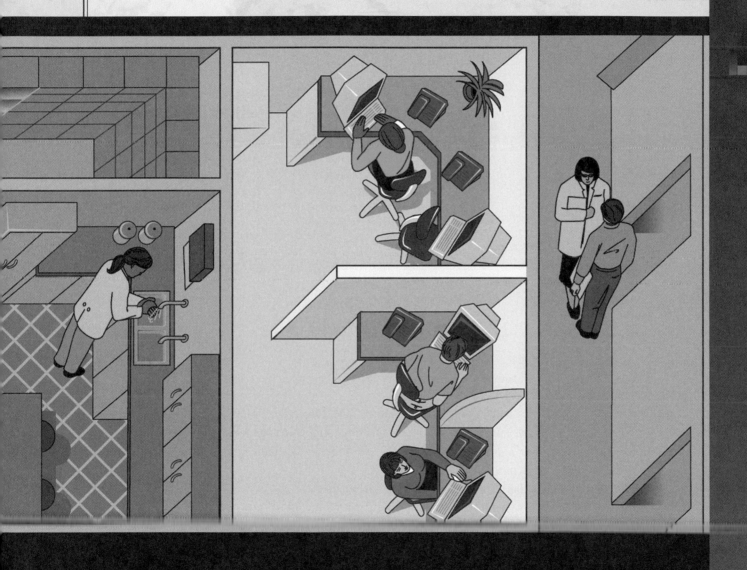

Legal Issues in the Workplace

Instructional Objectives

After completing this chapter, you will be able to do the following:

1. Define and spell the vocabulary words for this chapter.
2. Differentiate between constitutional law, statutory law, administrative law, international law, and common law.
3. Discuss implications of mandated reporting, licensure, and crimes for the medical office.
4. Differentiate between breach of contract, intentional torts, and unintentional torts.
5. Identify four defenses to intentional torts and three defenses to unintentional torts.
6. Describe the six phases of a civil lawsuit.
7. Explain the differences between a court case and arbitration.
8. Discuss limitations on a patient's right to sue if he or she participates in a managed care health insurance plan.
9. Describe various business forms used for medical practices, including sole proprietor, partnership, corporation, and vertical integration.
10. Describe how doctors and medical assistants are paid under various business forms.
11. List five types of insurance purchased by a medical practice to protect the business and/or employees.
12. Describe laws that protect employees and potential employees from discrimination in hiring, promotion, compensation, and firing.
13. Discuss the rights of employers and employees related to preemployment testing and disabilities.
14. Describe measures to protect the rights of employees related to drug testing and sexual harassment.
15. Explain how the Employee Retirement Income Security Act (ERISA) protects employee rights.

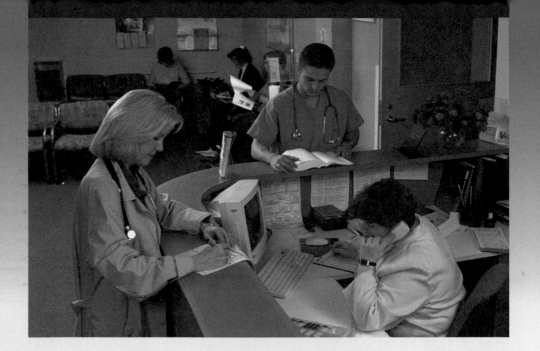

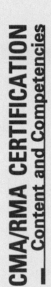

CMA/RMA CERTIFICATION
Content and Competencies

■ Legal guidelines/requirements for health care   ■ Perform within legal and clinical boundaries

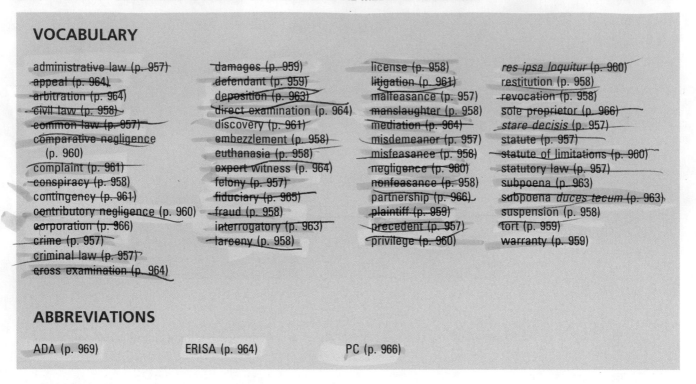

VOCABULARY

administrative law (p. 957)
appeal (p. 964)
arbitration (p. 964)
civil law (p. 958)
common law (p. 957)
comparative negligence (p. 960)
complaint (p. 961)
conspiracy (p. 958)
contingency (p. 961)
contributory negligence (p. 960)
corporation (p. 966)
crime (p. 957)
criminal law (p. 957)
cross examination (p. 964)

damages (p. 959)
defendant (p. 959)
deposition (p. 963)
direct examination (p. 964)
discovery (p. 961)
embezzlement (p. 958)
euthanasia (p. 958)
expert witness (p. 964)
felony (p. 957)
fiduciary (p. 965)
fraud (p. 958)
interrogatory (p. 963)
larceny (p. 958)

license (p. 958)
litigation (p. 961)
malfeasance (p. 957)
manslaughter (p. 958)
mediation (p. 964)
misdemeanor (p. 957)
misfeasance (p. 958)
negligence (p. 960)
nonfeasance (p. 958)
partnership (p. 966)
plaintiff (p. 959)
precedent (p. 957)
privilege (p. 960)

res ipsa loquitur (p. 960)
restitution (p. 958)
revocation (p. 958)
sole proprietor (p. 966)
stare decisis (p. 957)
statute (p. 957)
statute of limitations (p. 960)
statutory law (p. 957)
subpoena (p. 963)
subpoena duces tecum (p. 963)
suspension (p. 958)
tort (p. 959)
warranty (p. 959)

ABBREVIATIONS

ADA (p. 969)   ERISA (p. 964)   PC (p. 966)

The American legal system governs the way professional relationships and many personal relationships are carried out. The law has been mentioned throughout this book as it applies to specific instances discussed. In addition, some legal issues were discussed in chapter 4. The purpose of this chapter is to provide additional information about legal issues, especially as they apply to the office-based medical practice.

TYPES OF LAW

The law is an evolving system of governing relationships. The law today will not necessarily be the law tomorrow. As society grows and changes, the laws change to conform to realities and to try to govern future realities. There are five types of law:

1. Constitutional law
2. Statutory law
3. Administrative law
4. International law
5. Common law.

Constitutional Law

The United States Constitution describes the process for enacting and reviewing federal laws based on the three branches of the federal government:

1. Executive branch: The President, Vice President, Cabinet officers, and all of the various departments of the federal government.

2. Legislative branch: Members of the U.S. Senate and House of Representatives and the staffs of individual legislators as well as legislative committees and legislative research offices.
3. Judicial branch: The courts, including the U.S. Supreme Court, Courts of Appeals for the nine judicial regions, District Courts, as well as special courts.

The purpose of the Constitution is to articulate the way the federal government is organized, various rights held by U.S. citizens, and the relationships between the federal government and state governments, as well as between the federal government and each of its citizens. The Constitution also clarifies the relationship between the three branches of government.

The U.S. Constitution was drawn up by representatives of the original 13 states meeting at the Constitutional Convention in Philadelphia in 1787. Since then, there have been 27 amendments to the Constitution. The first 10 amendments, ratified in 1791, are collectively known as the Bill of Rights. The last amendment was ratified by the states in 1992.

Most of the 50 states have state constitutions, which lay out the rights and responsibilities of citizens of the particular state, as well as the way the state government is organized. States' executive branches have a governor as the highest officer, state legislatures may have one or two houses (unicameral or bicameral), and state court systems have a number of levels before reaching the highest appellate court.

Statutory Law

Statutory law is the body of laws enacted by a legislative body with the power to make law. An individual law or group of related laws is called a **statute**. On the federal level, statutes must be approved by both houses of Congress and signed into law by the president. States and local governments (cities, towns, counties, and special taxing districts for such services as schools or fire protection) follow established procedures to enact legislation.

No statutes passed at the state or local level can violate the rights of citizens as defined by the U.S. Constitution and its various amendments.

Administrative Law

Administrative law establishes administrative agencies of the federal government and describes their powers and procedures. Some agencies have their own special administrative law courts to hear disputes brought by individuals, groups, or companies against the agency.

For instance, the Internal Revenue Service (IRS) has a tax court to hear appeals by citizens or corporations disputing their tax bills; similarly, the Social Security Administration (SSA) has a large administrative court where citizens are allowed to dispute denial of Social Security disability benefits.

International Law

International law is based on treaties and other agreements between and among two or more countries.

Common Law

Before the establishment of the U.S. Constitution, many countries had a body of law established over centuries that was usually not written in the form of statutes, but rather as individual decisions of a court. This type of law is called **common law**. To make legal decisions, judges relied on decisions made in previous legal cases where similar circumstances existed.

This form of legal decision making is called *stare decisis,* which means "the previous decision stands." Many countries, such as England, still do not have written constitutions; common law in these countries is still the strongest form of law.

In the United States, judges base their decisions on a combination of statutory law (where statutes exist that clearly speak to the issue in dispute), interpretation of the U.S. Constitution or a state constitution, and principles of common law. When a decision made in the past is used as the basis for a decision in the present, it is called a **precedent**. These precedents, or interpretations of the law, lay a foundation for subsequent legal decisions.

CRIMINAL LAW

The branch of statutory law that describes offenses against the public welfare is called **criminal law**. As discussed in chapter 4, a **crime** is an offense in violation of a law that prohibits or requires certain behavior. Another term sometimes used to describe a criminal act is **malfeasance**—a wrongdoing that is illegal or contrary to official obligation.

When a person is convicted of a crime (or pleads guilty to a crime), punishment is imposed. The parameters of possible punishment are defined in statutory law. Corporal punishment, such as flogging, is not a part of the American system of punishment; punishments include imprisonment, payment of fines, restitution to the victim, a period of supervision called probation, or a term of service to the community. For certain murders, including the killing of a law-enforcement officer, many states have a death penalty, as does the federal government.

For a person to be found guilty of committing a crime, a judge or jury must find that the evidence presented against the individual proves guilt "beyond a reasonable doubt."

Types of Crimes

Crimes are defined as either felonies or misdemeanors.

Felony

A **felony** is a serious crime, punishable by death or imprisonment in a state or federal penal institution for more than one year. Felonies are described within the general law of the state, and are often described by degrees of seriousness. Murder, assault with a deadly weapon, and grand theft are examples of felonies.

Misdemeanor

A **misdemeanor** is a less serious crime, punishable by a fine or imprisonment for less than one year, often in a local or county penal institution. Petty theft is an example of a misdemeanor.

How Criminal Law May Affect the Medical Office

The medical assistant must be aware that participation in criminal activity makes him or her vulnerable to being named in a criminal action, even if the extent of involvement did not exceed going along with the actions of others in the office.

Mandatory Reporting

#3

As discussed in chapter 4, medical facilities must report to the police injuries that may be the result of criminal activities, including gunshot wounds, stab wounds, wounds that may have come from a beating or rape, and suspected abuse of a child or an elderly person. Also, certain communicable diseases such as AIDS must be reported to state or county health officials.

Failure to make a mandated report is a crime. When a report is required by law, the patient should be informed why the report is required and who the report will be made to.

Licensure

State laws regulate practitioners of certain professions by requiring specific credentials. Each state sets its own credentials, and issues a **license**—official permission to perform an activity or participate in a profession. All states require a license to practice medicine, although a doctor may practice in certain federal facilities and agencies with a license from a different state than the one in which the facility is located.

#4

Conviction of any crime, whether related to medical practice or not, is grounds for **revocation** (permanent cancelation) or **suspension** (temporary cancelation) of a doctor's license to practice. Practicing medicine without a license is also a crime. The seriousness and nature of the crime will influence the state medical board's decision about the length of time a person's license may be suspended.

Violent Crimes

#5

In the medical office, an employee is more likely to be the victim of a crime such as robbery than to be accused of a crime. Some health professionals have been accused and convicted of crimes such as a murder, attempted murder, or rape that occurred in the course of practice, but this is extremely rare. Occasionally, a doctor is charged with **manslaughter** (the unintentional causing of a death), wrongful death, or criminal negligence when a patient dies under treatment and there is a question of whether inappropriate treatment caused the death.

Although there is currently a movement trying to decriminalize assisted suicide, such an act is still defined as some type of murder in most states, as is **euthanasia** (mercy killing). Currently, abortion is legal in the United States, but state legislatures are continually enacting laws that try to restrict the circumstances under which an abortion can be performed.

Nonviolent Crimes

Two or more people who have joined together to commit an unlawful act may be accused of **conspiracy**; this may be applied to actions that are illegal in and of themselves, or actions to prevent detection of a prior crime.

Stealing another person's property (without violence) is called **larceny.** In the medical office, this may take the form of **embezzlement**—appropriating funds from a client, customer, or employer.

A growing problem in the health care industry is **fraud**—deliberate deception carried out to secure unfair or unlawful gain. Billing for services not provided, billing for services provided to imaginary patients, performing unneeded services, and even deliberately using codes from a higher level of service than that provided (so-called upcoding) are all forms of insurance fraud. Every instance of such a billing can be considered a separate act; the fraud will be considered either mail fraud or wire fraud depending on whether the reimbursement forms were submitted by mail or computer.

In the mind of an office employee, there may be a difference between billing an insurance company using a code for more complex service than was actually provided, "because they pay us so little anyway," and billing for procedures that were never performed. But from a legal perspective, both are considered fraud; if proved, both carry serious penalties.

Insurance companies and agencies of the federal and state government are victims of billions of dollars in fraudulent claims each year. They have increasing incentives to investigate health care facilities they suspect of fraudulent billing.

CIVIL LAW

Civil law is the branch of law that regulates relationships and interactions between individuals and other individuals or groups. Civil law is based both on statutory law and on common law. Two terms sometimes used for civil offenses are **misfeasance**—the improper execution of a lawful act—and **nonfeasance**—the failure to perform an act that is either an official obligation or a legal requirement. These two terms are related to the term "malfeasance," already introduced in the discussion of criminal acts.

Civil cases need to be proved only by a "preponderance of the evidence," which means that proof is more likely than not. The outcome of a civil case is usually **restitution**, a monetary award to the injured party or parties to compensate for the damage, or an agreement by the charged party never to engage in similar behavior again or to perform an obligation. The victim of a crime can also bring a civil action to recover damages that occurred as a result of the crime. Civil and criminal cases may be brought against an individual at the same time, or one after another.

Classification of Civil Law

There are three classifications of civil law:

Contract law governs contracts or legal agreements between or among parties.
Tort law governs acts that bring harm to a person.
Administrative law governs regulations by government agencies.

Breach of Contract

Breach of contract occurs when the terms of a contract are not kept by one or more parties to the contract. For example, if one party does not pay a bill for services provided by agreement, that party can be charged with breach of contract. If the court determines that a breach of contract has occurred, monetary compensation (called **damages**) is usually awarded to the injured party to make up for the losses incurred.

The party bringing the legal action, called a lawsuit, is called the **plaintiff.** The party against whom the lawsuit is brought is called the **defendant.** In the case of a breach of contract, the plaintiff must prove that a contract exists and that both parties agreed to its terms. This is easiest if there is a written contract.

In the medical office, patients may be sued for not paying bills. When elective surgery or an elective procedure is performed (i.e., surgery that is not medically necessary), the patient is usually required to sign a written contract that specifies the amount to be paid, and that payment is required whether or not the patient is satisfied with the results of the treatment. This avoids the implication of a **warranty,** or promise about the results of treatment.

The medical office can be sued for not paying its bills as well, for supplies, rent, equipment leases, and so on.

Contracts may be found to be invalid if one of the parties is a minor, mentally incompetent, or subject to undue influence at the time the contract was entered into.

Torts

A **tort** is a private wrong, other than breach of contract, for which a person can initiate a lawsuit. The purpose of the lawsuit is to restore the injured party or parties to his, her, or their position before any damage occurred.

This can include replacement of property (or a money award equal to the loss), compensation for medical expenses, compensation for loss of income, and compensation for less tangible damages such as pain and suffering.

Types of Torts

Intentional torts are torts committed with intent, such as assault and battery or a deliberate invasion of privacy. Unintentional torts include malpractice or negligence. Both types of torts were discussed in detail in chapter 4.

To prevail in a lawsuit alleging negligence or malpractice, usually the plaintiff must prove the so-called four D's of malpractice, as discussed in chapter 4. These are:

1. The defendant had a duty to the plaintiff.
2. The plaintiff failed to meet his or her duty.
3. Damage occurred.
4. The failure to meet the duty resulted directly in the damage.

In some instances, the plaintiff has no direct knowledge of the incident (for example, if the plaintiff is under general anesthetic). In such a case, a lawsuit may be allowed under the doctrine of *res ipsa loquitur*, discussed in detail in the box on the next page.

The medical assistant's position as a professional was discussed in detail in chapter 4, but it is worth reiterating here. Depending on the circumstances surrounding an allegedly negligent act, the medical assistant may or may not be considered a professional. A professional sued for malpractice is held to a higher standard of care than a lay person would be.

Suppose, for instance, a patient goes into respiratory arrest in the office and ends up with permanent impairment. If a medical assistant was working in the front office when no doctor was present and responded to the patient, he or she might be held to the standard of a reasonable person and sued for negligence if he or she delayed calling an ambulance. However, if a medical assistant was working in the clinical area, drawing blood or giving an injection to the person, he or she would probably be held to the standard of a professional, and might be sued for malpractice (which is sometimes called professional negligence) if the patient was injured during the procedure.

Defense to an Intentional Tort

The outcome of any lawsuit depends on what a judge or jury believes. There are a number of defenses against a charge of an intentional tort.

Doctrine of *Res Ipsa Loquitur*

There are cases where the plaintiff cannot have personal knowledge of how an injury due to negligence occurred; for example, the patient may be under general anesthesia at the time. For this type of case, the plaintiff's attorney will ask the judge to apply the doctrine of *res ipsa loquitur* (meaning the "thing speaks for itself").

Under this doctrine, the court assumes that the type of injury being presented could have occurred only by negligence. It is usually used in errors such as forceps, sponges, or other items left in the patient during surgery; or performing a surgery other than that which the plaintiff was supposed to have.

The plaintiff's attorney only has to establish that the defendant was responsible for the care that resulted in the injury. For example, if a patient went to surgery for a left-leg amputation and woke up to find that the right leg had been amputated, it is clear that someone made a mistake during surgery, even though the patient did not see who actually removed the wrong leg.

In such a case, the lawsuit would probably name the surgeon as the person responsible for the surgery, the hospital as the party responsible for having procedures in place to keep such a mistake from happening, and possibly also the person responsible that day for bringing patients into the operating room and completing the preoperative checklist.

#9 **Privilege** is a special right or permission granted to a certain group of individuals. For example, a hospital's policy and procedure manual may give doctors and medical residents (doctors in training) the power to order soft restraints or leather restraints for a patient in certain circumstances, and allow other professionals to apply them when a doctor's order has been written. If a patient is placed in restraints according to established procedures, he or she could not make a case for false imprisonment, an intentional tort, against those who had actually placed him or her in restraints.

Consent has been discussed in detail in many instances in this book. A patient scheduled for surgery will often be asked to consent to photographs being taken and published in a medical journal or textbook, or used as a slide in a lecture (without personal identifying information) for the purpose of providing education.

Self-defense or the defense of others is another defense against intentional tort. When physical contact occurs, a person accused of assault and/or battery may assert that he or she was defending against contact initiated by another person.

Error, rather than intent, is another defense. An injury caused by an intentional tort is willful; the defense may argue that the injury was unintentional or a mistake. For example, a person may argue that he lost his balance and bumped into a person, and did not mean for that person to fall and get hurt.

Defenses Against Charges of Negligence or Malpractice

#10 **Negligence.** An act that causes injury, without intent to cause harm, is negligence. If a negligent act is committed by a professional, it is called malpractice. Malpractice is discussed in detail in chapter 4. There are several defenses that can be used against a charge of negligence or malpractice.

Statute of Limitations. The **statute of limitations** is the law that limits the time period during which a person can sue. The period varies from one to three years, depending on the laws of the particular state and whether the suit is for negligence or malpractice (negligence usually has a shorter statute of limitations than malpractice).

The statute of limitations begins at one of three points, as defined in the state where the incident occurred:

1. When the injury occurs.
2. When the individual determines that an injury has occurred; for instance, if a hemostat is left in the body during surgery and is discovered by an x-ray taken at a later date for another reason.
3. When a minor reaches the age of majority (usually 18).

Contributory Negligence or Comparative Negligence. If the injured person has played a part in causing the injury, some states regard this as a complete defense (**contributory negligence**). Other states determine **comparative negligence**—how much of the negligence was caused by the professional and how much was caused by the injured individual. Judges and juries are asked to assess damages to the injured party depending on the percentage of the injury caused by the professional.

For example, following surgery a patient developed a wound infection that required additional surgery and resulted in an unsightly scar. The doctor's attorney brought out that the patient had failed to seek medical attention for several days after noting swelling, drainage from the wound, and a fever of 102° F. Prompt medical attention, the attorney argued, would have prevented the second surgery and minimized scarring.

In a state using contributory negligence, the patient would not collect any damages. In a state using comparative negligence, the judge or jury would determine the amount of negligence on the part of the doctor and award the patient that percentage of the total damages established by the court.

Assumption of Risk. A patient who does not follow medical advice becomes responsible for any problems that occur as a result of his or her decision. Hospitals obtain signatures if possible when a patient refuses to have side rails in place, or leaves the hospital against medical advice.

A complete note should be written in the patient's medical record if he or she refuses to follow medical advice, including the patient's exact words if possible, and the presence of any witness(es). If a patient frequently misses appointments, it is also an example of disregarding medical advice, and should be noted in the medical chart.

MALPRACTICE LITIGATION

Litigation (the process of taking a lawsuit or criminal case through the courts) is complex. It is important to understand the litigation process, even though fewer than five percent of all malpractice cases brought against medical professionals or medical institutions ever reach the stage of going to trial. Figure 40–1 summarizes the litigation process.

Initiation of a Lawsuit

A person who believes he or she has received inappropriate medical care consults an attorney, who obtains information from the patient, and usually tries to obtain copies of the relevant medical records. A letter containing a patient's authorization to send a copy of medical records to a lawyer may be the first indication to the medical office that the patient is actively contemplating a lawsuit.

In some states, medical offices are required to provide a copy of the record on request by a lawyer accompanied by a patient's authorization. In other states, medical offices may refuse to provide a copy until compelled to do so by a court order, which is issued after a formal lawsuit has been filed with the court.

Health care facilities, including doctors' offices, are allowed in most states to charge a copying fee for records sent to an attorney. This contrasts with the policy of sending copies of records without charge to another doctor or health care facility to provide continuity of care.

 At the time a lawsuit is actually filed, whether before or after the patient's medical records have been obtained by his or her attorney, the patient signs a document releasing the doctor from the requirements of patient confidentiality. This is necessary because information about the patient's medical record becomes part of the public record in the litigation process.

Whenever he or she obtains the patient's medical records, the attorney has them reviewed by doctors or other health professionals uninvolved in the patient's treatment to determine if a case can clearly be made for malpractice. Appropriateness of care is clearly the major issue in a suit for malpractice. However, incomplete, illegible, or altered records decrease the medical record's credibility, even if the care actually given was appropriate.

Most malpractice suits are accepted by attorneys on a **contingency** basis. In such a case, the individual filing the lawsuit only pays for the attorney's time and effort, or the expenses involved in litigation, if he or she collects an award from the party being sued. This is usually a percentage of the settlement or judgment amount. Contingency payments are often one-third to one-half of the amount collected if the suit goes to trial (even if a settlement is reached during the trial, or if a settlement is reached during any appeal process after the initial trial), and one-fourth to one-third the amount collected if the suit settles before the trial.

The first thing a doctor should do on being served with notice of a lawsuit is to inform the company that provides his or her malpractice insurance (the doctor should also inform the insurance company of a request by an attorney for medical records). If a suit is filed, the malpractice insurance provider will appoint an attorney to represent the doctor as a policy holder. The doctor may also wish to hire an independent attorney, since the doctor's interests are not always the same as the malpractice insurance carrier's.

To formally initiate a lawsuit, the patient's attorney files a **complaint**, a written statement listing the claim against the person or facility alleged to have performed acts of malpractice, and the amount of money desired as payment for damages caused by that malpractice. The person who files the complaint is called the plaintiff; and the person(s), corporation(s), organization(s), and/or institution(s) allegedly at fault is/are the defendant(s). It is possible, but not common, for staff in a medical office to be named as defendants in a malpractice lawsuit; usually, however, just the doctor (or doctors) who provided the care are named.

Notification of a complaint is given to the defendant(s), and attorneys for the defendant(s) are given time to file written responses to the complaint.

Formal Discovery

After the complaint has been filed and the initial response has been made, information is gathered by attorneys for both the plaintiff and defendant(s) in a process called **discovery**. The rules of discovery at both the federal and state levels define how information can be obtained by either side. There are three main ways of obtaining information during discovery:

ON THE JOB: ANALYSIS OF A MALPRACTICE SUIT

The plaintiff, Cynthia Herdrich of Bloomington, Illinois, was examined by her doctor, Lori Pegram, on March 1, 1991, complaining of midline abdominal pain. A week later, on March 8, the doctor found an inflamed mass about 6 by 8 centimeters in Herdrich's abdomen.

Dr. Pegram thought the mass was an ovarian cyst. Even though Herdrich had experienced discomfort and inflammation for a week, Dr. Pegram told her to wait another 8 days before having an ultrasound to determine the exact nature, size, and location of the mass. The reason was that Herdrich's insurance plan, Health Alliance Medical Plans, and Dr. Pegram's employer, Carle Clinic, required patients with "nonemergency" situations to wait 8 days for diagnostic ultrasound, assuming that some minor problems would resolve themselves and make testing unnecessary. In addition, the procedure would need to be done at a Carle Clinic affiliate in Urbana, 50 miles away.

During the 8-day waiting period, Herdrich's appendix ruptured, resulting in peritonitis (infection of the abdominal cavity). She required surgery to drain and cleanse the abdominal cavity. This surgery was performed in Urbana instead of a hospital closer to Herdrich's home.

Herdrich filed a complaint on October 21, 1992, alleging medical negligence against Dr. Pegram and Carle Clinic Association (Counts I and II). In 1994, she amended the complaint, claiming that Health Alliance Medical Plans itself breached its duty to those covered by the plan by depriving them of proper medical care in order to save money, and that it violated the Illinois Consumer Fraud Act by failing to notify plan members that doctors' income would be increased if they ordered fewer diagnostic tests (Count III). The state court dismissed the third count, but a trial was held on the first two counts.

Answer the questions below based on the summary of the case above (the full decision, by the Court of Appeals for the United States Seventh Circuit, No 97-1070 can be found at www.kentlaw.edu/7circuit/1998/aug/97-1070.html.)

QUESTIONS:
1. What questions should you ask to determine if this case meets the 4 D's of malpractice?
   a. duty
   b. derelict
   c. damage
   d. direct cause
2. Discuss if and how this case meets the 4 D's of malpractice:
   a. duty
   b. derelict
   c. damage
   d. direct cause
3. What questions should you ask to determine if there is evidence to support the following defenses to a malpractice action in this case?
   a. statute of limitations
   b. contributory negligence
   c. assumption of risk
4. Discuss whether you see evidence of any of the following possible defenses to a malpractice action in the case:
   a. statute of limitations
   b. contributory negligence
   c. assumption of risk
5. Discuss the monetary amount a jury might award to Herdrich if negligence occurred. Differentiate between general and special damages.

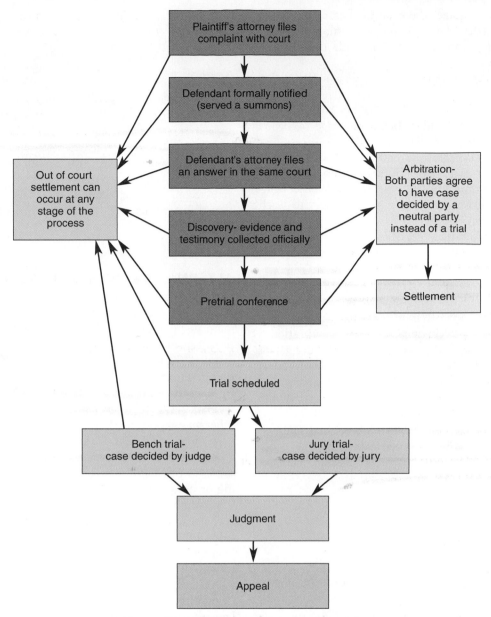

➤ **Figure 40–1** The process of litigation in a civil case.

1. An **interrogatory** is a written set of questions that must be answered, under oath as if in court, within a specific time period.
2. A **deposition** is oral testimony taken by a court reporter at a location outside the courtroom, subject to the same requirements for truth as court testimony. A judge is usually not present for a deposition, but the person being deposed may have an attorney present to provide counseling. If an individual does not agree to a request to be deposed, the court may issue a **subpoena**, a court order that requires the individual to make him- or herself available to be deposed.
3. Production of documents. During discovery, at-

torneys for the various parties request that certain documents be made available. Again, if a party refuses to make certain documents available, the court can issue a **subpoena** *duces tecum,* a court order requiring that the documents (or other material evidence) be made available.

Pretrial Conference

At some point, a judge or magistrate will convene a pretrial conference, at which point the plaintiff presents evidence to determine if the case has merit and the defendant asks for dismissal of the suit for lack of merit. Even if the case is weak and certain charges are not proven at this stage, the plaintiff has a legal right to take the case to trial. The judge or magistrate can narrow the trial's scope if he or she finds that there is no merit to certain aspects of the charge.

Trial Phase

A trial can be held either before a judge (a bench trial) or before a jury.

When the trial begins, an attorney for each side gives an opening statement, during which he or she outlines the case that will be presented and the conclusions his or her client wishes the judge or jury to reach from the evidence presented.

The plaintiff's attorney gets the first opportunity to call witnesses and produce evidence of the malpractice. Each witness is subjected to questions from the attorney who has requested (or demanded by subpoena) his or her testimony; this is known as **direct examination**. Following this are questions from the attorney representing the other party, known as **cross examination**.

When the plaintiff's case is complete, the defendant presents a case, with each defense witness being questioned in the same way, first on direct examination by the defense attorney, then on cross examination by the plaintiff's attorney.

Each side may request testimony from one or more **expert witness(es)**, uninvolved experts, such as other doctors, who are hired to give a professional opinion about the usual treatment of similar cases.

Judgment

As part of a judgment for a plaintiff, the judge or jury awards a specific amount of money, or damages.

1. Nominal damages are token amounts of money awarded when a legal right has been violated, but no actual injury has occurred requiring compensation.

2. Compensatory damages are awarded to compensate the plaintiff directly for an injury.

These may be general damages—for such items as medical bills, extended hospital stays, scarring, and pain and suffering—or special damages to compensate for indirect results of the malpractice, such as lost wages, cost of travel, or cost of future medical care to repair the injury.

3. Punitive damages are additional damages awarded as punishment for an act the judge or jury considers willful misconduct or wanton disregard for proper procedure. Punitive damages are rarely awarded in malpractice suits.

If a jury awards damages, the judge may either set aside the verdict if he or she believes the jury acted in error, or modify the award of damages, if he or she

believes the jury did not act appropriately in this regard.

Appeal

After a court decision, whichever party the decision has gone against can begin the appeal process. An **appeal** is a request for a hearing from a higher court, usually on the basis that the legal process in the lower court was faulty. Figure 40–2 summarizes the appellate process. Higher courts review cases submitted, and may accept or reject them after reviewing the record or after a formal hearing. The final court of appeals is the U.S. Supreme Court.

ALTERNATIVE DISPUTE RESOLUTION

Instead of a trial, both parties may agree to have their dispute decided by a neutral third party. This process can reduce time, expense, and publicity of a dispute. Such a process may take the form of mediation or arbitration.

Mediation uses a facilitator to help two parties in conflict settle their differences. This can be done in different ways; and if no settlement is reached, either party may find recourse in the court system.

Arbitration is a process whereby a neutral party settles the dispute. The arbitration can be either binding or nonbinding.

In nonbinding arbitration, the parties do not have to accept the decision, and one can proceed with a court case. In binding arbitration, the parties agree at the beginning to be bound by the decision of the arbitrator(s).

Various organizations provide lists of arbitrators, and depending on the circumstances and applicable state law, the parties in arbitration either select a mutually acceptable arbitrator or are assigned one from a list prepared during the arbitration process.

Arbitration is not very common in malpractice cases; it is far more common in commercial contract and labor contract disputes.

DISPUTES INVOLVING MANAGED CARE

The Employment Retirement Income Security Act of 1974 (**ERISA**) regulates employee benefit plans, including managed care health plans. ERISA has been interpreted by the federal courts as preventing patients of health maintenance organizations (HMOs) from suing their HMO for malpractice or breach of contract in cases where their doctor does not perform appropriate treatment because the HMO has rejected the treatment as unnecessary. They may, however, sue the doctor.

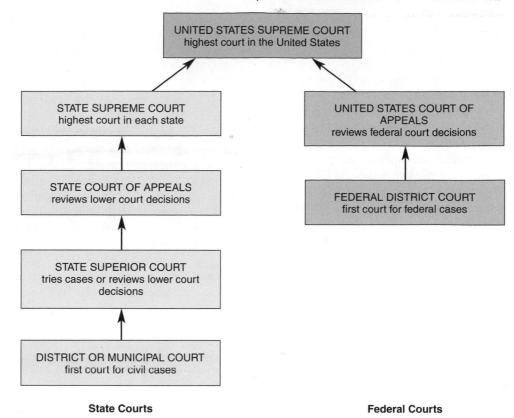

State Courts **Federal Courts**

➤ **Figure 40–2** The appellate process: After the initial trial, appeals usually progress systematically through the higher courts although sometimes one or more levels are skipped. The courts may have different names in some states.

Federally qualified HMOs are required to have a grievance procedure for patients to appeal rejections by HMO personnel of reimbursement for certain treatments. However, they do not have to have an external grievance-review process.

To date, many states have enacted legislation responding to this situation in different ways. As part of what has commonly been called the "Patients' Bill of Rights," legislators attempted in 1999 and 2000 to enact federal legislation to define the relationship among HMOs, doctors, and patients, and provide either a right for patients to sue HMOs when the HMO denies reimbursement for a treatment prescribed by a doctor whom it usually reimburses, or at least an outside review process of the internal HMO grievance process.*

The case of Cynthia Herdrich v. Lori Pegram, M.D., Carle Clinic Association, and Health Alliance Medical Plans, Inc., illustrates the issue clearly.

In 1992, Ms. Herdrich sued Dr. Pegram and the clinic where Pegram worked for negligence, alleging that she suffered a ruptured appendix and peritonitis

due to Dr. Pegram's negligence in failing to provide her with timely and adequate medical care.

In 1994, the court allowed Ms. Herdrich to amend her complaint. In the amended complaint, she added as a defendant Health Alliance Medical Plans, Inc., her HMO, and added a third count, charging the clinic and the HMO with state law fraud for breaching their responsibility to her as a plan beneficiary by depriving her of proper medical care and retaining the savings resulting for their own benefit.

The HMO had the case moved from the state court to the federal district court by arguing that it was not a state fraud case, but a case that should be decided under the ERISA statute.

The new charge in Ms. Herdrich's suit alleged that the owners of the health plan, the clinic, and the clinic doctors who receive financial incentives from the plan for limiting patient care breached their duty to her (and by extension to all plan members) by taking profits from the plan to the detriment of the best possible patient care.

The federal district court dismissed the third count, arguing that neither the clinic nor the HMO was a "fiduciary" to the participants in the plan. A **fiduciary** is a person or organization that has a responsibility to

---

*This legislation is under consideration by Congress again in 2001.

act in the best interests of those for whom it holds a relationship of trust.

Ms. Herdrich won a verdict on the negligence counts and an award of $35,000. She appealed the dismissal of the third count to the U.S. Court of Appeals, which issued its opinion in June, 2000.

In that opinion, the Court of Appeals ruled that the HMO and clinic were indeed fiduciaries to plan members, and ordered the federal district court to hear the third count of Ms. Herdrich's complaints on its merits.

However, the HMO appealed the Appeals Court decision to the U.S. Supreme Court, which reversed the decision without a hearing on September 12, 2000. In its reversal, the Supreme Court found that HMOs are business entities, with a right to make and keep profits, and that they cannot be sued under ERISA.

THE MEDICAL OFFICE AS A BUSINESS

Because a doctor's office is a business, there are a number of regulations that govern its operations and many activities that a medical assistant in charge of administration needs to perform for smooth operations. They fall into the areas of tax, insurance, and regulations.

Traditional Business Forms

Doctors can operate in any number of different business forms for the purpose of federal taxation and liability. The most common are:

Sole proprietor
Partnership
Corporation (doctor-owned)
Corporation (investor-owned)
Collection of personal corporations
Hospital owned (profit or not-for-profit)
Not-for-profit community health center.

Sole Proprietor

A **sole proprietor** is an individual who conducts business without being incorporated. A sole proprietor owns all of the business's assets (or leases them). A sole proprietor may have employees.

A sole proprietor files a federal tax Schedule C form to show the profit or loss from the business after all expenses are accounted for. Sole proprietors do not withhold taxes from any weekly or monthly pay (called a draw) they receive from the business's income; rather, they are responsible for filing quarterly estimates of taxes owed, then finalizing their tax payments by April 15 after the end of the calendar year (all sole proprietors keep tax records based on the calendar year).

A sole proprietorship affords its owner no liability protection; a lawsuit would be filed against the individual, and the individual would be responsible for any judgment or settlement.

Partnership

A **partnership** is a group of two or more individuals who conduct business together without being incorporated and share ownership of the business's assets. Partners split the business's profits after meeting all expenses, and each partner is responsible for meeting his or her own tax liabilities through quarterly estimated taxes and filing a federal income tax Schedule C form in April after the end of the calendar (and tax) year.

Partnership affords no liability protection. In fact, all partners can be held "jointly and severally" liable for the business actions of any partner, although generally not for any negligence or malpractice claim.

Historical Changes and New Forms of Business

Sole proprietors and partnerships were the traditional business forms medical practices took throughout most of the 20th century. Partnerships often hired young doctors on salary for a period of two to five years; then if the partners agreed to admit the new doctor to the partnership, he or she bought a share of the business's assets over time, usually through money withheld from his or her share of the profits. When a partner left, retired, or died, the other partners "bought out" the departing partner or the estate.

Corporation

Tax law changes in the 1970s and 1980s, as well as rapid increases in the cost of malpractice insurance for individual doctors and the ability to buy group liability policies less expensively, encouraged doctors to do one of two things, either to incorporate as a group practice or to become a personal corporation (**PC**). Changes in patient expectations, as well as changes in the method by which doctors are paid—the trend toward managed care—encouraged doctors to form larger groups, either as a group of personal corporations, or through merger of incorporated or unincorporated groups into larger doctor-owned corporations.

Incorporation does three things for a doctor or group of doctors.

First, it adds a layer of liability protection between a malpractice claim and an individual doctor. Only the assets of a corporation—even a personal corporation—are at risk if the corporation pays (and owns) the malpractice insurance policy. Doctors and their families are no longer personally at risk (at least up to the limits of the malpractice insurance coverage).

Second, becoming a doctor-owned corporation allows the business to take advantage of a number of federal tax breaks regarding employee benefits. Two are especially important.

Corporations are allowed to set up retirement plans where corporate executives (doctors) can receive larger benefits packages than other employees; under a sole proprietorship or partnership arrangement, all retirement plan contributions must be an equal percentage of salary. Also, the corporation can pay each doctor a salary, and at the end of the year any excess cash can be paid out as a dividend to shareholders (the doctors) without incurring a Medicare tax liability, since it is not salary.

Third, incorporation makes transfer of ownership easier. Doctors who are owners purchase shares in the corporation, and the annually audited books of the corporation serve as a way to value the corporation's assets. So if a new doctor is accepted as an investor, or if a former investor leaves, retires, or dies, shares are bought or sold at a price that is established in an objective way. There are fewer business hassles over valuation than with partnerships.

Finally, with more doctors owning the buildings they practice in, or a suite of offices in a medical condominium, it is easier for the corporation to own property than for a group of doctors (who may or may not include all of the partners).

Vertical Integration

Increasingly, doctors are working on salary for corporations in which they have no ownership interest. These corporations can either be for-profit or not-for-profit. Many health care providers, such as hospitals, closed-panel HMOs, and community health centers, are corporations.

Since the early 1990s, hospitals have moved to become vertically integrated corporations. This means that they own a top-to-bottom variety of businesses that are able to provide medical services to patients at any stage of that person's need. The move to vertical integration is also an outgrowth of competition for health care dollars in a system that is increasingly being driven by those who pay for care—managed care insurance companies and major employers. These third-party payers are shopping for the best price and the most comprehensive services with the least amount of administrative overhead cost.

To provide this, hospitals are focusing on their businesses as much as or more than their medical care, creating full "supply chains." For instance, a major medical center in a city of 300,000 people might also own two or three community hospitals within 20 miles of the city as well as a variety of formerly independent medical practices in the primary care specialties of pediatrics, internal medicine, family practice, and obstetrics/gynecology.

By owning these practices and community hospitals, the medical center knows that the salaried doctors in its various practices will admit a steady stream of patients to both the community hospitals and the medical center, depending on the level of care they need. By having the doctors from its practice also work part-time at the hospitals, it can reduce the number of full-time doctors at the hospital and, the argument goes, provide patients with a better continuity of care.

Within the city itself, the medical center might establish a set of primary care clinics, located either in a building near the hospital or in offices in neighborhoods around the city. Whether the hospital is part of a for-profit chain of hospitals or is a not-for-profit hospital affiliated with a university or with a religious organization is of no consequence to the doctor or the rest of the medical staff in terms of their employment (although there may be some practical issues, particularly around the issue of birth control and abortion at facilities owned by the Roman Catholic Church).

Compensation

Doctors are paid in one of three ways.

If they are sole proprietors or partners, they take a weekly, biweekly, or monthly draw from which they pay their personal bills, their federal and state income taxes, and their Social Security and Medicare taxes, together known as FICA taxes. They are also responsible for establishing, maintaining, and making payments to their retirement plan, and paying for their own health, life, and disability insurance plans.

If doctors have established a practice as a personal corporation (PC), or if they are shareholders in a doctor-owned corporation, they receive a weekly, biweekly, or monthly salary, just like other employees of the corporation. From this salary, income and FICA taxes are withheld.

Sometimes the corporation pays for health, life, and disability insurance. Other times the individual doctors pay all or part of these fees, having them withheld from their pay, again, like other employees. The same is true for payments into the retirement plan.

At the end of the year, the corporation's stockholders (the doctors) may declare a cash dividend to stockholders. They are personally responsible for any state and federal income taxes that must be paid on these dividends.

Doctors who work for investor-owned corporations such as closed-panel HMOs, for-profit hospitals, or for not-for-profit corporations such as religious- or university-affiliated hospitals or health care centers are also paid a salary, and are sometimes paid an additional productivity bonus. Sometimes these incentives are based on the number of patients seen in a week, month, or calendar quarter, or on how much care the doctor is able to provide in a primary care setting (thus saving the company money by not utilizing specialists). Not-for-profit entities pay productivity bonuses less frequently than for-profit businesses.

Medical assistants are usually paid an hourly wage, and may work either part-time or full-time. When they are full-time employees, they usually receive benefits such as paid vacation, medical insurance, and possibly participation in a retirement savings plan (a 401k or 403b plan, so-called for the section of the federal tax code that describes them). They may also be given some reimbursement for education, uniforms, parking, and possibly other benefits. An office manager may receive a salary and a larger benefits package; but in return, the office manager will probably work longer and more inconvenient hours.

INSURANCE TO PROTECT THE BUSINESS AND EMPLOYEES

A medical assistant who is responsible for business operations must maintain the company's insurance policies. The office manager or medical assistant in charge of administration should also make arrangements to store backup copies of all computerized financial and patient records outside the office so they can be reconstructed if the office is damaged or destroyed.

General Liability Insurance

Any property owner is responsible to the public for injuries that may occur in its space, be it an office, warehouse, or laboratory. Because the medical practice is a business, it has to have general liability insurance, which includes liability against injuries that occur on the property to a patient or a visitor (such as a fall in the waiting room). If the medical practice owns the building, it is also responsible for keeping stairways and corridors well lighted and not blocked, as well as for shoveling snow or ice from the walkways and around the entrances.

Property and Theft Insurance

The practice should carry general business insurance, which covers the practice against theft, fire, water damage, and other damage to the office. A separate policy (or a rider) might be necessary to cover computers and other expensive office equipment.

Criminal Loss Insurance

This insurance protects the business against loss from theft by employees. Policies may name individual employees who have access to company funds; these employees may sometimes be "bonded," meaning that the insurance company performs a background check and agrees to specifically cover any theft of company funds (embezzlement) the individual may carry out. Blanket policies cover any theft by any employee.

Malpractice Insurance

Malpractice insurance covers any judgment or settlement, as well as the cost of any lawsuit, against a charge of professional negligence.

Malpractice insurance is carried by hospitals, clinics, doctors, and other health professionals. Cost of the insurance depends on the medical specialty. Obstetricians and surgeons pay the highest malpractice premiums.

Medical assistants are generally covered by the doctor's policy, but a situation could arise where the medical assistant is named as a defendant in a lawsuit, in which case the medical assistant's interests may differ from the doctor's. A medical assistant can purchase malpractice insurance through one of the field's professional organizations, usually at a reasonable cost.

Workers' Compensation Insurance

Workers' compensation insurance covers the health needs of employees who are injured on the job or develop a job-related medical condition. Employers are required to pay premiums based on previous claims made by their employees. Premiums vary from state to state.

Accounts Receivable Insurance

A medical office can buy insurance to protect against loss of income if accounts receivable ledgers are lost due to fire, flood, other disaster, or theft. It requires the office to adhere to certain rules on safe storage, but it can be valuable protection in the case of unexpected disaster.

FEDERAL LAWS PROTECTING EMPLOYEES

Employee health and safety regulations are issued by the Occupational Health and Safety Administration (OSHA), which was discussed in detail in chapter 6. Other regulations regarding employees are issued by federal and/or state regulatory bodies.

Hiring and Firing

A person who works for an organization that has more than 15 employees is protected by federal Equal Opportunity Employment laws (Title VII of the Civil

Rights Act of 1964) and the Federal Age Discrimination Act of 1967, which make it illegal for a company to discriminate in hiring practices on the basis of race, sex, religion, national origin, or age. Some states also have legislation making it illegal to discriminate on the basis of sexual orientation. Complaints about discrimination in hiring are submitted to the federal Equal Employment Opportunity Commission (EEOC).

Employment policies must treat employees equally and cannot discriminate against any category of employees by paying one group (such as men) more than another group for the same job.

Preemployment Testing

Preemployment testing is only allowed to determine if the potential employee can do the job. The test must test skills and abilities pertinent to the job.

Americans with Disabilities Act

While most of the Americans with Disabilities Act (**ADA**) deals with the necessity of making public accommodations accessible to disabled individuals, part of the law discusses the need for employers to make "reasonable accommodations" to any individual with a physical or mental disability who is otherwise qualified to perform the tasks necessary in the job. The EEOC hears complaints about possible failure to comply with the workplace portions of the ADA.

Family and Medical Leave Act

The Family and Medical Leave Act of 1993 (FMLA) applies to employers with 50 or more employees. Under FMLA, employees are entitled to up to 12 weeks of unpaid leave to accommodate a serious health crisis of any family member, or the birth or adoption of a child. The employee must notify the employer before the beginning of the leave how much of the leave he or she intends to take. After the employee returns, he or she must be given former job and seniority status.

Drug Testing

Preemployment drug tests have been ruled legal for any position. However, random drug tests while on the job are legal only if the public safety outweighs the employee's right to privacy. Medical assistants are far more likely to be performing both preemployment and on-the-job drug tests (especially if they work in an occupational health setting) than they are to be subjected to drug tests themselves. Urine testing for drugs is discussed in chapter 24.

Sexual Harassment

Sexual harassment is defined as any unwanted physical or verbal sexual attention from anyone an individual interacts with on the job that causes that individual to fear reprisal if the attention is refused. Sexual harassment is not flirting. Flirting occurs when both parties engage in actions or verbal exchanges intended to attract or compliment the other. Harassment occurs when one party (most often a man) engages another party (most often a woman) in unwanted comments or physical contact of a sexual nature.

Minimum Wage and Overtime

The federal Fair Labor Standards Act regulates the minimum wage, although some states have a higher minimum wage than that set under federal law. The Fair Labor Standards Act also requires overtime pay of one-and-one-half the employee's regular rate of pay for time worked beyond 40 hours in one week. Professional and supervisory employees are exempt from the law. RNs and office managers are considered professional employees, but medical assistants are not, and are covered by the overtime rules.

Employee Retirement Income Security Act (ERISA)

The Employee Retirement Income Security Act of 1974 (ERISA), discussed above in the context of medical benefits and HMOs, also regulates pensions and other employee benefits. ERISA sets minimum standards for pension plans to prevent unfair denial of pension rights, and states that employee health plans cannot use health status or medical condition to deny certain employees the right to insurance.

STUDENT STUDY PLAN

To reinforce your understanding of the material in this chapter . . .

Complete *Complete* the **Review & Recall** questions.

Discuss *Discuss* the situation in **If You Were the Medical Assistant** with your classmates and answer the questions.

Answer *Answer* the **Critical Thinking Questions** and discuss them with your classmates.

Visit *Visit* the **Web sites** suggested and search for additional Web sites using the **Keywords for Internet Searches**.

Complete *Complete* the exercises in chapter 40 of the **Student Mastery Manual**.

 REVIEW & RECALL

1. Identify five different classifications of law and briefly describe each.

2. Distinguish between criminal law and civil law with respect to the basic definitions, types of offenses, standards of proof, and consequences for an individual if found guilty (or liable) by the court system.

3. For each of the following examples, identify if it is an example of a breach of criminal law, civil law, or contract law, and explain why. Name the type of offense.
   a. Accidentally burning an infant with a heating pad.
   b. Preparing insurance claims that are coded at a higher level than the services provided.
   c. A doctor taking a vacation on a day when he had scheduled a surgery.
   d. Leaving a sponge in a patient's abdomen during surgery.
   e. Impersonating a doctor and prescribing medication.

4. List four defenses to intentional torts and three defenses to unintentional torts.

5. How is arbitration used to settle legal differences? What is the difference between binding and nonbinding arbitration?

6. Describe four ways that a doctor or medical practice can be organized as a business.

7. What differences exist when employees are paid a salary versus an hourly wage?

8. Describe five types of insurance that can protect a medical practice from financial loss.

9. How do the federal Equal Opportunity Employment laws, the Americans with Disabilities Act, and the Family and Medical Leave Act protect the right of employees in a medical office?

10. Describe the purpose and provisions of the Employment Retirement Income Security Act.

 IF YOU WERE THE MEDICAL ASSISTANT

Medication errors occur more frequently than health professionals would like to admit. But many do not lead to lawsuits. Assume that you made a medication error by giving a 45-year-old male patient an intramuscular injection of hydrocortisone sodium succinate 200 mg instead of the 20 mg ordered by the doctor. You notice the error when you return to the medication preparation area. Identify as many reasons as possible why this error may not result in a lawsuit.

CRITICAL THINKING QUESTIONS

1. Discuss the implications of having information about settlements and successful malpractice lawsuits against doctors on the Internet. Do research to find out whether the licensing board in your state makes this information available.

2. Discuss the implications of laws regulating drug testing of employees from the point of view of individuals being tested, and from the point of view of the safety of the general public. Who do you think should have regular drug tests as part of their employment? Why?

3. Call your local board of health to determine exactly what diseases and conditions must be reported in your state and local area. Discuss how you should respond if a person with one of these conditions asked you not to report it.

4. Many states have passed legislation limiting the amount of monetary damages that can be awarded for malpractice lawsuits. Find out what legislation exists in your state. Discuss with your classmates how such limits can affect health care costs, the quality of health care, and the rights of the public.

 EXPLORE THE WEB

INTERNET WEB SITES

Physician licensing boards
www.fsmb.org/members.htm
www.docboard.org

American Health Lawyers Association
www.healthlawyers.org

KEYWORDS FOR INTERNET SEARCHES

Americans with
   Disabilities Act
drug testing
ERISA (Employment
   Retirement Income
   Security Act)

medical law
medical malpractice
preemployment testing

 ANSWERS TO ON THE JOB

1. a. Did the doctor have a duty to the patient?
  b. Was the doctor derelict in performing the duty?
  c. Did the failure to perform the duty adequately cause damage to the patient?
  d. Was the failure to perform the duty the direct cause of damage with nothing else intervening?

2. a. The doctor saw the patient twice in the office, establishing a doctor–patient relationship (if one had not existed before).
  b. The case hinges on what the jury believed about the doctor's decision to delay the diagnostic ultrasound test. Would another doctor in the same geographic area, with the same education and training, have delayed the test?

    An expert witness would probably testify that suspicion of an inflamed appendix requires an immediate test, whereas suspicion of an ovarian cyst does not. Would another doctor have suspected an inflamed appendix? The expert witness for the plaintiff would say Yes; the expert witness for the defense would say Not necessarily.

  c. An inflamed appendix is surgically removed as soon as possible to prevent it from rupturing and causing infection throughout the abdomen. A person's appendix could rupture before surgery even if the condition is diagnosed and treatment is begun promptly. In that case, it would not be the doctor's fault that resulted in the damage.

    In this case, however, the plaintiff can make a good case that prompt diagnosis would have prevented the appendix from rupturing and thus have simplified the treatment, shortened the recovery period, and decreased the risk of severe consequences.

  d. There is no evidence to suggest that anything other than delay caused Mrs. Herdrich's appendix to rupture.

3. a. Was the case filed in a timely manner?
  b. Did any action by the patient contribute to the damage?
  c. Did the patient knowingly fail to follow the doctor's advice?

4. a. The incident occured in March 1991, and the complaint was filed in October 1992, not later than the time allowed by the statute of limitations.
  b. There is no evidence that any action by the patient caused the appendix to rupture; nor did it cause any extra delay.
  c. The patient appears to have followed the doctor's advice.

5. General damages would be calculated on the patient's pain and suffering beyond that expected by a routine appendectomy, and extra medical costs because of the longer hospital stay. These must be costs incurred by the patient (not covered by insurance). Special damages would be calculated related to the cost of traveling farther to the hospital required by the health plan, and loss of income due to prolonged recovery. The actual award in this case was $35,000.

Chapter 41

Managing the Office

Instructional Objectives

After completing this chapter, you will be able to do the following:

1. Define and spell the vocabulary words for this chapter.
2. Place an ad in the classified section of a newspaper seeking to fill a position in the office.
3. Use communication techniques to interview a prospective employee.
4. Create a team environment.
5. Evaluate employee performance.
6. Maintain employee files.
7. Prepare payroll.
8. Manage office-based education or research programs.
9. Create an employee and procedure manual.
10. Create a professional environment.

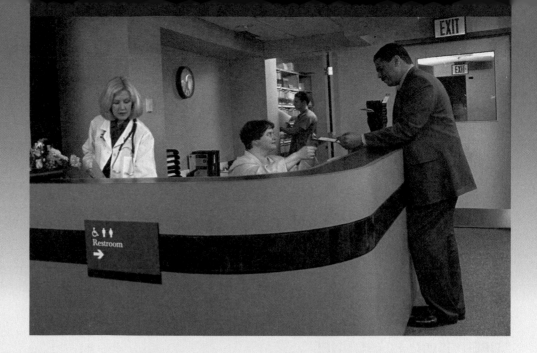

- Management and supervision of employees
- Meeting management
- Employee payroll

VOCABULARY

agenda (p. 974)   exit interview (p. 977)   minutes (p. 974)   procedure (p. 979)
bonded (p. (976)   gross pay (p. 978)   net pay (p. 978)   Social Security tax (FICA) (p. 977)
employee (p. 974)   memorandum (p. 974)   policy (p. 978)   W-4 (p. 976)

In smaller medical offices, a medical assistant may undertake the responsibilities that fall to an office manager in a larger office. These include supervising personnel, preparing an office procedure manual, running office meetings, and managing any research or conferences that the office runs.

SUPERVISING PERSONNEL

Personnel supervision involves more than simply guiding employees through their tasks. **Employees** are people who work for a business or professional service practice such as a medical office. Although him- or herself an employee of the practice, the supervising medical assistant is also responsible for the job performance of other employees whom she or he supervises.

The medical assistant who is in charge of supervising the office's personnel is responsible for managing, recruiting, interviewing, hiring, and evaluating employees. She or he must also manage the office's payroll, set the tone, and create an environment in which employees can work effectively as team members.

Creating an Environment for Teamwork

An environment that supports teamwork is one in which people are willing to help each other out, but are also willing to allow each individual to display her or his particular expertise. A supervisor sets the tone for such teamwork by showing respect for each employee and his or her skills, and pitching in for anyone who needs a little assistance during an especially busy time.

A good supervisor knows how to get the best effort from everyone, and how to make everyone feel appreciated for those efforts.

In a busy office where each person is performing specialized tasks, one of the ways a supervisor promotes teamwork is through regular staff meetings, as shown in Figure 41–1. These meetings should occur often enough—weekly or, at most, monthly—so situations that need to be corrected can be dealt with quickly.

The staff meeting should be used to share information or work through changes in office practice or procedures, to discuss ways to improve patient satisfaction and office performance, and to encourage staff to take advantage of opportunities to improve skills. Some skill improvement efforts can take place in the form of inservice training as part of the staff meetings; others can be opportunities to attend off-site seminars and workshops.

When planning a meeting, a written **agenda** (list of specific items of business to be covered) assists in focusing the meeting and ensuring that all important business is considered in an organized way. One person should be assigned the task of taking **minutes** (a record of the meeting's proceedings).

Written minutes are valuable because they assist individuals who attended a meeting to follow up on suggestions and decisions. The agenda should be prepared in advance; but except for a large, formal meeting, it need not be circulated until the meeting begins. Minutes, however, should be circulated. They should be distributed as soon as possible after the meeting, although they are not usually formally approved until the beginning of the next meeting.

A common way to communicate follow-up with staff is through the use of a **memorandum**, a form of written communication often used within an organization. Although a printed form can be used, it is not difficult to produce a template that can be used frequently in a given office. The title "Memorandum" or "Interoffice Memorandum" should appear at the top of the page.

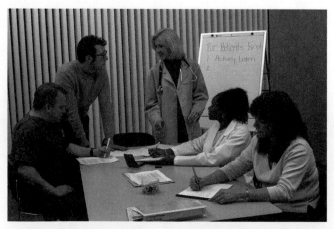

> **Figure 41–1** Focus and group participation allow meeting time to be productive.

INTEROFFICE MEMORANDUM

TO:	All Staff
FROM:	Howard Lawler, MD
DATE:	6/18/XX
SUBJECT:	Introduction of new office manager

- -

It is my pleasure to announce that effective July 1, Diane Janes, CMA will join our staff as office manager. Ms. Janes has had extensive experience in a variety of medical settings. Most recently she has been employed as office manager in a family care practice in Minnesota. With the relocation of her family to Wisconsin, Ms. Janes has become available to join our practice. I hope that you will join me in welcoming Ms. Janes over lunch in the office on Friday, June 28.

➤ **Figure 41–2** An interoffice memorandum is used for communication within a business.

Four headings commonly appear at the top of the memorandum:

- TO:
- FROM:
- DATE:
- SUBJECT:

The headings may be separated from the body of the memorandum by a line that extends from 2 inches to completely across the page. The message should be informative but succinct. The body of the memo is single-spaced. See Figure 41–2 for an example of a memorandum.

Recruiting Personnel

Recruiting personnel means finding the best people to fill the various roles that need to be performed in the office. In a small office, this may mean looking for a medical assistant who is a generalist, able to perform administrative, laboratory, and clinical tasks, and possibly even take on some of the supervision. In a larger office, it may mean looking for more specialized personnel, such as a receptionist, a laboratory technician, and/or a billing coordinator.

Recruitment can be undertaken in a number of ways. One is to ask the people who currently work in the office if they know of anyone with the necessary skills who might want to join the office's team. Another is to place an advertisement in the classified section of the local newspaper. Still another might be to advertise at a local school that trains the kind of personnel you need, or to ask faculty for their recommendations. Large organizations often have a special bulletin board where job openings are posted.

When preparing an advertisement for a newspaper or a job posting board—and when creating a job description for a position—make sure you include the following information:

1. A brief description of the activities that need to be carried out in the job.
2. Whether the job is part-time or full-time; if it is part-time, list specific days and times that must be worked or indicate a flexible schedule.
3. If previous experience is necessary, or desired.
4. Where to respond, and how (i.e., address, post office box, telephone, fax number, and e-mail address).
5. What materials should be sent (i.e., a resume, names of references).
6. The salary, or salary range, or a request for those responding to state what salary they would like.

If you are looking to hire for a newly created position, it is important to do some research first. Call around to other medical practices and see if they have such a position on their team. Ask how much they pay such a person, what kind of credentials the person in the position has, and how difficult it was to hire someone the last time they looked to fill the position.

If the position is for a specialist whose specialty has a national organization, call that organization to find out how to contact educational institutions that train people for the position. Inquire about a salary survey that shows about how much you should expect to pay for someone to fill the position in your region of the country.

Interviewing Prospective Employees

After you have collected responses from people interested in the job, you must interview those candidates who have the best backgrounds—work experience and/or education—combined with the best references. Figure 41–3 shows an interview.

Interviews should be conducted when you will be able to give the prospective employee your full attention. But the interview should occur during working hours, so the potential employee can observe the office's rhythm and see how members of the staff interact with one another. It is also helpful if members of the office team can meet potential colleagues, even if only for a moment.

Before conducting interviews, familiarize yourself with federal, state, and local laws regarding questions that cannot be asked in a job interview. For instance, it is illegal to ask about prior drug use or arrests, or whether a woman of childbearing age is planning to have children.

It is legal to have mandatory preemployment physical examinations and drug tests, but only if they are given to all new employees. It is also legal to perform preemployment background checks of criminal records, as long as all prospective employees are treated the same. If these policies are in effect, prospective employees must be notified at their employment interviews.

In an interview with a potential employee, you should review the individual's resume or list of previous experience, and discuss the job description and what is expected of an individual who fills the job. You should also discuss the potential for improving skills, starting salary, and policies regarding raises and/or bonuses based on both annual review and special recognition.

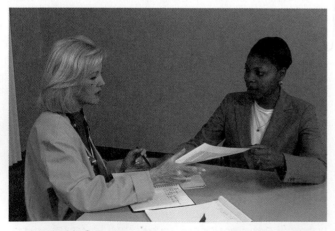

➤ **Figure 41–3** During a job interview, both employer and prospective employee try to get to know each other and determine if they could work together.

If the position requires the individual be licensed or certified, discuss the requirement(s) at this time. If the practice requires employees handling practice funds to be **bonded** (covered by insurance to reimburse the employer in the event of unforeseen financial loss because of the employees actions), inform the employee. A background check is usually required before an employee can be covered under bonding insurance.

If there is a skills test required, the prospective employee should be made aware of that before the interview. The testing should occur after some discussion. If the test can be scored quickly, discussion can continue after the test is taken and scored. If it takes longer to score the test, the test should be taken at the end of the interview.

At the end of the interview, let the potential employee know approximately when you will be making a decision about the best candidate to fill the position.

Hiring

Once you have decided whom to hire for the position, you must call that person to establish whether he or she will take the job. A specific salary is not usually offered until the position is offered. This may require some negotiation. Be sure that you know exactly how much you can offer for the position. You may have to discuss the prospective employee's salary request with one of the doctors. Salary negotiations are often handled in a second interview.

If the applicant accepts the position, establish when that person will begin work and explain the particulars of the orientation period and the probation period. If the position requires licensure or certification, make sure the new hire brings his or her paperwork on the first day of work.

After the individual has agreed to accept the position, you should call others whom you interviewed to thank them for applying, and for the time they took to come in for an interview. These phone calls should be followed up with letters. In addition, you should send a letter to individuals who were not interviewed informing them that the position has been filled and thanking them for their application.

On the first day of work, the new employee must fill out the necessary paperwork, including an Internal Revenue Service form **W-4,** which identifies the number of exemptions claimed for proper income tax withholding. Photocopy any licenses or certificates; put one copy in the employee's personnel file and send file copies to any malpractice and/or other insurers who may need them. Next give the new employee an orientation to the entire office and all of the office personnel, then ask the new employee's immediate supervisor to orient the new employee to the specific tasks he or she will be required to perform.

Evaluating Employees

All employees should receive a regular evaluation. Usually, the first evaluation comes at the end of a new employee's probation period. After that, annual evaluations can be given either on the anniversary of the employee's hiring or shortly before the annual salary adjustment for all employees. Performance evaluations should always occur before a salary change, not shortly after it.

Employees should always be evaluated against objective criteria—meaning a scale that everyone is measured against. They should not be measured against one another, except when the compensation represents a "pay for knowledge" situation (i.e., a person who can perform two sets of tasks well is paid more than a person who can perform only one set of tasks well). However, this is rarely, if ever, the case in a medical office environment.

An employee should be evaluated on the quality and quantity of his or her work, the general appearance he or she presents, dependability and discipline, and willingness and ability to work in a team environment. Any comments, positive or negative, that patients make about particular employees should also be taken into account.

Some offices, in an effort to improve "customer service," give patients cards on which to note if they were treated especially well by a particular member of the staff. Patients drop those cards off in a box at the reception desk on their way out. Such cards, known in the human resource field as "attaboys," have long been popular in retail and other businesses for personnel who deal with customers.

These patient compliments can be totaled up at annual review time. They can also be collected and totaled monthly so that small recognition gifts can be given to the employees who have received the most praise in that period.

Terminating Employees

Employees may leave their employment with a medical practice for a number of reasons. Voluntary termination is relatively simple to document. The employee should be asked to provide a letter of resignation for the personnel file, identifying the final date of employment.

An **exit interview** is usually scheduled to achieve a sense of closure. In this interview, the employee may be asked to describe aspects of the job that have been most and least satisfying, and to make recommendations about ways to improve the job satisfaction of his or her replacement. In addition, the employee may be given a letter of reference to show to prospective future employers.

Involuntary termination is a more difficult matter. If an employee performs poorly, or does not adhere to office policies and procedures, it may be necessary to evaluate the employee before the annual review.

Some companies use a device called "warnings" to notify employees that their performance is not meeting the expected standards. Any discussions with the employee regarding job performance (even though they may be called "verbal warnings") should be documented, and the employee should be asked to sign a statement that he or she has read any performance review or list of behaviors needing improvement.

The employee's signature should only indicate that he or she has been informed. A separate opportunity should also be provided for the employee to document the ways in which he or she does not agree with the performance review. The employee is usually given a specific time period in which to demonstrate improvement. If improvement does not occur, or is not adequate, the employee is dismissed.

For serious violations, such as theft, fraud, breach of confidentiality, and/or unsafe actions that place patients in jeopardy, an employee may be dismissed immediately.

When it is necessary to dismiss an employee, the practice manager should be sure to conduct the interview in private. There is an increasing trend to escort the employee from the premises as soon as he or she has gathered up any personal belongings. This prevents the disgruntled employee from initiating discussions with other staff members and from engaging in any other unacceptable activity in the office out of a desire for revenge.

Once the decision has been made to dismiss an employee, it is important to conduct the interview calmly, without trying to persuade the employee that the decision is a good one. A calm demeanor while informing the employee of the decision, combined with a willingness to listen to the employee's objections without arguing or becoming angry, allows the discussion to end in a reasonable amount of time, with the least unpleasant emotion.

PREPARING PAYROLL

Preparing a payroll is an increasingly complex task. Consequently, many offices—even those that have long done their own payroll—are switching to outside payroll services. The reasons for the complexity are many, including:

Social Security taxes (called **FICA**) (the national program of retirement benefits into which all workers pay 6.2 percent of the first $80,400 in

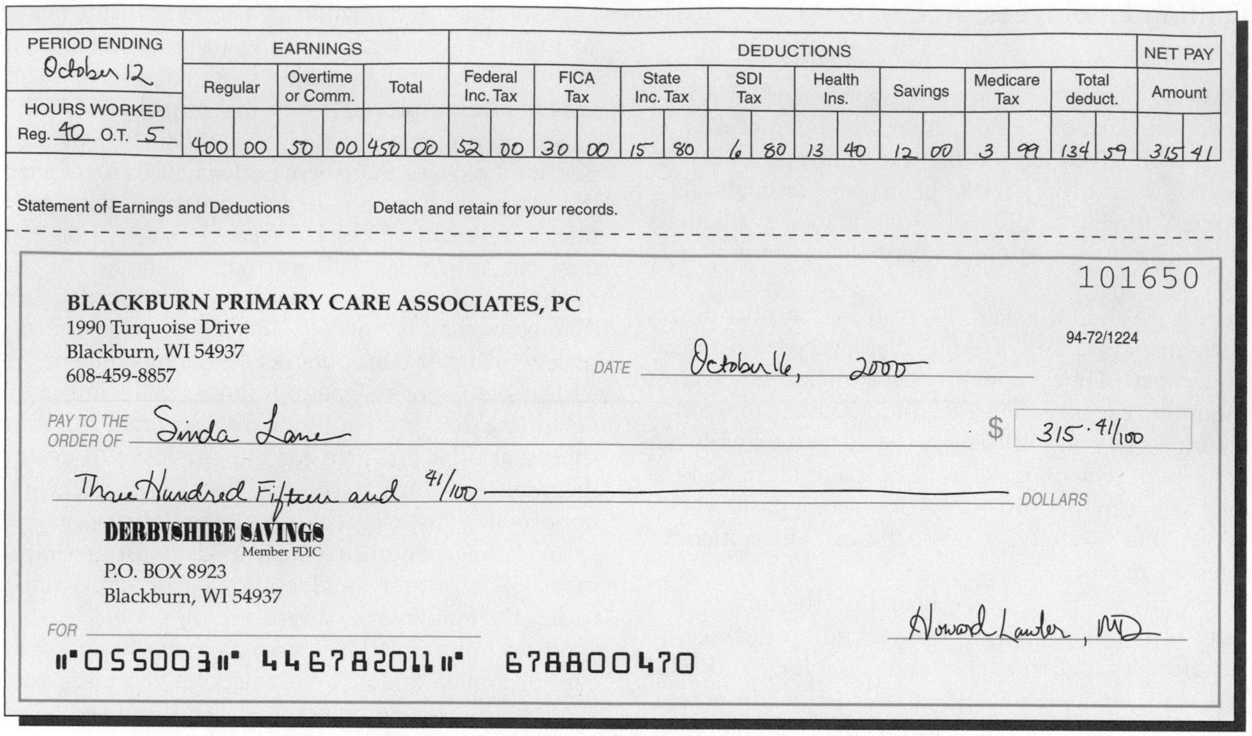

PERIOD ENDING	EARNINGS			DEDUCTIONS									NET PAY
October 12	Regular	Overtime or Comm.	Total	Federal Inc. Tax	FICA Tax	State Inc. Tax	SDI Tax	Health Ins.	Savings	Medicare Tax	Total deduct.	Amount	
HOURS WORKED Reg. 40 O.T. 5	400 00	50 00	450 00	52 00	30 00	15 80	6 80	13 40	12 00	3 99	134 59	315 41	

Statement of Earnings and Deductions   Detach and retain for your records.

- -

101650

BLACKBURN PRIMARY CARE ASSOCIATES, PC
1990 Turquoise Drive
Blackburn, WI 54937
608-459-8857

94-72/1224

DATE _October 16, 2000_

PAY TO THE ORDER OF _Sinda Lane_ _____ $ _315.41/100_

Three Hundred Fifteen and 41/100 _____ DOLLARS

DERBYSHIRE SAVINGS
Member FDIC
P.O. BOX 8923
Blackburn, WI 54937

FOR _____   _Howard Lawler, MD_

⑈055003⑈ ⑆44678201⑈ 678800470

> **Figure 41–4** The employer must keep track of all deductions taken from the employee's paycheck.

income for 2001) are withheld on a lower amount of income than are Medicare taxes. There is no ceiling for Medicare taxes for which workers pay 1.45% of all income.

Many state income taxes phase out at different income levels.

The amount of money withheld from pay to cover the employee's contribution to health insurance may or may not be tax-deductible, depending on whether the office has filed the proper forms.

If the office offers it, employees may or may not be taking advantage of a retirement savings plan by having money withheld from their paychecks before taxes are calculated.

If the office offers it, employees may or may not be taking advantage of pretax withholding for medical expenses not covered by insurance, and for care for children and other dependents.

If the payroll is being done in the office, the supervising medical assistant who does the payroll must gather time sheets or time cards if they are used; calculate wages, taxes, and other deductions for each employee; prepare the checks, such as those seen in Figure 41–4; and record five items of information in the payroll record for each employee:

1. Total wages for the pay period (gross pay).
2. Federal, state, and (sometimes) local income taxes, as well as Social Security and Medicare taxes

3. Other deductions, such as health insurance, uncovered medical expenses, dependent care, and retirement savings
4. **Net pay**, or take-home pay (pay after deductions)
5. **Gross pay**, or total pay, from January 1 to the end of the pay period being recorded.

Before calculating wages, the manager should review time sheets for accuracy. (If a time clock is used, the exact time of clocking in and clocking out is recorded.) If the payroll is being managed by a service outside the office, the supervising medical assistant is only responsible for collecting time sheets and transmitting to the payroll agency each employee's gross pay for the pay period.

The manager can make notes to speak to employees who have been tardy more than occasionally, or who are developing a pattern of absence.

MAINTAINING AND DEVELOPING OFFICE POLICY AND PROCEDURE MANUALS

Effective management of the medical office requires activities to meet all legal requirements and to maintain a high standard of patient care. A guiding principle for management of the office is called a **policy**.

Often an organization formulates its own statements (written policies) to help it adhere to laws or regulations and practice ethically. For example, a medical office might have written policies regarding sexual harassment, confidentiality, and honest and ethical billing, to name just a few.

These are collected in a policy manual, which can easily be reviewed by employees and regulatory agencies. It is the responsibility of the manager to review existing policies and implement changes if necessary.

In order to put policies into practice, an organization utilizes procedures. A **procedure** is a description of the steps to handle a specific situation or perform a certain task. Written procedure manuals are common in large organizations, but they can also benefit smaller medical offices, for several reasons.

They are excellent resources for new employees. They can also provide guidelines and information when a long-term employee suddenly becomes unavailable, either by changing jobs or becoming ill. They encourage office staff to reflect on the methods used to accomplish tasks and examine the reasons for specific actions.

Regular review of procedures is necessary to be sure that they are up-to-date and conform to changes in legal regulations and/or improvements in technology. There may be separate procedure manuals for clinical procedures and administrative procedures. But both are important.

Procedures that facilitate proper functioning of every area of the office should be available. New procedures should be written when they are missing or when new equipment or different supplies have changed how things are done. The manager oversees the job of setting the schedule to review or create procedures, obtaining written or verbal input from those who actually carry out the tasks, and finalizing the written procedures.

After the procedure manual has been created, the manager should encourage all personnel, especially new staff members or those with questions, to utilize the procedure manual as a reference. It often seems easier to ask questions of coworkers with experience, but it increases independence and individual capability if staff are encouraged to refer to comprehensive written procedures.

MANAGING OFFICE-BASED RESEARCH, PRESENTATIONS, AND OTHER PROGRAMS

Increasingly, community-based medical offices are performing research, especially patient-based research for drug companies seeking approval of new medications. In addition, many doctors serve on various committees and commissions, and sometimes are responsible for making presentations or hosting meetings.

Research

In offices where patient-based medication research (called a clinical trial) is being undertaken, the supervising medical assistant is responsible for making sure all records are being maintained properly for the pharmaceutical company or the contract research organization that is managing the clinical trial.

Presentations and Other Programs

For presentations, programs, or meetings that a doctor in the office is running or hosting, the medical assistant who manages the office may be called on to assist in setting up the presentations. This may include arranging for a site, such as a group of conference rooms at a local hotel, function hall, or the local medi-

ON THE JOB

You have just been hired by a practice as a managing medical assistant. The practice has three doctors and eight medical assistants. You want to introduce the team concept and establish professionalism in the environment. Prior to your hiring, the doctors managed the medical assisting staff.

QUESTIONS
1. You have found that there are no employee files. What do you need to have in each file?
2. When you met with individual employees, you discovered that there are no clear job descriptions for employees in this office. How can you help establish these?
3. After meeting with the employees you decide to hire an insurance specialist. What do you need to do next?
4. What information will you go over when you interview prospective employees for the job?

cal school; arranging for audiovisual and other equipment, materials, and refreshments for the meeting; and organizing personnel to help with logistics on the day of the meeting.

The medical assistant may also be asked to prepare an outline of the doctor's talk, and even do some of the background research. This research may be conducted using the office's own medical library or the local medical school or hospital library; it can also involve using an Internet search engine to find material from medical Web sites to which the office subscribes, medical journal archives, or medical organization libraries.

STUDENT STUDY GUIDE

To reinforce your understanding of the material in this chapter . . .

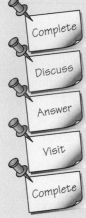

Complete the **Review & Recall** questions.

Discuss the situation in **If You Were the Medical Assistant** with your classmates and answer the questions.

Answer the **Critical Thinking Questions** and discuss them with your classmates.

Visit the **Web sites** suggested and search for additional Web sites using **Keywords for Internet Searches.**

Complete the exercises in chapter 41 of the **Student Mastery Manual.**

✔ REVIEW & RECALL

1. What information needs to be included in a classified employment ad?

2. What type of questions should be asked when interviewing a potential employee?

3. What type of questions cannot be asked when interviewing a potential employee?

4. What type of information must a new employee complete?

5. What are some of the purposes of having a staff meeting?

6. How is an employee evaluated?

7. What responsibilities does the medical assistant have to prepare payroll?

8. What is the purpose of written policy and procedure manuals in the medical office?

9. What types of activities would the medical assistant be expected to perform if the medical practice or one of the doctors hosts a program or meeting?

✔ IF YOU WERE THE MEDICAL ASSISTANT

You have been asked to organize a meeting for local office managers and doctors to explore the services offered by a new HMO that plans to expand into your area. Include the arrangements, time frames, and other activites that will make the meeting a success. Make a list of the tasks you will have to complete in order to plan a successful meeting. Arrange the list to identify those tasks that must be completed before details can be finalized or other tasks can be completed.

CRITICAL THINKING QUESTIONS

1. Two of your staff are having personality differences, which has become evident to patients. As the manager for the office, how should you handle this conflict?

2. You have been interviewing prospective employees for the administrative part of the practice. The responsibilities include creating and processing all written correspondance. What types of questions should you pose in the job interview?

3. Obtain the classified section of your local newspaper. Identify at least five advertisements that refer to positions in a medical office. Discuss how complete and informative the advertisements are, and identify how they could be improved.

4. Create an advertisement for a job opening for a clinical medical assistant at Blackburn Primary Care Associates.

EXPLORE THE WEB

INTERNET WEB SITES

Healthcare Information and Management System Society
www.himss.org

Medical Group Management Association
www.mgma.com

The American Academy of Medical Management
www.epracticemanagement.org

KEYWORDS FOR INTERNET SEARCHES

medical employee management
medical practice management

ANSWERS TO ON THE JOB

1. Each employee file needs to contain a photocopy of a completed W-4 form, application for employment, and current creditials, such as a license or certificate. The folder should also contain a copy of each annual review and a written summary of any disciplinary actions.

2. To develop job descriptions, you should first establish a list of job titles. After you have decided what the different jobs in the office are, you can enlist the help and cooperation of your staff in developing job descriptions. Ask them to write up a statement of what their job is, and what duties they are responsible for. Based on this information, you can develop formal job descriptions.

3. To hire an insurance specialist, you need to place an ad in the newspaper, list the experience required, education required, and job expectations. After receiving the resumes of prospective applicants, you interview the most qualified candidates.

4. When interviewing prospective employees, you need to review their previous work experience, educational qualifications, credentials and certificates, the responsibilities of the job they have applied for, the salary range, and the potential for growth or advancement offered by the position.

Chapter 42

Biomedical Ethics

Instructional Objectives

After completing this chapter, you will be able to do the following:

1. Define and spell the vocabulary words for this chapter.
2. Differentiate between deontological, teleological, and combination theories of ethics.
3. Discuss the relationship between law and ethics.
4. Correlate the concept of rights to specific rights in health care.
5. Correlate the concept of duties to the actions expected of health professionals.
6. Describe six steps that may be used to make ethical decisions.
7. Discuss several ways that ethical decisions may be made by individuals and/or groups.
8. Describe potential areas of conflict related to reporting health professionals who are dishonest or impaired.
9. Describe the process for scientific research and measures to protect the rights of research subjects.
10. Identify potential areas of ethical conflict related to genetic engineering.
11. List at least four ethical issues raised by abortion and the abortion pill.
12. Discuss the ethical problems of different types of infertility treatments.
13. Explain how individuals can preserve their right to make decisions about health care, even if their medical condition prevents actual participation in the decision-making process.
14. Describe the extent to which individuals are permitted to authorize treatment or procedures that might hasten their death.
15. Describe ethical implications for individuals and groups that result from scarce medical resources.

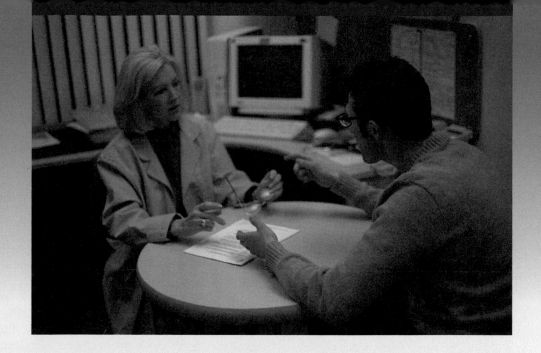

- Perform within ethical and legal boundaries
- Principles of medical ethics

- Ethical decision making

VOCABULARY

autonomy (p. 986)
beneficence (p. 987)
biomedical ethics (p. 984)
deontological (p. 985)
duty (p. 987)

ethics (p. 984)
etiquette (p. 985)
fee splitting (p. 991)
fidelity (p. 987)
gene therapy (p. 993)

ghost surgery (p. 991)
in vitro fertilization (p. 995)
nonmalfeasance (p. 987)
recombinant DNA techniques (p. 993)
right (p. 986)

surrogate (p. 995)
teleological (p. 985)
utilitarianism (p. 985)
veracity (p. 985)

INTRODUCTION TO ETHICS

What do we mean by ethics?

Ethics is the attempt to establish what is right and what is wrong by using systematic thinking. As an academic discipline, it is a branch of philosophy. Philosophy, in turn, uses logic as well as reason that is influenced by, but not confined to, any particular religious teaching or social ideology.

Biomedical ethics, or bioethics, looks at issues related to the science and practice of medicine and biomedical research and, using the principles of ethics, tries to determine what is proper and what is not.

Why do medical assistants need to study ethics? Although ethics is an abstract discipline, and medical assisting is firmly grounded in practice and procedure, medical assistants should study ethics for a number of reasons.

First, it is an important part of an individual's education to develop the intellectual skills to analyze complex problems and justify the choices made in particular situations. In the case of ethics, the choice is between alternative courses of action that have moral and social consequences.

Second, as society has become increasingly complex, average citizens are more aware that choices affect not only people living now, but those who will live in the future. People hesitate to allow only elected and appointed officials to deal with these choices. Learning about ethics and social issues may help ordinary people act to achieve ethical goals.

There is also a greater sense of world unity, sometimes called globalism, such that many individuals feel some level of responsibility for all human beings, and indeed for all living beings on the earth.

Third, in the specific realm of medicine and science, more sophisticated medical treatment and new technologies are constantly becoming available. However, society does not have unlimited resources to provide everything to everyone, even in the developed world. There is a need to make informed choices about what care will be provided to whom, and when, rather than simply responding to special interests.

Scientists are excited by the research itself, and business people see the opportunity to make money using these new technologies. But some groups are resistant

to change, and others question how such costs can be justified when so few people might be helped by each new technology.

Fourth, every year new biomedical research makes it possible to do more things that the world has no previous experience with. People need (1) to be able to think about the consequences; (2) to make decisions about what is the right (or wrong) way to go; and (3) to decide how to proceed. Society must have informed citizens who can analyze issues and guide the future. Within the health care system, health care workers, including medical assistants, need skills in considering ethical questions in order to improve health care for individuals and society.

Ethics Before the Modern Era

Ethical guidelines, or statements about how a person ought to behave, have existed for centuries. The sacred texts of various world religions contain ethical discussions, usually as they relate to broad areas of social behavior. Throughout much of history, religion and government were closely intertwined, and most societies were influenced by one dominant religion.

Guidelines for the practice of medicine have also existed for centuries. The earliest surviving written description of expected behavior for doctors is part of the Code of Hammurabi. Hammurabi was a Babylonian king who ruled from about 1792 to 1750 B.C.E. During his reign, the laws of Babylon, including those related to conduct of doctors, were carved on a stone column.

The Hippocratic Oath, discussed in detail in Chapter 4, which dates to around 400 B.C.E., is another surviving formulation of guidelines for the behavior of ancient doctors.

Theories of Ethics

Various theories of ethics have been developed in all cultures to guide the beliefs of members of a particular society about what kind of behavior is right and wrong. Ethical theories affect every part of the social structure. In modern Western societies, ethical theories are divided into three major categories:

CODES OF ETHICS

The word code comes from the Latin word *codex*, derived from the word for tree trunk. Trees are the source of boards, which were used to write on after stone, and later of paper used to produce writing tablets, manuscripts, and finally books.

Code can mean a set of symbols that stand for something else, such as Morse code, a system of dot-and-dash electrical impulses sent over wires that, when strung together, can be read as the letters in the alphabet. DNA is also called a code because it is a series of chemicals that can be arranged in various configurations to determine what proteins a cell will produce.

Another meaning of code is a set of principles that a group of people adhere to, such as a code of conduct for students at a school or college. The Code of Hammurabi, a set of ancient Babylonian laws, has sections that are related to modern ethical codes, such as those published by the American Medical Association (AMA) or American Association of Medical Assistants (AAMA), which describe principles of behavior for the professions of doctors and medical assistants, respectively.

1. Deontological theories
2. Teleological theories
3. Combination theories

Deontological Theories

One approach to thinking of ethics is to define rights and duties for an individual. These deontological theories come from the Greek stem *deont*, meaning that which is binding or needful.

Deontological theories identify underlying rules that determine how people should behave, and require the individual to make moral decisions largely without respect to the consequences. The social order depends on the expectation that everyone will follow such rules. The Chinese philosopher Confucius (551–469 B.C.E.) provided one of the most important influences on Chinese society, and indirectly on almost all Asian societies. He asserted that man's behavior must be moral in order to harmonize with the balance of forces within the universe.

Immanuel Kant (1724–1804), a German philosopher, is one of the best known European thinkers to follow this approach. He emphasized the inherent dignity of each individual, which entitles him or her to respect. In Kant's eyes, duties, such as **veracity** (telling the truth), are absolute; deviations, even the telling of white lies to ease social interactions, are always wrong.

Teleological Theories

While deontological theories begin with absolutes, **teleological** (from the Greek *teleos*, meaning complete or final) theories of ethics begin with the consequences of choices.

One of the best known of these theories is **utilitarianism**, developed by Jeremy Bentham (1748–1831) and John Stuart Mill (1806–1873), two English philosophers. The theory of utilitarianism, defines the best action as that which does the most good for the largest number of people. If there is more than one goal, the best action is the one that meets the most goals.

Applied strictly, this theory argues that the suffering of any individual is unimportant when compared to the good of the society in general. Problems arise with this way of thinking because the consequences of actions cannot always be accurately predicted, and because there may be a lack of consensus as to what constitutes a desirable outcome, or what constitutes greatest good.

Combination Theories

Combination theories consider the duties or virtues of the individual while projecting the consequences both for the individual and for society. In these theories, individuals consider rules for behavior, but they also explore the possible consequences when making decisions about what is the right thing to do in a given situation.

Most modern discussions of medical ethics fall into this combination category, although the particular emphasis varies, depending on the particulars of the problem being explored and the personal outlook of those participating.

Relationship Between Law and Ethics

Within a democracy, society tolerates a wide range of beliefs about what is moral, and uses the democratic process to create rules and laws that regulate public behavior. This process allows for change and flexibility because laws are continually reviewed through the judiciary process.

It is important to remember that society's beliefs about right and wrong precede laws and tend to influence their interpretation. Currently, opinions change rapidly, and accepted beliefs are questioned, putting considerable stress on the social structure.

There is also a wide diversity of beliefs about normal, acceptable behavior, sometimes called **etiquette**, or manners. Breaches of etiquette are far less important than failure to adhere to high ethical standards; they pose no true threat to the integrity of an individual or society. However, individuals may have just as strong an emotional reaction to what they see as bad manners as they would to a true ethical breach.

In the context of the medical office, an individual may feel that, even though the level of care being provided is satisfactory, being rushed by the doctor and treated "as a number, not a name" by the front-office staff is being treated without dignity, and therefore a reason to change providers.

ETHICAL CONCEPTS

Current thinking about biomedical ethics identifies several rights (very strong claims) for patients and duties (requirements) for the institutions and individuals who provide health care. There are several sources for these ideas, including:

Individuals who have developed ethical theories
Religious traditions
The social and belief systems
The Declaration of Independence (life, liberty, and the pursuit of happiness)
The U.S. Constitution and the Bill of Rights.

Rights

A **right** is a claim that is expected to be honored. It is stronger than a wish or a need.

The early leaders of the American government believed in natural rights; that is, rights of the individual granted by God (or nature) that are so important that any government has a duty to preserve and maintain them. These include:

1. Right to life
2. Right to privacy
3. Right to autonomy
4. Right to the means to sustain life

Life

One of the rights mentioned in the Declaration of Independence is the right to life.

Since the 1970s, the term "right to life" has come to be associated with the movement against abortion. But in a broader context, it reflects the belief that human beings may not kill others. The belief in the right to life is found in all major religions.

The right to life has many implications for medicine. Historically, doctors and other health care workers may not harm patients because this may threaten their lives. They may not assist with suicide; this is expressly stated in the Hippocratic Oath. In the United States today, however, many individuals want some control

over death, including the choice of suicide assisted by their doctor. The Hippocratic Oath also states that a doctor should not perform an abortion, but doctors' professional organizations no longer prohibit performing abortion.

Two important areas of conflict appeared in the middle of the 20th century.

First, advances in medical care made it possible to keep people alive who could not recover their health; sometimes, this sustaining of life came at the cost of prolonged suffering.

Second, the absolute right to life of an unborn fetus conflicts with the right of a woman to control her own reproductive capacity by using birth-control methods, including abortion if necessary, to control the size of her family, or employing artificial conception methods to become pregnant. Many women and their doctors have come to believe they have a right to make decisions related to reproduction, including using available technology, as they see fit.

Privacy

The Supreme Court has ruled that there is an implicit right to privacy in the Bill of Rights, specifically in the Fourth Amendment. A series of court decisions affirming a woman's right to use mechanical birth control and to have an abortion hinged on justices' perceiving this right to privacy.

Patient confidentiality, which has been upheld by courts, is another manifestation of the right to privacy. Patient confidentiality is discussed in detail in chapter 4.

Autonomy

Currently, medical ethics takes the position that an individual has the right to **autonomy**, which means the right to make decisions about his or her health care according to individual values and concerns, without constraint or coercion from others. This right is preserved even when the individual's decisions do not match the value of the medical community or the individual doctor. The right of autonomy is the basis for informed consent.

In order to support this right, health care professionals must provide complete information as a basis for patient decision making. And the patient must have the mental capacity to reason and consider alternatives. Because of this, the law limits the autonomy of children, or individuals with decreased mental capacity such as the mentally retarded, those acting under the influence of drugs or alcohol, those suffering senile dementia, and those experiencing transitory mental illness.

Respect for autonomy does not derive from the Hippocratic Oath. Rather, it comes from the thinking of

European philosophers such as Immanuel Kant and John Locke.

Means to Sustain Life

Every society must grapple with how to equitably distribute goods and services to its citizens, and how to regulate that distribution over time.

This is not a problem when the supply is adequate, or when no one wants the item in question—when supply is greater than demand. For instance, in ordinary circumstances the supply of oxygen is more than adequate to meet the needs of the entire population.

When the amount of a particular resource is less than the desire for that resources—when supply is less than demand—problems develop. In this case, resources are said to be scarce, and the society's organizing model—government—must determine who will have access to the scarce resource.

At a minimum, every individual should have access to what is necessary to sustain life and preserve human dignity—enough to meet the needs for the first two levels of Maslow's hierarchy. Consideration of justice in distribution and access is especially important in social and political movements. Any society must find ways to respond to need while also rewarding contribution and providing for stability within the social system.

Currently, in the allocation of health care resources in the United States, it is increasingly difficult to determine what is necessary for everyone, given the availability to a large number of expensive procedures, many of which have limited expectations for success.

Health care economists and nongovernmental organizations such as the World Health Organization are constantly engaging in this discussion, along with experts in biomedical ethics. For instance, for the same financial cost as one heart transplant, with its attendant postsurgical care and need for immunosuppressive drugs for years to come, thousands of children could receive basic immunizations.

Duties

A **duty** is a commitment to act in a certain way, based on religious beliefs, moral principles, or a particular professional code of conduct. There are five main duties of a health care professional:

1. Do no harm
2. Do the best possible
3. Be faithful to reasonable expectations
4. Tell the truth
5. Give each person a fair share.

Do No Harm

The concept of **nonmalfeasance** means, first of all, doing no harm in any treatment given. This duty is found in the Hippocratic Oath. It is not taken in a literal sense, because many treatments can have adverse effects. Rather, it is taken to mean that medical benefits should outweigh adverse effects.

This concept especially influences scientific research. Guidelines for ethical research not only require informed consent, but also restrict research with possible serious effects to those patients whose conditions are so serious that doing nothing is likely to be as dangerous as the treatment or procedure being studied.

Do the Best Possible

The concept of **beneficence**, doing the best possible, is seen in some concepts of ethics as a separate duty, while in others it is considered an extension of doing no harm. It is often difficult to pinpoint exactly what harm and good are; this may vary with a particular individual's viewpoint.

Be Faithful to Reasonable Expectations

The concept of **fidelity**, being faithful (in the case of medical practice, faithful to reasonable expectations), comes from the Latin term *fides*, which means faithful. Although patient expectations vary, there is general agreement that a patient can reasonably expect to be treated with dignity; treated by individuals who honor their agreements; treated by competent providers; and treated by individuals who adhere to the ethical standards of their profession, to statutory law, and to accepted medical and scientific practice.

Tell the Truth

The concept of veracity has increased in importance since the 19th century. Veracity is not found in the Hippocratic Oath. It is seen as a proactive duty—doctors and other health care professionals must provide truthful information without having to be asked. It is a tenet of modern science that scientific knowledge belongs to all: Results of experiments must be accurate and reviewed by other scientists to see if the results can be replicated, then published for the benefit of all.

Give Each Person a Fair Share

The concept of justice provides that each individual is given his or her due and deserves a fair share of resources. However, there is often an underlying feeling that an individual must contribute or bear a portion of the burden before being allowed to get certain resources.

Justice in the context of medical practice appears not only in terms of distribution of medical resources, but also in the belief in the right to compensation if a mistake is made.

Many Americans believe that everyone is entitled to the benefit of health insurance. But as a nation, we have not been able to agree on a means to provide universal health insurance. We try to provide emergency care to all, resulting in situations where people without insurance for various reasons need to wait until their health status deteriorates to the level of an "emergency" before they can receive care. To many, this seems not only unfair, but a poor way to manage health care resources as well.

Deciding what is "fair" is often a matter of the situation. In the United States, the tendency is to believe in "first come, first served." But in an emergency room, serious conditions must take precedence.

Ethical Conflict

Many issues become controversial when there is a disagreement within society about the relative hierarchy of certain rights and duties.

The issues surrounding infertility, contraception, and abortion are prime examples. In regard to pregnancy, some people feel that the duty to follow divine law takes precedence over an individual's right to autonomy, which would allow the use of "unnatural" means of preventing conception and becoming pregnant. And some argue that the fetus's right to life outweighs the woman's right to privacy in determining—with her doctor—the proper course of her medical care.

Making ethical decisions involves measures to respond to conflict between different values and their relative importance.

PROCESS USED TO MAKE ETHICAL DECISIONS

A person or group of people can confront a decision that has ethical implications in a situation where different choices carry moral weight. In this case, the decision may be difficult because different values conflict. In order to decide on a course of action, it is helpful to clarify the conflict and make a thoughtful choice.

A six-step process can be used to make sure that actions are well considered and in accordance with beliefs about what is right and wrong, rather than simply impulse reactions.

1. Gathering information
2. Identifying conflicting values, rights, duties, and desires
3. Determining the relative value of conflicting claims
4. Exploring alternatives
5. Choosing one alternative and justifying it
6. Implementing the decision.

Gathering Information

Information that needs to be gathered includes background about the situation; facts related to the specific medical problem; information about the people involved, their knowledge of the situation, and their mental capacity; and the impact of any laws or institutional policies that relate to the situation.

Identifying Conflicting Values

A conflict does not always involve lofty values. It may be as simple as one person's wish not to cause problems, to save time, or to avoid a hassle. However, this desire may conflict with professional duties or with another individual's right.

If a medical assistant is working in a facility that does not always follow established procedures—for example, does not always run controls for lab tests—the desire to go along with coworkers and avoid conflict may be strong; however, the duty to act with fidelity is not being met. The medical assistant may him- or herself be performing the needed controls, but the knowledge that others are not doing so creates a conflict between reluctance to violate the autonomy of a coworker and the duty of fidelity to patients.

Determining Relative Importance of Conflicting Claims

To determine the relative importance of these conflicting claims, an individual needs to clarify his or her goals and weigh the conflicting values.

In the situation discussed above, the patient's right to have tests performed correctly seems to outweigh the reasons for not performing controls (expense, time, and so on). In more complex situations, two or more positions may have almost equal weight.

It is important to remember that when values conflict, an individual or group makes a decision about importance that is valid within its own context, but may not conform with the values of other individuals or groups.

For example, in the case of abortion, some people believe that the right of a fetus to life outweighs all other rights. Others believe that a woman's right to autonomy in medical decisions about her body, and the consequences to a child of being unwanted, diminish or outweigh the absolute right to life, at least in the early stages of a pregnancy.

Exploring Alternatives

Once it has been established which values are more important, it is important to consider the possible outcomes of actions that may be taken. It is helpful to identify as many courses of action as possible, predict the consequences of each action, and project how dif-

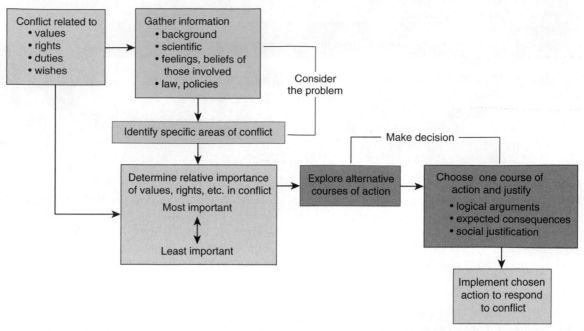

> ➤ **Figure 42–1** Process to decide a course of action when rights, duties, and/or personal wishes conflict.

ferent goals would be met or not met by following each possible course of action.

Choosing and Justifying One Alternative

Conflicting claims require choices. It is important to analyze hypothetical situations in detail in a classroom situation in order to construct some sort of personal framework for ethical decisions; once on the job, there is often little time to analyze each situation individually.

In the end, there are four ways to justify a decision.

1. By presenting logical arguments—deductions based on facts
2. By social justification—consideration of the larger consequences to society.
3. By projection of consequences—imagining what might happen if a given alternative is chosen
4. By refuting alternative claims—stating explicitly why alternative choices have less merit than the one you have chosen.

If it is possible to select any alternative that seems comfortable, or "right," the choice to do nothing becomes a chosen alternative rather than simply the avoidance of a decision.

See Figure 42–1 and On the Job.

Implementing the Decision

The final step in this process is to put the ethical decision into action.

WHO MAKES ETHICAL DECISIONS?

An ethical decision can be made by one of four parties:

1. An individual
2. A peer group
3. An ethics committee
4. Society, through the law.

Individual

Often, the person who is responsible for the consequences makes the decision. In a medical office, the medical assistant refers decisions related to patient care to the doctor.

This means that the medical assistant cannot ethically withhold from the doctor information given by the patient related to medical condition. Even if the medical assistant does not agree with how the doctor is managing a patient's care, the medical assistant cannot ethically (or legally) suggest another treatment plan for the patient.

On the other hand, the medical assistant makes decisions related to his or her own actions. This was discussed in chapter 4, in the situation when Stacy, the medical assistant, refused to discuss Brittany's medical problems with the office receptionist.

Consensus, Peer Support

When a decision affects more than one person, there is often a need for discussion and agreement from all parties. For example, when an office or organization changes policy, each department affected must agree to the change.

ON THE JOB

Videotape: *Legal, Ethical, and Professional Concepts, "Bulemia"*

The patient, a 17-year-old high school student named Brittany, is being interviewed by Stacy, a medical assistant at Blackburn Primary Care Associates. Brittany weighs 121 pounds today, but has lost 9 pounds since the last visit and 18 pounds in the last year. Stacy has been asking Brittany questions about her diet and eating habits. Brittany has admitted that sometimes she vomits after she eats.

Stacy: Do you eat a lot of food and then that's when you find yourself vomiting?
Brittany: Yeah, I guess so. You're not going to tell my parents, right? Or the doctor?
Stacy: Well, tell your parents what? What I'm trying to do is to get at what might be the problem here. What I think the problem is, is that maybe you're worried about your weight too much. And I'm just concerned. Because, you know, your weight loss, that's 18 pounds since about a year ago, that's just not healthy. Is there something going on you want to share with me?
Brittany: No.
Stacy: No? How about, have you ever made yourself vomit?
Brittany: Oh, yeah. That's usually how it happens.
Stacy: That's usually how it happens . . . you just go in right after you eat your meal, and kind of you just help it along, or it just comes up on its own?
Brittany: I just go to the ladies room after I eat.

After more discussion, Brittany says directly, "Don't tell the doctor. Don't tell my parents. I know they'll kill me." The questions below explore how Stacy might decide what to do in this situation.

QUESTIONS
1. Identify information that Stacy must have to make a decision about what she should do. Use the chart in Figure 42–1 to identify the areas of information to explore.
2. Identify the areas of conflict in this situation between rights, duties, and wishes of the people involved.
3. Using the values, right, duties, and wishes you identified in this situation, place them in order of importance, with the most important first and the least important last. What order do you think Stacy would place them in?
4. What should Stacy do?

A medical practice can look to a professional organization for guidance. Medical associations publish guidelines related to medical ethics. In addition to the basic principles of medical ethics (discussed in chapter 4), there is an entire document that describes medical ethics in detail: *Current Opinions of the Council on Ethical and Judicial Affairs* by the American Medical Association (AMA), issued in June 1996 and available on the AMA Web site.

Professional associations for medical assistants can also be a source of information and guidelines. (See the AAMA code of ethics, in chapter 4.)

The box on page 991 identifies some activities that have been identified as unprofessional for doctors by doctors' professional organizations. For problems affecting the medical office, a discussion by all office staff may assist in decision making. An office staff meeting is shown in Figure 42–2.

Ethics Committee

Hospitals and other health care institutions often form committees to review specific cases and decide on a course of action, and to establish institutional policies for situations that typically occur. The doctors in a medical office may be members of such ethics committees through hospitals or medical schools with which they are affiliated.

Unprofessional Conduct for a Doctor

Whether or not illegal, many activities are considered unprofessional for doctors, and by extension for their employees.

1. Payment for referrals to other doctors, laboratories, treatment centers, or pharmacies.

    Although doctors often make specific referrals, it is unethical for them to have arrangements to receive payments for those referrals, and especially to refuse to refer a patient unless a payment is made. This practice is sometimes called **fee splitting**. It is also unethical to charge a patient simply for being admitted to a hospital, without any other service being provided.

2. Prescribing medication or diagnostic tests for financial gain rather than because of the patient's need for the test.

    Although doctors may have financial interests in pharmacies or laboratories and may charge for diagnostic and lab tests performed in the office, it is considered unethical for a doctor to pressure patients to use the facility in which he or she has a financial interest. It is also unethical to prescribe medication, tests, or procedures that are not medically necessary. Billing an insurance company for unnecessary procedures is illegal.

    Doctors should not accept gifts from pharmaceutical companies or medical equipment manufacturers or suppliers in return for promoting the company's product or prescribing only the company's drug. They may accept inexpensive or educational gifts with the understanding that they have no obligation to promote the product.

3. Failing to disclose certain information to a patient.

    A doctor may not allow another doctor or surgeon to perform surgery without informing the patient. This is sometimes called **ghost surgery**. The patient has the right to know who is performing a procedure.

    A patient undergoing artificial insemination is entitled to know the source of sperm used for the procedure (husband, sperm bank, paid donor), and the doctor may not substitute sperm without informing the patient.

4. Failing to practice medicine appropriately.

    A doctor should not practice medicine under the influence of mind-altering drugs, alcohol, or any prescription medication that may impair mental function, alertness, or physical performance.

    A doctor should not allow an unlicensed person to practice medicine.

    A doctor should order a consultation for any medical problem that is beyond his or her personal experience and expertise. For example, a gynecologist should not treat a patient for renal failure.

5. Charging for missed appointments, or charging interest on unpaid bills, without informing patients that such a procedure is in effect.

    Patients must be notified about any policy related to charges for missed appointments or appointments canceled without 24 hours notice.

    Patients must be notified about interest charges on past-due accounts, in accordance with state laws.

    Information about a patient's medical care should not be withheld from another medical facility just because the patient has an outstanding bill.

6. Putting a patient at risk of HIV infection, or refusing to treat a patient who is HIV-positive.

    A doctor, or any other health care worker, who is HIV-positive, should not perform a procedure that might transmit the virus to a patient.

    A doctor who is qualified to treat a patient should not refuse service simply because the person is HIV-positive. The doctor can limit his or her practice to certain medical specialties, and can refuse to accept specific types of insurance.

7. Engaging in a sexual relationship with a patient.

    Something inherent in the relationship between two individuals in which one is perceived to be more influential than the other puts pressure on the "weaker" party to please the more powerful party. Because this makes it difficult to determine if consent is freely given, such a relationship should never be sexual in nature. Sexual relationships between professionals and the people they serve (e.g., doctor–patient, attorney–client, teacher–student) are thus considered unethical and unprofessional.

Law/Society

Society attempts to regulate behavior by passing laws. But on many issues, society is divided as to the proper ethical course. There may be no specific law, or the law may not reflect the ethical beliefs of all members of the society, as in the case of abortion.

Scientific discoveries introduce new ethical problems, and laws that respond to them may emerge slowly and be subject to review by state and federal courts.

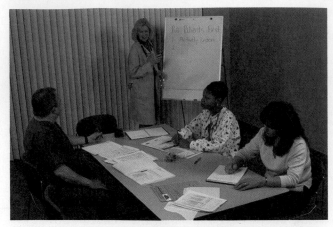

➤ **Figure 42–2** An office staff meeting may provide a forum for discussion of ethical questions.

INFORMING ON UNETHICAL COWORKERS (WHISTLEBLOWING)

Sometimes, doing the right thing and maintaining a friendship come into conflict. It should be a fairly easy decision to alert the proper authorities—a supervisor, an employer, or a regulatory agency—in the case of a colleague who is incompetent, impaired, or acting in an illegal manner. The decision becomes more difficult if the behavior in question is more a case of personal ethics.

Having a strong sense of personal ethics and maintaining ethical behavior can make this decision easier. In addition, some organizations—such as the AMA—make part of their ethical code the obligation to report colleagues who are violating ethical standards.

The term that has come to be used for going around employers to report unethical or illegal behavior in one's job is "whistleblowing." Congress has enacted laws to protect whistleblowers from retribution by employers, including firing, demotion, or other loss of privilege.

CURRENT ISSUES

Scientific research and discoveries often raise ethical questions, as do many new treatment protocols. Society must first decide what is right and wrong before laws can be passed to regulate conduct. When social attitudes and values change, new laws are passed. If a sharp division remains in society regarding an ethical issue, there is controversy about the law and legal challenges from many sides of the issues.

The remainder of this chapter considers ethical questions in five areas:

1. Research
2. Genetic engineering
3. Reproductive rights
4. The right to die and the right to refuse treatment
5. Scarce medical resources.

Research

There are a number of guidelines for scientific research that leads to new medical treatments. These guidelines have been developed by national and international bodies over the last half century. These include the following principles:

1. Scientific information must be made available to all. This has led to conflict between peer-review journals, which often take months to review and approve articles for publication, and the researchers who write for them. This issue came to a head in the early 1990s, when the *New England Journal of Medicine* waived its rule that authors could not discuss their research until it was published, or it would not be published. The journal waived its rule in the case of research on three possible treatments for AIDS, because the study showed that one treatment had proved to be much more effective than the other two. Researchers argued that to keep the information bottled up for the 4–6 months the journal normally took to referee an article would cause hardship—and possibly death—to many patients.
2. Medical treatments need to be studied scientifically before they can become "accepted medical practice." The medical community pressed for years for the National Institutes of Health to conduct scientific studies of alternative treatments such as acupuncture. Such studies have been carried out since the mid-1990s.
3. Patients must give informed written consent to participate in research. Patients may not be charged for treatments carried out as part of a research study.
4. Research studies must be carried out according to strict scientific methods and validated by other researchers before they are generally accepted.
5. Final approval in the United States for new treatments—whether medications or devices—rests with the Food and Drug Administration (FDA).
6. Between the time final documentation has been submitted to the FDA for approval and the time when the FDA makes the decision to approve or disapprove the drug or device for general use, those in any research studies may continue their treatment.

A controversial research issue surrounds the use of embryonic cells. Studies have shown that embryonic cells can be induced to develop into different types of cells. Embryonic cells may be used to reduce, or possibly even reverse, the symptoms of Parkinson's disease and other diseases.

The ethical conflict arises because a possible source of embryonic cells tissue is from aborted fetuses or fertilized ova not used for *in vitro* fertilization. Although researchers who use fetal tissue stress that they use only tissue from spontaneous abortions (miscarriages), anti-abortion advocates argue that if there is an increased need for fetal tissue, a time may come when women might be influenced in their decision whether or not to have an abortion if they could sell their fetus's tissue for research and/or treatment.

Genetic Engineering

A number of ethical issues surround the practice of genetic engineering (making, altering, or repairing genetic material).

One is the issue of genetically engineered crops and other food products, which have been dubbed "Frankenfoods" by those opposed to the practice. In fact, mankind has been "genetically engineering" crops since the first farmers in the Fertile Crescent of the Middle East domesticated particular wild grains and not others. Hardy strains of grain, rice, corn, and vegetables have been created by manipulating the seeds of various plants; they are often chosen because they will grow in particular climates and soil conditions.

Objections to today's genetic engineering arise because of the practice of manipulating plants and animals by using genetic material from other species. This encompasses practices as diverse as injecting milk cows with growth hormones in order to get them to produce more milk to incorporating material from bacteria into plant seeds.

Opponents argue that we cannot predict all of the possible effects of manipulating genetic material, and are likely to see unexpected and unwanted consequences to ourselves or other species.

Production of Human Insulin by Bacteria

Recombinant DNA techniques (inserting segments of genes from one species into the genetic material of another species) have been used to synthesize human insulin for the treatment of diabetes mellitus. Since the discovery of insulin in 1921 by Frederick Bantung, its primary source has been the pancreas of slaughtered cattle (bovine insulin) and pigs (porcine insulin).

Though chemically active, both forms of insulin are slightly different from human insulin, and can stimulate antibody formation in human beings. The synthesis of human insulin was achieved by inserting human genes for insulin into *E. coli* bacteria, which then produce insulin that is identical to human insulin; in addi-

tion, these modified bacteria can pass the genetic information on to their offspring.

Insulin is the only human protein that has been made whose structure is identical to that of the natural molecule. In the past 20 years, most diabetics in the United States and Europe have either been started on or switched over to genetically engineered human insulin. Only one form of animal insulin is still manufactured in the United States.

Some evidence suggests that diabetics have become less able to identify the onset of an episode of low blood sugar (hypoglycemia) when recieving human insulin than when receiving insulin derived from cattle or pigs. Several researchers have also studied deaths in diabetics with possible hypoglycemia. Most doctors have maintained that patients could be monitored carefully enough to prevent this from being an insurmountable problem.

Other patients have alleged that biosynthetic insulin has caused other symptoms, such as paralysis and bone and joint pain. In April 2000, a class action lawsuit was filed on behalf of Susan Kawulok and all other diabetics using products manufactured by an American pharmaceutical company (Eli Lilly) and a Danish pharmaceutical company (Novo Nordisk). This suit alleged that these companies continued to manufacture human insulin knowing that diabetics might have serious side effects, failed to warn diabetics about the lowered awareness of low blood sugar, and tried to prevent other companies from making animal-based insulins.

This lawsuit does not focus on the issue of genetically engineered human insulin per se, but rather on other ethical issues, such as how much responsibility a medical products manufacturer has to test extensively, to publish results of testing, and to keep the public informed of potential adverse effects from using the product, even if those actions lower the company's profits.

Gene therapy is a term used for experimental treatments that attempt to treat or cure disease by giving patients new genes or parts of genes that may have been synthesized in the laboratory, taken from human tissue, or engineered from genetic material of animals or other species. Experiments using gene therapy have indicated a possibility of many treatments for heart disease, stroke, complications from aneurysm rupture, Parkinson's disease, and other diseases.

The first patient known to have died as a result of gene therapy research, an 18-year-old named Jesse Gelsinger, was given genetically engineered viruses to treat an inherited liver disease. Gelsinger's family sued the University of Pennsylvania on the basis that federal research rules had not been followed. The lawsuit was settled out of court in November 2000.

In the Gelsinger case, there was less controversy about the gene therapy itself than other issues. The research study was criticized for several reasons: Informed consent forms did not contain information about monkeys that had died after receiving similar treatment; Gelsinger was given the treatment in spite of lab values that should have caused the treatment to be delayed; and one of the principal investigators in the study had a financial interest in a biotechnology company that stood to profit from the research.

The U.S. Food and Drug Administration (FDA) investigated the case and suspended all human gene therapy experiments at the research center, although research continues in animals.

Reproductive Issues

Perhaps no area of modern medicine is so fraught with ethical conflicts as reproductive issues. There are four major issues to focus on:

1. Abortion
2. RU-486, the so-called abortion pill
3. Infertility treatment
4. Surrogacy.

Abortion

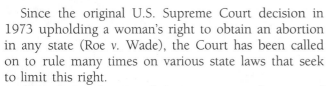

Since the original U.S. Supreme Court decision in 1973 upholding a woman's right to obtain an abortion in any state (Roe v. Wade), the Court has been called on to rule many times on various state laws that seek to limit this right.

Abortion in the United States is most often carried out in one of two general procedures: either by dilating the cervix and removing the fetus, or by introducing a toxic substance into the uterus to kill the fetus, which is then expelled through contractions similar to those in a spontaneous abortion.

Roe v. Wade established a woman's absolute right to an abortion until the age of viability (when the fetus can live outside the uterus). After the point of viability, the fetus is deemed to have legal rights, and courts must decide on an individual basis whether the mother's right outweighs the fetus's right.

Although neonatal intensive care techniques have changed much since Roe v. Wade, so that babies born as young as 24 weeks of gestation routinely live, the age of viability has never been defined any lower than approximately 28–32 weeks, when a fetus can be expected to live outside the uterus without medical intervention.

In 2000, the U.S. Supreme Court struck down state laws that would have outlawed late abortions performed using a procedure in which the brain is removed first so the skull can be made small enough to pass through the dilated cervix—a technique that anti-abortion advocates call "partial-birth abortion."

RU-486

The drug mifepristone, developed in France and popular in Europe since the 1980s, is used to induce an abortion for fetuses up to 49 days (7 weeks) after conception. This drug is still known by its research name, RU-486, in the United States.

Mifepristone, when given with a second drug, induces contractions and expulsion of the fetal tissue. Sometimes, it does not work completely and dilation of the cervix and curettage of the uterus is necessary.

In September 2000, the FDA approved mifespristone for use in the United States. Anti-abortion advocates had lobbied Congress and the FDA for years and had threatened boycotts of any pharmaceutical company that agreed to produce and market the drug in the United States.

Even after the FDA approved the treatment, anti-abortion advocates continued to lobby the FDA and Congress to restrict use of the treatment to doctors who are prepared to perform a traditional surgical abortion.

Those who advocate for abortion rights argue that this would make mifepristone treatment available only at abortion clinics, which would hurt the treatment's effectiveness greatly. They argue that the treatment should be available from any OB/GYN, family practice, or internal medicine practitioner trained in its use, which would allow a woman to receive abortion treatment without having to pass through the gauntlet of anti-abortion protesters who daily picket many abortion clinics throughout the country.

The situation was further complicated later in 2000 by controversy over misoprostol (Cystotec). Misoprostol was originally developed and approved by the FDA as an anti-ulcer medication. However, it also induces uterine contractions. It is given 2 days after RU-486 to induce uterine contractions and expel the uterine contents. The drug's developer, G. D. Searle, issued a statement on August 23, 2000, advising doctors not to use misoprostol as part of an abortion regimen because it might cause severe complications such as uterine rupture. For fear of legal liability (since the drug's manufacturer advised against it), most hospitals and clinics stopped using misoprostol.

Although other drugs can be used with RU-486, many doctors believe they carry similar or greater potential for harmful side effects than does misoprostol. Some people have speculated that Searle does not want to be associated with abortion, and therefore issued the health advisory.

Without a safe adjunct medication, it is likely that RU-486 will be used less frequently than it might have been, even after its approval as an abortion measure.

Another contraceptive treatment, the so-called morning-after pill, sometimes called Plan B, has also been controversial since being approved in the mid 1990s.

As of 2000, many states allow pharmacists trained in its use to provide it to a woman without a doctor's prescription. Again, anti-abortion advocates would like to see Plan B taken off the market.

Infertility

Artificial insemination, using sperm from a life partner or anonymous donor, is no longer a particularly controversial process. In terms of technique, sperm can be either fresh or thawed after having been frozen at a sperm bank. They can be introduced either into the vagina or, after being washed, directly into the uterus.

An area of controversy that remains active surrounds the use of artificial insemination by unmarried mothers, especially lesbian couples. Many groups oppose this activity within the larger context of concern for children being raised by openly gay couples.

In vitro **fertilization**, fertilization of an ovum by sperm in a laboratory and insertion into the uterus, is also usually seen as a private decision. Medication is used to stimulate ovulation of multiple eggs, which are harvested, combined with sperm, grown in the laboratory through the first few cell divisions, then implanted. Success rates vary.

The controversy arises around two issues. One is that multiple births often occur through this technique, including the rare cases of sextuplets (six live births), septuplets (seven), and even octuplets (eight). Techniques exist to abort some of the fetuses—a source of ethical conflict.

Should a woman be forced to carry multiple fetuses, knowing that the health risks to herself and the unborn children rise dramatically for each additional fetus beyond one? She and her family face the possibility that some or all may not survive, or may have physical and/or mental impairments.

On a societal level, the cost of pregnancy and delivery becomes extremely high. The children of multiple births are usually small and premature. After the children leave the hospital (assuming they live), the family faces enormous financial and psychological burdens in caring for a large number of children born at the same time.

On the other hand, to choose abortion for one or more of the fetuses often seems immoral and unfair for families who have struggled, often for years, to overcome infertility. Even though reducing the number of fetuses to two or three is likely to benefit the mother and surviving fetuses, a sort of random injustice seems to ocur when, within a group of fetal siblings conceived together, some will be selected to live while others must die.

A second area of ethical concern involves fertilized ova that are not reimplanted into the mother. Should they be destroyed, or retained, either to be used by the same woman or to be used by other women? If a couple later divorces, the disposition of frozen embryos may be contested, as has happened in several cases already.

Surrogacy and Egg Donation

Use of a **surrogate** involves a contract between a couple who cannot conceive and/or carry a pregnancy to term and a woman who agrees to carry a fetus for the couple and then give the child to them at birth. The fetus may be a product of the couple's ovum and sperm, or the surrogate's egg may be fertilized by the male partner's sperm. Alternatively, a woman may donate one or more ova to be fertilized by the male partner in a couple with fertility problems, and then be implanted in the uterus of the female in the couple.

Particularly in the case of surrogacy, legal problems have arisen because the surrogate has wanted to retain custody of the child after birth, claiming a heartfelt maternal bond. Disputes of this kind often hinge on the validity of the contract between the surrogate and the infertile couple, and over the state of mind of the individual woman who entered into a contract to become a surrogate.

In the case of Baby M, in New Jersey, the issue was even more complex because the surrogate was also the biological mother. She petitioned for custody after birth, and the case made its way through the courts to the New Jersey Supreme Court.

The Court ruled that the contract between the couple and the surrogate was not valid because the consideration offered by the surrogate (turning a baby over to the couple) and the consideration offered by the couple (money) constituted the act of selling a child. To allow such a contract, the Court ruled, was not consistent with good public policy.

The question of custody then arose, whereupon the court was forced to make its decision based on the child's best interests. In this instance, the court granted custody to the male partner in the couple, the baby's biological father, on the theory that a woman who would sell her baby should not be granted custody.

This case raised issues about the nature of parenthood, the right of a woman to have children even if she cannot bear them herself, and the proper compensation for a woman who has endured the physical and emotional stresses surrounding pregnancy when that pregnancy is undertaken for another couple's benefits. It also raises the issue of the government's ability to regulate such behavior, or the type of compensation provided within such an arrangement.

Right to Die, Right to Refuse Treatment

The right to refuse treatment is well established for adults. The 1990 Patient Self-Determination Act establishes the right of an adult to express his or her wishes related to health care, and to refuse treatment. The act also establishes the right of an individual to prepare an advance directive that specifies what treatments he or she would like to receive, and which he or she would not wish to receive, if the individual becomes incapable of making those decisions at a later time. Courts have held an individual's right to refuse treatment in such high regard that they have enabled mentally ill patients to refuse treatments for their mental illness.

In the case of life-saving or life-prolonging treatments, in the absence of an advance directive, an individual's family may bring to court a petition to remove life support. Such a petition must be supported by witnesses other than those who file the petition, stating that the incompetent individual made affirmative statements saying that he or she would not want to remain on artificial life support.

The first such case was brought in 1975 by the parents of Karen Ann Quinlan, a New Jersey woman injured years before in a car accident and existing in a persistent vegetative state. She was maintained on a ventilator and feeding tube. A federal court allowed doctors to remove the ventilator, but not the feeding tube. Quinlan lived until 1985.

Later court decisions have allowed doctors—at the family's request—to remove feeding apparatus from individuals with no hope of recovery, including patients in a vegetative state; that is, a patient who is medically viable but without any meaningful human interaction.

Physician-assisted suicide and euthanasia (literally, "good death"), sometimes called mercy killing, evoke fears that the power to take life will be abused—that it will be used more for the convenience of others than for the well-being of those who are dying. Advocates for the disabled have argued that allowing physician-assisted suicide or euthanasia could be the first step in society's determining that the severely disabled are too much of a financial and physical burden, and having them euthanized.

Throughout the 1990s, an individual doctor named Jack Kevorkian provided patients with degenerative, terminal illness a machine that used injection of lethal drugs to promote their death. In the early 1990s, Kevorkian did not himself press the plunger to send the drugs into an individual's vein, but he did help set up the IV drip to deliver the drug. And in the case of a woman with advanced amyotropic lateral sclerosis (ALS, or Lou Gehrig disease), Kevorkian actually modified the machinery to accommodate her greatly limited mobility. However, in 1998, Kevorkian was seen on television on the CBS magazine show "60 Minutes" giving a lethal injection to Thomas Youk. Kevorkian was convicted of second-degree murder in Michigan for causing Youk's death, and for giving a controlled substance in a state where he was not licensed. Kevorkian was sentenced to 10–25 years in prison, and

appealed the sentence. As of the end of 2000, the case was still being appealed.

In 1997, Oregon became the first state to legalize physician-assisted suicide, allowing doctors to write a prescription for a patient of a lethal dose of pain killer or other medication. The doctor must certify that he or she has treated the patient, that the patient has a terminal illness from which recovery is not possible, and that the patient has had an evaluation to rule out clinical depression.

A similar law failed to be approved in Maine in 2000.

A research study published in November 2000 revealed that many terminally ill patients surveyed wanted the option of doctor-assisted suicide to be available, but that fewer than 1 percent had actually considered suicide or desired doctor-assisted suicide for themselves. Experience in Oregon has shown that the phenomenon remains relatively rare, and has not been abused.

Scarce Medical Resources

The fact is that medical resources are not infinite.

Decisions must be made about who will receive what medical resources and who will not. These decisions are sometimes made on the basis of who can pay to obtain the resource, or who is the sickest. Occasionally, they are made on the basis of who is "worthy." These decisions must be made in four large contexts:

1. Transplants
2. Cost of treatment
3. Payment for expensive and/or experimental treatment
4. Conflict between business interests and interests of care.

Transplants

The sad fact is that most Americans who need an organ transplant will die before an organ becomes available. And others who might have survived if they had received an organ earlier die because their condition has degenerated so badly before they receive the organ.

The way the U.S. organ donation system is designed, the sickest patient within a geographic area in which an organ can be transported and remain viable is given the organ, provided tissue and blood matches are appropriate. This seems the fairest way to provide organs.

But what about situations in which personal behavior has led to the need for an organ transplant? Should an alcoholic whose liver has become sclerotic receive a new liver before an individual who developed primary sclerosing cholangitis secondary to a history of inflammatory bowel disease? Should a two-pack-a-day smoker receive a new heart instead of individual with a familial history of heart disease but who does not smoke or eat fatty food, and who keeps his weight down and exercises regularly?

Should there be age limits (as there currently are) beyond which a person will no longer be considered for a kidney transplant? Many people believe that such personal responsibility factors ought to be considered. But in practice, it is very difficult to establish guidelines and to obtain consensus, especially when any means of implementing them requires weighing several factors and is to some extent a subjective process.

Cost

The cost of medical treatment, and especially of medications, is causing a great deal of social controversy. Should the poor and the elderly be deprived of the most promising—yet expensive—new drugs, or does society have an obligation to provide its less fortunate with equal access to all treatments through taxpayer-financed health insurance (Medicare and Medicaid)?

And the issue goes beyond the United States. Many African, Asian, and Latin American countries are being decimated by AIDS. AIDS treatment can be extremely expensive. In the United States, an individual living with AIDS is usually able to obtain medication, either through private insurance or through Medicaid. Should the newest, most expensive AIDS drugs be made available to those in developing countries who live with AIDS? And if so, who should pay for them? Should drug companies accept lower profit margins in less developed countries? Is that fair to citizens in more developed countries?

On the other hand, should taxpayers pay for treatments that have a small likelihood of success, such as bone marrow transplants used to treat some types of cancers?

Payment

Who should pay for expensive experimental treatments? Should private insurance companies be mandated to provide such coverage in their policies? Or should the federal government agree to use taxpayer funds to pay for the treatment of a certain number of individuals while a particular treatment is experimental, only requiring insurance companies to pay for it after it has become approved for general use?

Today, most Americans have a feeling that the allocation of medical resources is unfair. However, the problem is so large and unwieldy that they have little idea how to create a comprehensive solution. The problem is like an underinflated balloon—as the federal and state legislatures press in one side to contain costs or increase access, the other side bulges.

The managed care movement, which began with an emphasis on preventive health care and better management of resources, is now seen by many consumers as a system that seeks to maximize income for insurance companies at the expense of patient care and patient/doctor relations.

In a similar way, patient research often seems to present a conflict between good patient care and profit. This can be seen when companies do not divulge health risks in a timely manner, such as tobacco and drug companies. It is also seen in the case of scientists who perform research at academic institutions, but are also involved in business development with the company on whose products they are conducting supposedly "unbiased" research.

Finally, the cost of new treatments sometimes seems more related to consumer interest in the medication, procedure, or device than to the actual cost of development and marketing.

There seems to be no end in sight to these contradictions and conflicts. The challenge of the 21st century will be for individuals and society to implement ethical choices to benefit targeted groups within society or society as a whole, in spite of continuing pressure from groups which are primarily motivated by self-interest.

STUDENT STUDY PLAN

To reinforce your understanding of the material in this chapter . . .

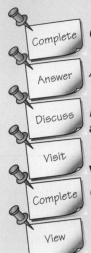

Complete the **Review & Recall** questions.

Answer the **Critical Thinking Questions** and discuss them with your classmates.

Discuss the situation in **If You Were the Medical Assistant** with your classmates and answer the questions.

Visit the **Web sites** suggested and search for additional Web sites using **Keywords for Internet Searches.**

Complete the exercises in chapter 42 of the **Student Mastery Manual.**

View the Legal and Ethical Professionalism **Videotape:** Part One, "Bulemia."

 REVIEW & RECALL

1. Give an example of a deontological, a teleological, and a combination theory of ethics.

2. Describe four important rights of citizens in the United States. How do these rights apply to health care?

3. Describe five duties of a health care professional and give an example of each.

4. Describe the six steps of the ethical decision-making process.

5. Identify measures to protect the rights of subjects who participate in scientific and/or medical research programs.

6. Describe briefly the ethical issues raised by the treatment of infertility, by abortion, and by oral medications to terminate pregnancy.

7. Define genetic engineering and explain why it raises ethical issues related to medical research.

8. What methods are available for individuals to influence decisions about health care if a person becomes unable to participate in the decision-making process?

9. To what extent is a person able to control his or her own death legally? ethically?

10. List ethical problems that arise because the supply of medical resources is limited.

 IF YOU WERE THE MEDICAL ASSISTANT

At Blackburn Primary Care Associates, one medical assistant is having personal problems. She is frequently tardy (from 10 minutes to 2 hours); and, on several occasions, she has called 10–15 minutes before she is scheduled to work to say she will be unable to come to work that day.

This assistant has been a steady and reliable employee for 6 years, and the office staff have been supporting her during her current difficulties. But the situation has begun to deteriorate: Some staff members have begun to resent having to cover for this employee, and sometimes her failure to come to work results in poor patient care. The office manager calls a meeting with the medical assistants to discuss how to deal with this situation.

1. Identify as many conflicting values, rights, duties, and desires as you can think of in this situation.

2. Choose the two areas you think are most important, and give at least one reason why you think these are the factors that should be weighted most heavily. Would you be comfortable presenting these at a staff meeting?

3. What could be done to resolve this situation? Try to identify at least four different alternatives. Identify the value, right, duty, or desire that each alternative addresses.

4. Which of the alternatives that you identified would you choose? Even though it is difficult to make a choice with inadequate information, choose an alternative that responds to the area you think is most important, and give at least three reasons why you think it is a good choice.

 ## CRITICAL THINKING QUESTIONS

1. Use the process for making ethical decisions to discuss with your classmates what would be the best action for the medical assistant in each of the cases below. Identify reasons why the medical assistant might take an action other than that which you think is best.

   a. A medical assisting student named Gail normally rides to her externship with JoAnne, another student in the same class whose current externship is at a different office in the same building as Gail's. One day, JoAnne, who was supposed to drive, does not pick her friend up and does not answer the telephone at her apartment. Gail waits about 45 minutes and tries to telephone several times. She also telephones the externship to explain that she has been delayed. Gail knows that JoAnne went to a party the evening before and suspects that JoAnne stayed at a friend's the previous night. Finally, she calls a neighbor to ask for a ride. When she arrives at her externship, her instructor is there on a supervisory visit. The instructor asks her why she is late. What explanation should Gail give?

   b. Gail suspects that JoAnne has not called her externship site to say she will be late or absent. Should Gail call? If so, what should she say?

   c. While working at the front desk of her externship, Gail is approached to check a patient who has a note on her medical record saying that the patient must speak to the office manager about her bill before she can be seen by the doctor. There are several people standing near the appointment window when the patient arrives. What should Gail do?

   d. While interviewing a patient in the examining room, a patient tells Gail that her bruises and black eye occurred when her boyfriend stabbed her in the leg with a knife, and she shows a 2-inch laceration. Discuss Gail's legal and ethical obligations.

2. Find out if mifepristone (RU-486) is available in your state, and if so, how it is being used. Discuss its use with your classmates, and discuss why its use is ethical or unethical, justifiable or not justifiable. Respect your classmates' opinions during the discussion, since all may not agree.

3. Do research to find out what kinds of health hazard may be caused by genetically engineered corn or other food products. Discuss the potential advantages and disadvantages of using genetic engineering to develop new agricultural products.

4. Find out if the Medicaid program in your state pays for infertility treatments and/or for bone marrow transplants. Discuss with your classmates whether this is a good use of taxpayer dollars and/or fair to Medicaid recipients.

EXPLORE THE WEB

INTERNET WEB SITES

American Medical Association: Council on Ethical and
Judicial Affairs
www.ama-assn.org

KEYWORDS FOR INTERNET SEARCHES

abortion
    artificial insemination
    fetal tissue research
    gene therapy

genetic engineering
infertility treatment
medical research
physician-assisted suicide
right to die
RU-486
surrogacy

ANSWERS TO ON THE JOB

1. **Background Information.** Stacy has obtained background information by weighing the patient, from the medical record, and through the interview. She knows that Brittany weighs 121 pounds, and has lost 9 pounds since the last visit and 18 pounds since last year. Brittany has admitted to vomiting after meals. Earlier in the interview, Stacy asked about heartburn, dental cavities, and physical activity, and found out that Brittany does have heartburn, has had four cavities recently, and is a cheerleader.

    Scientific and/or Medical Information. Stacy knows that wight loss can be caused by many conditions, and she asks questions about Brittany's eating habits specifically to determine if there is a possiblity of anorexia nervosa or bulimia.

    Dental cavities and regular vomiting are symptoms of bulimia. The vomiting prevents food from being digested and absorbed. Gastric juice in the vomit can cause destruction of tooth enamel, resulting in cavities. Stacy also knows that bulimia is a potentially serious condition that usually requires intervention (that is, it does not just go away by itself).

    Feelings and Wishes of Those Involved. Brittany has stated that she does not want her parents or the doctor to know about the vomiting. In order to treat Brittany, it is important to find out what kinds of feelings lead her to behave in a way that can harm her health.

    Brittany may not have a clear idea what patient confidentiality means. Stacy knows that she is interviewing the patient for the doctor, and she must give the doctor information related to the patient's health. Stacy believes that Brittany's behavior poses a health risk, and that it is important for Brittany to get help.

    Law, Policies. The right to obtain health care without a parent's consent is limited until age 18 to care for alcohol or drug abuse, pregnancy, or sexually transmitted diseases. In this case, Brittany came for a physical examination, but the doctor will probably feel that the parents have the right to be told about any additional serious medical problems such as bulimia.

    From an ethical standpoint, Brittany's right to privacy is considered less important than her parents' need for complete information in order to fulfill their duty as parents. The law is inflexible in order to be just (i.e., it establishes the same age of consent for all). Considering the situation from an ethical standpoint alone, it is important to determine the extent to which Brittany is able to be responsible for herself when evaluating her right to make decisions about her own health care.

2. Areas of ethical conflict:
    a. Stacy's desire to promise Brittany not to tell the doctor or Brittany's parents what Brittany said versus Stacy's concern for Brittany's health.
    b. Stacy's obligation to communicate patient symptoms to the doctor versus Brittany's right to confidentiality.
    c. Brittany's parents' duty to take care of her as their child versus their wish to foster independence and allow Brittany to make her own decisions.

3. From Stacy's point of view, the most important concern is probably Brittany's health. Since Brittany is under 18, she is not legally allowed to be totally responsible for health care decisions, so the law supports Stacy. Stacy's second most important value is her duty to communicate patient symptoms to the doctor.

Stacy does not consider that Brittany has a right to keep information regarding her health care strictly between Stacy and herself, because Stacy works with and for the doctor and cannot treat her health problems. If Brittany had told her something personal that did not relate to her health, Stacy could agree to keep that confidential.

Under the law, Brittany's parents' duty to care for her until she is 18 takes precedence over Brittany's right to confidentiality. In order to reverse this order, Brittany would have to assume responsibility for herself by becoming financially independent of her parents or getting married. On a personal level, Stacy might not agree. But as an employee in a medical office, she is obligated to work according to legal guidelines.

4. Stacy should express clearly to Brittany that she will have to tell the doctor about the symptoms and behavior Brittany has told her about because she works with the doctor and not independently. She should express clearly that she is concerned about Brittany's health and the possible consequences of Brittany's behavior. She should communicate the information to the doctor.

Chapter 43

Professionalism: From Externship to Employment

Instructional Objectives

After completing this chapter, you will be able to do the following:

1. Define and spell the vocabulary words for this chapter.
2. Describe how the medical assisting externship works.
3. List student responsibilities during the medical assisting externship.
4. Explain the importance of certification for a medical assistant.
5. Describe the process for becoming a certified medical assistant (CMA) or a registered medical assistant (RMA).
6. Identify two professional organizations to which a medical assistant may belong.
7. Identify benefits of joining a professional organization.
8. Describe the process for locating potential employers when looking for a job.
9. Discuss the steps in preparing a resume.
10. Describe how to write a cover letter.
11. Differentiate between information placed on a resume and information required in an employment application.
12. Prepare to answer questions commonly asked in a job interview.
13. Describe measures to prevent job burnout.
14. Explain how to prepare for job advancement or career change.

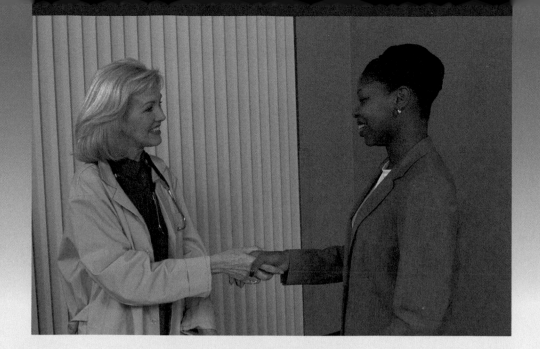

CMA/RMA CERTIFICATION
Content and Competencies

- Externship
- Job search

- Resume writing, interviewing techniques, and follow-up

VOCABULARY

burnout (p. 1018)
cover letter (p. 1012)

externship (p. 1004)
internship (p. 1004)

networking (p. 1008)

resume (p. 1008)

ABBREVIATIONS

CEU (p. 1007)

CMA (p. 1006)

RMA (p. 1006)

EXTERNSHIP

Some people are unfamiliar with the term **externship.** An externship is the practical experience a student receives in a medical office environment. To be called an externship, the practical experience must take place in a facility other than the facility in which the student is taught. (Practical experience within the institution is called an **internship.**)

To use an analogy, an externship is to a student of medical assisting what a student teaching assignment is to a student of education.

In order to be accredited by either the Commission on Accreditation of Allied Health Education Programs (CAAHEP) or the Accrediting Bureau of Health Education Schools (ABHES), a medical assisting education program must provide its students with an externship experience of at least 160 hours.

During this placement, you as a medical assisting student will have an opportunity to practice many of the skills learned in the classroom and laboratory in a real office or clinic setting. The externship is an important part of the transition from student to qualified medical assistant.

How Externship Works

Each site that hosts medical assisting students is selected by the faculty member who coordinates externships, and must be able to meet the student's instructional needs.

In some programs the students may spend their entire externship at one site; in other programs, students rotate from one site to another to get a feel for different types of offices or to obtain different types of experience. In either case, students have an opportunity to practice the skills they have learned in the administrative and clinical areas. The school has a contractual relationship with each externship site; if the site can no longer provide an appropriate educational experience, the school ends the relationship.

In an externship affiliated with an accredited medical assisting program, students are not paid. Although some students feel that they are doing "free work" for the office or clinic where they are on their externship, they must understand that the doctors and other personnel in the office are, in turn, providing "free teaching," offering the student a rich learning experience.

Because students are not employees, they must have their own health insurance and malpractice insurance (which is usually provided under the school's blanket policy). Before you begin your externship, you should check your health insurance status, and determine if the school covers you for malpractice.

Like other health care professionals, a medical assistant on externship should have current immunizations and a recent Mantoux test (for tuberculosis). It is strongly recommended that you complete a course of hepatitis B immunizations before beginning the externship. You have the legal right to refuse these immunizations, but many externship sites require them.

Some sites want to interview students who would potentially perform their externships at the facility. If this is the case, you may have to go for a personal interview, just like a job interview. (See the discussion later in the chapter on interviewing for a job.)

During your externship, you will be asked to keep records such as a log of your attendance and activities. The person at the site where you perform your externship will also keep such records. The externship coordinator from the school will also make regular visits to help supervise your performance. Staff at the site will also complete periodic written evaluations of your performance.

At the end of the externship, you may be asked to complete a form evaluating the site or sites where you did your externship. Externship evaluation, follow-up program evaluation, and graduate surveys are all very helpful to your program's externship coordinator and director in determining where to send students in the future and how to improve the program.

Student Responsibilities

During their externship, medical assisting students have an opportunity to improve their skills in a number of areas, including interpersonal communication with patients and other staff members, administrative skills, clinical competencies, and knowledge of situations with legal and/or ethical implications. Students receive a set of performance objectives for their externship similar to the performance objectives discussed in chapter 31.

There are seven keys to making the externship a successful experience:

1. Attendance
2. Appearance
3. Use the time as a learning experience
4. Stay busy
5. Take time and care in your work
6. Don't overstep your role
7. Don't gossip.

Attendance

As the comedian Woody Allen once said, "90 percent of life is just showing up."

Attendance and punctuality—being there, and being there on time—are indicators of reliability and dependability. In a medical office setting, your employer must be able to rely on the expectation that you and all the other employees will show up. Offices are staffed in such a way that everyone has work to do; if a person is absent, that means everyone else has more work to do.

Of course, employees get vacation time; and when one person is on vacation, colleagues know they will have extra work. And people do get sick. But frequent absence or tardiness is a problem, especially for small businesses such as a medical office.

Appearance

Medical assistants are expected to have a neat, clean, professional appearance. A professional appearance increases the confidence of patients and other office visitors in your skills and capabilities. In addition, during your externship, you represent your school, and your appearance sends a message to the doctors and other staff in the office about the quality of your educational program. You may need to review the guidelines for a professional appearance discussed in chapter 4.

Learning Experience

The externship can often be a cause for anxiety. It is a step to a new level, from classroom and laboratory work to "hands on" administrative and patient-based work.

Your externship may start off slowly, as you get a feel for the office and the office personnel get a feel for your abilities and your desire to learn. Many offices have their students shadow a medical assistant for a few days as he or she performs various tasks, as shown

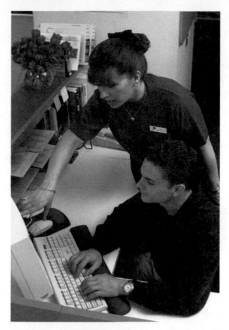

➤ **Figure 43–1** The medical assistant in an externship usually works closely with an experienced medical assistant.

in Figure 43–1. Other offices give students responsibilities right from the start, believing that people's abilities can not really be judged without seeing how they react to new situations.

You may find that the technique you have been taught for performing a particular task is not the technique used in the office you are assigned to. There is often more than one correct way to perform procedures and carry out tasks. Try to respond positively to any feedback, and do not take critiques of your technique personally. Discuss any serious problems with the externship coordinator from the school.

You should carry a small notebook in which to write down memory joggers for yourself, such as which doctors use which exam rooms, how doctors like patients to be dressed for the exam, and other working preferences. Also write down medications used in the office and unfamiliar terminology to look up during quiet moments or in the evenings. Identify things you would like to learn more about, and see if the office's contact person can help you arrange the time to learn it.

Be sure to locate emergency equipment, emergency exits, fire extinguishers, and emergency telephone numbers.

Stay Busy

Once the office is confident of your abilities to perform certain tasks, do them without being asked. Take advantage of the chance to observe and learn about unfamiliar procedures. Ask to be included and find out who among the staff—doctors and others—likes to teach. Try to spend more time with the people who enjoy teaching and who respond eagerly to questions.

Be careful, however, not to waste the time of office staff by asking questions to which you could easily find answers yourself, or requesting information that you have already been given. Use quiet periods to look up information. Avoid the temptation to concentrate on familiar tasks and activities as a way to escape from the challenge of learning those that are unfamiliar.

Take Time and Care in Your Work

A medical office may look hectic. Many staff members may look as if they are working very fast. But speed is not the most important thing. Accuracy is. Take the necessary time to do things right!

You may not be excited about filing patient charts, but take care to do it accurately. A misplaced chart can tie up large amounts of staff time. Students and/or new staff are often suspected when a file is missing; try not to take it personally if this happens. Offer to help find it. If it is a file you remember handling, think of ways you may have misfiled it—by the patient's first name instead of the last, for instance.

Do Not Overstep Your Role

Be sure you understand what you may and may not do in the particular office in which you are working. Different offices have different guidelines for what medical assistants, and medical assisting students, do.

If you believe you are not being allowed to do enough, consider the possibility that staff members think you have neither the ability nor the motivation. Let them know that you think you can do more. Ask for help if you are uncertain about a particular procedure, but if possible try to figure things out on your own. If you are uncertain about how to perform a particular task or procedure, arrange a session at your school.

Do Not Gossip

Avoid the temptation to gossip, especially to share any negative impressions you may have. If you express negative opinions about any part-time job you may have, or about an employer, office staff may wonder what you are saying about your externship experience when you are with others.

If you have a problem with a coworker, speak to that person directly rather than talking about the situation with other employees or with family and friends. Ask your externship coordinator for suggestions on how to handle difficult situations.

CERTIFICATION

Certification is a process by which an organization, often a national body, validates the credentials of an individual or a program. Certification is very important for health care professionals who are not licensed by their own state, because an unbiased national organization validates their knowledge and skills. Do not confuse a certificate given after completion of a specified number of hours at a particular school with certification or validation by a national organization.

Medical technologists, medical assistants, diagnostic sonographers, dental assistants, phlebotomists, and other health care professionals can be certified by various organizations. Certification provides a potential employer with a benchmark about a potential employee, saying that this person possesses a particular level of ability, proficiency, and education.

The two most prestigious credentials for medical assistants are those for the certified medical assistant (CMA) and the registered medical assistant (RMA).

Certified Medical Assistant

A certified medical assistant (**CMA**) has passed the certification examination given by the American Association of Medical Assistants (AAMA). In order to take the exam, the individual must have graduated from one of two types of accredited medical assisting programs: A program accredited by the Commission on Accreditation of Allied Health Education Programs (CAAHEP) or a program accredited by the Accreditation Bureau of Health Education Schools (ABHES).

The exam is given twice a year, on the last Friday of January and the last Saturday of June. Applications are due October 1 for the January exam and March 1 for the June exam. There are several testing locations in each state.

Application material can be obtained from the AAMA Certification Department, 20 North Wacker Drive, Suite 1565, Chicago IL 60606-2903; from the director of accreditation at the medical assisting program you attend; or from the AAMA's Web site, www.aama-ntl.org.

Passing this exam allows a medical assistant to use the title CMA after his or her name on all official documents, including office letterhead and business cards. An individual must be recertified as a CMA every five years, either by retaking the certification exam or by successfully completing the required continuing education programs.

Registered Medical Assistant

A registered medical assistant (**RMA**) has passed the examination given by the American Medical Technologists (AMT), an organization that certifies, in addition to medical assistants, medical technologists, medical laboratory technicians, phlebotomists, and other health professionals.

In order to take this exam, an individual must have (1) graduated from a medical assisting program accredited by the Accreditation Bureau of Health Education Schools/Programs (ABHES) or an organization approved by the U.S. Department of Education; (2) graduated from a formal medical services program of the U.S. armed forces; or (3) been employed in the profession of medical assisting for five years.

Applications for the RMA exam can be obtained from the Registrar's Office, American Medical Technologists, 710 Higgins Rd., Park Ridge, IL 60068-5765. Information about the exam can be obtained from the AMT's Web site, www.amt1.com. The RMA exam is given at Cogent testing center locations throughout the country on specific dates, or in many centers every week.

Passing this exam entitles the medical assistant to use the initials RMA after his or her name on all official documents.

In many areas, employers hire only medical assistants who are either CMAs or RMAs. As medical assistants perform more specialized clinical tasks, employers have become increasingly concerned about validating skills and knowledge before hiring them.

Obtaining Additional Training, Credentials

A medical assistant may need to validate specific skills as a condition of employment.

Training in cardiopulmonary resuscitation (CPR) is offered directly through the American Red Cross (ARC) and the American Heart Association (AHA) and by hospitals and other health care agencies. Like other health professionals, medical assistants recertify every two years to be sure their skills are current. Almost all health care facilities require current CPR credentials.

Medical assistants may also take courses in first aid, hearing tests, or other specialized tests, depending on the needs of the medical practice. In many areas, medical assisting certification or registration is a valid qualification to perform phlebotomy, but some states and/or institutions require separate certification in phlebotomy. This can be obtained through the AMT, the American Society of Clinical Pathologists (ASCP), or the American Society of Phlebotomy Technicians, Inc. Addresses and Web sites for these organizations are listed at the end of the chapter.

PROFESSIONAL ORGANIZATIONS

The AAMA and the AMT maintain professional organizations of medical assistants. For an annual membership fee, many benefits are available, including:

1. Peer support
2. Continuing education programs
3. Legislative advocacy on issues important to medical assistants
4. Publications and/or newsletters with information related to the profession of medical assisting.

Support of Peers

Through local and national meetings and workshops, medical assistants are able to enter a network of peers with whom they can share and from whom they can learn. They can also obtain insurance at reasonable cost, professional journals, and other sources of information important to the profession.

Continuing Education Units

With the constant change in the medical field, it is not merely important but necessary to keep skills up to date, attain new skills, and obtain new information about professional practices. Most health professions require a certain amount of continuing education for licensure or certification renewal. These are designed either as contact hours or continuing education units (**CEUs**).

Medical assisting contact hours and CEUs can be obtained from education programs that have been approved by the particular certifying agency. The AAMA validates continuing education programs given through the state and national organization. Home study programs are also available to obtain continuing education credit.

Legislation Affecting Medical Assistants

Another service provided by professional organizations is advocacy for pending state and federal legislation that may affect the medical assisting profession.

Changes in legislation require actions by many people. In some states, issues for medical assistants arise from actions taken by other professionals to limit procedures to their profession. As a result of such actions, medical assistants may no longer take x-rays in most states, and may not be permitted to administer injections or draw blood, depending on the state.

A future task for the medical assisting profession will be to organize and help draft legislation giving medical assistants the right to perform all skills in the workplace for which they have been trained. This can best be accomplished by working with the national professional organizations and their state chapters.

FINDING A JOB

Finding a job involves more than simply answering newspaper advertisements or responding to help-wanted notices on the school's career bulletin board. To find the right job, a student needs to do some research about the types of medical practices in the community in which he or she would like to work, then target specific employers for whom he or she would like to work.

Successful Job Hunting

Successful job hunting has two parts. The first is setting appropriate goals; the second is identifying potential employers that would allow you to attain your goals.

Setting goals means identifying the ideal job for your current circumstances. Do you want to work full-time or part-time? In what area of the country or region do you want to work? Do you want to work in a city? in the suburbs? in the country? Do you have a preference about the size of the organization you would like to work in? Are you interested in working in a particular medical specialty? What are your particular strengths and weaknesses? Do you want to perform all of the diverse tasks a medical assistant may perform, or do you want to specialize in either clinical or administrative duties?

After you have set your goals, it is time to begin identifying potential employers. This is done through scanning newspaper want ads to see what kinds of positions are being advertised, and also by looking through the Yellow Pages to see what kinds of practices there are in the community you want to work in. Many large organizations post job openings internally first; so if you have family or friends who work in such institutions, you need to ask them to keep an eye on the internal posting boards for you.

Larger institutions also often have personnel or human resource departments that keep files of potential employees to give to doctors or department administrators who need to fill a position. If you submit a resume or fill out an application for such a facility, that paperwork will stay on file for a period of time—usually six months or one year. After that, you must submit a new, updated application.

During the job-hunting period, it is important to set aside some time each day to look for a job. Cast your net wide. The more opportunities you explore, the more possibility not only of finding a job, but of finding the right job.

Do not underestimate the importance of **networking,** contacting people you know who may know of potential jobs. Your personal network should include former instructors, contacts you made during your externship, classmates, and your personal doctor. Maintain these contacts. Talk to them even when you are not looking for a job. If you stay in touch, they may call you in the future when they have an opening or know of one elsewhere for which you might be a "good fit."

Preparing a Resume

The primary purpose of a resume is to obtain an interview for an open position. A **resume** is a summary of information about a person that describes education, work experience, and other information that employers may find pertinent in deciding whether or not to hire an individual.

A resume is often important in making a first impression on a potential employer. It must be neat, professional, and informative. Employers who receive a lot of resumes for one position use the resume to create a list of people with the desired training and/or experience to call in for personal interviews.

A resume should describe your education, experience, and skills completely, but not in an exaggerated way. If possible, limit the resume to one typewritten sheet. If the resume is more than one page, make sure that information is especially pertinent to the job you are applying for appears on the first page. Some people who are applying for many different types of positions have many variations of their resume available, each one slanted toward the requirements of certain positions.

Do not include personal information on your resume, such as marital status, children, and so forth. Because it does not relate to your credentials for the position, the effect of such personal information is most likely to be neutral or negative, providing a reason *not* to grant you an interview if, for example, the employer is afraid children may result in excessive absence.

Resume Styles

In general, there are three styles of resumes: chronological, functional, and targeted.

A chronological resume contains a list of formal education, with degrees and certificates earned, followed by work experience. This is the most common type of resume for applicants with limited work experience, or those who are seeking work similar to their present work.

A functional resume categorizes experience according to skills or abilities, some of which may be a result of activities other than paid employment (such as volunteer work or unpaid work). A functional resume is useful for an individual who wants to change from one type of work to a different type of work, and wants to highlight how particular skills attained in one line of work can be helpful in the new position for which he or she is applying.

Susan Anderson
2314 May Avenue
West River, MU 00000
(666) 111-5555

EDUCATION/CERTIFICATION

1999-2001   West River Community College
A.S. Medical Assisting, June 2001

1998-1999   University of North Brook

Certified Medical Assistant: June, 2001
CPR for the Professional: January, 2001

RELATED EXPERIENCE

2001   **MEDICAL ASSISTING EXTERNSHIP** (160 hours)
John Smith Medical Associates, West River, MU
  • Prepared patients for examination, took vital signs and charted chief complaint.
  • Performed diagnostic tests including throat cultures, rapid strep test, EKG's,
    dipstick urinalysis
  • Performed clerical duties including answering telephones, filing, writing referrals,
    scheduling appointments
  • Data entry of patient information and insurance payments

1998-2001   **HOME HEALTH AIDE**
Medical Home Care, Newtown, MU

Performed personal care and took vital signs in private homes.

SPECIAL SKILLS

Fluent in Spanish,
Keyboarding 45 wpm
Microsoft Word, MediSoft, Practice Management Software (PMS)

OTHER EXPERIENCE
1996-1997   **CASHIER**
Fresh and Fine Supermarket, West River, MU

Responsible for checking groceries; weekend supervisor.

➤ **Figure 43–2** Sample resume of a recent graduate.

A targeted resume organizes information about an individual who has targeted a particular job opportunity in such a way as to highlight the skills and work experiences being called for in the new employment. This type of resume often begins with an employment objective that identifies the type of position the individual is seeking.

Information to Include

The basic pieces of information needed for a resume are personal demographics, objective, education, experience, skills, credentials, and references. Once you have gathered all of these bits of information (dis- cussed in more detail below), you must decide how to organize them.

A number of computer programs are available for preparing resumes. If you use one, be sure to learn enough about it so you can personalize your resume. It is also helpful to use some sample resumes as guides. Figures 43–2, 43–3, and 43–4 are sample resumes. Others can be found in your school's placement office or in resume-writing books.

Personal demographics include your name, address, telephone number, and e-mail address if you have one. It is usually placed at the top of the resume, either centered or flush left. Make sure the identifying information is in a larger type size, boldfaced, and/or in a

Patricia A. Saychelles

26 Gillian Street
West River, MU 00000
(666) 111-5555
saychelles@anyserver.com

Objective	To obtain a challenging position as a clinical medical assistant	
Education	1997-1998	West River Community College Certificate in Medical Assisting, June 1998
Related Experience	1997-1998	Family Health Care West River, MU Clinical Medical Assistant
		Duties include: preparing patients for examination; taking vital signs and completing growth charts; documenting chief complaint; taking EKG's; obtaining throat cultures; fingersticks; phlebotomy; performing lab tests including rapid strep tests, dipstick urinalysis, cholesterol, and glucose; assisting with procedures such as I & D, suture insertion, suture removal; instructing patients regarding diet and exercise; stocking exam rooms
Other Experience	1988-1997	Homemaker
	1994-1997	Library volunteer West River Elementary School
		Responsible for checking books in and out, reshelving, minor repairs of torn books
	1986-1988	Package Sorter United Parcel Service Newtown, MU
Other Credentials	Registered Medical Assistant; January 1999	
Activities	Member of the American Medical Technologists since 1998	
References	Available upon request	

➢ **Figure 43–3** Sample resume of a woman who stayed home with children for several years before training as a medical assistant.

different font than the body of the resume, so it stands out.

The objective is a statement of the type of position you are looking for. A medical assistant just graduating may be—even should be—flexible about the type of position being sought. If your objective is general, such as to obtain an entry-level position as a medical assistant, you may find better ways to use the limited space on a single-sheet resume. This becomes a matter of personal preference.

A medical assistant with a more focused goal may wish to use a statement such as: "To obtain a clinical medical assisting position in an office specializing in family practice or internal medicine." A specific objective reassures the potential employer that the candidate is interested in the position it is trying to fill, but it limits the positions you can apply for.

Under the education section, list institutions attended and degrees or certificates received, with the year, in chronological order, most recent first. You should list at least one program from which you received a degree, certificate, or diploma. Do not list your high school diploma unless you have not received any higher credential.

You can include the dates attended, or only the year in which the credential was awarded. If you are preparing a resume in anticipation of completing a program in the near future, you may list the credential you anticipate receiving and the date when it will be conferred (e.g., A.S. in Medical Assisting, anticipated June 200X).

You may also include your grade-point average (GPA) and any honors or awards you received from the educational institution.

In the section on previous experience, identify the job title, years of employment, employer's name, and the town and state in which the work was performed.

Describe the position's responsibilities. Give more detail for positions that relate to the type of job you are seeking. Use active verbs to describe responsibilities, and be sure to use a consistent style. (See the box on Describing Responsibilities on a Resume.)

Put only paid, relevant employment in the area for work experience. If you wish to list your externship or volunteer experience, place it under another heading, such as Related Health Care Experience.

Jobs outside of health care can be listed under Other Experience. Try not to list summer jobs; but if

---

John Davidson
19 Carriage Way
West River, MU 0000
(666) 111-3333
airman@anyserver.com

OBJECTIVE: Clinical medical assistant in an emergency care setting with full range of responsibilities from health care and procedures to management.

SUMMARY: More than ten years of providing professional military and civilian health care, specializing in emergency treatment, physical examination, aeromedical safety instruction and health awareness training.

1990 to present UNITED STATES NAVY

1994-2000 Hospital Corpsman First Class (E-6). *Squadron Medical Department Representative, Naval Air Station, Harbor Bay, MU.*
Responsible for 350 personnel in all areas of world wide medical organizational deployments, including electrocardiograms, x-ray, laboratory testing, occupational and preventative medicine, personnel health care and sanitary conditions. Trained in Federal Aviation Administration (FAA) conduction of aeromedical examinations, fixed wing aircraft rescue, emergency egress procedures for jet, propeller and helicopter aircraft, and aviation life support systems. Responsible for maintaining computerized records for over 3,00 physical examinations annually.

1990-1994 Hospital Corpsman Second Class (E-5). *Squadron Medical Department Representative, Naval Air Station, Harbor Bay, MU.*
Responsible for 250 personnel for rapid deployment to naval service ships around the world. Additionally trained in rotary wing aircraft rescue and shipboard/aircraft fire fighting. Received qualifications as Medical Assistant (MA), Nursing Assistant (NA), Emergency Medical Technician (EMT), Emergency Vehicle Operator (EVO) and Emergency Medical Dispatcher (EMD)

1988 to 1990 Medical Clerk, *State Department of Corrections, West River MU*
Responsible to assist with medical care of 600 inmates involving all aspects of health care and treatment, including scheduling appointments, admission of patients to the hospital ward, maintaining health records and instruction in personal hygiene and preventative care.

OTHER CREDENTIALS:
Instructor: Emergency Medical Technician (EMT-B)
Instructor: American Heart Association Cardiopulmonary Resuscitation
Prehospital Trauma Life Support provider
Advanced Life Support (ACLS) provider

EDUCATION: Attended West River Community College from 1987-1988 taking general education courses and introductory health courses

➤ Figure 43–4 Sample resume of a man who received health care training in the Armed Services.

Describing Job Responsibilities on a Resume

1. Use action verbs like those listed below to describe responsibilities concisely:

administer	distribute	prepare
analyze	document	process
arrange	establish	proofread
assist	file	propose
authorize	instruct	purchase
balance	list	reconcile
calculate	log	run
classify	mail	schedule
code	measure	send
collect	monitor	set up
compose	order	sort
contact	organize	stock
coordinate	perform	teach
copy	post	write
develop		

2. When using these words in the resume, use one of the two following styles consistently. Either can be written in sentence form or as a list with bullets.

Style 1 uses verb in past tense.

Sentence form:

Measured vital signs, prepared patients for examination, posted charges and payments, sent monthly bills . . .

Bullet form:

- Measured vital signs
- Prepared patients for examination
- Posted charges and payments
- Sent monthly bills

Style 2 uses a participle form of the verb.

Sentence form:

Responsible for measuring vital signs, preparing patients for examination, posting charges and payments, sending monthly bills . . .

Bullet form:

Duties included:

- Measuring vital signs
- Preparing patients for examination
- Posting charges and payments
- Sending monthly bills

---

you do not have an extensive work history, an employer will prefer to see at least summer work on a resume.

Medical assisting is a field in which a number of women choose to obtain training after spending time out of the work force raising children. If this is the case, it is recommended that you avoid showing a gap in work history; instead, identify these years and list "Homemaker" or "Full-time parenting" as a type of experience, as shown in the sample resume in Figure 43–3.

The special skills section describes skills learned in an educational program that may not be reflected in any direct experience, or that are usually not included in a medical assisting program. Even if the externship is included in the resume, a graduate of a medical assisting program may have special skills he or she did not have or use during the externship. These may include computer skills with particular programs, ability to perform specific diagnostic tests, or knowledge of or fluency in a language other than English.

In the section on activities and other credentials, you may include memberships in professional organizations such as the AAMA, a well as any other affiliations, and any specific certifications you have attained, such as CPR. Avoid lists of unrelated activities, hobbies, and interests on a professional resume.

In the section on references, traditional resumes included the statement that references will be furnished on request. Actual references are not included on the resume because the goal is to be interviewed before the potential employer checks your references. Most resumes today do not even include the statement about providing references, on the assumption that if an individual is granted an interview, he or she will provide references at that time.

Before using someone's name as a reference, be sure to get that person's permission. Bring all of the pertinent information about your references or original letters of reference with you to any interview. It is also polite to call your references and give them a "heads up" about the fact that you have given their names to a potential employer. That way, they will be ready to receive a phone call or written request for a reference.

For references, you should choose a balance of instructors, supervisor at the office in which you did your externship, other job supervisors, or those you have worked with in volunteer activities. Avoid using friends or family for references.

The resume should be formatted with 1-inch margins. Use a word processing program and a laser printer if possible, to provide a professional look. The resume should be laid out so that it looks balanced on the page.

Avoid sending copies. Either send a laser-printed original, or have the original professionally duplicated. You can use white, cream, or light gray paper, heavier than copier paper (stationary weight). Since you will be applying for a position in a fairly conservative segment of the job market, avoid using colored paper, unusual type fonts, or flashy formatting.

Writing a Cover Letter

Each time you send a resume, include a **cover letter** that explains briefly why the resume is being sent. The cover letter clarifies whether you are responding to an advertisement, whether an individual has referred you because he or she knows there is an opening or whether you are simply sending an open query about possible job opportunities.

Use the format for a business letter, and print it out on the same color paper as the resume. Address the letter either as directed in the advertisement you are responding to, or to the individual you want to contact. If you do not have the name of a specific individual, call the office to find out the name of the office manager or other person responsible for hiring medical assistants.

The letter should begin with your reason for writing the letter and sending the resume. This should be followed by a brief summary of the position you are seeking, and your qualifications for filling that position.

The final paragraph should be a request for an interview.

Personalize each cover letter, because this is the first thing the potential employer will see. Keep the letter short, and refer the reader to your resume for details. Figure 43–5 is a sample cover letter.

Keep a copy of all cover letters. You can either write the results of your inquiry (interview, second interview, job offer) on the copy, or you can set up a log of responses to avoid duplication.

Sending the Resume

It is recommended that you send resumes in 9 × 11-inch manila envelopes that allow you to send the

---

2314 May Avenue
West River, MU 0000
September 5, 200X

Denise Wilson, Office Manager
Medical Practice Associates
525 Main Street
West River, MU 00000

Dear Ms. Wilson:

I read your advertisement in the West River Daily Item for a medical assistant, and I would like to be considered for the position. I have an Associate in Science degree in Medical Assisting, and I have passed the certification exam given by the American Association of Medical Assistants.

The enclosed resume summarizes my education and experience. I am a self-motivated, and I get along well with people. My training in medical assisting included an externship in a physician's office, and I also have experience as a home health aide. I believe that I am well qualified for the position in your advertisement.

I can be contacted at (666)111-5555 during the late afternoon and evening, and I will respond promptly to messages. I am looking forward to hearing from you so that we can schedule an interview.

Sincerely,

Susan Anderson

Susan Anderson

Enclosure

➤ **Figure 43–5** Sample cover letter.

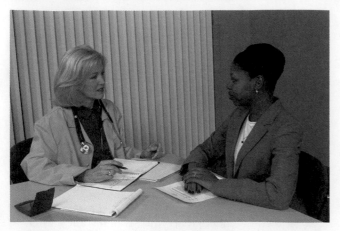

➢ **Figure 43–6** At a job interview, the medical assistant should look and act in a professional manner.

resume and cover letter without folding them. If you do use a standard No. 10 business envelope, make sure its color and weight match the paper you use for the resume and cover letter.

Increasingly, offices are requesting that resumes be faxed, or even e-mailed. If you do this, remember to fax or e-mail a cover letter as well.

The advantage of a faxed or e-mailed resume and cover letter is that the material arrives quickly, often within minutes of your making a telephone inquiry. The disadvantage is that a fax, or a print of an e-mail, does not look as crisp or professional as a mailed resume and cover letter. After sending the material by fax or e-mail, you can mail a backup copy that looks nicer.

A couple of days after you fax or e-mail a resume, or a couple of days after you believe a mailed resume should have arrived, you may call to see if the material did, indeed, arrive. You may also ask at this time if the person doing the hiring has an idea about the time frame in which a hiring decision will be made. However, do not call again after that, to avoid appearing too aggressive.

Filling Out an Employment Application

Most medical facilities ask you to complete an application in addition to providing a resume. In large facilities, you may need to do this before an interview is scheduled. In smaller offices, you may fill out the application at the time of the interview.

Be sure to bring information about previous employers, including the names and telephone numbers of supervisors, as well as the names, addresses, and telephone numbers of references. Also bring any letters of reference you have. The facility will make copies and attach them to your application.

On the application, answer all questions fully and truthfully. Print legibly or type. Do not refer the reader to your resume for answers, although the answers to questions may be there. If a question does not apply to you, write N/A or Not Applicable. Plan ahead of time what your response will be to the question of why you are leaving your current or previous employment (if you are employed). Avoid negative statements about your employer or supervisor.

Common reasons for leaving are returning to school, relocation for a spouse's job, end of a temporary position, or exploration of new career options.

Some health care facilities may require applicants for medical assisting positions to take a keyboarding test or other skills test.

Interview Techniques

An employment interview provides a potential employer with an opportunity to assess your interpersonal and communication skills, and also to assess your knowledge about the tasks encompassed by the job you are applying for.

But the interview also provides you with a chance to assess the potential employer. From the questions you are asked, the flow of the discussion, and responses to any questions you ask, you can get a feel for whether the position fits appropriately with your work style and personality.

If you wish to be offered a job, you must do well in the interview. Your skills as they appear on paper will not be enough. There are always a number of candidates who "look good on paper." The key for the employer is to find the person who seems to be the best fit for the position.

It is important to accept any job interview offered, even if you are not sure that you want the position. The more you interview, the more comfortable you will become with the job interview process. It is not appropriate, however, to accept more job interviews after you have accepted a position and before you start the job. Figure 43–6 shows a professional-looking candidate for a medical assistant position.

There are six important aspects to the job interview.

1. Preparing
2. Appearance and behavior
3. Responding to questions
4. Discussing salary and benefits
5. Asking appropriate questions
6. Determining the timeline for filling the position.

Preparing

It is important to do some research about the practice or facility where you will be interviewing. If you know someone who works there, talk to him or her. Check your network to find out if someone has worked there in the past, and why that person left.

When you are called for the interview, find out who will be interviewing you, what position(s) the interviewer(s) holds, and whether you will be interviewed by one person at a time or by a committee at one time.

Ask if there are any particular things about you that the interviewer(s) would like to know, and if you should bring any background materials with you. Ask if there are any key skills the facility or practice is looking to acquire with the person hired in this position.

Appearance and Behavior

As always, a professional appearance is important. For the position of medical assistant, it is not necessary to wear a business suit to an interview, although this is always a good choice.

A woman should wear tailored, professional-looking clothing, such as a suit or blouse and skirt, or dress slacks. Avoid denim skirts or pants for an interview. If you have long hair, wear it pulled back and off the collar, as you would at work. Avoid bulky jewelry;

2314 May Avenue
West River, MU 00000
September 5, 200X

Denise Wilson, Office Manager
Medical Practice Associates
525 Main Street
West River, MU 00000

Dear Ms. Wilson:

Thank you for giving me the opportunity to interview for the medical assisting position at Medical Practice Associates. After meeting with you, I believe that my skills and training would allow me to do an excellent job as your employee. In addition this position would allow me to grow in my professional career.

I was very impressed with the organization and high quality of care given by your practice. I hope to hear from you in about a week as we discussed. Please feel free to call me at (666)111-5555 if you think of any other questions. Thank you again for your time and consideration.

Sincerely,

Susan Anderson

Susan Anderson

Enclosure

➤ **Figure 43–7** Sample letter following an interview.

trim your nails; and if you wear polish, it should be clear polish without chips.

A man should wear a suit or dress slacks and sports coat or blazer, with a dress shirt and tie.

Never chew gum during an interview.

If you are sitting at a table for the interview, keep your feet flat on the floor under the table. If you are in a chair or on a couch facing the interviewer(s), cross your legs at the ankle or knee over knee. Try not to fidget. You may hold a pen in your hand to keep from playing with your clothing or hands. Have a note pad handy to write any additional information the interviewer(s) would like you to send; also note any questions they ask that seem especially important to you and that you might encounter in future interviews, so you can practice answering it later.

It is important to behave maturely, but not stiffly. Always try to be yourself, and let your personality come through to the interviewer. Although you will be on your best behavior, don't act like someone you're not.

Responding to Questions

Based on your experience at interviews and any suggestions from your friends about their experiences, try to prepare for questions the interviewer(s) will ask. Practice answering sample interview questions out loud with friends, family, or a roommate. See the box that lists some commonly asked questions, and discusses how to prepare appropriate responses.

Discussing Salary and Benefits

Specific salary is usually not discussed until a job is offered. But it is common for a salary range to be discussed. If the first interviewer does not state the salary range, it is acceptable to ask about it as the interview is winding down. If you ask about it early in the interview, the interviewer may feel that money is the most important thing to you about the job; but if you don't ask about it at all, the interviewer may think you don't really want the job.

It is also appropriate to ask a general question about benefits, such as how long an employee must work before becoming eligible for the benefits package and if health insurance is a benefit. Avoid asking specifically about vacation, sick days, and personal days until a job offer has been made.

If you are offered the job, a discussion of salary and benefits helps you make a decision about whether or not to accept the position. If you are unhappy about the amount being offered, ask for a specific time frame when your performance will be reviewed and a raise will be possible.

Often, especially in larger facilities with rigid salary structures, a position is limited to a particular salary range. But it is important to negotiate before accepting the position for a salary that allows you to meet your expenses. If the salary offered is not higher than you are currently earning, assuming you are working in the same field, that may be a point to help you negotiate a higher salary. On the other hand, the salary being offered may be substantially higher than your current salary, but apart from the low salary, you like your current job. In that ease, an offer of another position may encourage your current employer to increase your salary.

Asking Questions

A good interviewer will ask a candidate at the end of the interview if he or she has any questions. If the interviewer does not ask, and you do have questions, say so politely. You may ask about who supervises the position, ask the interviewer to clarify the job responsibilities if you are not clear about them, and ask about the availability of training programs in-house or financial support for outside training. Do not offer irrelevant personal information. Focus on what you have to offer the employer, not what you want or need.

Determining the Timeline for Filling the Position

If the interviewer or lead interviewer in a committee does not state the employer's time frame for making a decision about filling the position, you may ask about it. Employers know that people must seek employment at many facilities, and most are willing to tell you their time frame and get back to applicants who have been interviewed promptly.

Follow-up

The day of the interview, or the next day, write a short note thanking the interviewer or committee for the opportunity to interview and expressing your interest in the position. If you have been asked to provide additional information or materials regarding a question, send that material along with the note. Figure 43–7 is a sample follow-up letter.

If you have not heard from the interviewer by the date expected, you may telephone to ask if the position has been filled.

LIFELONG LEARNING

The field of health care is becoming more complex all the time. It is important for every member of the health care team to constantly improve his or her skills and stay up to date on new techniques in his or her field. A person can no longer end his or her education with one degree, diploma, or certificate. To provide

Responding to Common Interview Questions

1. **What can I tell you about my organization?** It is always important to have questions prepared. Ask about the history of the office or clinic and/or how long it has been in its present location. You should have found out how many physicians work there and what specialties are represented, but you can ask how many medical assistants are employed.

2. **What was your favorite subject in school?** Your answer should have some relation to the position you are applying for. Math, English, science, and medical assisting courses are good answers; avoid emphasizing the acting class you took to complete your degree requirements.

3. **Why did you choose medical assisting?** People who choose this field are usually interested in health, like people, like a job where they can be active, and believe that preventive care and early diagnosis are important components of health.

4. **What courses did you like least In school?** It is better to identify courses that were difficult for you (even if that does not directly respond to the question) than to say that you are totally uninterested in certain subjects. You can phrase your answer positively by saying that you found one subject more interesting than another.

5. **What campus activities did you participate in? What did you learn from them?** Prepare by thinking of the most interesting extracurricular activity you have ever participated in, even if you were not a member of any club or organized activity in school.

6. **Describe your responsibilities when you worked for XYZ company.** Identify your responsibilities, being sure to emphasize anything positive. For example, were you given extra responsibility during the evening or weekends, did you open or close, did you handle money, did you receive safety awards, and (especially) were you promoted?

7. **What types of problems have you encountered in your jobs? How did you handle them?** Focus on problems that might occur in a medical office, such as angry or unsatisfied people, telephones ringing off the hook, work backing up, being overwhelmed at first. Be sure you have a solution to offer.

8. **What would your instructors or previous supervisors tell me about you if I were to call them?** Identify your positive attributes and practice saying them calmly, even if it seems like bragging. "They would say that I work hard, I am organized, I catch on quickly, I am good with people, I try hard to be accurate" or whatever applies to you. Don't lie about yourself; just focus on the positive.

9. **What are some of your weaknesses or areas you need to work on?** Think carefully about weaknesses that may be seen in some lights as positive, or weaknesses that everyone is subject to. Being a perfectionist, not liking to stay home even if you are sick, checking and doublechecking your work are examples of weaknesses that employers usually like. Being nervous in a new situation, becoming frustrated when you don't have time to do your work as well as you would like, and hating to see others sitting around when there is much work to do are traits common to many people. If you are shy and reserved, this is a good opportunity to explain that you are shy in new situations but are able to open up once you feel comfortable.

10. **What are your long-term goals?** or **Where do you plan to be in five years?** The prospective employer is trying to get a sense of how long you plan to stay in your current job. In many areas turnover of medical assistants is rapid, but an employer would like to be able to count on you for at least two years. If your long-term plans include returning to school, let the interviewer know if you would be available for part-time work.

Questions you are not required to answer: If you are married, if you have or are planning to have children, your religion or ethnic background, your age (unless you must be a certain age by law to obtain the job). If the interviewer asks a question about any of these things, try to identify or respond to the underlying concern without directly refusing to answer the question. Then respond to the concern.

Interviewer: Do you live with your parents or are you married?

Applicant: Are you concerned about transportation or if I need health insurance?

high-quality patient care, every member of the health care team must engage in lifelong learning.

Staying Current

Medical assistants must keep their skills current. This means keeping abreast of new techniques, as well as learning how to utilize the latest technology.

On the administrative side, you may need to learn to use the latest computer software. You also need to keep up to date on changes in insurance coding and claim submission, an area that is constantly changing.

On the clinical side, you may need to learn how to use new diagnostic or laboratory equipment. You also have to stay current on administration of new medications and on regulations pertaining to the medical assistant's scope of practice in your state.

If you are asked to supervise others, you may need to attend classes or workshops in supervision, appraisal, conflict management, or other subjects.

If continuing education units (**CEUs**) are required for recertification, you should keep a file with the paperwork acknowledging your attendance at classes or workshops, together with the CEU credits approved for them.

Avoiding Burnout

Burnout is a constant worry, especially for those in repetitive, high-stress jobs. Burnout is a term that has come to mean disillusionment with work and inability to continue working; it is characterized by a loss of interest or enthusiasm and energy about work.

A person experiencing burnout may exhibit behavioral changes as well, including increased irritability, inability to empathize with patients, chronic fatigue, and poor relations with coworkers. Job burnout can be a precipitator for a clinical depression, and needs to be dealt with as a medical issue rather than a disciplinary problem.

Job burnout may also be a symptom of factors outside the job. If an individual's life is out of balance, or if the individual is having problems with relationships within the family, he or she may not have the necessary energy to expend at work; this may appear as burnout. In the medical community, where prescription medications and/or prescription pads are available, job burnout often manifests itself in substance abuse.

If you feel that you are at the point where job burnout is a concern, try to take action. If possible, reduce the hours you work, even if only for a three- or six-month period. Increase social activities. Increase exercise, and change your diet. Try to find a hobby to engage your mental and/or physical energies, something that helps you "decompress" from work.

If you are in a supervisory role and sense that an employee is suffering from burnout, try to get that person to assess the situation realistically and take one or more of these actions.

Sometimes, burnout is not recognized until the problems have progressed to such a degree that professional intervention is necessary. The individual suffering severe burnout may need counseling, therapy, or a job change; and if the individual has developed a substance abuse problem, he or she may even need inpatient rehabilitation. Many large facilities have in-house employee counseling.

Planning for Job Advancement or Career Change

One of the best ways to avoid job burnout is to chart a course of career advancement. There are four possible routes to go:

1. Advancing to management
2. Upgrading technical/clinical skills in the health care field
3. Transferring your skills to another field
4. Teaching.

Advancing to Management

If the administrative end of things is where you feel most at home, you will have significant opportunities to find a management position in the health care industry.

The larger the facility, the more the administrative and management tasks are broken into discrete parts, and the larger the management and administrative staff necessary.

If you are currently in such a facility, and would like to move up the management ladder, discuss your interest with the highest level of management to whom you have access. Ask about the possibility of rotating through the various departments to gain experience in finance, billing, marketing, public relations, or any other department. If you are working at a small facility or private practice, take the opportunity to learn all aspects of your practice. This makes you more versatile, and a more valuable employee. If you become bored or want to expand your skills, you can find a position in a larger facility.

Determine if there is any formal education that would be helpful. A number of colleges have both bachelor's and master's degree programs in health care administration. A degree in public administration or even in business management would also be appropriate.

Upgrading Technical/Clinical Skills

If you want to advance to a position of greater responsibility on the clinical side, you will probably need to return to school. Within the medical office setting, you might want to become a physician's assistant, a registered nurse, a medical technologist, or an x-ray technologist.

The opportunities become broader if you wish to work in a hospital or rehabilitation center. You should talk to people in the fields you might be interested in, determining what the education requirements are, and research education programs you can attend. You will need to see whether you have the financial support to pursue your education full-time or must pursue it part-time while continuing to work, either part-time or full-time at your present position. Many employers encourage education and pay all or part of an employee's education costs.

Transferring Skills

If in the course of your work you have developed exceptionally good computer skills, you may find opportunities to pursue in the computer field. From programming to doing business analysis using large databases, businesses of all kinds need proficient computer personnel.

The insurance industry also needs a huge number of people to process claims, to manage relationships with doctors and other providers, and to perform a host of other tasks in the health insurance field.

Pharmaceutical companies often hire people with medical office experience to do direct marketing of new drugs to doctor's offices, hospitals, clinics, and other health care facilities.

Teaching

This discussion would not be complete without a word about the enormous rewards that can come from teaching—transferring your knowledge and abilities to others who would like to become medical assistants.

With just your medical assisting degree or certificate, you may be able to get some work teaching a specific class related to medical assisting skills. If you are working in the region where you went to school, you can speak to the director of the program where you trained about teaching opportunities.

If you want to teach full-time, you will need to be certified and will probably need to get additional credentials. This might be a bachelor's degree and master's degree in a health care field, or in education. Depending on the financial resources available from a spouse or partner's income, family assistance, or scholarships and loans available, you may be able to return to being a full-time student; or you can pursue further education part-time while continuing to work, either part-time or full-time.

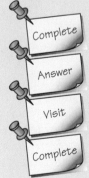

STUDENT STUDY PLAN

To reinforce your understanding of the material in this chapter . . .

Complete the **Review & Recall** questions.

Answer the **Critical Thinking Questions** and discuss them with your classmates.

Visit the **Web sites** suggested and search for additional Web sites using **Keywords for Internet Searches.**

Complete the exercises in chapter 43 of the **Student Mastery Manual.**

REVIEW & RECALL

1. What are the components of a medical assisting externship?

2. Describe student responsibilities during the medical assisting externship.

3. Identify two national organizations that certify medical assistants. What is the process for certification by each?

4. Describe the benefits of joining a professional organization for medical assistants.

5. List information that is usually included on a resume.

6. Why should a cover letter be sent with any resume? What information should it include?

7. What information is usually needed to fill out an employment application?

8. Describe how to prepare for an effective job interview.

9. Why is continuing education usually required to maintain credentials in a health profession?

10. Discuss the benefits of a commitment to lifelong learning.

CRITICAL THINKING QUESTIONS

1. Discuss the advantages and disadvantages for a medical assistant because most states do not require medical assistants to be licensed. Discuss the process of certification for students graduating from your educational program.

2. Develop a first draft of your own resume. Work with your classmates to refine and polish it. Try to create a resume that is professional and identifies as much information about your personal qualifications as possible. Proofread for spelling and punctuation errors.

3. Create templates for sample cover letters, one to answer an advertisement in a local paper and the other for resumes you send to several offices. Compare your letters with those composed by your classmates.

EXPLORE THE WEB

INTERNET WEB SITES

American Association of Medical Assistants
www.aama-ntl.org

American Medical Technologists
www.amt1.com

American Society of Clinical Pathologists
www.ascp.org

American Society of Phlebotomy Technicians
www.aspt.org

Resume links
www.studyweb/com/links/41.html

KEYWORDS FOR INTERNET SEARCHES

resume writing
job interview

Community Resources for the Medical Assistant

Professional Organizations Related to Medical Assisting

American Association of Medical Assistants

http://www.aama-ntl.org
20 North Wacker Drive
Suite 1575
Chicago, IL 60606-2963
(800) 228-2262

American Association for Medical Transcription

http://www.aamt.org
3460 Oakdale Road
Suite M
Modesto, CA 95355-0690
(800) 982-2182

American Medical Technologists

http://www.amt1.com
710 Higgins Road
Park Ridge, IL 60068-5765
(847) 823-5169

American Society of Phlebotomy Technicians, Inc.

http://www.aspt.org
Post Office Box 1831
Hickory, NC 28603
(704) 322-1334
(828) 294-0078

Agencies of the United States Government

Centers for Disease Control

http://www.cdc.gov
(Health Topics *http://www.cdc.gov/health/diseases.htm;*
National Immunization Program *http://www.cdc.gov/nip;*
National Prevention Information Network
    http://www.cdcnpin.org)
1600 Clifton Road
Atlanta, GA 30333
(404) 639-3311

Drug Enforcement Administration (DEA)
United States Department of Justice

http://www.dea.gov
Information Services Section
2401 Jefferson Davis Highway
Alexandria, VA 22301
(800) 882-9539

Food and Drug Administration (FDA)

http://www.fda.gov
5600 Fishers Lane
Rockville, MD 20857-0001
(888) 463-6332

Health Care Financing Administration

http://www.hcfa.gov
(Medicaid *http://www.hcfa.gov/medicaid/medicaid.htm;*
Medicare *http://www.hcfa.gov/medicare/medicare.htm;*
State Children's Health Insurance Program (SCHIP)
    http://www.hcfa.gov/init/children.htm)
7500 Security Boulevard
Baltimore, MD 21244
(410) 786-3000

National Institutes of Health

http://www.nih.gov
(List of Institutes that make up the NIH
    http://www.nih.gov/cd/; Toll Free Information Hotlines
    http://www.nih.gov/health/infoline.htm)
Bethesda, MD 20892
(301) 496-5787

Occupational Safety and Health Administration
U.S. Department of Labor

http://www.osha.gov
200 Constitution Ave NW
Washington, DC 20210
(800) 321-6742

U.S. Department of Health and Human Services

http://www.dhhs.gov
200 Independence Avenue, SW
Washington, DC 20201
(877) 696-6775

Other Health-Related Resources and Organizations

Alzheimer's Association
http://www.alz.org
919 N. Michigan Ave.
Suite 1100
Chicago, IL 60611-1676
(800) 272-3900

American Academy of Allergy, Asthma & Immunology
http://www.aaaai.org
611 East Wells Street
Milwaukee, WI 53202
(414) 272-6071

American Board of Medical Specialties
http://www.abms.org
1007 Church Street
Suite 404
Evanston, IL 60201-5913
(847) 491-9091

American Dietetic Association
http://www.eatright.org
216 W. Jackson Blvd
Chicago, IL 60606-6995
(312) 899-0040

American Geriatrics Society
http://www.americangeriatrics.org
350 Fifth Avenue, Suite 801
New York, NY 10118
(212) 308-1414

American Health Information Management Association
http://www.ahima.org
233 North Michigan Avenue
Suite 2150
Chicago, IL 60601-5800
(312) 233-1100

American Heart Association
http://www.americanheart.org
7372 Greenville Ave.
Dallas, TX 75231
(800) AHA-USA1 (Heart and Stroke Information)
(800) AHA-4-CPR (ECC information)

American Lung Association
http://www.lungusa.org
1740 Broadway
New York, NY 10199
(212) 315-8700

American Red Cross
http://www.redcross.org
431 18th Street NW
Washington, DC 20006
(202) 639-3520

Asthma & Allergy Foundation of America
http://www.aafa.org
1233 20th St. NW
Suite 402
Washington, DC 20036
(800) 727-8462

Joint Commission for Accreditation of Health Care Organizations (JCAHO)
http://www.jcahco.org
One Renaissance Boulevard
Oakbrook Terrace, IL 60181
(630) 792-5000

National Clearinghouse for Alcohol and Drug Information
http://www.health.org
P. O. Box 2345
Rockville, MD 20847-2345
(800) 729-6686

National Committee for Quality Assurance
http://www.ncqa.org
2000 L Street, NW
Suite 500
Washington, DC 20036
(888) 275-7585

Common Medical Abbreviations

Ab	abortion	CPR	cardiopulmonary resuscitation
ac	before meals	CPT	Current Procedural Terminology
ad lib	as desired	CPT-4	Current Procedural Terminology, 4th edition
AD	right ear		
ADL	activities of daily living	C&S	culture and sensitivity
AED	automated external defibrillator	C/S	Cesarean section
AFB	acid fast bacillus	CSF	cerebrospinal fluid
AFP	alpha-fetoprotein	CT	computed tomography
AIDS	acquired immune deficiency syndrome	CVA	cardiovascular accident
AM; am	morning		
amp	ampule	dB	decibel
amt	amount	DC, D/C	discontinue
AP	anteroposterior	DC	doctor of chiropractic
aq	aqueous	D&C	dilatation and curettage
AS	left ear	DEA	Drug Enforcement Agency
ASHD	arteriosclerotic heart disease	dL	deciliter
AU	both ears	DM	diabetes mellitus
AV	atrioventricular	DNR	do not resuscitate
A&W	alive and well	DO	doctor of osteopathy
		DOA	dead on arrival
bid	twice a day	DOB	date of birth
BM	bowel movement	DPM	doctor of podiatric medicine
BP	blood pressure	dr	dram
BPH	benign prostatic hypertrophy	DRG	diagnostic related groups
BSA	body surface area	DTaP	diphtheria, tetanus, adsorbed pertussis vaccine
BUN	blood urea nitrogen		
Bx	biopsy	DW	distilled water
		Dx	diagnosis
C	Centigrade	EBV	Epstein Barr virus
CA	carcinoma, cancer	ECG	electrocardiogram
CAD	coronary artery disease	EDC	estimated date of confinement
cap	capsule	EDD	estimated date of delivery
CAT	computed [axial] tomography	EKG	electrocardiogram
CBC	complete blood count	ELISA	enzyme-linked immunoabsorbent assay
CC	chief complaint	elix	elixir
CCMS	clean catch midstream urine	EMS	emergency medical services
CDC	Centers for Disease Control	EMT	emergency medical technician
CEA	carcinoembryonic antigen	ENT	ear, nose, throat (otorhinolaryngologist)
CHF	congestive heart failure	EOB	explanation of benefits
CIN	cervical intraepithelial neoplasia	EOM	external occular movements
CO_2	carbon dioxide	EPO	exclusive provider organization

ER	emergency room	lat	lateral
ESR	erythrocyte sedimentation rate	lb	pound
ET tube	endotracheal tube	LDL	low density lipoproteins
ext	extract	LEEP	loop electrosurgical excision and cryosurgery
F	Fahrenheit, female	LLQ	left lower quadrant
fax	facsimile	LMP	last menstrual period
FBS	fasting blood sugar	LP	lumbar puncture
FDA	Food and Drug Administration	LUQ	left upper quadrant
FEV_1	forced expiratory volume at one second	L&W	living and well
FH	family history		
fl	fluid	m, min	minim
ft	foot	mcg, μg	milligram
FUO	fever of unknown origin	MCH	mean corpuscular hemoglobin
FVC	forced vital capacity	MCHC	mean corpuscular hemoglobin concentration
Fx	fracture		
		MCV	mean corpuscular volume
g	gram	MD	medical doctor
GI	gastrointestinal	MDI	metered-dose inhaler
gr	grain	mEq	milliequivalent
gt(t)	drop(s)	MI	myocardial infarction
GYN	gynecology	mL	milliliter
		mm	millimeter
h, hr	hour	MMR	measles, mumps, rubella vaccine
Hb, Hgb	hemoglobin	MRI	magnetic resonance imaging
HBV	hepatitis B virus	MS	multiple sclerosis
HCFA	Health Care Finance Administration		
HCG	human chorionic gonadotrophin	NaCl	sodium chloride
HCPCS	Health Care Finance Administration Common Procedure Coding System	NEC	not elsewhere classified
		NIDDM	non-insulin dependent diabetes mellitus
Hct	hematocrit	NKA	no known allergies
HDL	high density lipoproteins	noc, noct	night
HEENT	head, eyes, ears, nose, throat	NOS	not otherwise specified
Hib	*H. influenzae* type b vaccine	NP	nurse practitioner
HIV	human immunodeficiency virus	NPI	national practice identification (number)
HMO	health maintenance organization	NPO	nothing by mouth (*non per os*)
HPI	history of the present illness	NS	normal saline
hs, HS	hour of sleep	NSF	not sufficient funds
ht	height	NST	non stress test
Hx	history	N&V	nausea and vomiting
I & D	incision and drainage	O_2	oxygen
ICD-9-CM	International Classification of Diseases, 9th ed., Clinical Modification	OD	right eye
		OH	occupational history
ID	intradermal	ophth	ophthalmic
IDDM	insulin dependent diabetes mellitus	OPV	oral polio vaccine
IM	intramuscular	ORIF	open reduction, internal fixation (of a fracture)
in	inch		
IPA	independent practice association	os	mouth
IPV	inactivated polio vaccine	OS	left eye
IU	international units	OT	occupational therapy, occupational therapist
IV	intravenous		
IVP	intravenous pyelogram	OTA	occupational therapy assistant
		OTC	over the counter
K	potassium	OU	both eyes
kg	kilogram	oz	ounce
L	liter, left	P	pulse

PA	physician assistant or posteroanterior
PAC	premature atrial contraction
PAT	preadmission testing
pc	after meals
PCV	pneumoccocal conjugate vaccine
PERRLA	pupils equal, round, react to light and accomodation
PET	postiron emission tomography
PH	past history
pH	potential of hydrogen (measure of acidity or alkalinity)
PI	present illness
PIN	personal identification number
PKU	phenylketonuria
pm, PM	afternoon
PO	by mouth (*per os*)
POL	physician office laboratory
POMR	problem oriented medical record
POP	plaster of Paris
POS	point of service
PPO	preferred provider organization
PPE	personal protective equipment
PRN	as needed
PSA	prostate specific antigen
pt	patient or pint
PT	physical therapy, physical therapist, prothrombin time
PTA	physical therapy assistant
PTT	partial thromboplastin time
PVC	premature ventricular contraction
q	every
q 2 h	every two hours
QA	quality assurance
QC	quality control
qd	every day
qid	four times a day
qs	quantity sufficient
R	respirations, right
RBC	red blood cells
RICE	rest, ice, compression, elevation
RLQ	right lower quadrant
R/O	rule out
ROM	range of motion
ROS	review of systems
RPM	revolutions per minute
RUQ	right upper quadrant
Rx	take, prescribe
SA	sinoatrial
SC, subq	subcutaneous
SH	social history
Sig	directions to patient
SIL	squamous intraepithelial lesion
SL	sublingual
SOAP	subjective; objective: assessment: plan (progress note format)

SOB	shortness of breath
SOF	signature on file
sol	solution
SOMR	source oriented medical record
SPECT	single photon computed tomography
STAT	immediately
supp	suppository
T	temperature
T, Tbsp	tablespoon
t, tsp	teaspoon
tab	tablet
TB	tuberculosis
TENS	transcutaneous electrical nerve stimulator
TIA	transient ischemic attack
tid	three times a day
tinc, tinct	tincture
TPR	temperature, pulse, respiration
TURP	transurethral resection of the prostate gland
U	units
UA	urinalysis
UCHD	usual childhood diseases
UCR	usual, customary, reasonable
ung	ointment
URI	upper respiratory infection
USP/NF	United States Pharmocopeia/ National Formulary
UTI	urinary tract infection
UV	ultraviolet
Var	Varicella (chicken pox) vaccine
VDRL	venereal disease research laboratory test
VO	verbal order
WBC	white blood cells
WDWN	well developed, well nourished
WNL	within normal limits
wt	weight

Symbols

aa	of each
c̄	with
p̄	after
s̄	without
s̄s̄,	half
ℨ	dram
♏	minim
℥	ounce
<	less than
>	more than
Δ	change
↑	increase
↓	decrease
♂	male
♀	female

AAMA Entry-Level Competencies for the Medical Assistant

From the 1999 *Standards and Guidelines*

Competency content in all areas (administrative, clinical & transdisciplinary) should be presented utilizing manual and state-of-the-art methods.

Invasive procedures must be taught to clinical competency.

Patient care **instructions** should encompass all phases of the life cycle: pediatric, adult and geriatric.

Adaptations for special needs patients should be addressed.

ADMINISTRATIVE

(1) Perform Clerical Functions
   a. Schedule and manage appointments
   b. Schedule inpatient and outpatient admissions and procedures
   c. Perform medical transcription
   d. Organize a patient's medical record
   e. File medical records
(2) Perform Bookkeeping Procedures
   a. Prepare a bank deposit
   b. Reconcile a bank statement
   c. Post entries on a daysheet
   d. Perform accounts receivable procedures
   e. Perform accounts payable procedures
   f. Perform billing and collection procedures
   g. Prepare a check
   h. Establish and maintain a petty cash fund
(3) Prepare Special Accounting Entries
   a. Post adjustments
   b. Process credit balance
   c. Process refunds
   d. Post NSF checks
   e. Post collection agency payments
(4) Process Insurance Claims
   a. Apply managed care policies and procedures
   b. Apply third party guidelines
   c. Obtain managed care referrals and precertifications
   d. Perform procedural coding
   e. Perform diagnostic coding
   f. Complete insurance claim forms
   g. Use a physician's fee schedule

CLINICAL

(1) Fundamental Principles
   a. Perform handwashing
   b. Wrap items for autoclaving
   c. Perform sterilization techniques
   d. Dispose of biohazardous materials
   e. Practice standard precautions
(2) Specimen Collection
   a. Perform venipuncture
   b. Perform capillary puncture
   c. Obtain throat specimen for microbiological testing
   d. Perform wound collection procedure for microbiological testing
   e. Instruct patients in the collection of a clean-catch mid-stream urine specimen
   f. Instruct patients in the collection of fecal specimens
(3) Diagnostic Testing
   a. Use methods of quality control
   b. Perform urinalysis
   c. Perform hematology testing
   d. Perform chemistry testing
   e. Perform immunology testing
   f. Perform microbiology testing
   g. Screen and follow-up test results
   h. Perform electrocardiograms
   i. Perform respiratory testing
(4) Patient Care
   a. Perform telephone and in-person screening
   b. Obtain vital signs
   c. Obtain and record patient history
   d. Prepare and maintain examination and treatment areas
   e. Prepare patient for and assist with routine and specialty examinations
   f. Prepare patients for and assist with procedures, treatments, and minor office surgery
   g. Apply pharmacology principles to prepare and administer oral and parenteral medications
   h. Maintain medication and immunization records
   i. Obtain CPR certification and first aid training

TRANSDISCIPLINARY*

(1) Communicate
   a. Respond to and initiate written communications
   b. Recognize and respond to verbal communications
   c. Recognize and respond to nonverbal communications
   d. Demonstrate telephone techniques
   e. Identify community resources
(2) Legal Concepts
   a. Identify and respond to issues of confidentiality
   b. Perform within legal and ethical boundaries
   c. Establish and maintain the medical record
   d. Document appropriately
   e. Perform risk management procedures

(3) Patient Instruction
   a. Explain general office procedures
   b. Instruct individuals according to their needs
   c. Instruct and demonstrate the use and care of patient equipment
   d. Provide instruction for health maintenance and disease prevention
(4) Operational Functions
   a. Perform an inventory of supplies and equipment
   b. Perform routine maintenance of administrative and clinical equipment
   c. Utilize computer software to maintain office systems

*May be addressed in clinical, administrative, or both areas.

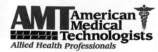

American Medical Technologists
REGISTERED MEDICAL ASSISTANT CERTIFICATION EXAMINATION CONTENT SUMMARY

I. GENERAL MEDICAL ASSISTING KNOWLEDGE
A. Anatomy and Physiology
  1. Body systems
  2. Disorders of the body
B. Medical Terminology
  1. Word parts
  2. Definitions
  3. Common abbreviations and symbols
  4. Spelling
C. Medical Law
  1. Medical law
  2. Licensure, certification, and registration
D. Medical Ethics
  1. Principles of medical ethics
  2. Ethical conduct
E. Human Relations
  1. Patient relations
  2. Other interpersonal relations
F. Patient Education
  1. Patient instruction
  2. Patient resource materials

II. ADMINISTRATIVE MEDICAL ASSISTING
A. Insurance
  1. Terminology
  2. Plans
  3. Claim forms
  4. Coding
  5. Financial aspects of medical insurance
B. Financial Bookkeeping
  1. Terminology
  2. Patient billing
  3. Collections
  4. Fundamental medical office accounting procedures
  5. Banking
  6. Employee payroll
  7. Financial mathematics
C. Medical Secretary Receptionist
  1. Terminology
  2. Reception
  3. Scheduling
  4. Oral and written communications
  5. Records management
  6. Charts
  7. Transcription and dictation
  8. Supplies and equipment management
  9. Computers for medical office applications
  10. Office safety

III. Clinical Medical Assisting
A. Asepsis
  1. Terminology
  2. Universal blood and body fluid precautions
  3. Medical asepsis
  4. Surgical asepsis
B. Sterilization
  1. Terminology
  2. Sanitization
  3. Disinfection
  4. Sterilization
  5. Record keeping
C. Instruments
  1. Identification
  2. Usage
  3. Care and handling
D. Vital Signs
  1. Blood pressure
  2. Pulse
  3. Respiration
  4. Height and weight
  5. Temperatures
E. Physical Examinations
  1. Problem oriented records
  2. Positions
  3. Methods of examination
  4. Specialty examinations
  5. Visual acuity
  6. Allergy testing
F. Clinical Pharmacology
  1. Terminology
  2. Injections
  3. Prescriptions
  4. Drugs
G. Minor Surgery
  1. Surgical supplies
  2. Surgical procedures
H. Therapeutic Modalities
  1. Modalities
  2. Patient instruction
I. Laboratory Procedures
  1. Safety
  2. Quality control
  3. Laboratory equipment
  4. Urinalysis
  5. Blood
  6. Other specimens
  7. Specimen handling
  8. Records
  9. Microbiology
J. Electrocardiography
  1. Standard, 12-lead ECG
  2. Mounting techniques
  3. Other ECG procedures
K. First Aid
  1. First aid procedures
  2. Legal responsibilities

TASK INVENTORY NOTE

The tasks included in this inventory are considered by American Medical Technologists to be *representative* of the medical assisting job role. This document should be considered dynamic, to reflect the medical assistant's current role with respect to contemporary health care. Therefore, tasks may be added, removed, or modified on an ongoing basis.

Virtual Medical Office Challenge CD-ROM

ABOUT THE PROGRAM

Through the use of case studies, *The Virtual Medical Office CD-ROM* allows students to practice the application of information provided in the textbook, and to use problem-solving, decision-making, and critical thinking skills. In addition, for specific administrative and clinical competencies, the learner's ability to use critical thinking and priority-setting skills during a clinical or administrative procedure can be challenged. This Appendix contains information on how to install and use the program. The *Student Mastery Manual* contains materials and forms used throughout the program, should students wish to refer to printed documents or complete any forms manually.

Minimum System Requirements

PC and PC-Compatible:	Computer:	80486/66, or Pentium CPU
	System:	Windows 95 or 98/Windows NT
	Memory:	24 MB RAM
	Other:	4× CD-ROM Drive
		256-color mode
		Sound card/speakers
		Mouse
		SVGA, or higher graphics
		640 × 480 screen resolution
Macintosh:	Computer:	Power PC Processor
	System:	7.6×, or higher
	Memory:	24 MB RAM
	Other:	4× CD-ROM Drive
		256-color mode
		Mouse
		640 × 480 screen resolution

LOGGING ON TO THE VIRTUAL MEDICAL OFFICE CHALLENGE

Logging on for the first time

To record the challenges that they complete, students will enter their first initial and last name as a single word (e.g., tsmith). See Figure 1. Students will then click **ENTER**. If students do not wish to record their progress, they will simply click **NEXT** and advance to the **MAIN MENU**.

Logging on after the first time

If students have entered their names during the first log on, the program will keep track of the challenges they have attempted, and those they have completed. If students enter their names the same way every time, the program will recognize them and give them the option to review the status of those challenges they have completed, or attempted, to date. Students can either review this status information or go straight to the **MAIN MENU**.

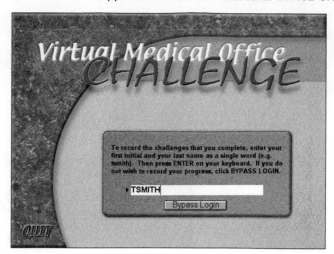

➢ **Figure 1**

- **Storing bookmarking to the hard disk.** If the installation is configured to store students' bookmarking on the hard drive, then the students will not need to insert a floppy into the diskette drive and can simply proceed to the **MAIN MENU** after selecting the hard drive option and logging on.

- **Storing bookmarking to a floppy disk.** If the installation is configured to store student bookmarking on data diskettes, the data diskette must be inserted into the diskette drive before logging on. If no diskette is detected, the program will prompt for it. *Note:* The program will accept blank, formatted data diskettes as student data diskettes. After inserting the data diskette into the floppy drive, students can then proceed to the **MAIN MENU** after selecting the A:\drive option and logging on.

USING THE MAIN MENU

The **MAIN MENU** is the navigational front door to the *Virtual Medical Office Challenge*. Through it, students can select to explore any one of four patient case scenarios, or go directly to either the Clinical or Administrative Skills Building section (see Figure 2). Students also have an option to check Challenge Status, which is a log of what interactions they have either completed or partially explored.

- **Selecting CASE STUDIES.** By selecting **CASE STUDIES** on the **MAIN MENU**, students will be directed to the **Patient Cases** screen, which allows them to select a particular case by patient name (see Figure 3). When the cursor rolls over the patient's name, a description of that case, and the administrative and clinical competencies that are challenged within that case, appears in the dialog box below. Students can then select a case by clicking on a patient case file folder, which will automatically advance them to the beginning of that case. A new case can be accessed at any time from anywhere in the program by first selecting **MAIN**

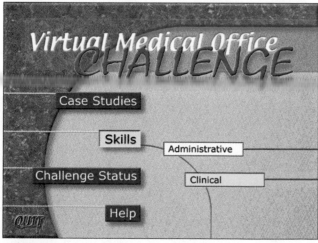

➢ **Figure 2**

➢ **Figure 3**

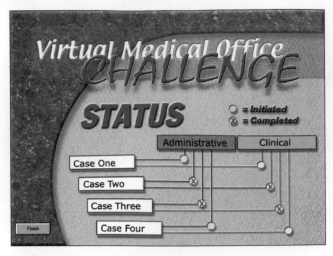

➤ **Figure 4**

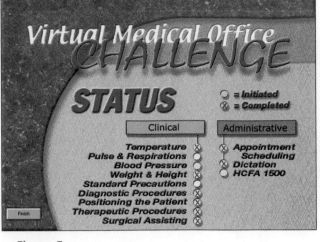

➤ **Figure 5**

MENU, then selecting **CASE STUDIES**, and a new case folder from the **Patient Cases** screen.

- **Selecting SKILLS.** By selecting **SKILLS** on the **MAIN MENU**, students will be directed to another screen that will then prompt them to select either **Clinical** or **Administrative**, which will take them through all the skills in either skill set, or they can select an individual skill to explore within either skill set. Skills can be selected from anywhere in the program by first selecting **MAIN MENU**, then selecting **SKILLS**.

- **Selecting CHALLENGE STATUS.** The *Virtual Medical Office Challenge* will keep track of where students have been in the program, and what areas are still left to be challenged. Selecting **CHALLENGE STATUS** on the **MAIN MENU** will bring up a list of what sections of the program have been partially completed and which have been fully completed. Separate screens will then show students what portions of the four patient cases have been completed, or partially completed (see Figure 4), and what portions of the **Clinical** and **Administrative** **Skills** have been fully, or partially, challenged (see Figure 5). Partially completed sections are marked with a circle that is filled in with color. Fully completed sections are filled in with the same color and marked with an X within the circle. The **CHALLENGE STATUS** can be accessed at any point in the program by first selecting **MAIN MENU**, then selecting **CHAL-LENGE STATUS**.

- **Selecting the DEMONSTRATION BUTTON.** It is recommended that all first-time log-on users review the **Demonstration Module** to familiarize themselves with the program before getting into the actual program. The **Demonstration Module** can be accessed from a permanent button on the **MAIN MENU** screen. It is self-running and requires no interaction on the student's part, and runs for approximately three minutes. This **Demonstration Module** will familiarize the first-time user with all program features, including interactions that will be required throughout. This **Demonstration Module** can be accessed at any time from anywhere in the program by selecting **MAIN MENU**, then selecting the **Demo** button.

PATIENT CASE SCENARIOS

Four patient case scenarios are presented in the *Virtual Medical Office Challenge* (see Table 1). Combined with the **ADMINISTRATIVE** and **CLINICAL** skills sections, they represent most of the key competencies students will need to master, as identified by the American Association of Medical Assistants (AAMA). In each of the cases, students will play the role of a medical assistant working in either the administrative or clinical area of a busy general practice medical office. The practice, which is called Blackburn Primary Care Associates, has three doctors and a broad mixture of patients with varying situations and needs. Students will be asked to play the role of one of four medical assistants, and will be asked to respond to simulated, realistic medical office situations. Students will receive feedback based on the choices they make, and can explore that feedback further to understand the rationale behind their correct or incorrect responses.

Table 1: Patient Case Studies

CASE ONE: Ivan Shapiro

A new patient, a 57-year-old white male with tightness in his chest, calls on the phone for an appointment. Competencies challenged include: telephone techniques and screening, scheduling appointments, prioritizing information, preparing medical records, completing insurance claim forms, taking history and vital signs, performing clinical procedures, documenting, obtaining specimens.

CASE TWO: Raymond Johnson

An established 32-year-old white male patient has an exacerbation of his asthma and calls on the phone for an appointment. Competencies challenged include: telephone screening, responding to emergencies, prioritizing, taking history and vital signs, preparing and giving medications, performing procedures, documenting.

CASE THREE: Robin Soto

A 4½-month-old Hispanic child is brought in for her immunizations after a missed appointment. Also she has not been given her vitamins for a week. Competencies challenged include: taking history and vital signs, performing developmental assessment, giving immunizations and patient instruction, completing insurance claim forms.

CASE FOUR: Lucille Ferguson

A 75-year-old black widow seeks her first appointment in the medical office. Due to her age and state of health, she is having difficulty functioning independently. Competencies challenged include: telephone techniques and confidentiality, scheduling appointments, preparing medical records, taking history and vital signs, positioning, examination procedures, performing diagnostic tests, patient instruction, completing insurance claim forms.

When you enter a patient case for the first time, you will start at the beginning of that case. If at any time during that case you wish to return to the main menu, click **MAIN** when you see the icon in the top left corner of the screen. This icon will appear each time you begin a new challenge throughout the case. If you have worked through part of the case previously, the program will bookmark which portion, or portions, you have completed. When you return to that case, it will ask you whether you would like to start at the **BEGINNING,** or your **PREVIOUS LOCATION,** which is the last challenge location you completed the last time you worked in that case.

To make the program as realistic as possible, all the patient situations have been selected from the files of practicing physicians. For confidentiality, all names, dates, places, and any other identifiable characteristics of physicians and patients have been carefully deleted, or changed. All forms are replicas of forms in current use. The four patient cases are described in Table 1.

ADMINISTRATIVE AND CLINICAL SKILLS

In addition to the four patient cases, students can select to work on individual skills in either the Administrative or Clinical areas. These can be accessed through the **MAIN MENU** by selecting **SKILLS,** then selecting which skill they wish to explore.

ADMINISTRATIVE SKILLS. Individual Administrative skills presented in this part of the program include:

> Schedule and Manage Appointments
> Complete Insurance Claim Forms

CLINICAL SKILLS. Individual Clinical skills presented in this part of the program include:

> Temperature
> Pulse and Respirations
> Blood Pressure

Weight and Height

Diagnostic Procedures

Standard Precautions

Positioning the Patient

Therapeutic Procedures

Surgical Assisting

USING THE GLOSSARY

The Glossary can be accessed from all screens in the software once students have selected an activity from the **MAIN MENU**. It can be accessed in one of two ways, either by clicking on any word in red type that appears within a dialog box, or by clicking on the **Glossary** icon button. A word can be selected within the **Glossary** from the alphabetical list provided by scrolling to search for a word. The definition appears in the Definition Box, and students can hear the word pronounced by selecting the **Pronunciation** button (see Figure 6). Clicking on the **RETURN** button on the **Glossary** screen returns students to their previous location.

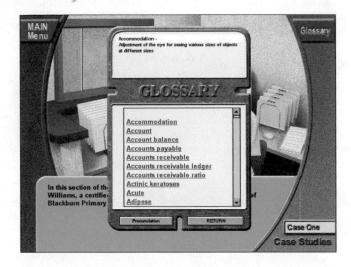

➢ **Figure 6**

PATIENT FORMS AND REFERENCE MATERIALS

Forms to complete activities on the CD-ROM will be found at the end of the *Student Mastery Manual* that accompanies this textbook.

Glossary

abandonment   Failure to continue to provide medical care to a patient without proper notification.

abduction   Movement away from the midline of the body.

abortion   Termination of a pregnancy before the fetus reaches the age of viability. May be spontaneous or induced.

abscess   A localized collection of pus.

abuse   Physical, emotional, or sexual injury.

accounts payable   Bills owed by a business such as a medical office.

accounts receivable   Money that is owed to the doctor for services performed.

accuracy   A measure of how close a laboratory measurement is to the true value.

acronym   A word formed from the initial letters of a series of words.

act   An enactment of a judicial body; often refers to a group of related laws.

acting out   To translate one's feelings into activity that is not appropriate.

active exercise   Muscle movements performed without assistance.

active immunity   Resistance to infection that develops as a response to exposure to antigens.

active listening   Careful and attentive listening.

addiction   A need to continue using a substance due to physiological or psychological dependence.

adduction   Movement toward the midline of the body.

adipose   Composed of fat.

administer   To give a dose of a medication as directed by a licensed practitioner who can prescribe.

advocate   A person who argues for or supports a cause or individual.

aerobic   Requiring oxygen to live.

aerosol   A wet mist; the medium in which medicated fluid is delivered to the lungs from a nebulizer.

affective   Refers to feelings or emotions, values, and attitudes.

agar   A culture medium obtained from seaweed

agglutination   The clumping of blood cells.

agranulocyte   A blood cell without granules.

airborne precautions   Special actions used for patients with a known diagnosis of illnesses transported by airborne droplet nuclei.

airway   Passageway for air to enter and leave the lungs.

allergen   An antigen that causes a hypersensitivity response.

Ambu-bag   A bag and mask that fit tightly over the individual's face.

ambulatory care   The patient coming to the care rather than the patient receiving care in a home or hospital setting.

amplitude   Size.

ampule   A small glass flask with a glass top that breaks off when appropriate pressure is applied, used to hold a single dose of medication.

anaerobic   Able to live without the presence of oxygen.

anaphylactic shock   Response to an allergen resulting in spasm of the bronchioles and lowered blood pressure.

anaphylaxis   A generalized hypersensitivity reaction that causes severe respiratory distress and circulatory system failure.

anemia   A decreased ability of red blood cells to carry oxygen.

aneroid   Without liquid. Used to describe sphygmomanometers that do not contain mercury.

answering service   An agency employed to answer the telephone for a business.

antagonism   When a drug binds to particular cells and blocks a sequence of biochemical events from happening.

antecubital   The area where the arm bends in front of the elbow.

anteroposterior (AP) projection   The x-ray beam passes through the patient from front to back before striking the film.

anthropometric   Measurements about the physical size of an individual.

antibody   Specific proteins produced by organisms that attach themselves to antigens, immobilize them, and target them for destruction.

antidote   A drug that can be given to counteract the effect of another drug.

antigen   A protein that is perceived as foreign by an organism.

antilipemics   Medications that decrease lipid levels of the blood.

anxiety   Vague apprehension, uneasiness, or feelings of dread.

apex   The pointed end of an object.

apnea   Absent respirations.

application software   A program on a computer allows the user to perform an activity.

approximated   Skin edges of a wound or surgical incision that have been brought together.

arbitrary   Based on a whim or subjective judgment.

arrhythmia   An abnormality of heart rate or heart rhythm.

arrythmia   Irregular heart beat.

artifact   A change in an EKG tracing that has not been made by the heart's electrical activity.

artificial immunity   Defense to microorganisms provided by antibodies of another individual or developed following immunization.

asepsis An environment in which microorganisms are controlled and eliminated to the greatest possible degree.

assessment Drawing conclusions based on data. The part of a SOAP progress note that contains the physician's impression of what is wrong with the patient.

assignment of benefits When the health care facility accepts payment directly from the insurance company.

asystole Lack of a heartbeat.

atherosclerosis A condition in which deposits of cholesterol and lipids occur along the walls of arteries and arterioles.

atrioventricular (AV) node The area of the heart where the electrical impulse is delayed before passing from the right atrium to the bundle of His.

atrium An upper chamber of the heart.

atrophy A wasting away of the muscle that often occurs when an extremity is in a cast.

audiometer The instrument that measures hearing.

aural Pertaining to the ear. Used for temperatures taken in the ear.

auscultation Listening with a stethoscope.

auscultatory gap A disappearance of Korotkoff sounds during blood pressure measurement.

autonomy Control.

avulsion The ripping off of a flap of tissue that may be completely severed or attached by one side.

axillary Pertaining to the armpit. Used for temperatures taken in the armpit.

axis A line that determines the direction of an organ or body.

B cells A type of lymphocyte produced in bone marrow and found in the spleen and lymph nodes.

back order A part of an order that is not delivered with the main part of the order.

back-up The process of saving copies of files to a disk in case of a system crash.

bacteria (singular: bacterium) Single-celled microorganisms that may or may not cause disease.

bandage A non-sterile material that is applied over the dressing to hold the dressing in place.

barriers to communication Elements that interfere with the exchange of thoughts or messages.

baseline The flat line on an EKG that signifies no electrical activity. A test or measurement that will be used for comparison to future tests or measurements.

basophil A type of white blood cell that stains blue.

benign A tumor with harmless cells.

bevel The slanted edge just behind the point, where the medication emerges from the needle.

biliruben A breakdown product of hemoglobin.

biohazard waste container A container for disposal of waste that is contaminated with blood or body secretions.

biohazard A product contaminated with blood or body fluids, which has the potential to spread disease.

biopsy An examination of tissue under a microscope to determine if cancerous cells are present.

blood chemistry A blood test to determine presence and amounts of chemicals in serum.

body language Communication through body position, muscle activity, facial expression and other nonverbal means.

body mechanics How the parts of the body interact for motion and movement.

boot To start up a computer.

bradycardia A pulse rate below 60 beats per minute.

bruit A rushing or blowing sound that can indicate narrowing due to atherosclerosis.

buccal Medication administered by placing it between the cheek and teeth until it dissolves.

bundle of His A group of specialized cardiac muscle fibers that help transmit electrical impulses through the heart.

byte Eight bits. Also the amount needed to display an alphanumeric character.

cachexia Weight loss with muscle wasting.

calibration The testing and adjustment of test equipment to provide the known relationship between the measurement response and the substance value measured by the test.

calorie The common term for amount of heat needed to raise the temperature of one kilogram of water by one degree centigrade. (In scientific terms this is a large calorie or kilocalorie.)

canthus The corner of the eye.

capillaries Microscopic blood vessels whose walls are so thin that nutrients can pass by osmosis between the circulatory system and the tissues.

capillary action Movement of liquid up the sides of a narrow tube.

capitation A type of payment in which primary care doctors provide all office care for patients for a set annual fee.

carcinoma in situ Cancerous changes of the surface cells that has not spread to surrounding tissues.

cardiogenic shock Failure of the heart to pump an adequate blood supply to the vital organs.

cast A hard covering for the area of a fracture.

casts Formed when protein accumulates in the kidney tubules and is deposited in the urine as it passes through the tubules.

catheter Narrow tube.

catheterization Use of a sterile tube to enter a part of the body such as an artery or the urinary bladder.

cell-mediated immune response Response to threat of infectious microorganisms through macrophages found in the tissues.

cellular telephone A telephone that communicates without telephone wires.

central processing unit (CPU) The main chip of a computer from which all of the main functions of the computer originate.

centrifuge A device used to "spin down" a substance by rapid rotation that separates the components of a liquid depending on their density.

cerebrovascular accident When an artery in the brain is blocked or ruptures, and blood flow to the brain is interrupted.

certificate of waiver A process by which a doctor's office can be granted permission under CLIA '88 to perform low-complexity tests.

certification A process by which a professional organization verifies a certain level or education and training.

cerumen Ear wax.

cervical intraepithelial neoplasia A term used to describe the presence of abnormal cells from the outer tissue layer of the cervix.

chemotherapy Treatment using anticancer drugs.

Cheyne-Stokes respirations A short period of apnea followed by gradually increasing rate and depth of respirations, respirations gradually slow and become more shallow until another period of apnea is reached. May occur during sleep in the elderly but may also be a sign of illness or impending death.

chief complaint (CC) The main problem that has brought a patient to see a doctor.

chloasma Brownish pigmentation of the face.

cholesterol A substance used by the body for the formation of bile and to produce certain hormones that can also be deposited in fatty plaques on the walls of the arteries.

circumference The measurement of size of the head or chest, measured around.

civil law The set of laws that deal with disputes between individuals or groups of people.

Clinical Laboratory Improvement Act of 1988 (CLIA '88) A set of regulations that controls the activities of medical laboratories.

clonus Regular, rapid alternation of muscle contraction and relaxation.

closed questions Questions for which you are looking for a one-word or short answer.

closed reduction Setting a fracture, or placing the bones into alignment without surgically opening the skin over the fracture.

clustering Scheduling medical appointments so that individuals with similar problems come in during the same time period.

cognitive Covers what a person knows as information, expressed primarily in words.

colonization Formation of colonies of bacteria in a specific tissue or area of the body.

colostrum Thick, yellowish fluid that nourishes a baby immediately after birth.

colposcopy Insertion of a tube to view the colon.

computer virus A program that stops the basic functions of a computer.

conception The union of a single sperm with an ovum, which starts pregnancy.

concussion A jarring injury to the brain in which the brain is shaken resulting in a period of loss of consciousness.

consensus Agreement about what has been observed or proven.

contact precautions Special actions used for patients with serious skin and wound infections.

continuity of care Continuing care based on knowledge of previous care.

continuous fever A fever that stays at about the same elevation all the time or returns to the same level about four hours after being treated.

contract A mutual agreement between two or more parties regarding a legal act.

contraction stress test Stimulation of mild contractions under fetal heart rate monitoring.

contraindicated Not indicated or not appropriate.

contrast medium A substance that absorbs x-rays and highlights a specific organ.

controlled substance A drug that has potential for addiction and abuse.

contusion Bleeding of the brain caused by injuring one or more blood vessels at the time of injury.

convulsion Seizure.

co-payment A fixed amount of money that the patient with managed-care insurance is required to pay each time he or she receives medical treatment or fills a prescription.

criminal law A term used to refer to the set of laws that protect society in a large sense.

cross index To file under one unit and to a file a guide or card under another unit that refers to the primary filing location.

cross sensitivity The ability of one antigen to cause an allergic response in a person who is sensitive to another antigen. The characteristic may be found in groups of antibiotics.

cryosurgery A technique in which tissue is frozen.

cryotherapy Treatment with cold.

crystals Unorganized components of urine sediment with no regular shape.

culture medium A substance rich in nutrients into which a culture is placed to see if bacteria grow.

culture A sample of body fluid to be tested for the presence of bacteria by encouraging bacterial growth.

curette An instrument used to scrape.

cursor The graphical representation of the insertion point in a document indicated by moving the mouse.

cyst An enlargement of tissue often caused by an oil duct in the body becoming clogged.

cytotoxic Cells that destroy foreign antigens.

data Files on the computer

data base The information about the patient in POMR charting, including the history and physical exam, laboratory data, and reports of diagnostic tests.

database A collection of information stored in a searchable form.

debridement The process of removing dead tissue.

decibel A measurement for intensity or loudness of sound.

defendant The person or entity who is charged with violating the law.

defibrillation Sending electric current through the patient's chest in order to depolarize the entire heart so that the SA node can reestablish a heartbeat.

defibrillator An instrument that provides an electric shock in order to depolarize all heart cells at once and allow a normal heartbeat to be reestablished.

dementia A condition of memory loss, confusion, and sometimes agitation and aggression.

demographic Information such as name, address, telephone number, and insurance information.

denial Failure to acknowledge the reality of a situation.

depolarize Suddenly changing the electrical charge of the cells, which allows an electrical impulse to begin to flow from one area to another.

desk top The opening screen seen on a computer, containing several icons.

development Intellectual skill, motor skill, and emotional change as a child grows.

diabetes mellitus A chronic illness caused by a lack of insulin in the body or the body's inability to use insulin effectively.

diabetic ketoacidosis A condition resulting from lack of insulin in which by-products of fat metabolism (ketones) build up in the blood and cause it to be more acidic than normal.

differential diagnosis Determining the exact nature of a disease or illness by performing tests to be sure that it could not be any other disease with similar symptoms.

diluent The liquid used to dilute a powder.

directory An organized listing of data or information.

disability Measurable loss of function.

disinfection To treat with chemicals or heat to kill pathogens.

disk drive A computer peripheral that reads disks and may also write information to disks.

dislocation The injury that occurs when a bone is displaced from the articular surface of the joint.

dispense To give a patient a supply of a medication to take later.

diurnal Daily.

doctrine A legal principle used as a basis for interpretation of law.

dosimetry The monitoring of an area and/or an individual's body to see how much radiation it has been exposed to over a period of time.

double booking Scheduling two patients for the same appointment time.

dressing A sterile covering that goes immediately over a wound or incision to protect the area and absorb drainage.

droplet precautions Special actions used for patients known to have or suspected of having illnesses transmitted by particle droplets.

drug abuse Continued desire for and willful misuse of a substance that is not medically indicated.

drug Medication or remedy.

durable power of attorney A document that gives a designated person the ability to make all legal decisions for another individual, including medical decisions.

dysplasia A term used to describe abnormal (but not cancerous) cells.

dyspnea Breathing difficulty.

eclampsia A serious condition of pregnancy that causes convulsive seizures, coma, and death if untreated.

ego defense mechanism Unconscious mental processes and behavioral strategies that offer psychological protection.

elective abortion Intentional termination of a pregnancy.

electrocardiogram Recording of the electrical activity of the heart using electrodes placed on the chest.

electrode Metal plates or metallic coated paper tabs that conduct electricity.

electrolyte An element that carries electricity when dissolved in solution.

elixir A liquid form of medication that traditionally used alcohol as a vehicle to dissolve the medication.

e-mail A message sent from one computer to another electronically.

embryo The products of conception, from weeks four through eight of pregnancy.

Emergency Medical System (EMS) The system used by most communities to receive and route calls for assistance in emergencies including fire, police, and ambulances.

emergency medical technician (EMT) Professionally trained provider of pre-hospital emergency care.

emetic A medication that causes vomiting.

empathy Objective awareness and sensitivity to the feelings and emotions of others.

empirical To determine a result through experimentation.

encounter form A charge slip.

endocervical curettage Scraping from within the cervical opening.

endoscopy A procedure in which a thin, flexible glass tube with a light source and camera lens is put into the mouth or in the anus.

endotracheal tube A tube that passes through the mouth or nose into the trachea to provide an airway when a person requires artificial ventilation.

enteric coated Containing a coating that will not be dissolved before the medication reaches the small intestine; used to prevent irritation of the gastric mucosa.

enunciation The way a person forms parts of words.

eosinophil A white blood cell whose granules stain red.

epilepsy A chronic condition characterized by frequent seizures.

episiotomy Incision made to enlarge the vaginal opening for birth.

epistaxis Nosebleed.

epithelial cells Skin cells.

Epstein-Barr virus A virus that causes infectious mononucleosis.

ergonomics The study of maximizing work efficiency by adapting the work environment for optimum physical and mental function.

erythrocyte   A red blood cell.

evacuated tube   A glass or plastic tube, sealed with a rubber stopper, which contains a vacuum.

eversion   Turning outward.

exacerbation   Time when symptoms increase.

expiratory reserve volume   The amount of air that can be forced out of the lungs after a voluntary expiration.

extension   Opening or widening the angle of a hinge joint.

family history (FH)   History of disease or illness and current medical status of family members.

fax (facsimile)   A method of sending printed communication via a telephone line.

fenestrated   Having an opening or hole.

fetus   The infant in utero, from the ninth week of pregnancy to birth.

fibrillation   An erratic heart rhythm that doesn't allow for sufficient blood to be pumped through the body.

fibrinolysis   The action that causes a fibrin clot to be removed.

file   A set of information containing one document, image, spreadsheet, etc. Also a manilla folder that holds material.

filtration   The act of straining out large particles the body desires to retain.

fixed appointment scheduling   An appointment scheduling method in which each patient is given a specific appointment time.

flexion   Bending or narrowing the angle of a hinge joint.

fluorescence   Use of ultraviolet light source to illuminate an object.

fluoroscope   A special x-ray machine used for fluoroscopy.

fluoroscopy   Continuous low-dose x-ray.

folder   A collection of computer files with the same directory path. Another name for manilla file folder.

fomite   An inanimate object that can pass microorganisms from one host to another.

forced expiratory volume   The amount of air that can be forcibly breathed out of the lungs after a normal inspiration.

forced vital capacity   The total amount of air that can be forcibly breathed out of the lungs after a maximal voluntary inspiration.

forceps   A tool used for grasping, pulling, compressing, or holding tissue or other instruments and supplies during surgery.

fracture   A break in the bone.

frostbite   Localized tissue freezing.

fundus   The base of the uterus, located opposite the cervix.

fungi (singular: fungus)   Plant-like organisms that exist on other organisms, including molds and yeasts. May be unicellular or multicellular.

gait belt   A strong piece of fabric used to tie around the waist of a patient for support when standing or walking.

gamma globulin   A specific protein that attaches itself to an antigen, immobilizes it, and targets it for destruction.

gauge   The diameter of the opening of a needle.

generic name   The general name of a drug, not the brand name.

geriatric   Old.

gestation   The length of time from conception to birth.

gigabyte (GB)   One thousand megabytes.

glomerulus   A tuft of very small capillaries that filter blood.

Good Samaritan Act   Law that protects health professionals from being sued for giving emergency care.

granulation   Filling in with granulated tissue instead of the original type of tissue.

granulocyte   A term that is used for white blood cells that contain granules.

gravida   The number that describes how many times a woman has been pregnant.

growth   Change in size over time.

guaiac   A chemical commonly used as a developer in tests for hidden blood.

handicap   The extent to which a person cannot perform normal activities.

hardware   Physical equipment that is vital to the function of a computer.

health insurance   A system by which a person or a person's employer pays an insurance company a yearly amount of money, and the insurance company pays some or most of the person's medical expenses for that year.

heat exhaustion   A less severe condition than heat stroke that occurs after prolonged exposure to high temperature and humidity.

heat stroke   A life-threatening emergency that occurs after prolonged exposure to high temperature and humidity.

hematoma   A large bruised area at a puncture site, caused by blood leaking into the tissue surrounding the vein.

hematopoiesis   Formation of blood cells.

hemiplegia   Paralysis on one side of the body. Also used for partial paralysis on one side.

hemoglobin   A protein containing iron molecules that carries oxygen in red blood cells.

hemostatis   Control of bleeding.

hepatitis B virus   The organism that causes the disease hepatitis B, which is passed by direct contact with the blood of an infected individual.

hernia   Protrusion of an organ through the abdominal muscle wall.

heterophile antibodies   A specific antibody seen in infectious mononucleosis.

hierarchy   Classified according to rank or importance.

high-density lipoproteins   The substance responsible for transporting cholesterol to the liver to assist in the manufacture of bile.

history of the present illness (HPI)   Description of the chief complaint including how long the person has been ill, signs and symptoms, and treatments that have been attempted.

hospice An organization that provides end-of-life comfort and care.

human immunodeficiency virus (HIV) The virus that causes AIDS (acquired immune deficiency syndrome).

humoral immune response Response to foreign proteins through cells found in the tissues that produce antibodies in response to remembered foreign proteins and microorganisms.

humoral immunity Production of antibodies.

hydrocephalus A condition in which there is increased cerebrospinal fluid in the brain cavity.

hyperextension Opening the joint beyond 180 degrees.

hyperopia Farsightedness.

hyperpnea Rapid and deep respirations.

hyperpyrexia Fever above 105° F; may cause convulsions, brain damage, and/or death.

hyperthermia A heat-related injury.

hypertonic solution Having higher osmotic pressure (more molecules per unit of volume) compared to another solution.

hypertrophy Increased size or growth.

hyperventilation Rapid, deep respirations that result in excessive loss of carbon dioxide.

hypoglycemia Acutely low blood sugar.

hypopnea Slow and shallow respirations.

hypothermia Abnormally low body temperature, usually due to exposure to a cold environment.

hypotonic solution Having lower osmotic pressure (fewer molecules per unit of volume) compared to another solution.

icon A small graphic that is used to represent a folder or file on a computer screen.

idiopathic Occuring for no known reason.

idiosyncratic Causing an individualized reaction.

immunoassay A test for the presence of a specific antibody.

immunoglobulins Specific proteins that attach themselves to antigens, immobilize them, and target them for destruction.

immunotherapy Cancer treatment using measures to stimulate the immune system.

impairment Disturbance of functioning that may be physical or psychological.

implied contract Not formally agreed on but obvious under the circumstances.

in vitro In the laboratory.

in vivo In the person.

incidence How frequently an event or condition occurs.

incision A cut in the skin made by a knife, scalpel, or other straight sharp object.

incision and drainage Cutting into an affected area in order to allow the collection of pus or sebum to drain out of the abscess or cyst in a controlled manner.

incubator A cabinet that maintains a constant temperature.

indexing unit Pieces of information used to identify the correct filing location of records.

infarction An area of tissue death due to interruption in blood supply.

infectious disease A disease caused by microorganisms and therefore able to pass from one individual to another.

informed consent Agreement to a medical test or procedure based on understanding of the procedure and its possible consequences and effects.

initiative The ability to begin or follow through on a plan.

inspection The visual observation of the body and its parts.

inspiratory reserve volume The amount of air that can be inspired into the lungs after a normal inspiration.

insulin reaction When the blood glucose level falls too low because there is more insulin in the bloodstream than the patient needs.

intermittent Not continuous, but rather coming and going.

intermittent fever A fever that rises and returns to normal in a regular pattern.

intimidation Using threats or fear to control the behavior of another individual.

intracervical insemination A procedure in which sperm are placed in the cervical canal.

intradermal Method of administering injections in which the medication is placed between the layers of the skin.

intramuscular Method of administering injections in which the medication is placed into the muscle.

intrauterine insemination A procedure in which sperm are placed directly into the uterus.

intravenous Method of administering injections where the medication is placed into a vein.

intravenous pyelogram An x-ray used to show the kidneys, ureters, and bladder following injection of a contrast medium.

invasion of privacy Release of information or photographs of a person without that person's permission.

invasive Entering a body cavity or penetrating through the skin.

inventory Lists information about equipment and/or supplies.

inversion Turning inward or toward the midline.

irrigation Application of a large amount of fluid to an area for the purpose of removing foreign material, cleaning, or removing a harmful substance.

ischemia Lack of oxygen to the tissue.

isolation precautions Used when there is a high risk of exposure to certain diseases.

isotonic Having the same concentration of electrolytes as body tissue.

Kaposi's sarcoma A rare type of skin cancer, often seen in patients who are HIV positive.

ketones The products of incomplete fatty acid metabolism that form when fat is burned.

keyboard A device used to communicate with the computer using a series of small buttons.

kilobyte (KB) One thousand bytes.

labor The process a woman's body goes through immediately preceding and during the birth of a baby.

laceration A cut or tear of the skin.

laryngoscope An instrument to view the larynx; used when an endotracheal tube is passed into the trachea.

lateral projection The x-ray beam passes through the patient from one side to the other before striking the film.

lead A reading of various combinations of electrodes.

learning objective Statements that describe behavior changes.

legislation The procedure of making laws or the laws made by such a procedure.

leukocyte A white blood cell.

liability Legal responsibility.

liaison A person who serves the purpose of communicating between individuals, groups, or units.

libel The release of false information about a person.

licensure The process by which the state examines a person's qualifications and gives permission to practice a certain profession.

life expectancy The expected length of life for a person at a given time.

ligate To tie off, so that it does not bleed.

liniment A liquid medication for external use, to be massaged or rubbed into the skin.

litigation A court case.

living will A document executed by an individual that gives medical professionals instructions about how that person wishes to be treated in the event he or she becomes incompetent.

log on (log in) To enter into a computer network or program.

low-density lipoproteins The substance that transports cholesterol to blood vessels and tissues.

lumen The diameter of the opening of a tubular structure.

magnetic resonance imaging Utilizes magnetic fields in combination with radio waves and sophisticated computer technology to create cross-sectional images of body parts.

malignant Cancerous.

malpractice Professional negligence.

mandated Required by law as for example reporting of suspected child abuse or neglect.

manipulation The passive movement of a limb to determine its range of motion.

matrix A rectangular or linear arrangement.

maturation Maturing, ripening.

Mayo stand A small table with removable tray top that can be positioned at different heights.

medical asepsis Aimed at removing pathogens and reducing transfer of microorganisms by cleaning any body part or surface that has been exposed to them.

medical model A term often used to describe how doctors and others trained in western medicine view health, disease, wellness, and treatment.

medical practice act Legislation that regulates the practice of medicine in each state.

medication Drug or remedy.

megabyte (MB) One thousand kilobytes.

meniscus The curved upper surface of a liquid in a cylindrical container.

menopause End of menstrual activity.

mensuration Measuring height, weight, blood pressure, temperature, head circumference, chest circumference, and leg or ankle diameter, to determine changes in measurements.

metastasis The spread of cancer from one part of the body to another.

metastasize To spread to distant parts of the body, via the circulatory or lymph system.

metazoa Multicellular parasites.

microhematocrit A measurement of the packed red blood cell volume.

miscarriage Common term for spontaneous abortion.

modem A device used with a computer to communicate with other computers via a phone line.

modified wave appointment system A system for making appointments that has some fixed appointments and some appointments in which patients with the same appointment time are seen in order of arrival.

monitor A device used to display to the user what is happening in a computer.

mordant A substance that holds stain onto a slide for microscopic examination.

mortality rate The rate of deaths in a certain number of instances.

motherboard The main area of the computer where different cards and/or chips are located.

mouse A device used to communicate with the computer.

multimedia Programs used by a computer that use colors and sound.

myocardial infarction Heart attack.

myocardium Heart muscle.

myopia Near-sightedness.

natural immunity Resistance to disease from natural processes.

nebulizer A device with a mouthpiece or mask through which a patient can receive inhalation treatment.

necrosis Destruction of tissue, from ulceration and infection.

neglect Failure to provide a child with the basic necessities of life.

negligence The failure to act, or refrain from acting as a reasonable person would act.

neoplasm Tumor.

nephron The kidney's microscopic filtration unit. Each kidney has over one million.

network A collection of computers connected by cables.

neurogenic shock Damage to the nervous system, which causes an inability to control the diameter of blood vessels.

neuropathy A lack of sensation due to reduced nerve function.

neutrophil A white blood cell whose granules do not absorb stain.

nitrites Salts of nitric acid whose presence in fresh urine indicates bacterial growth.

non-compliant Failure to follow a doctor's advice or regimen.

non-invasive Does not penetrate a body cavity.

non-stress test Test during which the mother's heart rate is monitored for several minutes to correlate the mother's heart rate to fetal movement and Braxton-Hicks contractions.

non-verbal Experienced without words through body posture, facial expression, etc.

normal flora Microorganisms that normally live in or on the body without causing disease.

no-show A person who simply does not show up for his or her appointment.

objective Not influenced by emotion or personal desire. A goal or intended outcome.

objectivity Not allowing what is going on in your life to distract you or change the way you understand and describe the patient's physical or emotional well being.

oblique projection The x-ray passes through the patient at an angle to the body part being x-rayed.

obstetrics The field of women's health that deals with pregnancy, childbirth, and the period immediately following childbirth.

obturator A smooth, rounded end that closes off the opening when a metal or plastic tube is inserted into a vessel or body structure.

occluder A device that covers one eye.

occult blood Hidden or invisible blood.

occupational history (OH) A history of the patient's employment.

Occupational Safety and Health Administration (OSHA) An organization that regulates workplace health and safety.

oil-immersion When a microscope lens is dipped in oil, enhancing magnification to 100×.

ointment A semisolid medication in an oily base, used externally.

opacity Cloudy or filmy.

open reduction Aligning bones after a surgical opening is made at the fracture site and often using screws, plates, or other hardware to hold bone fragments in place.

open-ended questions Questions that encourage the patient to open up and talk.

operating system The program that manages the basic functions of a computer.

opportunistic infection Infection that occurs because of a patient's decreased immunity.

oral Spoken; when referring to medication it means taken by mouth.

oral hypoglycemic A medication taken by mouth to lower blood sugar.

orthopnea Experiencing difficulty breathing except in the erect or upright position.

orthostatic hypotension Sudden low blood pressure that occurs when a person stands up.

osteoporosis Loss of bone mass of over 2.5 percent.

out guide Card used to mark the place of a manilla file folder that has been removed.

oxidation A chemical reaction in which a compound unites with oxygen, forming a new compound.

pager A device that beeps or vibrates to notify when a message has been received.

palliative Seeking to relieve or alleviate symptoms without curing the underlying condition.

palpation Use of the fingers and hands to feel or touch parts or organs.

para The number of pregnancies that went to the age of viability.

paraphrasing Attempting to put the words of another into your own words.

parasite An organism that lives on or in a host organism.

parenteral By injection.

passive exercise Exercise performed by another person who moves the limbs of a paralyzed or weak individual.

passive immunity Resistance to disease that is not the result of the organism forming its own antibodies; achieved by injection of antibodies or ingestion of antibodies through breast milk.

password A word used to enter into a protected system.

past history (PH) History of past illnesses, surgeries, or other medical problems.

pathogen A microorganism that can cause disease.

pathologist An MD who specializes in the study of disease processes.

pathology The scientific analysis of the cause and effects of disease.

percentage Whole number that expresses a part of 100.

perception The way a person believes things are.

percussion The tapping of the body with an instrument or the fingers.

peripheral Outside the center. Equipment of a computer system apart from the central processing unit.

personal protection equipment (PPE) Equipment used to protect from exposure to pathogens.

pH Parts hydrogen, a measure of acidity.

phagocytosis Engulfing cells and debris.

pharmacology The study of the sources, uses, and means of action of drugs.

phenylketonuria A metabolic condition in which an individual is missing the gene that codes for phenylalanine hydroylase and is unable to metabolize the amino acid phenylalanine.

phlebotomy Removal of a sample of blood, usually from a superficial vein.

physiologic need Basic biological need for survival.

pica Craving by a pregnant woman for non-food items such as starch, clay, and even dirt.

pinna Ear flap.

pipette A small glass or plastic vessel used to transfer fluid from one place to another.

plaintiff The person or entity that makes the complaint in a lawsuit.

plaque A deposit or accumulation of abnormal tissue.

plasma The liquid portion of blood.

platelet A cell that is needed for blood to clot.

pleuritic Painful, as in pleurisy (i.e. stabbing pain below the ribs, especially on inspiration or coughing).

point-of-service (POS) device A small machine in the doctor's office that is connected via telephone to the insurance company's data base.

polydipsia Extreme thirst.

polyphagia Extreme hunger.

polyuria Frequent urination.

positron emission tomography (PET) Use of positron-emitting radionuclides to produce diagnostic images.

posteroanterior (PA) projection The x-ray beam passes through the patient from back to front before striking the film.

postpartum The weeks and months immediately following the birth of a baby.

potentiation A situation where one drug's action either prolongs or multiplies the effect of a second drug.

precancerous A term used to describe a lesion or growth that is currently benign but may turn into cancer.

precision Measuring the testing method's capability to reproduce results.

precordial On the chest in front of the heart.

preeclamsia A complication of pregnancy characterized by hypertension, albuminuria, and edema of the lower extremities.

prenatal The time before birth.

presbyopia Difficulty with near vision associated with aging.

primary intention A wound in which the edges are approximated during the healing process.

printer A device used to take the information from the computer screen and change it into hard copy.

probe An instrument used to feel around inside an incision or measure the depth of a cavity.

problem list A list of each physical, social, or psychological problem the patient has or has had in the past.

problem-oriented medical record A record organized by the patient's particular problem.

professional liability The legal responsibility of a professional.

professionalism Behavior based on a body of knowledge and ethical standards to serve the public.

prognosis Outlook for future health.

projection To experience one's own feeling as the feeling of someone else.

pronation Turning the palm of the hand downward, to face the ground.

proportion Two equal ratios.

protozoa (singular: protozoon) Single-celled parasites.

psychogenic shock Unpleasant physical or emotional stimuli that cause low blood pressure and decreased oxygen to body tissues.

psychomotor Concerns itself with motor skills and the ability to perform tasks and processes.

puerperium The six-week period immediately following childbirth, when the mother's reproductive organs return to near pre-pregnancy state.

puncture A wound made by a pointed object.

purchase order (PO) The name for both the form used to order supplies and sometimes the order itself.

Purkinje fibers Nerve pathways that penetrate into both ventricles.

pyrexia Fever.

quadrant One quarter, or fourth of an area.

quality assurance The process of auditing records to make sure that the proper procedures have been followed and proper care has been given.

quality control A process used to insure the validity or accuracy of test results.

radiation therapy Cancer treatment using various types of radiation.

radiograph An x-ray.

radiologist A doctor who specializes in interpreting diagnostic radiology studies.

random access memory (RAM) The portion of computer memory that is available for use by software and that is erased when the computer is turned off.

range of motion Movement of the joints through all normal motions.

ratio A relationship between two numbers.

read-only memory (ROM) Computer or disk memory that cannot be altered.

reagent A substance that reacts with other substances.

reagent strip A strip impregnated with chemicals that reacts in a known manner when exposed to blood urine; also known as a dipstick.

reciprocal license Automatic issuance of a license in one state to the holder of a license in another state.

rectal By the rectum.

reduction Aligning bone ends.

reference laboratory Large laboratories, either privately owned or run by universities or research centers.

reflecting An attempt to catch the patient's emotion and meaning, then reflect it back to the patient.

refraction The ability of the eye's lens to bend light.

refractometer   An instrument that measures the refractive index of a solution.

relapsing fever   A fever that appears to go away, then returns.

remission   A period of time when symptoms disappear.

remittent fever   A fever that rises and falls but always remains above normal.

re-order point   A designation that indicates when the number of items remaining is low enough that they would have to be re-ordered.

repetition   Phenomena that can be induced to repeat themselves.

replicate   To perform repeatedly with the same result.

repolarize   The cells of the myocardium become able to contract again.

residual volume   The volume of air that remains in the lungs after maximal voluntary expiration.

resistance   The ability to defend against infection.

respondent superior   "Let the master answer." A doctrine of law that holds the employer responsible for the negligent actions of his or her employees.

reticulocyte   An immature red blood cell.

retractor   A surgical instrument used to hold open a flap of tissue in order for the doctor to view the area underneath.

review of systems (ROS)   A series of questions asked as part of the medical history progressing from head to toe to identify problems that the patient may have deemed insignificant.

risk management   The process of assessing risks and putting in policies that minimize them. The term is often used in the medical office related to the risks of lawsuits.

rotation   Movement around the axis of a ball and socket joint.

sanitizing   Washing with soap and water.

scalpel   A surgical knife.

scheduling   Setting up a prospective timetable of events.

sclerosed   Hardened.

secondary intention   A wound that heals by granulation.

sediment   Material left at the bottom of a test tube after centrifuging.

seizure   A sudden, violent series of involuntary muscle contractions caused by abnormal electrical discharges from neurons in the brain.

self-actualization   The fulfillment of each individual's potential.

senile   Having low mental functioning in the later years of life.

sensitivity   Antibiotic disks placed in culture medium to determine which antibiotic(s) will prevent growth of an offending bacterium.

septic shock   Widespread infection affecting the ability of the body to maintain blood pressure and provide adequate oxygen to the tissues.

septum   The wall between the left and right side of organs such as the heart or nose.

serum   The liquid portion of the blood after all the cells and clotting elements have settled and formed a clot.

service contract   A contract that allows for unlimited service calls within a specific period.

sexual harassment   When a person's actions, intentions, and clearly understood statements cause another person to feel that his or her job is at risk if advances are not accepted.

sharps   Needles, glass slides, scalpel blades, and other sharp biohazards.

sign   A manifestation of disease or illness that can be observed or measured.

sinoatrial (SA) node   The group of cells in the heart that initiate the heartbeat, also called the pacemaker.

slander   A term used for the release of false information about a person.

slough   Tissue that separates from healthy tissue.

SOAP charting   The type of chart used in the Problem Oriented Medical Record, in which each note refers to a specific problem and differentiates subjective and objective information, followed by an assessment and plan.

social history (SH)   The part of the medical history that includes the patient's habits and hobbies, and usually whether the patient smokes, uses alcohol, and/or abuses drugs.

solute   Substance that dissolves in solution.

solution   The liquid in which a solute is dissolved.

somatic tremor   An unnatural baseline deflection in an EKG caused by muscle tension or talking.

sorter   A device that facilitates placing documents in alphabetic or numerical order.

sound   An instrument used to measure the depth of a wound or body cavity.

source-oriented medical record   A record organized by what types of services were performed.

speculum   An instrument used to help view body cavities.

sphygmomanometer   A device used to measure blood pressure.

spirometry   The measurement of breathing.

splint   A device to immobilize a suspected fracture during transport.

spontaneous abortion   Natural expulsion of a fetus for unknown reasons.

spore   A dormant form of bacteria or mold that has formed a thick capsule around itself that is highly resistant to heat or chemicals.

spreadsheet   A table describing relationships that exist for performing calculations.

sputum   Bronchial secretions and saliva coughed up from the lungs.

squamous cell carcinoma   Cancerous changes of the surface that may have invaded the surrounding tissues or spread to distant sites.

squamous intraepithelial lesion   A term used to describe abnormal changes of the outer cells of the cervix.

standard precautions   Measures to prevent exposure to blood or body fluids that may spread disease.

standardization Placing a deflection on an electrocardiogram to show the amplitude of the heartbeat.

standards Norms that are generally agreed on.

statute of limitations A law limiting the time period for beginning a lawsuit for malpractice.

statute Law.

sterile Free from all microorganisms.

sterilization The process used to kill all microorganisms and bacterial spores.

stethoscope A device used to listen to body sounds.

stillbirth Birth of a dead fetus of the age of viability.

strain An injury to a muscle and the tendons that support the muscle, caused by over stretching.

stress The physical or mental experience of force or strain.

stress testing Electrocardiography performed during or immediately after exercise.

stylus A piece of pointed metal on an EKG machine.

subclinical Producing symptoms that are not noticed by the patient.

subcutaneous The method of administering injections where the medication is placed under the skin

subjective Perceived or experienced by an individual or influenced by personal interpretation.

sublingual Below the tongue.

subluxation Partial dislocation.

subpoena A legal document requiring an individual to appear in court.

subpoena *duces tecum* A legal document requiring that documentary evidence such as a medical record be presented in court.

superbill A charge slip that contains diagnosis and procedure codes.

superficial Toward the surface of the body; inconsequential.

supination Turning the palm of the hand upward, to face the sky.

supine hypotension syndrome Low blood pressure while an expectant mother lies on her back.

suppository Solid or semisolid form of medication at room temperature that will melt at body temperature. The medication is shaped to be placed into a body cavity.

surgical asepsis The destruction of all microorganisms, pathogenic and nonpathogenic, on an object and measures to keep sterile objects from coming in contact with nonsterile objects.

suspension An insoluble medication, which is contained in a liquid.

swaged Suture material that comes pre-packaged attached to a curved shaping needle.

symptom A manifestation of disease or illness that is experienced or felt by the patient but cannot be directly observed.

symptomatic Responding to symptoms.

syncope Fainting.

syndrome A group of signs and symptoms that are usually found together.

synergism A situation in which two drugs work to enhance each other.

syrup Liquid form of medication that is sweet in taste.

systemic Having effects on cells throughout the body.

T cells Lymphocytes that are produced by the thymus gland, or have passed through the thymus gland in order to mature.

tachycardia A pulse rate of over 100 beats per minute.

template A file that is used to make other files identical to it, but with different information.

teratogenic A side effect that may prevent a fetus from developing normally.

terminal When a patient is not expected to live more than six months.

terminal-digit filing A filing system in which numbers are considered a unit with the final or terminal group filed as the first unit.

tertiary intention Keeping a large wound open until the wound is clean, and suturing it.

therapeutic dose The amount of medication that will produce the desired effect.

thrombocyte Platelet.

tickler file A special file used to remind people about things that need to happen at a future time.

tidal volume The amount of air that is breathed in and out during normal breathing.

time-release A form of medication in which variation in coating allows some of the medication to be released more slowly, prolonging the overall effect.

titer A standard strength per volume of solution, used to test the presence of antibodies.

tolerance The tendency of some drugs to require a larger dose to achieve the same result, because the body has become used to the drug.

tomography A specialized radiological technique used to produce multiple images in selected planes of tissue.

topical Medication to be used on the skin or mucous membranes.

tort A wrongful act for which a civil suit can be initiated.

tourniquet A narrow strip of rubber that is wrapped around the upper arm to dilate the veins in the lower arm by preventing venous return during phlebotomy.

toxoid A harmful substance excreted by bacteria.

traction Using weight to pull on bone ends.

transdermal Through the skin.

transducer The instrument used to emit and receive sound waves for diagnostic and therapeutic ultrasound.

transient ischemic attack Small interruptions of blood flow to the brain.

triage The process of separating patients by their need of care.

triglycerides A form of lipid that can be metabolized for energy.

trimester Three-month period; there are three during pregnancy.

turbid Very cloudy.

tympanic The membrane also known as the ear drum. Used to measure body temperature.

ultrasound A procedure that uses high-frequency sound waves to create real-time or still images of soft tissue and internal organs.

universal precautions Measures used to prevent health care workers from having contact with pathogens.

urea Organic compound derived from the breakdown of protein metabolism.

ureter A long, cylindrical tube attached to each kidney to drain urine to the bladder.

urethra The tube-like structure that carries urine from the bladder to the outside of the body.

urinalysis Physical, chemical, and microscopic analysis of the urine.

urinary meatus The external opening of the urethra.

urinometer A small glass tube that floats in a container of urine.

urobilinogen Bilirubin converts to this substance by interaction with bacteria; it is then excreted in urine and feces.

urticaria Hives.

utilization review A process that identifies patients who no longer need to be hospitalized.

vaccine A substance used to immunize an individual.

valve A membranous structure that closes a vessel or organ to prevent backflow.

varicella Chicken pox.

vasoconstriction Narrowing of the lumen, or diameter, of blood vessels.

vasodilation Widening of the lumen, or diameter, of blood vessels.

vectors Insects or other animals that transmit disease.

vendor A person or company who sells an item.

venipuncture Removal of a sample of blood, usually from a superficial vein.

ventricle A lower chamber of the heart.

verbal Using words.

verbal contract A legal agreement that is not written.

viable An organism that can survive.

vial A small glass bottle, with a rubber stopper at the top, through which a needle can be inserted to draw out a dose of medication.

virulent Able to cause disease.

virus A microorganism smaller than a bacterium that contains DNA or RNA, but not both. It reproduces by taking over a cell and forcing it to produce the missing nucleic acid.

visual acuity The ability to see clearly.

vital capacity The amount of air that the lungs voluntarily inhale or exhale.

voice-mail An electronic system for managing telephone calls and taking messages.

wave appointment scheduling A method of scheduling appointments in which several patients are given the same appointment time and patients are seen in the order in which they arrive.

wheal Fluid-filled elevation of the skin.

word processing A computer program that displays and edits typed information.

written contract A legal agreement where the conditions are written and the agreement has been signed by the parties.

Index

Note: Page numbers followed by f indicate figures; those followed by t indicate tables; those followed by b indicate boxed material.

A

AAMA. *See* American Association of Medical Assistants (AAMA).
Ab. *See* Abortion(s) (Ab).
ABA number, 893
Abandonment, 69
Abbreviations
    common medical, 1023–1025
    for medications, 499, 500t
    for states, 865b
    in alphabetizing, 176
    in medical history, 258f
    metric, 502
Abdomen
    examination of, 310
    palpation of, 308, 309f
    percussion of, 308
    quadrants of, 310
Abdominal dressing, Montgomery straps for, 376
Abdominal reflex, 313f
Abducens nerve, 432f
Abduction, 834f, 835b
ABHES (Accreditation Bureau of Health Education Schools), 1004, 1006, 1007
ABO blood group antigens, 657–659, 660, 660f
Abortion(s) (Ab)
    elective, 722
    ethical issues of, 994–995
    for multiple gestations, 995
    in pregnancy history, 722
    legality of, 958, 994
    morning-after pill for, 994–995
    partial-birth, 994
    RU-486 for, 994
    spontaneous, 719, 722, 729t
Abrasion, 372f
Abruptio placentae, 729t
Abscess, incision and drainage of, 365–368, 370f
Absorbable sutures, 353
Absorbed poisoning, 790
Absorption, of drug, 495
Abuse
    child, 67, 694–695
    elder, 710–711, 710b
Abused drugs, 492–493, 492b–493b
AC (alternating current) interference, 400, 403f
Acceptance, in dying process, 747
Account aging, 943–946, 943f, 944b, 945b
Account aging record, 943, 943f, 944b
Account balance, 888t
Accounts payable, 18, 896, 900f
Accounts receivable, 18, 880–888
    charge slip for, 881–882, 882b, 884f
    day sheet for, 880, 884–888, 888t, 889f, 891b–892b
    fee schedule for, 884, 885f, 886b
    ledger for, 884, 886f, 887b–888b, 888t
    methods of maintaining, 880

Accounts receivable (*Continued*)
    pegboard system for, 140–141, 881, 881f, 882b, 890b, 893
    superbill (encounter form) for, 206, 207f, 882, 882f–883f, 886b
Accounts receivable control, 888t
Accounts receivable insurance, 968
Accreditation Bureau of Health Education Schools (ABHES), 1004, 1006, 1007
Accredited record technician (ART), 27t
Accrual method, of accounting, 885
Accuracy, 554
    of medical record, 168
Ace bandage, 473
Acetest, 587, 587b–588b
Achilles reflex, 313f
Acid spill cleanup kit, 559f
Acid-fast stain, 646, 648t
Acidity, of urine, 584, 584f
Acoustic nerve, 432f
Acquired immunity, 227, 228t
Acquired immunodeficiency syndrome (AIDS). *See* Human immunodeficiency virus (HIV) infection.
Acronyms, alphabetization of, 176
Act(s), legal, 65
Acting out, 40
Activated charcoal, in emergency box/crash cart, 767b
Active exercise, 833, 835b
Active immunity, 227
Active listening, 82, 82f, 83–84, 84t
Active records, 180
Active-assistive exercise, 835b
Activities of daily living (ADLs), 709, 805
Activities section, of resume, 1010f, 1012
Acupressure, 46t, 48–49
Acupuncture, 46t, 48–49, 49f
ADA (Americans with Disabilities Act), 21, 969
Addiction, 488
Adduction, 834f, 835b
Adhesive mock sutures, 353, 365, 366f
Adipose tissue, 829
Adjustment, 888t
ADLs (activities of daily living), 709, 805
Administration, of medication. *See* Medication(s), administration of.
Administrative area, 186–187, 186f
Administrative law, 957
Administrative procedures, 6
Administrative tasks, 2, 16, 17–18, 17f, 18f
Adolescent(s)
    growth and development of, 673t
    leaving alone of, 262
    patient teaching for, 804t
    physical examination of, 680
    pregnancy of, 718
Advance directives, 749–750, 750t
Adverse drug effects, 496–497, 513
Advertisements, 975

Advocate, 64
AEDs (automatic external defibrillators), 768
Aerobic exercise, 833
Aerobic organisms, 225, 643
Aerosol, 462
Affective domain, 801
Afferent arteriole, 572, 572f
African-American culture, 53
African-Caribbean culture, 53
Agar, 640
Age
    and drug metabolism, 496
    temperature variation with, 277
Aged. *See* Elderly.
Agenda, 974
Agglutination, 659, 660f
Agglutination tests, 657, 659–660, 660f
Aging. *See* Elderly.
Agonists, 495
Agranulocytes, 599
AIDS. *See* Human immunodeficiency virus (HIV) infection.
Air splints, 785.
Airborne pathogen precautions, 105
Air-lock technique, 533, 534f
Airway
    blocked, 772, 773b
    in emergency management, 767b, 768f, 770, 770f
Alanine aminotransferase (ALT), normal values for, 665t
Alarm reaction, 96–97, 97f
Albumin, normal values for, 665t
Albuminemia, during pregnancy, 725
Alcohol, source of, 486
Aldosterone, during pregnancy, 719–720
Alexander, F. M., 50
Alexander Technique, 50
Alkaline phosphatase (ALP), normal values for, 665t
Alkalinity, of urine, 584, 584f
Allergen, 775
Allergic reaction(s)
    emergency management of, 775–777, 777f
    to latex, 232, 234b, 235b
Allergist, 43t
Allergy(ies)
    drug, 497, 511, 513
    in present health history, 257
Allergy testing, 539, 540–543, 543f
Alliance for Quality Medical Imaging and Radiation Therapy, 447b
Allied health professionals, 27t
Allis tissue forceps, 348, 348f
Allowable charges, 926
ALP (alkaline phosphatase), normal values for, 665t
Alphabetic filing system, 175–177
Alpha-fetoprotein, maternal, 733
Alphanumeric filing system, 177

Revised Edition Updates

CHAPTER 6

Page 100, under *Protection from Exposure to Disease*

In 2001 OSHA revised the Bloodborne Pathogens Standard to include a requirement that employers select safer needle devices and employ needleless systems whenever possible. In addition, employees must be involved in identifying and choosing these safer devices. The revision also requires employers to maintain a log of injuries that occur as a result of needle sticks with contaminated sharps (see Figures A and B).

CHAPTER 7

Page 125, *Procedure 7-5: Activating the Emergency Medical Services (EMS) System*

Step 5: If possible, stay on the telephone line until an ambulance and medical personnel have arrived. If you cannot stay on the line, make sure to get the dispatcher's nonemergency number and call the dispatcher back soon to make sure emergency personnel arrived for the patient.

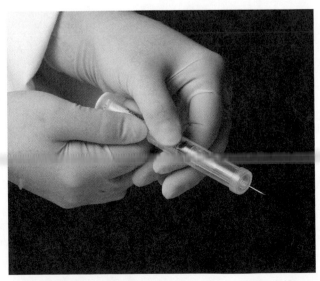

➤ **Figure A** Safety engineered syringe. (From Bonewit-West K: *Clinical procedures for medical assistants,* 6 ed. St Louis: Saunders, 2004.)

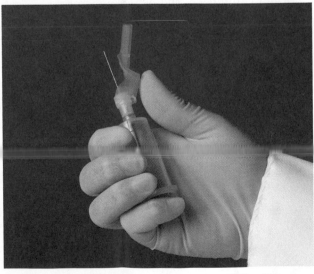

➤ **Figure B** Safety engineered phlebotomy device. (From Bonewit-West K: *Clinical procedures for medical assistants,* 6 ed. St Louis: Saunders, 2004.)

CHAPTER 13

Page 229, right column, under current subhead: *Handwashing*

Change subhead to: ***Handwashing and Hand Sanitizing***
After performing an initial aseptic handwash at the beginning of a work shift, many busy medical professionals use an alcohol-based hand-sanitizing solution to cleanse hands between patients or when putting on or taking off gloves. These solutions have been shown in studies to protect practitioners' hands from cracking and chapping, especially in winter and when working in dry, air-conditioned offices or hospitals. However, the sanitizing solution should be a name brand, with a high enough alcohol content to kill microorganisms. The sanitizing solution should be thoroughly rubbed into the hands, on the palms, between the fingers, and on the backs of the hands.

Students should note that in procedures subsequent to Procedure 13-1, when the box marked "wash hands" is checked, hands may be washed or sanitized using alcohol-based sanitizing solution in accordance with the regulations of the facility where they are working or training.

Page 232, right column, under *Proper Disposal of Hazardous Waste*

Hazardous waste is deposited in one of three containers. Linens that become soiled with potentially hazardous body fluids are put in a linen hamper with a biohazard sign on it to distinguish from linens that are generally soiled. Paper, latex, and soft plastic disposable goods ranging from straws to latex or other types of gloves to gowns and disposable bed pads are placed in hazardous waste trash bags, which are separate from general trash. Finally, "sharps," which consist of needles and syringes, vials, scalpels, or other hard disposable instruments, are disposed of in rigid biohazard containers often referred to as "sharps containers."

Page 238, *Procedure 13-3: Sanitizing Soiled Instruments*

Step 4: Students should remember not to plunge their hands into a tub full of soapy, sudsy water in which there are sharp instruments. Students should carefully feel for a rounded edge of a single instrument, gently lift it out of the water, and then begin to clean it with the scrub brush.

Page 241, left column, under *Sterilization Indicators*

Change in color of sterilization tape does not guarantee that instruments inside the pouch have been fully sterilized, only that the package has been autoclaved.

Right column, second paragraph
Change the first sentence to:
Sterilization strips should be placed in all packs to be sure that steam has penetrated.

Page 243, left column, under *Operating the Autoclave*

Students should note that **Procedure 13-5** discusses operating a manual autoclave. Automatic autoclaves, which have become more common in the past decade, usually fill, heat, steam, vent, and dry automatically after the desired cycle has been selected.

Page 244, *Procedure 13-5: Operating the Autoclave*

Step 9: Students should be reminded that color change to outside indicator tape does not guarantee effective sterilization of the items in the packet, only that the packet has been successfully heated in the autoclave.

CHAPTER 15

Page 272, *Procedure 15-1: Measuring Height*

Step 12: Discard paper towel used under patient's feet, or clean scale plate if paper towel was not used. Also, clean the measuring bar, which has touched the top of the patient's head.

Page 273, left column, under *Balance-Beam Scale Bar*

The final sentence should read:
Immediately after taking the measurement, be sure to clean the measuring bar and lower it to the closed position so no one gets hurt.

Page 278, right column, under *Types of Thermometers*

The use of glass-mercury thermometers has been discontinued over the past few years in almost all medical offices. Some patients still have glass-mercury thermometers at home, but medical practitioners are cautioning patients not to use them and to discard them at local hazardous waste disposal sites. New thermometer technology, including mercury-less thermometers, is being developed for in-office and in-home use. Glass non-mercury thermometers are available, however, and although not common, they are used in essentially the same way as glass-mercury thermometers (Figure C).

Readers should substitute "glass non-mercury" for "glass mercury" in this edition of *Fundamentals of Medical Assisting,* specifically in these references:
- Table 15-1, page 276
- Narrative, from the bottom of page 278, right column, to the top of page 279, right column
- Figures 15-4 and 15-5 on page 279
- Procedure 15-3 on pages 280-281
- Reference to not use oral glass-mercury with young children on page 280
- Reference to lubricating glass tip for rectal reading on page 282
- Procedure 15-7, page 285, specific references
- Narrative, subhead: Glass-Mercury Thermometers, on page 286, left column to top of right column
- Procedure 15-8, page 287, specific references
- Figure 15-7, page 288

Page 300, *Procedure 15-12: Measuring Blood Pressure*

Step 5. Make sure the proper size of blood pressure cuff is used. A too-small cuff can cause an artificially high blood pressure reading, and a too-large cuff can cause an artificially low reading.

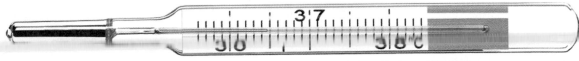

> **Figure C** Glass non-mercury thermometer. (Courtesy of Geratherm Medical.)

CHAPTER 16

Page 329, *Procedure 16-4: Ishihara Test of Color Vision*

Step 6: The patient has 3 seconds in which to respond.
Step 7: Some of the plates have a line that runs across the plate in the same color as the numbers on the other plates. Ask the patient to trace the line with the eraser-tip of a pencil, a cotton swab, or a plastic stylus.

CHAPTER 17

Page 355, *Procedure 17-4: Opening a Sterile Surgical Pack*

Step 2: Change last two sentences to:
Check date on the outside tape to make sure pack has been sterilized within the last month. Check sterilization indicator inside the outer packing to make sure that the inner pack has been sterilized.

Pages 378-379, *Procedure 17-9: Changing a Sterile Dressing*

Students should note that the charting example at the end of the procedure should state on which elbow the dressing has been changed.

Page 380, *Procedure 17-10: Suture Removal*

Students should note that the charting example at the end of the procedure should include where on the body the incision is.

CHAPTER 19

Page 429, *Procedure 19-4: Performing Sperm Washing*

Students should disregard this procedure. CAAHEP does not include this procedure in its list of competencies, and the procedure is rarely if ever performed in a general medical office.

CHAPTER 21

Page 456, *Procedure 21-1: Performing an Eye Irrigation*

Readers should note that in the photos, the medical assistant should be wearing gloves.

Page 461, *Procedure 21-3: Performing an Ear Irrigation*

Readers should note that in the photo, the medical assistant should be wearing gloves.

Page 467, *Procedure 21-6: Applying Warm Moist Compresses*

Readers should note that in the charting example, reference should be made to which elbow was treated.

CHAPTER 22

Page 512, box: *The "Five Rights" of Correct Medication Administration*

Although traditionally there are "five rights" of correct medication administration, various authors have added additional "rights" in the past few years. For example, it is important to administer medication using the "right technique." One right technique is proper preparation of the skin before administration of an injection, including proper cleaning technique. Another is "palming a label" when pouring a medication; the label should always be in the palm of the hand so no medication drips down the outside of the bottle and obscures the label; an unreadable label necessitates discarding the medication. Yet another right technique is to have a second person check to make sure the dosage is correct, especially when giving medications such as heparin (a blood thinner) or insulin.

It is also important to provide the right documentation. Documentation includes the date and time the medication is given, the dose, the route of administration, the site used for injections, and the name of the person who gives the medication.

Page 521, *Procedure 22-2: Drawing Up Medication from an Ampule*

Step 17: Readers should note that if the medication is a controlled substance, proper procedure must be observed when discarding, and the note regarding discarding must be cosigned. Any medication that needs to be counted and signed out on a controlled substance record must be documented by two individuals at the time it is discarded. If another person is discarding the medication and asks you to cosign, do not do so unless you actually see the medication being discarded appropriately.

Page 537, *Procedure 22-8: Administering a Z-Track Injection*

Step 10: Readers should note that in the rationale, the word **intramuscular** (IM) should be substituted for the word **subcutaneous**. Z-track injections are always IM injections.

CHAPTER 24

Pages 585–588, under *Clinitest and Acetest*

Readers should note that the Clinitest and the Acetest are no longer performed. The only confirmatory test still in use is the Ictotest. Please disregard narrative beginning on page 585 regarding Clinitest and Acetest, and disregard **Procedure 24-5** (page 586) and **Procedure 24-6** (pages 587–588).

CHAPTER 25

Page 604, *Table 25-1: Evacuated Tube Arranged in Correct Order of Draw,* **and subhead:** *Order of Draw*

The recommended order of draw of the Clinical and Laboratory Standards Institute (formerly NCCLS) of 2003 is as follows:
1. Sterile tubes for blood cultures
2. Citrate tubes (light-blue–capped tubes)
3. SSTs—tubes that contain silica gel
4. Serum tubes (glass or plastic red-capped tubes)
5. Heparin tubes (green-capped tubes)
6. EDTA tubes (violet-capped tubes)
7. Flouride tubes (gray-capped tubes)

Pages 606-609, *Procedure 25-1: Drawing Blood Using the Evacuated-Tube Method*

Step 4: Readers should be aware that a confused patient may answer to a name other than his or her own. Depending on the setting in which you are working (private office, skilled-care nursing facility, hospital, etc.), you may need to use another means to confirm a patient's identity. This may be looking at an identification bracelet or confirming with a patient's family member or other person that the patient is indeed the patient on whom you are to perform the blood draw. (This is also true for step 4 in **Procedure 25-2** and step 5 in **Procedure 25-3.**)

Step 25: Readers should note that some facilities ask that all collection tubes be fully labeled before the blood draw is performed. This is especially true in a busy laboratory where more than one individual is drawing blood, so that staff do not mix up samples before they are labeled. If this is the case, labeling the tubes would be placed between the current steps 5 and 6. (This is also true in **Procedure 25-2**, where step 19 may move to between steps 5 and 6, and in **Procedure 25-3**, where step 18 may move to between steps 6 and 7.)

CHAPTER 27

Page 688, *Procedure 27-6: Measuring the Respirations of an Infant*

Add at end of Step 8:
Irregularities may include wheezing, rales, or rhonchi.

Pages 687-691, under *Immunizations and Immunization Schedule, Table 27-3: Childhood Immunizations and the Diseases They Protect Against,* and *Table 27-4: Recommended Schedule for Immunizations*

Immunization schedules are updated every year by the Centers for Disease Control. Currently only the IPV is recommended for polio vaccination. Annual influenza immunizations are recommended after 6 months of age, and meningococcal vaccine is now recommended at age 11–12 years. For the most current immunization recommendations or requirements, see the website of the CDC (http://www.cdc.gov/nip) or your state's department of public health website.

CHAPTER 29

Page 737, *Procedure 29-3: Assisting with Postpartum Visits*

Step 5: Disregard the words, "If office policy includes assessment." All offices conduct an assessment of these issues at the postpartum visit.

CHAPTER 31

Page 777, right column, under *Thermal Burns.*

Remember, ice packs should not be placed directly on the skin, especially in the case of a burn. An ice pack should be wrapped in a soft cloth covering.

Page 780, *Procedure 31-4: Caring for Burns*

Step 2: This assessment generally will be made by a doctor or nurse.
Step 4: Assessment of how deep the burn is will have been made by a doctor or nurse.

CLINICAL PROCEDURES

In the following Procedures, substitute "sanitize hands" for "wash hands":

Procedures 13-1 to 13-4
Procedure 14-1
Procedures 15-1 to 15-12
Procedures 16-1 to 16-7
Procedures 17-1 to 17-10
Procedures 18-1 to 18-2
Procedures 19-1 to 19-3, 19-5, 19-6
Procedures 21-1 to 21-9
Procedures 22-1 to 22-10
Procedures 24-2 to 24-8
Procedures 25-1 to 25-9
Procedures 26-1 to 26-9
Procedures 27-1 to 27-7
Procedures 29-1 to 29-3
Procedures 31-2 to 31-5, 31-7
Procedures 33-1 to 33-3

Note: The reader is advised to refer to the CDC website for the Fact Sheet regarding hand hygiene.